SCIENTIFIC AMERICAN

MEDICINE

POCKET EDITION

SCIENTIFIC AMERICAN

MEDICINE

POCKET EDITION

Edward Rubenstein, M.D., M.A.C.P.
*Professor of Medicine and Associate Dean for
Postgraduate Medical Education,
Stanford University School of Medicine*

Daniel D. Federman, M.D., M.A.C.P.
*The Carl W. Walter Professor of Medicine
and Medical Education and Dean for Medical
Education, Harvard Medical School*

Scientific American, Inc., New York

Library of Congress Cataloging-in-Publication Data

Scientific American medicine / Edward Rubenstein, editor in chief;
Daniel D. Federman, editor. — Pocket ed.
p. cm.
Includes index.
ISBN 0-89454-013-0
1. Internal medicine—Handbooks, manuals, etc. I. Rubenstein, Edward, 1924 -
II. Federman, Daniel, D., 1928 - . III. Title: Medicine
[DNLM: 1. Medicine. WB 100 S416]
RC55.S37   1993
616—dc20
DNLM/DLC   92-48973
For Library of Congress   CIP

Publisher   Hilary Evans
Project Editor   Toby Bilanow
Production   Mark Flanagan
Copy Editor   Ozzievelt Owens
Art and Design   Elizabeth M. Klarfeld
                            Janet Betries
Electronic Composition   Diane Joiner
                            Sal Terillo

Printed in the United States of America
International Standard Book Number: 0-89454-013-0

Scientific American, Inc.
415 Madison Avenue, New York, NY 10017

The authors, editors, and publisher have conscientiously and carefully tried to ensure that recommended measures and drug dosages in these pages are accurate and conform to the standards that prevailed at the time of publication. The reader is advised, however, to check the product information sheet accompanying each drug to be familiar with any changes in the dosage schedule or in the contraindications. This advice should be taken with particular seriousness if the agent to be administered is a new one or one that is infrequently used. SCIENTIFIC AMERICAN *Medicine* describes basic principles of diagnosis and therapy. Because of the uniqueness of each patient and the need to take into account a number of concurrent considerations, however, this information should be used by physicians only as a general guide to clinical decision making.

Cover: Wood engraving from *De humani corporis fabrica (On the Fabric of the Human Body),* by Andreas Vesalius, a Flemish anatomist and physician. Written in 1543, when Vesalius was 28 years of age, *De humani corporis fabrica* laid the foundation for modern anatomy and has been referred to as one of the greatest medical books ever written.

List Of Contributors

RONALD A. ARKY, M.D.
Charles S. Davidson Professor of Medicine, Harvard Medical School, and Chairperson, Department of Medicine, Mount Auburn Hospital

WILLIAM M. BENNETT, M.D.
Professor of Medicine and Pharmacology and Co-Head, Division of Nephrology, Hypertension, and Clinical Pharmacology, Oregon Health Sciences University

ROBERT M. BLACK, M.D.
Associate Professor of Medicine, University of Massachusetts Medical School, and Director, Division of Nephrology, Saint Vincent Hospital

GEORGE F. CAHILL, JR., M.D.
Professor of Biological Sciences, Dartmouth College, and Professor of Medicine Emeritus, Harvard Medical School

GEORGE P. CANELLOS, M.D.
William Rosenberg Professor of Medicine, Harvard Medical School, and Chief, Division of Medical Oncology, Dana-Farber Cancer Institute

BART CHERNOW, M.D.
Physician in Chief, Department of Medicine, Sinai Hospital of Baltimore

ROBERT W. P. CUTLER, M.D.
Professor of Neurology and Neurological Sciences and Senior Associate Dean for Faculty Affairs, Stanford University School of Medicine

ROMAN W. DESANCTIS, M.D.
Professor of Medicine, Harvard Medical School, and Director of Clinical Cardiology, Cardiac Unit, Massachusetts General Hospital

MARK B. EFFRON, M.D., F.A.C.C.
Director of Coronary Care Unit and Director of Cardiovascular Research Laboratory, Sinai Hospital of Baltimore

GARY M. GRAY, M.D.
Professor of Medicine, Division of Gastroenterology, and Director, Digestive Disease Center, Stanford University School of Medicine

PETER B. GREGORY, M.D.
Professor of Medicine (Clinical), Division of Gastroenterology, and Associate Dean for Clinical Affairs and Medical Director, Faculty Practice Program and Stanford University Clinic, Stanford University School of Medicine

EDGAR HABER, M.D.
Elkan R. Blout Professor of Health Sciences and Director, Division of Biological Sciences, Harvard School of Public Health, and Physician, Massachusetts General Hospital

E. WILLIAM HANCOCK, M.D.
Professor of Medicine (Cardiology), Stanford University School of Medicine

CYRUS C. HOPKINS, M.D.
Associate Professor of Medicine, Harvard Medical School, and Hospital Epidemiologist and Clinical Director, Infectious Disease Unit

ADOLPH M. HUTTER, JR., M.D.
Associate Professor of Medicine, Harvard Medical School, and Physician in Medicine and Chairman, Medical Intensive Care Coordinating Committee, Massachusetts General Hospital

ROLAND H. INGRAM, JR., M.D.
Professor of Medicine and Director, Pulmonary and Critical Care Division, Emory University Medical School, and Chairman of Medicine, Crawford Long Hospital

ADOLF W. KARCHMER, M.D., F.A.C.P.
Associate Professor of Medicine, Harvard Medical School, and Chief, Infectious Disease Division, New England Deaconess Hospital

JAMES W. LEATHERMAN, M.D.
Assistant Professor of Medicine, Department of Medicine, University of Minnesota Medical School, and Pulmonologist, Division of Pulmonary Medicine, Hennepin County Medical Center

ANDREW B. NEWMAN, M.D., F.C.C.P.
Clinical Assistant Professor of Medicine (Respiratory Medicine), Stanford University School of Medicine

PETER O'HANLEY, M.D., Ph.D.
Assistant Professor, Department of Medicine (Infectious Diseases and Geographic Medicine) and Department of Microbiology and Immunology, Stanford University School of Medicine

ANDREW J. PERLMAN, M.D., Ph.D.
Senior Director of Clinical Research, Genentech, Inc.

EUGENE D. ROBIN, M.D., F.A.C.P.
Professor of Medicine and Physiology, Stanford University School of Medicine

DWIGHT R. ROBINSON, M.D.
Professor of Medicine, Harvard Medical School, and Physician, Massachusetts General Hospital

EDWARD RUBENSTEIN, M.D., M.A.C.P.
Associate Dean for Postgraduate Medical Education and Professor of Medicine, Stanford University School of Medicine

ROBERT H. RUBIN, M.D., F.A.C.P., F.C.C.P.
Associate Professor of Medicine, Harvard Medical School, and Chief, Transplantation Infectious Diseases, and Director, Clinical Investigation Program, Massachusetts General Hospital

JEREMY N. RUSKIN, M.D.
Associate Professor of Medicine, Harvard Medical School, and Director, Cardiac Arrhythmia Service, Massachusetts General Hospital

STANLEY L. SCHRIER, M.D., F.A.C.P.
Professor of Medicine and Chief, Division of Hematology, Stanford University School of Medicine

HARVEY B. SIMON, M.D., F.A.C.P.
Assistant Professor of Medicine, Harvard Medical School, and Physician, Massachusetts General Hospital

EVE ELIZABETH SLATER, M.D.
Vice President, Clinical and Regulatory Development, Merck Research Laboratories, and Associate Clinical Professor of Medicine, Columbia University College of Physicians and Surgeons

SUZANNE K. SWAN, M.D.
Clinical Pharmacology Fellow, Department of Medicine, Indiana University

MORTON N. SWARTZ, M.D., F.A.C.P.
Professor of Medicine, Harvard Medical School, and Chief, James Jackson Firm, Medical Services/Infectious Disease, Massachusetts General Hospital

NINA E. TOLKOFF-RUBIN, M.D.
Associate Professor of Medicine, Harvard Medical School; and Director, Hemodialysis and Continuous Ambulatory Peritoneal Dialysis Units, and Medical Coordinator for Renal Transplant Program, Massachusetts General Hospital

JOANNE H. VAN WOERT, M.D.
Specialist in Internal Medicine in Clinical Nutrition

PETER F. WELLER, M.D., F.A.C.P.
Associate Professor of Medicine, Harvard Medical School; Associate Physician, Beth Israel Hospital; and Associate Physician, Brigham and Women's Hospital

DOUGLAS W. WILMORE, M.D.
Frank Sawyer Professor of Surgery, Harvard Medical School, and Medical Director, Nutrition Support Service, Brigham and Women's Hospital

HARVEY S. YOUNG, M.D.
Assistant Professor of Medicine, Department of Gastroenterology, Stanford University School of Medicine, and Chief, Gastrointestinal Endoscopy, Stanford University Medical Center

Preface

In publishing a pocket edition of *Scientific American Medicine*, we are responding to requests from physicians, and physicians in training, who often find themselves in need of immediate bedside access to reliable, comprehensive, and up-to-date information about the management of life-threatening disorders.

There is no lack of manuals, handbooks, or outlines for physicians. But there is a large problem that needs to be addressed – the proliferation and diffusion of the medical literature. Standard textbooks are excellent vehicles for learning the basic principles of medical practice, but they are inevitably several years out of date at the time of their publication, and their rapid obsolescence renders them unsuitable for use in patient management, especially when the physician is dealing with serious illnesses. Housestaff manuals do not meet the broader needs of practicing physicians, on whose shelves they quickly become tucked away amid the stacks of unread journals. Electronic information retrieval systems have been useful in providing practitioners with answers to specific questions, especially about narrowly defined, arcane issues. But these systems often inundate the user with a sea of irrelevancies and do not provide a balanced view of emerging or controversial topics.

Scientific American Medicine, or *SAM* as it is affectionately called by so many of its users, was created to overcome these problems. It goes beyond an electronic information system. Its 70 authors employ electronic means to continuously collect new information, which they then assess in the light of other reports and findings as well as on the basis of their experience and expertise. If they decide to incorporate the new information, it is placed within the context of the ever-changing knowledge base that is *SAM*. Needless to say, these editorial steps are also accomplished electronically. Although *SAM* is most widely used in a printed, looseleaf format that is updated monthly, it is also available in a CD-ROM version, formerly known as CONSULT, now called SAM-CD™. Neither of these formats is suitable for the coat pockets of physicians or the backpacks of physicians in training. The pocket edition of *Scientific American Medicine*, another descendant of *SAM*, has been created for this purpose. It is a compilation of selected current chapters of *SAM* that are relevant to the management of patients on the medical services, intensive care units, and emergency departments of teaching hospitals. We have chosen these chapters because we believe they describe the care of the vast majority of patients encountered in these settings. None of the text has been deleted, but some tables have been revised and many figures are not included. The constraints of size inherent in the design of a pocket book force editors to make difficult decisions. The coverage is not complete; we are aware of these limitations.

It now seems likely that, in time, *SAM* will be available in an electronic pocket version. Until then, we hope that this pocket edition will prove to be a good companion to its owners. We are prepared to modify it continuously in response to their advice.

Edward Rubenstein, M.D., M.A.C.P.
Daniel D. Federman, M.D., M.A.C.P.

Table of Contents

1 Shock

MARK B. EFFRON, M.D.
BART CHERNOW, M.D.

Classification

Shock is a leading cause of morbidity and mortality in hospitalized patients. It can be defined as a state of inadequate tissue perfusion and oxygen delivery to critical organs. Shock may develop either acutely (e.g., hemorrhagic shock resulting from a gunshot wound) or more insidiously (e.g., cardiogenic shock resulting from chronic congestive heart failure).

There are four major types of shock: distributive (including septic, spinal, anaphylactic, and anaphylactoid), cardiogenic, hypovolemic, and obstructive. Each type has multiple potential causes [*see Table 1*]. Often, patients experience two or more types of shock at one time. Thus, a patient with severe heart failure and cardiogenic shock may also be in distributive shock (e.g., from sepsis), hypovolemic shock (e.g., from gastric hemorrhage), or both.

Hypovolemic Shock

The clinical conditions that cause hypovolemic shock include acute and subacute hemorrhage and dehydration. More than 30 to 40 percent of blood volume must be lost before compensatory mechanisms fail and shock develops. If this vascular volume is not replaced within approximately 90 minutes, an irreversible shock state may ensue. This irreversible state is probably caused by the release of cardiotoxic substances or insufficient coronary artery blood flow, resulting in myocardial ischemia.

Fluid loss into an extravascular compartment (the so-called third space) can significantly reduce intravascular volume and result in nonhemorrhagic hypovolemic shock. Acute pancreatitis, loss of the enteral integument (from conditions such as burns, surgical wounds, trauma, bullous dermatologic disease, or abdominal ascites), or occlusive or dynamic ileus can all induce oligemic hypotension as a result of extravasation of fluids into the extracellular compartment. Other forms of water and solute loss, such as diarrhea, hyperglycemia (leading to glucosuria), diabetes insipidus, salt-wasting nephritis, protracted vomiting, adrenocortical failure, acute peritonitis, and overzealous use of diuretics can also lead to decreased intravascular volume and hypovolemic shock.

Distributive Shock

Distributive shock is characterized by an abnormal distribution of intravascular volume that is attributable to stimulation by endogenous vasodilators and vasoconstrictors that alter regional vascular resistance. Sepsis, anaphylaxis and anaphylactoid reactions, certain endocrinologic disorders, microcirculatory impairment, metabolic factors, and selected neurologic disorders all may affect the distribution of blood flow and induce hypotension. Because of peripheral vasodilatation, the skin is usually well perfused; accordingly, this type of shock is known as warm shock. Cardiac output may be either normal or increased. If it is increased, the patient is considered to be in high-output shock.

Septic shock is usually the result of infection by microorganisms that trigger the release of mediators that act as vasodilators and myocardial depressants. Gram-negative bacteria release endotoxins, whereas gram-positive bacteria release exotoxins; the exotoxins released from staphylococci are present in toxic shock syndrome.[1-3] It is currently believed that in gram-negative infection, the release of endotoxin into the circulation leads to the activation of macrophages and monocytes, which, in turn, release cytokines such as tumor necrosis factor

Table 1 Causes of Shock

Hypovolemic	Hemorrhagic intravascular depletion Nonhemorrhagic intravascular depletion (vomiting, diarrhea, dehydration, diabetic ketoacidosis, diabetes insipidus, adrenocortical insufficiency, peritonitis, pancreatitis, burns, ascites, villous adenoma, pheochromocytoma)
Distributive	Sepsis, or endotoxemia Metabolic factors (acute respiratory failure, acute renal failure, hepatic failure, severe acidosis or alkalosis, drug overdose) Endocrinologic disorders (diabetes mellitus with ketoacidosis, hyperosmolar nonketotic hyperglycemic coma, adrenal insufficiency, hypothyroidism, diabetes insipidus, hypoglycemia) Microcirculatory impairment (polycythemia vera, hyperviscosity syndrome, sickle cell anemia, fat emboli) Neurogenic factors Anaphylaxis
Obstructive	Cardiac tamponade, constrictive pericarditis, aortic coarctation, pulmonary embolism, pulmonary hypertension

Cardiogenic	Arrhythmias
	Cardiac mechanical factors
	  Regurgitant lesions (acute mitral or aortic regurgitation, ventricular septal defect, left ventricular aneurysm, ventricular free wall rupture)
	  Obstructive lesions
	    Left ventricular outflow obstruction (valvular aortic stenosis, idiopathic hypertrophic subaortic stenosis)
	    Left ventricular inflow obstruction (mitral stenosis, left atrial myxoma and other cardiac tumors, left atrial thrombosis)
	Cardiomyopathies
	  Impaired left ventricular contractility (acute myocardial infarction, usually of the left ventricle but occasionally of the right ventricle; congestive cardiomyopathy)
	  Impaired left ventricular compliance (cardiac amyloidosis, idiopathic hypertrophic subaortic stenosis)

(cachectin) and interleukins. These cytokines trigger cascade reactions that lead to the clinical and biochemical manifestations of the sepsis syndrome. The understanding of this sequence of events has led to the development of novel therapeutic approaches to the sepsis syndrome, such as the use of monoclonal antibodies directed against endotoxin.[4-7]

Obstructive Shock

Factors that prevent adequate left or right heart filling markedly decrease stroke volume (and therefore cardiac output as well) and result in obstructive shock. Diseases of the pericardium (e.g., cardiac tamponade and constrictive pericarditis) can result in inadequate ventricular filling. Pulmonary emboli, primary pulmonary hypertension, or peripheral pulmonary artery stenosis may result in decreased left ventricular filling, as may other causes of pulmonary hypertension. Increasing right ventricular volume overload may shift the interventricular septum toward the left ventricle and compromise left ventricle filling. Although rare, tumors (both intrinsic and extrinsic) can cause decreased ventricular (left or right) filling that results in shock. Severe aortic or mitral stenosis may cause shock by obstructing outflow of blood from the heart. An acute obliterating ascending aortic dissection may also cause obstructive shock.

Cardiogenic Shock

Insults to the myocardium of the left ventricle, such as ischemia, infarction, toxic myopathy, or inflammatory diseases, may produce severe systolic dysfunction that leads to decreased cardiac output and cardiogenic shock. The most common cause of cardiogenic shock is an acute myocardial infarction. Shock is especially common when infarction results in loss of more than 40 percent of left ventricular mass.[8] The usual indicator of heart failure leading to cardiogenic shock is low cardiac output, high pulmonary arterial occlusion pressure (pulmonary arterial wedge pressure), and increased systemic vascular resistance. Occasionally, severe right heart failure from an extensive right ventricular infarction results in low cardiac output, normal or decreased pulmonary arterial occlusion pressure, and increased central venous pressure.

Mechanical factors may also give rise to cardiogenic shock. Examples of mechanical factors are mitral regurgitation (which may be acute in onset as a result of papillary muscle dysfunction or rupture), myocardial rupture, and acute aortic regurgitation.

Other causes of left ventricular dysfunction, such as acute myocarditis, severe congestive cardiomyopathies, and myocardial damage during surgery, may be responsible for cardiogenic shock. Left ventricular diastolic dysfunction, such as that seen in hypertrophic cardiomyopathy or amyloidosis, may, on rare occasions, cause shock through inadequate ventricular filling and subsequent decreased cardiac output.

Pathophysiology

Although many factors contribute to the pathophysiology of the shock state [see Figure 1], hypoperfusion of vital organs with inadequate cellular oxygen delivery is the final common pathway. Inadequate tissue perfusion results in inadequate delivery of oxygen and nutrients and local accumulation of the toxic end products of anaerobic metabolism; decreased oxygen and substrate delivery results in abnormal cellular metabolism and function.

Adequate delivery of oxygen to the tissues is primarily determined by three factors: cardiac output, oxygen-carrying capacity of the blood, and oxygen saturation. If red cell mass is decreased by factors such as blood loss or decreased red cell production, the oxygen-carrying capacity of the blood (i.e., the hemoglobin concentration) is decreased. Various metabolic effects of circulatory shock, such as acidosis, hypercapnia, hyperthermia, and increased levels of 2,3-diphosphoglycerate (2,3-DPG), shift the oxyhemoglobin dissociation curve to the right; as a result, oxygen is bound less tightly to the hemoglobin. Therefore, for any given oxygen tension, the capability for oxygen transport to the tissues is decreased because of decreased oxygen content. Hypothermia, alkalemia, reduced 2,3-DPG concentrations, and hypocapnia shift the curve to the left and thereby impair oxygen release from hemoglobin to the cells. Frequently, the three factors (cardiac output, oxygen-carrying capacity, and oxygen saturation) are simultaneously impaired in the shock state, which markedly reduces oxygen delivery to vital organs.

When shock develops, there is an imbalance between oxygen demand and oxygen delivery. Normally, oxygen consumption remains constant over a wide range of oxygen delivery values; that is, it is independent of oxygen supply. When oxygen delivery decreases below 15 ml/min/kg,[9] as in hypovolemic, cardiogenic, and obstructive shock, oxygen consumption becomes dependent on oxygen delivery. In distributive shock, oxygen consumption becomes dependent on oxygen extraction. In septic shock, oxygen demand is increased by several different mechanisms. Fever and inflammatory reactions create a greater metabolic demand, which leads to increased oxygen transport; however, altered oxygen extraction by the tissues limits the amount of oxygen the cells

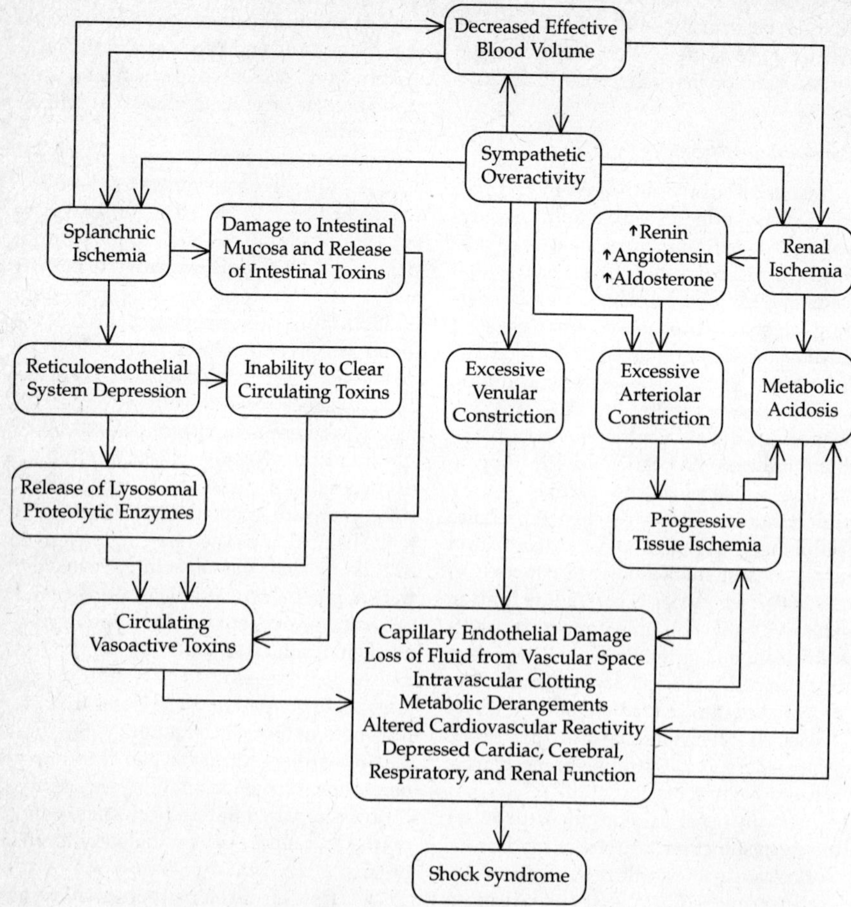

Figure 1 *Many factors interact to produce shock. Those indicated in blue are considered the most important factors in the pathogenesis of shock.*

can take up to meet the increased demand. The result is an increase in anaerobic metabolism, which generates lactic acid and leads to lactic acidosis. The decreased oxygen delivery associated with hypovolemic, cardiogenic, and obstructive shock also produces anaerobic metabolism and an increase in lactate production.

The adrenergic nervous system plays an important role in shock. A decrease in blood pressure stimulates the baroreceptor reflex, causing the release of epinephrine and norepinephrine into the circulation.[10] Epinephrine and norepinephrine bind to specific alpha- and beta-adrenergic receptors on the cell surface. The alpha-adrenergic receptors (alpha$_1$ and alpha$_2$) influence vascular tone by inducing vasoconstriction of arterioles and veins. These actions appear to be mediated by a second messenger system, known as the phosphatidylinositol protein kinase C cascade. The binding of alpha-adrenergic ligands to the alpha$_1$ adrenoreceptor causes hydrolysis of the phosphatidylinositols, a class of lipids that reside in the cell membrane. Hydrolysis of phosphatidylinositol, in turn, releases diacylglycerol and an inositol, 1,4,5-triphosphate (IP_3). Diacylglycerol increases the affinity of protein kinase C for intracellular calcium, and IP_3 mobilizes calcium from nonmitochondrial intracellular stores (usually in the sarcoplasmic reticulum). The increase in intracellular calcium activates protein kinase C as well as the calcium-calmodulin complex–dependent protein kinase that catalyzes the phosphorylation of myosin light chains and produces smooth muscle contraction.

Beta-adrenergic receptors are also divided into two classes: $beta_1$ receptors primarily regulate cardiac function, lipolysis, renin release, amylase secretion, and intestinal smooth muscle relaxation, whereas $beta_2$ receptors mediate smooth muscle and bronchial muscle relaxation. Beta-adrenergic receptors stimulate the production of cyclic adenosine monophosphate (cAMP), which then phosphorylates myosin-light-chain kinase. Phosphorylation of myosin-light-chain kinase prevents the phosphorylation of myosin light chains and the subsequent interaction of actin and myosin, thus resulting in relaxation of smooth muscle.

Dopaminergic receptors mediate vasodilatation of the splanchnic, renal, coronary, and cerebral arterioles and mediate venoconstriction as well. Dopaminergic receptors have been found in the zona glomerulosa of the adrenal cortex, where aldosterone is produced. In low doses, dopamine inhibits aldosterone synthesis and secretion, thus contributing to natriuresis.[11] This hormonal action is important because critically ill patients are thought to have secondary hyperaldosteronism.

Catecholamine receptors function abnormally in shock. Shock stimulates catecholamine release; with prolonged catecholamine excess, receptors down-regulate, and the tissue becomes less responsive to catecholamine stimulation.[12] Down-regulation is thought to be attributable to inadequate generation of replacement receptors.[12]

Catecholamine receptors on cells are also modulated by adrenergic agonists and antagonists, denervation, glucocorticoids, thyroid hormones, estrogen and progesterone, ischemia, aging, hypertension, heart failure, diabetes mellitus, alcohol withdrawal, and psychotropic drugs. Hepatic and vascular $alpha_1$-adrenergic receptors are down-regulated in experimental chronic sepsis.[13] The failure of norepinephrine or so-called alpha dosages (dosages high enough to have alpha-adrenergic effects) of intravenously infused dopamine to increase blood pressure in vasodilated septic patients may be explained by decreased receptor density resulting from such down-regulation.

The renin-angiotensin-aldosterone (RAA) system also plays a major role in regulating vascular tone. Stimuli that increase production of catecholamines also increase the release of renin. Increased renin release leads to elevated levels of angiotensin I, which is converted into the potent vasoconstrictor angiotensin II. Aldosterone levels are also increased via the RAA system, causing retention of sodium and more subsequent salt loading. Increased salt retention results in increased intravascular volume and venous pressure. This increased volume may help correct fluid losses in patients with hypovolemic shock or may further exacerbate problems with left ventricular preload in patients with cardiogenic shock.

In hypovolemic and cardiogenic shock, the circulating concentrations of catecholamines and angiotensin rise, leading to vasoconstriction, or cold shock (so called because of the cold extremities noted on physical examination). Distributive shock is manifested in an opposite manner, as a consequence of the release of endotoxin and endogenous vasodilators (e.g., endorphins, histamine, and prostacyclin) that induce peripheral vasodilatation, or warm shock, in which the patient has warm extremities despite hypotension. In cold shock, peripheral vasoconstriction occurs because hypoperfusion has stimulated the release of catecholamines and renin. In warm shock, however, the alteration in vascular tone (in this instance, peripheral vasodilatation) is the source of hypoperfusion rather than the response to it.

Other substances that have been demonstrated to alter vascular tone in shock include serotonin, eicosanoids, endorphins, and endothelial-dependent factors. Serotonin may have differential effects on the vascular system. In the presence of functional endothelium, serotonin causes the release of endothelial-dependent relaxing factors (EDRF, thought to be primarily nitric oxide), which results in vasodilatation; however, in certain vascular beds or in the absence of endothelium, serotonin causes vasoconstriction. Therefore, a high serotonin concentration may be either a cause or an effect of the shock state. The eicosanoids comprise the prostaglandins, the thromboxanes, and the leukotrienes. The prostaglandin prostacyclin is a vasodilator released by endothelium. By contrast, thromboxanes are potent vasoconstrictors that can be released from activated platelets, and leukotrienes are vasoconstrictors that are released from activated leukocytes and other cells.[14] The interaction of thromboxane and prostacyclin in septic shock is complex: whereas thromboxane causes platelet aggregation and sludging, endothelial damage, and pulmonary arteriolar vasoconstriction, prostacyclin causes peripheral vasodilatation and increased capillary permeability. In experimental endotoxic shock, cyclooxygenase inhibitors, which prevent formation of prostacyclin and thromboxanes, improve short-term survival and hemodynamic variables by increasing total peripheral resistance. Leukotriene levels are increased in experimental shock; treatment of animals with leukotriene synthesis inhibitors during experimental shock has protective effects.

Cytokines play a major role in the etiology of septic shock. Tumor necrosis factor (TNF) is made by macrophages and can be released by endotoxin; it produces hemodynamic collapse and multiple organ dysfunction when released into the circulation. Monoclonal antibodies to TNF have prevented death in animals given a lethal dose of endotoxin. Interleukin-1 (IL-1) activates T cells, stimulating cytokine release and subsequent hypotension. Interleukin-2 (IL-2) has been shown to decrease blood pressure and systemic vascular resistance and cause associated increases in heart rate and cardiac output (similar to those seen in sepsis) when used as an antitumor agent in cancer patients. IL-2 has also produced decreased left ventricular contractility and increased left ventricular volume (again, similar to findings in septic shock). IL-1 and TNF have been shown to be synergistic in animal studies: when applied simultaneously, they were effective in doses that were ineffective when the substances were given separately.

Endogenous glucagon is released into the circulation after the onset of shock. Elevated glucagon levels lead to hyperglycemia, increased cardiac output, and increased heart rate. Experimentally, the tachycardic effects of glucagon are blocked by verapamil but are not altered by beta blockers, which suggests that glucagon can facilitate the movement of calcium into the cell through calcium channels.[15] Glucagon has also been found to be useful in patients with hypotension caused by beta-blocker therapy[16]; increases in heart rate and blood pressure occur because glucagon's inotropic action is not affected by beta-adrenergic receptor blockade.

Calcium is required for normal cardiovascular and neurovascular function and is an important regulator of cellular homeostasis. Serum levels of total calcium and of ionized calcium have been found to be low in 64 percent and 12 percent of critically ill patients, respectively.[17] Calcium concentrations are maintained in a narrow range by parathyroid hormone in conjunction with vitamin D metabolites. Parathyroid glandular dysfunction or vitamin D insufficiency may occur in septic shock.[18] Therefore, in hypotensive patients in shock, the serum ionized calcium concentration should be measured and calcium homeostasis restored if clinically important hypocalcemia is identified.

Hypomagnesemia is seen in approximately 20 to 60 percent of critically ill patients.[19] Serum magnesium is important in the regulation of cardiovascular, endocrinologic, and neurologic homeostasis. Magnesium deficiency may predispose patients to tachyarrhythmias, sudden death, and heart failure, probably because of decreased intracellular potassium levels caused by functional impairment of the Na^+-K^+-ATPase pump. Magnesium deficiency may result from loss from the gastrointestinal tract, renal excretion, endocrine and metabolic causes, burns, hypothermia, and the administration of nephrotoxic agents such as aminoglycosides, cisplatin, cyclosporine, and amphotericin.

Other endocrine abnormalities are also noted in shock. For instance, adrenocorticotropic hormone (ACTH) secretion and plasma cortisol concentrations are typically increased by the physical stress associated with shock. One study, however, reported inappropriately low serum cortisol concentrations in almost one third of a group of severely stressed patients.[20]

Clinical Picture

Determining that shock is present is relatively easy; determining the etiology of the shock state is often more difficult. The clinical picture largely depends on the cause and severity of shock. Cardiogenic, hypovolemic, and obstructive shock are usually characterized by clinically important vasoconstriction, which makes the skin cool and clammy to palpation and mottled in appearance. Peripheral systolic arterial blood pressure is typically less than 90 mm Hg and may be significantly lower, which usually results in poor cerebral perfusion manifested by agitation, obtundation, and confusion. In the elderly, it is not uncommon for the symptoms of decreased cerebral perfusion to be mistaken for general agitation and to be inappropriately treated with sedatives.

Blood lactate determinations have proved to be useful markers in shock pa-

Table 2   Alterations in Selected Hemodynamic Indices in Shock

Type of Shock	Cause	PAOP	CO	SVR
Hypovolemic shock	Hemorrhagic intravascular depletion	↓↓	↓↓	↑↑
	Nonhemorrhagic intravascular depletion	↓↓	↓↓	↑↑
Distributive shock	Sepsis	↓ or 0	↑↑, 0, or, rarely, ↓	↑ intially, then ↓↓
	Anaphylaxis	↓ or 0	↑ or 0	↓↓
Obstructive shock	Pericardial tamponade	↑↑	↓ or ↓↓	↑
	Pulmonary embolism	0 or ↓	↓↓	↑
	Aortic dissection	↑	↓ or ↓↓	↑
Cardiogenic shock	Myocardial dysfunction	↑↑	↓↓	↑↑
	Mechanical dysfunction			
	Acute ventricular septal defect	↑↑	↓↓	↑↑
	Acute mitral regurgitation	↑↑	↓↓	↑↑
	Right ventricular infarct	↓ or 0	↓↓	↑↑

PAOP—pulmonary arterial occlusion pressure   CO—cardiac output   SVR—systemic vascular resistance
↑—increased   ↓—decreased   0—no change

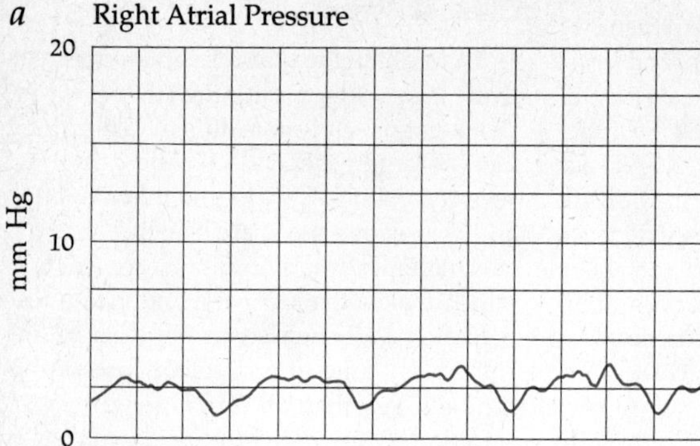

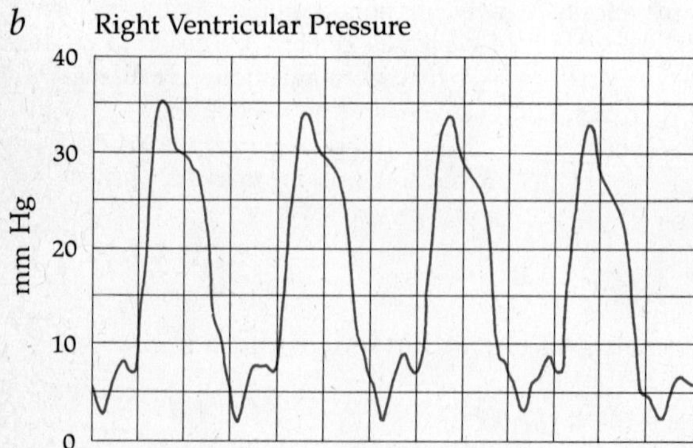

Figure 2 *To obtain the pulmonary arterial wedge (occlusion) pressure, which reflects left ventricular filling pressures and helps guide treatment of shock patients with left ventricular dysfunction, a balloon-tipped Swan-Ganz catheter is advanced through the chambers of the heart and positioned in the pulmonary artery. The progress of the catheter is guided by monitoring pressures in the right atrium (a), the right ventricle (b), and the pulmonary artery*

tients. Several studies have demonstrated that increased blood lactate values (2.5 mmol/L) are correlated with decreased oxygen delivery.[21-23] These studies also show that mortality from shock is increased in patients with an increased serum lactate concentration.

There are various other signs and symptoms of shock that are often reflective of the etiology of the shock state. In hypovolemic shock caused by hemorrhage, evidence of gross blood loss, either internal or external, is usually present. Hypovolemic shock caused by diarrheal illness can usually be detected by means of the history. Diabetic patients may be hypovolemic as a result of excessive glucosuria; however, these patients usually are very thirsty and therefore have a high intake of fluids. Septic shock is frequently associated with fever, rigors, an increased leukocyte count (with a shift to the left in the differential count), and, if infection is present, localizing signs of an infection. In cardiogenic shock, there is frequently an acute cardiac event, such as an arrhythmia, myocardial infarction, or congestive heart failure, that provides the diagnosis.

Urine output tends to be decreased (30 ml/hr) in shock states because of decreased renal perfusion; however, if glucosuria is present, that diagnostic clue is lost. The urine tends to be concentrated, and sodium values tend to be very low (20 mEq/L). When shock has persisted for a critical period, acute tubular necrosis may develop.

The hemodynamic picture in shock is variable. Systolic blood pressure and mean arterial blood pressure are usually low;

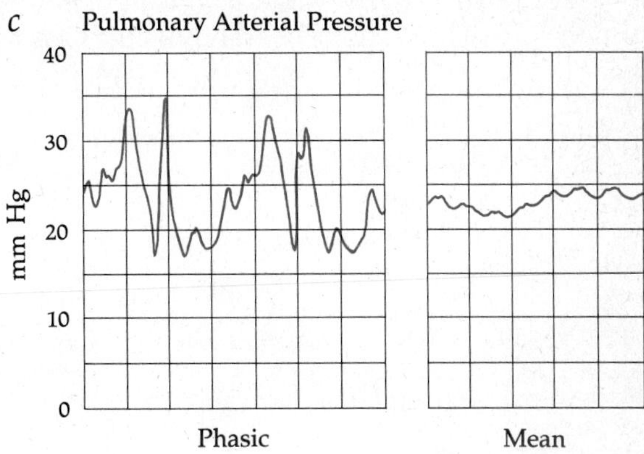

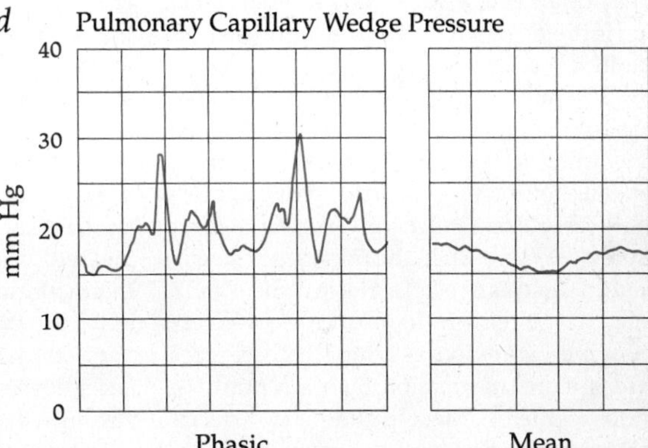

(c) as the catheter is advanced into the wedge position (pressures shown are representative of those encountered during this procedure). When the catheter is resting in the pulmonary artery, the balloon is inflated and the pulmonary arterial wedge pressure is recorded (d). Note that the mean pulmonary arterial wedge pressure, though minimally elevated, is slightly lower than the mean pulmonary arterial pressure

however, a normal blood pressure may, in a sense, reflect hypotension in a patient who is mildly hypertensive. Cardiac output is usually diminished, with an associated increase in systemic vascular resistance [*see Table 2*]; however, in septic and neurogenic shock, peripheral vascular resistance usually is markedly decreased, and cardiac output may be increased.

Therapy

Success in the treatment of shock is dependent on the early recognition that shock is present, the identification of its etiology, and the institution of appropriate therapeutic measures. Although the shock state itself may be transiently corrected with drugs and fluids, the circulatory disturbance may persist as long as the causative factor is still present.

Monitoring

All patients diagnosed as being in shock should be admitted to an ICU or to another special care unit where close observation can be maintained. Placement of an indwelling intra-arterial catheter allows close monitoring of blood pressure and provides access for blood sampling. Placement of a central venous catheter facilitates volume replacement and allows access for catheters to monitor cardiac function.

In patients with normal heart and lungs, volume status may be adequately determined by using a central venous catheter for central venous pressure assessment. Central venous pressure, however, is governed by several factors, including venous tone, venous capacitance, and right ventricular load. Under conditions in which these factors

Table 3 Hemodynamic Classification
of Shock Patients

Class	PAOP	Cardiac Index	Type of Shock
I	< 18 mm Hg	> 2.2 L/min/m^2	Distributive
II	> 18 mm Hg	> 2.2 L/min/m^2	Obstructive
III	< 18 mm Hg	< 2.2 L/min/m^2	Hypovolemic
IV	> 18 mm Hg	< 2.2 L/min/m^2	Cardiogenic, obstructive*

PAOP—pulmonary arterial occlusion (wedge) pressure

*Classic cardiogenic shock comprises hypotension, increased PAOP, and decreased cardiac index. Obstructive problems such as pericardial tamponade or constrictive pericarditis may be associated with a high PAOP and low cardiac index.

may be altered, a pulmonary arterial catheter is preferred for monitoring intravascular fluid status.

The pulmonary arterial catheter is more useful than the central venous catheter for determining the load on the left ventricle because pulmonary arterial occlusion pressure (PAOP) is a reflection of left atrial pressure [*see Figure* 2]. In the presence of severe mitral stenosis or a left atrial myoma, PAOP may not be reliable. In most cases of shock, however, a pulmonary arterial catheter provides more information than a central venous catheter. Most pulmonary arterial catheters are designed to permit measurement of cardiac output. If right atrial pressure, systemic blood pressure, and cardiac output are known, systemic vascular resistance can be calculated, and this parameter may aid in the diagnosis of the shock state as well as provide a yardstick for monitoring therapy.

Monitoring of cardiac output is helpful. The Fick method determines cardiac output by determining oxygen consumption per minute and dividing by the arteriovenous oxygen difference across the lungs. Because oxygen consumption is difficult to measure directly, approximations are derived on the basis of the oxygen-carrying capacity of hemoglobin and the hemoglobin content. Another method employs a dye indicator dilution technique. Indocyanine green dye is injected into the pulmonary artery and sampled in a peripheral artery. A plot of the changes in dye concentration over time is then obtained, and cardiac output is determined from this curve. The green-dye method, although relatively difficult to use, has the advantage of being able to discover intracardiac shunts by the more rapid appearance of the dye at the detector in the peripheral artery. The most common method of assessing cardiac output is the thermodilution technique. Cold saline is injected through the proximal port of a pulmonary arterial catheter into the right atrium and is then sampled by a thermistor downstream in the pulmonary artery. Knowledge of the blood temperature, the injectate temperature, and the transit time permits calculation of cardiac output. Recent technology has made possible the continuous sampling of mixed venous oxygen saturation. From the Fick equation, cardiac output is directly related to mixed venous oxygen saturation if it is assumed that oxygen consumption and arterial oxygen saturation are constant. Continuous monitoring of mixed venous oxygen saturation provides a continuous assessment of cardiac output, as opposed to the intermittent assessment obtained by means of the thermodilution technique.

Monitoring of cardiac output and pulmonary arterial occlusion pressure permits classification of shock patients into four categories [*see Table 3*], which is useful for patient management. Appropriate treatment with fluids, diuretics, vasopressors, or afterload-reducing agents normalizes both cardiac output and pulmonary arterial pressure, leading to improved tissue perfusion.

It is also important to monitor oxygen delivery to the tissues. Oxygen consumption is strongly dependent on oxygen delivery when oxygen delivery significantly decreases in the shock state. Oxygen delivery can be monitored by measuring both the oxygen saturation of blood and the cardiac output. Oxygen saturation is best measured directly through arterial blood gas sampling. The pulse oximeter provides a noninvasive method of monitoring oxygen saturation by sampling blood flow through an ear or a fingertip. Use of pulse oximeters has facilitated continuous monitoring of oxygen delivery and has decreased the amount of blood needed for repeated laboratory testing.

A leading cause of blood loss in critically ill patients is frequent aspiration of blood for analysis in monitoring their progress. Microchemical techniques have been developed that permit rapid analysis of blood gas and electrolytes in small samples. Moreover, because of technological improvements, it is now possible to reduce the amount of blood lost when specimens are obtained. Autologous blood replacement during surgery has also lessened the need for transfusion of blood, blood products, or nonblood products during surgical procedures.

Specific Measures

Initial therapy for patients in shock should be directed at basic life support. A patent airway must be established and maintained to provide adequate oxygen delivery. Supplemental oxygen and mechanical ventilation may also be necessary to ensure adequate oxygen delivery to cells. Noncardiogenic pulmonary edema (adult respiratory distress syndrome, or ARDS) may be present as a result of increased capillary permeability in the pulmonary vascular bed. The use of positive end-expiratory pressure is useful in this situation.[24]

Volume Replacement

In patients in early shock who have good left ventricular function, volume replacement is mandatory and may reverse the shock syndrome if given early enough in the course of the illness. Pharmacotherapy is more effective when intravascular volume is adequate. Before the administration of intravenous fluids, there are several maneuvers aimed at increasing central venous return that should be considered. Putting the patient into the head-down position (Trendelenburg's position) causes gravity-mediated return of blood from the periphery to the core. Military antishock trousers (MAST) also cause a large venous return from the periphery; however, a prospective, randomized study showed no benefit from MAST in patients with hypotension from trauma and, in fact, found that patients with cardiac and thoracic vascular injury who were treated with MAST had a worse outcome than patients who were not.[25]

Once a large-bore intravenous line has been established, normal saline, lactated Ringer's solution, or solutions containing colloids or blood products may be given to expand volume.

The use of blood products in the treatment of the shock state has become controversial because of the transmissible illnesses associated with their administration. In patients with hypovolemic shock of hemorrhagic origin, blood should be given to increase the red cell mass and to ensure adequate oxygen-carrying capacity. Substitutes for blood and red cells, such as perfluorocarbons and polymerized pyridoxylated hemoglobin solutions, are still under investigation.[26,27] Albumin administration is controversial but may be useful for its effects on oncotic pressure.[28] Colloids may also be given in an attempt to maintain oncotic pressure when large quantities of fluids are needed for resuscitation. For volume replacement in hypovolemic patients, there is little evidence that utilization of colloids offers sufficient advantage over crystalloids to justify their increased cost. Specific therapeutic measures to be taken depend in part on the etiology of the shock state [*see Table 4*].

Table 4 Treatment of Shock

Diagnosis	Etiology	Therapeutic Interventions
Hypovolemic shock	Hemorrhagic intravascular depletion	Fluid replacement (crystalloid, blood products, colloid); control of bleeding site and prevention of further bleeding
	Nonhemorrhagic intravascular depletion	Fluid replacement (crystalloid, colloid); treatment of underlying disease
Distributive shock	Sepsis	Antibiotics; fluid replacement; vasopressors; inotropic agents; possibly immunotherapy
	Anaphylaxis	Epinephrine; steroids; other vasopressors; removal of offending agents
Obstructive shock	Pericardial tamponade	Fluid replacement; pericardiocentesis
	Pulmonary emboli	Thrombolytic agent; surgical removal of thrombus; oxygen; prevention of further embolism
	Aortic dissection	Surgical repair; antihypertensive therapy
Cardiogenic shock	Myocardial dysfunction	
	Primary cardiomyopathy	Diuretics; afterload reduction; inotropic agents; intra-aortic balloon pump
	Acute myocardial infarction	Thrombolytic agent; intra-aortic balloon pump; inotropic agents; afterload reduction; coronary angioplasty
	Mechanical dysfunction	
	Acute ventricular septal defect	Afterload reduction; inotropic agents; intra-aortic balloon pump; possibly surgical repair
	Acute mitral regurgitation	Afterload reduction; inotropic agents; intra-aortic balloon pump; possibly surgical repair
	Right ventricular infarct	Fluid replacement; inotropic agents

After blood volume has been replaced, measures to stop the primary process must be initiated. Hemorrhage should be controlled by tourniquets, insertion of a Sengstaken-Blakemore tube (for esophageal variceal bleeding), or direct ligation of a bleeding vessel. Antibiotics should be given if septic shock is present or suspected. In cases of anaphylactic shock, the offending agent must be removed. Diuretics, inotropic agents, and vasodilators have been found to be useful in cardiogenic shock. Mechanical support with intra-aortic balloon counterpulsation, or so-called rescue coronary angioplasty, has also been useful.

Pharmacotherapy

Adrenergic agents After airway maintenance and volume replacement, adrenergic agents are the next therapeutic intervention [*see Table 5*]. The adrenergic agents are peripheral vasoactive drugs that bind to alpha-adrenergic, beta-adrenergic, and dopaminergic receptors.

Epinephrine is primarily a beta-adrenergic agonist, although it has alpha-adrenergic activity at high doses. Epinephrine causes cutaneous vasoconstriction (through alpha receptors), vasodilatation in skeletal muscle (through $beta_2$ receptors), and increased cardiac inotropy (through $beta_1$ receptors). Epinephrine acts mainly by increasing inotropy and shunting blood to the core by means of peripheral vasoconstriction; it has significant chronotropic actions as well. However, epinephrine also decreases the refractory period and accelerates ectopic foci, predisposing to arrhythmias.

Table 5 Sympathomimetic Amines Commonly Used in Shock

Drugs	Usual I.V. Dosage	Adrenergic Effects				Electrophysiological Effects		
		α	β₁	β₂	Dopamine	HR	AV Conduction	VEA
Norepinephrine	2–8 µg/min	+++	+	0	0	↑ or 0	↑ or 0	↑
Epinephrine	1–4 µg/min	+++	+++	+++	0	↑	↑	↑
Dopamine	1–4 µg/kg/min	+	0	0	++++	0	0	↑
	≥ 10 µg/kg/min	++	+	+	++++	↑	↑	↑
	10–20 µg/kg/min	++++	+++	++	++++	↑↑	↑	↑↑
Dobutamine	2–20 µg/kg/min	+	+++	+	0	↑ or 0	0	↑
Phenylephrine	5–20 µg/min	+++	+	0	0	↓	↓	0
Isoproterenol	0.5–4.0 µg/min	0	+++	+++	0	↑	↑	↑
Metaraminol	8–15 µg/kg/min	++	0	0	0	↑, ↓, or 0	0	↑
Methoxamine	8–15 µg/kg/min	+++	0	0	0	↓	↓	0

Note: adapted from references 50 and 51.

HR—heart rate AV—atrioventricular VEA—ventricular ectopic activity

0 = no effect + = slight effect ++ = moderate effect +++ = marked effect ++++ = greatest effect

Norepinephrine is released from post-ganglionic sympathetic nerves and, to a lesser degree, from the adrenal cortex. It is primarily an alpha-adrenergic drug but also stimulates beta₁ receptors. By producing significant vasoconstriction, norepinephrine elevates blood pressure; however, it may also decrease renal blood flow by constricting the renal vasculature. Norepinephrine increases not only cardiac contractility and chronotropism but also myocardial work and oxygen demand. Other alpha-adrenergic drugs, such as phenylephrine, also improve blood pressure and tissue perfusion by means of vasoconstriction.

Isoproterenol is a pure beta-adrenergic agonist. It increases heart rate and myocardial contractility while inducing peripheral vasodilatation; however, the vasodilatation tends to occur in skin and muscle vascular beds, which results in diversion of blood from key organs. For this reason, isoproterenol is rarely used now, except in patients who have isoproterenol-responsive bradycardia, with or without hypotension. Agents that have both alpha- and beta-adrenergic effects (e.g., norepinephrine) may be more useful because these agents increase cardiac contractility without causing vasodilatation.

Dopamine is the immediate precursor of norepinephrine in the endogenous biosynthetic pathway of catecholamines and is derived from the adrenal glands and the kidneys. It stimulates different receptors, depending on the dose infused and the rate of infusion.[11,29] At low infusion rates (0.5–2.0 µg/kg/min), dopamine usually stimulates dopaminergic receptors, causing diuresis through dilatation of renal arteries and inducing natriuresis by suppressing aldosterone. At slightly higher infusion rates (2–10 µg/kg/min), dopamine stimulates beta₁ receptors, resulting in increased myocardial contractility and mild peripheral vasodilatation. At infusion rates higher than 10 µg/kg/min, dopamine's predominant action is alpha-adrenergic stimulation and consequent vasoconstriction. Because dopamine causes dilatation of renal, splanchnic, coronary, and cerebrovascular beds at lower doses, it is used as the first-line agent in many shock patients and is continued in low doses even after shock is reversed. In our

Table 6 Vasodilator Drugs Commonly Used in Shock

Drug*	Usual Dosage	Mechanism of Action	Comments
Sodium nitroprusside (Nipride)	10–80 µg/min I.V.	Direct relaxing effect on vascular smooth muscle	Very potent vasodilator; rapidly inactivated; may have cardio-accelerator effect
Nitrates Nitroglycerin Isosorbide dinitrate	10–200 µg/kg/min I.V. or 0.3–0.6 mg sublingually q 1–2 hr 2.5–5.0 mg sublingually q 1–3 hr	Direct relaxing effect on vascular smooth muscle	—
Phentolamine (Regitine)	1–2 µg/kg/min I.V.	Alpha-adrenergic blocking agent	May be given as loading dose of 0.5 mg/min I.V. until either the desired effect is achieved or a total of 5 mg is given

*Whenever any of the drugs listed are given, the cardiac filling pressures and systemic arterial pressure must be closely monitored. Use of vasodilators may precipitate the need for volume. Intravenous nitroglycerin, 20–80 µg/min, and phenoxybenzamine (Dibenzyline), 1 mg/kg, have also been used to produce vasodilatation.

experience, this response to dopamine administration varies from patient to patient.

Dobutamine is a synthetic beta-adrenergic agent that promotes increased myocardial contractility and vasodilatation. Dobutamine is particularly helpful for patients in cardiogenic shock when myocardial failure and increased peripheral vascular resistance are present. For a given degree of enhancement of myocardial function, dobutamine causes less tachycardia than either dopamine or isoproterenol. The increased inotropy and vasodilatation usually preserve blood pressure and tissue perfusion, although a small decrease in blood pressure often occurs. This improvement in cardiac function leads to lower pulmonary arterial occlusion pressures and increased renal perfusion. Dobutamine also increases the cardiac index in patients in septic shock, thereby increasing oxygen delivery to tissues.

Other inotropic agents Phosphodiesterase III inhibitors increase myocardial contractility in normal hearts by increasing cAMP levels; they also cause vasodilatation by increasing cAMP levels in smooth muscle [*see* Pathophysiology, *above*]. Clinically, phosphodiesterase III inhibitors have been shown to enhance cardiac function in patients with acute and chronic heart failure.[30-32] It is thought that the major benefit of phosphodiesterase III inhibitors in heart failure derives from their ability to unload the heart by means of vasodilatation. Studies show that these agents act synergistically with dobutamine.[33,34]

Digoxin has been used for many years in the treatment of cardiogenic causes of low-output states (e.g., congestive heart failure and shock). There is some controversy regarding the benefit of digoxin in patients with heart failure who are in sinus rhythm.[35] In acute situations, digoxin may augment the release of norepinephrine and angiotensin, and the resulting vasoconstriction may have a detrimental effect on afterload.[36] In such situations, digoxin is primarily useful as a means of controlling supraventricular arrhythmias, especially atrial fibrillation with a rapid ventricular response. Thus, there appears to be no role for digoxin in the acute management of cardiogenic shock unless control of supraventricular arrhythmias is needed. Studies aimed at determining the utility of digoxin in the treatment of chronic heart failure are in progress.

Morphine Morphine is useful for patients with myocardial infarction or acute pulmonary edema. Its main actions are relief of pain and alleviation of anxiety; there is a resultant decrease in the level of circulating catecholamines. Morphine also increases venous capacitance, thereby decreasing venous return and reducing preload. The increase in venous capacitance results in decreased wall stress and myocardial oxygen consumption, which means that myocardial efficiency is improved.

Vasodilators Intravenous vasodilators such as sodium nitroprusside and nitroglycerin are useful adjuncts in the management of cardiogenic shock [*see Table 6*]. Sodium nitroprusside dilates peripheral arteries and veins, reducing preload and afterload and thereby decreasing left ventricular wall stress and left ventricular work as well. However, sodium nitroprusside also causes further arterial hypotension; the decrease in both the arterial and venous pressure may cause a decline in coronary artery perfusion, leading to ischemia. Nitroglycerin is a preferential venodilator, although it also dilates arteries at higher doses. Therefore, nitroglycerin may preserve coronary artery perfusion better than sodium nitroprusside does and may be more useful in ischemic states.

Corticosteroids Corticosteroid use is controversial in septic shock.[37,38] Corticosteroids are thought to preserve cellular membranes and endothelial integrity, stabilize lysosomal membranes, inhibit activation of complement, and interfere with release of myocardial depressant factors. One study[39] found that corticosteroid use lowered mortality from septic shock, but later randomized studies showed no benefit.[40,41]

Naloxone Naloxone inhibits endogenous endorphins and reverses experimental endotoxin-mediated hypotension[42-45]; however, confirmation of naloxone's clinical efficacy is yet to be obtained.

Antibiotics Antibiotics play a critical role in the management of septic shock. Initial therapy should employ broad-spectrum antibiotics until the offending organism is defined and can be eradicated by a single agent.

Monoclonal antibodies Immunotherapy is proving to be successful in the treatment of septic shock. Early studies focused on the use of a monoclonal antibody to the endotoxin core glycolipid of *Escherichia coli*.[4,5] Use of this antibody in septic shock demonstrated that it could reverse established shock and decrease death from gram-negative bacteremia.[4,5] Prophylactic immunization with the monoclonal antibody did not affect the infection rate in surgical patients but did decrease the serious consequences of gram-negative infections.[5] Subsequent studies showed that a monoclonal IgM antibody that binds to the lipid A domain of endotoxin (HA-1A) prevents death from septic shock in both laboratory animals and humans.[6,7] In a randomized, double-blind study,[7] patients in septic shock who were treated with HA-1A had a mortality of 33 percent, compared with a mortality of 57 percent in patients who were given a placebo ($P = 0.017$). Major complications of sepsis resolved more completely in the HA-1A group than in the placebo group (62 percent versus 42 percent; $P = 0.024$). In another study, a monoclonal antibody, MAb 60.3, that binds to the adhesive protein complex (CD11/CD18) on the cell membrane of polymorphonuclear neutrophils prevented death from hemorrhagic shock in Rhesus monkeys.[46] MAb 60.3 prevents polymorphonuclear neutrophils from adhering to

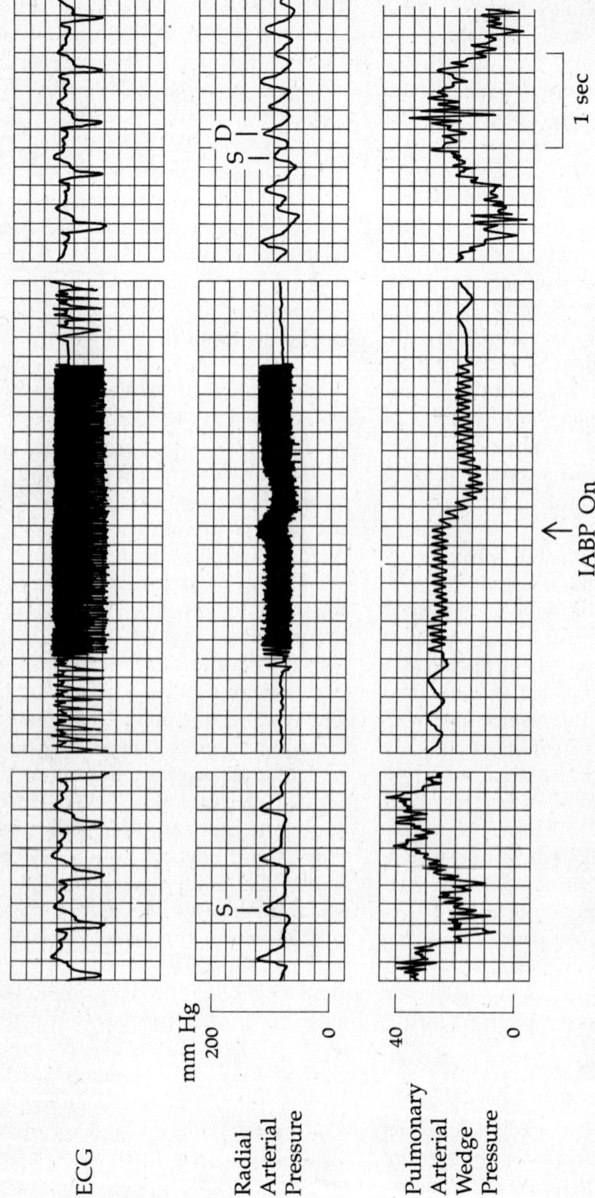

Figure 3 Pressure tracings show effects of intra-aortic balloon counterpulsation in a patient in cardiogenic shock (the paper speed has been slowed in the center panel). After the intra-aortic balloon pump (IABP) is turned on (arrow), the pulmonary arterial wedge (occlusion) pressure drops almost immediately from a mean of about 25 mm Hg to 18 mm Hg (bottom strip). Counterpulsation also reduces the arterial systolic pressure (S) and augments the diastolic pressure (D), as revealed by tracing of radial arterial pressure (middle strip, right). Inflation and deflation of the balloon are regulated by means of a surface-monitored electrocardiogram (top strip).

the vessel walls, thereby averting endothelial damage and subsequent vascular dysfunction. These forms of immunotherapy are awaiting approval by the Food and Drug Administration.

Mechanical Therapy

Mechanical therapy is primarily used for circulatory support in cardiogenic shock patients. Of the many devices that have been developed or are undergoing investigation, the most effective to date is intra-aortic balloon pump (IABP) counterpulsation [*see Figure 3*]. The intra-aortic balloon pump is inserted through the femoral artery and placed into the descending thoracic aorta. The balloon is programmed from the electrocardiogram to deflate just before systole and to inflate in diastole. Presystolic deflation reduces aortic impedance, allowing ejection of blood from the left ventricle at a decreased work load. Inflation of the balloon during diastole augments coronary artery blood flow by increasing coronary perfusion pressure.

Thrombolytic therapy for acute myocardial infarction has decreased the incidence of cardiogenic shock but has not improved survival in patients with cardiogenic shock.[47] The intra-aortic balloon pump, however, has been shown to improve survival in patients with acute myocardial infarction and cardiogenic shock. Placement of an intra-aortic balloon pump followed by emergency percutaneous transluminal coronary angioplasty may yield an even better outcome in these patients.[48,49] Intra-aortic balloon pump therapy has palliated cardiogenic shock in patients in whom mechanical lesions (e.g., rupture of a papillary muscle or the interventricular septum) complicate a myocardial infarction. These patients can then be stabilized until cardiac surgery can repair the lesion and revascularize the heart.

The intra-aortic balloon pump has also been useful in supporting patients awaiting cardiac transplantation who have cardiogenic shock from congestive heart failure caused by a dilated cardiomyopathy. Left ventricular assist devices (LVADs), the total artificial heart, and cardiac myoplasty utilizing the latissimus dorsi muscle have also been used as a bridge to cardiac transplantation in patients with severe heart failure.

Prognosis

Despite recent advances, the prognosis for patients in shock remains poor: for example, the mortality in patients presenting with cardiogenic shock from an acute myocardial infarction is still higher than 50 percent. Septic shock is a major cause of death in hospitalized patients and is the 10th leading cause of death among elderly Americans. With more aggressive therapy, it may be possible to decrease mortality from shock. As the technology available for resuscitation from shock improves, however, the cost of resuscitation will increase dramatically. Future management decisions may have to take into account not only the question of which diagnostic and therapeutic methods should be used in patients in shock but also the question of whether use of advanced technology in these patients is associated with an acceptable cost-benefit ratio.

References

1. JAMA 257:1053, 1987
2. Engl J Med 317:146, 1987
3. N Engl J Med 321:1, 1989
4. Proc Natl Acad Sci USA 82:1790, 1985
5. Lancet 2:59, 1985
6. Clin Res 35:619A, 1987
7. N Engl J Med 324:429, 1991
8. N Engl J Med 285:133, 1971
9. Crit Care Med 19:664, 1991
10. J Trauma 24:229, 1984
11. J Clin Endocrinol Metab 63:197, 1986
12. N Engl J Med 310:1570, 1984
13. Shock 19:185, 1986
14. FASEB J 1:186, 1987
15. Circ Shock 19:393, 1986
16. Ann Intern Med 105:65, 1986
17. Crit Care Med 10:848, 1982
18. Ann Intern Med 107:36, 1987
19. Crit Care Clin 7:225, 1991
20. Lancet 1:1414, 1982
21. Am J Cardiol 67:565, 1991
22. Clin Chem 36:1544, 1990

23. Crit Care Med 17:719, 1989
24. Crit Care Clin 5:157, 1989
25. J Trauma 29:1104, 1989
26. Ann Emerg Med 15:1423, 1986
27. Ann Emerg Med 15:1416, 1986
28. JAMA 237:460, 1977
29. N Engl J Med 275:1389, 1966
30. N Engl J Med 299:1373, 1978
31. N Engl J Med 314:290, 1986
32. N Engl J Med 314:349, 1986
33. Circulation 74:367, 1986
34. Am Heart J 119:891, 1990
35. Circulation 73:14, 1986
36. J Clin Endocrinol Metab 58:76, 1984
37. N Engl J Med 311:1137, 1984
38. Arch Surg 119:537, 1984
39. Ann Surg 184:333, 1976
40. N Engl J Med 317:659, 1987
41. N Engl J Med 317:653, 1987
42. Lancet 1:1363, 1985
43. Crit Care Med 13:28, 1985
44. Crit Care Med 13:972, 1985
45. Crit Care Med 11:650, 1983
46. Surgery 108:206, 1990
47. Am J Cardiol 55:871, 1985
48. Eur Heart J 10:958, 1989
49. Am Heart J 121:895, 1991
50. Cardiology. Parmley WW, Chatterjee K, Eds. JB Lippincott Co, Philadelphia, 1988, p 17:1
51. Harrison's Principles of Internal Medicine, 12th ed. Wilson JD, Braunwald E, Isselbacher KJ, et al, Eds. McGraw-Hill Book Co, New York, 1991, p 232

2 Cardiac Tachyarrhythmias: Basic Aspects and Pharmacologic Therapy

ADOLPH M. HUTTER, JR., M.D.

Physiologic Basis of Arrhythmias

Precipitating Factors

Two physiologic mechanisms account for most ectopic arrhythmias: reentry and enhanced automaticity. Reentry is precipitated by a variety of alterations in refractoriness, impulse formation, and conduction [see Chapter 3]. Enhanced automaticity leads to repetitive firing from a single focus within the heart. Factors underlying arrhythmias associated with either mechanism include hypoxia, electrolyte and acid-base abnormalities, ischemia, myocardial fiber stretch, altered sympathetic tone, bradycardia, and the use of certain drugs. Triggered activity associated with afterdepolarization, which presumably gives rise to repetitive electrical activity, may be a mechanism for some tachyarrhythmias.

In treating the patient with cardiac arrhythmias, it is important to consider reversible precipitating factors that might be corrected. Hypoxia can induce arrhythmias, and acidosis lowers the threshold for ventricular fibrillation. It is not commonly appreciated, however, that alkalosis is even more likely than acidosis to produce ventricular arrhythmias. Thus, establishment of a physiologic Po_2, Pco_2, and pH can be of major therapeutic benefit in some patients. Hypokalemia predisposes to ventricular arrhythmias and must be suspected in any patient who is taking diuretics. The correction of hypokalemia is of prime importance in the treatment of arrhythmias caused by digitalis toxicity. Hypomagnesemia, which is associated with diuretic use, and hypercalcemia may also provoke digitalis-induced arrhythmias.

Myocardial ischemia is commonly associated with ventricular arrhythmias.[1] About 60 percent of patients with ischemic heart disease die suddenly, presumably as a result of ventricular fibrillation. Variant angina, which is characterized by pain during rest and ST segment elevation, is particularly arrhythmogenic. Appropriate treatment of myocardial ischemia—for example, with nitrates, beta blockers, or calcium channel blockers—may alleviate arrhythmias in these patients. Enlargement of a failing left ventricle stretches individual myocardial cells and can thereby enhance automaticity. Reduction of left ventricular volume by the administration of digitalis, diuretics, or vasodilators helps control arrhythmias that are precipitated by this mechanism.

Increased sympathetic activity,[2] whether the result of anxiety, exercise, exogenous catecholamines, acute myocardial infarction, or congestive heart failure, can lead to ectopic ventricular and atrial activity. Part of the antiarrhythmic action of propranolol is probably related to its beta-blocking capabilities, although the drug also suppresses arrhythmias by a direct quinidinelike effect. Interestingly, orthostatic changes that decrease venous return to the right ventricle result in a shortening of the effective refractory period (ERP) for the right ventricle. This effect is mediated by beta-adrenergic mechanisms and is blocked by propranolol.[3] Exercise-induced ventricular tachycardia can be controlled with beta blockers[4] and verapil.[5] Vagal tone may protect against ventricular fibrillation in an acutely ischemic myocardium. Thus, atropine might induce ventricular tachycardia in an ischemic myocardium not only by precipitating excessive sinus tachycardia, which intensifies the ischemia, but also by its vagolytic action. Clinically, this phenomenon is more likely to occur when high doses (1.0 mg I.V.) are used but is rare when lower doses (0.50 to 0.75 mg

"

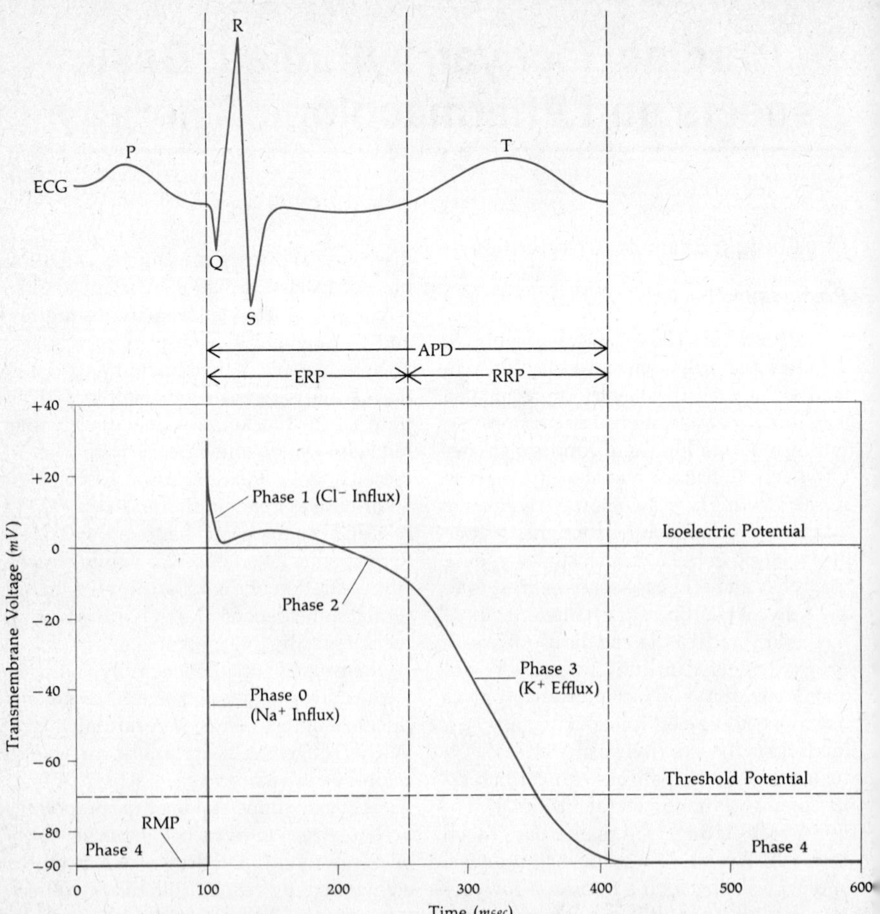

Figure 1 *A transmembrane action potential generated by a single ventricular cell is correlated with a simultaneously recorded electrocardiogram. When excitation occurs, the massive influx of sodium ions causes depolarization (phase 0). During subsequent repolarization (phases 1, 2, and 3), the early influx of chloride ions (phase 1) and the later efflux of potassium ions (phase 3) act to restore the original resting membrane potential (RMP, phase 4). The effective refractory period (ERP) plus the relative refractory period (RRP) constitutes an action potential duration (APD). During the ERP, no impulses, regardless of intensity, can be conducted by the heart; during the RRP, only stimuli of higher than normal intensity will be propagated. The relation of these periods to the characteristic ECG waves and to the phases of depolarization and repolarization is also indicated.*

I.V.) are given to treat bradyarrhythmias in acute myocardial infarction.[6]

Bradycardia itself can lead to ventricular arrhythmias by causing a temporal dispersion of refractory periods among Purkinje fibers, thus creating an electrical gradient between adjacent cells. Appropriate treat-ment with atropine or cardiac pacing to increase the heart rate may be essential in the management of patients with bradycardia. Overdrive pacing at a rate of 90 to 110 beats/min may also be effective in abolishing persistent ectopic tachyarrhythmias in patients with normal resting heart rates.[7]

Prolongation of the QT interval results in a dispersion of refractory periods and is associated with ventricular tachycardia and ventricular fibrillation.[8] *Torsade de pointes* is a polymorphic ventricular tachycardia that is characterized by alternating electrical polarity. The electrical mechanism may be related to dispersion of repolarization or to triggered activity associated with after-depolarizations.[9] *Torsade de pointes* is typically seen in patients with prolonged QT intervals [*see Chapter 3*]. A prolonged QT interval may be congenital or acquired. The congenital form is sometimes associated with congenital nerve deafness. Acquired causes of prolonged QT intervals include hypokalemia, hypomagnesemia, and the use of certain antiarrhythmic drugs, such as quinidine, disopyramide, or amiodarone.[10] Management of acquired forms of prolonged QT interval syndromes is directed at removal of the etiologic agent and the administration of certain antiarrhythmic drugs, including phenytoin, propranolol, or bretylium. Intravenous magnesium sulfate can be effective for the treatment of *torsade de pointes*.[11] Overdrive ventricular pacing, which reduces dispersion of refractory periods, is also very effective.[7] Isoproterenol can be given to increase the heart rate and to shorten the QT interval, but this drug may be dangerous in patients with ischemic heart disease and may be arrhythmogenic itself.

Cardiac Electrophysiology and Action of Antiarrhythmic Drugs

In many patients, correction of identifiable precipitating events is not sufficient to suppress cardiac ectopic arrhythmias, and therefore, specific antiarrhythmic drugs must be employed. Such agents act directly to alter the electrophysiologic characteristics of the Purkinje and myocardial fibers. Knowledge of basic cardiac electrophysiology aids in understanding the mechanism of action of these antiarrhythmic agents.[12]

The resting transmembrane electrical potential (RMP) of the cardiac cell is determined mainly by the concentration gradient for potassium and sodium ions across the cell membrane. Inside the resting cell, there is a relative excess of potassium; outside the cell, there is an excess of sodium. This gradient is maintained by active metabolic processes, including the Na^+ pump, which transports sodium ions to the exterior. An electrical stimulus produces a sudden increase in the permeability of the cell membrane to Na^+, resulting in a massive influx of Na^+ and consequent depolarization (phase 0) [*see Figure 1*]. After phase 0 depolarization, repolarization occurs in three phases (phases 1 through 3); there is also a resting membrane potential (phase 4) between action potentials. In nonpacemaker cells, phase 4 is flat. In pacemaker cells, spontaneous slow depolarization occurs in phase 4 until the threshold membrane potential is reached and another action potential is generated. This spontaneous phase 4 depolarization, which is termed automaticity, can be enhanced by increasing the slope of phase 4 depolarization or by reducing the resting membrane potential.

Antiarrhythmic drugs may be classified on the basis of their electrophysiologic properties [*see Table 1*].[13] Class I antiarrhythmic drugs block the fast inward sodium current and can decrease the rate of phase 0 depolarization. Drugs with antisympathetic activity, such as the beta blockers, are included in class II. Class III agents block potassium channels and prolong the action potential duration (APD) without affecting the rate of phase 0 depolarization. Class IV drugs are calcium channel blockers, such as verapamil.

Class I antiarrhythmic agents can be further divided into three subgroups. Class IA drugs depress phase 0 depolarization, prolong the APD, and slow conduction velocity; quinidine, procainamide, and disopyramide are included in this group. Class IB drugs shorten the APD and have little effect on phase 0 depolarization. Lidocaine and its orally administered derivatives, mexiletine and tocainide, as well as phenytoin, moricizine, and aprindine are included in class IB. Class IC drugs markedly depress phase 0 depolarization, minimally affect the APD,

Table 1   Electrophysiologic and Electrocardiographic Effects of Common Antiarrhythmic Drugs

	Antiarrhythmic Drug					
Effect	Class I			Class II	Class III	Class IV
	Class IA	Class IB	Class IC			
	Quinidine Procainamide Disopyramide	Lidocaine Mexiletine Tocainide Phenytoin Moricizine Aprindine	Flecainide Encainide Lorcainide Propafenone	Propranolol	Amiodarone Sotalol Bretylium	Verapamil Diltiazem
Depolarization rate (phase 0)	↓	— or ↓	↓↓	—	—	—
Conduction velocity	↓	— or ↓	↓↓	↓	↓	—
Effective refractory period (ERP)	↑↑	↓	↑	↑	↑↑	—
Action potential duration (APD)	↑	↓	?↑	—	↑↑	↓
Automaticity	↓	↓	↓	↓	↓	—
PR duration	—	—	↑	— or ↑	↑	— or ↑
QRS duration	↑	—	↑↑	—	↑	—
QT duration	↑ Procainamide ↑↑ Quinidine ↑↑ Disopyramide	— or ↓ Lidocaine — or ↓ Mexiletine — or ↓ Tocainide ↓↓ Phenytoin	↑	↓	↑↑	—

— = no effect; ↑ = increased effect; ↓ = decreased effect

and profoundly slow conduction velocity; flecainide, encainide, lorcainide, and propafenone are included in this group. Moricizine, aprindine, and lorcainide (all class I) and sotalol (class III) are not available for clinical use in the United States.

Class IA drugs prolong the ERP more than they prolong the APD. Class IB drugs shorten the ERP less than they shorten the APD. Thus, both class IA and class IB drugs prolong the ERP relative to the APD. All of the class I drugs depress automaticity, depress conduction in bypass tracts, and have a depressant effect on phase 0 depolarization at increased heart rates.

Quinidine

Quinidine, a class IA drug, may prolong the QRS complex and the QT interval, may lower T waves, and may cause the appearance of U waves [*see* Physiologic Basis of Arrhythmias, *above*]. The presence of a prolonged QT interval suggests that quinidine might be causing, rather than reducing, ventricular irritability.

Although quinidine slows conduction through the atrium, the AV node, and the His-Purkinje system by its direct action, it also exerts a vagolytic action that overrides its direct effects on the AV node at clinical dosage levels. Thus, quinidine will enhance conduction through the AV node in patients with atrial fibrillation and increase the ventricular rate. In patients with atrial flutter, quinidine may slow the flutter rate via its direct effect on atrial conduction while increasing the AV conduction by means of its vagolytic effect; one-to-one conduction may thereby occasionally be established and the ventricular rate increased.

Quinidine depresses the myocardium minimally and to a lesser extent than procainamide in equivalent doses. On the other hand, quinidine, because of its alpha-adrenergic blocking effects, can cause a greater degree of peripheral vasodilatation than can procainamide. This effect on peripheral blood vessels may contribute to hypotension in some patients taking quinidine. Rarely, severe vasodilatation occurs, which is probably related to an idiosyncratic reaction to quinidine. Patients thus affected require peripheral pressor support until the reaction subsides.

Quinidine is metabolized for the most part in the liver. Several instances of drug interactions involving quinidine have been observed. The concurrent administration of phenytoin, phenobarbital, or rifampin may lower blood levels of quinidine by enhancing liver clearance. Quinidine, on the other hand, may raise serum digoxin[14,15] and digitoxin levels[16] in patients receiving these glycosides. Combined therapy with quinidine and verapamil has led to increased quinidine blood levels in one patient,[17] and in others it has caused hypotension, which is probably the result of an additive blockade of alpha-adrenergic receptors by the two drugs.[18]

Therapeutic blood levels of quinidine range from 1.2 to 4.0 µg/ml, as determined by high-pressure liquid chromatography. In addition to body size and individual metabolic and excretory rates, a very important factor in establishing a therapeutic blood level for a given patient is the extent to which the agent is absorbed by the gastrointestinal tract. For example, a patient with splanchnic congestion caused by congestive heart failure may absorb the drug poorly and therefore have low blood levels.

Quinidine is effective in the suppression of atrial tachyarrhythmias; in the chemical conversion of atrial fibrillation, atrial flutter, and paroxysmal atrial tachycardia to normal sinus rhythm; and in the suppression of ventricular tachyarrhythmias.

Quinidine sulfate is usually given orally in a dosage of 200 to 400 mg four times daily; it cannot be given parenterally. Quinidine gluconate can be given orally in a dosage of 324 mg four times daily or, because of its slower absorption, in a dosage of 648 mg twice daily. It is also supplied as a solution containing 80 mg/ml, which can be administered intramuscularly in a dosage similar to that given orally. Quinidine lactate is also available for parenteral use. Intravenous bolus injection of quinidine is dangerous, but an intravenous infusion can yield adequate blood levels when administration by other routes has not produced satisfactory blood levels. Quinidine gluconate or quinidine lactate can be infused at a rate of 50 to 75 mg/hr (1,200 to 1,800 mg/day).

A useful semiloading oral or intramuscular regimen consists of 300 mg of quinidine every three hours for three doses and then 200 mg every six hours. With this program, therapeutically effective levels begin to appear within six to 12 hours (mean, nine hours), and a peak level occurs at 48 hours.[19] Quinidine sulfate costs less than quinidine gluconate. However, quinidine gluconate may be preferable for patients whose intestinal symptoms are dose limiting; it does not cause gastrointestinal irritation as frequently. Because quinidine is completely absorbed by the gastrointestinal tract, a change can be made from oral to intramuscular administration without varying the dosage.

Toxic Effects

The major side effects of quinidine are gastrointestinal disturbances, with diarrhea being the most frequent manifestation. Usually, this effect is dose related, but it may be idiosyncratic and develop after the ingestion of just a few tablets. Nausea and vomiting are less common. Paradoxic ventricular tachycardia can occur occasionally and is usually, but not necessarily, heralded by excessive prolongation of the QT interval. Therefore, it is important to measure the QT interval when the dose reaches the therapeutic range. On the other hand, a dangerous proarrhythmic effect is extremely rare in patients with reasonable left ventricular function, and thus the drug can be initiated safely in appropriate outpatients.[20] Allergic reactions, such as drug fever and rash, may occur in some patients. Quinidine fever is occasionally associated with a leukocytosis or a marked left shift in the white blood cell count.[21] Rarely, thrombocytopenia and hemolytic anemia are caused by an allergic response to quinidine. Thrombocytopenia can be quite severe and can lead to clinically

significant bleeding. Granulomatous hepatitis[22] and reactive lymphadenopathy[23] have been reported with the use of quinidine. Another possible toxic reaction is dementia. Arthralgias and even arthritis may occur in the absence of detectable antinuclear antibodies. A few cases of quinidine-induced lupus erythematosus have been reported.[24] Rarely, pleurisy and pericarditis may develop. I have seen one patient in whom acute skeletal myositis developed during treatment with quinidine. The clinical picture of muscle pain, fever, and elevated muscle enzyme levels was later reproduced by a single-dose challenge of the drug. Idiosyncratic responses include dizziness, shock, cyanosis, diaphoresis, or respiratory arrest. High blood levels of quinidine may produce signs of cinchonism (vertigo, tinnitus, headache, fever, and visual disturbances).

Procainamide

Although procainamide, a class IA antiarrhythmic drug, possesses an electrophysiologic action similar to that of quinidine, it produces less prolongation of the QT interval. As a result, paradoxic ventricular tachycardia is a rare feature of procainamide therapy. Procainamide depresses the myocardium modestly but to a greater degree than quinidine in comparable therapeutic doses, although it causes less peripheral vasodilatation. Thus, hypotension that results from procainamide is more likely to be caused by cardiac depression than by peripheral vasodilatation. Procainamide also has no vagolytic action and therefore can be used in patients with atrial fibrillation to suppress ventricular irritability without increasing the ventricular rate. Like quinidine, procainamide may prolong the QRS complex and cause ST and T wave changes. Because the major route of excretion is renal, the dosage must be altered when renal function is impaired.

Procainamide is as effective as quinidine for the treatment of ventricular tachyarrhythmias but is not as effective in abolishing atrial tachyarrhythmias. It is completely absorbed, and therefore, comparable doses may be given orally or intramuscularly. The therapeutic blood level is 4 to 8 µg/ml. When renal function is normal, therapeutic levels can be achieved by administering procainamide every three hours in a dosage based on the patient's weight: 250 mg for a patient weighing less than 120 lb (54 kg), 375 mg for a patient weighing between 120 and 200 lb (54 and 91 kg), and 500 mg for a patient weighing more than 200 lb. If the first maintenance dose is combined with a loading dose of 500 mg, therapeutic blood levels can be achieved in most persons after about nine hours.[25] The dose and frequency of administration must, however, be significantly reduced in patients with renal dysfunction. In urgent situations in which a therapeutic blood level must be achieved rapidly, part or all of the initial dose can be given intravenously at a rate not exceeding 100 mg every five minutes. The ECG and blood pressure should be carefully monitored throughout the procedure. Procainamide can also be given as a continuous intravenous infusion at a rate that would provide a dose comparable to that given by the above oral or I.M. schedule (usually 2 to 3 mg/min).

A sustained-release form of procainamide can be given every six hours up to a total daily dose equal to that of standard preparations. Thus, a patient whose renal function is normal and who weighs less than 120 lb should receive 500 mg, a person weighing 120 to 200 lb should receive 750 mg, and a person weighing more than 200 lb should receive 1,000 mg.

Toxic Effects

The most common early noncardiac manifestations of procainamide toxicity are gastrointestinal disturbances; anorexia, nausea, and vomiting occur more often than diarrhea. Like many drugs, procainamide can cause drug fever or allergic rash. Although agranulocytosis is rare,[26] leukopenia and thrombocytopenia may be seen following chronic use of procainamide, often in association with a lupus erythematosus–like syndrome. Like systemic lupus erythematosus, procainamide-induced lupus has features that reflect serositis, such as arthritis, pleurisy, or pericarditis. Procainamide-induced lupus does not exhibit the same vascular features as systemic lupus erythematosus, such as renal vasculitis. Patients in whom the lupuslike syndrome develops all have positive antinuclear antibody (ANA) tests, and eventually, a positive lupus erythematosus cell preparation will develop in most patients. The diagnosis of procainamide-induced lupus must be seriously questioned if ANA tests are negative. However, the clinical syndrome does not develop in all patients who have a positive ANA test. Because it is highly unlikely that procainamide alone will produce a full-blown lupus vasculitis, therapy with the drug probably need not be stopped when a positive test for ANA develops, unless clinical manifestations of serositis are bothersome to the patient. Manifestations usually start insidiously: mild, early-morning joint stiffness or mild chest discomfort with coughing or deep breathing may be the first symptom. Only later does the full clinical picture of arthritis, pleurisy, or pericarditis, or any combination of the three disorders, gradually develop. The syndrome will reverse with cessation of procainamide therapy but may take months to subside if the drug was continued for an extended period after the initial manifestations of toxicity appeared.

Disopyramide

Disopyramide, a class IA antiarrhythmic drug, is comparable to quinidine in effectively suppressing atrial and ventricular tachyarrhythmias. Absorption of oral disopyramide is almost complete, resulting in peak blood levels within two hours after administration. In healthy individuals, 50 percent of the drug is excreted unchanged in the urine, 30 percent is excreted in the form of metabolites in the urine, and 10 percent is excreted in the feces. Generally, therapeutic plasma levels of disopyramide are in the range of 2 to 4 µg/ml.

Disopyramide is supplied in 100 mg and 150 mg capsules. The usual dosage of disopyramide is 150 mg every six hours for an average-sized adult with good renal function. Lesser dosages (100 mg every six or eight hours) should be used for smaller individuals and for patients who have renal insufficiency or congestive heart failure. A controlled-release form of disopyramide is also available in 100 mg and 150 mg capsules.

The most common side effects of disopyramide are dry mouth and urinary hesitancy, both of which are caused by the drug's anticholinergic activity. Slow-release pyridostigmine, a cholinesterase inhibitor, selectively reverses the anticholinergic side effects of disopyramide without affecting its electrophysiologic or antiarrhythmic properties.[27] Some patients taking disopyramide also experience blurred vision or nausea. In addition, marked prolongation of the QT interval and paradoxic ventricular tachycardia (similar to the side effects of quinidine) can occur. The drug should be administered cautiously if patients have conduction defects. Disopyramide has a marked myocardial depressant effect that is greater than that of propranolol[28] and can precipitate congestive heart failure[29] and hypotension. Disopyramide should therefore be used cautiously in patients who have myocardial decompensation.

Lidocaine

In usual therapeutic doses, lidocaine, a class IB antiarrhythmic drug, has no significant effect on either the QRS or QT interval or on AV conduction. In high doses, however, the drug can decrease conduction in the AV node as well as in the His-Purkinje system. It depresses myocardial contractility less than any other effective agent commonly used for ventricular arrhythmias. In very high doses, lidocaine can have a negative inotropic effect, but this is not usually seen clinically. The drug is metabolized in the liver.

Lidocaine is very effective in the treatment of ventricular arrhythmias, acting to decrease ectopic activity and to increase the ventricular fibrillation threshold.[30] It is not very effective in the treatment of supraventricular tachyarrhythmias. In patients with normal cardiac output and normal hepatic function and blood flow, an initial intravenous bolus of 2 mg/kg followed by an infusion at the rate of 55 µg/kg/min should provide therapeutic lidocaine levels at all times after the initial injection.[31] A healthy 70 kg person would require a loading dose of 140 mg followed by an infusion at a rate of about 4 mg/min. In patients with acute infarction or low cardiac output, however, an initial injection of 1.5 mg/kg followed by a 30 µg/kg/min infusion is recommended, which corresponds to a 100 mg loading dose followed by a 2 mg/min infusion in a 70 kg person. It is preferable to give the initial loading dose in divided increments to avoid toxic effects on the central nervous system. An initial dose of 50 to 75 mg can be given and followed in five minutes by the remainder of the loading dose. A second bolus, given 20 to 30 minutes after the initial dose, may be necessary [*see Chapter 5*]. Lidocaine should always be injected over a period of several minutes because rapid injection can lead to transiently high plasma levels and can induce seizures. Continued intravenous administration can lead to reduced lidocaine clearance, as can coadministration of either propranolol[32] or cimetidine.[33] In patients with markedly reduced cardiac output, a loading dose of no more than 0.075 mg/kg followed by an infusion of 10 to 20 µg/kg/min should be given. In a 70 kg person, this would correspond to a total loading dose of about 50 mg followed by an infusion of 1 mg/min. In patients with significant liver disease, the lidocaine dose must also be reduced.

Lidocaine can also be administered intramuscularly. A dose of 4 mg/kg (about 300 mg for a 70 kg person) injected into the deltoid muscle can produce therapeutic levels lasting for one to two hours. The intramuscular route may be convenient for treating a patient being transported to the hospital after an acute myocardial infarction.[34] Lidocaine cannot be administered orally.

Toxic Effects

Cardiac toxicity is negligible at therapeutic levels; the major toxic effects are neurologic. The usual manifestations of toxicity are confusion, seizures, and, rarely, respiratory arrest and coma. The CNS effects usually disappear as soon as the lidocaine blood level falls after cessation of the drug. In general, the blood level falls within 30 to 60 minutes in patients who have been taking the drug for less than 24 hours, but it may remain elevated for a longer period in patients who have been on a long-term program.

Mexiletine and Tocainide

Mexiletine, a derivative of lidocaine, provides effective oral therapy for ventricular tachyarrhythmias of many causes. It is available in 150 mg, 200 mg, and 250 mg capsules. The drug is usually administered in an initial dosage of 300 mg every six hours for four doses and then reduced to 200 mg every six hours. The chronic maintenance dose is usually 150 mg or 200 mg every eight hours, although some patients may require 200 mg every six hours or, rarely, 300 mg every six hours.[35,36]

Epigastric burning may occur with mexiletine administration and is often relieved by taking the medication with meals. Constipation may also occur. Neurologic side effects include tremulousness, diplopia, dizziness, and, occasionally, slurred speech. Side effects often show improvement after a reduction in the dosage.

Tocainide, another derivative of lidocaine, is as effective as mexiletine and has similar side effects.[37,38] However, tocainide has also caused severe bone marrow depression (i.e., leukopenia, anemia, and thrombocytopenia) and pulmonary fibrosis, which are not seen with mexiletine. In addition, it causes cardiac depression when given to patients with severe congestive heart failure.[39] Tocainide is available in 400 mg and 600 mg tablets. The dosage is usually 400 or 600 mg given every eight hours, but some patients require and tolerate 800 mg given every eight hours. When the same patients were treated separately with mexiletine and tocainide, the patients had a concordant response of only 53 percent. Thus, failure to respond to one of these drugs does not necessarily mean that the patient will fail to respond to the other drug; the two drugs should be assessed individually.[40]

Phenytoin

Phenytoin, like lidocaine, is a class IB antiarrhythmic drug. Phenytoin exerts a greater effect on the electrocardiographic QT interval than lidocaine and shortens the QT interval more than any of the other antiarrhythmic agents in common use. Phenytoin has no significant effect on the ST and T waves or on the QRS complex. It does not significantly depress the myocardium in usual doses but may cause hypotension or cardiac arrest after rapid intravenous administration in large doses.

Therapeutic blood levels range from 10 to 18 µg/ml. Because phenytoin is metabolized by the liver, impaired hepatic function may lead to higher than normal blood levels. Blood levels can be lowered by drugs, such as barbiturates, that enhance the rate of metabolism of phenytoin. Warfarin, disulfiram, phenylbutazone, isoniazid, and sulfaphenazole may inhibit its metabolism and increase blood levels. Uremia increases the amount of so-called free phenytoin in the blood relative to the amount of phenytoin that is bound to plasma proteins.

Phenytoin is effective in controlling ventricular tachyarrhythmias that are caused by digitalis toxicity. It is also effective—although to a lesser extent than lidocaine, quinidine, or procainamide—in the treatment of ventricular arrhythmias from other causes. It can be very helpful in the treatment of paradoxic ventricular tachycardia or *torsade de pointes* that is associated with prolonged QT intervals. Phenytoin is not very effective in the treatment of atrial tachyarrhythmias.

Phenytoin can be given orally or intravenously. The usual oral dosage is 100 mg four times a day, which will yield a peak level in six to 12 days. A semiloading oral program may consist of 600 mg a day for two days and then 400 mg a day; a peak level will be achieved on such a regimen in four to five days. Because of its long half-life, phenytoin can be given to many patients in a single daily dose of 300 or 400 mg once a maintenance level has been established. It may also be given intravenously as a 100 mg bolus every five minutes until a dose of 300 to 700 mg is achieved. This gradual accumulation of the drug will permit the phenytoin blood level to rise at a reasonable rate. A large bolus, such as 300 mg, can lead to hypotension and cardiac arrest. Therapeutic levels can usually be achieved by the intravenous administration of 700 to 1,000 mg during the first 24 hours.[41] A loading program of 400 to 600 mg (depending on body weight) and then 100 mg every six hours is reasonable. Because phenytoin can precipitate in five percent dextrose in water, it is preferable to give the drug via a line carrying normal saline.

Toxic Effects

Phenytoin toxicity most commonly manifests as central nervous system disturbances, especially cerebellar disturbances. Symptoms include nystagmus, ataxia, slurred speech, vertigo, drowsiness, and mental confusion. Cerebellar symptoms and findings correlate well with phenytoin blood levels in excess of 18 µg/ml, and such findings can be used as a bedside indicator of high blood levels. The CNS effects can be reversed by adjusting the dose. Phenytoin can cause nausea, vomiting, and constipation, but these symptoms are usually not major problems. A skin rash, usually measleslike in appearance, can occur. Rarely, serious types of dermatitis, including exfoliative dermatitis, have been observed in patients receiving phenytoin. Leukopenia, granulocytopenia, and thrombocytopenia have been found and reflect marrow toxicity. A megaloblastic anemia can occur and usually responds to folic acid. Gingival hyperplasia can develop from long-term use of phenytoin; rarely, revers-

ible lymph node hyperplasia, polyarthropathy, and hirsutism occur. Phenytoin partially inhibits insulin secretion and may lead to increased blood glucose levels in patients who are hyperglycemic.

Flecainide, Encainide, and Propafenone

Flecainide, a class IC antiarrhythmic agent,[42] commonly prolongs the QRS complex by 25 percent or more and, to a lesser extent, the PR interval. It has little effect on the JT interval (QT minus QRS). In comparative studies, flecainide was more effective in suppressing ventricular premature beats, ventricular couplets, and runs of ventricular tachycardia than quinidine and disopyramide. However, its ability to suppress the inducibility of ventricular arrhythmias by programmed electrical stimulation is much less than that of the other two agents. Flecainide is also effective for the treatment of atrial tachyarrhythmias.[43] Because it delays conduction in the bypass tracts, flecainide can be effective for the treatment of tachyarrhythmias associated with the Wolff-Parkinson-White syndrome.

Oral flecainide is almost completely absorbed, and the plasma level peaks about three hours after dosing. The half-life is about 20 hours. It is excreted in the urine; elimination is reduced in patients with congestive heart failure or renal failure. Flecainide may increase the plasma level of digoxin by 13 percent and of propranolol by 30 percent. The therapeutic plasma level ranges from 0.2 to 1.0 µg/ml. Flecainide has a moderate negative inotropic effect and a proarrhythmic effect in seven to 10 percent of patients. The proarrhythmic effect is more likely to occur in patients with sustained ventricular tachycardia and a reduced ejection fraction.[44] The drug is available as a scored 100 mg tablet. Flecainide should be started at a dosage of 100 mg twice daily. If a therapeutic effect is not achieved with this dosage, each dose should be increased by a 50 mg increment every four to seven days (which is the interval required for the drug to achieve a steady state) until a therapeutic effect is obtained. The usual effective dosage is 100 to 200 mg twice daily. Occasionally, a patient will require up to 300 mg twice daily.

The most commonly observed side effects of flecainide are dizziness, blurred vision, and spots before the eyes (scotoma). Less frequent side effects are nausea, headaches, anxiety, ataxia, and metallic taste.

Encainide, a class IC agent, is similar to flecainide in its electrophysiologic effects,[45] clinical efficacy,[46,47] and side effects.[48] Encainide is almost completely absorbed, and the plasma level peaks 30 to 90 minutes after dosing. A steady-state plasma level of the active drug and its even more active metabolites is attained over three to five days. Clearance of encainide is reduced in the presence of liver disease and renal failure. The drug is available in 25 mg and 35 mg capsules. It should be started at a dosage of 25 mg three times daily. The dosage can be increased after three to five days to 35 mg three times daily, and depending on the clinical response, after another three to five days it can be increased to 50 mg three times daily. Occasionally, dosages as high as 50 mg four times daily are needed.

In the Cardiac Arrhythmia Suppression Trial (CAST), postinfarction patients with asymptomatic ventricular arrhythmias responsive to encainide or flecainide were randomized to one of those drugs or to a placebo. In April 1989, CAST reported a twofold increase in mortality with each drug and therefore discontinued their use. The FDA and the manufacturers of flecainide and encainide therefore recommend that the two drugs be reserved for treatment of life-threatening arrhythmias.[49] Such arrhythmias might include ventricular tachycardia and dangerous supraventricular tachycardias in patients with the Wolff-Parkinson-White syndrome.

Despite the results of CAST, there is no evidence that encainide or flecainide need be stopped in a patient who has not had a previous myocardial infarction, who has normal left ventricular function, and in whom either drug has already demonstrated control of symptomatic arrhythmias

for six months without side effects. The decision whether to continue flecainide or encainide should be made on an individual basis.

Propafenone is a class IC agent with weak beta-adrenergic blocking and calcium channel blocking activity.[50] Like flecainide and encainide, propafenone is effective in the treatment of ventricular and atrial tachyarrhythmias. Propafenone is well absorbed after oral administration, and peak plasma levels occur about three hours later. The drug is metabolized in the liver.

Even though 90 percent of patients metabolize propafenone efficiently, the dose should be individually titrated because higher blood levels of propafenone will develop in the 10 percent of patients who metabolize the drug poorly. Steady-state plasma levels are achieved after four to five days. With chronic dosing, clearance may decrease. The usual starting dosage is 150 mg every eight hours. After three to four days, the dosage may be increased to 225 mg every eight hours and, if necessary, up to 300 mg every eight hours after another three to four days.

Dizziness, disturbances in taste, and blurred vision are the most frequent side effects. Nausea, vomiting, and constipation are less common. Rarely, cholestatic hepatitis or worsening of asthma can be seen. A positive ANA titer may develop. Agranulocytosis is rare. Propafenone depresses the myocardium and may cause conduction abnormalities such as sinus slowing, atrioventricular block, or bundle branch block. Like the other class IC agents, propafenone may be proarrhythmic, especially in patients with poor left ventricular function and sustained ventricular tachycardia.

Propranolol

Propranolol, a beta-adrenergic blocker and therefore a class II antiarrhythmic drug, decreases conduction through the atrioventricular node and thus may prolong the PR interval. Consequently, it is an effective agent for slowing the ventricular response in patients with atrial fibrillation and atrial flutter. It has little effect on the ST and T wave changes, although it may tend to shorten the overall QT interval. The beta-adrenergic blocking action of propranolol makes the drug effective in treating arrhythmias caused by increased levels of catecholamines, which may occur during conditions such as emotional stress. It slows the sinus rate as a direct effect of its beta-blocking capabilities; indeed, the extent of this effect is the major determinant of the dosage. Effective beta blockade is usually achieved in an otherwise normal person when the resting sinus rate is 55 to 60 beats/min. Propranolol can depress the myocardium not only by beta blockade but also by a direct depressant action on cardiac muscle.

Propranolol is an effective agent for stabilizing atrial electrical activity and for controlling the rate of ventricular response in patients with atrial fibrillation and atrial flutter; it is also useful for chemical cardioversion of atrial flutter and paroxysmal atrial tachycardia, both of which are caused by a circus movement mechanism. Propranolol is useful in the treatment of digitalis-induced ventricular arrhythmias. The drug also is effective in the treatment of ventricular arrhythmias in patients with mitral valve prolapse, who often have high catecholamine levels. In addition, propranolol may be effective in controlling ventricular arrhythmias in patients with coronary artery disease by preventing ischemia-induced ventricular irritability.

The oral dosage usually ranges from 10 to 80 mg every six to eight hours, although an occasional patient requires far higher dosages. The total daily dose is determined by the physiologic effects of propranolol on the heart rate and blood pressure. The usual intravenous dose is 0.05 mg/kg (3 to 6 mg), which is best given in 1 mg increments every five minutes. The onset of action after intravenous administration occurs within two to five minutes, and the drug exerts its peak effect on the atrioventricular node at 10 to 15 minutes. Hence, a program in which the drug is administered at five-minute intervals will allow a reasonably safe accumula-

tion in most patients. In patients with marginal blood pressure or left ventricular dysfunction, propranolol must be used very cautiously, and initial intravenous doses should be reduced to 0.25 mg. The intravenous maintenance dosage of propranolol is usually 1.0 to 3.0 mg every four hours.

Toxic Effects

The major toxic effects of propranolol are related to its beta-blocking activity, which may precipitate excessive sinus bradycardia, congestive heart failure, or, in patients with bronchospastic disease, bronchial asthma. The direct depressant effect of the drug on the myocardium may accentuate congestive heart failure. Propranolol may cause drug fever, an allergic rash, and gastrointestinal side effects, commonly nausea or increased eructations. Abdominal cramping and diarrhea are less common. The drug may increase esophageal reflux. Rarely, agranulocytosis, nonthrombocytopenic purpura, or thrombocytopenic purpura may be seen. The most common central nervous system side effects are mental depression and lethargy, although visual disturbances, hallucinations, and acute disorientation have been reported. Fatigue is frequently experienced and may be related to excessive bradycardia or to a direct central nervous system side effect. Impotence and loss of libido are relatively common side effects, appear to be dose related, and are related to the high lipid solubility of the drug. Reversible alopecia can also occur.

Amiodarone

Amiodarone, a class III antiarrhythmic drug, has proved to be effective for the treatment of supraventricular and ventricular tachyarrhythmias.[51,52] The drug prolongs the effective refractory period in all cardiac tissues, including the sinus node, atrium, atrioventricular node, His-Purkinje system, ventricle, and, in the case of Wolff-Parkinson-White syndrome, bypass tracts. It has an antisympathetic effect; in addition, it has a minor negative inotropic effect, which may be offset by the drug's potent vasodilating properties.

Amiodarone suppresses supraventricular tachyarrhythmias in 80 percent of patients and ventricular tachyarrhythmias in about 66 percent of patients. It is effective for tachyarrhythmias associated with the Wolff-Parkinson-White syndrome because it depresses conduction in the atrioventricular node and in the bypass tracts. Electrophysiologic testing is useful for identifying those patients taking amiodarone who are at high risk for arrhythmia recurrences.[53]

Amiodarone has a reduced clearance rate, a low bioavailability, a large volume of distribution, and a very long half-life. The drug may persist in the body for more than two months after cessation of long-term therapy. A loading dose is required. A useful regimen consists of 1,200 mg a day for one week (600 to 800 mg may be given intravenously, and the remainder may be given orally), 1,200 mg a day in divided oral doses for the second week, and 600 to 800 mg a day given orally for the following two to four weeks, followed by a maintenance dosage. Although some electrophysiologic effects occur after two weeks of administration, a 10-week regimen is needed for the class III drugs to produce a maximal effect.[54] The maintenance dosage can usually be gradually reduced to about 400 mg a day for ventricular tachyarrhythmias and 200 mg a day for supraventricular tachyarrhythmias. Therapeutic blood levels appear to be between 1.0 and 3.5 µg/ml.

In one study, intravenous amiodarone, administered via a central line in a loading dose of 5 mg/kg over a period of 30 minutes, followed by a continuous infusion of 1 g every 24 hours for 72 hours, was effective in 70 percent of patients with recurrent drug-refractory sustained ventricular tachycardia or ventricular fibrillation.[55] The majority of patients who responded did so within the first two hours of therapy, and all who responded did so within 84 hours.[55]

Amiodarone potentiates the anticoagulant effect of warfarin and increases the serum concentration of digoxin, quinidine, procainamide, phenytoin, and flecainide. It may have a synergistic effect with drugs that depress the sinus and atrioventricular nodes, such as beta blockers or calcium antagonists.

Side effects are common, especially when dosages exceed 400 mg a day; the total cumulative dose may correlate better with the incidence of side effects than the daily dose or duration of therapy.[51] Thus, the lowest effective maintenance dose should be used. Skin reactions include photosensitivity, a slate-gray pigmentation, and, less commonly, a red rash. Gastrointestinal effects are usually mild and often consist only of constipation. Hepatitis is rare. Corneal deposits almost always occur during amiodarone therapy; their severity depends on the dosage and duration of treatment. Visual symptoms, however, are uncommon. Rarely, patients complain of seeing halos around bright lights. Neurologic toxicity may manifest as peripheral neuropathy, tremors, sleep disturbance, headaches, or proximal muscle weakness.

The most serious side effect is probably pulmonary alveolitis; fortunately, it is uncommon.[51] Affected patients complain of dyspnea and a nonproductive cough. The chest x-ray may show diffuse interstitial changes of diffuse alveolar infiltrates. The symptoms and chest x-ray are the best clinical means of detecting serious pulmonary toxicity. An isolated fall in carbon monoxide diffusion capacity is not a reason in itself for discontinuing amiodarone.[56]

Amiodarone contains iodine and has many effects on thyroid hormone metabolism, including decreased production of triiodothyronine (T_3) and decreased clearance of thyroxine (T_4) and reverse triiodothyronine (rT_3).[57] Iodine-induced hyperthyroidism may occur and is associated with low iodine intake. Iodine-induced hypothyroidism is more frequent and is associated with adequate iodine intake. Hyperthyroidism may be best detected by the finding of elevated serum T_3 or elevated free T_3 levels. Hypothyroidism is best diagnosed by an increased serum TSH (thyrotropin) level.

Patients should be carefully monitored for manifestations of thyroid disturbances, which may develop insidiously.

Like quinidine and disopyramide, amiodarone may prolong the QT interval, which may lead to an increased incidence of ventricular tachyarrhythmias, including *torsade de pointes*.

Bretylium

Bretylium can be given parenterally for treating serious ventricular tachyarrhythmias.[58] Bretylium has been shown to increase the ventricular fibrillation threshold[28] and to prolong the action potential duration and effective refractory period. It does not suppress phase 0 depolarization. Although bretylium is often classified as a class III agent, its antiarrhythmic action may be largely derived from its effects on adrenergic nerve terminals. Bretylium causes a direct early release of norepinephrine from adrenergic nerve terminals. Later, it restricts the release of norepinephrine from these nerve endings. Bretylium also potentiates the action of norepinephrine and epinephrine on adrenergic receptors by inhibiting the uptake of catecholamines into the nerve endings. Bretylium is excreted intact by the kidneys.

Use of bretylium should generally be restricted to the treatment of serious ventricular arrhythmias refractory to a first-line drug such as lidocaine or procainamide. However, it is frequently used as the initial drug in the treatment of ventricular fibrillation. Available only for intramuscular or intravenous administration, bretylium may be given in a dosage of 5 mg/kg (infused over a 10-minute period) every six hours.[58] Patients with renal dysfunction should receive a reduced dose. Hypotension related to peripheral vasodilatation is common after administration of bretylium; therefore, patients should be kept supine early in the course of treatment. Because of the initial release of norepinephrine, transient hypertension and increased ventricular irritability may occur after the first few doses, especially in patients receiving digitalis. Nausea

and vomiting are the other major adverse reactions.

Verapamil and Diltiazem

The calcium antagonists (class IV antiarrhythmic drugs) inhibit the flux of calcium across the slow channels of vascular smooth muscle cells and cardiac cells. The four major calcium antagonists, verapamil, nifedipine, nicardipine, and diltiazem, have different clinical effects. Of these agents, verapamil has the greatest efficacy in the therapy for arrhythmias.[59] It has a major depressant effect on the atrioventricular node and a negative chronotropic effect on the sinoatrial node; diltiazem has similar but less potent effects on the sinoatrial and atrioventricular nodes.[60] Verapamil has a negative inotropic effect on cardiac muscle and produces a moderate vasodilatation of the coronary and systemic arteries. Because of its marked effect on the atrioventricular node, verapamil has proved to be highly effective in terminating paroxysmal supraventricular tachycardia, a reentrant tachycardia whose pathway usually includes the atrioventricular node. It also effectively controls the ventricular rate in most instances of atrial flutter and fibrillation. Verapamil, however, does not have a depressant effect on bypass tracts; thus, it will not slow the ventricular rate in cases of atrial fibrillation or flutter in which the impulses are conducted over such pathways. In fact, verapamil may cause reflex sympathetic activity that enhances conduction over these bypass tracts and speeds up the ventricular rate, an effect similar to that of digitalis. The drug has little efficacy in the therapy for ventricular ectopy.

A 5 mg (0.075 mg/kg) bolus of verapamil may be infused intravenously over a two-minute period. Its effect is almost immediate and lasts for one to two hours. If necessary, a repeat dose can be given five minutes later. The administration of 1 g of intravenous calcium gluconate five minutes before verapamil is infused may reduce verapamil-induced hypotension without affecting verapamil's antiarrhythmic properties.[61]

Oral verapamil is available as 80 mg or 120 mg tablets and may be useful for the prevention of paroxysmal supraventricular tachycardia and for control of ventricular rate in atrial fibrillation or atrial flutter. The dosage is usually started at 80 mg three times a day and may be gradually increased to 120 mg four times a day as required and tolerated. A sustained-release preparation, available in 180 mg and 200 mg scored tablets, provides therapeutic levels in the blood for 24 hours.

By decreasing blood flow to the liver, cimetidine may elevate verapamil blood levels when given concurrently. Verapamil, like quinidine, may raise serum digoxin levels in patients receiving this glycoside. In general, verapamil is quite well tolerated, but occasional significant side effects occur, the most serious of which are severe hypotension, bradycardia, and the aggravation of congestive heart failure. Constipation, nausea, vomiting, headache, and dizziness have also been reported. Contraindications to the use of verapamil include severe hypotension or cardiogenic shock; severe congestive heart failure, unless the failure is occurring secondary to the tachycardia; and sinus node dysfunction or second- and third-degree AV block, unless a ventricular pacemaker is in place. Adverse reactions have also been reported when intravenous verapamil and propranolol are given simultaneously because both drugs act to depress atrioventricular conduction, sinus node automaticity, and cardiac contractility.

Digitalis

Digitalis is an excellent antiarrhythmic agent for the stabilization of atrial electrical activity and the prevention of atrial tachyarrhythmias. Because of its vagotonic effect, this agent also decreases conduction through the AV node and therefore slows the ventricular response in patients with atrial fibrillation. In combination with diuretics, digitalis may be useful in the treatment of ventricular arrhythmias that are caused by an enlarged heart and congestive heart failure.

Adenosine

Adenosine is an endogenous nucleoside that, when given intravenously, slows conduction in the atrioventricular node. Its use has been approved by the FDA for the treatment of paroxysmal supraventricular tachycardia, including that associated with bypass tracts such as those in the Wolff-Parkinson-White syndrome. It is not effective in atrial fibrillation, atrial flutter, or ventricular tachycardia.[62,63] It has a half-life of 10 seconds and is almost immediately removed from the circulation. Thus, adenosine must be given as a rapid I.V. bolus injection directly into a vein or proximally into an I.V. line followed by a saline flush. The usual dose is 6 mg followed, if necessary, by a bolus injection of 12 mg three minutes later. Side effects include facial flushing, headache, chest pressure, dyspnea, sweats, lightheadedness, tingling, and nausea. Adenosine may produce a brief atrioventricular block. The drug is antagonized by methylxanthines, such as caffeine and theophylline, and is potentiated by dipyridamole.

Proarrhythmic Effects

Antiarrhythmic drugs may at times cause or exacerbate dangerous ventricular arrhythmias.[44,64] One type of proarrhythmic ventricular arrhythmia is the classic *torsade de pointes*. This arrhythmia is seen most often with the class IA drugs quinidine and disopyramide and with the class III drug amiodarone. *Torsade de pointes* is more likely to occur in the setting of prolonged QT intervals, hypokalemia, hypomagnesemia, bradycardia, and poor left ventricular function. The second type of proarrhythmic ventricular arrhythmia is an incessant uniform ventricular tachycardia that may occur with either class IA or IC drugs and is probably caused by a reentry phenomenon. This type is more likely to occur with high doses of class IC agents and in patients with previous sustained ventricular tachycardia and poor left ventricular function. The proarrhythmic effect of flecainide may be indicated by its effect on the QRS duration, especially during exercise.[65] Beta-adrenergic blockade may suppress the proarrhythmic effect of flecainide and encainide.[66] The decision to treat any cardiac arrhythmia must be made after weighing such factors as the risks of the arrhythmia and the efficacy of therapy against the side effects and risks of therapy.

References

1. Am J Cardiol 60:1246, 1987
2. JAMA 257:2064, 1987
3. J Am Coll Cardiol 12:1488, 1988
4. Am J Cardiol 53:751, 1984
5. Am J Cardiol 56:292, 1985
6. Am J Med 63:503, 1977
7. Ann Intern Med 99:651, 1983
8. Circulation 78:1365, 1988
9. J Am Coll Cardiol 14:172, 1989
10. Circulation 79:674, 1989
11. Circulation 77:392, 1988
12. Heart Disease: A Textbook of Cardiovascular Medicine, 3rd ed. Braunwald E, Ed. WB Saunders Co, Philadelphia, 1988, p 581
13. J Clin Pharmacol 24:129, 1984
14. Ann Intern Med 92:605, 1980
15. Am J Cardiol 47:1052, 1981
16. Ann Intern Med 94:35, 1981
17. Am J Cardiol 57:706, 1986
18. N Engl J Med 312:167, 1985
19. N Engl J Med 285:979, 1971
20. Am J Cardiol 56:585, 1985
21. Am J Med 77:345, 1984
22. Arch Intern Med 146:526, 1986
23. Am J Med 82:143, 1987
24. Ann Intern Med 108:369, 1988
25. N Engl J Med 281:1253, 1969
26. Ann Intern Med 100:197, 1984
27. J Am Coll Cardiol 10:633, 1987
28. Circulation 61:938, 1980
29. N Engl J Med 302:614, 1980
30. Am Heart J 110:938, 1985
31. Circulation 50:1217, 1974
32. N Engl J Med 303:373, 1980
33. Ann Intern Med 98:174, 1983
34. N Engl J Med 313:1105, 1985
35. N Engl J Med 316:29, 1987
36. Am J Cardiol 60:1276, 1987
37. N Engl J Med 315:41, 1986
38. Circulation 73:143, 1986
39. Circulation 81:860, 1990
40. J Am Coll Cardiol 7:338, 1986
41. Circulation 38:363, 1968
42. N Engl J Med 315:36, 1986
43. Am J Cardiol 59:1337, 1987
44. Ann Intern Med 111:101, 1989
45. Am J Cardiol 58:18C, 1986
46. Am J Cardiol 63:73, 1989
47. J Am Coll Cardiol 14:992, 1989
48. Ann Intern Med 110:505, 1989
49. N Engl J Med 321:406, 1989
50. N Engl J Med 322:518, 1990
51. N Engl J Med 316:455, 1987
52. J Am Coll Cardiol 13:442, 1989
53. Am J Cardiol 61:1024, 1988
54. Circulation 80:34, 1989
55. J Am Coll Cardiol 12:1015, 1988
56. Am J Med 86:2, 1989
57. J Am Coll Cardiol 9:175, 1987
58. N Engl J Med 300:473, 1979
59. Am J Cardiol 59:153B, 1987
60. Circulation 73:316, 1986
61. Ann Intern Med 107:623, 1987
62. Am J Cardiol 64:1310, 1989
63. Am J Med 88:337, 1990
64. Circulation 80:1063, 1989
65. Circulation 79:1000, 1989
66. Circulation 80:1571, 1989

3 Disturbances of Cardiac Rhythm and Conduction

ROMAN W. DESANCTIS, M.D.

JEREMY N. RUSKIN, M.D.

Classification of Arrhythmias

Disturbances of cardiac rhythm generally can be classified according to three broad categories: passive arrhythmias, automatic or ectopic arrhythmias, and reentrant arrhythmias.

Passive arrhythmias occur when the automaticity, excitability, and conduction properties of the structures responsible for the initiation and propagation of the cardiac impulse become depressed. They are manifested as bradyarrhythmias and as disturbances of atrioventricular (AV) and intraventricular (IV) conduction.

Automatic or ectopic arrhythmias are due to enhanced automaticity of a focus within the heart that is capable of undergoing spontaneous depolarization during diastole. This ectopic focus thereby acts as a pacemaker cell in a manner analogous to the sinus node. Such foci may reside in the atria, the AV node and junction, or the His-Purkinje system of the ventricles. If an ectopic focus attains threshold potential, the result may be single or multiple premature beats. If there is rapid and repetitive firing, sustained tachycardia can occur.

Reentrant arrhythmias account for the majority of premature beats and tachyarrhythmias. Reentrant tachycardias are also referred to as reciprocating tachycardias. An understanding of the mechanisms of reentry is absolutely fundamental to an understanding of cardiac arrhythmias [*see Figure 1*]. Although there are many variations, certain basic conditions for reentry are generally present:

1. Two pathways must exist over which the cardiac impulse is conducted. These pathways are usually contiguous but may be widely separated. The pathways may be either physiologic or anatomic. Dual physiologic pathways are produced by localized metabolic or pathologic changes that alter electrical properties at the sites of reentry. Examples of true anatomic dual pathways are the Kent bundles that bridge the atria and ventricles in the Wolff-Parkinson-White syndrome. In reentry, one pathway carries the impulse forward (antegrade); the other pathway conducts the reentering impulse backward (retrograde).

2. Conduction velocities across the two pathways differ. Conduction across the antegrade tract may be delayed, accelerated, or normal. In the retrograde arm of the reentry circuit, antegrade conduction is usually blocked or else severely delayed, but retrograde conduction remains intact.

3. Recovery of excitability occurs proximal and distal to the reentry sites, allowing perpetuation or establishment of the reentrant circuit.

Thus, reentry involves a crucial relationship between antegrade and retrograde conduction velocities and between refractory periods of the dual pathways and the adjacent myocardium. Slight changes in these temporal relationships brought about by pharmacologic, physiologic, or pathologic factors may facilitate the development of reentry or conversely may cause the termination of reentrant arrhythmias or prevent their initiation.

Attention has also been focused on triggered activity as a mechanism for the origin of cardiac arrhythmias. Triggered activity is defined as repetitive electrical activity arising from delayed afterdepolarizations. Arrhythmias associated with delayed afterdepolarizations differ from automatic rhythms in that

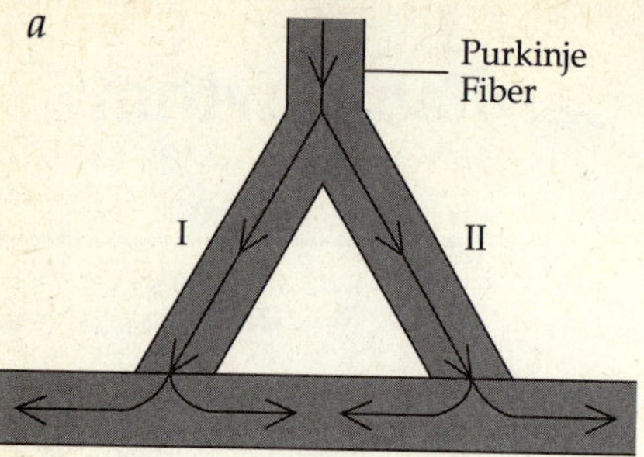

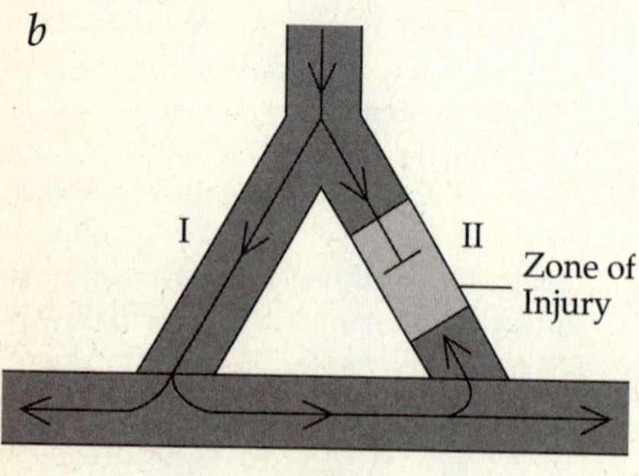

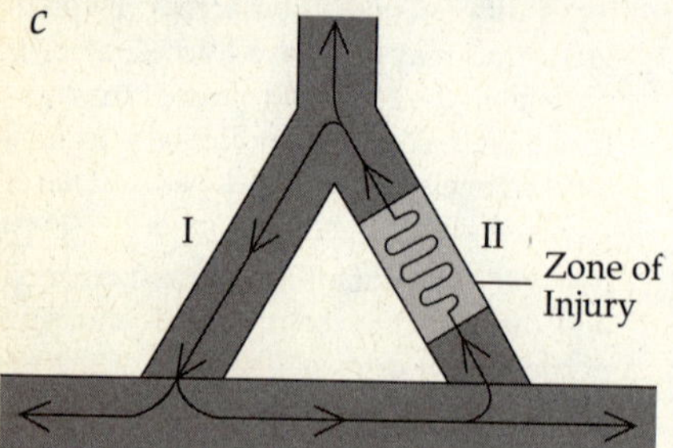

Figure 1 *Reentrant ventricular ectopy can occur as a result of myocardial injury from any of a number of different causes. In normal impulse conduction (a), the Purkinje network bifurcates into two pathways, I and II, that carry the impulse into the ventricular myocardium. Uniform depolarization and repolarization occur at all points. A zone of injury along pathway II (b) will impair impulse transmission, causing antegrade block. Consequently, the ventricle is activated only through pathway I, although the injured pathway can still conduct a retrograde impulse. The retrograde impulse from pathway II may cause repeat depolarization along the already repolarized pathway I (c). Frequently, atrial activation occurs as well. The reentry process may operate for only a single beat, or it may be sustained and cause ventricular tachycardia.*

they require a preceding action potential for their initiation. Microelectrodes have been used to study triggered activity mainly in isolated cardiac tissues. The ionic changes responsible for delayed afterdepolarizations are not fully understood. Although the mechanism of origin of some digitalis-induced arrhythmias is consistent with triggered activity, the importance of this phenomenon as a cause of arrhythmias has not yet been clearly established.[1]

General Approach to the Patient with Arrhythmias

When examining the electrocardiogram of any patient with a disturbance of cardiac rhythm, especially tachyarrhythmias but bradyarrhythmias as well, five basic questions should be asked:

1. Are P waves present, or is there any other evidence of atrial activity, such as flutter waves or fibrillatory waves?
2. What is the relationship between the atrial activity and the QRS complexes?
3. Are the QRS complexes wide or narrow (i.e., greater than or less than 0.10 sec)?
4. Is the ventricular rhythm regular or is it irregular?
5. Are any early beats or pauses observed that require explanation?

On the regular 12-lead electrocardiogram, atrial activity is usually seen most clearly in leads II, III, aVF, or V1. Special leads, such as the CR lead, may show P waves better. In the CR lead, the right-arm electrode becomes an indifferent electrode, and the left-arm electrode is used as an exploring precordial electrode while the electrocardiogram is recorded on lead I. Intracardiac recordings provide more definitive atrial and ventricular potentials than the standard electrocardiogram [*see Figure 2*]. Such intracardiac tracings can be obtained by passing an electrode from a peripheral vein into the right heart chambers under constant electrocardiographic monitoring [*see Figure 3*].

Physical examination may yield important information regarding an arrhythmia.

For example, evidence of AV dissociation characteristic of ventricular tachycardia is often more readily detected at the bedside than from the electrocardiogram. AV dissociation will produce such physical signs as intermittent cannon waves in the jugular venous pulses, fluctuation in the systolic blood pressure, and marked variation in the intensity of heart sounds; intermittent third and fourth heart sounds are also associated with AV dissociation. In contrast, paroxysmal supraventricular tachycardia and other arrhythmias that exhibit a fixed relationship between atrial and ventricular contraction are generally characterized by uniformity of heart sounds.

The physician must always judge the danger posed by an arrhythmia, especially a tachyarrhythmia, and hence the urgency with which it must be terminated. There are three major factors that determine how well a patient will tolerate a rhythm disturbance: the heart rate, the duration of the arrhythmia, and the presence and severity of associated underlying cardiac disease.

Passive Arrhythmias: Disorders of Sinus Node Function

Sinus Bradycardia

Sinus bradycardia, defined as a resting heart rate of less than 60 beats/min in an adult, is normally present in physically active people. Distance runners, for example, routinely have resting pulse rates that range between 40 and 50 beats/min.

There are, however, many conditions in which the discharge rate of the sinus node is abnormally slow. One common cause is excessive vagal tone. An increase in vagal tone may be spontaneous and transient, such as in vasovagal syncope and in acute myocardial infarction, particularly diaphragmatic infarction. Vagal tone may also be increased by severe pain or various stimuli, such as carotid sinus pressure, vomiting, and the Valsalva maneuver. It can be induced by parasympathomimetic drugs, such as edrophonium chloride and neostigmine, and by many tranquilizing drugs, particularly the phenothiazines. Digitalis glycosides have a modest vagotonic effect.

Although many drugs slow the rate of the sinus node by stimulating the vagus nerve, others act directly to depress its automaticity. In particular, beta-adrenergic blocking agents have a powerful depressant effect on sinus node function. The calcium entry blocking drugs verapamil and diltiazem depress sinus node automaticity and may cause profound slowing of the sinus rate when used in conjunction with beta-adrenergic blocking drugs.

Hypothermia, hypothyroidism, and severe icterus are all associated with slowing of the sinus rate.

Occasionally, syncope follows marked sinus slowing

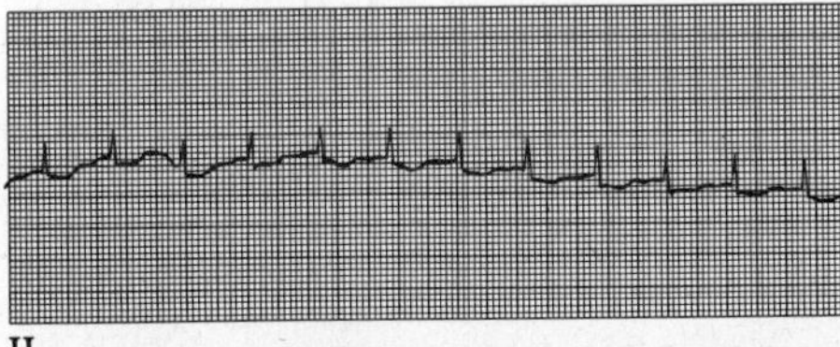

II

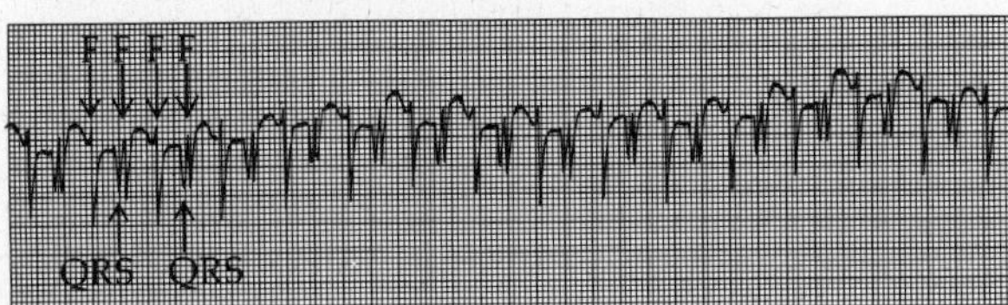

Atrial Wire

Figure 2 *Lead II of a surface electrocardiogram (top panel) recorded in a patient with atrial flutter and 2:1 AV block reveals a supraventricular tachycardia at a rate of 140 beats/min, but atrial activity is not clearly seen. Electrogram recorded from an electrode in the right atrium (bottom panel) clearly shows the atrial flutter. The flutter waves (F) are actually larger than the QRS complexes on which they are superimposed.*

Superior Vena Cava

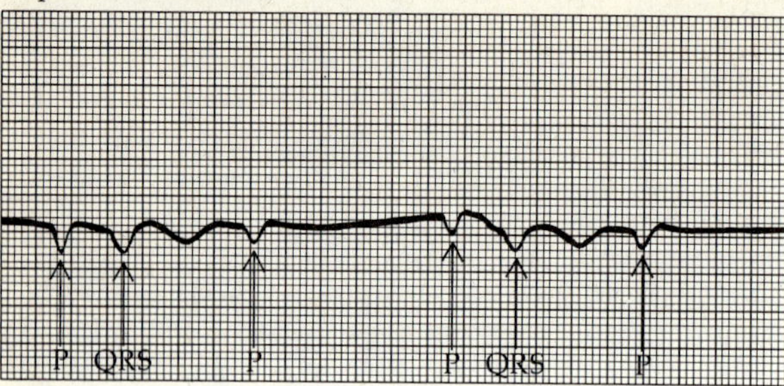

Right Atrium

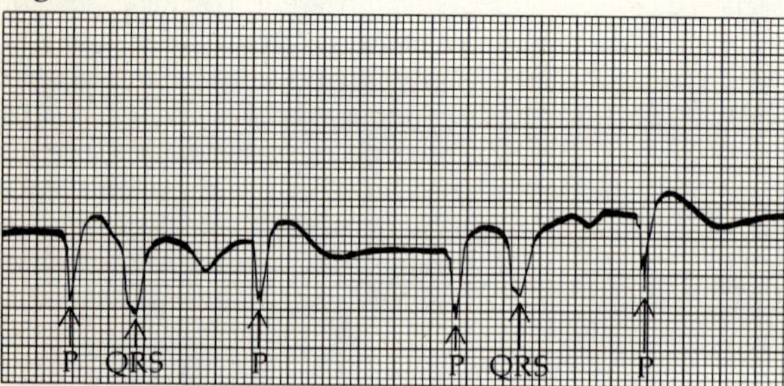

Right Ventricle

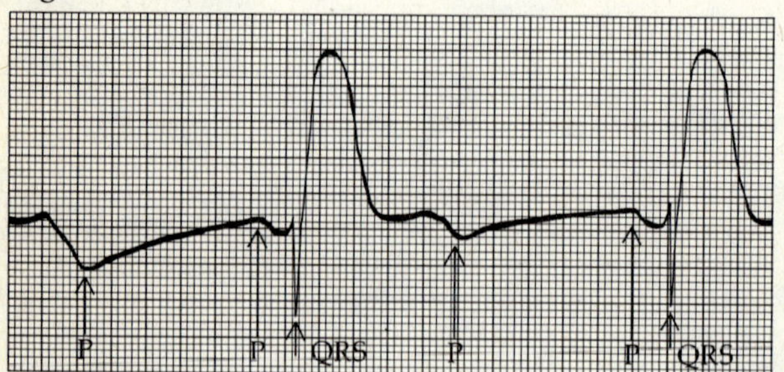

Figure 3 *Representative electrocardiographic potentials have been recorded from an intracardiac electrode placed at various sites (the superior vena cava, the right atrium, and the right ventricle) in a patient who had 2:1 heart block, with a long PR interval of 0.32 sec on the conducted beat. In the superior vena cava, the P waves and the QRS complexes are about equal in size and quite diminutive. In the right atrium, the P waves have a sharp, narrow negative configuration and are actually larger than the QRS complexes. In the right ventricle, the QRS complexes and the ST segments dwarf the P waves, which are virtually invisible in this recording.*

secondary to a hypersensitive carotid sinus reflex.[2] In addition to bradycardia, patients with carotid sinus hypersensitivity may also develop hypotension as a response to carotid sinus pressure. This so-called vasodepressor response may be the primary cause of syncope, or it may facilitate the development of syncope caused by the bradycardia.[3] Classically, this type of syncope develops when a tight collar is worn, when the neck is twisted, or when the carotid sinus is compressed in some other way. The carotid sinus becomes increasingly sensitive with advancing age, a sensitivity enhanced by digitalis glycosides. Carotid sinus hypersensitivity can be documented by gently compressing the carotid sinus while monitoring the electrocardiogram. If bruits are present, pressure should not be applied. Great care should be taken in assessing patients suspected of having carotid sinus hypersensitivity because the simple act of touching the carotid sinus is often sufficient to cause prolonged asystole.

Sick Sinus Syndrome

Etiology

During the past two decades, increasing attention has been focused on a group of patients who exhibit unexplained inappropriate sinus bradycardia, often associated with varying degrees of sinoatrial (SA) exit block and even sinus arrest.[4,5] Sinoatrial exit block, sinus pauses, or sinus arrest is usually transient, but permanent sinus arrest can occur [*see Figure 4*]. Often, the bradycardia is punctuated by episodes of supraventricular tachycardia, especially paroxysmal atrial fibrillation, paroxysmal atrial flutter, and less frequently, paroxysmal supraventricular tachycardia. In addition to sick sinus syndrome, these disturbances of cardiac rhythm have been described by a variety of terms, such as chronic sinoatrial node disorder, inadequate sinus mechanism, and when associated with tachycardia, the bradycardia-tachycardia syndrome. The reasons for the development of supraventricular tachyarrhythmias in many patients with sick sinus syndrome are not entirely clear. However, evidence of atrial disease manifested by prolonged and nonuniform refractoriness of atrial myocardium has been found in several individuals with sick sinus syndrome who had paroxysmal atrial flutter or fibrillation.[6] Such changes could facilitate the development of supraventricular tachyarrhythmias.

In the sick sinus syndrome, the sinus node is basically depressed and thus becomes more vulnerable to other exogenous influences, such as vagotonia and certain drugs.

Patients with the sick sinus syndrome are usually elderly, although a number of cases—sometimes associated with cardiomyopathies—have been reported in young patients. A group of otherwise healthy young people with idiopathic obliterative disease of the artery to the sinus node has been described who have experienced sudden cardiac death, usually during athletic activities.[7] Trauma to the sinus node sustained during cardiac surgical reparative procedures, especially correction of transposition of the great arteries, may also lead to disorders of sinus node function.[8]

A wide variety of underlying pathologic processes has been found in patients with the sick sinus syndrome. Fibrosis and degenerative changes within the sinus node are common and may occur either as primary events or as a consequence of obliterative disease of the sinus node artery.[9] In many patients, degenerative fibrotic changes are also present in other parts of the cardiac conduction system. In fact, about half of all patients with the sick sinus syndrome have disorders of AV and IV conduction, such as first- or second-degree heart block, complete heart block, right or left

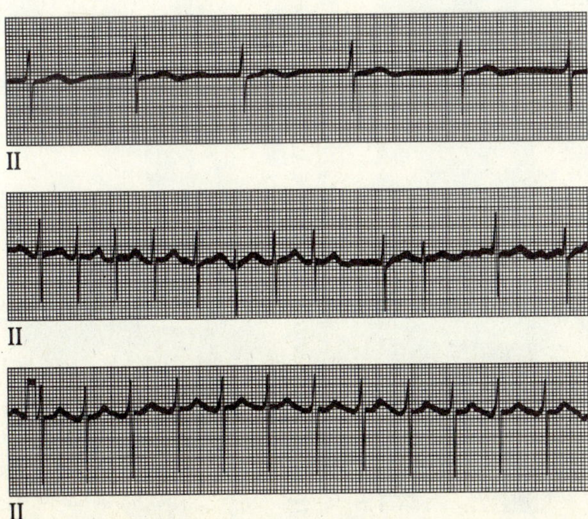

II

II

II

Figure 4 *Different electrocardiographic patterns are observed during a two-week period in a patient with the bradycardia-tachycardia variant of the sick sinus syndrome. An electrocardiogram displaying sinus arrest with a junctional escape rhythm at a rate of 50 beats/min (upper panel) is succeeded three days later by one that shows atrial flutter fibrillation in association with an irregular ventricular response (middle panel). Eight days later, electrocardiogram reveals a regular supraventricular tachycardia at a rate of 130 beats/min (bottom panel).*

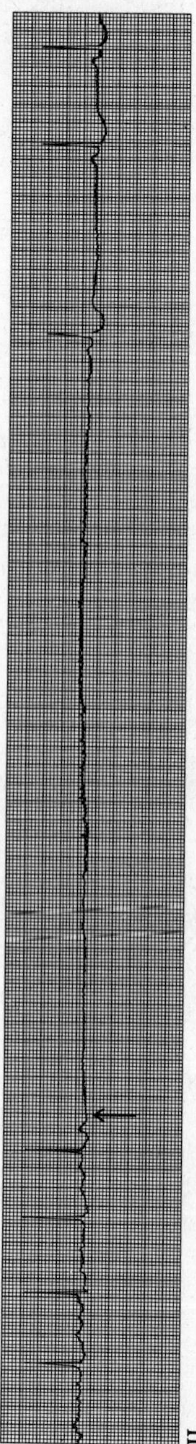

Figure 5   At the beginning of this electrocardiogram, taken from a Holter recording of a 72-year-old physician with syncope, the patient is in atrial fibrillation. After cessation of the atrial fibrillation (arrow), there is a period of asystole lasting nine seconds before the sinus node recovers.

bundle branch block, or bifascicular blocks.[5] Conversely, a very high incidence of sinus node disease can be found in patients with bifascicular and trifascicular conduction disease and bundle branch blocks.[10]

Clinical Features

Patients with sick sinus syndrome may be asymptomatic, but symptoms such as syncope and palpitations are commonly encountered. Syncope occurs under three different circumstances:

1. Following spontaneous sinus arrest without an adequate escape focus.
2. During episodes of supraventricular tachycardia. Although supraventricular tachycardia rarely causes syncope, it may degenerate into ventricular tachycardia or ventricular fibrillation, especially in patients with coronary disease, which can lead to loss of consciousness and even death. In some instances, however, supraventricular tachycardia alone may cause presyncope or syncope; this is due to the presence of extremely rapid heart rates or simultaneous atrial and ventricular contraction (as occurs in AV nodal reentry), both of which may result in inadequate cardiac filling and a precipitous fall in cardiac output.
3. At the termination of an episode of supraventricular tachycardia (the most common form of syncope). Tachycardia further depresses sinus node automaticity, and after cessation of the attack, there may be a long period of asystole before escape occurs [*see Figure 5*]. If the asystolic period exceeds six or seven seconds, the patient faints.

The slow heart rate may contribute to the development of congestive heart failure in patients with associated myocardial disease. Palpitations, which generally result from tachycardia, are present in the bradycardia-tachycardia syndrome. Tachycardia can also precipitate angina in patients with coronary artery disease. A significant complication of the bradycardia-tachycardia syndrome is systemic embolism, which eventually develops in as many as 10 to 20 percent of such patients.[5,11]

Diminished automaticity of the sinus node in the sick sinus syndrome may be demonstrated by physiologic, pharmacologic, and electrical methods. In exercise tests, the heart rate response of patients with the sick sinus syndrome is significantly lower than that of patients with normal hearts at the same exercise levels.[12] The degree to which the heart rate increases secondary to intravenously administered atropine is also blunted. When these patients are paced rapidly from the right atrium, the recovery time of the sinus node when pacing is halted abruptly may be markedly prolonged.[13] Normal sinus node recovery time after a period of atrial pacing at a rate of 150 impulses/min is about one to two seconds. In patients with the sick sinus syndrome, recovery times of three to four seconds are common, although there is considerable overlap between recovery times of patients with normal hearts and those with the syndrome. In addition to possible prolonged sinus node recovery time, the automaticity of lower escape foci, such as the AV junction and the ventricles, may also be diminished.

Other electrophysiologic abnormalities frequently demonstrable by intracardiac pacing studies and sinus node electrograms include prolongation of sinoatrial conduction time[14] and increase in the functional and effective refractory periods of the atria. These abnormalities indicate disease not only in the sinus node but also in the atria and the pathways leading out of the sinus node. However, physiologic, pharmacologic, and electrophysiologic studies are of limited value in diagnosing the sick sinus syndrome. For example, up to one third of patients with symptomatic sinus pauses have a normal sinus node recovery time during electrophysiologic testing. Thus, although electrophysiologic testing may be of diagnostic value in cases in which it detects abnormal sinus node function, a normal study does not exclude the presence of clinically significant sinus node disease. In the final analysis, the most important diagnostic information is provided by the clinical history and electrocardiographic monitoring, especially long-term monitoring of ambulatory patients,[15] which may provide a correlation between clinical symptoms and electrocardiographically recorded arrhythmias [*see* Ambulatory Electrocardiographic Monitoring, *below*].

Therapy for Sinus Bradycardia and Sick Sinus Syndrome

Vagolytic drugs, such as atropine 0.5 to 1.5 mg intravenously, may be useful transiently, especially when sinus slowing follows an increase in vagal tone. Similarly, beta-adrenergic stimulating drugs, such as isoproterenol or epinephrine, can be used to induce a faster heart rate in an emergency; usual dosages are 1 to 4 μg/min intravenously. Cardioaccelerator drugs, however, are virtually useless for the long-term treatment of bradycardia in patients with the sick sinus syndrome.

In the treatment of recurrent tachycardia, digitalis glycosides may be effective both in helping to suppress episodes of arrhythmia and in controlling ventricular rates during attacks.[5] Digitalis glycosides may also be necessary for the treatment of congestive heart failure. They may have the beneficial effect of shortening sinus node recovery time in the sick sinus syndrome.[16] As a general rule, digitalis glycosides can be used safely in patients with this syndrome. In occasional patients, however, sinus node automaticity may be seriously depressed by the digitalis drugs.[17] Digitalis toxicity must be scrupulously avoided, and the physician should be aware of potential oversensitivity to even ordinary therapeutic dosages of the digitalis drugs.

Other antiarrhythmic drugs, especially quinidine and to a lesser extent disopyramide and procainamide, may also be effective in suppressing recurrent tachycardia. However, these drugs may exacerbate preexisting abnormalities of sinus node function. Propranolol and other beta-blocking drugs are useful antiarrhythmic agents if a pacemaker is in place; otherwise, they must be used with extreme caution because of their severe depressive action on the sinus node. If a pacemaker is not in place, those calcium entry blockers that suppress the sinus node (i.e., verapamil and diltiazem) must also be avoided.

The onset of permanent atrial fibrillation sometimes brings about significant clinical improvement in patients with the bradycardia-tachycardia syndrome.[18]

Electrical pacing is the treatment of choice for symptomatic bradycardia caused either by spontaneously occurring sinus pauses or sinus arrest or by prolonged episodes of bradycardia after episodes of tachycardia. If AV conduction is normal, pacing may be initiated from the atrium, using either a right atrial or a coronary sinus electrode. If AV conduction is prolonged or if a higher degree of AV block is present, then ventricular or AV sequential pacing using any of several pacing modes is necessary [*see* Pacemakers and Automatic Defibrillators for Arrhythmias, *below*].

Although electrical pacing eliminates the symptoms of bradycardia, the success of this form of treatment in suppressing tachycardia has been much less predictable. Perhaps one explanation for this circumstance is that the abnormalities of atrial repolarization in patients with sick sinus syndrome do not seem to be corrected by rapid atrial pacing.[6] With pacing, the safety of beta-adrenergic blocking drugs, calcium entry blockers, and digitalis is considerably enhanced. Thus, pacing combined with larger doses of antiarrhythmic agents often reduces the frequency of attacks.

In very rare instances of incapacitating intermittent tachycardia, a radical approach entailing surgical interruption of the common bundle and the insertion of a ventricular pacemaker has been used to eliminate attacks. Because it now appears that the delivery of large bursts of electrical energy through transvenous electrodes can successfully ablate conduction over the bundle of His, the requirement for a thoracotomy may be eliminated.[19-22]

Because of the high incidence of embolism in patients who have bradycardia-tachycardia syndrome, we favor long-term anticoagulation with warfarin if there is no contraindication.[5,11] The effectiveness of antiplatelet agents is unproved [*see Chapter 7*].

Passive Arrhythmias: Atrioventricular and Fascicular Blocks

Two important developments have added much to our understanding of the mechanisms of AV conduction and the physiology of heart block. The first is an elegant correlation of the anatomy of the cardiac conduction system with electrophysiologic and electrocardiographic data, which has led to the concepts of fascicular blocks (hemiblocks).[23] The second development is the use of intracavitary electrodes for recording the potentials generated by the specialized structures of the cardiac conduction system, especially the bundle of His (His bundle electrocardiography).[24,25]

Conduction of the Normal Cardiac Impulse

The cardiac impulse originates in the sinus node and travels rapidly across the atria over three atrial bundles (internodal pathways) to the AV node [*see Figure 6*]. The major delay in transmission of the impulse from the atria to the ventricles takes place at the level of the AV node. Once the impulse crosses the AV node, the bundle of His is depolarized, and the impulse is propagated rapidly along the right and left bundle branches to activate the ventricles by way of the Purkinje network.

The right bundle branch is a relatively thin structure, about one fourth the width of the left bundle branch, and it traverses the right side of the anterior interventricular septum from the bifurcation of the common bundle into the right ventricle. In contrast, the anatomy of the left bundle branch is not so clearly defined. Usually, the left bundle divides into two branches: an anterior (superior) fascicle, which runs along the left side of the interventricular septum to activate the anterior left ventricle, and a larger posterior (inferior) ramus, which dips dorsally and fans out to activate the posterior septum and the posterolateral left ventricular wall. Some persons appear to have a third septal division of the left bundle, and in still others, the branching pattern of the left bundle is simply not very clear.[26]

His Bundle Electrocardiography

In His bundle electrocardiography, an electrode catheter is advanced, under fluoroscopic control, from a femoral vein up the inferior vena cava and across the tricuspid valve until it touches the interventricular septum. From this electrode catheter, intracavitary cardiac potentials can be recorded [*see Figure 7*]. Depolarization of the low septal right atrium causes a fairly large deflection, designated "A." A smaller and more rapid biphasic or triphasic deflection is registered on depolarization of the bundle of His (H spike). This spike is followed by another large deflection (V), which represents depolarization of the ventricular myocardium.

The AH interval, which approximates AV nodal conduction time, is generally measured from the first rapid deflection of the low atrial electrogram (A) to the onset of the His bundle deflection (H). The HV interval, a relatively precise indicator of conduction time within the His-Purkinje system, is measured from the onset of the His bundle deflection to the earliest point of ventricular activation, as observed either on the His bundle electrogram (HV) or on the surface ECG (HQ).

Because slight differences are observed in the values reported for AH and HV intervals from various laboratories (as a result of minor variations in recording and measurement), an exact range of normal limits cannot be rigidly defined. It is generally accepted, however, that during normal sinus rhythm in a resting state the normal AH interval in adults ranges from 60 to 140 msec and the normal HV interval ranges from 30 to 55 msec. Prolongation of the AH

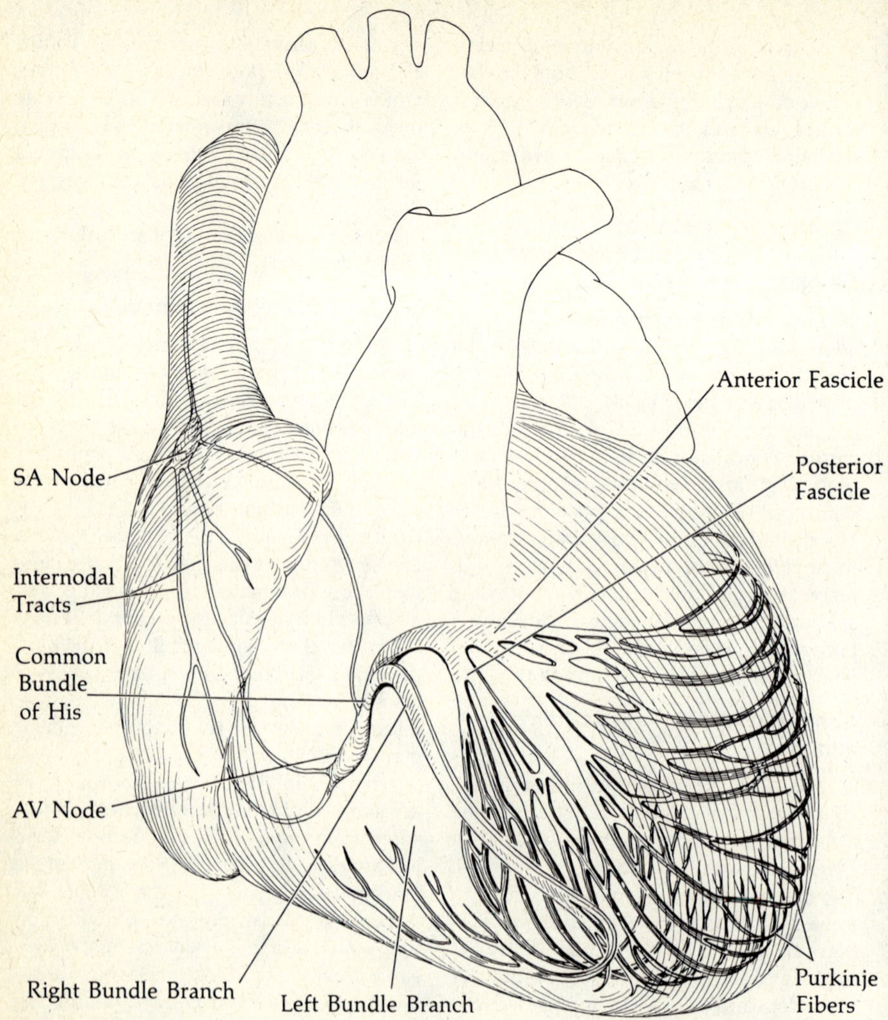

Figure 6 *Diagram depicts the cardiac conduction system. The cardiac impulse originates in the sinus node and is conducted to the ventricles via the internodal tracts, the AV node, the bundle of His, and the right and left bundle branches, which terminate in the network of Purkinje fibers. The left bundle branch subdivides into an anterior and a posterior fascicle.*

interval reflects delayed conduction within the AV node, whereas prolongation of the HV interval indicates block or delayed conduction within the His-Purkinje system. His bundle electrocardiography thus affords a precise mechanism for localizing the sites of conduction disturbances and for determining their severity.

The coupling of programmed electrical stimulation and intracardiac electrocardiography has dramatically advanced knowledge of the physiology and mechanisms of origin of cardiac arrhythmias and has greatly facilitated their diagnosis and treatment. These techniques are used in the following ways:

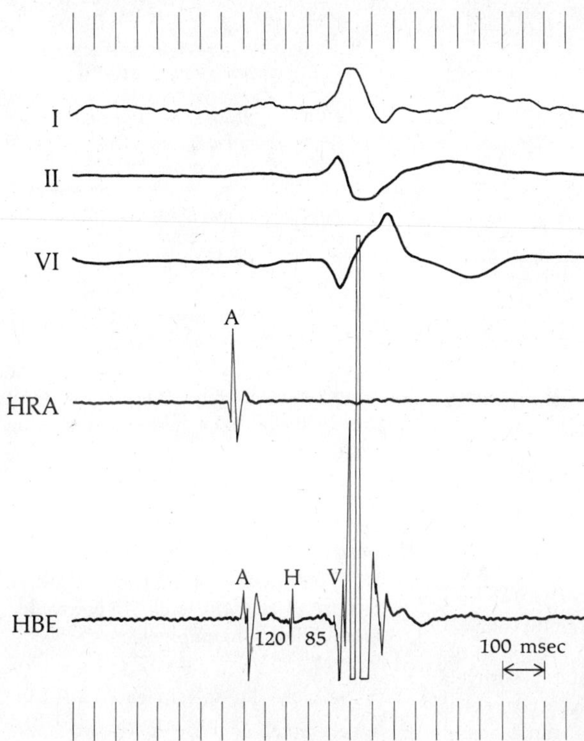

Figure 7   A His bundle electrogram (HBE) is recorded simultaneously with a conventional electrocardiogram (leads I, II, and V1) and a high right atrial (HRA) electrogram in a patient with right bundle branch block, left axis deviation, and first-degree AV block. The AH interval, that is, the time elapsed between atrial depolarization (A) and the onset of the His bundle spike (H), is 120 msec, which is normal. The HV interval, which extends from the onset of the H spike until ventricular depolarization (V), is 85 msec; this interval is prolonged and indicates that the delay in AV conduction is infranodal.

1. To assess sites of impulse formation and pathways of impulse propagation and to determine the mechanisms of initiation and termination of ectopic and reentrant tachycardias.[27] Such studies are very useful in the assessment of the preexcitation syndromes and of paroxysmal supraventricular and ventricular tachycardias. They are essential in the evaluation and management of those rare patients who have disabling tachycardias and in whom non-pharmacologic therapies such as surgery, antitachycardia pacing, and transcatheter electrical ablation are being considered.

2. To determine the effects of drugs on impulse formation and propagation. Such data may help guide therapy in many conditions, especially the preexcitation states, incapacitating paroxysmal supraventricular arrhythmias, and ventricular tachycardia.

Unifascicular Block

Despite some argument as to the validity of the fascicular block concepts, there is no doubt that they provide a useful theoretic framework for viewing abnormalities of AV and IV conduction.

Block of the left anterior (superior) division of the left bundle (left anterior hemiblock) causes a distinctive electrocardiographic abnormality characterized by marked left axis deviation [see Figure 8]. The impulse enters the left ventricle by way of the left posterior division, and the initial QRS forces are directed inferiorly and posteriorly. The following electrocardiographic features are characteristic of left anterior hemiblock:

1. The frontal plane QRS axis is negative, at least -45°. No other cause for marked left axis deviation can be present.

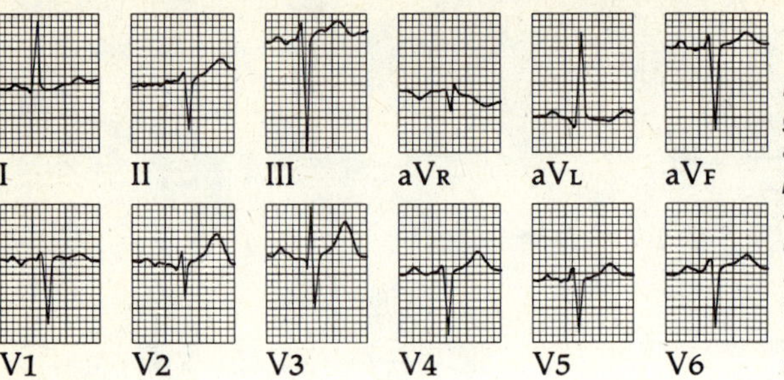

Figure 8 In an electrocardiogram from a patient with left anterior hemiblock, the frontal plane QRS axis is -50° . The small Q wave in lead V3 is the result of the hemiblock. The rS configuration (clockwise rotation) in leads V4, V5, and V6 is frequently seen in patients with this block.

2. QRS duration is usually normal, although there may be a slight widening of the QRS complex of up to 0.02 sec above normal.

3. A small R wave followed by a large S wave is present in leads II, III, and aVF, and small Q waves are seen in leads I and aVL.

In addition, because the initial QRS forces are directed posteriorly, small Q waves that are not indicative of myocardial infarction may be present in the right precordial leads (V1 to V3) in patients with left anterior hemiblock. Although the concept of left anterior hemiblock as a cause of isolated left axis deviation is generally accepted, left axis deviation may be associated with other disorders, including pulmonary emphysema, kyphoscoliosis, and various congenital heart diseases.[28] The natural history of isolated left axis deviation has generally been quite benign.

Block of the left posterior fascicle is much rarer than block of the anterior fascicle because the left posterior fascicle is substantially larger and better perfused and therefore less susceptible to damage. Isolated left posterior hemiblock may be difficult to recognize electrocardiographically. This block is most accurately diagnosed when it occurs as an intermittent pattern. It is characterized by the following features [*see Figure 9*]:

1. There is right axis deviation, generally more positive than +110° , in the absence of any other cause for right axis deviation, such as right ventricular hypertrophy, lateral infarction, emphysema, or pectus excavatum.

2. rS complexes are seen in leads I and aVL.

3. A very small Q wave is followed by a large R wave in leads II, III, and aVF.

As with left anterior hemiblock, the QRS width is normal or minimally prolonged in patients with left posterior hemiblock, and small Q waves may appear in anterior leads in the absence of myocardial infarction.

Bifascicular Block

The most common pattern of bifascicular block is that of right bundle branch block

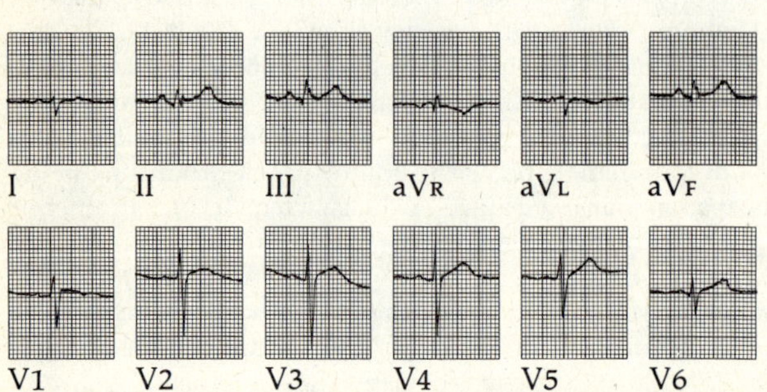

Figure 9 The QRS axis in a patient with isolated left posterior hemiblock (a 57-year-old man with coronary artery disease) is 120°, and small Q waves can be seen in leads II, III, and aVF. The pattern was present intermittently.

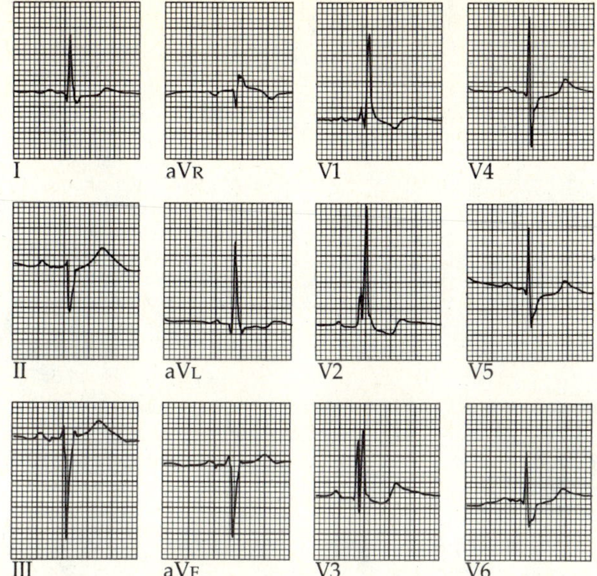

Figure 10 *Left axis deviation is apparent in electrocardiogram from a patient with right bundle branch block and left anterior hemiblock; the frontal plane QRS axis is -60° .*

with left anterior hemiblock, which is manifested electrocardiographically as right bundle branch block and marked left axis deviation [*see Figure 10*]. This pattern is observed in approximately one percent of electrocardiograms recorded in adults; it is routinely part of the electrocardiographic picture of congenital defects in the area of the AV canal. When disease is present in both the right bundle and left anterior fascicle, the development of block in the left posterior fascicle will, of course, result in complete heart block.

The combination of right bundle branch block with left posterior hemiblock is only about five percent as frequent as the combination of right bundle branch block with left anterior hemiblock. When the former combination does occur, however, it is manifested as right bundle branch block with otherwise unexplained marked right axis deviation [*see Figure 11*] and often leads to complete heart block.

In a sense, left bundle branch block represents a form of bifascicular block. The anatomic lesions responsible for this block, however, may occur in the common bundle before the bifurcation, in the left bundle before it divides into anterior and posterior fascicles, or as diffuse disease of the distal portions of the left bundle. Unless first- or second-degree AV block is also present, left bundle branch block is less likely to progress to complete heart block than is bifascicular block involving the right bundle branch.

Bilateral bundle branch disease is manifested as right bundle branch block with left anterior or posterior hemiblock or as alternating right and left bundle branch block [*see Figure 12*].

In patients who have bilateral branch disease and prolongation of the PR interval, the delay in AV conduction may occur either at the level of the AV node or distal to it. His bundle electrocardiography must be used to distinguish the site of the block [*see Figure 7*]. Although the evidence is somewhat conflicting, it appears that if the delay is infranodal (indicated by a prolonged HV interval) the likelihood of progression to complete heart block is much higher than if the delay occurs at the level of the AV node.[29,30] However, in a long-term follow-

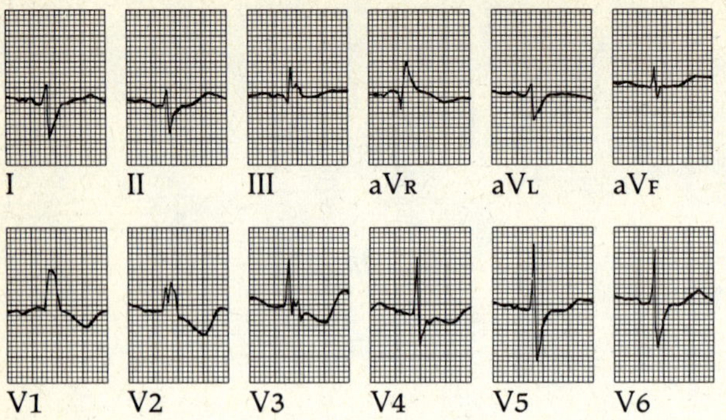

Figure 11 *Electrocardiogram from a patient with the combination of right bundle branch block and left posterior hemiblock demonstrates right axis deviation; the frontal plane QRS axis is 130° . The small Q wave in lead V1 is also probably the result of the hemiblock.*

up study of 554 patients with various types of chronic bifascicular and trifascicular block who were considered to be at high risk for complete heart block, the incidence of progression to complete heart block over five years was only approximately one percent per year.[31] Survival rate was related more to whether such factors as advanced age, associated coronary artery disease, and congestive heart failure were present than to the conduction abnormality. Insertion of pacemakers was recommended in patients who have chronic fascicular blocks only if symptomatic bradyarrhythmias could be documented.

Atrioventricular Block

AV block may be classified in two ways: (1) anatomically, based on the site of block as determined by His bundle electrocardiography, and (2) clinically, based on the routine electrocardiogram.[32,33] The three classic clinical types are first-, second-, and third-degree (or complete) AV block.

Anatomic classification recognizes three levels of block in relation to the bundle of His. These three levels and their electrophysiologic features are as follows:

1. Supra-Hisian (AV nodal) block is indicated by a prolonged AH interval. The HV interval is normal. When AV block occurs, the atrial potential is not followed by a His bundle deflection. Escape beats are preceded by an H spike, and the escape focus is in the AV junction. The QRS complexes of conducted beats are usually narrow unless associated bundle branch block is present. The AV node is the site of block in most cases of first-degree block and type I second-degree block.

2. Intra-Hisian (intranodal) block occurs within the bundle of His. The electrophysiologic finding is that of two His

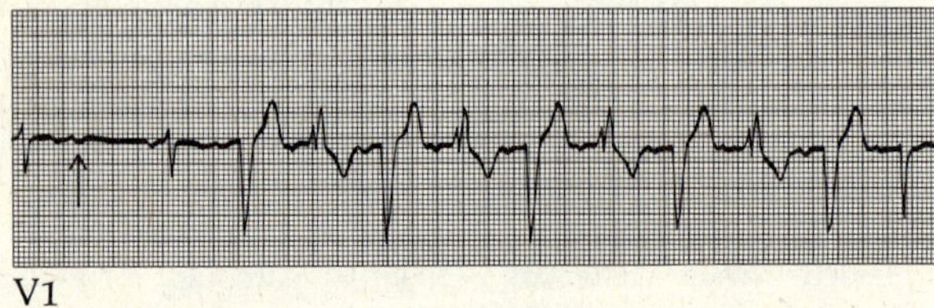

Figure 12 *A patient with calcific aortic stenosis shows evidence of bilateral branch disease, manifested in lead V1 as alternating right and left bundle branch block. The beat indicated by the arrow is blocked. The blocked beat is followed at first by a normally conducted beat and then by a series of beats showing left alternating with right bundle branch block. The final beat in the sequence is conducted normally. Such evidence of bilateral bundle branch disease is generally regarded as an indication for a permanent pacemaker.*

bundle deflections (also called split His potentials), designated H1 and H2 on intracardiac recordings. The A-H1 interval is usually normal, although it may be prolonged, and the H2-V interval is normal or short. The blocked beats show the H1 deflection but not the H2 spike. Escape beats originate in the bundle of His and are preceded by a His bundle (H2) spike. QRS complexes are usually narrow. Clinically, this type of block is virtually impossible to diagnose from the surface electrocardiogram. It is uncommon, and its behavior tends to resemble that of type II clinical block.

3. Infra-Hisian (infra-nodal) block occurs at some distal point, even though the impulse is propagated through the His bundle. When AV block is absent, the HV interval is usually long. When block occurs, nonconducted supraventricular beats show a His bundle spike, whereas escape beats do not. The QRS complexes of escape beats are wide.

Most decisions related to pacemaker therapy in heart block are based on clinical criteria, although His bundle electrocardiography can be helpful in some cases. Any clinical type of heart block can be caused by block at any anatomic level, and multiple levels of anatomic block may exist in any given patient.[33]

First-Degree AV Block

First-degree AV block is arbitrarily defined as a PR interval greater than 0.20 sec at a heart rate of 70; as the heart rate rises, the upper limit of normal decreases progressively to 0.17 sec at a rate of 115. When the QRS complex is of normal duration (less than 0.10 sec) or only unifascicular block is present, prolongation of the PR interval almost invariably is caused by a delay at the level of the AV node. When bundle branch block is present, conduction may be delayed either at the AV node or distal to it, and His bundle electrocardiography is required to pinpoint the site of the block.

Etiology Commonly, a prolonged PR interval is the result of degenerative changes in the AV conduction system caused by aging. Digitalis, exaggerated vagal tone, ischemia affecting the AV node (such as that which may occur with diaphragmatic infarction), and inflammation of the heart (such as myocarditis or acute rheumatic fever) are among the many other causes of a prolonged PR interval. First-degree heart block is found in a variety of cardiomyopathies, both primary and secondary, and is common in severe aortic regurgitation.

Clinical findings Normally, except for a soft first heart sound, no distinctive abnormalities or unusual symptomatology is apparent on physical examination of patients with first-degree AV block. The relatively benign course and good prognosis of most cases of first-degree AV block have been confirmed by the findings of a large study.[34]

Second-Degree AV Block

Two types of second-degree AV block have been distinguished. Type I (also called Wenckebach and Mobitz I) block is caused by AV nodal conduction delay, whereas type II (Mobitz II) block is the result of infranodal block. The causes and distinctive features of the two types of second-degree block have considerable importance [*see Table 1*]. Type I block is typified by Wenckebach second-degree block in which there is a progressive prolongation of the PR interval until a beat is finally blocked. Once a dropped beat occurs, the sequence begins again. Conversely, type II block is manifested as a sudden interruption of AV conduction without prior prolongation of the PR interval. Type II block carries a more ominous prognosis than does type I block and frequently progresses to complete heart block.

Third-Degree (Complete) AV Block

In third-degree, or complete, heart block, all atrial beats are blocked, and the ventricles are driven by an escape focus distal to the site of block. When the block is nodal, the

Table 1   Differences between Type I and Type II Second-Degree AV Block

Feature	Type I (Mobitz I, Wenckebach)	Type II (Mobitz II)
	ECG recorded in patient with Mobitz type I, or Wenckebach, block shows progressive prolongation of the PR interval until a P wave is completely blocked and a ventricular beat is dropped (broken arrow). The PR interval of the next conducted beat is shorter than the preceding PR interval.	In a patient with Mobitz type II block, a blocked beat (solid arrow) occurs suddenly and is not preceded by a change in the duration of the PR interval. Patient is equipped with a pacemaker, which cuts in (at broken arrow) to sustain a regular ventricular rhythm.
Site of block	Usually AV nodal (supra-Hisian)	Infranodal (intra- or infra-Hisian)
QRS complex	Usually normal in width	Usually wide (bundle branch block) with infra-Hisian block; narrow with intra-Hisian block
Causes	Degenerative changes in AV node; diaphragmatic myocardial infarct; digitalis toxicity; myocarditis; rheumatic fever; increased vagal tone	Extensive anterior myocardial infarct; degenerative changes in His-Purkinje system; massive calcification of mitral or aortic valve anulus

Feature	Type I (Mobitz I, Wenckebach)	Type II (Mobitz II)
ECG	PR interval lengthens progressively until ventricular beat is dropped PR interval shortens after dropped beat RR interval narrows progressively up to the dropped beat RR interval after the blocked beat is always less than twice the RR interval of conducted beats	PR interval is usually normal in duration and constant in length; if PR interval is prolonged, the duration of prolongation is fixed Blocked beats occur suddenly, without progressive lengthening of PR interval RR interval of conducted beats is constant or a multiple of a basic RR interval cycle length
Effect of carotid sinus pressure	May increase degree of block	No effect
Effect of atropine	Frequently shortens PR interval and increases AV conduction	No effect
Consequences of progression to complete heart block	Escape focus usually junctional: narrow QRS complex; rate > 45 beats/min; Adams-Stokes attacks uncommon	Escape focus infrajunctional (usually ventricular): wide QRS complex; rate < 45 beats/min; Adams-Stokes attacks common Junctional escape may be present with intra-Hisian block
Findings on His bundle electrocardiography	Prolonged AH interval; normal HV interval; His bundle spike absent on blocked beats	Prolonged HV interval; normal AH interval; rarely, split His bundle potentials AH interval usually normal; with intra-Hisian block, split His bundle potentials with normal HV interval; with infra-Hisian block, long HV interval; blocked beats show His bundle deflection, but second deflection (H2) is absent with infra-Hisian block.

escape rhythm arises in the AV junction and has a QRS width of normal duration; the ventricular rate, 45 to 55 beats/min, is somewhat faster than that seen in cases of infranodal block. Conversely, when the block is infranodal, the escape focus is in the common bundle or the ventricles, a wide QRS complex is seen on the electrocardiogram, and the pulse rate (30 to 40 beats/min) is slower than in AV nodal block. In general, because of its slower escape rate, infranodal block is potentially more hazardous than AV nodal block.

Etiology The most common cause of complete heart block in adults is simple fibrous degenerative changes in the conduction system that result from aging (Lenegre's disease). Fibrotic and degenerative changes in tissue located adjacent to the mitral anulus can also interrupt the common bundle (Lev's disease). Although coronary artery disease may contribute to heart block, the primary underlying disorder in most cases is degeneration of the bundle branch system.

In acute myocardial infarction, AV nodal block tends to occur with inferior or posterior infarction, whereas infranodal block is usually the result of damage to the His-Purkinje system sustained during a massive anterior wall infarct.

The conduction system may be interrupted by a number of infectious and inflammatory processes, such as abscesses, tubercles, tumors, infiltrative diseases of the myocardium, sarcoid nodules, and gummas. Transient AV block may result from infectious and inflammatory diseases, such as myocarditis and rheumatic fever, or from drugs, such as digitalis. Complete heart block is common in patients with ankylosing spondylitis, and there is evidence that the histocompatibility antigen HLA-B27 is associated with complete heart block independent of its relation to spondylitis.[35] Cardiac surgery, especially when performed in the region of the AV canal, may also precipitate heart block.

Congenital heart block, which is almost invariably AV nodal, is encountered occa-

sionally.[36] In about one fourth of the cases of congenital block, there is no other inherited cardiac anomaly, whereas in the remainder, some other cardiac defect is present. Particularly prevalent in association with congenital complete heart block are such anomalies as corrected transposition of the great arteries and defects of the AV canal. Congenital complete heart block in infants is also associated with a very high incidence of maternal antibody to the soluble ribonucleoprotein antigen Ro (or SS-A). Although some mothers who carry this protein show signs of systemic lupus erythematosus or another rheumatic disease, many appear healthy [*see Chapter 40*].

Clinical features The symptoms of complete heart block are those associated with Adams-Stokes attacks and occasionally congestive heart failure. Often, these two conditions occur simultaneously. Adams-Stokes attacks are caused by either sudden asystole or the development of ventricular tachyarrhythmias, such as transient ventricular tachycardia or ventricular fibrillation, that lead to circulatory arrest. Adams-Stokes syncope is usually sudden in onset, although some patients experience symptoms of impending syncope.

If adequate cerebral perfusion is restored promptly, patients recover consciousness rapidly and are almost immediately awake and oriented. This response contrasts with the somnolent, disoriented state that usually follows a seizure of central nervous system origin. Sometimes, patients have very mild near syncopal attacks before major fainting spells occur. The bradycardia associated with complete heart block may lead to congestive heart failure in patients with myocardial disease.

Signs of complete heart block are those that characterize bradycardia with AV dissociation. Such signs include variation in the systolic blood pressure, variation in the intensity of the first heart sound, intermittent cannon waves in the jugular venous pulses, and variable third and fourth heart sounds—all of which depend on the relation between atrial and ventricular systole. When atrial fibrillation is present, signs of AV dissociation are absent.

Treatment of Heart Block

Medical Treatment

For the most part, electrical pacing has rendered medical therapy for AV block obsolete. First-degree block and type I second-degree block sometimes respond to atropine, 0.5 to 1.5 mg intravenously, but such therapy is usually reserved for the reversal of transient excessive vagal tone in a medical emergency, such as acute myocardial infarction. In patients with complete heart block who have a very slow ventricular rate, sympathomimetic drugs, particularly isoproterenol or epinephrine, can be given until pacing can be established. The usual dose is 1 to 4 µg/min intravenously.

In patients with Adams-Stokes attacks secondary to repetitive ventricular tachycardia or fibrillation, the administration of antiarrhythmic agents is a common practice. Use of these drugs in patients with underlying complete heart block, however, is extremely dangerous because they tend to suppress lower escape foci; in general, antiarrhythmics are contraindicated unless an electrical pacemaker is in place.

The Use of Pacemakers in AV and Fascicular Blocks

Indications Pacemakers are being implanted in ever-increasing numbers of patients because of the simplicity of pacemaker insertion and the improved reliability and longevity of the units. Generally accepted indications for permanent pacing include the following:

1. Second- or third-degree AV block, either congenital or acquired, or bifascicular block that is associated with symptoms of syncope or near syncope suggestive of Adams-Stokes attacks. Pacemakers are clearly indicated for those patients in whom symptomatic bradycardia has been documented.

2. Asymptomatic complete heart block with ventricular ectopy. The more rapid pacing rate usually suppresses the ventricular premature beats and also ensures safer administration of antiarrhythmic drugs.

3. Complete heart block with congestive heart failure, with or without syncope. The increase in cardiac output induced by the faster rate may alleviate congestive failure. In addition, new modes of pacing that couple atrial and ventricular contractions may be especially helpful in patients with complete heart block, congestive heart failure, and underlying sinus rhythms.

4. Evidence of marked instability of conduction in the His-Purkinje system—for example, alternating right and left bundle branch block [*see Figure 12*]. The indications for pacing are less clear in patients with bifascicular block and first-degree AV block. This group includes individuals who have an abnormally prolonged PR interval and left anterior or posterior hemiblock combined with right bundle branch block, as well as those who have a long PR interval with left bundle branch block. Such patients should receive pacemakers if they experience symptoms of dizziness or syncope consistent with intermittent complete heart block. Pacemakers are also recommended for asymptomatic patients in whom transient complete heart block has been documented by electrocardiographic monitoring. Some investigators have suggested that prolongation of the HV interval for longer than 70 msec delineates a group of patients with a high risk of developing subsequent heart block[29,30]; others, however, have not found measurement of His bundle intervals to be helpful.[31] Thus, prophylactic pacing is not generally recommended for patients with first-degree block and bifascicular block who are asymptomatic or do not have documented transient periods of higher degrees of AV block, regardless of the HV interval.[26]

5. Complete heart block that persists after acute anterior myocardial infarction.

6. Bifascicular block that persists after acute anterior myocardial infarction, if the patient experienced transient complete heart block while having the myocardial infarct.[37]

We generally recommend permanent pacing even in asymptomatic patients with nodal or infranodal block if the escape rate falls below 40 beats/min because slowing of the heart rate frequently is a precursor of Adams-Stokes attacks.

If the PR interval is normal in patients who have right bundle branch block and left anterior hemiblock, pacing is not generally indicated, unless the patient has had symptoms suggesting Adams-Stokes attacks or if, as previously mentioned, transient AV block has been present following a myocardial infarction. The use of pacemakers designed to control tachyarrhythmias will be discussed later [see Pacemakers and Automatic Defibrillators for Arrhythmias, below]. Additional guidelines for pacemaker implantation have been developed by a joint task force of the American Heart Association and the American College of Cardiology.[38]

Pacing techniques Temporary pacemakers, which are required for the management of symptomatic bradycardia in many different circumstances, can be inserted either from the jugular or subclavian vein or from a femoral vein. A relatively comfortable and effective external pacing device has also been developed that is suitable for use in emergency situations.[39]

Most permanent pacemaker implantations now take advantage of the pervenous technique, whereby an electrode is inserted either through a cephalic or external jugular vein into the apex of the right ventricle and attached to a subcutaneous power source buried just inferior to the clavicle. A second electrode can be inserted through the same or a nearby site into the right atrium for dual chamber pacing. Some physicians still prefer to use direct epicardial electrodes. Such electrodes are attached to the ventricle through a small midline thoracotomy, and the pulse generator is implanted subcutaneously in the epigastric area.[40] This method is preferred for patients with prosthetic tricuspid valves.

The availability of complex and multiprogrammable dual chamber pacemakers has underscored the need for a uniform terminology for the description of various pacing modalities. At present, the Inter-Society Commission on Heart Disease (ICHD) five-position pacemaker code is the only classification scheme that has achieved widespread acceptance [see Table 2].[41] This code assigns one position to each of five major characteristics of an implantable pacemaker as follows: the chamber(s) paced (position I), the chamber(s) sensed (position II), the mode of response(s) to a sensed event (position III), programmable functions (position IV), and special tachyarrhythmia functions (position V). In practice, only the first three positions describe the commonly used pacemakers. For example, a pacemaker that paces the ventricle, senses in the atrium, and is triggered by a sensed atrial event would be classified as a VAT pacemaker. A standard ventricular demand (inhibited) pacemaker is classified as VVI. A pacemaker that paces and senses in both the atrium and the ventricle and that is triggered by an atrial event and inhibited by a ventricular event is classified as DDD.

Rapid refinements in electrode design, the development of more efficient circuitry, and especially, the introduction of new power sources have reduced the size and markedly prolonged the life of pacemaker pulse generators. The development of lithium batteries with a projected longevity of eight to 20 years has marked a signal advance in the pacing field. Lithium batteries have rendered the older mercury-zinc cells virtually obsolete. Lithium batteries have also drastically reduced the need for implantation of nuclear-powered sources, although those still offer the longest pulse-generation life. Most centers now use lithium pacemakers exclusively.

Table 2 Five-Position Pacemaker Code (ICHD)

Position Category	I Chamber(s) Paced	II Chamber(s) Sensed	III Mode of Response(s)	IV Programmable Functions	V Special Tachyarrhythmia Functions
Letter code	**V** = Ventricle **A** = Atrium **D** = Double **S** = Single chamber†	**V** = Ventricle **A** = Atrium **D** = Double **O** = None **S** = Single chamber†	**T** = Triggered **I** = Inhibited **D** = Double[*] **O** = None **R** = Reverse	**P** = Programmable (rate or output, or both) **M** = Multi-programmable **O** = None	**B** = Bursts **N** = Normal rate competition **S** = Scanning **E** = External

Note: in practice, only the first three positions are used to describe most existing pacemakers.

[*]Atrial triggered and ventricular inhibited.

Because the cost of a pacemaker generally increases in direct proportion to its expected longevity and complexity, pacemakers should be chosen wisely and tailored to the activity and anticipated life span of the recipients.

Different types of pacemakers yield characteristic electrocardiographic patterns [*see Figure 13*]. For ventricular pacing, some type of demand pacemaker is invariably used so as not to compete with the patient's own rhythm if AV conduction should return or with ventricular premature beats if they are present. The most frequently implanted demand pacemaker is the R wave–inhibited (VVI) type, which ceases to pace if it senses a conducted or premature beat but discharges again when the patient's ventricular rate drops below the previously set rate of the pacemaker. The ventricular-triggered (VVT) pacemaker discharges harmlessly in the QRS complexes of conducted or premature beats but otherwise functions as a demand pacemaker if no impulse is detected. Because the ventricular-triggered pacemaker deforms conducted QRS complexes, it is difficult to interpret the underlying electrocardiogram in patients with AV conduction who have this unit.

AV synchronous (VAT or VDD) and AV sequential (DVI) pacemakers are appropriate for patients who require a coordinated atrial contraction immediately preceding ventricular systole to maintain an adequate cardiac output. Both of these modes require pulse generators with two pacing chambers and permanent electrodes in both the atrium and the ventricle. The AV synchronous pacemaker senses the P wave resulting from spontaneous sinus beats and discharges a ventricular stimulus for each P wave sensed. Thus, the patient's underlying sinus node rate determines the pacemaker discharge rate. This mode may be particularly advantageous in individuals who wish to be physically active and who are limited by AV block but not by sinus node dysfunction. The major drawback of this mode of pacing is that AV synchronous pacemakers do not sense ventricular events, and thus, potential competitive pacing can ensue if there is ventricular ectopic activity. The AV sequential unit paces both the atrium and ventricle in sequence and senses the ventricle. The disadvantage of this pacemaker is that it may cause competition with the sinus node. The newest dual chamber pacemakers, known as DDD units in the pacemaker code, have substantial advantages over both the AV synchronous and AV sequential pacemakers because of their ability to sense and stimulate both the atrium and ventricle and because of their remarkable programming versatility.[42,43] If problems arise with the DDD mode, these units can be simply programmed to almost any other pacing system. Pacing that preserves the atrial and ventricular contraction sequence is referred to as physiologic pacing.[44]

In addition to providing enhanced cardiac output in patients with impaired ventricular function, dual chamber pacemakers are helpful in patients in whom standard ventricular pacing alone results in retrograde atrial conduction and a symptomatic fall in cardiac output, the so-called pacemaker syndrome. This is especially likely to occur when pacing is undertaken in the absence of AV block, as is often the case in

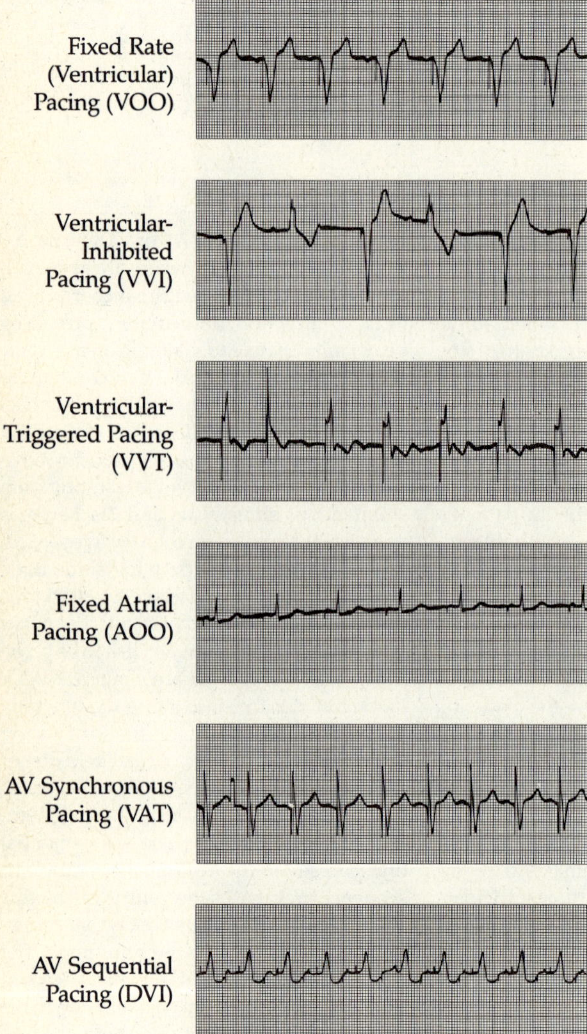

Figure 13 *Characteristic patterns of electrocardiographic activity are observed in patients who are outfitted with different types of pacing units, depending on the site (or sites) of electrode placement and whether the pacemaker is of the fixed rate (asynchronous) or demand type. Electrocardiograms representative of various types of pacing are shown above. The current ICHD terminology is given. Those pacemakers that have the designations VOO, AOO, VAT, and DVI could be different, depending on other sensing and response modes.*

patients with sick sinus syndrome. The symptoms of the pacemaker syndrome can usually be eliminated by conversion from ventricular pacing to physiologic pacing.[45]

The use of printed microcircuits has led to the development of more compact pacemakers endowed with many new capabilities. Many functions of the implanted pacemakers can be easily adjusted by using a magnetically activated potentiometer held externally in proximity to the pulse generator.[43,46] The most important programmable pacemaker functions are the discharge rate and the energy output. In newer pacemakers, the refractory period and sensing threshold of the pulse generator can also be altered. In fact, literally millions of programmable permutations of pacemaker functions are possible in currently available units. In addition, microcircuitry allows the storage and transmission of all sorts of information. For example, the precise electronic settings of new pacemakers can be called for and printed out on demand. Soon, pacemakers will be available that will record intracardiac electrical activity, store data for later recall and examination, and even carry a brief medical history of the patient.

A new generation of pacemakers that will respond to physiologic changes is under active development. For example, one unit that is now available contains a sensor that monitors the signals made by skeletal muscle contraction. When muscle noise increases, as during exercise, the pacemaker responds with an increase in the discharge rate.[47] The increment in rate may be graduated according to the amount of skeletal muscle activity that is sensed, and the rate response can be programmed to almost any level that the physician deems appropriate. Although these units have still not been perfected, they offer considerable flexibility to patients in whom the pacemaker discharge rate cannot be linked to an atrial signal, such as those who have atrial fibrillation. Other physiologic parameters that might be used to alter pacemaker rates are blood temperature, pH, oxygen saturation, and respiratory rate.

Although the programmable units contain a good deal of electronic excess, they are valuable in the management of many patients. For example, in patients with sick sinus syndrome and intact AV conduction, the pacemaker can be set at a slow rate so as not to compete with the patient's intrinsic rhythm. In a patient with possible myocardial infarction, a programmable pacemaker facilitates confirmation of the diagnosis. It is virtually impossible to diagnose myocardial infarction on a pacemaker electrocardiogram because pacing distorts QRS complexes. But if the pacing rate is slowed with a programmer, then conducted beats may emerge. Patients with myocardial disease or with angina may benefit from changes in heart rate and ideally should have programmable pacemakers. Variation in pacemaker discharge rates also may be important in terminating or suppressing arrhythmias. In other specific cases, alteration of the energy output, refractory period, and sensing threshold of the pulse generator may be important if pacemakers malfunction.

Pacemaker problems Early pacemaker failures (i.e., within six months of implantation) are usually due to electrode displacement or breakage, whereas later failures are due to premature battery depletion or faulty pulse generators. The burgeoning use of both atrial and ventricular electrodes increases the potential for the development of problems with sensing, pacing, or electrode displacement. Component failures are increasingly rare, as are breaks in electrodes.

A number of clinics are now available to which patients can transmit their pacemaker impulse by telephone to a signal recorder, and small changes in the discharge rates of the pacemakers can thereby be detected. Slowing of the discharge rate by as little as 25 msec may afford an early clue to pulse generator failure. Such changes are so small that they cannot be detected by examining routine electrocardiograms or by counting the patient's pulse rate. Demand pacemakers may be overridden by the patient's intrinsic heart rate if this rate is rapid. The physician can, however, momentarily convert such a pacemaker to an asynchronous mode by placing a magnet externally over the pulse generator and thereby obtain an accurate measurement of the pacemaker discharge rate.

A variety of arrhythmias related to pacemakers, particularly to the dual chamber pacemakers, have been reported. Such arrhythmias are perhaps most frequently due to difficulties in QRS complex sensing, which can cause asynchronous pacing and precipitate potentially serious ventricular arrhythmias. If retrograde (VA) conduction is present, retrograde atrial activation can ensue, with the production of reciprocating tachycardias.[48-50] Dual chamber pacemakers have also created a series of arrhythmias that are intrinsic to their mode of operation. Dual chamber sensing and pacing may produce asynchronous stimulation of either cardiac chamber and essentially create an artificial bypass tract.[48] The resulting arrhythmias may occur even when the pacemaker is functioning normally, and they can usually be terminated by reprogramming the units.[48,49]

In addition, pacemakers may be vulnerable to external electrical fields generated by such sources as microwave ovens, electrocautery, or diathermy, all of which can shut off ventricular-inhibited pacemakers; patients with pacemakers also cannot be subjected to nuclear magnetic resonance imaging. With improved shielding of pacing units, however, such problems are now rare. Many pacemakers are now designed so that external electrical fields will change the pacemaker rhythm to an asynchronous mode rather than shut off the unit completely. Some pacemakers have been turned off by the sensing of myopotentials arising from the use of the arm and shoulder girdle muscles.

Infection, thromboembolism, perforation of the ventricle by the electrode, dislodgment of the electrode, and diaphragmatic stimulation related to pacing are uncommon but bothersome problems.[51]

Overall, the use of pacemakers has dramatically improved the outlook of patients with complete heart block. Whereas the one-year mortality after the first Adams-Stokes attack was about 50 percent prior to the use of pacemakers, most patients with permanent pacemakers now die of a cause other than heart block.

Supraventricular Arrhythmias

Arrhythmias that arise in the atria or AV node or junction constitute supraventricular arrhythmias.

Atrial Premature Beats and Junctional Premature Beats

Atrial premature beats and junctional premature beats are common in patients with and without heart disease and are inconsequential except for the fact that they may precede the development of atrial or junctional tachyarrhythmias. Atrial premature beats may be aberrantly conducted or blocked.

When atrial premature beats occur before the bundle branch systems have fully recovered, aberrant ventricular conduction results. Because the refractory period of the right bundle is ordinarily longer than that of the left bundle, the electrocardiographic configuration of aberrantly conducted beats is usually that of right bundle branch block. The differentiation of aberrant conduction from ventricular ectopy is discussed later [see Ventricular Arrhythmias, Differentiation of Supraventricular Arrhythmia with Aberrancy from Ventricular Arrhythmia, *below*].

Atrial premature beats with aberrant ventricular conduction can mimic premature ventricular beats. Such premature atrial beats can be identified by uncovering the ectopic P wave, which is usually buried in the ST segment or in the T wave that precedes the aberrant beat [see *Figure 14*]. An additional distinguishing characteristic is that atrial premature beats, unlike ventricular premature beats, are not usually followed by a full compensatory pause. Blocked atrial premature beats mimic sinus pauses [see *Figure 15*] and are the most common cause of pauses in individuals with sinus rhythm.

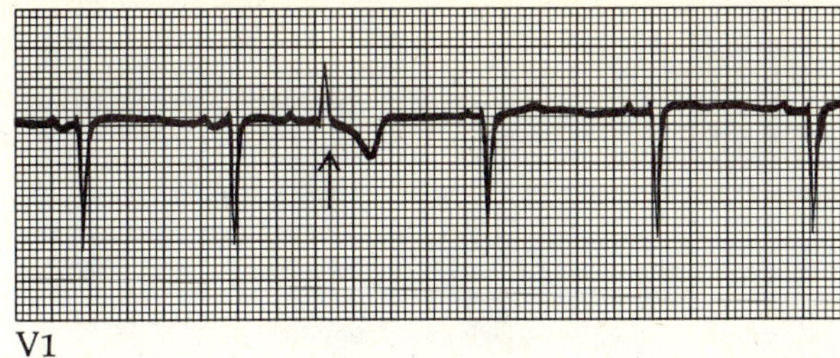

V1

Figure 14 *At the arrow, an atrial premature beat with aberrant ventricular conduction is noted. The electrocardiographic pattern is that of right bundle branch block, the usual configuration in cases of aberrant conduction.*

Junctional premature beats exhibit the same QRS configuration as do normally conducted beats, although like atrial premature beats, they also may be aberrantly conducted. A retrograde P wave, the result of retrograde atrial activation, may follow, be incorporated into, or immediately precede the QRS complex, depending on the speed of retrograde atrial activation. Junctional premature beats have no special significance and rarely require suppression.

Generally, atrial and junctional premature beats do not require treatment, although suppression is occasionally warranted for bothersome palpitations. Quinidine is the best suppressive drug. Disopyramide or procainamide may be used if the patient has an intolerance to quinidine. Beta-adrenergic blocking agents are also quite effective as suppressive drugs, but they are contraindicated in patients who are prone to bradycardia or who have congestive heart failure. Occasionally, atrial premature beats may be effectively suppressed by administration of digitalis glycosides or calcium channel blockers.

Sinus Tachycardia

Sinus tachycardia is not a true cardiac rhythm disturbance but merely an accelera-tion of the normal discharge rate of the sinus node. Sinus tachycardia is invariably secondary to conditions that drive the heart at a faster rate, such as fever, hypotension, pain, anxiety, drugs, thyrotoxicosis, and a host of other disorders. Transient sinus tachycardia is occasionally the result of a rebound phenomenon following the discontinuation of beta-adrenergic blocking drugs.

In sinus tachycardia, the heart rate rarely exceeds 160 beats/min, except in infants and children and in adults who are engaging in maximum physical effort. Sinus tachycardia is usually regular but may be slightly irregular because of sinus arrhythmia. At rapid heart rates, sinus arrhythmia is usually lost.

In sinus tachycardia, the P wave is often incorporated into the T wave of the preceding beat, which poses a problem in diagnosis. A constant deformity inscribed (often subtly) on the T wave indicates the P wave of the sinus beat [*see Figure 16*]. Also, examination of earlier electrocardiograms recorded at slower heart rates may reveal that by comparison the recently recorded T waves are more peaked because of the combination of the P and T waves. Carotid sinus pressure may produce transient slowing, so that the P wave may emerge from the T wave. Slowing is always gradual with carotid sinus pres-

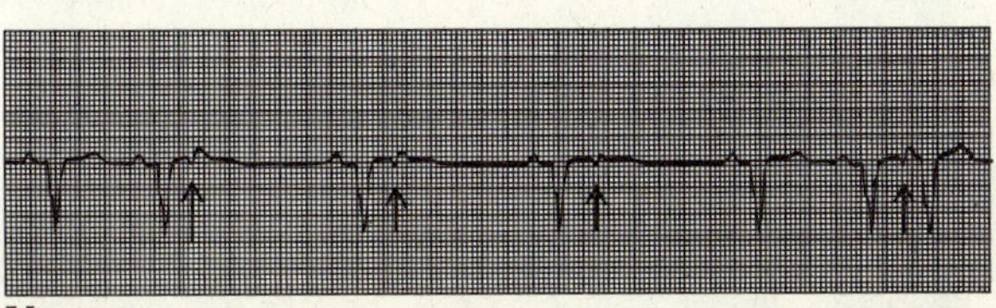

V1

Figure 15 *Frequent blocked atrial premature beats (indicated by arrows) are interspersed among normally conducted beats. The final atrial premature beat is conducted.*

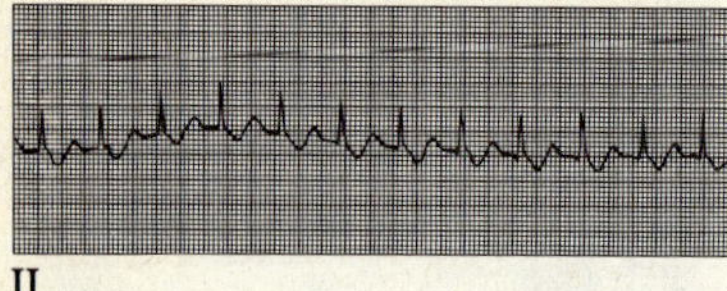

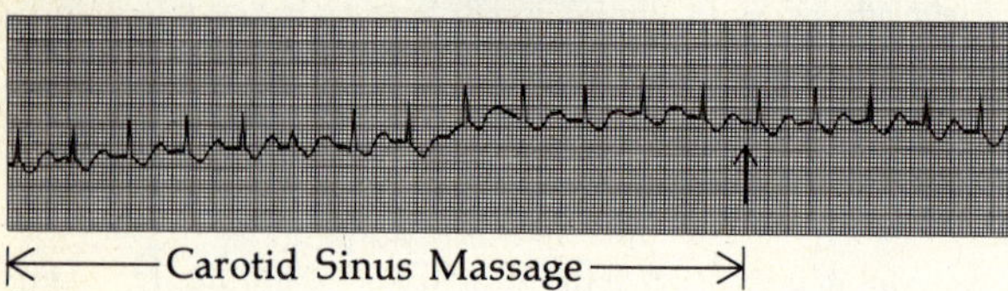

Figure 16 *Sinus tachycardia at a rate of 135 beats/min is present in a patient with first-degree AV block (upper panel). When carotid sinus massage is applied (bottom panel), the sinus rate slows gradually to a rate of 100 beats/min, producing a separation of the T and P waves. After carotid sinus pressure is released (at arrow), the rapid rate resumes.*

sure, and on release, the heart resumes its prior rate. If premature beats are present, the sinus P wave may be seen in the beat after the compensatory pause.

Therapy

With rare exceptions, treatment is directed at the underlying cause of the disorder rather than at the heart rate. Digitalis glycosides are not indicated unless sinus tachycardia is associated with congestive heart failure. An exception to this rule may be patients with angina or acute myocardial infarction in whom the rapid heart rate produces an undesirable increase in myocardial oxygen consumption. In such patients, slowing of the sinus rate by the cautious use of beta-adrenergic blocking drugs may be beneficial if there are no contraindications to their use.

Paroxysmal Supraventricular Tachycardia

Paroxysmal supraventricular tachycardia refers to a group of ectopic tachyarrhythmias that are characterized by sudden onset and abrupt termination; they are usually initiated by a supraventricular premature beat. Included in this category are those arrhythmias that traditionally have been classified as paroxysmal atrial tachycardia and paroxysmal junctional tachycardia.

Electrophysiologic studies that combine programmed atrial stimulation with His bundle electrocardiography have demonstrated that about 85 percent of cases of paroxysmal supraventricular tachycardia are caused by reentry at one of three sites: (1) in the AV node in about 60 to 65 percent of cases, (2) over a concealed, extranodal accessory bypass tract in 10 to 15 percent of cases (although reported in 50 percent of one series[52]), and (3) in the sinus node or atria in five to 10 percent of cases. Reentry over a concealed accessory bypass tract is not evident on the surface electrocardiogram as in Wolff-Parkinson-White or other preexcitation syndromes, because these concealed bypass tracts are usually only capable of retrograde impulse transmission. Another five percent of instances of paroxysmal supraventricular tachycardia are automatic in mechanism; in about 10 percent, the exact mechanism cannot be delineated.[53]

Electrocardiographic Features

Paroxysmal supraventricular tachycardia is manifested as an absolutely regular rhythm at a rate between 130 and 220 beats/min. Those episodes caused by reentry have abrupt onset and cessation. Automatic rhythms may show some variation in rate, especially as they begin and end.

The surface electrocardiogram may afford some useful clues as to the site of reentry and nature of the arrhythmia. In the case of reentry through the AV node or over a concealed bypass tract, the atria are always activated in a retrograde fashion; P waves are therefore inverted in leads II, III, and aVF. Reentry in the sinus node or atria is associated with normal P wave direction. Several points should be noted about the P wave configuration and its relation to the QRS complex in paroxysmal supraventricular tachycardia[52]:

1. Absence of a visible P wave during the tachycardia implies simultaneous atrial and ventricular activation and thus strongly suggests AV nodal reentry. Such activation can occur only if the reentrant circuit is confined within the region of the AV node.
2. Inverted (retrograde) P waves in the inferior leads with an RP interval less than one half the RR interval occur either in AV nodal reentrant supraventricular tachycardia (about 30 percent of all cases) or in reentry over a concealed bypass tract. All patients with concealed bypass pathways show this pattern. In such cases, the ventricles are always activated by antegrade conduction via the AV node; the atria are discharged by retrograde conduction of the impulse through the accessory pathway.
3. Patients with retrograde P waves and long RP intervals (greater than one half the RR interval) usually have an atypical and often incessant form of AV nodal reentry.
4. Patients with a PR interval appropriate for the rate of tachycardia may have sinus nodal reentry if the P wave is identical to the sinus P wave. If the P wave differs from the sinus P wave but is not retrograde, the arrhythmia is usually an automatic or reentrant atrial tachycardia.

Most accessory bypass pathways are left-sided. The retrograde atrial activation is so extreme that occasionally inverted P waves are seen in lead I—an important clue to the presence of a concealed bypass pathway.[54] Functional bundle branch block, usually of the left bundle, is a common feature of reentry using concealed AV bypass tracts.[53-55]

In general, reentrant arrhythmias utilizing concealed accessory bypass pathways tend to be considerably faster than AV nodal or sinoatrial reentry. There are several characteristic features that can aid in distinguishing among the four types of paroxysmal supraventricular tachycardias [*see Table 3*].

Etiology

Paroxysmal supraventricular tachycardia is very common and is often experienced by people with structurally normal hearts. It is frequently seen in preexcitation syndromes [*see* Preexcitation Syndromes, *below*] and in association with certain congenital abnormalities, such as atrial septal defect and Ebstein's anomaly of the tricuspid valve. Patients with concealed accessory bypass tracts appear far more likely to have otherwise normal hearts than persons with AV nodal or sinoatrial reentry.[53]

Clinical Findings

Patients usually tolerate paroxysmal supraventricular tachycardia well, but occasionally, it may precipitate congestive heart failure or hypotension, especially if underlying heart disease is present. As with most tachyarrhythmias, patients are usually aware of a rapid heart beat. Polyuria has been reported to occur during attacks. Cardiac auscultation reveals monotonously uniform heart sounds. When atrial and ventricular contraction coincide, constant cannon waves may be seen in the jugular venous pulses.

Therapy

Regardless of the mechanism of paroxysmal supraventricular tachycardia, initial therapy for the acute attack consists of maneuvers aimed at increasing vagal tone, particularly carotid sinus massage. Because carotid sinus massage is often applied improperly, some guidelines for its use are worthwhile.

The carotid arteries should be examined by auscultation in order to ensure that no occlusive bruits are present; if bruits are heard, carotid sinus pressure should not be applied. If no such contraindications are

Table 3   Features of the Four Types of
Paroxysmal Supraventricular Tachycardias

	AV Nodal Reentry	Concealed Accessory Bypass Tract	Sinus Nodal or Atrial Reentry	Automatic
Associated organic heart disease	Common	Rare	Common	Common
Heart rate	120–220 beats/min (average ~160)	170–230 beats/min (average ~190)	120–220 beats/min (average ~160)	120–220 beats/min (average ~150)
P wave in relation to QRS	Simultaneous (may be invisible) or immediately after QRS; rarely precedes QRS	Follows QRS	Precedes QRS	Precedes QRS
P wave direction and configuration	Retrograde; inverted in II, III, and aV_F	Retrograde; inverted in II, III, and aV_F; may be negative in I	Normal; in sinus nodal reentry, P wave identical to sinus P wave; in atrial reentry, P wave configuration slightly different	Variable, depending on site of ectopic focus
Functional bundle branch block	Rare	Common	Absent	Absent
AV block	Very rare	Never	Possible	Possible
Onset	Abrupt; initiated by crucially timed atrial premature beat	Abrupt; initiated by crucially timed atrial premature beat	Abrupt; initiated by crucially timed atrial premature beat	Unpredictable; no relation to atrial premature beats
Cessation	Abrupt	Abrupt	Abrupt	Unpredictable
Critical AV conduction time needed for initiation	Yes	Yes	No	No

present, the patient's head and neck should be extended slightly by placing a small pillow under the shoulders when the patient is supine. The head is next rotated very slightly away from the side to be massaged. The carotid sinus is then located by palpation; it lies at the point of maximum pulsation of the carotid artery in the neck, usually just lateral to the thyroid cartilage. Under constant electrocardiographic surveillance, firm pressure is applied for 10 to 20 sec and then released.

In terminating paroxysmal atrial tachycardia, right carotid sinus massage is more likely to be successful than left carotid sinus massage. If massage of the right carotid sinus does not work, left carotid sinus pressure should be attempted; however, the carotid sinuses should never be compressed simultaneously.

Additional vagal maneuvers include the induction of gagging by touching the posterior pharynx with a tongue blade. A Valsalva maneuver successfully terminates the tachycardia in many patients [*see Figure 17*].

If these simple approaches fail, pharmacologic or electrical therapy is necessary. The following measures are recommended in descending order of preference:

1. Intravenous verapamil. This calcium channel blocker is currently the treatment of choice for termination of acute episodes of paroxysmal supraventricular tachycardia.[56] The drug is effective in more than 90 percent of cases of reentry involving the AV node alone or the AV node in conjunction with retrograde conduction over a concealed, extranodal bypass tract. Verapamil terminates supraventricular tachycardia in these situations by producing block in the antegrade AV nodal limb of the reentry pathway.

   Verapamil should be administered in a dose of 5 to 10 mg (0.075–0.15 mg/kg) as an intravenous bolus over one to three minutes. Conversion to sinus rhythm usually occurs within 10 minutes. If no effect is observed, vagal maneuvers should be repeated, and if ineffective, the same dose may be repeated in 30 minutes. The blood pressure as well as the heart rate and rhythm should be observed closely during administration of the drug. Cardiovascular side effects associated with the use of verapamil include sinus bradycardia and transient asystole on conversion (especially in patients with preexisting sinus node dysfunction), AV block, hypotension, and exacerbation of heart failure. The drug should not be used intravenously in conjunction with beta-adrenergic blocking agents, in patients with sick sinus syndrome (unless a pacemaker is in place), or in patients with heart failure unrelated to the rapid heart rate.

2. Intravenous propranolol. This drug is given in an initial dose of 1 mg, with increments of 1 mg every five minutes until conversion occurs or a total dose of 0.1 mg/kg (5 to 10 mg in the average adult) has been administered.

3. Rapid intravenous digitalization. Commonly used cardiac glycosides are digoxin, 0.5 mg; lanatoside C, 0.8 mg; or ouabain, 0.5 mg. If tachycardia persists, then vagal maneuvers should be repeated 10 to 30 minutes after administration of the drug. Digitalis should be used cautiously if the surface ECG suggests a high likelihood of antegrade conduction over an extranodal bypass tract. In such patients, digitalis can block conduction through the AV node while decreasing refractoriness of the bypass pathway; rapid conduction down the accessory

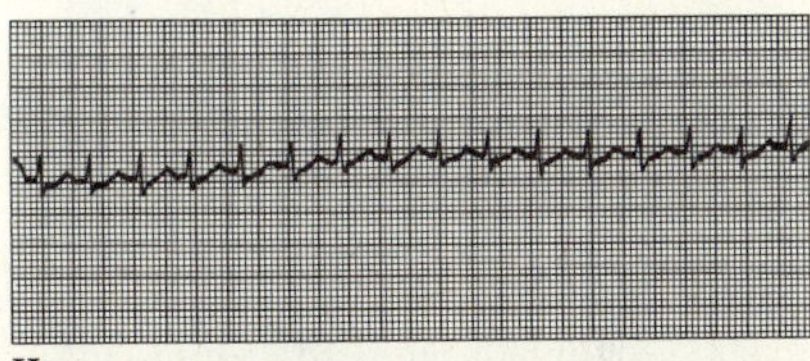

II

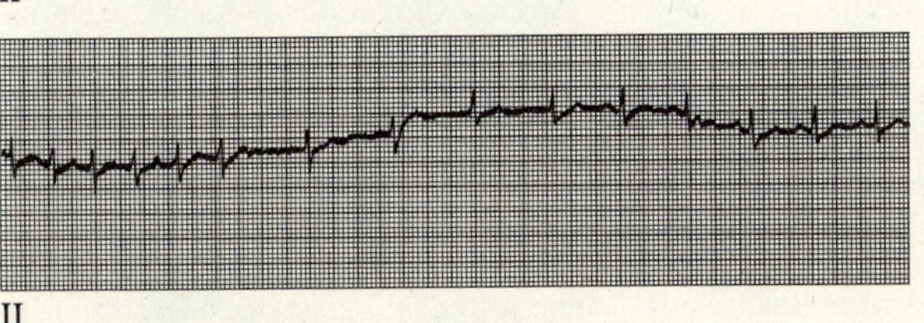

II

Figure 17 *A paroxysm of supraventricular tachycardia (upper panel) is terminated by a Valsalva maneuver, the duration of which is indicated by an arrow in the lower panel. After conversion, there is a transient junctional rhythm followed by a sinus tachycardia.*

pathway is facilitated, and occasionally, ventricular fibrillation can result.

4. Edrophonium chloride. The usual dose is 5 to 10 mg intravenously. This drug exerts its peak effect in one to three minutes and is generally dissipated in 10 to 15 minutes. Some patients experience nausea, cramps, increased salivation, or hypotension as manifestations of increased parasympathetic activity and should be informed of their possible occurrence before the drug is given.

5. Other antiarrhythmic drugs. Other antiarrhythmics, including lidocaine and procainamide, are occasionally successful in converting paroxysmal atrial tachycardia. Lidocaine, 1 mg/kg, may be given as an intravenous bolus; intravenous procainamide, 100 mg every two minutes to conversion or to a total dose of 2 g, may also be tried. The experimental drug adenosine appears to be a highly specific and effective agent for terminating acute episodes of reentrant supraventricular tachycardias.[57] Adenosine is administered intravenously and acts by producing selective conduction delay and block within the AV node. Although it also commonly causes transient sinus arrest, this action is not usually a problem, because the drug is rapidly metabolized and the effect of a single bolus injection dissipates within seconds.

6. Vasopressors. It is possible, by abruptly increasing arterial blood pressure pharmacologically, to stimulate the carotid sinus reflex and thereby terminate the arrhythmia. Vasopressors used to treat paroxysmal supraventricular tachycardia include phenylephrine, 0.5 to 1.5 mg, or methoxamine hydrochloride, 5 to 10 mg, in a direct intravenous injection for a period of two minutes. Alternatively, a more dilute sustained infusion of a vasopressor drug may permit better control of the increasing blood pressure than would direct intravenous injection. For example, metaraminol bitartrate, 100 mg in 500 ml of five percent dextrose in water, may be administered in this manner and the infusion titrated against the blood pressure.

The therapeutic goal is to raise the blood pressure to normal or slightly above normal levels; for example, a systolic pressure of 150 to 160 mm Hg with a diastolic pressure of 90 to 100 mm Hg. The vasopressor must be stopped immediately if conversion occurs or if the blood pressure becomes excessively elevated. Blood pressure must be monitored very carefully, and an alpha-adrenergic antagonist, such as phentolamine, 1 to 3 mg, should be available for instant intravenous use to counteract any potentially dangerous hypertension. A common consequence of an excessive blood pressure response to vasopressors is severe occipital headache; fatal intracerebral hemorrhages have occurred from their use. For these reasons and because of the availability of safer therapeutic alternatives, the use of vasopressors is not recommended for the treatment of paroxysmal supraventricular tachycardia.

7. Electrical therapy. Synchronized external cardioversion [*see* Cardioversion, *below*] will almost always convert paroxysmal supraventricular tachycardia when other measures fail, although it is exceedingly rare that the interventions listed above, either singly or in combination, will not terminate this group of arrhythmias. Cardioversion is the initial treatment of choice in those rare instances in which paroxysmal supraventricular tachycardia is associated with marked hypotension, severe angina, or cardiovascular collapse. It is contraindicated when digitalis toxicity is suspected as a cause of arrhythmia.

Premature or rapid atrial stimulation using an external stimulator and a temporary transvenous atrial electrode is also often effective in terminating most forms of paroxysmal supraventricular tachycardia. This technique may be used as an alternative to elective cardioversion, particularly in hospitalized patients in whom frequent episodes of tachycardia occur within a short interval of time.

There are many recommended therapies for the long-term suppression of paroxysmal supraventricular tachycardia. Oral verapamil may be used in doses ranging from 80 to 160 mg three or four times a day. Because of its depressant effects on ventricular function, AV nodal conduction, and sinus node automaticity, verapamil should be used with caution in the presence of beta-blockers; its use with disopyramide is contraindicated. Verapamil may be used in conjunction with digitalis, but careful monitoring is indicated, particularly during the initiation of therapy. Studies indicate that chronic oral administration of verapamil may increase digoxin blood levels. Verapamil blood levels are increased by the concomitant use of beta-blocking agents or cimetidine, both of which slow the metabolism of verapamil by decreasing hepatic blood flow. Noncardiac side effects that may be seen during chronic oral therapy include headache, dizziness, nausea, constipation, and skin rash.

Other agents that may be effective for long-term suppression of paroxysmal supraventricular tachycardia include digitalis glycosides, quinidine, procainamide, disopyramide, beta blockers, flecainide, and amiodarone; because of its toxicity, however, amiodarone should be used only in highly selected patients in whom the benefits of the drug clearly outweigh its risks. These drugs can be used singly or in combination. The addition of a beta blocker to a class IA drug such as quinidine, procainamide, or disopyramide frequently enhances the antiarrhythmic action of the latter and also blunts the effects of sympathetic neural stimulation on the rate of supraventricular tachycardia.

Electrophysiologic studies may be important adjuncts to therapy in patients with frequently disabling recurrent paroxysmal supraventricular tachycardia, in those who have particularly fast heart rates during the tachycardia (e.g., 180 to 230 beats/min), or in those who have experienced syncope during attacks. By the use of programmed electrical stimulation combined with intracardiac recordings, it is usually possible to reproduce the attacks, to determine sites of reentry and direction of conduction, to measure refractory periods and conduction velocities of the pathways participating in the reentry, and to assess the effects of various drug regimens in suppressing the ability to induce and sustain the attacks.[27,52] In patients with drug-resistant paroxysmal supraventricular tachycardia, electrophysiologic studies may be used to try to select appropriate patients for antitachycardia pacemaker therapy [*see* Pacemakers and Automatic Defibrillators for Arrhythmias, *below*]. In patients with extranodal bypass tracts and life-threatening arrhythmias, electrophysiologic studies may also indicate the location of the bypass tract and whether interruption of the aberrant bundle is indicated.[55]

Transcatheter electrical ablation has been employed by several centers to produce AV block in selected, highly symptomatic patients with drug-resistant supraventricular tachyarrhythmias, such as atrial flutter or fibrillation. This technique involves the delivery of high-energy electrical discharges between one pole of an electrode catheter positioned near the bundle of His and a second electrode on the body surface. The procedure produces high-degree AV block and thereby achieves rate control in a large majority of patients. Permanent pacemaker implantation is required following this procedure.[58-60] Low-energy transcatheter electrical shocks can eliminate or favorably modify AV conduction in patients with drug-resistant supraventricular tachyarrhythmias. It appears that the low-energy shocks may favorably influence the spontaneous tachycardia without producing complete heart block and pacemaker dependency; they may also be safer than high-energy shocks.[22] At present, however, permanent pacemakers are inserted in patients who have received low-energy shocks because the long-term stability of their AV conduction is uncertain.

Paroxysmal Atrial Tachycardia With Block

Paroxysmal atrial tachycardia with block is manifested as an automatic atrial tachycardia with varying degrees of AV block [*see Figure 18*]. Sometimes, the AV block is latent and is elicited by carotid sinus pressure. The atrial rate is generally between 130 and 200 beats/min; the ventricular rate is dependent on the degree of block. Carotid sinus pressure either has no effect on the arrhythmia or increases the AV block. P waves are usually seen best in precordial leads. The atrial rhythm may be slightly irregular, and a clear-cut flat base line usually follows the ectopic P waves, in contrast to the constant base-line activity characteristic of atrial flutter.

Etiology

About three quarters of all cases of paroxysmal atrial tachycardia with block are the result of digitalis toxicity. Patients with chronic obstructive lung disease are particularly prone to develop this arrhythmia, usually as a manifestation of digitalis toxicity. In the absence of digitalis intoxication, this arrhythmia may arise if paroxysmal atrial tachycardia develops in persons who also have disease of the AV node.

Therapy

When paroxysmal atrial tachycardia with block is caused by digitalis toxicity, the drug should of course be stopped immediately, and the serum potassium level should be brought to an upper normal range (4.5 to 5.0 mEq/l). Intravenous phenytoin is very effective in converting paroxysmal atrial tachycardia with block caused by digitalis toxicity. It is given in a dosage of 100 mg intravenously every five minutes until the arrhythmia is converted or a total of 600 mg has been given. Intravenous phenytoin is dissolved in a solution that is very caustic and should be administered at a very slow rate, preferably in normal saline. Intravenous propranolol may also be effective in converting paroxysmal atrial tachycardia with block caused by digitalis toxicity, although its use is generally contraindicated in patients with obstructive lung disease.

When paroxysmal atrial tachycardia with block is not caused by digitalis toxicity, the therapy is generally the same as that outlined earlier [*see* Paroxysmal Supraventricular Tachycardia, *above*].

Nonparoxysmal AV Junctional Tachycardia

Nonparoxysmal AV junctional tachycardia is an automatic rhythm caused by discharge of an ectopic focus in the area of the AV node and junction. Because the atria and ventricles are discharged simultaneously, the arrhythmia closely mimics paroxysmal supraventricular tachycardia that is due to reentry in the AV node. Thus, QRS com-

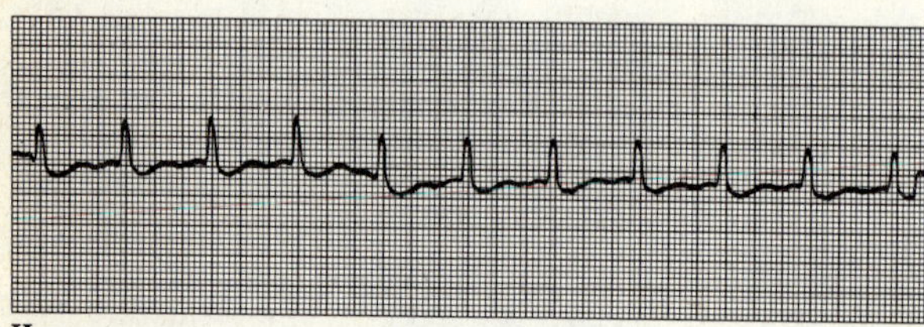

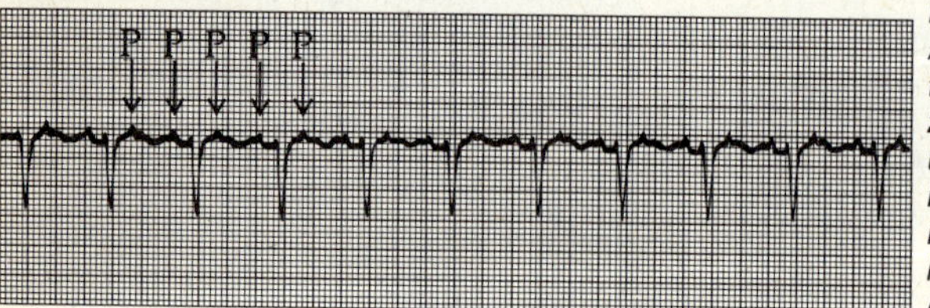

Figure 18　*Electrocardiogram demonstrates paroxysmal atrial tachycardia with 2:1 AV block in a patient with digitalis toxicity. The atrial rate is 200 beats/min, and the ventricular rate is 100 beats/min. As is usually the case, the arrhythmia is more easily seen in one of the precordial leads (lead V1, bottom) than in a limb lead (lead II, top).*

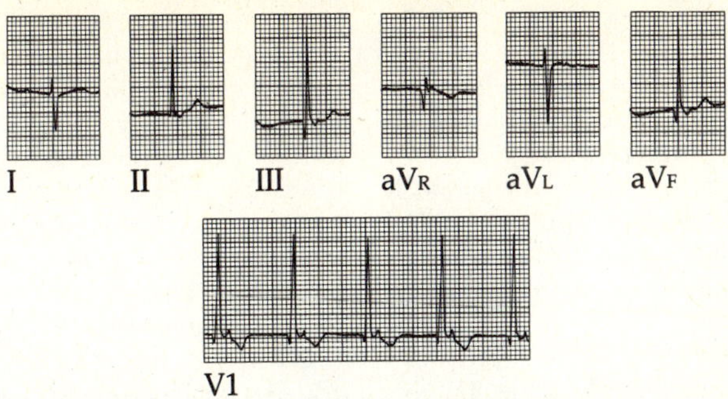

Figure 19   *Chronic accelerated AV junctional rhythm (95 beats/min) was detected in a 10-year-old child who, as an infant, had undergone a Mustard procedure for complete transposition of the great vessels. Presumably, the sinus node was injured as a result of the operation. P waves immediately follow the QRS complexes. The frontal plane P wave axis is approximately -90° , and leads II, III, and aVF show inverted P waves.*

plexes are of normal duration unless there is preexisting bundle branch block. P waves are retrograde and closely related to the QRS complexes [*see Figure 19*]. The rate of nonparoxysmal AV junctional tachycardia tends to be slow—between 70 and 150 beats/min—and the discharge rate of the ectopic focus may vary greatly. The arrhythmia may come and go in a haphazard fashion. It is not usually responsive to vagal maneuvers.

Etiology

Nonparoxysmal AV junctional tachycardia is usually encountered as a consequence of an acute ischemic, infectious, or inflammatory process involving the heart, such as acute myocardial infarction or acute myocarditis. It sometimes develops after cardiac surgery and is an occasional cardiac manifestation of drug toxicity, especially from the digitalis glycosides.

Clinical Manifestations

Because the rate of nonparoxysmal AV junctional tachycardia is slow in comparison with other tachyarrhythmias, it is usually well tolerated. However, since it is often encountered in patients with significant cardiac dysfunction, the loss of atrial contraction may cause a significant fall in cardiac output. Constant cannon waves are usually present in the venous pulses. Heart sounds are uniform.

Therapy

Treatment of the arrhythmia is usually directed at the underlying disorder: for example, treatment would consist of withholding digitalis and potassium replacement if the arrhythmia results from digitalis toxicity. Antiarrhythmic drugs, such as quinidine, procainamide, or beta-adrenergic blocking drugs, can effectively suppress the ectopic focus. If suppression is warranted, these antiarrhythmic agents can be used. If hemodynamic compromise is present, atrial pacing may suppress the ectopic focus and restore atrial transport.

Multifocal Atrial Tachycardia

Multifocal atrial tachycardia is characterized by an irregular supraventricular rhythm, at rates between 100 and 200 beats/min. The atrial activity is totally chaotic, and the morphology of the P waves varies from beat to beat, as does the PR interval [*see Figure 20*]. Each QRS complex, however, is preceded by a P wave. As is the case with paroxysmal atrial tachycardia, multifocal atrial tachycardia may also exist with varying degrees of AV block. The arrhythmia is unaffected by carotid sinus pressure.

Etiology

Multifocal atrial tachycardia is generally found in patients who are seriously ill with other diseases, particularly elderly patients who are experiencing respiratory failure; it may also occur following a major surgical procedure.[61] Rarely, multifocal atrial tachycardia is a manifestation of digitalis toxicity.

Therapy

Therapy is best directed at the underlying disease. The arrhythmia itself usually does not cause any significant consequences. Digitalis is not indicated unless the patient's underlying problem—for example, congestive heart failure—also warrants its administration. Verapamil can be administered if treatment of the arrhythmia itself is considered necessary. This drug reduces both the atrial and ventricular rates and occasionally converts multifocal atrial tachycardia to sinus rhythm.[62]

Atrial Flutter

Atrial flutter exhibits an absolutely regular atrial rate at 250 to 320 beats/min, with varying degrees of AV block. In untreated atrial flutter, 2:1 block is usual [*see Figures 2 and 21*].

The base line of the electrocardiogram in flutter displays a continuous movement (producing a sawtooth configuration). The axis of the flutter waves is generally -30° to -60°, and flutter is best seen in leads II, III, and aVF. This arrhythmia differs from paroxysmal atrial tachycardia with block, with which it may be confused, in that the atrial rate is faster. Another differential point is that in paroxysmal atrial tachycardia with block the base line after nonconducted P waves is usually flat and the P waves are usually upright in leads II, III, and aVF.

When patients with atrial flutter are treated with antiarrhythmic drugs, such as quinidine, the atrial rate may slow to less than 200 impulses/min. The arrhythmia then closely resembles paroxysmal atrial tachycardia with block, although the base line still shows continuous motion rather than discrete P waves.

Etiology

Atrial flutter may occur as a paroxysmal arrhythmia in persons with normal hearts. It has been associated with chronic obstructive lung disease, pulmonary embolism, alcoholism, thyrotoxicosis, and mitral valve disease and has been reported to result from myocardial infarction and thoracic and cardiac surgery.

Clinical Manifestations

When atrial flutter first develops, it generally presents as an absolutely regular rhythm with a ventricular rate of 125 to 150

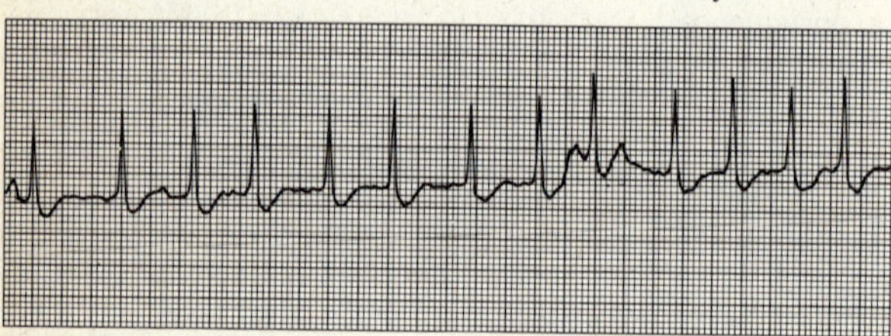

II

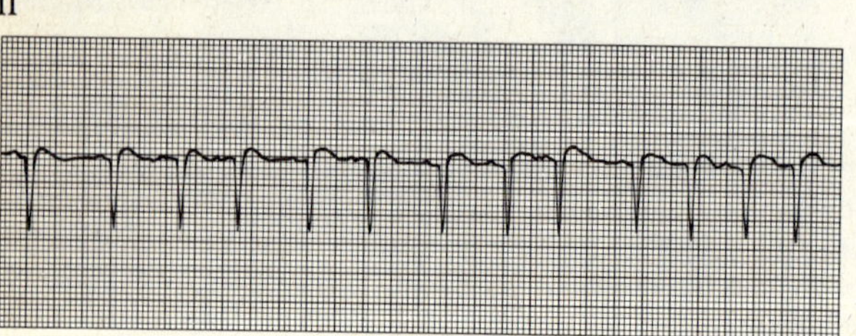

V1

Figure 20 *Electrocardiogram in a patient with pneumonia and an old anterior wall infarct shows evidence of multifocal atrial tachycardia. Leads II (upper panel) and V1 (lower panel) reveal an irregular rhythm at a rate of approximately 100 beats/min with P waves of varying morphology and changing PR intervals.*

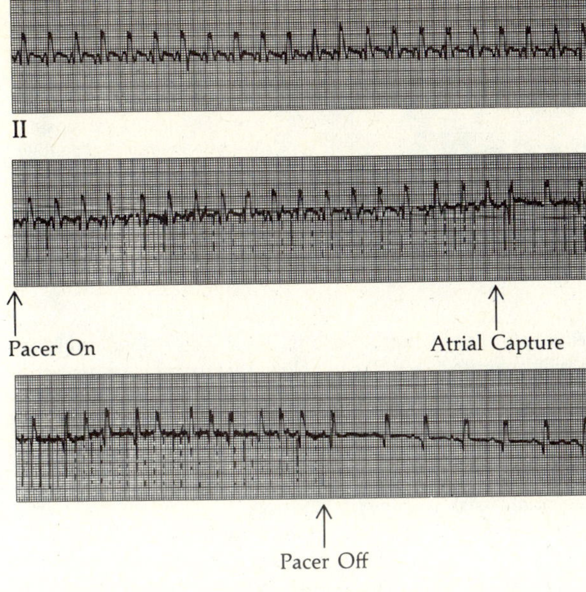

Figure 21 *Atrial flutter with 2:1 AV block is terminated by rapid atrial stimulation. The flutter (upper panel) developed after open heart surgery; prior to stimulation, the atrial rate is 280 beats/min and the ventricular rate is 140 beats/min. In the middle panel, atrial pacing is initiated (first arrow) at a rate of 180 impulses/min and then increased to 360 impulses/min. At the second arrow, the ventricular response becomes irregular, indicating that the arrhythmia has been broken. In the lower panel, the pacer is discontinued (arrow), followed by the emergence of sinus rhythm at a rate of 85 beats/min.*

beats/min. Close inspection of the jugular venous pulses sometimes reveals the presence of flutter waves occurring at a rate of 250 to 320 beats/min. Because atrial flutter results in a somewhat coordinated atrial contraction, a fourth heart sound may be heard. Carotid sinus massage either has no effect or increases the degree of AV block.

Therapy

Atrial flutter can pose a challenging management problem, and treatment of combined atrial flutter and 2:1 block is particularly difficult. Therapy may be aimed at conversion of the arrhythmia or at control of the ventricular rate. If the arrhythmia is paroxysmal, therapy should be directed at conversion. If conversion of the arryhthmia is impossible or if the arrhythmia is recurrent, an effort should be made to control the ventricular rate pharmacologically.

In the initial management of paroxysmal atrial flutter, it is our policy to give a short-acting digitalis glycoside intravenously (such as digoxin, 0.5 mg; ouabain, 0.5 mg; or lanatoside C, 0.8 mg) with the hope of converting the arrhythmia.[63] Intravenous pro-

pranolol or intravenous verapamil (used separately) may be added [*see* Paroxysmal Supraventricular Tachycardia, *above*] if there is no contraindication to its use. This pharmacologic approach may be successful either in converting the arrhythmia or in increasing the degree of AV block. With the above drugs, paroxysmal atrial flutter can be converted in about one fourth of cases.

If the initial pharmacologic efforts at conversion are unsuccessful, rather than administering additional digitalis to control the ventricular rate, we prefer to proceed directly to cardioversion. A synchronized direct-current shock, often at low-energy levels (25 to 100 watt-sec), is almost invariably successful in stopping atrial flutter.

When flutter is recurrent or when it cannot be terminated electrically, an attempt should be made to achieve control of the ventricular rate by giving increments of digitalis glycosides, with or without propranolol or verapamil. Frequently, large quantities of digitalis may be needed to slow the ventricular rate. Sometimes, carotid sinus massage can offer a useful clue as to whether adequate rate control is near. As the

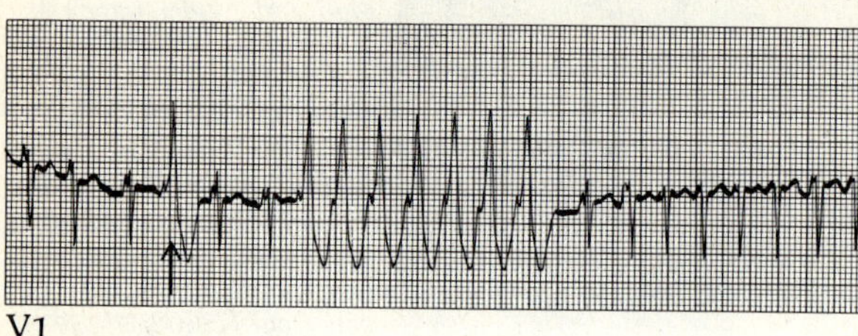

Figure 22   *Aberrant ventricular conduction is seen in a patient with atrial fibrillation and a rapid ventricular response. The first aberrant beat (arrow) follows a slight pause, as does the run of aberrantly conducted beats. Note that the slight irregularity of the underlying atrial fibrillation persists during the run.*

dosage of digitalis approaches the effective range, carotid sinus massage will begin to provoke AV block; slowing of the heart rate will soon follow the administration of additional digitalis.

Rapid atrial stimulation may be successful in the treatment of paroxysmal atrial flutter. In this technique, the right atrium is stimulated at a rate between 180 and 1,200 impulses/min. Rapid atrial stimulation may convert atrial flutter either to sinus rhythm [*see Figure 21*] or to atrial fibrillation—an arrhythmia that allows better control of the ventricular rate and that often reverts spontaneously to normal sinus rhythm. This approach is especially useful in the management of flutter in cardiac surgical patients, most of whom have temporary atrial electrodes. It may also be valuable in patients who are not candidates for cardioversion, such as those who exhibit digitalis toxicity. In such cases, an electrode can be guided into the right atrium for rapid atrial stimulation. It is crucial to ensure that the electrode is in the right atrium and not in the right ventricle because ventricular stimulation at these rates could be fatal.

For the prevention of recurrent atrial flutter, an oral digitalis preparation alone may suffice. Additional antiarrhythmic therapy, however, such as quinidine, 200 to 300 mg every six hours, disopyramide, 100 to 250 mg every eight hours, or propranolol, 20 to 60 mg every six hours, may be necessary.

Atrial Fibrillation

Atrial fibrillation is manifested as totally chaotic atrial activity at a rate of 350 to 500 impulses/min, with a correspondingly irregular but slower ventricular response. In untreated atrial fibrillation, the ventricular rate is frequently 140 to 170 beats/min.

In cases of atrial fibrillation, regularization of the ventricular response or the presence of a slow ventricular rate with ventricular premature beats should raise the question of digitalis toxicity.

Atrial fibrillation is occasionally associated with the Ashman phenomenon, which is manifested by aberrant conduction of the beat following a beat that has been preceded by a long pause [*see Figure 22*]. The Ashman phenomenon almost invariably exhibits the configuration of right bundle branch block. The electrophysiologic explanation of the Ashman phenomenon lies in the fact that the refractory period of the bundle branches is increased by the long pause, with that of the right bundle being prolonged more than that of the left. The impulse after the pause is conducted normally, but the next impulse finds the right bundle branch refractory and so is conducted with a pattern of right bundle branch block.

Because Ashman beats can be confused with ventricular premature beats, their identification is important. The differentiation can normally be made by the usual criteria for distinguishing aberrant ventricular conduction from ventricular ectopy [*see* Ventricular Arrhythmias, Differentiation of Supraventricular Arrhythmia with Aberrancy from Ventricular Arrhythmia, *below*]. In addition, the coupling intervals between normally conducted and aberrant beats will vary considerably in the Ashman phenomenon, with the beats falling into the irregular pattern of the underlying atrial fibrillation.

Etiology

Atrial fibrillation is often part of the bradycardia-tachycardia syndrome. It is common in the elderly and in patients with rheumatic mitral valve disease, coronary artery disease, cardiomyopathy, or thyrotoxicosis. It often occurs after thoracic and cardiac surgery. Alcohol increases the vulnerability of the heart to the electrophysiological induction of atrial flutter and fibrillation.[64]

Clinical Manifestations

There are no symptoms that are unique to atrial fibrillation. When this arrhythmia starts, patients are often aware of a rapid heartbeat. Because atrial contractions are not coordinated, the jugular venous pulses do not show evidence of atrial activity. The cardiac rhythm is irregular, and the intensity of heart sounds and associated murmurs varies greatly because of this irregularity. Signs of the underlying heart disease are often noted, particularly those associated with mitral valve disease.

The loss of atrial transport, combined with the rapid heart rate, may substantially reduce cardiac output and even precipitate congestive heart failure in patients with atrial fibrillation. In certain diseases, such as hypertrophic cardiomyopathy, in which atrial contraction is especially important for proper ventricular filling, the onset of atrial fibrillation is often tolerated very poorly.

Antiarrhythmic Therapy

Initial therapy for atrial fibrillation should be digitalization; preferably, the digitalis should be given intravenously. Because digitalis increases AV block, the ventricular rate is a good guide to the adequacy of digitalization. Ordinarily, a ventricular rate of 70 to 90 beats/min is considered adequate. An attempt should be made to keep the heart rate during exercise below 140 to 150 beats/min. Allowance should be made for factors that might drive the heart at a faster rate. For example, in a seriously ill patient, a resting heart rate of 110 to 130 beats/min may represent adequate rate control.

Propranolol may be used in combination with digitalis glycosides to control the acute and the long-term ventricular rate. For intravenous use, propranolol is given in doses of 0.025 to 0.1 mg/kg. For long-term oral therapy, initial dosages are 10 to 60 mg every six hours. Other beta blockers may be as effective as propranolol but little use has been made of them in the treatment of atrial fibrillation. Intravenous verapamil may also be effective in slowing the ventricular rate acutely; it is given in a dose of 0.075 to 0.15 mg/kg over two to three minutes. Oral verapamil (80 to 120 mg q 6 to 8 hr) can also be used for long-term control of the ventricular rate when digitalis glycosides alone are inadequate.

In the conversion of atrial fibrillation to normal sinus rhythm, initial digitalization is successful about 20 percent of the time in patients not previously in atrial fibrillation, and propranolol may enhance the success rate. If fibrillation persists, cardioversion or pharmacological conversion to sinus rhythm, with quinidine being the drug of choice, is recommended.

Quinidine may be given in a variety of ways, but our preference is to prescribe 200 mg orally every two hours for five doses on the first day and 300 mg every two hours for five doses on the second day. On each day, the first dose of quinidine is given at 7:00 A.M. and the last at 3:00 P.M. Some cardiologists consider this method to be antiquated, but an advantage of this approach is that any problems caused by the use of quinidine occur during the part of the day when the largest number of personnel equipped to handle such problems are available. Furthermore, if conversion does not ensue and no adverse reaction has developed, an extra dose of 200 to 300 mg of quinidine can be given between 7:00 and 8:00 P.M.

Under an alternate schedule, 200 mg of quinidine is given every four hours for one day and, if conversion has not occurred, 300 mg is given every four hours for a second day. If atrial fibrillation does not respond to these amounts of quinidine, cardioversion should be undertaken because this method is far safer than the administration of still higher doses of quinidine.

Several other antiarrhythmic drugs, including procainamide, disopyramide, flecainide, and amiodarone, may be used in selected patients for the conversion of atrial fibrillation and for long-term prophylaxis. Guidelines for these drugs, which are approved primarily for the treatment of ventricular arrhythmias, are discussed later.

Many cardiologists use cardioversion as the initial method of choice in converting atrial fibrillation. Several factors appear to favor success both in the initial conversion and in the subsequent maintenance of sinus rhythm. These factors include atrial fibrillation of less than six months' duration, small left atrial size, mitral stenosis rather than mitral regurgitation if mitral valve disease is the underlying problem, and an onset after cardiac or thoracic surgery [see Cardioversion, below].

Antithrombotic Therapy

A potentially serious problem in patients with atrial fibrillation is systemic embolism. Patients with nonrheumatic atrial fibrillation have a five times greater risk of stroke than the general population.[64a]

In one randomized, controlled but unblinded study of nonrheumatic atrial fibrillation, long-term, low-dose warfarin therapy (average duration, 2.2 years; prothrombin time increased to an INR of 1.5 to 2.7) reduced the risk of stroke by 86 percent.[64b] Specifically, two strokes occurred among 212 patients in the warfarin group, compared with 13 strokes among 208 patients in the untreated control group. An antithrombotic effect of aspirin was not identified in this study. (Only patients in the control group were free to take aspirin.) Eight of the 13 strokes in the control group occurred among patients taking aspirin, seven of whom took at least 325 mg/day. The frequency of bleeding was the same in the two groups.

A preliminary study comparing warfarin and aspirin found a similar reduction in risk with warfarin (INR of 2.0 to 3.5).[64c] The 1,244 patients in this randomized, placebo-controlled study of nonrheumatic and non–prosthetic valve atrial fibrillation were followed for an average of 1.13 years. Aspirin (325 mg/day) benefited patients younger than 75 years.

It is recommended that patients with atrial fibrillation who have suffered systemic embolism should receive warfarin therapy at a dosage that achieves an INR of 3.0 to 4.5.[65] However, decisions regarding the use of antithrombotic therapy should be based on consideration of the patient's comorbid conditions as well as assessment of the patient's overall health.

Atrial fibrillation and valvular heart disease Long-term warfarin therapy should be used in patients with atrial fibrillation and associated mitral valve disease.

Atrial fibrillation and nonvalvular heart disease Long-term oral warfarin therapy to prolong the prothrombin time to an INR of 2.0 to 3.0 should be instituted in patients with cardiomyopathy-associated atrial fibrillation. Long-term warfarin therapy to prolong the prothrombin time to an INR of 2.0 to 3.0 may be considered in young patients who are not at increased risk for hemorrhagic complications. When congestive heart failure is present in patients with nonvalvular heart disease complicated by atrial fibrillation, long-term warfarin to prolong the prothrombin time to an INR of 2.0 to 3.0 should be considered because of the increased risk of pulmonary embolism and left ventricular mural thrombi.

Atrial fibrillation and thyrotoxic heart disease Warfarin therapy to prolong the prothrombin time to an INR of 2.0 to 3.0 should be instituted in patients with atrial fibrillation and thyrotoxicosis, and therapy should be continued for four weeks after conversion to sinus rhythm and the reestablishment of the euthyroid state.

Idiopathic (lone) atrial fibrillation Patients with idiopathic atrial fibrillation without associated heart disease (so-called lone AF) should not receive long-term antithrombotic therapy.

Atrial fibrillation and cardioversion Warfarin therapy to prolong the prothrombin time to an INR of 2.0 to 3.0 should be given for three weeks before elective cardioversion of patients who have been in atrial fibrillation for more than two days and should be continued until normal sinus rhythm has been maintained for at least four weeks. Antithrombotic therapy is not recommended for cardioversion of atrial flutter or supraventricular tachycardia or for cardioversion of patients who have been in atrial fibrillation for less than three days unless other risk factors for systemic embolism are present.

Preexcitation Syndromes

Since the late 1960s, spectacular advances have been made in elucidating the mechanisms of preexcitation syndromes and in delineating the genesis and treatment of the associated arrhythmias.

Preexcitation has been defined as a condition in which all or some portion of the ventricle is activated by atrial impulses earlier than if the impulses were to reach the ventricles by way of the normal cardiac conduction pathways.[66] Although this definition covers most cases of preexcitation, it appears that a few instances are caused by accelerated conduction within the AV node itself. Classically, the electrocardiogram shows a short PR interval followed by a wide QRS complex with a slurred initial deflection, or delta wave, that represents early ventricular activation. This electrocardiographic pattern characterizes the Wolff-Parkinson-White syndrome, but many variations of preexcitation have been observed.

Incidence

The incidence of preexcitation has been estimated at between 0.1 and three percent of the population.[67] The Wolff-Parkinson-White syndrome is associated with certain congenital cardiac defects, particularly Ebstein's anomaly of the tricuspid valve and corrected transposition of the great vessels. A familial form of the Wolff-Parkinson-White syndrome also has been reported and may be associated with congestive or hypertrophic cardiomyopathy.[68]

Etiology and Mechanism

Preexcitation can occur through a number of different pathways [*see Figure 23*]. The major accessory bypass tracts along which preexcitation occurs include:

1. Kent bundles, which are probably the most common preexcitation pathways, are electrically active muscular fibers bridging the atria and ventricles; they are usually situated near the surface of the heart, close to the anuli of the AV valves.[69] They can be located at just about any point where the atria and ventricles are contiguous. Most often, they occur posteriorly, connecting the left atrium and left ventricle.
2. James fibers. Presumably continuations of the internodal pathways that connect the sinus node and the AV node, the James fibers bypass the AV node and terminate in the common bundle or in the muscle of the interventricular septum.[70] These fibers shunt impulses around the AV node, circumventing the locus at which the major delay in AV conduction occurs.
3. Mahaim fibers. These are fibers that can pass from the AV node, the bundle of His, or either of the bundle branches directly into the interventricular septum. They short-circuit the cardiac impulse, causing it to deviate from its normal course and activate the septal muscle mass prematurely.

Electrocardiographic Characteristics

A variety of electrocardiographic patterns result from preexcitation. Two major patterns associated with the Wolff-Parkinson-White syndrome have been distinguished and are commonly designated as

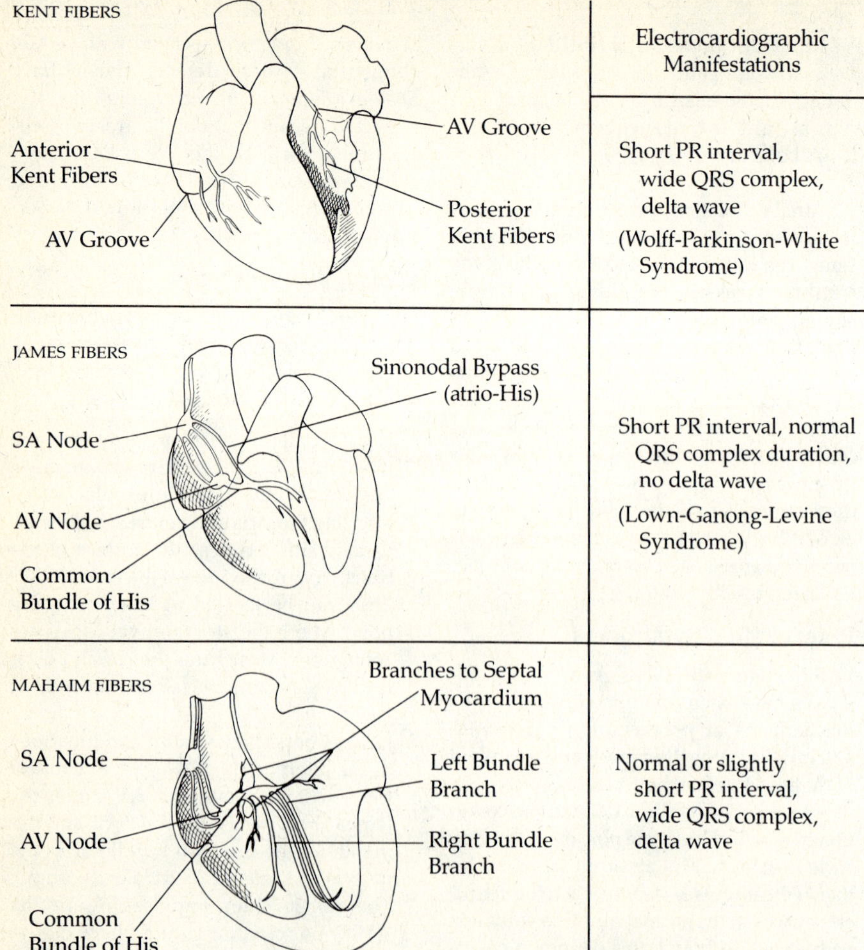

Figure 23 *Preexcitation may result from conduction of the cardiac impulse via any one of the three major anomalous pathways shown at left: the Kent fibers, the James fibers, or the Mahaim fibers. The electrocardiographic manifestations of this syndrome differ depending on the specific mechanism of preexcitation. The Kent fibers are electrically active muscular bridges that connect the atria and the ventricles. These tracts may be located anywhere on the circumference of the heart but most frequently are found posteriorly, bridging the left atrium and left ventricle. Less commonly, they connect the right atrium and right ventricle. The James fibers short-circuit the AV node and attach to the common bundle. Finally, Mahaim fibers are structures that shunt the impulse from the common bundle or either bundle branch into the interventricular septal myocardium.*

type A and type B. The classic alphabetic terminology for the electrocardiographic patterns (i.e., type A or B), however, is being gradually replaced by a more specific designation based on the anatomic location of the accessory pathway (e.g., left posterior, right anterior, left septal). A left-sided bundle of Kent that activates the posterosuperior portion of the left ventricle causes a delta wave that is directed anteriorly and rightward, and the electrocardiographic pattern mimics that of right bundle branch block (type

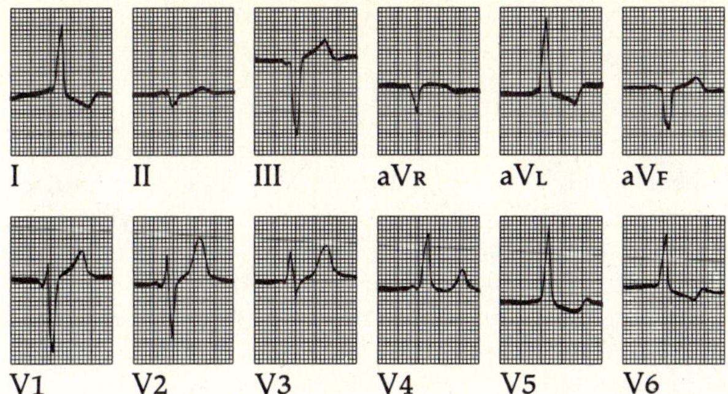

Figure 24   *The electrocardiographic pattern in patients with the Wolff-Parkinson-White syndrome type B resembles left bundle branch block. The anomalous pathway connects the right atrium and the right ventricle. The ST segment and T wave abnormalities are meaningless in the presence of the aberrant conduction.*

A). Conversely, when preexcitation is caused by impulse conduction over an anterior bundle of Kent, the anterosuperior portion of the right ventricle is the first area of ventricle to be activated; the delta wave is thus pointed posteriorly and to the left. The electrocardiographic pattern [*see Figure* 24] resembles that of left bundle branch block (type B). At the same time that the ventricle is being activated by the anomalous pathway, the normal cardiac impulse travels over the AV node and the His-Purkinje system. Therefore, the terminal portion of the QRS complex often represents later ventricular activation by way of the normal pathways, and the final impulse is a fusion beat: a beat that represents fusion of the delta wave that results from early ventricular depolarization with the QRS complex of normal AV conduction.

If the atrial impulse is conducted to the common bundle over James fibers, a short PR interval with a QRS complex of normal duration (Lown-Ganong-Levine syndrome) will result. Accelerated conduction directly through the AV node will give a similar pattern. If the impulse crosses the AV node normally but is diverted into the septal musculature over the Mahaim fibers, the PR interval will be normal or nearly so, but a ventricular complex initiated by a delta wave will be inscribed; the configuration of the delta wave will depend on the location of the Mahaim fibers. Finally, it is theoretically possible for an impulse to be conducted from the atrium to the common

bundle over the James fibers and then to the ventricles by way of Mahaim fibers, producing the classic Wolff-Parkinson-White pattern: a short PR interval, delta wave, and wide QRS complex.

Clinical Features

It is unknown exactly how many patients with preexcitation have arrhythmias, but one study of the Wolff-Parkinson-White syndrome reported an incidence of 13.3 percent.[67] The incidence, however, may be even higher. The most frequent arrhythmias are paroxysmal supraventricular tachycardias, although atrial fibrillation and atrial flutter also commonly occur.[71]

Usually, the arrhythmias are sporadic and well tolerated, even when ventricular rates are as fast as 250 to 300 beats/min. They are well tolerated because the patients are often young and their hearts are otherwise normal. At times, the frequency and severity of the arrhythmias can be disabling. Also, serious ventricular arrhythmias may result from the supraventricular arrhythmias, and occasionally, sudden cardiac death occurs in patients with the Wolff-Parkinson-White syndrome.

The patients who are most likely to develop ventricular fibrillation in the Wolff-Parkinson-White syndrome usually have a history of both atrial fibrillation and reciprocating (reentrant) tachycardias; they demonstrate rapid conduction over an accessory pathway during atrial fibrillation; and they frequently have multiple accessory bypass pathways that can be demonstrated electrophysiologically.[72]

Electrophysiology of Preexcitation

The electrocardiogram in the Wolff-Parkinson-White syndrome represents a very intricate balance between conduction across normal and anomalous pathways. For example, if the atrium is stimulated electrically near the anomalous pathway, the entire sequence of ventricular activation may take place via the anomalous route. In fact, antegrade conduction across concealed bypass tracts may occasionally be revealed if an area of the atrium immediately adjacent to the pathway is paced.[54] The preexcitation pattern may come and go, and in one series,[67] 47 percent of the patients exhibited it intermittently. Any factor that changes the balance of conduction between the anomalous pathway and the AV node may either augment or abolish the pattern. Increased vagal tone delays conduction across the AV node but has little if any effect on the anomalous pathway. Hence, the administration of a vagolytic drug, such as atropine, may normalize AV conduction. The conduction abnormality may also disappear with exercise.

Cardiac depressants and antiarrhythmic agents have variable effects on normal and abnormal pathways.

It appears that most instances of paroxysmal supraventricular tachycardia associated with preexcitation syndromes are reciprocating in nature.[72,73] The arrhythmias almost invariably are initiated by premature beats that arise in the atria, the AV junction, or the ventricles. Impulses originating in the atrium or junction activate the ventricles via the normal pathway. When the ectopic impulse, regardless of its point of origin, reaches the aberrant pathway, there is antegrade block because of a longer refractory period in the bypass tract than in the AV node. The premature impulse is conducted with delay over the normal conduction system to the ventricles and is then transmitted retrogradely to the atrium via the anomalous pathways, thereby setting sets up a self-propagating tachycardia. A reentry path is thus established involving the atrium, AV node, ventricle, and anomalous pathway [*see Figure 25*].

Because antegrade conduction occurs more readily over the anomalous pathway than over the AV node, tachyarrhythmias in which antegrade conduction to the ventri-

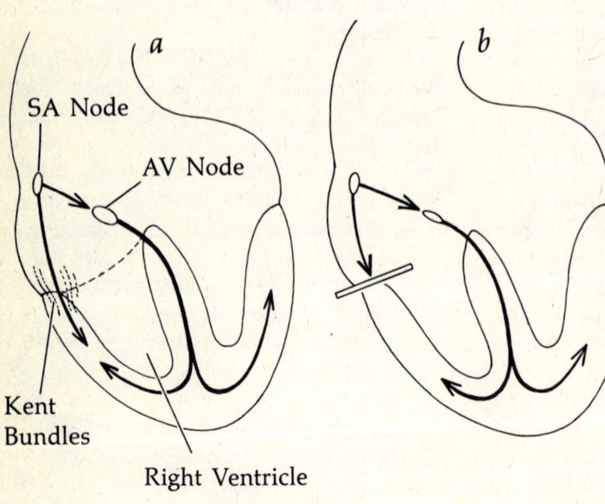

Figure 25 *An atrial premature beat may induce a reentrant supraventricular tachycardia in an individual with conduction over an anomalous pathway. In a, the sinus impulse is conducted antegrade over the Kent bundle and over normal and anomalous pathways via the AV node. The resultant QRS complex would have the Wolff-Parkinson-White configuration. In b, an atrial premature beat is conducted across the AV node but is blocked at the level of the Kent bundle because of the prolonged refractory period of this anomalous pathway. The impulse activates the ventricle along normal conduction pathways.*

cles takes place over the accessory paths may be characterized by exceedingly rapid ventricular rates. This is particularly true in cases of atrial fibrillation, in which rates of 200 to 300 beats/min are common. Because the impulses traverse the anomalous pathways, the conducted beats demonstrate the bizarre Wolff-Parkinson-White QRS pattern [*see Figure 26*]. Many patients with atrial fibrillation have been shown to possess multiple accessory pathways.[73]

Although antegrade conduction over the aberrant pathway may be more rapid than over the AV node, the antegrade refractory period of the accessory pathway is usually longer than that of the AV node. When this is the case, it is almost always possible to produce reciprocating tachycardias by inducing premature atrial beats. Because of the accessory pathway's longer refractory period, the induced premature atrial impulse traverses the receptive AV node rather than the still refractory anomalous bundle. When the impulse finally reaches the Kent bundle, however, the bundle has recovered sufficiently for retrograde conduction to the atrium to occur, and a reciprocating tachycardia ensues [*see Figure 25*].

Application of programmed atrial stimulation and His bundle electrocardiography has yielded a great deal of valuable information about patients with the preexcitation sydrome, particularly about those who suffer from recurrent attacks of tachycardia. By comparing normally conducted beats with paced beats, it is possible to ascertain whether preexcitation is actually present, what portion of the observed ventricular complex is the result of conduction via the anomalous pathway, the effective refractory period of the accessory AV pathway and its contribution to the genesis of arrhythmias, and the location of the accessory pathway. Most important, by introducing programmed atrial beats, it is usually possible to initiate episodes of tachycardia as well.[74,75] These techniques permit assessment of the relative effects of various drugs on conduction over normal and accessory pathways—information that may be valuable clinically.

Which patients with Wolff-Parkinson-White syndrome should undergo electrophysiologic studies? A dogmatic answer cannot be given, but such studies generally should be undertaken in patients who give a history of syncope during attacks; patients who are capable of rapid anomalous path-

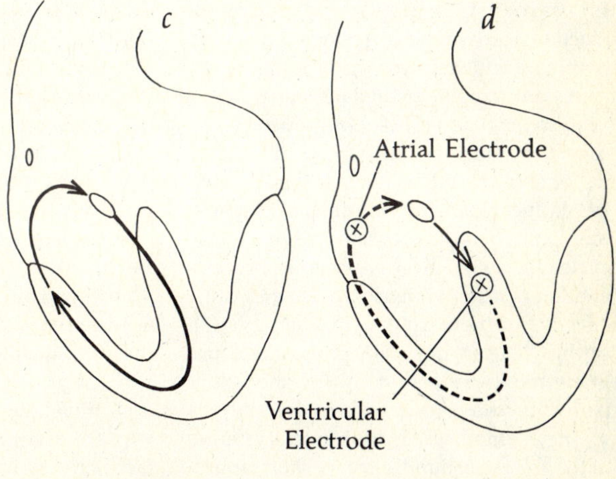

In c, the impulse arrives at the Kent bundle and is transmitted retrograde to the atrium. A reciprocating tachycardia is thus set up involving the atria, AV node, ventricles, and Kent bundle; the electrocardiogram would show a QRS complex of normal configuration. A premature impulse arising in the AV junction or either ventricle could initiate a similar cycle. In d, properly timed electrical stimuli delivered via an electrode placed in either the atrium or the ventricle could interrupt the reentry rhythm by terminating the circus movement.

Reciprocating
Tachycardia

Electrode Placement

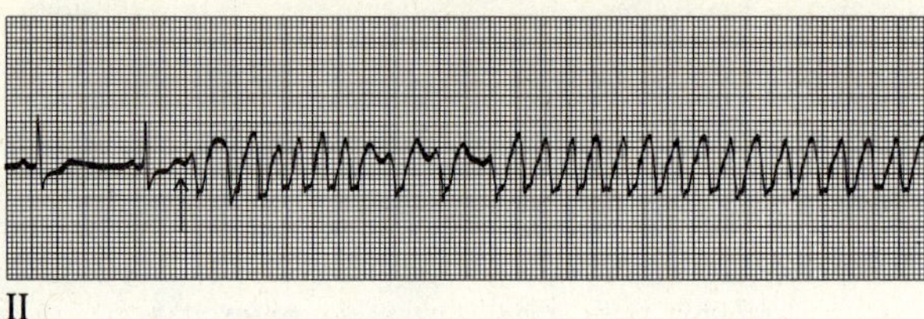

Figure 26 *Atrial fibrillation with conduction over an aberrant pathway is seen in a patient with the Wolff-Parkinson-White syndrome. The run is initiated by an atrial premature beat (arrow), and the ventricular response exceeds 300 beats/min in some portions of the electrocardiogram. Note the slowing and irregularity of the response in the middle of the strip, which is characteristic of atrial fibrillation. This arrhythmia could easily be confused with ventricular flutter.*

way conduction during episodes of atrial fibrillation or flutter—for example, ventricular rates above 180 beats/min; and patients with medically refractory paroxysmal reciprocating tachycardias. Electrophysiologic studies are clearly mandatory if surgical therapy for arrhythmia is contemplated.

Therapy

Fortunately, in most patients with tachycardia complicating the Wolff-Parkinson-White syndrome, the episodes of tachycardia are relatively infrequent and are easily terminated and suppressed. In patients with reentry paroxysmal atrial or paroxysmal junctional tachycardias, it may be possible to terminate and suppress the arrhythmias by using propranolol or digitalis, either singly or in combination. These drugs increase the refractory period of the AV node, thus reducing or abolishing the ability of the AV node to conduct premature impulses across normal pathways and breaking the reentry cycle. Drugs such as quinidine, procainamide, and disopyramide are also frequently effective in preventing reciprocating tachycardias. These drugs act by prolonging retrograde refractory periods in the anomalous pathways, thus preventing reentry.

In patients in whom the refractory period of the accessory bundle is very short, appropriately timed ventricular premature beats may occasionally initiate supraventricular tachycardia. Reciprocating tachycardias initiated in this way are best treated by procainamide or quinidine, or both, because these drugs seem to prolong refractoriness in the accessory pathway.[76,77] In some patients, propranolol appears to be effective because it slows AV nodal conduction; the drug evidently has minimal effect on the anomalous bundle.[78]

In the pharmacologic management of patients with the Wolff-Parkinson-White syndrome, the physician must bear in mind an exceedingly important fact: digitalis will not slow AV conduction in instances of atrial fibrillation in which there is antegrade conduction via the anomalous pathway. In fact, digitalis glycosides may actually shorten the antegrade refractory period of the accessory pathway and thereby accelerate AV conduction in many patients. Hence, for all practical purposes, digitalis is contraindicated in patients with atrial fibrillation or flutter and rapid ventricular rates caused by AV conduction across an anomalous pathway. The treatment of choice in such cases is quinidine or procainamide. Electrical conversion is sometimes necessary and is the initial therapy of choice if the patient is hemodynamically compromised by the arrhythmia.

Intravenous verapamil has proved to be very effective in the termination of reentrant tachycardias involving the AV node. The usual dose is 0.075 to 0.15 mg/kg given over two to three minutes. However, verapamil may also accelerate conduction over anomalous pathways. Therefore, it is not indicated for slowing the ventricular rate in atrial flutter or atrial fibrillation when impulses are conducted to the ventricle by way of bypass tracts.[79]

The following is a summary of opinions regarding drug therapy in the Wolff-Parkinson-White syndrome:

1. Intravenous verapamil or propranolol is the drug of choice in the acute therapy for regular reciprocating supraventricular tachycardia with normal QRS complexes. Propranolol is the drug of choice for chronic suppression of these arrhythmias. Alternative agents include quinidine, procainamide, and disopyramide. Digitalis glycosides or verapamil should be used chronically only when they have been shown by electrophysiologic testing to produce a long refractory period in the bypass tract.
2. Intravenous procainamide is the drug of choice for the acute treatment of tachyarrhythmias characterized by AV conduction over anomalous pathways and wide QRS complexes. Quinidine also may be effective. Digitalis is contraindicated. Verapamil, propranolol, and lidocaine either accelerate conduction or have no effect on the aberrant pathway and thus should not be used.[80] Quinidine, procainamide, or disopyramide is preferred for chronic suppression of these arrhythmias. Two new antiarrhythmic drugs, flecainide and amiodarone, also show promise in chronic therapy.

In occasional patients with reciprocating tachycardias, the reentry cycle can be broken by inducing an electrical discharge and depolarizing either the atrium or the ventricle. The depolarizing impulse can be administered via an implanted pacemaker that is externally activated during episodes of tachycardia. This approach seems particularly useful in patients with type A of Wolff-Parkinson-White syndrome.[81]

Of great interest has been the pioneering work on the surgical treatment of the Wolff-Parkinson-White syndrome.[82] By using epicardial mapping at the time of surgery, the sequence of ventricular activation can be precisely delineated in patients with this syndrome and the location of anomalous pathways determined. A surgical incision is made into the AV groove. The incision often extends into the anulus of the tricuspid valve in the case of a right-sided anomalous pathway or of the mitral valve in the case of a left-sided bundle. This procedure is designed to interrupt the abnormal pathways and thereby prevent recurrence of the tachycardia. Cryosurgical techniques have also been used to ablate the Kent bundles.[83] The results of such carefully planned and performed techniques are excellent: about 90 percent of treated patients are arrhythmia free.[84] Transcatheter delivery of electrical shocks is another technique that has been used to ablate posteroseptal accessory pathways in selected patients.[85] Although promising, the technique is considered highly investigational at present.

Rarely, sectioning of the common bundle had been used to produce complete heart block in patients with otherwise refractory and totally incapacitating episodes of supraventricular tachycardia; a ventricular pacemaker was then inserted to maintain a normal ventricular rate. Transcatheter electrical ablation techniques, however, have now replaced surgery in these highly selected patients.[58-61]

Surgery is generally reserved for those patients with the Wolff-Parkinson-White syndrome who are seriously disabled by episodes of tachycardia or in whom the arrhythmias are life-threatening. Furthermore, surgery should be undertaken only in centers that possess the necessary technology and personnel for carrying out careful epicardial mapping.

Ventricular Arrhythmias

Ventricular Ectopic Beats

Ventricular ectopic beats often occur in persons with otherwise apparently normal hearts. Studies of random population samples of actively employed American males have demonstrated the presence of one or more ventricular premature beats on six- to 24-hour electrocardiographic recordings in approximately 20 percent of men 35 to 40 years of age. This incidence increases steadily with age, reaching 80 percent in males 60 to 65 years of age.[86] Similarly, the frequency of ventricular premature beats in such recordings also increases progressively with age. The occurrence of frequent ventricular premature beats (more than 10 per hour or 10 per 1,000 recorded complexes) in middle-aged males is generally associated with the presence of clinically apparent coronary artery disease, hypertension, chronic obstructive lung disease, or other forms of heart disease.

Ventricular ectopic beats are more common in patients with cardiac disease, especially ischemic heart disease and the cardiomyopathies. They occur in as many as 95 percent of patients with acute myocardial infarction. In chronic ischemic heart disease, the presence of ventricular ectopy is directly correlated with the severity of coronary arterial involvement[87] and with the severity of left ventricular dysfunction.[88] Ventricular ectopic beats are also frequently encountered in patients with myocarditis and the mitral valve prolapse syndrome. Cardiac stimulants, such as alcohol, caffeine, cocaine, and sympathomimetic drugs, may lead to ventricular ectopic beats. Other causes are digitalis toxicity; various other drugs, such as those of the thioridazine family; hypokalemia; hypoxia; hyperthyroidism; and mechanical irritation of the ventricles with cardiac catheters and electrodes.

Ventricular extrasystoles are characterized by wide, often bizarre QRS complexes. Traditionally, it has been assumed that ventricular premature beats arising from the left ventricle show a pattern of right bundle branch block, whereas right ventricular extrasystoles produce left bundle branch block. This distinction may be important because right ventricular arrhythmias appear to have a more benign prognosis.[89] Studies using intracardiac recordings that localize the origin of ventricular ectopy suggest that beats with a right bundle branch block pattern do indeed arise in the left ventricle; beats with a left bundle branch block configuration, however, can arise from either ventricle.[90]

Classification and Mechanisms

Ventricular ectopic beats can generally be separated into three categories: reentrant, parasystolic, and escape. Reentrant and parasystolic beats are premature and therefore terminate cycles shorter than the cycle of the underlying dominant rhythm; escape beats terminate cycles longer than those of

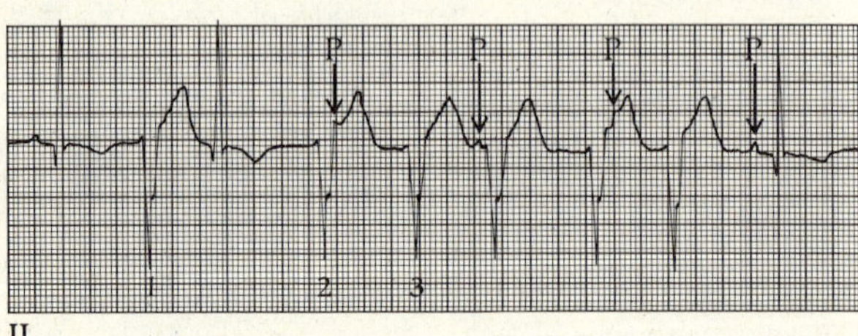

Figure 27   *In an electrocardiogram (lead II) of a patient with a parasystolic ventricular rhythm, the coupling interval of the first extrasystolic beat (1) is 0.16 sec shorter than that of the second extrasystolic beat (2). The interval between ectopic beats 1 and 2 is just about twice that between beats 2 and 3. Note that the first ectopic beat is interpolated between two normally conducted beats. The P waves march through the brief run of parasystolic rhythm.*

the dominant rhythm. Typical reentrant extrasystolic beats bear a constant relationship, termed fixed coupling, to preceding beats of the dominant rhythm. Parasystolic beats share a common interectopic interval with each other but bear no relationship to the dominant rhythm and therefore exhibit variable coupling intervals [*see Figure 27*]. Escape beats occur at a relatively constant interval in relation to the last beat of the dominant rhythm. Sometimes, ventricular ectopy cannot be easily classified.

A vulnerable period exists in diastole, corresponding roughly to the middle third of the T wave and occurring at a time when there is maximum dispersion of refractoriness within the ventricles. This dispersion of refractoriness creates an electrically unstable myocardium and promotes the development of reentrant arrhythmias. Ventricular premature beats that occur within or near the vulnerable period in diastole may initiate repetitive ventricular responses, ventricular tachycardia, or ventricular fibrillation.

In the normal heart, the duration of the vulnerable period is short, and there is little variation in the dispersion of recovery of excitability in different areas of the ventricles. Therefore, the risk of an early ventricular premature beat initiating a sustained ventricular arrhythmia is extremely low. In the diseased heart, however, the duration of the vulnerable period may be extremely long and the magnitude of dispersion of refractoriness within the ventricles may be great. Ventricular premature beats are therefore far more likely to initiate reentrant arrhythmias in the diseased heart than in the normal heart. The most common conditions in which abnormal electrical properties predispose to sustained and life-threatening ventricular arrhythmias include acute ischemia, acute or remote myocardial infarction, valvular heart disease causing pressure or volume overload of one or both ventricles, cardiomyopathies, myocarditis, electrolyte imbalances, and medications. Other less common clinical conditions associated with electrical instability of the myocardium and malignant ventricular arrhythmias include

the long QT interval syndromes, myocardial tumors, and mitral valve prolapse. In addition, some patients appear to suffer from an idiopathic so-called electrical heart disease in which a wide range of ventricular tachyarrhythmias may occur in association with exercise or emotional stress, without apparent provocation and without any evidence of structural heart disease. Many agents, including all known antiarrhythmic drugs, occasionally precipitate new or exacerbate preexisting ventricular arrhythmias. This phenomenon, termed a proarrhythmic effect, is unpredictable and may occur whether or not the drug prolongs the QT interval.

The Lown classification system for ventricular premature beats, which is based on electrocardiographic monitoring,[90] defines the following categories:

Grade 0: No ventricular arrhythmia

Grade 1: Fewer than 30 ventricular premature beats/hr

Grade 1A: Maximum of one ventricular premature beat/min

Grade 1B: Period(s) of two or more ventricular beats/min

Grade 2: 30 or more ventricular premature beats/hr

Grade 3: Multiform ventricular premature beats

Grade 4: Repetitive ventricular ectopy

Grade 4A: Ventricular couplet(s)

Grade 4B: Ventricular tachycardia of three or more beats

Grade 5: R-on-T ventricular premature beats

Although the Lown classification is widely used, it has many limitations. For example, the system implies a more serious degree of ventricular ectopy with higher grades and tends to discount the importance of the frequency of ventricular premature beats. One study found that in Lown grades 4 and 5 the risk of sudden death increased with the frequency of ventricular extrasystoles.[92] The Lown classification places great prognostic emphasis on R-on-T premature beats, but paired ventricular extrasystoles and ventricular tachycardia appear to be more serious prognostic indicators than R-on-T occurrence of ventricular premature beats.[92]

Clinical Features

Patients with ventricular premature beats may be totally asymptomatic or may be aware of a skipping or fluttering sensation in the chest. Sometimes, the actual premature beat is felt; at other times, the forceful beat after the compensatory pause is sensed. Premature beats are particularly likely to occur after meals or when the patient changes position; they commonly increase in frequency as a result of excitement and tension.

In general, benign ventricular premature beats tend to disappear with exercise. Exercise may also abolish ventricular premature beats in abnormal hearts, but an increase in their frequency with exercise is generally considered indicative of a cardiac abnormality.

Therapy

Treatment of ventricular premature beats is an area of great interest, controversy, and uncertainty. In general, ventricular premature beats are undesirable, particularly in patients with underlying cardiac disease. However, all of the drugs currently available for suppression of ventricular extrasystoles have potentially serious side effects, including even exacerbation of the ventricular ectopy itself. Thus, the treatment is often worse than the disease, and the decision to initiate therapy for ventricular premature beats must not be made lightly, especially in asymptomatic patients.

The crucial issue of whether the suppression of complex ventricular ectopy reduces the risk of sudden cardiac death remains unresolved.[93] Although no data from controlled prospective trials are available, it appears that antiarrhythmic therapy directed at the suppression of advanced grades of ventricular ectopy affords protection against recurrent ventricular arrhythmias and sudden death in patients with recurrent ventricular tachycardia or ventricular fibrillation.[91]

It is commonly agreed that unifocal ventricular premature beats in persons with otherwise normal hearts are usually benign and thus do not warrant treatment. Furthermore, even untreated complex ventricular ectopy is associated with an excellent long-term prognosis when it occurs in asymptomatic individuals who do not have evidence of heart disease.[94,95]

Although we generally recommend antiarrhythmic drug therapy for complex ventricular ectopy (particularly repetitive forms of ectopy) in patients with impaired ventricular function, the ability of such therapy to reduce the risk of sudden death is unproved. Several studies have examined the predictive value of electrophysiologic testing in patients with complex ventricular ectopy. Preliminary results suggest that this technique may be helpful in identifying two groups of patients: the minority who are at particularly high risk for sustained ventricular arrhythmias and sudden death and, equally important, the large majority who do not require antiarrhythmic therapy.[96-99] It appears that patients in whom ventricular arrhythmias are noninducible with programmed electrical stimulation have a good long-term prognosis.

We usually do not use the R-on-T phenomenon as an indication for therapy except in patients with long QT interval syndrome [*see Torsade de Pointes* and Long QT Interval Syndromes, *below*] or in patients with beats that have been clearly identified as ones that initiate ventricular tachyarrhythmias.

In particular, an attempt at the suppression of frequent repetitive ventricular ectopy seems indicated in patients with the following problems:

1. Coronary artery disease with angina pectoris or acute or remote myocardial infarction.

2. Clinically significant valvular heart disease.

3. Hypertrophic or dilated cardiomyopathies.

4. Mitral valve prolapse syndromes that are associated with symptoms such as ventricular tachycardia or syncope.

5. Repetitive ventricular ectopic activity associated with severe symptoms even in the apparent absence of heart disease.

Even though complex ventricular ectopy and left ventricular dysfunction tend to occur together and may be pathophysiologically related, complex ventricular ectopy has been established as an independent predictor of risk for sudden cardiac death in the patient with impaired ventricular function.[88] Whether aggressive antiarrhythmic therapy can reduce the risk for sudden death in patients with significantly impaired ventricular function remains to be determined.

In the United States, the drugs that are used to suppress ventricular arrhythmias are lidocaine, mexiletine, tocainide, phenytoin, quinidine, procainamide, disopyramide, flecainide, encainide, several beta-adrenergic blocking drugs, bretylium, and amiodarone [*see Chapter 2*]. Intravenous lidocaine is the drug of choice for the suppression of ventricular premature beats in acute conditions, such as myocardial infarction.

Quinidine is effective in suppressing ventricular premature beats and is given in an oral dosage of 200 to 400 mg every six hours. The major side effects associated with its chronic administration are gastrointestinal problems, manifested as diarrhea, cramps, and nausea. Less common adverse reactions to quinidine are fever, rash, and thrombocytopenia.

A rare but important adverse effect of quinidine is a paradoxic increase in ventricular irritability; quinidine-induced syncope may ensue from ventricular tachycardia or ventricular fibrillation. This increase in ventricular irritability is ascribed to prolongation of the QT interval by quinidine, an action that may lengthen the vulnerable phase of the cardiac cycle and predispose to the occurrence of *torsade de pointes*. Like other antiarrhythmic drugs, quinidine may also unpredictably exacerbate ventricular arrhythmias without markedly prolonging the QT interval.[100,101]

Procainamide is effective in suppressing ventricular premature beats and is given in an oral dosage of 250 to 1,000 mg every three to four hours. This drug is also available in a sustained-release preparation that may be given less frequently. There is a high incidence of adverse reactions during long-term procainamide therapy. Approximately 50 percent of patients receiving procainamide develop either a positive antinuclear antibody titer or a positive lupus erythematosus preparation. The development of these serologic abnormalities does not necessitate discontinuation of procainamide, but if symptoms such as fever, arthritis, or polyserositis occur, the drug must be stopped. Occasionally, procainamide causes rash and agranulocytosis.

Disopyramide is effective in suppressing ventricular ectopy and is administered in an oral dosage of 100 to 250 mg every six to eight hours. Its major side effects are anticholinergic, consisting of blurred vision, dry mouth, and in males, urinary retention. Disopyramide may exert a marked negative inotropic effect and should be avoided in patients who have left ventricular failure.

Propranolol and allied beta-adrenergic blocking drugs are moderately effective in suppressing ventricular premature beats. Because these agents may also simultaneously relieve angina, they may have particular value in patients with angina or ischemic heart disease. Beta blockers may also be useful in patients with ventricular arrhythmias related to exercise or mitral valve prolapse. Because beta blockers have a marked propensity for slowing the discharge rate of the sinus node, their bradycardic action sometimes offsets their antiarrhythmic properties, causing a paradoxic increase in ventricular ectopy. Several beta blockers have also been shown to improve the long-term prognosis of patients following myocardial infarction, apparently by prevention of sudden cardiac death.[102,103]

Several new drugs have been approved for the treatment of symptomatic ventricular arrhythmias. Two of these agents, mexiletine and tocainide,[104,105] are related to lidocaine in structure and electrophysiologic effects. Both drugs are moderately effective in the treatment of ventricular arrhythmias, and both have a significant incidence of troublesome side effects, including rare reports of agranulocytosis and pulmonary fibrosis after tocainide administration [*see Chapter 2*]. Mexiletine is administered orally in a dosage that usually ranges from 100 to 300 mg every six to eight hours, but it is sometimes effective when given in a twice-daily regimen. Tocainide is usually administered in an oral dosage of 400 to 600 mg every eight hours, although even lower doses may sometimes be effective.

Mexiletine or tocainide exhibits significantly enhanced antiarrhythmic efficacy when combined with a beta blocker or another antiarrhythmic drug such as quinidine or procainamide; because of this apparent synergistic effect, the dosage of mexiletine or tocainide can be lowered and the incidence of adverse side effects decreased. Both mexiletine and tocainide may be used safely in patients with left ventricular dysfunction. Phenytoin, which is generally placed in the same class as lidocaine, mexiletine, and tocainide, is only infrequently effective in suppressing ventricular arrhythmias,[106] but it is highly effective in the treatment of ventricular arrhythmias caused by digitalis toxicity.

Flecainide and encainide, both of which are classified electrophysiologically as class 1C drugs, are effective in suppressing ventricular ectopy, with an efficacy that is comparable to that of quinidine and procainamide.[107] Flecainide is administered in a dosage of 100 to 200 mg twice daily. It is usually well tolerated and has few side effects [*see Chapter 2*]. Flecainide does, however, possess significant potential for cardiac toxicity, including proarrhythmic effects in patients with advanced heart disease and left ventricular dysfunction. The drug should not be administered to patients with advanced AV conduction system dis-

ease or sinus node dysfunction unless a pacemaker is in place. Because it can exacerbate congestive heart failure, flecainide should be used with caution in patients with moderate left ventricular dysfunction and avoided in patients with severe left ventricular dysfunction. Like many other antiarrhythmic drugs, flecainide should not be used with beta blockers or calcium blockers in patients with sinus node dysfunction, AV conduction system disease, or significant left ventricular dysfunction. Encainide appears to have less myocardial depressant action than flecainide, but the same general precautions advised in the use of flecainide pertain to encainide. Encainide is given in a dosage of 25 to 50 mg every eight hours.

In April 1989, the FDA issued a warning on the use of flecainide and encainide on the basis of preliminary findings from a study of the use of antiarrhythmic drugs in survivors of acute myocardial infarction.* In the study, termed the Cardiac Arrhythmia Suppression Trial (CAST), postinfarction patients with asymptomatic ventricular premature beats shown to respond to encainide or flecainide were randomized into four treatment groups for long-term follow-up. In three of the groups, patients received either encainide, flecainide, or a third, experimental drug; in the fourth group, patients were given a placebo. A review of interim data showed a mortality in the flecainide- and encainide-treated groups that was more than twice that of the placebo group. On the basis of these data, the FDA has recommended that flecainide and encainide be used only in the treatment of life-threatening ventricular arrhythmias, such as sustained ventricular tachycardia. We would emphasize that these data pertain to a restricted group of patients—namely, those who have had a myocardial infarction. These data cannot be readily extended at this time to patients with ventricular ectopy and other types of heart disease or to pa-

---

* Enkaid and Tambocor use in non-life-threatening arrhythmias halted. FDA Talk Paper (T89-22). Food and Drug Administration, Rockville, Maryland, April 25, 1989

tients with apparently normal hearts. The authors have many such patients who have done very well on these drugs. Nevertheless, prudence in the use of class 1C drugs is presently urged.

Amiodarone, approved as a drug of last resort for the treatment of life-threatening ventricular arrhythmias, exceeds most other agents both in antiarrhythmic efficacy and toxicity.[108,109] Its complex pharmacokinetics, extremely long half-life, and potential for serious toxicity make amiodarone a difficult drug to administer and argue for its use only by experienced cardiologists. We reserve amiodarone for patients with life-threatening arrhythmias that are unresponsive to conventional and investigational antiarrhythmic drugs. The drug is generally administered in a loading dose [*see Chapter 2*] for several weeks, followed by a maintenance dosage of 200 to 400 mg daily. The use of Holter monitoring or electrophysiologic testing to demonstrate the antiarrhythmic efficacy of amiodarone is mandatory. The use of amiodarone is associated with a high incidence of adverse reactions, including pulmonary fibrosis, hyperthyroidism and hypothyroidism, hepatitis, corneal microdeposits, gastrointestinal and neuromuscular toxicity, photosensitivity, and various adverse electrophysiologic effects. Amiodarone interacts with many other drugs, causing significant increases in the serum levels of digoxin, phenytoin, quinidine, and procainamide; in addition, amiodarone raises the prothrombin time in patients receiving warfarin.

Various antiarrhythmic drugs are now under active investigation in the United States. These agents include indecainide, recainam, ethmozin, pirmenol, propafenone, and sotalol. The availability of at least some of these agents within the next few years will broaden the alternatives for the treatment of ventricular arrhythmias.

Spontaneous variability in the frequency of ventricular ectopic activity may make it difficult to assess the efficacy of antiarrhythmic drug therapy in individual patients. The problem of spontaneous variability of ven-tricular ectopic activity has been examined using sequential ambulatory ECG recordings in the absence of drugs.[110] If only single 24-hour control and 24-hour treatment recordings were compared, then a greater than 83 percent reduction in ventricular extrasystoles was required to distinguish a reduction in ventricular premature beat frequency caused by a therapeutic intervention from that caused by biologic or spontaneous variation alone.[110]

Ventricular Tachycardia

Ventricular tachycardia is defined as three or more consecutive beats of ventricular origin at a rate greater than 120 beats/min. As is the case with ventricular ectopic beats, there are also at least two kinds of ventricular tachycardia: reentrant, which is initiated by premature beats and propagated through a reentry pathway, and automatic, in which a focus discharges autonomously. Whereas abnormal or enhanced automaticity and, possibly, triggered activity are operative in some forms of ventricular tachycardia (e.g., that which is associated with digitalis intoxication), reentry accounts for the majority of cases.

QRS complexes are wide and often bizarre, and the heart rate is between 120 and 280 beats/min. In about 85 percent of cases of spontaneously occurring ventricular tachycardia, AV dissociation is present [*see Figure 28*]. Ventricular tachycardia may be slightly irregular, and occasionally, an exit block may be present.

Because of the very wide QRS complexes, there is often very little base line available on which to detect dissociated P waves. In such cases, intracardiac tracings are very helpful in demonstrating the pattern of atrial activity. On occasion, if the rate of the ventricular tachycardia is slow enough, atrial capture or fusion beats are found; fusion beats represent combinations of normally conducted sinus beats and ventricular ectopic beats.

Wellens and coworkers first described the use of programmed cardiac stimulation

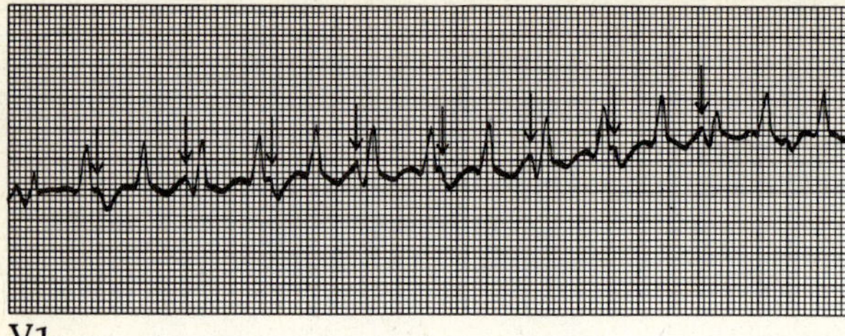

Figure 28 *Dissociated sinus P waves (arrows) can be observed in electrocardiogram recorded in a patient who has ventricular tachycardia at a rate of 160 beats/min with AV dissociation.*

techniques in the evaluation of ventricular tachycardia.[111] The ability of critically timed premature ventricular extrastimuli to initiate and terminate ventricular tachycardia supports the postulate that reentry is the mechanism responsible for its origin. In addition, subsequent studies suggest that sustained ventricular tachycardia associated with chronic ischemic heart disease and remote myocardial infarction is reentrant in mechanism and that the reentrant pathway is located within a small region of the endocardium.[112]

Etiology

Ventricular tachycardia is common in patients with ischemic heart disease, particularly after an acute myocardial infarction. In such patients, this arrhythmia is also associated with heart failure and can occur as a complication of a ventricular aneurysm. Ventricular tachycardia is common in cardiomyopathies and is sometimes seen in patients with mitral valve prolapse. A cardiomyopathy termed right ventricular dysplasia, which selectively involves the right ventricle,[113] may present as a ventricular tachycardia of right ventricular origin (left bundle branch block configuration).

Any inflammatory or infectious disease of the heart may cause ventricular tachycardia, as may tumors, infiltrative diseases of the myocardium, and mechanical irritation of the heart by extraneous devices such as catheters. Metabolic derangements, such as hypokalemia, hypercalcemia, hypomagnesemia, and hypoxia, can also lead to ventricular tachycardia.

Many drugs, including antiarrhythmic agents, may initiate ventricular tachycardia. Occasionally, arrhythmia occurs as a consequence of digitalis toxicity and may be precipitated by the thioridazine drugs used in the treatment of psychiatric illness. Cardiac stimulants, such as sympathomimetic amines, may also cause ventricular tachycardia. On occasion, ventricular tachycardia occurs in patients whose hearts appear to be otherwise completely normal.

Clinical Features

Ventricular tachycardia is generally considered the most serious of all tachyarrhythmias, perhaps because in large measure it is frequently associated with serious underlying cardiac disease. Patients with ventricular tachycardia often present with concomitant hypotension, congestive heart failure, syncope, or cardiac arrest, although the arrhythmia can be well tolerated.

Signs of AV dissociation are often better detected by physical examination than by the electrocardiogram. Independent and asynchronous atrial and ventricular contraction produce the following signs: (1) variation in the systolic blood pressure as measured peripherally, (2) variation in the intensity of heart sounds, (3) intermittent cannon waves in the jugular venous pulses caused by the simultaneous contraction of the atria and the ventricles, and (4) extra heart sounds, such as third and fourth heart sounds. These signs are absent when atrial fibrillation is present or if there is constant retrograde atrial activation. In the latter case, constant cannon waves are seen in the jugular venous pulses.

Because of asynchronous activation of the right and left ventricles, the first and second sounds are widely split in patients with ventricular tachycardia, especially in those patients who have left ventricular tachycardia with a right bundle branch block pattern.

Therapy

The treatment of choice in a patient who has serious hemodynamic compromise as a result of ventricular tachycardia is immediate electrical cardioversion [*see* Cardioversion, *below*]. A firm thump delivered to the precordium with the clenched fist is occasionally successful in terminating the arrhythmia and can be given while cardioversion is being prepared. If the arrhythmia is well tolerated, lidocaine, 1 mg/kg, can be administered as a rapid intravenous bolus. This dose can be repeated every five minutes until the arrhythmia has been terminated, until side effects appear, or until a total dose of 5 mg/kg has been given.

In general, oral drugs have no role in the acute therapy for ventricular tachycardia. Procainamide, however, may be given intravenously, 100 mg every two minutes either to conversion or up to a total dose of 2 g, if the patient is tolerating the arrhythmia well. When procainamide is given in this way, the patient must be observed closely for the development of hypotension, and the physician should be ready to institute electrical conversion immediately if necessary.

In hospitalized patients with either recurrent ventricular tachycardia that progresses rapidly to ventricular fibrillation or recurrent ventricular tachycardia that is associated with cardiovascular collapse, intravenous bretylium may be effective when lidocaine and procainamide fail to suppress the arrhythmia. Bretylium should be administered intravenously in a dose of 5 mg/kg, to be repeated in one to two hours if the initial dose is ineffective. Rapid intravenous administration of the drug commonly results in hypotension, nausea, vomiting, and in some instances, a transient increase in ventricular arrhythmias. These side effects can generally be avoided by diluting 5 mg/kg of bretylium in 50 to 100 ml of five percent dextrose and water or normal saline and administering the dose slowly during a

period of 30 to 45 minutes. If subsequent doses of bretylium are required to stabilize the cardiac rhythm, the drug should be administered by slow intravenous infusion at 1 to 2 mg/min or as a 3 to 5 mg/kg dose in 50 to 100 ml of five percent dextrose and water or saline during a period of 30 to 45 minutes at six- to eight-hour intervals. All patients receiving bretylium should be monitored closely for hypotension, with the drug dosage adjusted accordingly. The dosage of bretylium should be reduced in patients with impaired renal function.

In patients with recurrent ventricular tachycardia, suppressive therapy is necessary [*see* Ventricular Ectopic Beats, *above*]. In all such patients, it is necessary to seek out and correct underlying disorders, such as hypoxia, hypokalemia, hypomagnesemia, or digitalis toxicity.

An unusual form of ventricular tachycardia has been described that occurs in young patients who have apparently normal hearts.[114] The arrhythmia shows the configuration of right bundle branch block and left axis deviation and responds to intravenous verapamil.

In patients with refractory ventricular arrhythmias, the first obvious, yet frequently overlooked, step is to ascertain that the antiarrhythmic agents that the patient is receiving are in fact being administered in optimal dosages. The measurement of plasma drug concentrations is very important in ensuring that the correct dosage is being administered and absorbed. However, in some cases, antiarrhythmic drugs may themselves contribute to the problem: discontinuation of these drugs has resolved arrhythmias in approximately five percent of patients referred to us for the treatment of recurrent refractory ventricular tachycardia.

Programmed electrical stimulation of the heart combined with intracardiac electrograms has provided a powerful new tool for understanding the mechanisms of ventricular tachycardia and for assessing the effectiveness of treatment in patients with ventricular tachycardia resistant to usual therapy.[115] The objective of these techniques is to initiate ventricular tachycardia reproducibly by delivering programmed electrical stimuli to the heart and then to intervene with drugs that will render the arrhythmia noninducible [*see Figure 29*]. Studies have demonstrated that suppression by antiarrhythmic drugs of recurrent, life-threatening ventricular tachyarrhythmias that were electrically inducible before drug therapy is highly predictive of freedom from recurrent episodes.[115-120] In one long-term study in a large population of patients with recurrent ventricular tachyarrhythmias, multivariate regression analy-

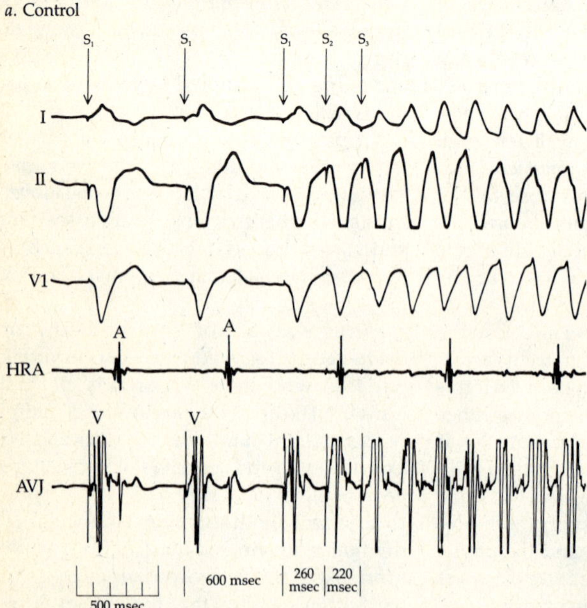

Figure 29 *The successful treatment of inducible ventricular tachycardia with quinidine is shown in this series of panels. In panel A, tracings (top to bottom) represent surface ECG leads I, II, and V1 and intracardiac recordings from the high right atrium (HRA) and the AV junction (AVJ). Two ventricular extrastimuli (S₂ and S₃) delivered to the right ventricular apex during fixed-rate ventricular pacing (S₁–S₁) initiate sustained ventricular tachycardia. In panel B, all tracings represent surface ECG lead II. During maintenance therapy with quinidine, repeat programmed ventricular stimulation with double extrastimuli at two close coupling intervals fails to initiate ventricular tachycardia.*

ses demonstrated that the two strongest predictors both of sudden death and of cardiac death were (1) higher New York Association functional class and (2) failure to identify effective therapy at electrophysiologic study.[121]

In addition to providing information about the mechanisms of ventricular tachycardia and assessing the effectiveness of treatment, electrophysiologic techniques also provide a means of assessing the possible role of pacemaker therapy in patients with drug-resistant ventricular arrhythmias. Rapid atrial or ventricular pacing may suppress recurrent ventricular arrhythmias. In rare instances, implantable patient-activated or automatic antitachycardial pacemakers have been used in the treatment of recurrent, drug-resistant ventricular tachycardia. However, in the near future, these devices will be supplanted by highly sophisticated automatic implantable arrhythmia-control systems with backup defibrillation [*see* Pacemakers and Automatic Defibrillators for Arrhythmias, *below*].

The indications for determining which patients with ventricular tachyarrhythmias should be subjected to electrophysiologic studies vary from institution to institution, but we select patients for electrophysiologic testing based on the nature of the ventricular tachycardia. In patients with frequently occurring symptomatic *nonsustained* ventricular tachycardia, empiric antiarrhythmic therapy can be initiated. Therapy should be directed toward the complete elimination of nonsustained ventricular tachycardia, both at rest and during exercise; in addition, if possible, therapy should aim toward a 75 percent or greater reduction in the frequency of ventricular extrasystoles on a 24-hour electrocardiogram. Electrophysiologic testing in patients with symptomatic nonsustained ventricular tachycardia is reserved for those patients in whom the frequency of the spontaneous arrhythmia is not high enough to assess the effectiveness of empiric antiarrhythmic therapy.

We currently recommend electrophysiologic testing in patients with chronic recurrent *sustained* ventricular tachycardia if the arrhythmias have been associated with life-threatening sequelae as a result of either hemodynamic compromise during ventricular tachycardia or degeneration of ventricular tachycardia to ventricular fibrillation. In patients in whom the sustained ventricular tachycardia is frequently recurring, comparatively slow, electrocardiographically stable, and hemodynamically well tolerated, a reasonable course of action would be to begin empiric trials with a series of antiarrhythmic drugs administered under continuous monitoring in the hospital in an attempt to define an effective agent or combination of agents. Ambulatory electrocardiographic monitoring and electrocardiography stress testing are used to judge the efficacy of such treatment if the frequency of spontaneous arrhythmias is high. If the arrhythmias occur sporadically, electrophysiologic testing provides a rapid and cost-effective means of defining effective therapy in most cases.

In any group of patients with documented ventricular tachycardia or fibrillation studied by programmed stimulation techniques, there will be some patients who will manifest no inducible ventricular arrhythmias. The number of such patients depends in part on the patient population studied, the stimulation techniques used in the evaluation, and the definition of inducible ventricular tachycardia. The optimal management of this patient subgroup is ill defined. Our experience suggests that the prognosis for these patients is variable and depends on the nature of the underlying heart disease. In particular, patients with coronary artery disease and well-preserved ventricular function who are treated aggressively with anti-ischemic therapy (either medical or surgical) have a favorable prognosis without antiarrhythmic drug therapy.[122] However, contrary findings have been reported, and further observations are required to clarify the prognosis and optimal management for these patients.[123]

Surgical therapy represents an important new approach to recurrent life-threatening ventricular tachycardia.[124,125] It has long been known that resection of a ventricular aneurysm or large myocardial scar in a patient with acute or remote myocardial infarction sometimes eliminates recurrent ventricular tachycardia. The technique of map-guided endocardial resection has been developed in an effort to improve the results of such surgery for ventricular tachycardia.[125] Crude localization of the area of origin of the tachycardia is established using electrode catheter mapping studies. At the time of surgery, ventricular tachycardia is initiated by programmed electrical stimulation, and an exploring electrode is used to identify the region of earliest activation on the endocardial surface. The endocardium is then dissected in this area, and a piece measuring roughly 1 to 3 mm in depth and roughly 5 to 10 cm^2 in size is resected.

The superiority of map-guided scar resection over surgery without mapping has not yet been proved by prospective randomized studies. However, considerable clinical evidence indicates that routine left ventricular aneurysm resection alone, without map-guided endocardial resection, is much less effective in eliminating ventricular tachycardia or fibrillation.[126]

Map-guided endocardial resection is not universally applicable. Automatic ventricular tachycardia or any ventricular tachycardia that cannot be initiated reproducibly by programmed cardiac stimulation cannot be treated by this method unless the arrhythmia is incessant. Our experience with this technique has also demonstrated that surgical mortality is unacceptably high in patients in whom left ventricular reserve is minimal as judged by systolic function in the non-aneurysmal segments of the left ventricle. Postsurgical survival is excellent in patients who have at least moderate preservation of systolic ventricular function, and such patients generally remain free from recurrent arrhythmias.[127] Thus, patients who are candidates for map-guided endocardial resection and aneurysmectomy should be carefully selected on the basis of both hemodynamic and electrophysiologic data obtained prior to surgery. At present, we reserve this type of surgery for patients who are unresponsive to or intolerant of medical therapy and who have evidence of discrete myocardial scars or an aneurysm. We also undertake map-guided resection in patients with ventricular tachycardia who require cardiac surgery for a cause other than arrhythmias.

Occasionally, coronary artery bypass surgery has eliminated refractory ventricular irritability in patients with significant coronary arterial obstruction and no anginal symptoms. The true effectiveness of this mode of therapy, however, has not been established. In our experience, coronary artery bypass surgery has been effective mainly in patients who develop dangerous ventricular arrhythmias during bouts of ischemia. Needless to say, coronary artery bypass surgery is combined with resection of a ventricular aneurysm and subendocardium when necessary.

Torsade De Pointes *and Long QT Interval Syndromes*

Torsade de pointes, which literally means twisting of the points, refers to an unusual form of ventricular tachycardia characterized by undulating rotations of the QRS complexes around the electrocardiographic base line, producing a very polymorphic type of arrhythmia[128,129] [*see Figure 30*]. This arrhythmia is initiated by a ventricular premature beat in the setting of abnormal ventricular repolarization characterized by prolongation of the QT interval. The prolonged QT interval can be either congenital or acquired. The congenital form was first described in association with congenital nerve deafness (Jervell and Lange-Nielsen syndrome), although it was subsequently noted as an isolated abnormality without deafness (Romano-Ward syndrome). The underlying mechanism of the repolarization abnormality is unknown, but at least in some patients, it appears to be caused by dominance of left-sided over right-sided cardiac sympathetic activity.[130]

In congenital long QT interval syndromes, the arrhythmias tend to abate with advancing age. Because there is a potential

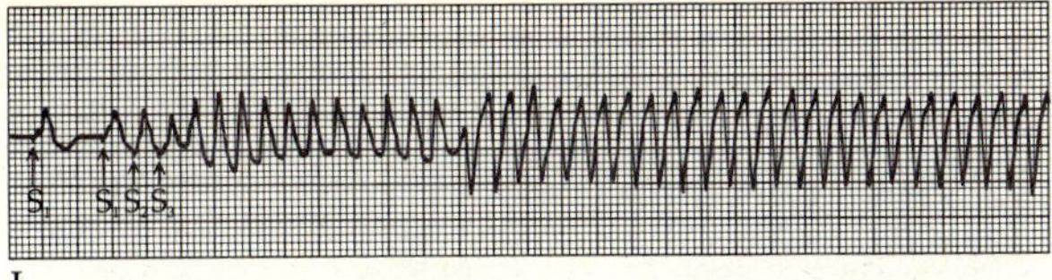

I

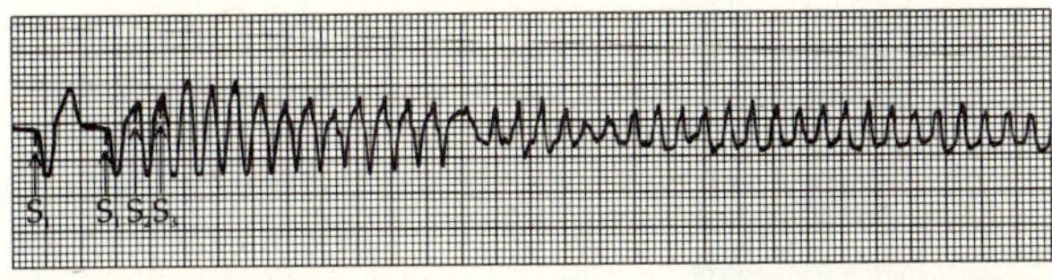

II

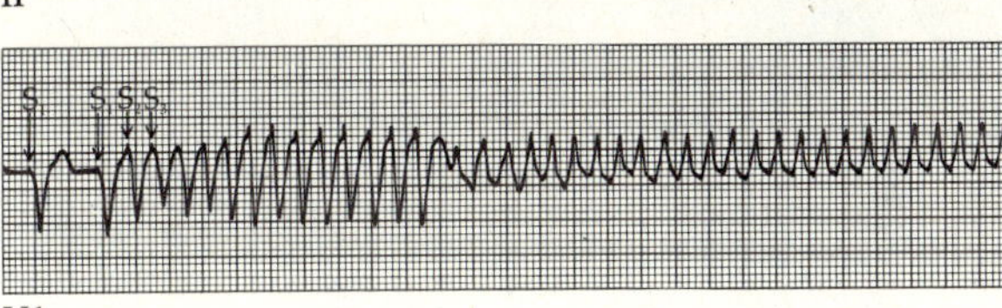

V1

Figure 30 *Simultaneous recordings of surface ECG leads I, II, and V1 from a patient with recurrent* torsade de pointes *are shown. The ventricle is being paced regularly (S_1); at the arrows, two rapid stimuli are delivered prematurely, initiating the tachycardia. Note the continuous change in the QRS complex amplitude and axis that is characteristic of* torsade de pointes.

for hereditary transmission (the Romano-Ward syndrome is autosomal dominant), close family members of patients with these disorders should have electrocardiograms.

There are many causes of acquired long QT interval syndromes.[131] Prominent among these are quinidine and other antiarrhythmic drugs that prolong repolarization. In fact, most cases of quinidine-induced syncope are attributable to the effect of this drug in prolonging ventricular repolarization. Other important causes of the long QT interval syndromes and *torsade de pointes* ventricular tachycardia are as follows:

1. Psychotropic drugs, such as the phenothiazines, thioridazines, tricyclics, and lithium.

2. Electrolyte imbalances, especially hypokalemia and hypomagnesemia. Some sudden deaths that have occurred in patients on liquid-protein diets and in anorexia nervosa are probably due to this arrhythmia caused by the metabolic derangements from the diet or starvation.

3. Central nervous system lesions, such as subarachnoid or intracerebral hemorrhage, head trauma, and cerebral tumors.

4. Myocarditis and myocardial ischemia.

5. Marked bradycardia, particularly in patients with complete heart block.

6. Mitral valve prolapse syndromes.

Patients with long QT interval syndromes are prone to recurrent dizziness or syncope from the ventricular tachycardia. Sudden auditory stimuli, such as the ringing of a telephone at night or the slamming of doors, may initiate *torsade de pointes* in certain vulnerable individuals with a long QT interval syndrome.[129] Fortunately, the arrhythmia usually terminates spontaneously. However, *torsade de pointes* ventricular tachycardia may lead to fatal ventricular fibrillation and must be taken very seriously.

The treatment of acquired forms of prolonged QT interval syndromes is that of the underlying disorder—for example, repletion of potassium and magnesium, discontinuation of offending drugs, and so forth. In the idiopathic forms of the disease, drugs such as propranolol, lidocaine, or phenytoin—all of which either shorten or do not affect ventricular repolarization—may be helpful. Quinidine and antiarrhythmic drugs with similar electrophysiologic ac-

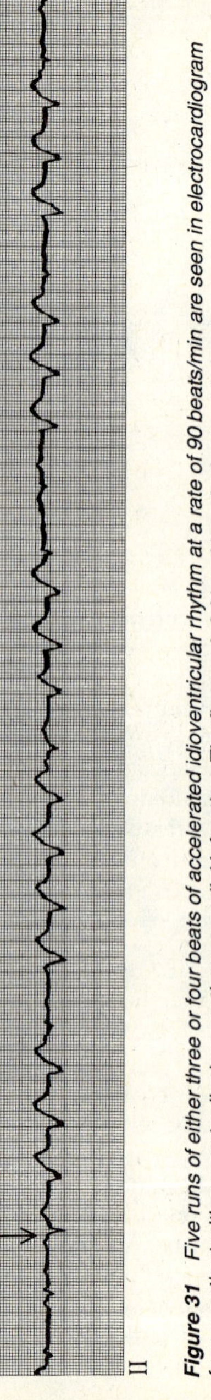

Figure 31   Five runs of either three or four beats of accelerated idioventricular rhythm at a rate of 90 beats/min are seen in electrocardiogram from a patient with an acute diaphragmatic myocardial infarction. The first run is initiated by a fusion beat (arrow).

tions should not be used. Rapid cardiac pacing may suppress episodes of tachycardia and may be used acutely for emergency treatment of the arrhythmia. Because of the possibility that some cases of this arrhythmia are due to excessive left-sided sympathetic activity, ablation of the left stellate ganglion has been attempted and reported to be effective in some patients.[132]

Accelerated Idioventricular Rhythm

Accelerated idioventricular rhythm is characterized by an ectopic focus that discharges the ventricles at a rate between 60 and 100 beats/min. Occasionally, the accelerated focus is in the AV junction. The arrhythmia usually occurs in the setting of sinus bradycardia, which allows the more rapid idioventricular focus to escape and capture the ventricles. Onset is usually in late diastole, and the arrhythmia is frequently initiated by a fusion beat between the ventricular impulse and the normally conducted beat [*see Figure 31*]. Although the rhythm can be sustained, it is usually episodic and typically lasts from four to 30 impulses.

Etiology

Accelerated idioventricular rhythm is quite common in acute myocardial infarction, especially diaphragmatic infarction, which is more likely to be associated with bradycardia than is anterior infarction. This arrhythmia may also be a manifestation of myocarditis or of digitalis toxicity and is sometimes found in apparently healthy people, especially athletes with slow sinus rates.

Clinical Features

In general, accelerated idioventricular rhythm is a benign rhythm that is well tolerated. In fact, patients with this arrhythmia are usually asymptomatic. Rarely, the loss of the atrial contraction that occurs secondary to the arrhythmia may cause transient hypotension. Because of its association with bradycardia, accelerated idioventricular rhythm is likely to emerge during sleep.

Therapy

Because of its benign nature, accelerated idioventricular rhythm rarely warrants treatment. In our experience, however, it occurs as an isolated arrhythmia only about half of the time. In the remaining instances, accelerated idioventricular rhythm is accompanied by ventricular premature beats, which can lead to ventricular tachycardia. If the rhythm is uncomplicated, no therapy is necessary. When premature beats accompany the arrhythmia, they should be suppressed, by administering lidocaine, by accelerating the underlying heart rate using atropine or a similar drug, or by electrical pacing.

Differentiation of Supraventricular Arrhythmia with Aberrancy from Ventricular Arrhythmia

One of the greatest challenges in the diagnosis of arrhythmias is that of distinguishing between supraventricular arrhythmias with aberrant IV conduction (or bundle branch block) and ventricular arrhythmias [*see Table 4*]. Intracardiac electrocardiography may be very helpful in making this distinction, as may His bundle electrocardiography. If these techniques reveal that each of the QRS complexes is preceded by a His bundle deflection and an HV interval of normal duration, then the arrhythmia must arise at or above the level of the AV junction.

Ventricular Fibrillation

Ventricular fibrillation is fatal unless it reverts spontaneously or is converted either by a chest thump or by electrical countershock. Ventricular fibrillation is of two types: primary and secondary. Primary ventricular fibrillation occurs suddenly and unexpectedly in patients with otherwise good cardiac function. This type of fibrillation is common in the early phase of acute myocardial infarction. Resuscitation of such individuals is highly successful if they are treated promptly. Secondary ventricular fibrillation occurs as the terminal event in a severely failing heart. Resuscitation of patients with secondary ventricular fibrillation is seldom successful.

Table 4   Diagnostic Clues That May Help Differentiate Ventricular Ectopy from Supraventricular Beats with Aberrancy or Bundle Branch Block

Feature	Ventricular Ectopy	Supraventricular Beats with Aberrancy
Right bundle branch block morphology of QRS complex	Present in 60%–70% of cases	Present in > 90% of cases
Configuration of right bundle branch block*	Monophasic; if biphasic or triphasic, R is taller than R′	Triphasic (RSR′) with R smaller than R′
Direction of initial 0.02 sec of QRS complex†	Almost always different from that of normally conducted beats	Same as that of normally conducted beats
QRS axis	Markedly leftward (-60° to -120°)	Usually -30° to +60°
QRS duration	Often > 0.14 sec	Usually < 0.14 sec
	Ventricular Tachycardia	*Supraventricular Tachycardia with Aberrancy or Bundle Branch Block*
Regularity	Usually regular, but slight variation in cycle length of up to 0.02–0.03 sec may occur	Quite regular unless atrial fibrillation or AV block is present
Relation of P waves to QRS complexes (if apparent)	AV dissociation in 85%; retrograde P waves following QRS complexes seen in most of remainder	1:1 relation unless varying degrees of AV block are present
Capture or fusion beats, or both	Diagnostic, if present	Absent
Relation of QRS complex morphology to that seen prior to or following the arrhythmia	Resembles that of ventricular premature beats, if present	Resembles either that of bundle branch block or that of aberrantly conducted beats, depending on which is present
Effect of carotid sinus massage	Rarely converts the arrrhythmia; usually no response	May convert the arrhythmia or increase the AV block
Findings on His bundle electrocardiography	No relation between His bundle deflections and QRS complexes, except when retrograde activation is present; in this case, a His bundle spike follows each QRS complex	His bundle deflection before every QRS complex

Note: the first five items apply to individual beats; the final six relate to the distinction between ventricular tachycardia and supraventricular tachycardia with aberrant conduction.

*If a QRS complex with right bundle branch block is biphasic with R > R′ or monophasic, the beat is almost always of ventricular origin. The converse, however (i.e., a triphasic complex with R < R′), is less specific for a supraventricular origin; about 30 to 40 percent of beats of ventricular origin also show this configuration.

†To be certain of the direction of the initial QRS forces, more than a single lead, and preferably all 12 standard leads, should be examined.

The high incidence of recurrent ventricular fibrillation and sudden death in survivors of out-of-hospital cardiac arrests underscores the need for an effective approach to long-term antiarrhythmic prophylaxis in these patients. Until recently, there were little data on the effect of various therapeutic interventions on recurrent cardiac arrest and survival in this patient population. Observations by one group of investigators suggest that antiarrhythmic drug therapy directed against advanced grades of ventricular ectopy affords protection against spontaneous sustained arrhythmias.[91] Another group has found a high incidence of complex ventricular ectopy in survivors of sudden cardiac death up to six months after the cardiac arrest, and this finding was a predictor of subsequent sudden death.[133] Other data suggest that some antiarrhythmic drugs, if present in therapeutic concentrations, may prevent fatal ventricular arrhythmias, whether or not advanced grades of ventricular ectopic activity are suppressed.[134]

Observations from our laboratory as well as others have demonstrated that invasive electrophysiologic testing identifies survivors of out-of-hospital cardiac arrest who require antiarrhythmic therapy and accurately predicts the efficacy of electrophysiologically guided drug regimens in preventing recurrent cardiac arrest.[116,120,135,136] At present, we advise patients who have a history of out-of-hospital cardiac arrest to undergo electrophysiologic testing combined with serial antiarrhythmic drug testing when ventricular arrhythmias can be reliably initiated. In addition, exercise testing is carried out both prior to and following the selection of an antiarrhythmic drug regimen to confirm that protection against exercise-induced ventricular arrhythmias is adequate.

The use of implantable defibrillators in recurrent refractory ventricular fibrillation is discussed below.

Pacemakers and Automatic Defibrillators for Arrhythmias

A variety of pacing techniques may be helpful in controlling recurrent supraventricular and ventricular tachyarrhythmias that are refractory to pharmacologic therapy. Pacemakers may be used either to prevent an arrhythmia or in more refractory cases to terminate arrhythmias [*see Figure 32*]. One or more of the following mechanisms are operative in the prevention or termination of cardiac tachyarrhythmias by pacing: (1) overdrive suppression, (2) interruption of reentrant and possibly triggered rhythms, and (3) conversion to a less refractory rhythm (e.g., the conversion of atrial flutter to atrial fibrillation) that reverts spontaneously to sinus rhythm.

Increasing sophistication in pacemaker design allows a number of different pacing modes to be used. Pacemakers can be programmed to sense a tachycardia and to deliver automatically a wide range of stimuli at virtually any rate and for any duration [*see Figure 32*]. Stimuli generated from an external radio frequency pacemaker can also be delivered by way of subcutaneously implanted receivers and electrodes. Such units may be activated by the patient at the time of an attack of tachycardia.

Reentrant supraventricular tachycardias may be terminated with single premature stimuli in many patients, particularly those patients who incorporate accessory pathways into the arrhythmia since their circuits are anatomically large and usually easily penetrated by paced extrastimuli. By contrast, AV-nodal and ventricular tachycardias are usually associated with small circuits that are often surrounded by slowly conducting tissue. In these circumstances, unless the tachycardias are extremely slow (<160 beats/min), they often cannot be penetrated and terminated by single premature stimuli, even when the stimulating electrode is positioned as closely as possible to the reentry circuit. By using two or more closely coupled extrastimuli or brief bursts of stimuli at rates in excess of the tachycardia, it is possible to abbreviate the refractory periods of surrounding tissues and penetrate the reentry circuit. The use of multiple extrastimuli or burst pacing facilitates the termination of atrial and AV-nodal reen-

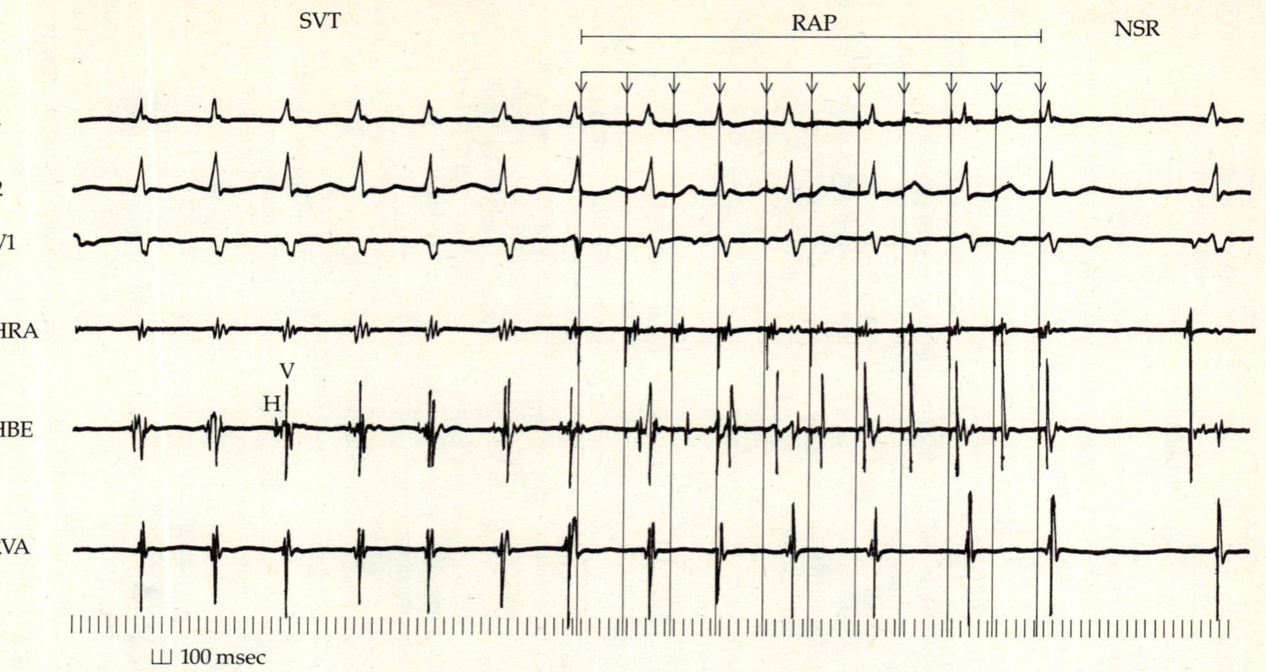

Figure 32   *Termination of sustained supraventricular tachycardia (SVT) by automatic burst atrial pacing is illustrated. Shortly after the onset of sustained supraventricular tachycardia at a rate of 150 beats/min, a burst of pacing applied from the right atrial appendage at a rate of 250 beats/min by an automatic antitachycardia pacemaker interrupts the arrhythmia and the heart is returned to normal sinus rhythm (NSR).*

trant tachycardias, atrial flutter [*see Figure 21*], reentrant tachycardias using accessory pathways, and most sustained ventricular tachycardias. However, burst pacing in the atrium may sometimes induce atrial fibrillation. This arrhythmia is potentially dangerous in the presence of the Wolff-Parkinson-White syndrome with rapid antegrade conduction over an accessory pathway. The risk of pacing-induced atrial fibrillation precludes the use of burst pacing in patients with this form of the syndrome. Furthermore, the use of multiple extrastimuli or burst pacing in the ventricular position during ventricular tachycardia is associated with the common and unpredictable phenomenon of pacing-induced acceleration of the tachycardia rate. This life-threatening complication, as well as the less common phenomenon of pacing-induced ventricular fibrillation, makes automatic antitachycardia pacing unacceptable for the treatment of ventricular tachycardia in the absence of backup defibrillation. The response of any tachycardia to antitachycardia pacemakers should be thoroughly proved in the electrophysiology laboratory before the unit is implanted.

In occasional patients with refractory ventricular arrhythmias, overdrive electrical pacing may be beneficial, particularly if the basic heart rate is slow. Pacing may be instituted either from the atrium, if AV conduction is intact, or from the ventricle. Pacing may be used transiently if the factors responsible for the arrhythmia are evanescent, although at times permanent pacemakers may have to be implanted for long-term rapid pacing.[137]

An implantable automatic cardioverter defibrillator (AICD) has been developed that senses ventricular fibrillation and ventricular tachycardia and delivers a synchronized corrective 25 joule electrical discharge.[138] The device consists of a 300 g pulse generator and three lead electrodes that are used for sensing and defibrillation. The rate-sensing electrode system employs either a transvenous right ventricular endocardial bipolar lead or two sutureless myocardial leads. For defibrillation, two additional electrodes are used: a patch electrode that is placed over the epicardial surface of the left ventricle and either a second patch over the right ventricle or a transvenous spring electrode positioned at the junction of the right atrium and the superior vena cava. The AICD is capable of delivering approximately 100 shocks on one set of batteries, after which the pulse generator must be replaced.

The AICD was approved by the FDA in 1985 for use in patients who have had a cardiac arrest due to ventricular tachycardia or fibrillation unassociated with acute myocardial infarction. Electrophysiologic testing is required prior to implantation to demonstrate the presence of inducible ventricular tachycardia or fibrillation that is unresponsive to antiarrhythmic drug therapy. The AICD has already been implanted in more than 1,200 patients worldwide at centers that specialize in the treatment of cardiac arrhythmias and the use of electrophysiologic techniques. At present, implantation of the device requires general anesthesia and a thoracotomy for lead placement. The pulse generator is implanted in a subcutaneous paraumbilical pocket. Periodic follow-up is performed with an external monitoring device. With the aid of a magnet, this device determines the number of shocks that have been delivered to the patient, the battery strength (charge time), the status of the pulse generator, and the integrity of the sensing function.

The AICD appears to have markedly reduced mortality in the high-risk group of patients in whom it has been implanted.[139] The incidence of arrhythmic deaths in recipients of the AICD is reported to be two percent at one year and four percent at two years. Expected arrhythmia mortality, defined as actual arrhythmia mortality plus appropriate defibrillator discharges (assuming that the patients who received those shocks would have died had the AICD not actively intervened), is reported to be 25 percent at one year and 45 percent at two years.

It is likely that future devices of this type will be smaller and more versatile than the

AICD. These new devices will function as multiprogrammable arrhythmia control systems rather than as single-function defibrillators. Such systems will have algorithms for a hierarchy of responses, including pacing for the prevention and termination of tachycardia, low-energy cardioversion, and defibrillation. The enhanced versatility and safety as well as the reduced size of the implantable arrhythmia control systems that are currently being developed will make them applicable to large numbers of patients with life-threatening ventricular arrhythmias.

Cardioversion

The electrical cardioversion of tachyarrhythmias, which is accomplished by delivering a dc discharge of short duration (2 to 3 msec) to the external thorax, represents a major therapeutic advance. Because of its short duration, the shock can be programmed to be discharged by the R wave of the electrocardiogram, so that the current is delivered in or near the QRS complex. This ensures that the discharge will not occur during the vulnerable phase of the cardiac cycle when an electrical stimulus might induce serious ventricular ectopy.

The arrhythmias most responsive to cardioversion are atrial flutter, atrial fibrillation, and ventricular tachycardia, but any ectopic tachycardia unresponsive to usual therapy can be successfully terminated with this technique. In patients with these arrhythmias who show serious decompensation—for example, those who are hypotensive or in severe congestive heart failure—cardioversion should be the initial therapy and may have to be performed as an emergency measure.

The only circumstance in which cardioversion is contraindicated is in arrhythmias due to digitalis intoxication. Such toxic arrhythmias are refractory to cardioversion, and cardioversion frequently triggers more serious ventricular rhythm disturbances.

In preparation for elective cardioversion, all evidences of digitalis glycoside excess should be resolved. The serum potassium level should be brought within a normal range, particularly in patients who have been receiving chronic diuretic therapy. Cardioversion carries the risk of systemic embolization in patients with atrial fibrillation, and there is some controversy about the indications for anticoagulation prior to cardioversion in such patients.[140] In 1986, a national conference sponsored by the American College of Chest Physicians and the National Heart, Lung and Blood Institute issued specific recommendations regarding the use of antithrombotic therapy prior to cardioversion in patients with atrial fibrillation[65] [*see* Supraventricular Arrhythmias, Atrial Fibrillation, *above*].

When cardioversion is performed electively, premedication with intravenous diazepam, 5 to 10 mg, is both effective and safe. Methohexital sodium, a short-acting barbiturate that induces transient sleep, is even more effective but should be administered by an anesthetist. An anesthetist should always be present when elective cardioversion is undertaken. Resuscitation equipment should be readily available.

The discharge is delivered by means of two electrode paddles placed anteriorly and posteriorly on the thorax, which appears to be more effective than an anterior and lateral placement. Cardioversion should be attempted initially with energy levels of 50 to 100 watt-sec; if unsuccessful, the level should be raised in increments of 50 to 100 watt-sec until either conversion is achieved or energy levels of 300 to 400 watt-sec are reached. High-energy levels are often needed in thick-chested patients, such as those with emphysema. If there is any suspicion of digitalis intoxication, the initial shocks should be in the range of 5 to 10 watt-sec in order to determine whether the electrical discharge will produce any serious rhythm disturbances.

Arrhythmias are common after delivery of the electrical shock. Lidocaine, 70 to 100 mg, should be readily available for immediate intravenous infusion should dangerous ventricular ectopy be initiated. Similarly, intravenous atropine, 1 to 2 mg, should be available in the event of bradycardia. If the existence of an underlying sinus node dysfunction is suspected, equipment for emergency pacing should be at hand or inserted prior to initiation of cardioversion.

Other than arrhythmias, complications of cardioversion are few. There are rare reports of unexplained pulmonary edema following cardioversion, and systemic emboli ensue in about one percent of patients after conversion of atrial fibrillation. Even when repeated shocks are delivered, there does not appear to be a major risk of inflicting significant damage to the myocardium.

Ambulatory Electrocardiographic Monitoring

Although it has long been possible to record the electrocardiogram of ambulatory patients on magnetic tape continuously over several hours for later playback and interpretation (Holter monitoring), only within recent years has this technique been widely applied. As recording and playback systems using semiautomated analysis have advanced, ambulatory ECG monitoring has assumed a major role in the management of cardiac patients.

The ambulatory electrocardiographic recording is useful in tracking down the nature of any cardiac arrhythmia but is especially helpful for certain problems:

1. Ascertaining the etiology of dizzy spells or syncope when a cardiac origin is suspected [*see Figure* 4].
2. Determining the nature of palpitations or episodes of tachycardia described subjectively by patients.
3. Searching for potentially malignant ventricular arrhythmias, particularly in patients who have ischemic heart disease, mitral valve prolapse syndromes, or cardiomyopathies.

4. Assessing the effectiveness of antiarrhythmic therapy in the treatment of ventricular arrhythmias.

5. Evaluating patients with chronic bifascicular or complete heart block for asymptomatic but potentially life-threatening arrhythmias, such as those found in periods of asystole or ventricular irritability. Such episodes may justify the use of a pacemaker or antiarrhythmic drug treatment, or both, even in the absence of symptoms.

Several investigators have described the frequent occurrence of episodes of asymptomatic ST segment depression, termed silent myocardial ischemia, on ambulatory electrocardiograms.[141,142]In patients with known coronary artery disease and angina pectoris, such episodes are frequently associated with objective evidence of ischemia by radionuclide scintigraphy. Although the precise clinical significance of asymptomatic ST segment depression has not yet been defined, it is likely that ambulatory ECG monitoring will assume an increasingly important role in the evaluation of patients who have ischemic heart disease.

In addition to the numerous long-term and event-triggered electrocardiographic recording systems that are available, transtelephone transmission of the electrocardiogram also may be useful to delineate the nature of arrhythmias that occur sporadically or infrequently. Many such systems are now available commercially.

References

1. Ann Intern Med 94:794, 1981
2. Am J Med 77:561, 1984
3. Circulation 71:927, 1985
4. Circulation 47:635, 1973
5. Circulation 46:5, 1972
6. Circulation 60:404, 1979
7. Ann Intern Med 67:1013, 1967
8. Mayo Clin Proc 60:667, 1985
9. Am Heart J 93:735, 1977
10. Circulation 60:413, 1979
11. N Engl J Med 295:190, 1976
12. Am J Med 62:330, 1977
13. Circulation 45:140, 1972
14. Circulation 66:864, 1982
15. Am J Cardiol 40:189, 1977

16. Am J Cardiol 41:318, 1978
17. Am J Cardiol 43:983, 1979
18. Br Heart J 39:160, 1977
19. Int J Cardiol 2:507, 1983
20. Lancet 1:1280, 1984
21. Ann Intern Med 101:234, 1984
22. Am J Cardiol 58:959, 1986
23. Am Heart J 78:450, 1969
24. Circulation 39:13, 1969
25. Circulation 39:287, 1969
26. Prog Cardiovasc Dis 26:333, 1983
27. Circulation 57:845, 1978
28. Circulation 60:12, 1979
29. Circulation 64:1265, 1981
30. Am J Cardiol 50:1316, 1982
31. N Engl J Med 307:137, 1982
32. Am J Med 50:146, 1971
33. Arch Intern Med 131:663, 1973
34. N Engl J Med 315:1183, 1986
35. Br Heart J 51:184, 1984
36. Am J Cardiol 48:1098, 1981
37. Circulation 58:689, 1978
38. Circulation 70:331A, 1984
39. N Engl J Med 309:1166, 1983
40. Prog Cardiovasc Dis 23:435, 1981
41. Circulation 68:227A, 1983
42. Prog Cardiovasc Dis 23:393, 1981
43. N Engl J Med 311:1671, 1984
44. Br Heart J 50:109, 1983
45. Mayo Clin Proc 58:452, 1983
46. Prog Cardiovasc Dis 23:401, 1981
47. PACE 8:52, 1985
48. Ann Intern Med 99:354, 1983
49. Am J Cardiol 52:88, 1983
50. Circulation 35:1170, 1967
51. N Engl J Med 312:1428, 1985
52. Am J Cardiol 41:1123, 1978
53. Am J Cardiol 41:1045, 1978
54. Am J Cardiol 41:1052, 1978
55. Am J Med 64:214, 1978
56. Ann Intern Med 93:875, 1981
57. Circulation 68:1254, 1983
58. JAMA 248:851, 1982
59. N Engl J Med 306:194, 1982
60. Circulation 70:1024, 1984
61. N Engl J Med 279:344, 1968
62. N Engl J Med 312:21, 1985
63. Circulation 45:681, 1973
64. J Am Coll Cardiol 1:816, 1983
64a. Neurology 28:973, 1978
64b. N Engl J Med 323:1505, 1990
64c. N Engl J Med 322:863, 1990
65. Chest 89(suppl):68S, 1986
66. Am J Cardiol 25:690, 1970
67. N Engl J Med 278:492, 1968
68. Am J Med 43:951, 1967
69. Circulation 41:375, 1970
70. Am Heart J 62:756, 1961
71. Arch Intern Med 143:760, 1983
72. N Engl J Med 301:1080, 1979
73. Am J Cardiol 37:93, 1976
74. Ann Intern Med 90:153, 1979
75. Circulation 56:409, 1977
76. Circulation 50:114, 1974
77. Circulation 55:15, 1977
78. Am J Cardiol 41:1061, 1978
79. Ann Intern Med 104:791, 1986
80. Circulation 63:435, 1981
81. Circulation 43:99, 1971
82. Prog Cardiovasc Dis 20:285, 1978
83. Circulation 74:525, 1986
84. J Thorac Cardiovasc Surg 90:490, 1985
85. Circulation 72:170, 1985
86. Am J Cardiol 24:629, 1969
87. Circulation 52(suppl):III-170, 1975
88. Circulation 69:250, 1984
89. Am Heart J 97:159, 1979
90. Circulation 57:440, 1978
91. Am J Cardiol 50:437, 1982
92. Br Heart J 45:717, 1981
93. Ann Intern Med 91:480, 1979
94. N Engl J Med 312:193, 1985
95. N Engl J Med 312:238, 1985
96. Circulation 70:43, 1984
97. Am J Cardiol 53:1275, 1984
98. J Am Coll Cardiol 7:71A, 1986
99. Am Heart J 111:860, 1986
100. Circulation 65:886, 1982
101. N Engl J Med 309:1302, 1983
102. Am Heart J 107:189, 1984
103. N Engl J Med 310:830, 1984
104. J Am Coll Cardiol 6:780, 1985
105. Ann Intern Med 103:387, 1985
106. Circulation 43:420, 1971
107. N Engl J Med 315:36, 1986
108. J Am Coll Cardiol 3:1059, 1984
109. N Engl Med 316:455, 1987
110. Circulation 58:408, 1978
111. Circulation 46:216, 1972
112. Circulation 57:431, 1978
113. Circulation 65:384, 1982
114. Am J Cardiol 54:1131, 1984
115. Am J Cardiol 43:631, 1979
116. Prog Cardiovasc Dis 23:81, 1980
117. N Engl J Med 303:607, 1980
118. N Engl J Med 303:1073, 1980
119. Am J Cardiol 45:725, 1980
120. Am J Cardiol 50:452, 1982
121. N Engl J Med 308:1436, 1983
122. J Am Coll Cardiol 7:195A, 1986
123. Circulation 66(suppl):II-75, 1982
124. Circulation 71:413, 1985
125. Circulation 60:1430, 1979
126. J Thorac Cardiovasc Surg 80:527, 1980
127. Am Coll Cardiol 8:201, 1986
128. Ann Intern Med 93:578, 1980
129. Mod Concepts Cardiovasc Dis 51(6):103, 1982
130. Circulation 59:769, 1979
131. Mod Concepts Cardiovasc Dis 51:85, 1982
132. Circulation 71:17, 1985
133. Am J Cardiol 49:928, 1982
134. Circulation 59:855, 1979
135. Am J Cardiol 57:113, 1986
136. Circulation 74(suppl 2):482, 1986
137. Ann Intern Med 80:380, 1974
138. Ann NY Acad Sci 382:371, 1982
139. J Am Coll Cardiol 6:461, 1985
140. Am Heart J 100:881, 1980
141. Am J Cardiol 56:34E, 1985
142. Am J Cardiol 57:1010, 1986

Acknowledgments

Figure 1 Dana Burns.

Figure 2 Al Miller.

Figure 3 Carol Donner.

Figures 4 and 5 Al Miller.

Figure 6 Carol Donner.

Figure 7 Al Miller. Photograph provided by Dr. Jeremy N. Ruskin, Cardiac Unit, Massachusetts General Hospital.

Figures 8 and 9 Al Miller.

Figure 10 Andy Christie.

Figures 11 and 12 Al Miller.

Figure 13 Al Miller. Photograph provided by Dr. J. W. Harthorne, Massachusetts General Hospital.

Figures 14 through 16 Al Miller.

Figure 17 Al Miller. Electrocardiogram provided by Dr. Peter M. Yurchak, Massachusetts General Hospital.

Figures 18 through 22 Al Miller.

Figure 23 Carol Donner.

Figures 24 through 28 Al Miller.

Figures 29 and 30 Hank Iken. Modified from "Ventricular Arrhythmias," by Jeremy N. Ruskin, in *Practice of Cardiology*, edited by R. Johnson. Little, Brown & Company, Boston, 1980. Used by permission.

Figure 31 Andy Christie.

Figure 32 Dana Burns.

Table 2 From "Implantable Cardiac Pacemakers: Status Report and Resource Guidelines," by V. Parsonnet, S. Furman, and N.P.D. Smyth, in *American Journal of Cardiology* 34:487, 1974. Used by permission.

Text on pages 72–73 excerpted from "Antithrombotic Therapy in Atrial Fibrillation," by M. Dunn, J. Alexander, and R. De Silva. A National Conference sponsored by the American College of Chest Physicians and the National Heart, Lung and Blood Institute. Reprinted from *Chest* 89(suppl):68S, 1986. Used by permission.

4 High Blood Pressure

EDGAR HABER, M.D.

EVE ELIZABETH SLATER, M.D.

High blood pressure is the most significant risk factor for cardiovascular disease[1] and a major cause of heart failure, renal failure, and stroke. Despite the fact that hypertension contributes to the development of these disorders, its detection and treatment have often been neglected by both physicians and patients. Three factors have accounted for this neglect: the etiology of the disorder is poorly understood, the treatment is lifelong, and the condition is generally asymptomatic until complications develop.

Fortunately, worldwide efforts aimed at hypertension detection and follow-up have begun to change prevailing attitudes. Prior to 1970, only one quarter of the estimated 60 million Americans with hypertension were aware of their condition, and only one quarter of those diagnosed were adequately treated. As of 1984, one half of the hypertensive population were properly diagnosed, and one third were receiving some form of antihypertensive therapy.[2] Evidence suggests that intensive patient education has resulted in improved compliance.[3] Moreover, the wide array of antihypertensive agents that have become available will permit most patients to find a regimen that is both effective and free of bothersome side effects.

Pathogenesis

Blood pressure is normally regulated by a series of feedback loops. Changes in blood pressure are sensed by baroreceptors located throughout the circulation. These receptors relay information to the central nervous system; when blood pressure is low, autonomic output produces direct vasoconstriction and cardiac adaptations, as well as secretion of a variety of agents to restore homeostasis.

Derangements of this system can produce hypertension. Primary, or essential, hypertension has no identifiable cause and affects well over 90 percent of hypertensive patients. Secondary hypertension, by definition, has an identifiable etiology [*see Table 1*].

For the past two decades, research efforts have focused primarily on the measurement of vasoactive hormones and peptides by radioimmunoassays to determine the role of these factors on central and peripheral neurogenic control of the heart, vascular resistance, and renal electrolyte transport.

The Renin-Angiotensin-Aldosterone System

Of all the hormones responsible for blood pressure control, renin has been studied the most extensively. Renin is a proteolytic enzyme produced by modified

---

Table 1 **Causes of Secondary Hypertension**

Coarctation

Cushing's syndrome

Drugs and hormones
 Amphetamines, oral contraceptives, estrogens, steroid or thyroid hormone excess

Increased intracranial pressure

Pheochromocytoma

Primary aldosteronism
 Conn's syndrome, idiopathic hyperaldosteronism

Renal parenchymal disease
 Chronic pyelonephritis, congenital renal disease, diabetic nephropathy, glomerulonephritis, interstitial nephropathy, obstructive uropathy, polycystic disease, renin-secreting tumors, vasculitis

Renovascular hypertension

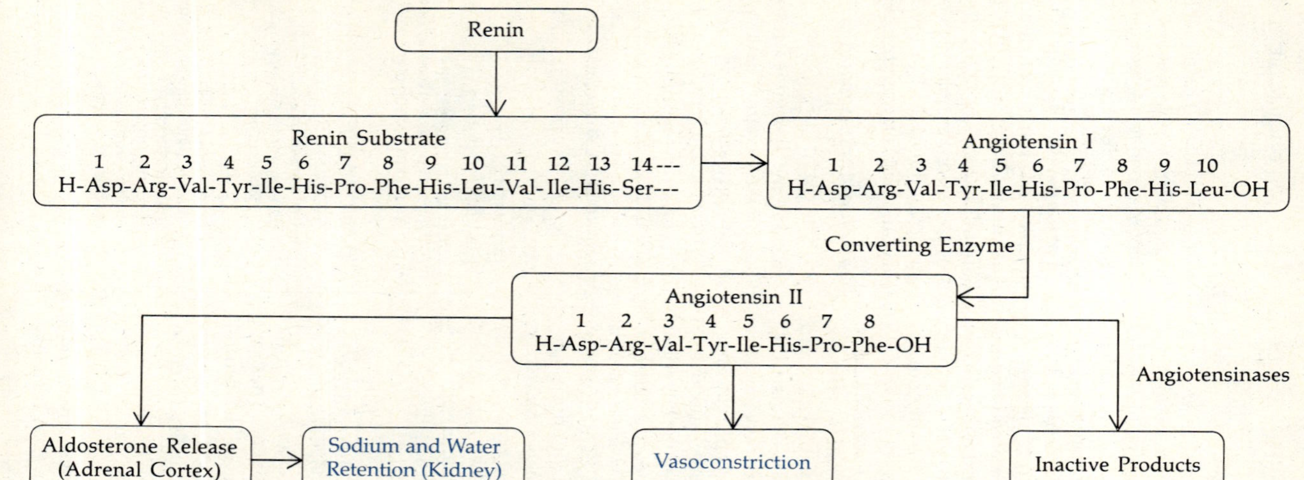

Figure 1   *Renin cleaves renin substrate, a plasma protein, to yield angiotensin I, a decapeptide. Angiotensin I, on passage through the pulmonary circulation, is cleaved by a membrane-bound converting enzyme, which removes two amino acids to yield the octapeptide angiotensin II, a very powerful vasoconstrictor. Angiotensin II stimulates the production of aldosterone by the adrenal cortex and is eventually degraded by enzymes termed angiotensinases. Aldosterone reduces renal excretion of sodium and water, thus increasing intravascular volume.*

afferent arteriolar smooth muscle cells in the juxtaglomerular apparatus. Although reninlike enzymes have been identified at other anatomic sites, their physiologic role in blood pressure regulation has not been ascertained.

Once released into the circulation, renin acts on renin substrate, an alpha globulin synthesized in the liver, to release angiotensin I. Angiotensin I is a decapeptide with no apparent physiologic effect. In a single passage through the pulmonary circulation, angiotensin I is cleaved by a membrane-bound converting enzyme to produce angiotensin II, a very potent vasoconstrictor and regulator of renal sodium reabsorption. Angiotensin II is also the primary stimulus for adrenocortical production of aldosterone, a mineralocorticoid that promotes the reabsorption of sodium and water by the renal tubules. This biochemical cascade has been termed the renin-angiotensin-aldosterone (RAA) system [see Figure 1]. Aldosterone increases intravascular volume and elevates cardiac output; these effects, in combination with angiotensin II–induced vasoconstriction, raise blood pressure. Increased blood pressure, increased angiotensin II, and increased fluid volume signal directly to the juxtaglomerular apparatus to shut off renin release, a process termed negative feedback. Angiotensin II may also cause the central nervous system to decrease autonomic output by a direct effect.

Renin release is subject to an intricate control system. Renal perfusion pressure, sodium concentration, and beta-adrenergic stimulation are considered to be the chief regulating factors. The net effect of these physiologic controls is to render renin production inversely proportional to effective blood volume. Therefore, anything that decreases effective blood volume stimulates renin release, and anything that increases effective blood volume suppresses the release of renin.

Renin Levels in Various Disease States

Plasma renin activity (PRA) levels in various disease states can be predicted from knowledge of the physiology of the renin system [see Table 2].

Renal artery stenosis raises renin production by decreasing renal perfusion pressure. Hypertension is then mediated by the direct vasoconstrictive effect of angiotensin II and by fluid retention secondary to adrenocortical aldosterone. Both PRA and aldosterone levels are usually elevated.

In primary hyperaldosteronism (Conn's syndrome or idiopathic hyperaldosteronism), autonomously secreted aldosterone induces sodium retention, expanded plasma volume, and consequent hypertension. Renin production is suppressed, and PRA is usually undetectable.

Rarely, renal tumors or cysts mimic renal artery stenosis by causing extrinsic compression of the renal vasculature, which gives rise to an elevated PRA. These tumors or cysts can be distinguished from stenotic lesions by arteriography. Benign renal hemangiopericytomas that secrete renin are exceedingly rare.[4] Three case reports exist of renin-secreting adenocarcinomas of the lung, ovary, and pancreas.[5]

Reduced PRA is found in patients with a renin-deficiency syndrome that is characterized by hyperkalemia, postural hypotension, and below-normal aldosterone levels in the presence of otherwise normal adrenal function.[6] Patients tend to be elderly, to have evidence of prior renal disease with diminished creatinine clearance, or to be diabetic. The renin deficiency may be caused by an acquired abnormality of the juxtaglomerular apparatus, which may be related to a deficiency in either atrial natriuretic peptide or prostacyclin.[7,8] Hyporeninism should be considered in the differential diagnosis of hyperkalemia. Agents that inhibit renin activity or renal prostaglandin production, such as angiotensin converting enzyme (ACE) inhibitors, beta blockers, calcium channel blockers, or nonsteroidal anti-inflammatory agents, should be discontinued for patients with this condition. Salt repletion and, if necessary, mineralocorticoid administration are effective treatments.

Table 2   Renin and Aldosterone Levels in Certain Disease States

Disease State	Renin Level	Aldosterone Level	Confirmation of Diagnosis
Renovascular hypertension	↑ or —	↑ or —	Differential venous renin measurements Angiography
Primary aldosteronism	↓ (near 0)	↑	Aldosterone determination Venography
Renal tumors, cysts	↑	↑	Angiographic appearance of lesion
Essential hypertension	↑ or — or ↓	↑ or — or ↓	
Low-renin state	↓	↓	↓ Creatinine clearance Clinical setting
Bartter's syndrome	↑	↑	Patient normotensive Clinical setting

Bartter's syndrome is a condition that is characterized by juxtaglomerular cell hyperplasia, hyperreninemia, hyperaldosteronism, hypokalemia, and normal blood pressure. Responsiveness to infused angiotensin II or to norepinephrine is subnormal, and proximal tubular reabsorption of sodium by the kidney is diminished. It is probable that all of these defects, including hyperreninemia, are mediated by increased renal synthesis of prostaglandin E_2 (PGE_2).[9] Traditional therapy, which consists of propranolol, spironolactone, and potassium supplements, is being replaced by aspirin and other anti-inflammatory agents that suppress PGE_2 synthesis.

Renin in Essential Hypertension

The fact that renin plays an integral role in blood pressure homeostasis and in the pathogenesis of hypertension has long been appreciated.[10] A classification system of essential hypertension based on PRA was devised in 1972 by Brunner and associates.[11] The system has been criticized as imposing arbitrary divisions on what many believe is a continuous spectrum. We agree that hypertensive patients need not be classified on the basis of PRA and that the PRA level does not predict the risk of vasculotoxic events.[12,13] Thus, PRA determination is not recommended at present for large-scale patient screening. However, when a renin-related form of secondary hypertension is suspected or a search for secondary hypertension is advisable, PRA is a valuable screening parameter that can identify patients with renovascular disease or primary aldosteronism.[14]

The effectiveness of ACE inhibitors in the treatment of primary hypertension suggests that the RAA system plays a major role in the disease [*see* Treatment, *below*]. At present, research is directed toward developing renin inhibitors for clinical use; currently renin inhibitors are peptides that are unsuitable for oral use.[15]

Renin Measurement

Renin is quantified by measuring the rate of generation of angiotensin I, as determined by a radioimmunoassay. PRA is expressed as nanograms of angiotensin I per milliliter per hour.

PRA is exquisitely sensitive to variations in sodium balance and posture. Commonly used antihypertensive drugs also alter PRA [*see Table 3*]. Thus, PRA is usually measured when the patient is eating a normal diet and is not receiving antihypertensive medication. Two methods yield a more accurate assessment of a patient's renin status than that obtained by random PRA determination: PRA measurement with simultaneous 24-hour urine sodium determination and measurement of both stimulated and suppressed renin values. The stimulated PRA value alone is a simple and sufficient screen for renin-related forms of secondary hypertension [*see Table 4*].[14]

The Renal Kallikrein–Kinin System

Kallikrein is a renal enzyme that acts on kininogen, a plasma substrate, to release bradykinin. Bradykinin is a small peptide with vasodilator properties. Bradykinin in turn is degraded by kininases, one of which is identical to the enzyme that converts angiotensin I to angiotensin II. The kallikrein-kinin system affects water and electrolyte excretion by influencing renal blood flow, by mediating prostaglandin release, and possibly, by exerting a direct effect.[16]

In humans and animals, renal kallikrein excretion decreases in certain forms of hypertension.[17] Ongoing studies seek to determine whether decreased kallikrein excretion is a pathogenetic factor in these forms of hypertension or in renal disease. Because the angiotensin converting enzyme

Table 4 **Plasma Renin Activity (PRA) Determination**

Prerequisites	Normal diet
	Antihypertensive medication discontinued for three weeks
	Oral contraceptives discontinued for at least six months
	Iced, unclotted plasma specimen
Methods of measurement	PRA with 24-hr urine sodium determination (useful only when dietary Na^+ < 100 mEq/day)
	or
	Suppressed PRA (patient supine for > 30 min)
	plus
	Stimulated PRA (40–80 mg furosemide p.o. followed by 4 hr upright or 40 mg I.V. followed by 30 min upright)*

*Sufficient to screen for secondary hypertension.

degrades bradykinin, it is possible that the antihypertensive action of the angiotensin converting enzyme inhibitors may include potentiation of kinin activity.

Vasopressin

Vasopressin, or antidiuretic hormone, is a more potent vasoconstrictor than angiotensin II in vitro, but it appears to participate only in rapid, short-term control of arterial pressure when autonomic reflexes and the RAA system become maximally stressed, as in hemorrhage.[18] Vasopressin may also play a role in certain volume-dependent forms of hypertension.[19] Research, however, has been hampered by the lack of a widely available radioimmunoassay for vasopressin.

Natriuretic Factors

Atrial Natriuretic Factor

It has long been recognized that dilatation of the atrium results in natriuresis, and this observation has led to the isolation of a

Table 3 **Effect of Antihypertensive Drugs on Renin**

Renin Inhibition	*Renin Stimulation*
Beta blockers	Angiotension converting enzyme inhibitors
Clonidine	
Guanabenz	Calcium entry blockers
Labetalol	Diuretics
Methyldopa	Guanadrel
Prazosin	Guanethidine
Reserpine	Vasodilators

powerful vasodilatory and natriuretic peptide from atrial extracts.[20,21] This peptide, termed atrial natriuretic factor (ANF), appears to promote natriuresis by increasing the glomerular filtration rate; it also inhibits aldosterone production and renin secretion. ANF may thus serve as an endogenous antagonist to the RAA system. Because of the considerable potency of ANF, it will likely prove to have a significant role in cardiovascular homeostasis. ANF or a derivative drug might eventually be applied in therapy. Thus far, aberrant ANF secretion has not been linked to hypertension.

The existence of a hormone with ouabainlike properties, which may emanate from the hypothalamus, has been demonstrated in the circulation of volume-expanded animals and a few hypertensive patients.[22] Such a factor, although promoting renal sodium excretion, might also cause increases in vascular sodium and, in turn, calcium. The increased calcium would raise vascular resistance.[23] Counteraction of this effect might explain the efficacy of calcium entry blockers in the treatment of certain forms of hypertension [*see* Treatment, *below*].

Other Renal Factors

Decreased renal sodium excretion and increased vascular resistance have been shown to occur early in the course of essential hypertension.[24] In addition, in about one half of patients with essential hypertension, renal blood flow does not increase in response to sodium loading. This failure has been linked to defective adrenal and renal responses to angiotensin II. These defects, which are corrected by ACE inhibitors [*see* Treatment, *below*],[2] suggest the presence of an undefined renal abnormality in some patients with essential hypertension. Interestingly, some cases of essential hypertenison have been corrected by renal transplantation.[26]

A major step in the understanding of essential hypertension could be made if abnormalities in membrane ion transport could be correlated with abnormalities in renal sodium handling. (Such ion transport defects could result from altered renal ion transport function, aberrant innervation, or hormonal influences.)

A role for abnormal electrolyte transport is suggested by the finding of abnormalities in leukocyte sodium content, in erythrocyte Na^+, K^+, Cl^{-2} cotransport, or in Li^+, Na^+ countertransport in hypertensive patients. These latter abnormalities appear to follow a hereditary pattern in families with hypertensive members.[27-29] An inverse relation between erythrocyte Li^+, Na^+ countertransport and fractional lithium clearance in the kidney (a measure of proximal tubular sodium resorption) has been reported in patients with essential hypertension.[30] However, the correlation was weak, fractional Na^+ clearance was unchanged, and only a few patients were studied. Studies that further define these abnormalities and their hereditary pattern are under way.

Diagnosis

Certain commonly held beliefs regarding diagnosis have been challenged by epidemiologic data, such as those generated by the Framingham study.[1] Contrary to former teaching, casual blood pressure levels seem to be more reliable than basal levels in predicting long-term cardiovascular risk. This finding is not surprising if we accept the fact that a person in whom anxiety-provoked hypertension develops in a physician's office is equally likely to respond to the stresses of daily life with hypertension that is labile.

There is no critical level of blood pressure that appears to delineate excess risk, and therefore, the definition of hypertension remains an arbitrary one. Morbidity and mortality increase linearly with increasing levels of either systolic or diastolic blood pressure. Even modest elevations carry substantial risks.[1]

We define as hypertensive those blood pressure levels that are associated with a greater than 50 percent increase in mortality: 130/90 mm Hg for men younger than 45 years; 140/95 mm Hg for men 45 years of age and older; and 160/95 mm Hg for all women. Systolic hypertension is present when the systolic blood pressure exceeds

140 mm Hg and the diastolic pressure is less than 90 mm Hg. Borderline hypertension is defined as intermittent elevation of systolic or diastolic pressure exceeding the accepted normal value for the person's age and sex.

Criteria for children and adolescents have been published by the National Heart, Lung, and Blood Institute.[31] The following levels are associated with significant risk: 116/76 mm Hg (three to five years of age); 122/78 mm Hg (six to nine years of age); 126/82 mm Hg (10 to 12 years of age); 136/86 mm Hg (13 to 15 years of age); and 142/92 mm Hg (16 to 18 years of age).

Clinical Examination

Blood pressure is properly measured in both arms while the patient is comfortably seated. Tradition holds that the arm is straight while the hand is supine. The cuff should be placed as high as possible on the arm, and the arm should be held so that the cuff is level with the heart. If blood pressure is measured with the arm dependent or with an inadequately sized cuff, falsely elevated values may be obtained.[32] The cuff width should be greater than two thirds of the arm's diameter; the length of the inflatable portion should be greater than two thirds of the arm's circumference. The average of two successive measurements in each arm is recorded. Diastolic pressure is determined by the point at which sound disappears (Korotkoff 5), rather than by the point at which sound changes in quality (Korotkoff 4). The patient who, on two separate occasions, demonstrates a pressure equal to or greater than those levels listed above is classified as hypertensive. A diastolic pressure of 90 mm Hg or greater should be confirmed within two months; a diastolic pressure between 105 and 114 mm Hg should be retested within two weeks.[33]

Hypertension caused by severe atherosclerosis, or so-called pseudohypertension, is generally seen in patients older than 70 years who have elevated cholesterol levels. Intra-arterial blood pressure measurement is the only reliable method for detecting pseudohypertension in such patients.[35]

Evaluation of the hypertensive patient includes a careful interview emphasizing the following points:

1. Family history of high blood pressure, diabetes, or cardiovascular disease.
2. Age at onset of elevated blood pressure.
3. Diet and salt intake.
4. The presence of other cardiovascular risk factors.
5. Symptoms of cardiovascular disease, such as angina, dyspnea, or claudication.
6. Use of agents associated with hypertension, such as oral contraceptives, estrogens, steroids, topical mineralocorticoids, thyroid hormones, anorectics or decongestants that contain amphetamines, or large quantities of licorice. Increasing use of over-the-counter cold and diet pills that contain alpha- and beta-adrenergic agonists requires greater attention to this point.[35]
7. Symptoms of secondary hypertension—for example, headache, excessive perspiration, and palpitations (prominent symptoms of pheochromocytoma); muscle cramps, weakness, and polyuria (which suggest hyperaldosteronism); or leg claudication (found in coarctation).
8. Renal disease or history of flank trauma.

The physical examination focuses on weight measurement, funduscopy, thyroid evaluation, careful cardiopulmonary examination, and evaluation of the peripheral vasculature. The last consists of arm and leg blood pressure measurements, simultaneous radial-femoral pulse palpation, auscultation of extremities for bruits, and abdominal palpation and auscultation. A search for the stigmata of Cushing's syndrome, polycystic kidney, chronic renal failure, or neurofibromatosis and a complete neurologic evaluation are also important.

The utility of the classical Keith-Wagener-Barker funduscopic grades for predicting hypertensive vascular damage is controversial. Most patients with established hypertension of several years' duration will exhibit narrowing of the arteriolar lumina (grade I) and obscuring of veins as

Table 5 Costs in 1988 for Evaluation of Hypertension

Determination or Procedure	Approximate Cost ($)*
Complete blood count†	8.55
Urinalysis†	4.00
Serum potassium (K^+)†	3.00
Blood urea nitrogen†	5.25
Fasting blood glucose†	5.25
Serum cholesterol†	3.00
Serum uric acid†	3.00
Electrocardiogram†	35.00
	67.05
Urine culture and sensitivity	23.50
Serum sodium	3.00
Serum chloride	3.00
Serum carbon dioxide	3.00
Serum creatinine	3.00
Serum triglycerides	10.00
Urine potassium	3.00
Urine creatinine	8.65
Urine metanephrine	24.55
Urine vanillylmandelic acid	23.70
Plasma renin activity (PRA)	40.00
Plasma catecholamines	59.80
Plasma aldosterone	45.00
Plasma cortisol	24.00
Urine catecholamines	46.40
Chest roentgenogram	57.00
Intravenous pyelogram	258.00
Radioisotope renal scan	362.00
Abdominal CT scan	462.00
Abdominal ultrasound	201.00
Digital subtraction angiography	340.00
Renal arteriography (includes aortography and selective injections of the renal arteries)	1,800.00‡
Selective renal or adrenal vein catheterization	324.00‡

Note: estimates do not include the cost of hospitalization.

*These estimates may vary considerably by region.

†Essential tests.

‡Costs are variable depending on the complexity of the procedure.

they cross behind the arteries (grade II). More serious disease is indicated by the appearance of flame hemorrhages and large, ill-defined exudates (grade III), which may eventually progress to increased intracranial pressure and papilledema (grade IV). Ill-defined exudates must be distinguished from the well-circumscribed, small exudates seen in patients with atherosclerosis.

Laboratory Evaluation

Arguments in favor of conducting an elaborate laboratory evaluation of hypertensive patients have been tempered by the finding that surgically correctable disease is much less prevalent than anticipated. A Mayo Clinic study estimated that annually 0.23 percent of all hypertensive patients require surgery for secondary hypertension (assuming that 16.4 percent of the adult population is hypertensive).[36]

Although it has been argued that increasing laboratory costs may eventually limit the extent to which hypertensive patients can be evaluated, it is becoming clear that extensive workup is necessary in only a small subset of the hypertensive population. One who exercises good clinical judgment and follows the guidelines outlined here will neither miss treatable disease nor contribute to excessive medical costs.

Tests that are essential in the routine evaluation of hypertension are a complete blood count; urinalysis; determinations of serum potassium, blood urea nitrogen or serum creatinine, fasting blood glucose, serum cholesterol, and serum uric acid; and an electrocardiogram [*see Table 5*]. These tests usually provide sufficient information regarding both the presence of end-organ damage from hypertension and the likelihood that complications will develop from the blood pressure elevation. The total cost of these tests is approximately $67. For most patients, evaluation is complete at this point.

Patients at high risk for secondary hypertension should clearly receive a more thorough diagnostic evaluation. Such patients include those younger than 35 years because these patients have a higher incidence of secondary disease. Also included are patients with abrupt onset of hypertension and those without a family history of essential hypertension because these factors are atypical of essential hypertension. Patients who have severe elevation of blood pressure, who are at exceptional cardiovascular risk (see below), or whose hypertension has not responded to empiric therapy also need further study. The screening program for such patients includes, in addition to routine tests, a chest x-ray, measurement of urine metanephrine or vanillylmandelic acid, a rapid-sequence intravenous pyelogram or a renal scan, and determination of stimulated PRA.

In some patients, a specific form of secondary disease is suspected because of certain clinical clues, and diagnosis is simplified. Patients with Cushing's syndrome can easily be identified by appearance. Patients with coarctation can be diagnosed by arm and leg blood pressure measurements. The patient's history often provides evidence that supports a diagnosis of pheochromocytoma or drug-induced disease. Hyperaldosteronism is usually suspected on the basis of hypokalemia apparent on a routine serum potassium measurement. Renovascular disease should be looked for in young hypertensive patients or in older patients who experience abrupt onset of hypertension and have no history of familial hypertension. In such cases, simple and relatively inexpensive tests can usually confirm or rule out the diagnosis [see Special Topics, *below, and Table 6*].

Risk Factors

For assessment of cardiovascular risk in hypertensive patients, we advise reliance on the Framingham study data.[1] This study has identified five simple variables that appear to accurately predict the risk of cardiovascular complications: blood pressure, serum cholesterol, cigarette smoking, glucose intolerance, and electrocardiographic evidence of left ventricular hypertrophy with strain. Other contributing factors such as family history, obesity, hypertriglyceridemia, and hyperuricemia, although significant, were shown to exert their influence through one of the five major risk determinants. Other risk factors may yet be identified; the inverse correlation between high-density lipoprotein cholesterol concentration and coronary artery disease is widely accepted.[37] High cardiovascular risk clearly lowers the threshold at which hypertensive patients should be treated.

Treatment

Whom Should We Treat?

Patients with Diastolic Blood Pressure of 105 mm Hg or Greater

Patients with diastolic blood pressure of 105 mm Hg or greater should be treated aggressively. Therapy significantly reduces morbidity and mortality from congestive heart failure, renal failure, stroke, and ischemic cardiac events.[38,39] The goal of therapy in these patients is reduction of diastolic

Table 6 Screening Tests for Secondary Hypertension

Suspected Diagnosis	Test
Coarctation	Chest roentgenogram
Cushing's syndrome	Plasma cortisol after suppression with dexamethasone (1 mg)
Pheochromocytoma	Urine metanephrine or vanillylmandelic acid Clonidine suppression test
Primary aldosteronism	Serum K^+ Stimulated PRA Urine K^+
Renovascular hypertension	Intravenous pyelogram or renal scan Suppressed or stimulated PRA Digital subtraction angiography (if diagnosis highly suspected)

blood pressure to less than 90 mm Hg with minimal adverse effects. However, even partial reduction of blood pressure has been shown to significantly reduce any hypertensive complications.[40]

Patients with Diastolic Blood Pressure between 90 and 104 mm Hg

Four large clinical trials—the Australian Management Committee study,[41] the Oslo study,[42] the Hypertension Detection and Follow-up Program of the National Heart, Lung and Blood Institute,[43,44] and the Medical Research Council study[45]—have demonstrated that patients whose diastolic blood pressure ranges from 90 to 104 mm Hg benefit from treatment. All four studies showed a significantly reduced incidence of cerebrovascular events (including stroke), aortic dissection, heart failure, and cardiac hypertrophy in treated patients. The first and third studies also demonstrated significant reductions in mortality in treated patients.

The Hypertension Detection and Follow-up Program (HDFP) of the National Heart, Lung and Blood Institute has provided the most striking support for intervention in patients with diastolic blood pressure of 90 to 104 mm Hg.[43,44] Hypertensive patients were randomized and then either given aggressive drug treatment or referred for customary medical care. After five years, mortality was 17 percent lower in the aggressively treated group than in the referred group; the difference was even larger when only patients with a diastolic pressure between 90 and 104 mm Hg were compared. Aggressively treated patients also demonstrated a dramatic reduction in stroke and other cardiovascular events.

A similar study, the Multiple Risk Factor Intervention Trial (MRFIT), tested the efficacy of an intervention program aimed at reducing hypertension, cigarette smoking, and elevated blood cholesterol levels.[46] Risk factors and subsequent mortality were reduced significantly in the regular-care control group, whose members remained in the care of their physicians, and even more so in the special-intervention group. The difference in mortality between the two groups was not significant. This similarity may be accounted for by the substantial reduction in risk factors in the control group and by a surprisingly high mortality among hypertensive patients in the intervention group who had an abnormal resting ECG. It is postulated that arrhythmias triggered by hypokalemia secondary to high-dose diuretic therapy may be responsible for this latter finding. However, aggressively treated patients who had an abnormal resting ECG in the HDFP study experienced no increase in mortality.[47] Thus, we believe that aggressive reduction of risk factors is still mandatory and that any degree of diuretic-induced hypokalemia must be avoided, especially in patients with other cardiovascular disease.

The International Prospective Primary Prevention Study in Hypertension (IPPPSH) provided important information about the use of beta blockers as antihypertensive agents.[48] The study evaluated oxprenolol, a nonselective beta blocker. A reduction in coronary events was seen only in nonsmoking males.

Research is being directed at the effects of antihypertensive therapy on end-organ damage. Effective blood pressure control reduces hypertensive left ventricular enlargement, as determined by echocardiography,[49] and retards the decline in creatinine clearance that is seen in diabetic patients who have mild hypertension.[50]

Patients with Systolic Hypertension

Indications for treatment of systolic blood pressure elevation in the absence of diastolic hypertension are less clear. Even though epidemiologic data point to an increased risk associated with systolic hypertension, benefits from treatment have not yet been shown. Thus, current recommendations are conservative. Treatment is indicated for the following individuals: those younger than 35 years who have a systolic pressure greater than 140 mm Hg, those 35 to 59 years of age who have a systolic pressure greater than 150 mm Hg, and those older than 60 years who have a systolic pressure greater than 160 mm Hg.

Systolic hypertension is often difficult to control, especially in the elderly; our treatment goal is a gently achieved 10 percent reduction of systolic blood pressure. Pharmacotherapy carried to the point at which the patient experiences uncomfortable side effects is rarely indicated. Systolic hypertension caused by high cardiac output states such as aortic regurgitation or anemia should not be treated with antihypertensive drugs.

Patients with Intermittent Elevation of Systolic or Diastolic Blood Pressure

Fixed essential hypertension develops in patients who have borderline hypertension more commonly than it develops in normal persons.[51] Attention has focused on these patients in attempts to identify in its earliest stages the abnormality that leads to essential hypertension. Evidence for autonomic nervous system dysfunction has been demonstrated in certain patients. Patients who manifest enhanced sympathetic activity with an elevated heart rate and increased cardiac output respond well to therapeutic intervention with beta-blocking drugs, although the ultimate impact of treatment on disease progression and on prognosis has yet to be determined. The decision to treat such patients may be facilitated by the use of a 24-hour recording device to determine blood pressure levels during normal activity.

Elderly Patients

The elderly are particularly susceptible to the side effects of antihypertensive therapy, and it has been suggested that the threshold for treating high blood pressure in such patients be raised. Initial results of a study by the European Working Party, however, indicate that mortality in hypertensive patients older than 60 years can be reduced by therapy.[52] In the study, 840 patients with diastolic pressure between 90 and 119 mm Hg and systolic pressure between 160 and 239 mm Hg were randomly assigned to treatment, either with a thiazide and triamterene (or methyldopa when the patients did not respond to those two drugs) or with a placebo. The number of deaths from cardiovascular events was significantly lower in the treated group, except in those older than 80 years.[53] The approach to antihypertensive therapy in the elderly has been reviewed.[54]

Summary

Our recommendations for identification of patients who require treatment parallel those of the Joint National Committee on Detection, Evaluation, and Treatment of High Blood Pressure.[34]

In certain patients, vigorous dietary and behavioral modifications (see below) may be attempted before instituting pharmacologic therapy or as an adjunct to such therapy. Patients in whom such alternatives may be advisable are those whose diastolic blood pressure consistently remains between 90 and 100 mm Hg, who have no apparent cardiovascular risk or family history of hypertension, and who exhibit a high degree of motivation.[55] The World Health Organization currently recommends continued observation of such patients and initiation of drug therapy only after the diastolic blood pressure exceeds 95 mm Hg.[56]

Diet and Behavioral Modifications

A low-salt diet must be maintained by all hypertensive patients regardless of the pharmacotherapy chosen. The FDA has published an accessible and comprehensive guide to sodium and calorie content of most common foods.[57] We have found this list to be invaluable. Patients also should be instructed on how to lose weight, if indicated. Weight reduction has been shown not only to lower blood pressure in hypertensive patients but also to decrease left ventricular mass, presumably by reducing obesity-related increases in preload.[58] Moreover, data derived from the Dietary Change in Hypertension Group of the Hypertension Detection and Follow-up Program demonstrate that approximately 70 percent of mildly hypertensive individuals receiving rigorous single-drug therapy who achieve effective weight loss (mean reduction of 10 lb) or sodium reduction (mean reduction of 54 mEq/day) can remain off medication once it is stopped.[59]

Increasing attention is being focused on the role of dietary electrolytes in essential hypertension. There is evidence that a high-potassium–low-sodium diet can lower resting blood pressure in some, but not all, hypertensive individuals.[60] In addition, potassium supplementation in patients receiving diuretic therapy for hypertension resulted not only in a decreased tendency toward tachycardia but also in a significant further reduction in mean blood pressure.[61] A retrospective analysis of the dietary histories of adult Americans has demonstrated a correlation between reduced calcium intake and higher blood pressures.[62] Magnesium supplementation for patients receiving chronic diuretic therapy was shown in one study to significantly reduce both systolic and diastolic pressure[63]; however, the benefits of calcium or magnesium supplementation have not been proved, and potential long-term adverse effects have not been evaluated.[64-67]

Increasing evidence shows that vigorous exercise in combination with weight reduction can significantly ameliorate both systolic and diastolic blood pressure in certain individuals with borderline or established high blood pressure.[68,69] Being physically fit may also forestall the development of hypertension.[70] Highly motivated patients should be considered for these interventions as adjuncts to pharmacologic therapy. Selected patients appear to benefit from therapy designed to improve the ability to respond to stress.[71,72]

Improved understanding by the patient of the pathophysiology, therapy, and consequences of high blood pressure is important in enhancing cooperation and compliance. Home blood pressure units have proved useful in enlisting patients' active participation in their therapy. As an additional motivation for compliance, insurance companies will now reduce premiums for patients whose hypertension has been successfully controlled for several years.[73]

Drugs

Drugs used to treat hypertension include diuretics, sympatholytics, vasodilators, angiotensin converting enzyme inhibitors, and calcium entry blockers [*see Table 7*]. Although it has often been argued that hypertension therapy is largely empiric, factors such as disease severity or drug side effects frequently dictate therapeutic choices.

Diuretics

Diuretics are commonly used to initiate and maintain antihypertensive therapy. To augment compliance, relatively inexpensive agents and those that need be taken only once daily are preferred.

Significant diuretic-induced hypokalemia is a side effect that occurs frequently. It results most commonly from excessive salt intake or, rarely, from mineralocorticoid hypertension. The diuretic's duration of action is apparently a major determinant of its tendency to cause hypokalemia: the longer-acting agents induce more continuous kaliuresis. This effect should be considered when hypokalemia arises. It is wise to measure serum potassium soon after diuretic therapy has been initiated. If hypokalemia ($[K^+] \leq 3.6$ mEq/l) develops, supplementary potassium or a potassium-sparing diuretic should be administered.

Strong arguments favor avoidance of hypokalemia in almost every patient. The weakness associated with even mild hypokalemia often limits compliance. Prolonged hypokalemia will impair glucose metabolism.[74] Moreover, a high incidence of ventricular irritability has been related to diuretic-induced hypokalemia in patients with or without manifest cardiac disease.[75] Thus, hypokalemia must be avoided, especially in patients who have coronary artery disease, who are receiving digitalis, or who have ventricular irritability.

Hypercalcemia is rarely caused by thiazides and should prompt a search for hyperparathyroidism. In several studies, patients taking thiazides maintained small but significant and reversible increases in LDL cholesterol and triglyceride levels[76]; however, the HDL cholesterol level and the ratio of total cholesterol to HDL cholesterol remained unchanged. Whether these minor changes contribute to cardiovascular risk is unknown.

Because of their higher cost and shorter duration of action, the potent diuretics furosemide, ethacrynic acid, and bumetanide are best reserved for patients who show evidence of renal insufficiency (creatinine clearance < 20 to 30 percent of normal), in whom thiazides are ineffective, and for patients who have documented allergy to thiazides. The strength of 1 mg of bumetanide is equivalent to 40 mg of furosemide. Each of these three agents should be administered twice a day. Metolazone may also be effective in those patients who have reduced creatinine clearance.

Potassium-sparing diuretics are less potent than other diuretics. These drugs, however, are especially useful in patients who have mineralocorticoid hypertension, thiazide hypersensitivity, or gout. For individuals in whom hypokalemia is a special risk, such as those who receive digitalis or who have ventricular irritability, the potassium-retaining properties of the distal tubular diuretics are advantageous, whether the agents are given alone or in combination with thiazides.

In contrast, because there is a risk of hyperkalemia, extreme caution should be exercised when using a distal tubular diuretic alone in diabetic patients, in patients who have impaired renal function, or in patients receiving an angiotensin converting enzyme inhibitor (see below). Triamterene should be avoided in patients who have kidney stones or in those with a history of kidney stones.

Sympatholytic Agents

Beta blockers Beta blockers are commonly used as initial therapeutic agents in the treatment of hypertension or as second-ary agents when diuretic therapy alone fails to control hypertension.

An increasing number of physicians have been initiating therapy with beta blockers rather than with diuretics. Single-drug therapy with a beta blocker appears to be most effective in young and middle-aged patients. More than 75 percent of patients younger than 40 years respond to beta blockade, whereas only 50 percent of patients 40 to 49 years of age and 25 percent of those 50 to 59 years of age respond.[77] The practice of commencing therapy with a beta blocker is recommended for younger patients and for patients with special needs, such as those with concomitant angina pectoris.

Treatment with beta blockers involves certain risks. When used as initial therapy in patients with volume-dependent hypertension, beta blockers may give rise to paradoxic increases in blood pressure. In addition, many beta blockers, used either alone or in combination with diuretics, may produce adverse changes in cholesterol levels, including an increase in the ratio of total cholesterol to HDL cholesterol. Beta-selective agents alone, however, do not affect the HDL cholesterol level.[76] Patients with heart failure, bradycardia, second- or third-degree heart block, or asthma usually cannot tolerate more than modest doses of beta blockers.

There are eight beta-blocking agents from which to choose. Although propranolol has been in use the longest, a number of the other available beta-blocking agents have more desirable properties (see below).

Beginning dosages of propranolol are modest (20 to 40 mg twice a day), and subsequent dosages are gradually increased until the desired fall in blood pressure is achieved. Propranolol acts by a dose-related mechanism. At low doses (160 mg/day or less), beta-blocking effects predominate; at high doses, a renin-independent, central nervous system effect is probably more important, and side effects generally become significant. We therefore rarely exceed doses of 240 to 360 mg/day.

Nadolol, a nonselective beta-blocking agent with a prolonged duration of action,

Table 7 Antihypertensive Drugs

Drug	Trade Name	Initial Dose/Maximum Dose (mg/day)	Frequency of Dosage	Approximate Daily Cost ($)* (dose in mg)
Thiazides				
Bendroflumethiazide	Naturetin	2.5/5	q.d.	0.35 (5)
Benthiazide	Exna / Aquatag	25/50	b.i.d.	0.12 (50)
Chlorothiazide	Diuril	250/500	q.d.	0.09 (250)
Chlorthalidone	Hygroton	25/50	q.d.	0.36 (50)
Cyclothiazide	Anhydron	1/2	q.d.	0.22 (2)
Hydrochlorothiazide	Esidrix / HydroDIURIL / Oretic	25/50	q.d.	0.12 (50)
Hydroflumethiazole	Saluron	25/50	b.i.d.	0.28 (50)
Indapamide	Lozol	2.5/5	q.d.	0.40 (2.5)
Methyclothiazide	Enduron	2.5/5	q.d.	0.22 (5)
Metolazone	Zaroxolyn	2.5/5	q.d.	0.23 (5)
Polythiazide	Renese	2/4	q.d.	0.29 (2)
Trichlormethiazide	Naqua / Metahydrin	2/4	q.d.	0.31 (4)
Loop diuretics				
Bumetanide	Bumex	0.5/10	b.i.d.	0.15 (0.5)
Ethacrynic acid	Edecrin	50/200	b.i.d.	0.29 (50)
Furosemide	Lasix	40/160	b.i.d.	0.13 (40)

SIDE EFFECTS: $\downarrow$ serum K^+, alkalosis, $\uparrow$ uric acid, $\uparrow$ blood glucose, $\uparrow$ Ca^{++}, $\uparrow$ LDL cholesterol, dermatitis, photosensitivity, $\uparrow$ PRA, possible $\downarrow$ GFR, pancreatitis, impotence, $\downarrow$ lithium clearance in patients receiving lithium therapy. Uncommon side effects: inappropriate ADH secretion, $\downarrow$ platelets, $\downarrow$ WBC, $\downarrow$ RBC, GI or hepatic toxicity. Combination with a potassium-sparing diuretic is advised for patients with an abnormal ECG. Antihypertensive effect may be blunted by indomethacin, ibuprofen, and other nonsteroidal anti-inflammatory agents.[182]

Drug	Trade Name	Initial Dose/Maximum Dose (mg/day)	Frequency of Dosage	Approximate Daily Cost ($)* (dose in mg)
Potassium-sparing diuretics				
Amiloride	Midamor	5/10	q.d.	0.31 (5)
Spironolactone	Aldactone	50/100	t.i.d.	0.40 (50)
Triamterene	Dyrenium	50/100	q.d.	0.28 (100)

SIDE EFFECTS: $\uparrow$ serum K^+, rash, hyperpigmentation, megaloblastic anemia (triamterene), $\uparrow$ PRA, $\downarrow$ GFR, nephrolithiasis (triamterene), two reported cases of acute renal failure when combined with indomethacin (triamterene),[182] nausea, vomiting, diarrhea, menstrual irregularities, gynecomastia (spironolactone), impotence, drowsiness, ataxia. Diabetics, elderly patients, those with impaired renal function, and those using angiotensin converting enzyme inhibitors should use with caution.

Drug	Trade Name	Initial Dose/Maximum Dose (mg/day)	Frequency of Dosage	Approximate Daily Cost ($)* (dose in mg)
Amiloride and hydrochlorothiazide	Moduretic	1–2 tablets (5 mg amiloride, 50 mg hydrochlorothiazide)	q.d.	0.33 (1 tablet)
Spironolactone and hydrochlorothiazide	Aldactazide	1–4 tablets (25 mg spironolactone, 25 mg hydrochlorothiazide)	b.i.d.	0.49 (2 tablets)

Note: lists of side effects may be incomplete. Consult package insert before prescribing.

*Cost to pharmacist for mean doses indicated in parentheses, based on listings in the *1988 Drug Topics Redbook*; average wholesale price used.

Diuretics

	Drug	Trade Name	Initial Dose/Maximum Dose (mg/day)	Frequency of Dosage	Approximate Daily Cost ($)* (dose in mg)
Diuretics (continued)	Triamterene and hydrochlorothiazide	Dyazide Maxzide	1–2 capsules (50 mg triamterene, 25 mg hydrochloro-thiazide)	b.i.d.	0.29 (1 capsule)
			or		
			1 tablet (75 mg triam-terene, 50 mg hydrochloro-thiazide)	b.i.d.	0.43 (1 tablet)
	Potassium supplements	K-Lyte/CI	20–25 mEq	q.d. to q.i.d.	0.42 (25 mEq)
		Potassium Glu-conate Elixir			0.08 (20 mEq)
		Slow-K			0.30 (24 mEq)
		Klorvess			0.48 (20 mEq)
Sympatholytics	Beta blockers				
	Acebutolol	Sectral	200/800	q.d.	0.44 (200)
	Atenolol	Tenormin	25/100	q.d.	0.52 (50)
	Metoprolol	Lopressor	50/300	b.i.d.	0.46 (100)
	Nadolol	Corgard	20/480	q.d.	0.68 (80)
	Oxprenolol	Trasicor	80/480	q.d. to b.i.d.	No price available
	Pindolol	Visken	10/60	b.i.d.	0.42 (10)
	Propranolol	Inderal	40/480	b.i.d. to q.i.d.	0.43 (80)
	Timolol	Blocadren	10/60	b.i.d.	0.65 (20)

SIDE EFFECTS: Nausea, vomiting, diarrhea, constipation, bradycardia, weight gain, congestive heart failure, bronchospasm, insomnia, depression, paresthesias, Raynaud's phenomenon, claudication, masking of hypoglycemia, masking of thyrotoxicosis, impotence, sedation, possible precipitation of angina with abrupt discontinuation of drug, $\downarrow$ PRA possible, $\downarrow$ GFR (propranolol), $\uparrow K^+$, $\downarrow$ HDL, $\uparrow$ tricyclerides, positive ANA (rare).[183,184] Antihypertensive effect may be blunted by indomethacin, ibuprofen, and other nonsteroidal anti-inflammatory agents.[182] Selective beta$_1$ blockers (acebutolol, atenolol, metoprolol) given in low dosages reportedly produce less bronchospasm, less masking of hypoglycemia, and less reduction of peripheral vascular blood flow than do nonselective beta blockers and cause no change in the HDL cholesterol level.[76] Beta$_1$ blockers are preferred agents for patients with pulmonary disease, insulin-dependent diabetes, or symptomatic peripheral vascular disease. The intrinsic sympathomimetic effect of acebutolol, oxprenolol, and pindolol is advantageous for patients with bradycardia and possibly for those with heart failure, peripheral vascular insufficiency, or pulmonary disease. Metoprolol, propranolol, and timolol are cardioprotective.

	Drug	Trade Name	Initial Dose/Maximum Dose (mg/day)	Frequency of Dosage	Approximate Daily Cost ($)* (dose in mg)
	Beta and alpha blocker				
	Labetalol	{ Normodyne Trandate }	200/1,200	b.i.d.	0.62 (400)

SIDE EFFECTS: Paresthesias (scalp tingling), headache, bradycardia, orthostatic hypotension, voiding difficulty, urinary retention, ejaculation failure, dyspepsia, pruritus, nausea. Cardiovascular side effects, fatigue, insomnia, depression, and withdrawal complications are reported to be less likely with this agent than with the beta blockers. Incidence of bronchospasm similar to that seen with atenolol or metoprolol. Causes symptomatic aminotransferase elevations. Rare side effects: fever,[185] leukopenia, tremor, nightmares, toxic myopathy, positive ANA, and drug-induced lupus erythematosus. Labetalol metabolites in the serum can lead to the false diagnosis of pheochromocytoma.[152]

Note: lists of side effects may be incomplete. Consult package insert before prescribing.

*Cost to pharmacist for mean doses indicated in parentheses, based on listings in the *1988 Drug Topics Redbook*; average wholesale price used.

Table 7   (continued)

Drug	Trade Name	Initial Dose/Maximum Dose (mg/day)	Frequency of Dosage	Approximate Daily Cost ($)* (dose in mg)
Clonidine	Catapres	0.1/2.4	b.i.d.	0.84 (0.4)
Guanabenz	Wytensin	4/32	b.i.d.	0.48 (8)
Methyldopa	Aldomet	250/2,000	q.d. to t.i.d.	0.46 (500)

SIDE EFFECTS: Drowsiness (usually transient), depression, dry mouth, constipation, orthostatic hypotension (greater with methyldopa [186]), weakly positive Coombs' test (usually without clinical hemolysis), impotence, sudden rebound hypertension with abrupt discontinuation of drug (clonidine, guanabenz), ↓ PRA. Unchanged GRF. Efficacy diminished by tricyclic antidepressants. Causes mild reductions in cholesterol and triglyceride levels. Uncommon side effects: flulike syndrome (methyldopa), drug fever, hepatotoxicity, myocarditis (methyldopa), exacerbation of parkinsonism (methyldopa), bradycardia or atrioventricular block (clonidine), impaired glucose tolerance (clonidine). A transdermal form of clonidine is available.[88]

Drug	Trade Name	Initial Dose/Maximum Dose (mg/day)	Frequency of Dosage	Approximate Daily Cost ($)* (dose in mg)
Guanadrel	Hylorel	10/150	b.i.d.	0.29 (10)
Guanethidine	Ismelin	10/300	q.d.	0.52 (25)

SIDE EFFECTS: Orthostatic hypotension (in A.M.), weakness, bradycardia, diarrhea (dose related), nasal congestion, sedation (rare), impotence (retrograde ejaculation). ↑ PRA. Efficacy diminished by tricyclic antidepressants.

Drug	Trade Name	Initial Dose/Maximum Dose (mg/day)	Frequency of Dosage	Approximate Daily Cost ($)* (dose in mg)
Prazosin	Minipress	2/20	b.i.d. to t.i.d.	0.71 (4)

SIDE EFFECTS: Dizziness, drowsiness, headache, weakness, depression, palpitations, tachycardia, orthostatic hypotension, syncope (may occur suddenly after first dose), nausea, diarrhea, constipation, impotence, ↓PRA. Causes mild reductions in cholesterol and triglyceride levels. Uncommon side effects: edema, dyspnea, rash, pruritus, dry mouth, blurred vision, urinary frequency or incontinence, hallucinosis.

Drug	Trade Name	Initial Dose/Maximum Dose (mg/day)	Frequency of Dosage	Approximate Daily Cost ($)* (dose in mg)
Reserpine	Serpasil / Sandril	0.1/0.5	q.d.	0.07 (0.25)

SIDE EFFECTS: Drowsiness, nasal congestion, increased appetite, bradycardia, depression (can be severe), nightmares, ↑ gastric acidity (may be ulcerogenic), impotence. Uncommon side effects: parkinsonian rigidity, galactorrhea, postural hypotension, ?breast cancer (causative relation doubtful).

Drug	Trade Name	Initial Dose/Maximum Dose (mg/day)	Frequency of Dosage	Approximate Daily Cost ($)* (dose in mg)
Hydralazine	Apresoline	50/300	b.i.d. to q.i.d.	1.07 (200)

SIDE EFFECTS: Headache, tachycardia, palpitations, fever, weight gain, edema, lupus erythematosus-like syndrome (rare if dosage < 200 mg/day), exacerbation of coronary insufficiency, one reported case of pancytopenia and obstructive jaundice, ↑ PRA, ↑ or unchanged GFR.

Drug	Trade Name	Initial Dose/Maximum Dose (mg/day)	Frequency of Dosage	Approximate Daily Cost ($)* (dose in mg)
Minoxidil	Loniten	5/100	b.i.d.	0.55 (10)

SIDE EFFECTS: Severe hypotension, headache, tachycardia, palpitations, exacerbation of coronary insufficiency or heart failure, sodium and water retention, hemodilution, pericardial effusion, nonspecific T wave changes on ECG, hypertrichosis, coarsening of facial features, ↑ PRA, ↑ GFR. Uncommon side effects: rash, ↑ alkaline phosphatase.

Sympatholytics (continued) · *Vasodilators*

Note: lists of side effects may be incomplete. Consult package insert before prescribing.

*Cost to pharmacist for mean doses indicated in parentheses, based on listings in the *1988 Drug Topics Redbook*; average wholesale price used.

	Drug	Trade Name	Initial Dose/Maximum Dose (mg/day)	Frequency of Dosage	Approximate Daily Cost ($)* (dose in mg)
Angiotensin converting enzyme inhibitors	Captopril	Capoten	25/150	b.i.d. to t.i.d.	0.99 (100)
	Enalapril	Vasotec	10/40	q.d.	0.95 (20)
	Lisinopril	Prinivil / Zestril	5/40	q.d.	No price available

SIDE EFFECTS: Hypotension, hyperkalemia (because both agents cause potassium retention, their use with distal tubular diuretics or potassium supplements must proceed cautiously), cough, and rhinorrhea. Uncommon side effects: urticaria, angioedema (0.1%). Contraindicated in pregnant women and in patients with bilateral renal artery stenoses, unilateral stenosis of a solitary kidney, or transplant stenosis. ↑ PRA, ↓ angiotensin II, and no change in GFR. *Captopril:* rash,[187] taste loss or alteration. Uncommon side effects: fever, tongue ulceration, stomatitis, proteinuria, membranous glomerulonephritis, acute renal failure, granulocytopenia, hemolytic anemia, cholestatic jaundice, and zinc deficiency.[188] Antihypertensive effect may be blunted by indomethacin, ibuprofen, and other nonsteroidal anti-inflammatory agents.[189] One case of eosinophilia with Coombs'-positive hemolytic anemia and renal failure has been reported. *Enalapril:* uncommon side effects: rash, granulocytopenia; experience in patients with renal failure limited.

	Drug	Trade Name	Initial Dose/Maximum Dose (mg/day)	Frequency of Dosage	Approximate Daily Cost ($)* (dose in mg)
Calcium entry blockers	Diltiazem	Cardizem	120/240	t.i.d. to q.i.d.	1.68 (240)
	Nifedipine	Procardia	30/180	t.i.d. to q.i.d.	1.94 (60)
	Verapamil	Calan / Isoptin	240/480	t.i.d. to q.i.d.	0.85 (320)

SIDE EFFECTS: *Nifedipine:* dizziness, flushing, nausea, edema, headache, fatigue, tachycardia, constipation. Uncommon side effects: rash. Verapamil: bradycardia, arrhythmias, syncope, diarrhea. Uncommon side effects: exacerbation of congestive heart failure or heart block, elevation of liver enzymes or creatine kinase. Extreme caution is advised in concomitant use with beta blockers or digitalis because of risk of bradycardia or congestive heart failure. The side effects of diltiazem are similar to those of nifedipine and verapamil.

Note: lists of side effects may be incomplete. Consult package insert before prescribing.

*Cost to pharmacist for mean doses indicated in parentheses, based on listings in the *1988 Drug Topics Redbook*; average wholesale price used.

is similar to propranolol in efficacy and side effects. Nadolol dosages are identical to those of propranolol, except that nadolol can be administered once daily.

Timolol, another nonselective beta blocker, is given in dosages of 10 to 30 mg once or twice a day. Its efficacy and side effects also resemble those of propranolol. Timolol is approved for use in prevention of second myocardial infarctions [*see Chapter 5*]; a large-scale Norwegian study demonstrated its so-called cardioprotective effect.[78] A similar study demonstrated the cardioprotective effect of propranolol. As stated above, however, when beta blockers are used for primary prevention, their cardio-protective effects have been shown to occur only in nonsmoking males.

Metoprolol and atenolol are selective beta$_1$ antagonists with efficacies comparable to that of propranolol. Because these two agents in low dosages involve less risk of exacerbating bronchospasm than the other beta blockers, they are better tolerated by patients with asthma or obstructive pulmonary disease. Selective beta$_1$ antagonists in low dosages may also be preferred in patients with insulin-dependent diabetes because they interfere less with the beta-mediated response to hypoglycemia than the nonselective beta antagonists. They may also be advantageous in patients with symptomatic peripheral vascular disease because they apparently do not raise systemic vascular resistance. A 50 mg dose of metoprolol is equivalent to a 40 mg dose of propranolol; therapy usually begins with 50 mg twice a day. Atenolol is initially given at a dosage of 50 mg once a day (25 mg/day for mild hypertension) and is increased to a maximum of 100 mg once a day. As dosages are increased, both agents show less beta[1] selectivity.

Pindolol and oxprenolol are nonselective beta blockers with intrinsic sympathomimetic activity (ISA).[79,80] Acebutolol is beta[1] selective and has weak ISA.[81] ISA does not seem to influence the beta-blocking efficacy of pindolol, oxprenolol, or acebutolol; these agents also produce less bradycardia than other beta blockers, so they may be safer for patients with this complication. Moreover, ISA should, in theory, be advantageous for patients with a history of congestive heart failure, peripheral vascular insufficiency, or asthma. These advantages have yet to be proved in large-scale clinical trials. The starting dosage of pindolol is 5 mg twice a day; of oxprenolol, 80 mg twice a day; and of acebutolol, 200 mg once a day.

Atenolol and nadolol are less lipid soluble than the other beta blockers. Because of this, they appear to be associated with fewer central nervous system side effects, and patient acceptance of both drugs has been high.

Use of a beta blocker as an antihypertensive is different, in terms of dosage intervals, from its use as an antianginal. In patients with angina, inadequate serum drug levels for any period involve considerable risk. In contrast, increasing dosage intervals in patients with mild to moderate hypertension often improves compliance and is relatively safe. For patients who have hypertension and angina, we advise strict adherence to the shorter dosage intervals. The serum half-lives of the beta blockers are as follows: acebutolol, eight to 13 hours; atenolol, six to nine hours; metoprolol, three to four hours; nadolol, 20 to 24 hours; oxprenolol, two hours; pindolol, three to four hours; propranolol, two to three hours; and timolol, four to five hours.

A retrospective study in Sweden reported an increased incidence of diabetes in hypertensive women taking diuretics or beta blockers.[82] The incidence was further increased in women taking both drugs. Another study reported a worsening of glucose control in hypertensive patients with maturity-onset diabetes who received the combination of propranolol and a thiazide diuretic.[83] A third study noted an increase in the level of glycosylated hemoglobin in type II diabetics after 20 months of therapy with propranolol, atenolol, or nadolol; the increase was greatest with propranolol.[84] Although an association between diabetes and long-term diuretic usage has been previously known, a relation between diabetes and beta-blocking agents, if it exists, would be a new finding.

We thus recommend that physicians be aware of the potential development or worsening of glucose intolerance in patients who are on long-term antihypertensive therapy, especially in those taking diuretics or beta blockers.

Labetalol Labetalol is the first approved drug in a new class of agents that combine both alpha- and beta-blocking properties.[85] In addition, labetalol appears to have a direct vasodilatory effect.[86] Its differences derive primarily from its alpha-blocking effects, which may result in less bradycardia and negative inotropy than that caused by beta blockers. These alpha-blocking properties, however, lead to side effects such as postural hypotension and retrograde ejaculation. Its beta-blocking properties have been reported to induce bronchospasm and other side effects associated with the beta blockers at an incidence comparable to that seen with the nonselective beta blockers. Unusual side effects, such as scalp tingling, tremulousness, nausea, and elevation of aminotransferase levels, have been reported. Dosage begins at 100 mg twice a day. An intravenous form should prove useful in treating hypertensive emergencies.

Methyldopa Methyldopa has been used safely and reliably for a long time. We believe, however, that it is a drug of second choice to the beta blockers because it has many compliance-limiting side effects, including orthostatic hypotension, decreased alertness, and depression. Methyldopa acts by producing a false neurotransmitter. Increased therapeutic efficacy is rarely observed with doses greater than 2 g/day. Although usually prescribed in multiple daily doses, methyldopa is often effective when given once a day.

Clonidine Clonidine can be extremely effective, especially in patients with severe hypertension or renin-dependent disease. Clonidine acts by decreasing sympathetic output from the CNS. Side effects resemble those of methyldopa, although orthostatic hypotension is not usually a complication. Rebound hypertension may occur on rapid discontinuation of therapy but does so only rarely in patients with mild to moderate hypertension. This side effect appears to be most prevalent in patients with high levels of plasma renin activity,[87] and it is independent of dose or duration of therapy. Rebound hypertension is best treated by readministration of clonidine. In severe cases, treatment should be the same as that for pheochromocytoma crisis [*see* Hypertensive Emergencies, *below*]. The availability of transdermal clonidine patches designed for weekly administration may improve compliance, but a relatively high incidence of pruritus has limited patient acceptance.[88]

Guanabenz Guanabenz, like clonidine, is a central alpha$_2$-adrenergic agonist. It appears to be similar in efficacy to clonidine. Although the incidence of side effects for guanabenz is said to be less than that for clonidine, dry mouth, drowsiness, and rebound hypertension can occur. The usual dosage is 4 to 8 mg twice a day. Like clonidine and prazosin (see below), guanabenz mildly lowers serum lipid levels.

Guanethidine and guanadrel Although its popularity has waned because of side effects such as orthostatic hypotension and diarrhea, guanethidine is still administered. The advantages of the drug include a wide dose-response range and a relative freedom from sedation. The pharmacologic profile of guanadrel is similar to the profile of guanethidine.[89]

Reserpine Because reserpine may be associated with sudden severe depression, it should be administered only to emotionally stable patients and only after adequate warning to both patient and family. Because of its single daily dosage and low cost, reserpine may be useful in patients unable to tolerate other antihypertensive agents.

Prazosin Prazosin blocks smooth muscle postsynaptic alpha$_1$ receptors. Thus, it does not usually induce reflex increases in cardiac output and renin release. We have successfully used prazosin in combination with a diuretic and another sympatholytic agent, particularly in patients with some degree of peripheral vascular disease. When prazosin is used as a single agent in mild to moderate disease, it appears to be less effective than a thiazide diuretic. However, when used as a secondary agent in combination with a diuretic, prazosin is quite effective for the treatment of young patients with moderately severe hypertension.

Patient acceptance of prazosin has been relatively high. Rarely, after the first dose of prazosin, a patient may experience sudden syncope that is usually postural and is often dose related; the mechanism remains unexplained. Therefore, an initial trial dose of 1 mg taken in the physician's office or at bedtime is recommended. Prazosin has been effectively used to relieve the vasospasm of Raynaud's phenomenon. Prazosin has been associated with short-term reduction in serum lipid levels; the significance of this observation is unclear.

Vasodilating Agents

Hydralazine Hydralazine is most commonly used in combination with a beta blocker and a diuretic. When given in combination, its efficacy is impressive and its side effects are minimal. Hydralazine may produce a lupus erythematosus–like syndrome; the syndrome is extremely rare when the daily dose is below 200 mg.[90]

Minoxidil Minoxidil is a more potent vasodilator than hydralazine. Used with furosemide and either a beta blocker or another potent sympatholytic, minoxidil is effective in treating the severest forms of hypertension (e.g., hypertension associated with transplant rejection, bilateral renovascular disease, or renal failure). Minoxidil may prove to be the agent of choice for combination therapy in patients with refractory hypertension and compromised renal function because it preserves renal blood flow.[91] Such adverse effects as significant volume retention and possible overshoot hypotension dictate cautious initiation of this therapy. Initial experience with minoxidil has been very encouraging, and acceptance by patients has been high. The most limiting side effects have been hypertrichosis, which is especially bothersome to children and women, and fluid accumulation in serous cavities, including the pericardium.

Angiotensin Converting Enzyme Inhibitors

Captopril Captopril, the first approved member of its class, inhibits the enzyme that converts angiotensin I to angiotensin II.[92] It apparently reduces peripheral resistance without changing cardiac output or glomerular filtration and, therefore, also reduces afterload in congestive heart failure. Use of captopril in patients with all forms of hypertension has been very successful.[93]

The recommended dosage of captopril for mild to moderate hypertension is 25 mg twice or three times a day, which can be increased to 50 mg twice or three times a day when needed in all but severely hypertensive patients, who may require as much as 300 mg/day.[94,95] The starting dose should be reduced to 12.5 mg/day and dose titration should be slower in patients with myocardial or renal dysfunction or in those receiving concomitant antihypertensive therapy. For all patients, the dose should not exceed 450 mg/day. Ideally, if diuretics are being given, they should be stopped several days before captopril is begun.

Side effects have included rash or pruritus in approximately 10 percent of patients and alteration or loss of taste (dysgeusia) in two to four percent.[94] Proteinuria occurs in about one percent of patients, almost all of whom exhibit renal disease prior to antihypertensive therapy or receive doses in excess of 150 mg/day. In one study, granulocytopenia occurred in 0.01 percent of patients with normal renal function, in 0.2 percent of patients with a serum creatinine level greater than 1.6 mg/dl, and in 3.7 percent of those with collagen vascular disease or impaired renal function.[94] Most cases of granulocytopenia and proteinuria were reversible on discontinuation of the drug; however, 13 percent of the cases of granulocytopenia were fatal.[94] Nearly all patients in whom granulocytopenia developed were seriously ill and receiving many other drugs.

Because of the side effects of captopril, we recommend that patients be monitored for proteinuria and leukopenia prior to and during the first year of treatment; white blood cell counts should be obtained twice a month for three months if creatinine levels are greater than 1.6 mg/dl, if the dose exceeds 150 mg/day, or if collagen vascular disease is present. Patients should be told to promptly report any sign of infection (e.g., sore throat or fever). Captopril should be immediately discontinued if abnormalities appear.

Although it has been argued that certain side effects of captopril are related to its molecular structure (specifically, its free sulfhydryl group), the role of this functional group can be resolved only after further experience is gained with enalapril, an ACE inhibitor that lacks a free sulfhydryl group. Certainly, the serious side effects of captopril noted earlier have been minimized with lower dosage regimens; the incidence of rash and dysgeusia, however, has not been diminished significantly with reduced dosage.

Enalapril The mechanism of action of enalapril is identical to that of captopril. Clinical experience includes its use in approximately 1.2 million patients with all forms of hypertension. Data indicate that it is an effective antihypertensive agent that is extremely well tolerated.[96,97] Thus far, renal insufficiency and severe granulocytopenia have occurred less often with enalapril than with captopril.[98,99]

Enalapril is begun at 5 mg/day; the dose can be increased to 40 mg/day.[98] Although enalapril is effective when taken once a day, twice-daily administration increases its effectiveness in some patients.[99] As is the case with captopril, patients who have myocardial or renal dysfunction or collagen vascular disease should receive a lower starting dose of 2.5 mg/day and should undergo slower titration of the dose; diuretics should be stopped several days before therapy is started.

Lisinopril Lisinopril is a newer ACE inhibitor that has properties and a dosage schedule very similar to that of enalapril.

Selection of ACE inhibitors ACE inhibitors represent a major advance in the treatment of all forms of hypertension, based on their potency and minimal side effects. A multicenter trial that compared captopril, methyldopa, and propranolol in the treatment of hypertension concluded that captopril, with or without a diuretic, was better tolerated and was associated with superior quality of life, as evaluated by work performance and measures of well-being.[100]

Preliminary data suggest that ACE inhibitors are more effective and possibly safer than other antihypertensive drugs for the treatment of hypertension in diabetics.[101,102] Because ACE inhibitors interfere with production of the major stimulus of aldosterone release, they may produce hyperkalemia, especially in patients with renal insufficiency or underlying hypoaldosteronism (see

above) or in those receiving potassium supplements or potassium-sparing diuretics. We recommend discontinuation of these other agents when ACE inhibitors are begun.

ACE inhibitors should be used cautiously or avoided altogether in patients with suspected bilateral renal artery stenosis, renal artery stenosis in a solitary functioning kidney, or stenosis of a vessel perfusing a transplanted kidney. In these patients, renal perfusion is highly dependent on angiotensin II.[103-105]

Both captopril and enalapril have been associated with urticaria or angioedema in less than 0.1 percent of cases. With enalapril, the risk of urticaria or angioedema has been shown to be highest during the first week of therapy and significantly lower thereafter.[106] Occasionally, angioedema caused by captopril or enalapril has produced respiratory distress and laryngeal obstruction. Although the cause of angioedema is unknown, it is probably related to inhibition of kinin degradation by ACE inhibitors (ACE also degrades bradykinin). Physicians and patients should be aware that angioedema is a potential complication of ACE inhibitor therapy. If angioedema is suspected, therapy with the ACE inhibitor should be halted immediately and an antihypertensive agent from another class should be substituted. If respiratory distress develops, we advise prompt injection of epinephrine (0.3 to 0.5 ml of a 1:1000 dilution).

Calcium Entry Blockers

Although calcium entry blockers were introduced and approved as second-line agents for the treatment of angina pectoris and, in the case of verapamil, for supraventricular tachyarrhythmias, their hypotensive effects will inevitably result in their use as antihypertensives.[107] For practical purposes, they can be considered arteriolar vasodilators. Nifedipine is the most potent agent in this regard. When it or diltiazem is administered, reduced peripheral vascular resistance and increased cardiac output ensue. Side effects commonly associated with vasodilators, such as tachycardia, headache, flushing, and edema, can occur. Verapamil has significant negative inotropic and chronotropic effects, and thus, its use results in bradycardia. Caution is dictated if verapamil is prescribed with another bradycardic agent. We favor diltiazem or nifedipine because of verapamil's bradycardic potential. Diltiazem may have the fewest side effects. Dosage for diltiazem is 30 mg three times a day initially. More widespread use is limited by high frequency of dosage.

It has been suggested that increased levels of calcium in vascular smooth muscle may mediate at least several forms of hypertension; therefore, it has been proposed that treatment with a calcium entry blocker may specifically counteract this mechanism and thus prove beneficial for therapy.[108] These drugs have been particularly successful in treating hypertension in elderly patients. Nifedipine may be used for hypertensive emergencies (see below).

Choice Of Drugs

The wide array of antihypertensive drugs now available allows considerable flexibility in tailoring an effective regimen with minimal side effects. However, it imposes a complexity that demands considerable pharmacologic sophistication. Nevertheless, we believe that the treatment of hypertension can proceed in a logical manner [*see Figure* 2].

Traditionally, either a diuretic or a beta blocker is used initially, followed by a combination of the two if blood pressure is not effectively reduced. However, enalapril and low-dose captopril are safer and have fewer side effects, which justifies initiation of treatment with one of these two agents either alone or in combination with a diuretic for greater control. These combinations are likely to become the preferred treatment for most hypertensive patients.

Initial therapy with diuretics is waning in popularity because of concern about their hypokalemic and plasma lipoprotein–raising potential. We still find them useful as single-agent therapy for elderly and black patients; benefits include low cost, low frequency of dosage, and greater effectiveness in black patients. The beta blockers, particularly atenolol, which is both long acting and cardioselective, have been extremely popular for single-drug therapy, especially among the young; however, they will probably be displaced by the ACE inhibitors for single-drug therapy or combination drug therapy. The calcium entry blockers have been proposed for initial therapy in the elderly; however, we believe that the associated side effects and the frequent dosages argue against the initial use of these agents.

We believe that two-drug therapy is best accomplished by the combination of an ACE inhibitor with a diuretic. If this combination does not reduce hypertension, the formerly preferred combination of a diuretic with either a beta blocker or a calcium entry blocker (in patients who are intolerant of or insensitive to beta blockers) is advised. The formerly used combinations would be preferred over the first combination in patients with concomitant angina or coronary artery disease. The calcium entry blockers might be more effective in treating elderly patients with primary systolic hypertension; alternative sympatholytic agents are less desirable because of their side effects.

Severe hypertension is best treated by several possible combinations of drugs: a diuretic and a high-dose ACE inhibitor; a diuretic and a beta blocker combined with either an ACE inhibitor, an alternative vasodilator such as hydralazine or prazosin, or a calcium entry blocker; or a diuretic combined with one or more potent sympatholytics, such as clonidine, guanabenz, or a beta blocker. It should be noted that labetalol is equivalent to certain fixed dosages of a nonspecific beta blocker combined with prazosin.

For patients with refractory hypertension, additional combinations must be devised. The potent vasodilator minoxidil or a high-dose ACE inhibitor can be combined with a diuretic and a sympatholytic. Alternatively, two sympatholytics that act by different mechanisms, such as a beta blocker

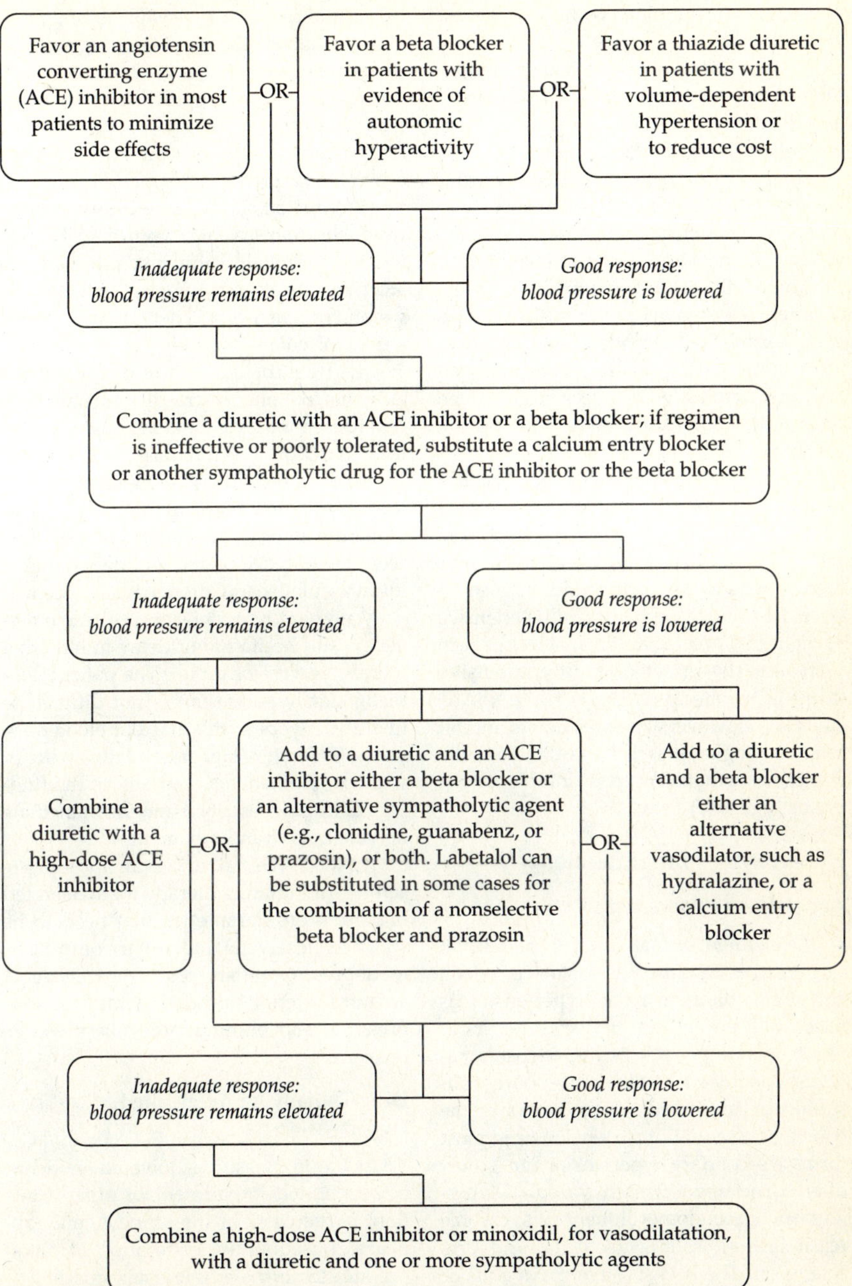

Figure 2   *A simplified approach to treating high blood pressure is diagrammed.*

and either prazosin, clonidine, or guanabenz, can be combined with a diuretic and a vasodilator.

Lastly, it should be noted that requirements for therapy can change. It is reasonable to attempt controlled drug reduction in patients with stable blood pressure.

Long-term use of antihypertensive drugs is safe and well tolerated. In a five-year study of 5,485 hypertensive patients coordinated by the National Heart, Lung and Blood Institute, no deaths attributable to therapy were reported, fewer than one percent of patients were hospitalized for side effects, and only about nine percent of the participants had definite or probable side effects from a given drug that were severe enough to require withdrawal of that drug.[109]

It should be noted that certain nonsteroidal anti-inflammatory drugs (NSAIDs), such as indomethacin, ibuprofen, and naproxen, which are available as over-the-counter medications for arthritic conditions, can reduce the efficacy of many antihypertensive agents; renal prostaglandin synthesis, which increases the effect of antihypertensive drugs, is inhibited by NSAIDs.[110] The NSAID sulindac, however, appears not to inhibit renal prostaglandin synthesis at therapeutic doses (doses that completely inhibit platelet cyclooxygenase).[111]

Hypertensive Emergencies

Accelerated Hypertension

Accelerated, or malignant, hypertension can best be described as a state in which end-organ damage from hypertension is telescoped into a brief period. It occurs in less than one percent of hypertensive patients, usually when disease is poorly controlled or untreated. It can occur in the course of essential hypertension or in most forms of secondary hypertension but is most often associated with renovascular hypertension, acute glomerulonephritis, chronic renal failure, renal vasculitis, and pre-eclampsia. The RAA system plays a major role in pathogenesis, but disease can occur in patients with normal PRA levels.[10]

Accelerated hypertension is manifested by a rapid increase in diastolic blood pressure (usually to 130 mm Hg or higher) and the appearance of either grade III or IV retinopathy. However, papilledema is an unreliable physical sign of malignant hypertension and is not required for diagnosis.[112,113] Symptoms may include restlessness, confusion, somnolence, blurred vision, headache, nausea, and vomiting. Hypertensive encephalopathy, a syndrome characterized by severe hypertension, loss of vision, focal neurologic deficit, seizure, and stupor or coma, may develop [*see Chapter 36*]. Left ventricular failure or myocardial ischemia, or both, may result and may progress to pulmonary edema or acute myocardial infarction. Renal damage is inevitable. Proteinuria, hematuria, and red cell casts in the urine sediment are often observed; azotemia develops early, and oliguria is often seen. Hemolytic anemia and disseminated intravascular coagulation may also occur.

Malignant hypertension is a true emergency, and hesitation or delay in initiating therapy is a major pitfall. The patient with malignant hypertension is not difficult to identify: anyone with a diastolic blood pressure of 130 mm Hg, retinopathy with or without papilledema, and any of the findings hitherto described merits immediate hospitalization and treatment.

An intensive care unit is an appropriate setting for initiating therapy for accelerated hypertension. Parameters that need to be watched closely include urinary output, arterial pressure (often recorded by means of an intra-arterial cannula), central venous pressure, and pulmonary capillary wedge pressure.

Drug Therapy for Accelerated Hypertension

As blood pressure is lowered, evidence of accelerated impairment of organ function, particularly of the kidneys, may appear. Consequently, restoration of blood pressure to normotensive levels must be carried out slowly, with continued attention to urine output and other parameters of renal function. Moreover, many patients in hypertensive crisis have reduced intravascular volume and may be very sensitive to overly rapid vasodilatation or diuresis. The goals of therapy are to resolve symptoms, to reduce diastolic blood pressure to at least 100 mm Hg, and to maintain urine output greater than 20 ml/hr. Fulfillment of all of these criteria may not be possible. For example, a reduction of blood pressure that is sufficient to relieve hypertensive encephalopathy or pulmonary edema may lead to such complications as oliguria or anuria. In such cases, peritoneal dialysis or hemodialysis is indicated.

For patients with life-threatening accelerated hypertension, such as when it is accompanied by encephalopathy, intracranial hemorrhage, or pulmonary edema, admission to an intensive care unit and blood pressure titration with sodium nitroprusside are advised. When acute monitoring is not required or feasible, sublingual nifedipine, parenteral labetalol, or intravenous diazoxide is recommended. When it is safe to allow 30 to 60 minutes to achieve blood pressure control, parenteral hydralazine, captopril, or clonidine may be used instead [*see Table 8*].[114]

Sodium nitroprusside When continuous monitoring is available, sodium nitroprusside is the safest and most effective drug for use in hypertensive emergencies.[115] This potent smooth muscle relaxant is particularly useful in patients with ischemic heart disease because it does not impair myocardial blood flow.

Sodium nitroprusside is metabolized to cyanide and thiocyanate. Prolonged use, therefore, may lead to cyanide toxicity, which is manifested by metabolic acidosis, or to thiocyanate toxicity, which is manifested by muscle weakness, hyperreflexia, confusion, delirium, or coma.

When an immediate effect is desired, the recommended maximum dosage is 1.0 mg/kg over the first three hours (or approximately 300 µg/min for a 70 kg person). The maximum dosage for extended therapy is 200 µg/min (or approximately 0.2 mg/kg/hr). Blood thiocyanate levels should be determined frequently; levels less than 10 mg/dl are generally well tolerated. If thiocyanate toxicity develops, it can be treated with hemodialysis.

Trimethaphan Trimethaphan is a rapidly acting and powerful ganglionic blocking agent, but it is rather difficult to use, for a few reasons: tachyphylaxis prevents prolonged efficacy, severe hypotension is common as a result of difficulties in dose titration, and the side effects of systemic ganglionic blockade are difficult to control. Because it combines potent hypotensive and negative inotropic properties, trimethaphan is the alternative of choice for the treatment of dissecting aortic aneurysm when the preferred treatment, a combination of sodium nitroprusside and beta blockers, cannot be tolerated (see below).

Nifedipine Nifedipine, a calcium entry blocker that has been approved for treatment of angina, has not received FDA approval for treatment of hypertension. Nevertheless, preliminary experience with this drug in hypertensive emergencies (10 to 20 mg given sublingually or orally as a broken or chewed capsule) demonstrated that it effectively lowered blood pressure within five to 30 minutes.[116,117] Because nifedipine is a vasodilator, overshoot hypotension in hypovolemic patients is a potential problem. Nifedipine also increases heart rate somewhat, but coronary insufficiency has not been associated with its use because of its coronary vasodilator properties. Nifedipine, administered as described, may well prove to be the drug of choice for rapid lowering of blood pressure when constant monitoring of patients is unavailable.

Diazoxide Diazoxide, a potent vasodilator structurally related to the thiazides, rarely causes overshoot hypotension unless administered along with other nondiuretic antihypertensives. Continuous blood pressure monitoring, therefore, is usually not

Table 8   Drugs Used in the Treatment of Hypertensive Emergencies

Drug	Administration	Onset of Action	Mechanism of Action	Side Effects	Indications/ Contraindications
Sodium Nitroprusside (Nipride)	Prepare 50–100 mg/500 ml 5% dextrose in water; administer at rate of 25–50 μg/min and titrate (solution is light sensitive and should be covered with aluminum foil) Patient needs constant monitoring	Immediate	Vasodilatation	Nausea, restlessness, disorientation, severe hypotension, thiocyanate toxicity (check blood levels every 48 hr; discontinue if levels exceed 10 mg/dl), hypothyroidism or methemoglobinemia (rare), ↓ platelet adhesiveness, intracranial hypertension	Especially useful in patients with ischemic heart disease, aortic dissection (combined with a beta blocker), or intracranial hemorrhage
Trimethaphan (Arfonad)	Prepare 500 mg/500 ml 5% dextrose in water; administer 1 mg/min initially and titrate Patient needs constant monitoring	Immediate	Ganglionic blockade	Severe hypotension, tachyphylaxis, orthostatic effect, sympathetic blockade (urinary retention, constipation, ileus, pupillary dilatation), respiratory arrest (> 5 mg/min)	Second-choice agent in patients with aortic dissection, intracranial hemorrhage, or ischemic heart disease when sodium nitroprusside cannot be used
Nifedipine (Procardia)	Administer 10–20 mg sublingually or orally as a broken or chewed capsule	5–30 min	Calcium entry blocker	Hypotension, tachycardia, flushing	Drug of choice for hypertensive emergencies when invasive monitoring is not required; contraindicated in patients with aortic dissection; not yet approved by FDA as antihypertensive

CO—cardiac output   HR—heart rate

Drug	Administration	Onset of Action	Mechanism of Action	Side Effects	Indications/ Contraindications
Labetalol (Trandate, Normodyne)	Administer 20–80 mg I.V. at 10-min intervals (maximum cumulative dose 300 mg)	Immediate	Nonselective beta blocker and alpha$_1$ blocker	Pressor response after previous beta-blocker treatment, nausea, paresthesia, headache, hypotension, bradycardia, bronchospasm, urinary retention, ? congestive heart failure	Experience limited; contraindicated for patients with asthma, heart failure, heart block greater than first degree, or bradycardia
Diazoxide (Hyperstat)	Give 150–300 mg rapid I.V. push or 50–150 mg I.V. every 5 min; to minimize overshoot hypotension, use 7.5–30 mg/min constant I.V. infusion instead Each dose after the first 300 mg should be preceded by furosemide, 40 mg I.V.	Immediate	Vasodilatation	$\uparrow$ CO, $\uparrow$ HR, $\uparrow$ blood glucose, $\uparrow$ uric acid, Na$^+$ retention; may precipitate angina and cardiac ischemia, nausea, postural hypotension, painful extravasation	Hypertensive encephalopathy, accelerated hypertension, eclampsia; not to be given to patients with ischemic heart disease, intracranial hemorrhage, or aortic dissection

CO—cardiac output HR—heart rate

required. Rapid I.V. injection acts faster than continuous I.V. infusion; however, the latter is effective within 20 minutes.[118] Side effects include fluid retention, best counteracted by a loop diuretic; hyperglycemia; and reflex stimulation of heart rate and cardiac output. Diazoxide can thus precipitate angina pectoris or myocardial infarction and is contraindicated in patients with coronary artery disease or dissecting aortic aneurysm.

Hydralazine Parenteral hydralazine is an intermediate agent for moderately ill patients or for those with eclampsia. Onset of action is 20 minutes after administration, and overshoot hypotension may occur. Administration of hydralazine alone is contraindicated in patients with ischemic cardiac disease; lower doses (10 mg) are recommended for elderly patients to avoid overshoot hypotension.

Labetalol Intravenous labetalol is useful for rapid reduction of blood pressure when it is administered in doses of 20 to 80 mg at 10-minute intervals, especially in patients who have coronary artery disease or impaired hemodynamic function.[119] Caution is urged in the use of labetalol because of its beta-blocking properties; its possible side effects include bradycardia, bronchospasm, heart failure, and delayed conduction of cardiac impulses. Labetalol's alpha-blocking effects may cause postural hypotension. Rebound hypertension may be seen in patients who were previously receiving other beta-blocking agents.[120]

Captopril Anecdotal experience has reported the use of single-dose captopril (12.5 to 50 mg orally or sublingually) to lower blood pressure during a 60- to 120-minute period (30 to 60 minutes sublingually) in patients with accelerated hypertension unaccompanied by life-threatening complications.[121] We await further studies confirming this experience.

Clonidine Clonidine is effective during a two- to five-hour period.[122] An initial dose of 0.1 to 0.2 mg of oral clonidine is administered, followed by 0.1 mg hourly up to a total dose of 0.7 mg or until the desired blood pressure is reached.

Maintenance After control of blood pressure has been achieved, an appropriate combination of antihypertensive drugs may be instituted. We caution that use of nifedipine, labetalol, captopril, or clonidine in hypertensive emergencies does not conform to published FDA guidelines.

Management of Hypertension-related Emergencies

Acute Pulmonary Edema

Hypertension associated with acute pulmonary edema is often resolved with treatment directed at congestive heart failure. Sodium nitroprusside should be reserved for those patients with persistent severe hypertension that is unaffected by the usual therapies for heart failure.

Acute Myocardial Infarction

Although myocardial infarction associated with systolic hypertension has a worse prognosis than myocardial infarction accompanied by normal blood pressure, there is no conclusive evidence that reduction of blood pressure either improves outcome or reduces infarct size. Nevertheless, judicious reduction of systolic blood pressure under careful monitoring can effect dramatic clinical improvement, especially when heart failure is also present. Trimethaphan, sodium nitroprusside, and more recently, the beta blockers and calcium entry blockers have been used effectively in this setting.

Aortic Dissection

Most patients with aortic dissection have a history of hypertension. Moreover, acute hypertension is often seen at presentation, especially in dissections involving the descending aorta.[123] Therapy is aimed at containing the progression of the hematoma by reducing blood pressure and by lessening the velocity of myocardial contraction (dp/dt). A combination of sodium nitroprusside and I.V. propranolol is most often used to achieve these effects. Propranolol diminishes cardiac dp/dt and also prevents reflex tachycardia and increased cardiac output, which might otherwise be produced in response to the vasodilatation induced by sodium nitroprusside.

Therapy should begin in an intensive care unit with complete monitoring, including measurement of pulmonary capillary wedge pressure. A 0.5 mg I.V. test dose of propranolol should be slowly infused and followed by repeated 1.0 mg doses, each given during a five-minute period, until the desired effect is achieved or up to a total dose of 0.15 mg/kg. Oral therapy begins later.

If sodium nitroprusside does not control hematoma progression, trimethaphan should be substituted. If beta blockers cannot be tolerated, trimethaphan should be used instead of the combination of sodium nitroprusside and I.V. propranolol. Alternatively, reserpine (1 to 8 mg I.M. every four to eight hours following a test dose of 0.25 mg) can be used instead of propranolol. Reserpine increases gastric acidity, which can be counteracted by simultaneous administration of an H_2-receptor–blocking drug (i.e., cimetidine, ranitidine, or famotidine). Management of aortic dissection has been reviewed.[124]

Pheochromocytoma Crisis

Pheochromocytoma crisis and its analogues, which include severe hypertension caused by tyramine ingestion in patients receiving monoamine oxidase inhibitors, rebound hypertension that may occur after abrupt clonidine withdrawal, and trauma to the central nervous system, are best treated initially by the alpha-adrenergic blocking agent phentolamine (Regitine).[125] A dose of 2 to 5 mg is given intravenously every five minutes until blood pressure is controlled. After adequate alpha blockade has been achieved, beta blockade is started. Beta blockade is delayed so as not to interfere with beta-mediated vasodilatation in the setting of alpha-adrenergic vasoconstriction. The combination of sodium nitroprusside and adrenergic blocking agents has reportedly been used successfully in the management of pheochromocytoma crisis.

Toxemia of Pregnancy

Toxemia of pregnancy is best prevented by adequate prenatal care. Treatment of established toxemia is unsatisfactory, and the syndrome is resolved only after parturition. The rapid correction of extreme hypertension in patients with eclampsia can further compromise placental blood flow, thereby aggravating the syndrome.

Hypertension should be treated urgently with pharmacologic agents if the diastolic pressure reaches 105 mm Hg.[126] Intravenous administration of hydralazine is the preferred approach. An initial dose of 5 mg is used; if the diastolic pressure is not lowered to the desired level within 20 minutes, an additional 5 to 15 mg is injected. A total dose of 5 to 20 mg almost always achieves the desired effect. The injection is repeated whenever the diastolic pressure rises to 105 mm Hg. Diazoxide has been advocated for the treatment of intrapartum hypertensive emergencies; the dose is titrated with small boluses of 30 to 60 mg I.V. There have been reports, however, of severe hypotension, maternal hyperglycemia, and fetal hypoglycemia from diazoxide use. Moreover, diazoxide may interrupt uterine contractions, which must then be stimulated by an oxytocic agent.

A number of drugs are contraindicated during pregnancy, such as sodium nitroprusside, which may cause fetal cyanide poisoning; ganglionic blocking agents, which may cause meconium ileus; and angiotensin converting enzyme inhibitors, which may cause fetal death. Magnesium sulfate (an I.V. loading dose of 2 to 4 g for 15 minutes, followed by a continuous infusion of 1 to 2 g/hr or more if necessary) is still the preferred agent for control of eclamptic seizures and should be administered for 12 to 24 hours after childbirth [*see* Special Topics, Hypertension Associated with Pregnancy, *below*].[127]

Cerebral Disease

Hypertension secondary to cerebral hemorrhage cannot be treated effectively with drugs. Hematomas in the putamen, subcortical white matter, and cerebellum are treated by surgical evacuation, whereas those in the thalamus and pons are usually managed conservatively [*see Chapter 36*]. The hypertensive patient with subarachnoid hemorrhage is usually managed with bed rest and, when necessary, gentle reduction of blood pressure by use of oral agents. Reserpine has been favored for this purpose because it simultaneously decreases vascular spasm; however, nifedipine may become the drug of choice. Likewise, oral agents should be used to carefully lower blood pressure in patients with a thrombotic or embolic stroke and severe hypertension, especially when anticoagulation is being considered. Rapid reduction of blood pressure in a patient who has a cerebral thrombosis can often aggravate the neurologic deficit if a major obstruction to blood flow exists. Sodium nitroprusside has been favored by neurosurgeons for treating hypertensive emergencies that complicate cerebral catastrophes.[128] In general, if vasodilator therapy is contemplated in any of the circumstances described, concomitant use of a beta blocker is advised.

Special Topics

Routine Surgery

Questions often arise regarding the proper use of antihypertensive agents during routine surgery and in the perioperative period. In patients with hypertension and diastolic pressure less than 110 mm Hg, surgery is generally safe provided that antihypertensive medications are continued prior to surgery and a skilled anesthesiologist and good monitoring facilities are available.[129] If diastolic blood pressure is greater than 110 mm Hg, surgery should be delayed in most instances until control of blood pressure is achieved.

There is good evidence that the beta blockers can be continued throughout surgery without ill effects. Because guanethidine and guanadrel potentiate the effect of norepinephrine, they should be replaced by another agent. Similarly, the monoamine oxidase inhibitors should be withdrawn and replaced. Clonidine and guanabenz, neither of which is available in a parenteral form in the United States, should be tapered and replaced by an agent that can be continued throughout surgery. Because perioperative hypokalemia often occurs in patients receiving diuretic therapy and can be life threatening, we generally advise discontinuation of thiazide therapy one week prior to elective surgery, if possible, or vigorous potassium replacement in all other patients to achieve a blood level greater than 4.0 mEq/l. If emergency surgery is required, potassium can be replaced at a maximum rate of 1 mEq a minute, provided simultaneous monitoring is available.

Severe perioperative hypertension is best managed with sodium nitroprusside. Reinstitution of antihypertensive therapy in the postoperative period is dictated by blood pressure levels. Intravenous hydralazine, reserpine, methyldopa, propranolol, or sublingual nifedipine may be used if a patient cannot take oral medications. Those with a nasogastric tube can receive oral preparations via the tube. The goal during the perioperative period should be to adjust blood pressure to the preoperative level rather than to an ideal level.

Coarctation

Aortic coarctation in adults usually involves the portion of the aorta located just below the left subclavian artery. Symptoms of headache, cold feet, and fatigue of the lower extremities may be ignored by the patient for many years. Physical examination reveals hypertension of the upper extremities and a 20 mm Hg or greater reduction of systolic blood pressure in the legs. A delay in the femoral pulse, best detected by simultaneous palpation of the radial and femoral pulses, is a very suggestive sign. A bruit is often heard in the back over the narrowed aortic segment or from blood flow in dilated intercostal vessels. Associated abnormalities may include a bicuspid aortic valve, ventricular septal defect, or Turner's syndrome. Chest roentgenograms may reveal cardiomegaly, rib notching, or the so-called figure three, a silhouette made by coarctation at the aortic knob. Diagnosis is confirmed by angiography.

Surgical correction is almost always indicated. Early reports suggest that balloon angioplasty is as effective as surgery for patients with coarctation or its postoperative recurrence.[130] Untreated coarctation may be complicated by heart failure, aortic dissection or rupture, bacterial endocarditis, or intracranial hemorrhage. Hypertension may persist after surgical correction but is less likely to continue if the defect is corrected at an early age.[131] Preoperative and postoperative medical therapy is best accomplished with a sympatholytic agent and, if necessary, a diuretic. We find beta blockers most effective in this situation.

Adult-type aortic coarctation is most often congenital in origin, but Takayasu's arteritis may account for more cases of aortic coarctation than has been appreciated.[132] Paradoxic hypertension is often observed immediately after surgical coarctation resection, and it can occasionally be associated with mesenteric arteritis.

Cushing's Syndrome

Hypertension is one of the manifestations of Cushing's syndrome.

Hypertension Associated With Estrogen-containing Contraceptives

Elevation of both systolic and diastolic blood pressure occurs in almost all patients receiving prolonged estrogen therapy.[133] No correlation is apparent between the specific estrogen compound used and the degree of elevation, but compounds with large amounts of estrogen are probably associated with an increased risk of hypertension. Five percent of patients receiving estrogen therapy become overtly hypertensive, and approximately half of these patients remain hypertensive after the medication is discontinued.

Factors that predispose to the development of hypertension during estrogen administration include family or personal history of high blood pressure, chronic renal disease, and hypertension during pregnancy. A patient should be given oral contraceptives or estrogen therapy only after a careful history has been obtained to exclude these factors. Continued blood pressure monitoring for the duration of therapy is indicated. A rise in blood pressure of 15/10 mm Hg or more or the development of overt hypertension warrants immediate cessation of estrogen therapy.

Hypertension Associated With Pregnancy

Hypertension that develops during pregnancy may represent either preeclampsia or exacerbation of preexisting essential hypertension. Preeclampsia is characterized by a diastolic blood pressure of 85 to 90 mm Hg or higher, edema, and proteinuria, all of which appear after the 26th week. The typical patient is a very young primigravida. Multiple fetuses, diabetes, and hydatidiform mole are frequently associated factors. On the other hand, exacerbation of preexisting essential hypertension begins before 20 weeks of gestation; blood pressure is often higher than in preeclampsia; and end-organ damage may be evident. The patient who has chronic hypertension is usually a multigravida.

Normal blood pressure during early pregnancy is low. Between weeks 17 and 20, a resting blood pressure greater than 110/75 mm Hg with the patient in a sitting position or greater than 100/65 mm Hg with the patient in the left lateral position may indicate a risk of developing preeclampsia.[134] Between weeks 28 and 32, a primigravida should be considered at risk if her diastolic blood pressure rises by 20 mm Hg or more when she rolls from left lateral recumbency to the supine position.[135] The results of one study indicate that pregnant women who receive calcium supplementation (2 g/day as calcium carbonate, commencing in the 20th week of gestation) have a reduced risk of gestational hypertension (7.2 percent versus 10.7 percent) and preeclampsia (2.6 percent versus 3.9 percent).[135a] The mechanism of these effects is unknown. Further studies of the risks and benefits of calcium supplementation are under way.

Hypertensive patients who become pregnant should continue receiving antihypertensive therapy. Several commonly used agents have been given without adverse effect on mother or fetus; methyldopa and hydralazine have been used most successfully.[136] An increasing number of reports on the use of beta blockers in pregnant hypertensive patients suggest that these agents improve the likelihood of the birth of a normal infant.[137,138] Angiotensin converting enzyme inhibitors are contraindicated because fetal deaths have been caused by these drugs in certain animal species. Data are too preliminary to recommend use of the calcium entry blockers or labetalol during pregnancy.

If preeclampsia is diagnosed, bed rest is indicated.[126] If this measure does not adequately control blood pressure, hospitalization and cautious drug therapy are required to prevent the development of eclampsia, especially in patients whose diastolic blood pressure rises above 85 mm Hg. In contrast to treatment of preexisting hypertension, it is inadvisable to restrict salt or to administer diuretics or sedatives in preeclampsia. Labor is induced if hypertension cannot be controlled and poses severe risk to the mother.

A placebo-controlled, double-blind study suggests that low-dose aspirin (60 mg a day), administered to high-risk pregnant patients during the second and third trimesters, decreased the incidence of preeclampsia without producing adverse effects on the fetus.[139] These data need to be confirmed.

Hypertension during Lactation

As an increasing number of mothers breast-feed their infants, the management of hypertension during lactation must be considered.[140] Diuretics are contraindicated because they decrease milk production. Of the various beta blockers, propranolol, timolol, and oxprenolol are least concentrated in milk and are, therefore, preferred over other beta blockers. Captopril also appears to be safe. Other hypertensive agents, such as the sympatholytics and vasodilators, may be acceptable for use during lactation, but data are lacking.

Hypertensive Hypertrophic Cardiomyopathy of the Elderly

Elderly patients with long-standing hypertension and heart failure who manifest with severe concentric cardiac hypertrophy (revealed by echocardiography), a small left ventricular cavity, and above-average indices of systolic function, such as elevated ejection fraction, respond well to beta blockers or calcium entry blockers. However, such patients develop severe hypotension in response to many vasodilators, including captopril, hydralazine, nitrates, and prazosin.[141]

Pheochromocytoma

Although pheochromocytoma is traditionally characterized by paroxysmal hypertension, one half to two thirds of patients who have the disease show sustained hypertension.[142] Classic symptoms, whether sustained or intermittent, include headache, excessive perspiration, and tachycardia. Also encountered are signs of hypermetabolism such as weight loss, nervousness, orthostatic hypotension, and glucose intolerance. Laboratory evaluation may reveal increased blood sugar, a rise in hematocrit, and an elevated leukocyte count with an increase in the number of band cells. Familial syndromes such as multiple endocrine adenomatosis type 2 with medullary carcinoma of the thyroid, neurofibromatosis, von Hippel–Lindau disease, or neuroblastoma have a high incidence of associated pheochromocytoma. Patients with primary epinephrine-secreting tumors may present with paradoxic hypotension (primarily caused by increased beta stimulation) and may even present with shock or cardiomyopathy as prominent manifestations of the disease.[143,144]

Ten percent of pheochromocytomas are bilateral; bilateral tumors are especially frequent in familial syndromes. One to three percent are extra-abdominal, and are usually located in the thoracic para-aortic areas. Five to 15 percent of pheochromocytomas are malignant and have the potential to metastasize.

Not all patients with hypertension need to be screened for pheochromocytoma. The disease will rarely be missed if looked for in (1) patients with hypertension who are younger than 35 years, (2) patients who have hypertension and headache, perspiration, or tachycardia, (3) patients who have paroxysmal hypertension, and (4) patients who have a fixed diastolic pressure of 130 mm Hg or higher.

Screening for pheochromocytoma is performed most reliably by determining the metanephrine level in a 24-hour urine collection.[144] The levels of urine vanillylmandelic acid and urine catecholamines are less reliable indicators because they are altered by various medications. A second reliable screening test compares the levels of metanephrine and creatinine in a single voided urine specimen[145]; more than 1 μg of metanephrine per mg of creatinine suggests possible pheochromocytoma and the need for further diagnostic studies. Proper measurement of plasma catecholamine levels appears to be the most sensitive test and is coming into widespread use.[146] Prior to the test, patients should fast overnight and should remain supine for 30 minutes; venipuncture should be performed 20 minutes prior to plasma sampling. The diagnostic yield of each of these determinations is enhanced when samples are obtained during a hypertensive attack. Such results are so reliable that they obviate hazardous provocative or inhibitory tests.

The clonidine suppression test may be used in conjunction with determination of plasma catecholamine levels.[147] This test involves administration of 0.3 mg of clonidine. In patients with pheochromocytoma, elevated plasma norepinephrine levels measured three hours after clonidine is given are unaffected. In contrast, in patients with essential hypertension, plasma norepinephrine levels are suppressed to less than 500 ng/l. The sensitivity and specificity of the clonidine suppression test are quite good. A radioimmunoassay for chromogranin A, a catecholamine storage protein, appears to be useful and may soon become available.[148]

Computed tomography (CT) is safer than angiography and is an accurate means of localizing tumors that exceed 0.5 cm in diameter. In complicated cases, however, angiography may be needed. When extra-adrenal tumors are suspected, the guanethidine analogue ^{131}I-metaiodobenzylguanidine may be useful for scintigraphic localization.[149]

Differential diagnosis includes a syndrome characterized by anxiety and essential hypertension that is often associated with high-normal plasma catecholamine levels and low plasma conjugated catechol levels; this syndrome responds to beta-blocking therapy.[150] Posterior fossa lesions, including strokes, abnormal vascular loops, tumors, and aneurysms, can also mimic pheochromocytoma. They do so by stimulating the medullary sympathoadrenal pathway, which causes paroxysmal hypertension and elevated catecholamine levels.[151] Detection of labetalol metabolites can lead to an erroneous diagnosis of pheochromocytoma.[152]

Surgery offers the potential for cure of hypertension in most cases of pheochromocytoma. Preoperative stabilization is essential to reduce the risk of surgery; it includes prior treatment with alpha blockade followed by beta blockade. Beta-mediated vasodilatation must not be inhibited before satisfactory alpha inhibition has been achieved. Beta blockade is then used to prevent sinus tachycardia and catecholamine-induced arrhythmias. An appropriate program begins with phenoxybenzamine (Dibenzyline), administered initially at a dosage of 10 mg orally twice a day; the dose is increased until adequate blood pressure control is achieved. A low-dose, short-acting beta blocker (e.g., propranolol, 10 mg orally four times a day) is then given, and the dose is gradually increased until a normal pulse rate is obtained. Although anecdotal reports attest to the ability of calcium entry blockers, prazosin, or labetalol to control blood pressure in patients with pheochromocytoma,[153,154] we prefer the specific and potent adrenergic blocking regimen described above.

Surgery should be undertaken only when blood pressure is completely controlled and blood volume is replete. Careful monitoring during surgery is essential. Manipulation of the tumor may cause severe hypertension and tachyarrhythmias, even in a patient who has been well prepared. After the tumor has been removed, hypotension may occur. The anesthesiologist must be prepared to treat such fluctuations in blood pressure with intravenous solutions of propranolol, phentolamine, norepinephrine, sodium nitroprusside, or volume expanders. The measures used in the treatment of pheochromocytoma crisis are discussed earlier [*see* Hypertensive Emergencies, *above*].

Primary Aldosteronism

High blood pressure that results from increased aldosterone production is the classic example of volume-related hypertension. Aldosterone promotes renal sodium retention while increasing urinary loss of potassium and hydrogen ions, resulting in hypokalemic alkalosis. Hypokalemia, in turn, can produce insulin resistance with glucose intolerance, renal tubular damage with polyuria, muscle weakness, and cardiac arrhythmias. Although hyperaldosteronism leads to salt and water retention, the ultimate mechanism that sustains hypertension is unknown.[155]

Primary aldosteronism results from benign adrenal adenoma (Conn's syndrome) or from bilateral adrenal hyperplasia (idiopathic hyperaldosteronism). Conn's syndrome occurs about four times as often as idiopathic hyperaldosteronism. Idiopathic hyperaldosteronism may have several etiologies, one of which may involve a pituitary factor.[156]

Because hypokalemia eventually appears in almost all patients with primary aldosteronism, screening for this disease need be undertaken only in patients who exhibit either unprovoked or significant diuretic-induced hypokalemia despite dietary sodium restriction. Screening tests include stimulated PRA, which yields a very low result in primary aldosteronism, and a 24-hour urine K^+ determination, which yields a result of 30 mEq/24 hours or higher when hypokalemia and primary aldosteronism are present. Plasma aldosterone levels will fail to show a normal level of suppression after the oral administration of 25 mg of captopril.[157] The definitive diagnosis of primary aldosteronism is made by demonstrating elevated aldosterone levels that do not decline or that decline only slightly after sodium loading. Hypokalemia must be corrected before measuring aldosterone levels. Plasma and urine aldosterone levels are best determined by radioimmunoassay; sensitivity is enhanced by measuring plasma levels at 8:00 A.M. Localization of the lesion is most commonly accomplished by CT scanning and by selective sampling of blood from both adrenal veins for aldosterone. Absence of a visible tumor on CT scanning and bilateral elevation of aldosterone levels implicate idiopathic hyperaldosteronism and differentiate this condition from Conn's syndrome.[158]

Distinguishing between the two forms of hyperaldosteronism is important in choosing therapy. Simple adenomas are best removed surgically, and excellent results are usually obtained; patients in whom an anomalous postural fall in aldosterone is induced are the most likely to benefit from surgery.[159] Adrenal venous sampling during continuous ACTH infusion is a sensitive method for localizing the adenoma.

Idiopathic hyperaldosteronism is better managed medically because bilateral adrenalectomy has reversed hypertension in only one third of these patients. Spironolactone, an aldosterone antagonist, is used to treat idiopathic hyperaldosteronism and to treat Conn's syndrome during the presurgical period or in patients who are ineligible for surgery.

Excessive licorice ingestion (< 0.45 kg/wk) can produce a condition called pseudo–primary hyperaldosteronism because licorice contains glycyrrhizic acid, which has salt-retaining properties. A case of pseudo–primary hyperaldosteronism caused by glycyrrhizic acid in chewing tobacco has also been described.[160]

Renal Artery Stenosis

The role of the renin-angiotensin-aldosterone system in the pathogenesis of renovascular hypertension has already been described [*see* Pathogenesis, *above*]. Renal artery stenosis arises either from fibroplasia of arterial tissue or from atherosclerosis. Fibroplasia is seen predominantly in women 20 to 30 years of age, whereas atherosclerosis of the renal arteries generally appears in patients older than 45 years who have evidence of diffuse atherosclerosis. Rarer causes of renovascular hypertension are renal artery dissection, embolization, or thrombosis; the last may be suspected in patients receiving oral contraceptives.[161] Physical examination of patients with renal artery stenosis is unremarkable except for the inconstant presence of an abdominal bruit, which is heard in 50 percent of these patients; it is audible in only 10 percent of patients without the disease.[162] Candidates for renal artery stenosis screening are patients who are younger than 35 years or older than 45 years at the onset of hypertension and who are eligible for surgical correction. A negative family history for hypertension or the presence of an abdominal bruit favors a diagnosis of renal artery stenosis. The incidence of renovascular hypertension in patients with severe hypertension (diastolic blood pressure ≥ 125 mm Hg with funduscopic evidence of grade III or IV retinopathy) is 31.0 percent, in contrast to a 0.1 to 1.0 percent incidence in the entire hypertensive population.[163] Other patients who should be screened for renal artery stenosis are those with refractory hypertension who have a sustained elevation of serum creatinine (greater than 1.5 mg/dl).[164] A history of cigarette smoking may correlate with both the fibromuscular and atherosclerotic types of renal artery stenosis.[165]

There is no simple, reliable screening protocol for renal artery stenosis. Both suppressed and stimulated PRA values may be markedly elevated in renal artery stenosis, but they may also be normal. A more sensitive measure is the presence of reactive hyperreninemia, demonstrated by measurement of PRA values after angiotensin blockade using either an angiotensin II antagonist or an angiotensin converting enzyme inhibitor.

Digital subtraction angiography (DSA), a procedure that entails intravenous injection of contrast material, is the method of choice for visualizing the renal arteries.[166] DSA should be avoided if sensitivity to the contrast material is anticipated—for example, in patients with an allergy to contrast agents or in those with diabetes; it should not be used for routine screening because of its risks and cost (see below). When digital angiography is unavailable, radioisotope renal scanning or intravenous pyelography (IVP) is used for diagnosis of renovascular hypertension. Compared with IVP, scanning is thought to be slightly more sensitive but less specific. Scanning is the procedure of choice for patients in whom IVP or DSA poses risks. Such patients include those with hypersensitivity to contrast agents, compromised renal function, dysproteinemia, or diabetes.

When stenosis is strongly suspected, differential renal venous catheterization for renin determination is indicated. If renal artery constriction is seen on angiography, if the PRA ratio between the two renal venous samples is greater than 2 : 1, and if the PRA from the uninvolved renal venous effluent is suppressed, the probability of cure is high.[167] Maximally stimulating PRA can enhance the diagnostic accuracy of differential renal venous sampling. Stimulation of PRA enhances specificity and does not introduce false positive results. For this purpose, we prefer the vasodilator hydralazine (10 mg I.M. or I.V.) or single-dose captopril (12.5 mg orally) rather than a diuretic, which can cause dehydration and enhance the risk of dye-induced renal failure in patients who are about to receive contrast material. If an angiotensin converting enzyme inhibitor is used, care must be taken to avoid severe hypotension.[168]

The optimal surgical treatment is arterial repair or bypass rather than nephrectomy. Revascularization for left renal artery stenosis appears to be most appropriately performed by means of the splenorenal arterial anastomosis. Autogenous tissue is employed, and only a single anastomosis is required. The spleen continues to be nourished by the short gastric arteries. This technique minimizes the incidence of postoperative renal failure by obviating aortic cross-clamping and avoids the difficulties often encountered when grafting to an atherosclerotic aorta.[169] Hepatosaphenous bypass for lesions on the right side and mesenterorenal bypass to repair either kidney have been used with good short-term success.

Utilization of newer operative techniques along with sophisticated perioperative care and, when it is indicated, prophylactic coronary or carotid bypass grafting in symptomatic patients is resulting in much improved success rates.[170] Moreover, there is increasing evidence that such surgery can and should be undertaken not only to ameliorate hypertension but also to preserve or salvage renal tissue. One study indicates that late revascularization of totally occluded renal arteries in patients with kidneys greater than 9.5 cm in length can restore renal function, regardless of the preoperative functional level.[171] Renin production is a valuable measure of the reversibility of ischemia.

Percutaneous transluminal angioplasty, a potentially simple and relatively non-invasive and inexpensive procedure, has also been used extensively in treating renovascular hypertension. This technique entails percutaneous balloon catheter dilatation of the renal artery to compress atherosclerotic or fibromuscular lesions. On two-year follow-up, more than 80 percent of patients experienced improved blood pressure control, and roughly half required no further antihypertensive medication. The two-year patency rate is approximately 70 to 80 percent for patients with fibromuscular dysplasia and only about 50 percent for patients with atheromas; a patency rate of approximately 80 to 90 percent has been reported following surgical intervention.[172]

The limitations of angioplasty are anatomic. Certain lesions are so severely stenotic that they do not admit passage of a balloon catheter; others are so calcified and rigid that they resist dilatation. The complications are similar to those of percutaneous angiography. Those that occur with a frequency of one to five percent include infection, arterial rupture or dissection, false aneurysm formation, local or retroperitoneal bleeding, thrombosis, subsegmental renal infarction, and balloon rupture with embolization or with femoral artery occlusion.[173] Although it has been argued that angioplasty is the preferred treatment of patients at high risk from general anesthesia and surgery, it should be cautioned that several of the complications of angioplasty require immediate surgical intervention. Thus, balloon catheter dilation of the renal artery should be attempted only in centers that have had extensive experience in percutaneous angiography and angioplasty of peripheral vascular lesions. A vascular surgical team should be immediately available to deal with any complications resulting from this procedure.

Dilation is advised only for discrete lesions that appear amenable to compression and, moreover, for lesions demonstrated to be associated with ipsilateral increased renin production; increased renin production on the involved side is the most sensitive index of reversible renal ischemia.

We currently favor an attempt at angioplasty in the following patients[174]: those with an intrarenal stenosis, in whom surgical repair might necessitate sacrifice of renal tissue; patients younger than 30 years with severe hypertension and fibromuscular lesions because such lesions are progressive; patients with relative but not absolute contraindications to surgery; patients with bilateral renal artery stenoses and poorly controlled hypertension or evidence of diminished renal function; patients with a single functioning kidney and decreasing renal function believed caused by an extrarenal arterial stenosis[175]; and patients with hypertension caused by transplant stenosis. For patients with bilateral disease, angioplasty can serve as part of a stepwise approach to improving renal perfusion and controlling blood pressure prior to surgical or balloon catheter repair of the contralateral lesion. Some argue that angioplasty should be tried first in all candidates for surgical repair of renovascular disease. We do not favor such an approach at this time. Randomized clinical trials are needed to establish the long-term complications of angioplasty and the length of time and degree to which renal arteries will remain patent after its use.

It has been argued that potent drugs, the angiotensin converting enzyme inhibitors in particular, may serve as effective alternatives to surgery. We agree that these agents can be used to control blood pressure in patients with unilateral, but not bilateral, stenosis[103,104] [see Treatment, *above*]. Conversely, the risk of anatomic progression of stenotic lesions with loss of renal function militates strongly in favor of surgical correction in all affected patients except those in whom surgery poses unacceptable risk. In this regard, two studies support the finding that a satisfactory decline in blood pressure in response to long-term therapy with an angiotensin converting enzyme inhibitor predicts a favorable surgical result.[176,177] A large percentage of patients with renovascular hypertension are refractory to drug therapy and must undergo surgical correction of the stenotic lesion. Renovas-

cular hypertension is the subject of two recent reviews.[178]

Renal Parenchymal Disease

In 80 to 90 percent of patients with hypertension and end-stage renal disease, the hypertension is volume dependent and can be effectively controlled by salt restriction and potent diuretic therapy. In 10 to 20 percent of patients with hypertension and renal parenchymal disease, the hypertension is associated with elevated renin activity; these patients respond well to therapy aimed at decreasing PRA, such as the use of beta blockers. Use of the vasodilator minoxidil has been shown to forestall the need for nephrectomy and transplantation or dialysis, which may ultimately be required to achieve blood pressure control. The belief that correction of hypertension often worsens renal function is incorrect. The treatment of malignant hypertension with renal parenchymal involvement, for example, can result in improved renal function.[179] Nevertheless, in treating such cases, antihypertensive agents that increase the glomerular filtration rate (e.g., minoxidil) are preferred [*see Table* 7]. Patients who have undergone unilateral nephrectomy, such as kidney donors, should be carefully monitored for hypertension.[180]

Transplantation Hypertension

Hypertension can develop after renal transplantation and may result from a number of factors, including renal artery stenosis at the site of anastomosis, renin secretion by the host kidney, renal dysfunction associated with rejection, and renal toxicity caused by immunosuppressive agents.

Surprisingly, hypertension occurs quite often after cardiac transplantation. The pathogenesis is not well understood, but the condition most likely results from cyclosporine-related renal dysfunction and volume retention rather than major alterations in the catecholamine or the RAA systems.[181]

References

1. Am J Cardiol 37:269, 1976
2. Hypertension 7:457, 1985
3. N Engl J Med 293:65, 1975
4. Hypertension 2:714, 1980
5. N Engl J Med 307:993, 1982
6. N Engl J Med 287:573, 1972
7. N Engl J Med 314:1015, 1986
8. N Engl J Med 314:1041, 1986
9. Am J Med 61:43, 1976
10. N Engl J Med 291:389, 446, 1974
11. N Engl J Med 286:441, 1972
12. JAMA 238:611, 1977
13. Clin Sci 64:273, 1983
14. Ann Intern Med 82:27, 1975
15. N Engl J Med 311:1631, 1984
16. Klin Wochenschr 56(suppl 1):113, 1978
17. Circ Res 31(suppl):II-125, 1972
18. Fed Proc 43:103, 1984
19. J Hypertens 3:557, 1985
20. Life Sci 28:89, 1981
21. Hypertension 7:469, 1985
22. Br Med J 300:847, 1981
23. Hypertension 6:445, 1984
24. Fed Proc 44:2846, 1985
25. J Clin Invest 75:1285, 1985
26. N Engl J Med 309:1009, 1983
27. Hypertension 4:795, 1982
28. N Engl J Med 310:1191, 1984
29. N Engl J Med 314:222, 1986
30. N Engl J Med 314:198, 1986
31. Pediatrics 79:1, 1987
32. Br Med J 288:1574, 1984
33. Arch Intern Med 144:1045, 1984
34. N Engl J Med 312:1548, 1985
35. JAMA 252:1898, 1984
36. Mayo Clin Proc 52:549, 1977
37. Circulation 55:767, 1977
38. JAMA 202:1028, 1967
39. JAMA 213:1143, 1970
40. N Engl J Med 291:329, 1974
41. Lancet 1:1261, 1980
42. Am J Med 69:725, 1980
43. JAMA 242:2562, 1979
44. JAMA 242:2572, 1979
45. Br Med J 291:97, 1985
46. JAMA 248:1465, 1982
47. Circulation 70:996, 1984
48. J Hypertens 3:379, 1985
49. Lancet 1:467, 1982
50. Lancet 1:1175, 1983
51. JAMA 126:829, 1944
52. Lancet 1:1349, 1985
53. Lancet 2:589, 1986
54. JAMA 256:70, 1986
55. Ann Intern Med 102:359, 1985
56. J Hypertens 4:383, 1986
57. JAMA 248:537, 1982
58. N Engl J Med 314:334, 1986
59. JAMA 253:657, 1985
60. Ann Intern Med 98:770, 1983
61. N Engl J Med 312:746, 1985
62. Science 224:1329, 1984
63. Br Med J 286:1847, 1983
64. Ann Intern Med 103:825, 1985
65. Lancet 1:359, 1986
66. Ann Intern Med 105:947, 1986
67. Lancet 2:703, 1986
68. JAMA 249:54, 1983
69. Lancet 2:473, 1986
70. JAMA 252:487, 1984
71. Lancet 1:289, 1974
72. Br Med J 290:1103, 1985
73. JAMA 251:756, 1984
74. Am J Med 75:553, 1983
75. Am J Med 70:762, 1981
76. Drugs 32:335, 1986
77. Am J Cardiol 36:653, 1975
78. N Engl J Med 304:801, 1981
79. N Engl J Med 308:940, 1983
80. Am J Cardiol 52:1D, 1983
81. Cardiovascular Reviews and Reports 6:979, 1985
82. Br Med J 289:1495, 1984
83. Lancet 1:123, 1985
84. Br Med J 290:322, 1985
85. Med Lett Drugs Ther 26:83, 1984
86. Ann Intern Med 99:553, 1983
87. JAMA 238:1734, 1977
88. Med Lett Drugs Ther 27:95, 1985
89. Cardiovascular Reviews and Reports 5:281, 1984
90. Semin Arthritis Rheum 5:83, 1975
91. J Cardiovasc Pharmacol 2:S131, 1980
92. Science 196:441, 1977
93. Ann Intern Med 90:19, 1979
94. Capoten. Physicians' Desk Reference, 41st ed. Medical Economics Co, Oradell, NJ, 1987, p 1940
95. Med Lett Drugs Ther 27:103, 1985
96. J Hypertens 2(suppl):S75, 1984
97. Lancet 1:872, 1986
98. Vasotec. Physicians' Desk Reference, 41st ed. Medical Economics Co, Oradell, NJ, 1987, p 1347
99. Medical Letter 28:53, 1986
100. N Engl J Med 314:1657, 1986
101. Br Med J 293:467, 1986
102. Br Med J 293:471, 1986
103. N Engl J Med 308:373, 1983
104. N Engl J Med 308:377, 1983
105. NZ Med J 100:6, 1987
106. JAMA 260:967, 1988
107. Drugs 25:154, 1983
108. Lancet 2:22, 1983
109. JAMA 253:3263, 1985
110. Hypertension 3:23, 1981
111. N Engl J Med 310:279, 1984
112. Br Med J 292:233, 1986
113. Br Med J 292:235, 1986
114. Medical Letter 27:22, 1985
115. Ann Intern Med 91:752, 1979
116. Am Heart J 105:865, 1983
117. Arch Intern Med 144:2357, 1984
118. Am Heart J 103:390, 1982
119. Am J Cardiol 49:1267, 1982
120. Br Med J 2:737, 1977
121. N Engl J Med 314:181, 1986
122. Cardiovascular Review and Report 6:1249, 1985
123. Am J Med 60:625, 1976
124. Aortic Dissection. Doroghazi RM, Slater EE, Eds. McGraw-Hill Book Co, New York, 1983
125. JAMA 230:1692, 1974
126. N Engl J Med 313:675, 1985
127. Am J Obstet Gynecol 148:162, 1984
128. Current Concepts of Cerebrovascular Disease/Stroke 12:7, 1977
129. Ann Intern Med 98:504, 1983
130. Am J Cardiol 57:828, 1986
131. Am J Cardiol 37:769, 1976
132. N Engl J Med 299:1002, 1978
133. JAMA 237:2499, 1977
134. Lancet 1:1273, 1977
135. Am J Obstet Gynecol 120:1, 1974
135a. N Engl J Med 325:1399, 1991
136. Lancet 1:647, 1982
137. N Engl J Med 305:1323, 1981
138. Lancet 1:431, 1983
139. Lancet 1:1, 1986
140. Hypertension 6:297, 1984
141. N Engl J Med 312:277, 1985
142. Mayo Clin Proc 39:281, 1964
143. Am J Med 47:648, 1969
144. Am Heart J 83:688, 1972
145. N Engl J Med 311:1298, 1984
146. Arch Intern Med 137:190, 1977
147. N Engl J Med 305:623, 1981
148. N Engl J Med 311:764, 1984
149. J Clin Endocrinol Metab 61:769, 1985
150. Hypertension 3:347, 1981
151. Neurology (NY) 31:1560, 1981
152. J R Soc Med 78:588, 1985
153. Lancet 2:711, 1983
154. Br Med J 280:1300, 1980
155. N Engl J Med 289:1330, 1973
156. N Engl J Med 311:94, 1984
157. J Clin Endocrinol Metab 57:892, 1983
158. N Engl J Med 303:1503, 1980
159. Ann Intern Med 90:386, 1979
160. N Engl J Med 302:784, 1980
161. Ann Intern Med 90:939, 1979
162. JAMA 220:1209, 1972
163. N Engl J Med 301:1273, 1979
164. N Engl J Med 311:1070, 1984
165. Lancet 2:765, 1983
166. JAMA 254:388, 1985
167. Am J Med 55:402, 1973
168. JAMA 251:56, 1984
169. Surgical Rounds 1(3):18, 1978
170. JAMA 257:498, 1987
171. Surgery 88:753, 1980

172. AJR 135:961, 1980
173. Radiology 159:201, 1986
174. Br J Surg 73:91, 1986
175. Ann Intern Med 91:684, 1979
176. Am J Med 76:398, 1984
177. Am J Cardiol 51:1317, 1983
178. Annu Rev Med 35:665, 1984
179. N Engl J Med 277:57, 1967
180. Mayo Clin Proc 60:367, 1985
181. Am J Cardiol 56:927, 1985
182. Clin Sci 64:407, 1983
183. NZ Med J 96:833, 1983
184. Am J Med 66:405, 1979
185. JAMA 256:619, 1986
186. N Engl J Med 313:596, 1985
187. J Clin Pharmacol 22:151, 1982
188. Nephron 34:196, 1983
189. Hypertension 3:168, 1981

Acknowledgments

Figure 1   Dana Burns. Data on the biochemistry of the renin system adapted from "The Renin-Angiotensin System," by S. Oparil and E. Haber, in *The New England Journal of Medicine* 291:389, 1974. Used by permission.

Figure 2   Sally Black.

Table 8   Modified from "Hypertension," by S. G. Sheps and R. A. Kirkpatrick, in *Mayo Clinic Proceedings* 50:709, 1975.

5 Acute Myocardial Infarction

E. WILLIAM HANCOCK, M.D.

Epidemiology

The term myocardial infarction refers to the death of myocardial tissue that results from a relative or an absolute insufficiency of blood supply. The term usually implies a classic clinical syndrome with sudden onset of characteristic symptoms, followed by serial electrocardiographic changes and transient rises in the serum levels of enzymes released from the myocardium. In the classic syndrome, a sudden, total occlusion of a major coronary artery by thrombosis causes infarction involving virtually the full thickness of the left ventricular wall in the specific region supplied by the affected artery. In other instances, however, the occlusion of the artery is less sudden or less complete, and the resulting infarction occurs during a period of hours or days and is less localized. Often, only a portion of the left ventricular wall is involved.

In a wider sense, the term myocardial infarction also applies to deaths that occur instantaneously or within minutes after the onset of ischemic symptoms, before acute myocardial necrosis can be demonstrated histologically. Myocardial infarction may also be used to describe myocardial fibrosis that develops during a period of months or years in patients with coronary artery disease who do not experience acute clinical episodes.

In the United States, myocardial infarction occurs in approximately 1,300,000 persons annually, of whom 800,000 are hospitalized and 500,000 die suddenly outside of the hospital.[1] The disease is much more prevalent in men than in women up to the age of 70, and the occurrence increases steeply with age in both sexes.

Pathogenesis

Coronary artery thrombosis almost always occurs at the site of an atheromatous plaque, usually a plaque that has already produced severe narrowing of the lumen. Thrombus formation is probably initiated by an acute event such as endothelial ulceration, formation of a fissure in the intimal lining, or hemorrhage within the plaque.[2] The first response to endothelial injury is aggregation of platelets. The platelets then release thromboxane, which promotes further platelet aggregation, coronary vasoconstriction, reduction of blood flow, and, ultimately, formation of a true thrombus. Occasionally, the mere presence of severe narrowing of the lumen, perhaps augmented by local vasospasm, may promote the initial platelet aggregation. Coronary spasm or embolism involving a non-diseased coronary artery is a rarer cause of acute coronary occlusion.[3,4] Aortic dissection or primary dissection of a coronary artery are also rare causes of coronary occlusion.[5]

Myocardial infarction may also arise from a sudden severe disparity between myocardial oxygen supply and demand in the absence of acute changes in the caliber of the coronary arteries. For example, a sudden reduction in oxygen supply caused by a drop in blood pressure during anesthesia and surgery may precipitate myocardial infarction. An acute increase in oxygen demand resulting from such stresses as heavy exertion, acute hypertension, or an excess of catecholamines may also precipitate myocardial infarction. Cocaine abuse, increasingly recognized as a cause of acute myocardial infarction, can produce a sudden increase in oxygen demand similar to that caused by catecholamine excess and may also cause spasm of the coronary arteries.[6,7]

In classic acute myocardial infarction, the infarct-related artery is totally occluded in about 85 percent of patients who are studied within six hours after the onset of symptoms but in only two thirds of those who are studied between six and 12 hours after the onset. These findings suggest that spontaneous lysis of the thrombus occurs frequently. Such spontaneous lysis, however, does relatively little to reverse the process of myocardial necrosis, which is largely completed within three to six hours after onset. Necrosis is largely irreversible after an even shorter period if the occlusion has been sudden and complete and there is no collateral circulation.

Clinical Features and Diagnosis during Initial Phase

Symptoms

The first symptom of acute myocardial infarction is usually chest pain, typically similar to angina pectoris but more severe, more persistent, and unrelieved by nitroglycerin. Radiation of the pain or its localization to the neck, jaw, shoulder, or left arm occurs as in angina; pain in the epigastrium, simulating that of indigestion, is particularly frequent. Marked sweating, almost from the onset of pain, is characteristic, and nausea and vomiting are also common.

Premonitory symptoms occur within a month before the onset of acute myocardial infarction in about two thirds of all cases.[8] These symptoms usually manifest as brief, mild episodes of new-onset angina pectoris or an abrupt progression of previously existing angina. Other premonitory symptoms are nonspecific, including unexplained fatigue noted by many patients.

The presentation of acute myocardial infarction in patients in the community differs from that in patients who are seen in the hospital. Almost one in four myocardial infarctions that occurred in patients in the Framingham study was unrecognized clinically and was detected only by the appearance of diagnostic Q waves in annual routine ECGs.[9] Half of the previously undiagnosed myocardial infarctions were associated with atypical symptoms, but the other half were truly asymptomatic.

Myocardial infarction that occurs after noncardiac surgery affects approximately 0.1 percent of the general adult population, but it affects about five to six percent of patients who have had a previous infarction.[10] Its incidence is particularly high after thoracic or abdominal surgery or when surgery is performed within six months after an infarction. Postoperative infarction is difficult to recognize because of concurrent medical circumstances such as pain and the use of analgesic drugs, but mortality in such cases is high, especially for those patients who have had previous infarctions.

Myocardial infarction in elderly patients presents in the classic manner in fewer than half of all instances.[11] The most frequent manner of onset is sudden dyspnea or exacerbation of chronic congestive heart failure. Acute confusion, dizziness, syncope, or stroke may also be the presenting symptom or sign.

Physical Examination

Physical examination typically reveals a patient with continuing chest pain who prefers to lie quietly in the supine position and is in evident acute distress. The skin is usually cool, moist, and pale. The pulse may be rapid or slow, and the blood pressure may be elevated or reduced. The changes in pulse and blood pressure depend on whether there is a predominance of excessive sympathetic or of excessive parasympathetic neural activity in response to the acute myocardial injury.[12] Exaggerated sinus arrhythmia is another indication of excessive parasympathetic activity.[13] The heart sounds are often faint, and an S_4 is often present. An S_3, inspiratory rales, and elevated jugular venous pressure are signs of congestive heart failure and are observed in only a minority of patients at the initial presentation. Pericardial friction rubs are rarely heard initially.

Electrocardiography

Almost any patient who had a previously normal ECG will show serial changes during acute myocardial infarction.

In about two thirds of such cases, the changes include development of pathologic Q waves and serial ST segment and T wave changes, patterns that are virtually diagnostic in themselves. In the remainder, the changes are limited to the ST segments and T waves. These patterns were formerly termed subendocardial or nontransmural infarction but are better described as non–Q wave infarction because the presence or absence of Q waves correlates poorly with the extent of the infarct across the left ventricular wall.

In cases of acute myocardial infarction associated with localized ST segment elevation in the initial ECG, the occluded artery can be identified with considerable accuracy by analyzing this ECG.[14] ST segment elevation in chest leads V1 through V4 indicates occlusion of the left anterior descending artery [*see Figure 1*]. When the lateral leads are involved as well, the left anterior descending artery is also usually the occluded artery, but the infarct is more extensive and is often caused by a more proximal site of occlusion [*see Figure 2*]. ST segment elevation in leads II, III, and aVF signals occlusion of the right coronary artery in about 80 percent of cases and of the left circumflex in about 20 percent [*see Figure 3*]. Other ECG findings can help distinguish between these two possibilities. Inferior infarcts with posterior involvement, manifested as an abnormally prominent R wave in lead V1, are more likely to be caused by occlusion of the circumflex artery [*see Figure 4*]. Right ventricular infarction, manifested as ST segment elevation in the right precordial leads or in leads V1 through V4 in the presence of an acute inferior infarct, is likely to be caused by occlusion of the right coronary artery in its most proximal portion [*see Figure 5*].[15,16] Infarcts in the lateral wall, which are caused by occlusion of nondominant circumflex arteries, often do not produce characteristic ECG abnormalities.[17] This finding reflects the fact that such infarcts are usually small and that the lateral wall is activated relatively late and its activation is represented in the latter part of the QRS complex rather than the initial part.

ST segment depression in leads opposite those that show the infarct pattern may represent either reciprocal changes or additional ischemia in a region remote from the infarct. In either case, a marked degree of such remote or reciprocal ST segment depression tends to indicate a more extensive infarct and a high likelihood of more than one diseased coronary artery [*see Figure 6*].[18]

Echocardiography

Two-dimensional echocardiography is readily able to demonstrate the abnormality in left ventricular wall motion that occurs in acute myocardial infarction, even when performed within the first few hours after the onset.[19] The procedure is therefore useful in the initial evaluation of the patient, especially when the ECG is not diagnostic and the diagnosis is in doubt. The extent of the wall motion abnormality is also helpful in assessing the initial prognosis and likelihood of complications. Abnormal bulging of the atrial septum toward the left atrium in patients with acute inferior myocardial infarction is a reliable indicator of right ventricular infarction. This finding reflects the fact that the right atrial pressure is higher than the left atrial pressure as a result of right ventricular failure.[20]

Prognosis in the Early Phase

The prognosis during the early phase of acute myocardial infarction, at the time of hospitalization, can be determined with considerable success from simple clinical observations. It is useful to distinguish four grades of congestive heart failure, termed Killip classes, on the basis of clinical criteria [*see Table 1*]. The Killip class and the age of the patient are strongly correlated with the patient's prognosis at the time of initial presentation. The initial ECG also provides an important guide to prognosis. Mortality is less than one percent for patients with ECGs that show no acute changes at the time of initial presentation in the emergency room.[21]

Additional features that correlate with mortality include a history of angina or previous myocardial infarction and the location

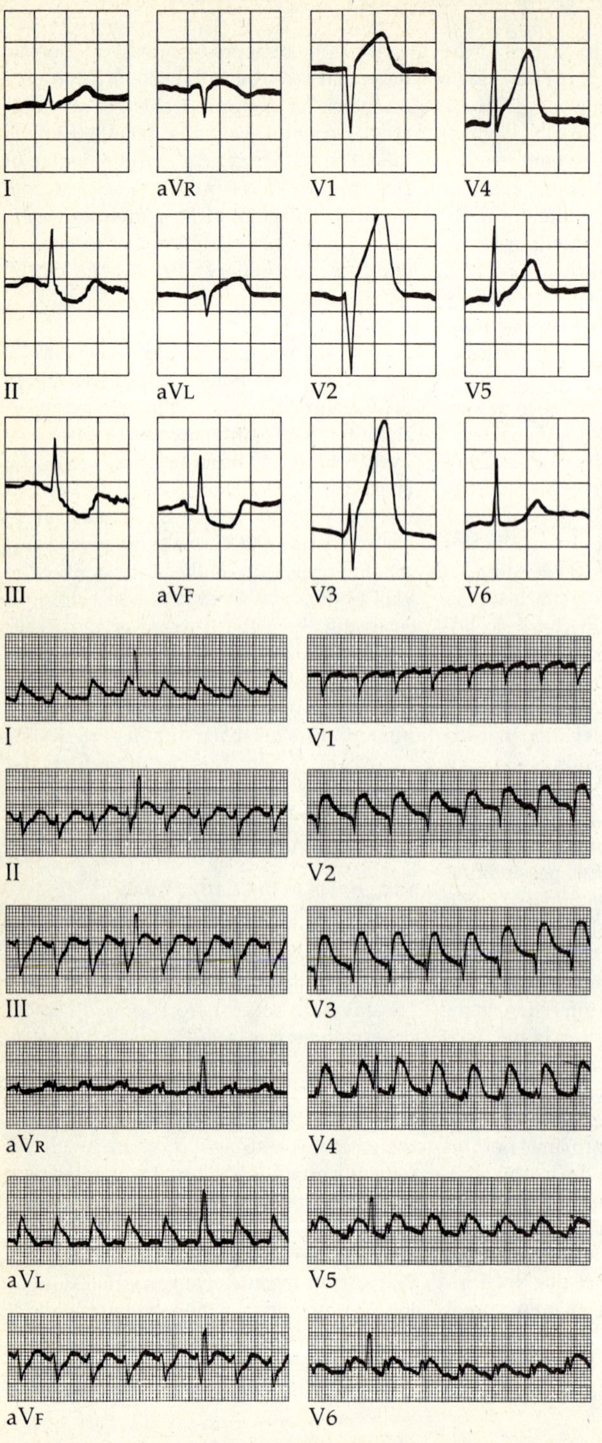

Figure 1 *Electrocardiogram from a patient with acute myocardial infarction caused by occlusion of the left anterior descending coronary artery was recorded 30 minutes after the onset of chest pain. ST segment elevation in leads V1 to V4 is associated with tall peaked T waves (so-called hyperacute T waves), a feature of very early acute myocardial infarction.*

Figure 2 *Electrocardiogram from a patient with acute myocardial infarction caused by occlusion of the left anterior descending coronary artery reveals ST segment elevation in the anterolateral leads and reciprocal ST segment depression in the inferior leads. The sinus tachycardia reflects sympathetic overactivity.*

of the infarct (as determined by the ECG). The Norris prognostic index is based on an assessment of these features as well as age, blood pressure, and severity of congestive heart failure.[22]

Initial Treatment

The treatment of patients in the early phase of acute myocardial infarction presents many issues. Guidelines for the management of such patients have been developed by a task force of the American College of Cardiology and the American Heart Association.[23]

Relief of Pain

The severe pain of acute myocardial infarction should be treated with sublingual nitroglycerin initially; the dose is repeated twice at five-minute intervals, unless the patient is hypotensive.[24] If the drug is ineffec-tive sublingually, an intravenous infusion should then be started. Nitroglycerin should be infused at a rate of 5 µg/min initially, and the dose should be increased progressively, as permitted by the blood pressure. Morphine sulfate (2 to 4 mg I.V. every 10 minutes to a total dose of 20 mg, if necessary) is also effective and should be used initially unless therapy with thrombolytic agents or intravenous beta-adrenergic blocking drugs is to be used.

Beta-adrenergic Blocking Therapy

Beta-blocking drugs, which are administered intravenously as soon as possible after the onset of acute myocardial infarction, have been found to reduce mortality and infarct size in several controlled trials.[25] By blocking the often excessive sympathetic nervous system activity in patients with myocardial infarction, the work of the heart

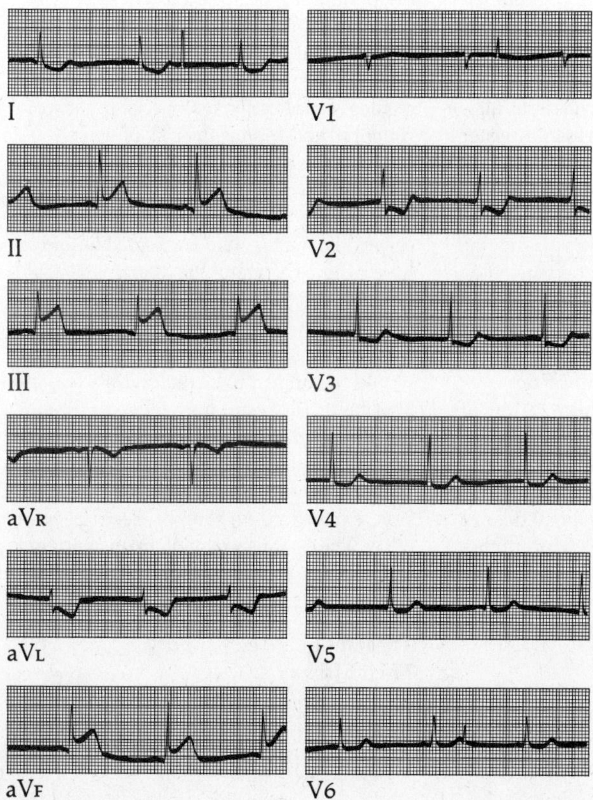

Figure 3 *Electrocardiogram from a patient with acute myocardial infarction caused by occlusion of the right coronary artery reveals ST segment elevation in the inferior leads and reciprocal ST segment depression in the anterior and lateral leads. The sinus bradycardia reflects parasympathetic overactivity.*

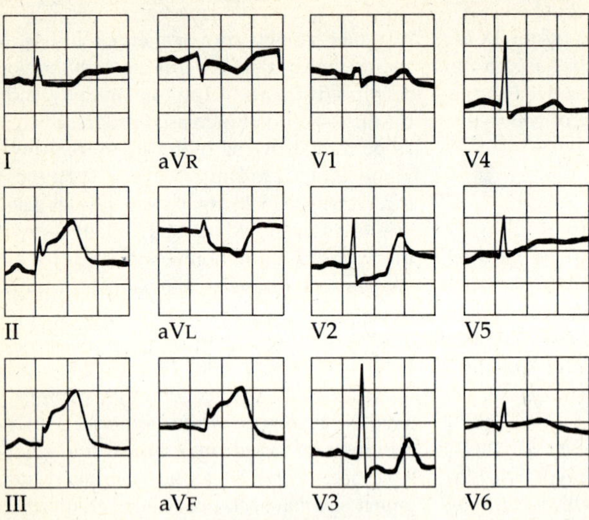

Figure 4 *Electrocardiogram from a patient with acute myocardial infarction caused by occlusion of a dominant left circumflex coronary artery reveals ST segment elevation in leads II, III, and aVF, indicating inferior wall injury. In addition, the Rs waveform in leads V1 and V2, with upright T waves, indicates infarction of the posterior wall.*

is reduced and arrhythmias are less likely. In one large study, it appeared that the reduction in mortality associated with beta-blocker therapy was attributable chiefly to prevention of cardiac rupture and ventricular fibrillation.[25] Except in patients with overt pulmonary congestion, bradyarrhythmia, or hypotension, it is reasonable to administer a beta-adrenergic blocking drug intravenously in the emergency room as soon as the diagnosis of acute myocardial infarction is evident. Beta-blocker therapy is particularly valuable in patients with hypertension and sinus tachycardia. Several agents are available that show comparable efficacy and safety. Propranolol may be given in a dosage of 0.1 mg/kg divided into three doses and administered at five-minute intervals. Metoprolol may be given in a dosage of 15 mg divided into three doses and administered at two-minute to five-minute intervals. Atenolol may be given in an initial dose of 5 mg over five minutes, followed by another 5 mg 10 minutes later. The beta blocker may then be continued orally, starting 30 to 60 minutes after the intravenous infusion.

Thrombolytic Therapy

Thrombolytic therapy is now widely considered to be indicated in patients who are seen in the early stage of acute myocar-

dial infarction and who do not have specific contraindications to this form of therapy.[26-29] Reopening the occluded artery and restoring perfusion to the ischemic or infarcted region by thrombolytic therapy can prevent or limit the myocardial necrosis and thereby reduce complications, preserve myocardial function, and reduce the risk of death.

These objectives are feasible primarily in patients in whom the artery can be reopened very soon after the onset of the occlusion, especially in those who are treated within the first hour. Thrombolytic therapy also appears beneficial when it is administered later, during the period six to 24 hours after the onset, when limitation of infarct evolution would not appear to be biologically feasible. This favorable result may relate to the slow development of infarction in many instances, or it may be that establishing perfusion helps prevent further complications such as extension, expansion, rupture, or electrical instability. The establishment of an open artery is now widely accepted as an optimal goal of therapy in acute myocardial infarction.[30]

Thrombolytic Agents and Their Efficacy

Several thrombolytic agents are now approved for use in the treatment of acute myocardial infarction in the United States [*see Table 2*], and new agents, combinations of agents, and dosing schedules are being actively investigated.[31,32] The earliest agent to be widely used was streptokinase. Its efficacy was demonstrated in a study done in Italy that involved 11,806 patients at 176 hospitals.[33] The intravenous administration of 1.5 million units of streptokinase was associated with a mortality after 21 days of 10.7 percent, compared with 13.0 percent in a control group. Statistically significant reductions in mortality were found for patients younger than 65 years who were treated within six hours after the onset of chest pain and who had anterior infarcts of class 1 or 2 on the Killip scale and no previous infarction. The largest reduction in mortality occurred in those who were treated within the first hour after the onset of pain. Another large multi-institutional trial that included patients with merely suspected as well as proven acute myocardial infarction showed similar overall results. The findings of this trial also suggested that thrombolytic therapy was beneficial when given up to 24 hours after the onset of chest pain.[34]

Alteplase (recombinant tissue plasminogen activator, or rtPA) was introduced with the goal of providing a thrombolytic agent that would be specific for the fibrin clot itself and that would be less likely than streptokinase to induce a systemic thrombolytic state. The efficacy of alteplase was established in an Anglo-Scandinavian study, in which the mortality at one month was 7.2 percent in the treated patients and 9.8 percent in the control group.[35]

Anistreplase (anisoylated plasminogen streptokinase activator complex, or APSAC) was synthesized in an effort to produce an agent with a longer duration of action than either streptokinase or alteplase. In a large randomized clinical trial in which 1,258 patients were given either anistreplase or placebo, the treated group had a 30-day mortality of six percent, as compared with 12 percent in the control group.[36]

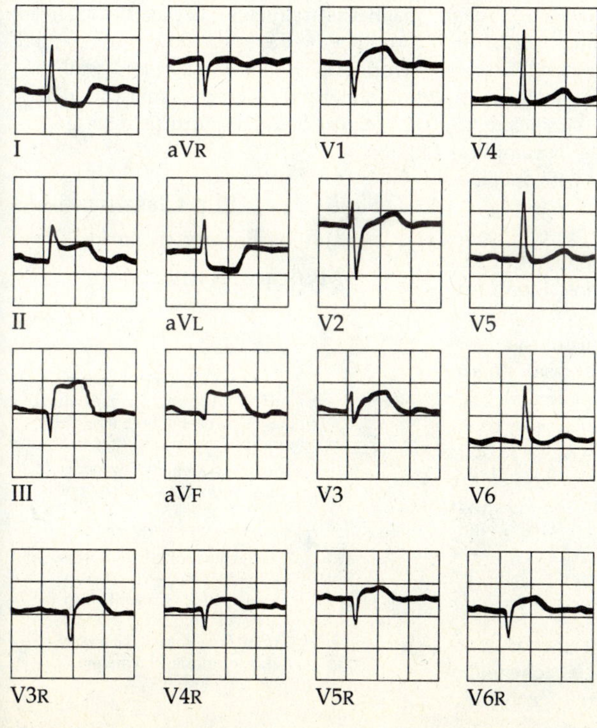

Figure 5 *Electrocardiogram from a patient with acute myocardial infarction caused by proximal occlusion of the right coronary artery demonstrates ST segment elevation in leads II, III, and aVF, indicating inferior wall injury. In addition, ST segment elevation in the right-sided precordial leads indicates infarction of the right ventricle.*

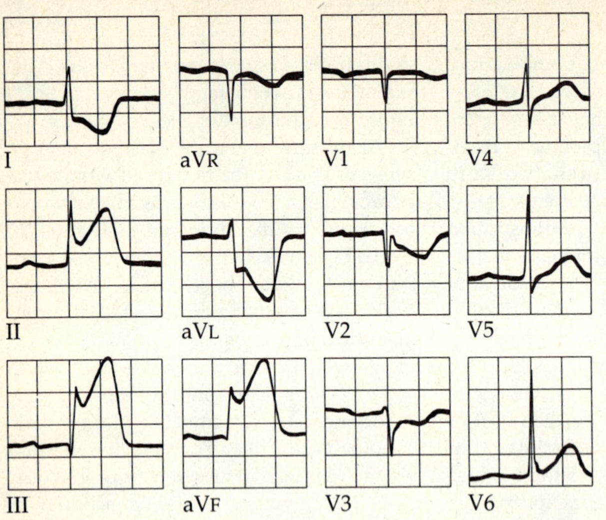

Figure 6 *Electrocardiogram from a patient with acute myocardial infarction caused by occlusion of a dominant right coronary artery shows ST segment elevation in leads II, III, and aVF, with reciprocal ST segment depression in leads I and aVL, indicating inferior wall injury. In addition, ST segment depression in leads V2 and V3 indicates an extensive infarct, probably involving the posterolateral region of the left ventricle.*

Choice of Thrombolytic Agent

Alteplase has proved somewhat more effective at reopening the infarct-related artery than streptokinase. This difference is probably more important when the thrombolytic agent is administered later than three hours after the onset. On the other hand, the reocclusion rate appears to be slightly higher after alteplase than after streptokinase. A large clinical trial showed no significant difference in mortality or in bleeding complications between groups treated with alteplase and those treated with streptokinase.[37]

Anistreplase has not been directly compared with alteplase or streptokinase with regard to mortality in large clinical trials, but it is probably equivalent to alteplase in most respects. One advantage of anistreplase therapy is ease of administration because the agent is given as a single intravenous injection.[38]

Because of the much higher price of alteplase and anistreplase [*see Table* 2], it is reasonable to employ streptokinase as the thrombolytic agent of choice in most circumstances.

Left Ventricular Function after Thrombolysis

Evidence that thrombolytic therapy is associated with improved left ventricular function has been difficult to interpret, but it appears likely that such therapy helps preserve myocardial function when it is administered within 30 minutes of the onset. In general, the ECG pattern of infarction in treated patients evolves in nearly the same manner as in patients who have not received thrombolytic therapy.[39] Studies of the left ventricular ejection fraction and wall motion show only slight, if any, differences between treated and control patients. Exper-

Table 1 **The Killip Classification of Heart Failure in Acute Myocardial Infarction**

Class I	No signs of heart failure
Class II	Mild or moderate heart failure: rales can be heard over as much as 50 percent of both lung fields
Class III	Pulmonary edema: rales can be heard over more than half of both lung fields
Class IV	Cardiogenic shock: blood pressure by cuff < 90 mm Hg; signs of inadequate peripheral perfusion are evident, including reduced urine flow, cold and clammy skin, cyanosis, and mental obtundation

Table 2 Comparison of Thrombolytic Agents Used in Acute Myocardial Infarction

	Streptokinase	*Alteplase*	*Anistreplase*
Half-life	23 min	8 min	90 min
Dose	1.5 million units infused over 1 hr	100 mg (or 1.25 mg/kg for patients who weigh less than 65 kg) infused over 3 hr (6–10 mg over 2 min, 50–54 mg over the next 58 min, 20 mg over the second hour, and 20 mg over the third hour)	30 units over 2–5 min
Expected success in reperfusion	50%–70%	60%–80%	60%–80%
Hypotensive Effect[*]	2+	1+	1+
Allergic reactions	Yes	No	No
Cost[†]	$186	$2,332	$1,700

[*]Based on a scale of values ranging from 0 to 4+.

[†]Cost to the pharmacist for a single course of therapy.[36]

imental and clinical studies indicate that the severely ischemic myocardium may show contractile dysfunction for a prolonged period after perfusion has been restored, a condition that has been termed stunned myocardium.[40] A related concept, termed hibernating myocardium, has been advanced to describe chronic but reversible myocardial dysfunction caused by ischemia.[41] Stunned myocardium may in turn exhibit a condition termed no-reflow, in which severe impairment of perfusion of an injured or infarcted area may persist after occlusion has been resolved in the affected artery. Furthermore, there is evidence that early reperfusion may have deleterious effects on the myocardium. Such damage, termed reperfusion injury, may appear as hemorrhage, edema, washout of intracellular enzymes, intracellular calcium overload, or alterations of myocardial ultrastructure.[42,43] It is possible that no-reflow, arrhythmias, and contractile impairment are all aggravated by reperfusion injury, which appears to be mediated by oxygen free rad-

icals. These various phenomena make it difficult to determine whether recanalization of acutely occluded coronary arteries truly preserves myocardial function when the thrombolytic agents are given more than 30 minutes after the attack.

Emergency Angioplasty after Thrombolysis

Because a severe stenosis of the infarct-related artery usually persists after lysis of an acute coronary arterial thrombus, it is logical to consider routinely performing coronary arteriography immediately after thrombolytic therapy. Immediate balloon angioplasty could then be carried out in an effort to restore more nearly normal blood flow and prevent reocclusion. However, trials of routine immediate balloon angioplasty have demonstrated no better, and perhaps even less favorable, clinical outcomes than trials in which angioplasty has been carried out only for individualized specific indications.[44,45] There are no simple clinical indicators that can consistently determine whether thrombolytic therapy has been successful in opening the infarct-related artery. It is reasonable to consider immediate coronary arteriography in patients with apparently large infarcts in whom thrombolytic therapy has not relieved the pain or produced prompt resolution of the ST segment elevation.

Bleeding Complications

Thrombolytic therapy carries a major risk of bleeding complications. Hematomas commonly occur at arterial puncture sites, and gastrointestinal and retroperitoneal bleeding has also been noted. The complication of greatest concern, however, is intracerebral hemorrhage, which has occurred in up to 0.5 to one percent of cases and is likely to be fatal.[46,47] The level of fibrinogen in the circulating blood is typically reduced to 10 to 20 percent of normal for as long as 24 hours after intravenous streptokinase administration. Although alteplase lowers fibrinogen levels to a much lesser extent than streptokinase, the incidence of hemorrhagic complications with alteplase is not demonstrably lower than with streptokinase. Cerebral hemorrhage has occurred more frequently with alteplase than with streptokinase. Bleeding complications from thrombolytic therapy are not well correlated with the degree of reduction in the fibrinogen level but instead appear to be more closely correlated with the presence of localized vascular injury.[48]

The principles of the management of bleeding complications after thrombolytic therapy in patients with acute myocardial infarction have been outlined in one study.[49] According to this approach, heparin and aspirin are discontinued first. Then, the administration of cryoprecipitate and fresh frozen plasma is considered. Finally, if bleeding persists, platelet transfusion (if the bleeding time is prolonged) or the administration of antifibrinolytic drugs may be considered.

Selection of Patients for Thrombolytic Therapy

The ideal candidate for thrombolytic therapy is one in whom the drug can be administered within approximately three hours after the onset of the infarction and in whom the clinical features indicate that the infarct will be large and complications likely.[50,51] In such cases, an electrocardiographic pattern of distinct regional ST segment elevation is typically present. It is not clear whether thrombolytic therapy is useful in patients with less specific electrocardiographic patterns that involve only ST segment depression or T wave inversion. It also is not clear whether patients with inferior infarcts should be treated, because inferior infarcts are often smaller and less life-threatening than anterior infarcts. It is reasonable to consider the patient's age and the degree of reciprocal ST segment depression in leads V1 through V3 when deciding whether to use thrombolytic therapy in patients with acute inferior infarcts.[52]

There are several general contraindications to thrombolytic therapy that should be kept in mind [*see Table 3*]. Age alone is not necessarily a contraindication, but experience with thrombolytic therapy has been unfavorable in patients older than 75 years, particularly in women who have diabetes or hypertension.[53]

Only about one in four patients who present with acute myocardial infarction are younger than 76 years, are seen earlier than four hours after the onset, and have diagnostic initial ECGs. Because some of these patients have other contraindications to thrombolytic therapy, the use of such criteria would limit the treatment to only about 15 percent of cases.[50] Therefore, more liberal criteria would have to be employed before thrombolytic therapy could have a major impact on mortality. However, such expanded criteria would lead to the administration of thrombolytic drugs to some patients who do not have acute myocardial infarction.

Primary Angioplasty or Bypass Surgery

Balloon angioplasty can be used to open the infarct-related artery as primary treatment without thrombolytic therapy, and

Table 3 Selected Contraindications to Administration of Thrombolytic Agents

Absolute Contraindications

Active bleeding

Surgery, trauma, cerebrovascular accident, or neurosurgical procedures within previous six months

Gastrointestinal bleeding or biopsy predisposing to bleeding within previous two weeks

Traumatic or prolonged cardiopulmonary resuscitation within previous two weeks

Allergy to specific thrombolytic agent selected for use

Relative Contraindications

Age > 75 years

Severe systemic arterial hypertension

Abnormal hemostasis

Severe hepatic or renal disease

Major malignant disorder

Proliferative diabetic retinopathy

Pregnancy or menorrhagia

Hemorrhagic pericarditis

emergency coronary artery bypass surgery can also be used as primary initial therapy.[54-56] No controlled trials of these approaches, however, have been reported. Emergency coronary artery bypass surgery is indicated in certain patients with acute myocardial infarction and critical multivessel disease, especially disease of the left main coronary artery, and in whom thrombolytic therapy, angioplasty, or both have been unsuccessful or are not considered feasible.

Antithrombotic Therapy

Because the incidence of reocclusion after the institution of thrombolytic agents is relatively high (about 20 percent), antithrombotic therapy with heparin or aspirin is usually started immediately after this procedure.[57] A collaborative, randomized study has been reported comparing the efficacy of ad-

junctive antithrombotic therapy with either heparin or aspirin in 205 patients treated with recombinant tissue plasminogen activator for acute myocardial infarction.[57a] Patients received either intravenous heparin (an initial bolus of 5,000 units followed by continuous infusion of 1,000 U/hr) or low-dose oral aspirin (80 mg immediately and 80 mg daily thereafter). Arterial patency was determined seven to 24 hours later by coronary angiography. Arteries were patent in 82 percent of the patients given heparin but only in 52 percent of those given aspirin. Of the arteries that were patent at the initial angiogram, 88 percent remained open after seven days in the group receiving heparin and 95 percent in the group receiving aspirin.

These results suggest that early concomitant heparin therapy is more effective than early concomitant aspirin therapy for achieving immediate arterial patency, at the doses employed in this study. The two treatment regimens did not appear to produce a significant difference in the reocclusion rate one to seven days later. The incidence of hemorrhagic and recurrent ischemic events was similar in the two groups.

Diagnosis during Acute Phase

Laboratory Evaluation

Serum Enzymes

Necrosis of myocardial tissue allows certain intracellular enzymes to pass through the damaged plasma membrane and reach the interstitial spaces and the circulating blood, where their transient rise in activity provides the most useful confirmatory laboratory test for acute myocardial infarction.[58] Creatine kinase (CK) and its MB molecular subtype (CK-MB) are the most useful enzymes for this purpose. CK-MB is present in significant amounts only in cardiac muscle; the MM and BB subtypes may also be released from skeletal muscle and other organs.

It is possible to detect an increase in the blood level of CK within three hours after the onset of pain in a typical case of acute myocardial infarction. The peak level is reached about 12 hours later and is followed by a decline to normal levels after another 12 to 24 hours. When the occluded artery has been recanalized promptly, the peak enzyme level occurs earlier because the increased blood flow washes out the enzyme more rapidly.

The peak level of CK or CK-MB correlates with the size of the infarct and therefore with the prognosis and the likelihood of complications. Thus, it is useful to follow the enzyme levels even when the diagnosis of acute myocardial infarction is not in doubt. Sampling at 0, 12, and 24 hours is usually sufficient.[59]

Measurements of CK-MB by highly accurate methods indicate that some patients with acute myocardial infarction exhibit a serial rise and fall in the CK-MB level even though the total CK level remains within the normal range.[60] Useful criteria for myocardial necrosis include a peak CK-MB level that is higher than 13 IU/L and that has risen at least 50 percent during the four to 12 hours after onset of symptoms or a peak CK-MB level that is more than twice the upper normal limit.[58]

Another useful measurement is the lactic dehydrogenase (LDH) assay. LDH rises later than the CK and remains elevated for up to a week or even longer after the onset of acute myocardial infarction. It is necessary to assay both the fraction 1 (cardiac) and fraction 2 isoenzymes of LDH for this test to be specific for myocardial infarction. LDH is particularly useful when patients are first seen more than 24 hours after the probable time of onset of the acute myocardial infarction.

Radionuclide Imaging

Technetium-99m stannous pyrophosphate is taken up selectively by areas of recent myocardial necrosis and provides a so-called hot spot imaging technique for acute myocardial infarction.[61] The imaging agent is complexed with albumin, and the complex binds to calcium, which is deposited in abnormal amounts within irreversibly damaged myocardial cells. The pyrophosphate scan can be done with single-photon emission computed tomography (SPECT) to permit an assessment of the size of the infarct.

Thallium-201 (^{201}Tl) scanning visualizes myocardial perfusion, which may be abnormal in patients with either acute or old myocardial infarction. The scan is generally positive during the first 24 hours, but it may be negative after 24 hours because of the establishment of collateral blood flow.

Magnetic Resonance Imaging

Magnetic resonance imaging (MRI) that is synchronized to the ECG to avoid motion artifacts provides useful images of acute myocardial infarction. Infarcts appear as regions of high signal intensity and prolonged T_2 relaxation time.[62] Such studies are as yet impractical for routine clinical use.

Routine Management in the Coronary Care Unit

Routine Hemodynamic Management

Acute myocardial infarction is usually accompanied by some degree of left ventricular failure.[63] Left ventricular end-diastolic pressure (LVEDP) is raised in most patients, and pulmonary arterial wedge pressure is also frequently elevated. Pulmonary congestion is often revealed in the chest radiograph, and many patients show arterial hypoxemia secondary to the congestion. Echocardiographic and radionuclide studies indicate that the left ventricular contractile abnormalities are established during the first 24 hours of infarction and change little during the next two weeks.

Clinical signs of congestive heart failure are less frequent than abnormal hemodynamic measurements. S_4 may indicate only an elevated LVEDP. S_3, pulmonary rales, and elevated jugular venous pressure indicate more advanced degrees of congestive failure. Hemodynamic monitoring, by means of a pulmonary arterial thermodilution catheter (Swan-Ganz), will permit a more accurate assessment of the patient's hemodynamic status. It should not be used routinely, however, because clinical evidence alone is usually sufficient to plan appropriate therapy and the indwelling catheter carries a risk of sepsis and other complications.

Routine Arrhythmia Management

Because of the high risk of ventricular tachycardia (VT) or ventricular fibrillation (VF) during the first few days after acute myocardial infarction, continuous ECG monitoring should be routine. The administration of a lidocaine infusion prophylactically in all patients reduces the incidence of VT and VF, but it does not reduce mortality, because the arrhythmic episodes are successfully treated in the coronary care unit.[64,65] In addition, lidocaine causes central nervous system toxicity, and it also may inappropriately suppress ventricular escape rhythms that compensate for atrioventricular block or pathologic sinus slowing. Thus, the routine use of prophylactic lidocaine infusions in all acute myocardial infarction patients is not advisable.

Medically Treatable Complications

Recurrent Ischemic Pain

Recurrent ischemic pain at rest or with light activity occurs frequently during the first week after acute myocardial infarction. Some episodes are precipitated by stress and are associated with an increase in heart rate or blood pressure. Transient changes in the ST segments and T waves may appear during episodes of ischemic pain. Occasionally, the Prinzmetal phenomenon occurs. The appearance of ischemic pain calls for careful evaluation, because it suggests a high risk of recurrence or extension of infarction.

ST segment depression that occurs during episodes of ischemic pain in leads that correspond to myocardial regions other than the recently infarcted region is particularly significant because it suggests multivessel disease.[66]

Mild angina that occurs only occasionally during the in-hospital recovery phase does not necessarily indicate an adverse prognosis and can often be managed conservatively with oral nitrates, beta blockers, or calcium channel blockers.[67] More severe cases should be treated with intravenous infusions of nitroglycerin or verapamil. In critical cases, intra-aortic balloon counterpulsation may be necessary. Coronary arteriography is usually indicated in patients with frequent or severe pain, because coronary angioplasty or bypass surgery can be used effectively for this problem.[68,69]

Extension and Expansion of Infarction

The term extension of infarction refers to a new episode of acute myocardial infarction that occurs within two to three weeks after a previous acute infarction, usually in the same electrocardiographic region. A new episode may occur in any patient with acute myocardial infarction, often with little or no warning. Extension is often accompanied by new complications such as arrhythmia or congestive heart failure and may end in death. Studies using multiple precordial lead ECG maps and frequent radioimmunoassays of CK-MB indicate that extension of infarction during the first 24 to 48 hours occurs in as many as 30 percent of patients. These more subtle extensions are often unaccompanied by new symptoms or ECG changes.

The specific pathologic basis for extension of infarction is unknown and may involve various processes. In some cases, acute infarction evolves gradually during a period of one to two weeks. Postmortem examination often shows areas of infarction that have occurred during a period of one to three weeks in patients who have died after only a few days of symptoms.

Many instances of apparent extension actually represent expansion of the infarcted area resulting from disruption of the necrotic muscle architecture, which leads to thinning of the ventricular wall and dilation of the chamber.[70] This process has been termed remodeling of the ventricle.[71] Remodeling that involves dilation of the noninfarcted regions has an important prognostic implication because such dilation produces the equivalent of chronic volume overload and contributes to later congestive heart failure.

Thromboembolic Complications

Left Ventricular Mural Thrombus

A mural thrombus forms on the endocardial surface of the left ventricle at the site of recent myocardial infarction in about 30 percent of patients with anterior infarcts, generally those that are large enough to cause a major region to be akinetic.[72] Patients with anterior infarcts who have Q waves in lead aVL as well as in the precordial leads have mural thrombi in more than 50 percent of instances.[73] The thrombi are well visualized by echocardiography. Mural thrombi form despite the use of thrombolytic therapy.[74] Systemic arterial embolism occurs in only about 15 percent of all patients in whom mural thrombi can be detected, but in those in whom the thrombus is large and mobile, long-term anticoagulation is indicated.[75] Warfarin has generally been used for this purpose, but aspirin has also been reported to be beneficial in such cases.[76]

Venous Thromboembolism

Early ambulation in patients with acute myocardial infarction has greatly reduced the prevalence of deep venous thrombosis and pulmonary embolism.[77] However, patients who are likely to be at high risk for these complications because of prolonged immobilization should be treated with a low dose of heparin (5,000 U subcutaneously twice a day).

Pericarditis and Dressler's Syndrome

Pericarditis is a frequent complication of acute myocardial infarction, particularly in patients with larger infarcts that are truly transmural.[78] The incidence of pericardial friction rubs in pericarditis is high, but their detection depends on how frequently one listens for them. Pericarditis causes anterior chest pain that is often severe and easily confused with the continuing or recurring pain of myocardial ischemia. The pain of pericarditis is worsened by inspiration and in some instances by lying flat. Pericarditis may be accompanied by the ECG finding of diffuse ST segment elevation, in addition to the regional ST segment elevation that results from the infarct itself.

Pericardial effusion, usually relatively small, occurs in approximately one third of patients with acute myocardial infarction.[79] Its presence or absence has little correlation with the presence or absence of chest pain or a pericardial friction rub.

Pericarditis in acute myocardial infarction rarely requires specific treatment other than aspirin. Prednisone and nonsteroidal anti-inflammatory drugs such as ibuprofen or indomethacin should be avoided because they may promote thinning and rupture of the infarct.[80]

Dressler's postinfarction syndrome is a delayed form of acute pericarditis that occurs after the first week of infarction and up to many months later. Its relation to pericarditis of the first week is obscure. It is considered an immunologic reaction but is poorly understood.

Bradyarrhythmias and Conduction Disorders

Sinus bradycardia, sinus arrest, and various forms of atrioventricular (AV) block constitute the important bradyarrhythmias that occur in patients with acute myocardial infarction. One element in their production is the increased vagal tone that is often present in the early phases of infarction. The reason for the increased vagal tone is not fully known. Ischemia of the specialized conducting tissues is another factor leading to bradyarrhythmias. Both the sinus node and the AV node are supplied by specific arterial branches that may be compromised by acute coronary occlusion. The His bundle and the Purkinje tissues have a dual blood supply from the right and left coronary arteries through the ventricular septum. In general, these tissues become significantly ischemic only in cases of extensive anteroseptal infarction.

Sinus bradycardia in the early phase of acute myocardial infarction usually responds well to atropine given intravenously in a dose of 0.4 mg, repeated in 30 minutes if necessary. Sinus bradycardia may not require treatment unless hypotension is present or unless the slow ventricular rate appears to be predisposing to ventricular arrhythmias.

The most common type of AV block in acute myocardial infarction occurs at the AV node or the prenodal atrial myocardium, mainly in patients with inferior infarcts caused by occlusion of the right coronary artery.[81] AV nodal block usually appears in a graded fashion, beginning with a prolonged PR interval, followed by the Wenckebach type of second-degree AV block, and then higher degrees of block, including complete AV block. The escape rhythm usually arises in the AV junction and is typically stable at a rate of 50 to 60 beats/min.

AV block of the nodal type is frequently transient, and no treatment may be required. Atropine is effective, particularly when the block develops within six hours after the onset of infarction. AV nodal block that develops more than six hours after the onset of infarction is more likely to be ischemic in origin and is apt not to respond as well to atropine. In severe cases, particularly those associated with heart failure, syncope, or ventricular arrhythmia, a temporary transcutaneous or transvenous pacemaker may be needed. The development of high-grade AV nodal block usually indicates a relatively large infarction, with a higher risk of complications and death, but the AV block itself has little effect on the prognosis when appropriately treated.[82]

AV block in the His-Purkinje system is a far more serious complication than AV nodal block. It is usually associated with extensive anteroseptal infarction and results from infarction of the several bundle branches. Typically, bundle branch block with normal AV conduction occurs first. A phase with a prolonged PR interval or an incomplete AV block of the Mobitz type II pattern may follow. Complete heart block, however, is likely to appear suddenly, with a slow and unstable idioventricular escape rhythm [*see Figure 7*]. Progression to a Mobitz type II block is particularly frequent in patients who have right bundle branch block and left anterior fascicular block with a prolonged PR interval or a combination of right bundle branch block and left posterior fascicular block, even if the PR interval is normal [*see Figure 8*].[83] The mortality in such cases is high, even when a pacemaker is used to circumvent the heart block, because the infarcts responsible for His-Purkinje block are large and frequently lead to congestive heart failure and cardiogenic shock. For this reason, pacemakers probably do relatively little to improve survival in such cases, even if they do prevent death from the AV block itself.

Complete heart block that develops during acute myocardial infarction rarely persists as permanent complete heart block, although bundle branch block often persists. Permanent pacemakers have been advocated for persistent bundle branch block to prevent sudden death from late development of complete AV block, but this approach is recommended only for patients who have transient, complete AV block during the acute phase of myocardial infarction.[84]

Ventricular Tachyarrhythmias

Incidence and Mechanism

Ventricular ectopic beats occur in more than 90 percent of patients with acute myocardial infarction, ventricular tachycardia in about 10 percent, and ventricular fibrillation in about 15 percent. Several electrophysiologic mechanisms are involved in the genesis of ventricular arrhythmia.[85] Ventricular arrhythmias that occur in the first few minutes after coronary occlusion appear to be caused by a reentrant mechanism that is related to delayed recovery of excitability in acutely ischemic tissues, with little slowing of conduction. In the next few hours, the principal mechanism of arrhythmia appears to be slowing of conduction velocity in the severely damaged periphery

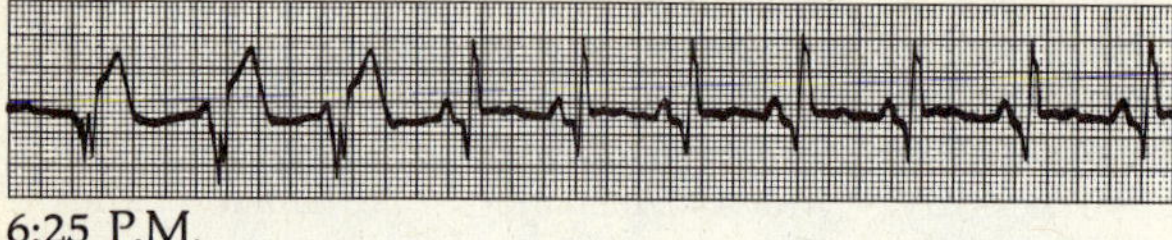

6:25 P.M.

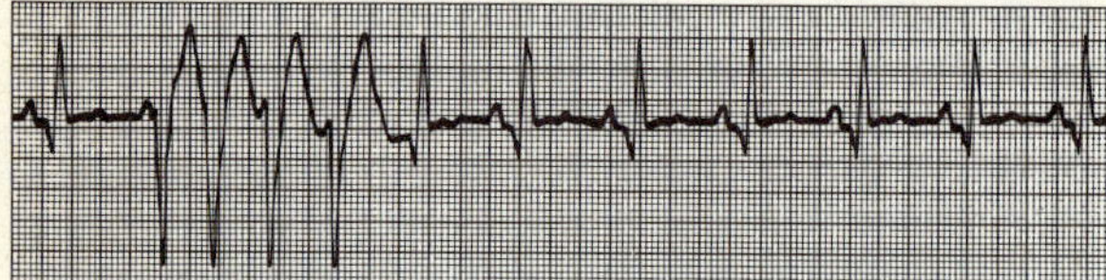

3:30 A.M.

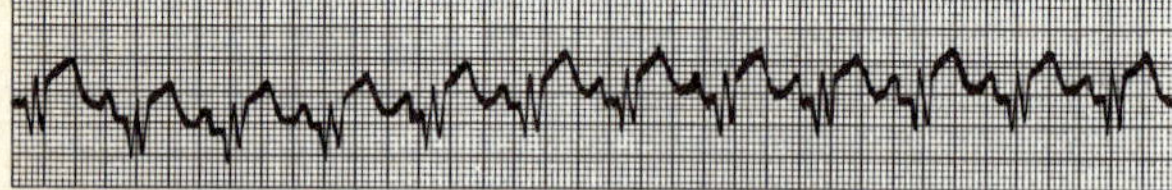

3:45 A.M.

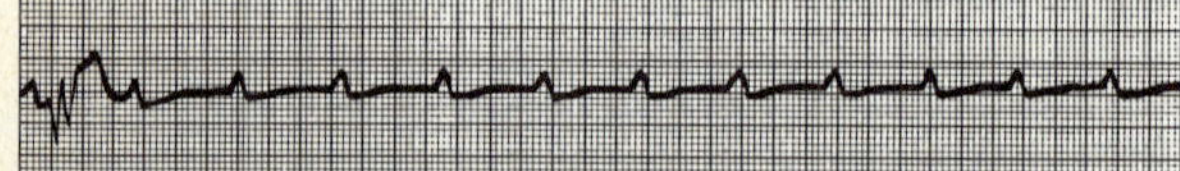

6:28 A.M.

Figure 7 *Successive ECGs reveal different arrhythmias in a patient during the first 24 hours after the onset of symptoms. At 6:25 P.M., a brief period of accelerated idioventricular rhythm terminates. At 3:30 A.M., there is a brief period of ventricular tachycardia. Fifteen minutes later, there is a normal sinus rhythm at a rate of 98 beats/min, with a PR interval of 0.15 second. In the bottom ECG, made at 6:28 A.M., only P waves can be seen. The sudden appearance of complete heart block with ventricular asystole occurred without any intervening incomplete AV block. This is one mode of onset of the Mobitz type II complete AV block at the His-Purkinje tissue level in acute anteroseptal infarction.*

of the infarcted area; the delayed conduction also promotes arrhythmia by a reentrant mechanism.

Premature beats may arise as a result of markedly different repolarization rates in adjacent areas of myocardium. This condition causes a local potential difference to exist near the end of the T wave, creating a premature cardiac impulse. There may also be a true enhancement of intrinsic automaticity resulting from the inability of injured myocardial cells to maintain the normal negative transmembrane potential in diastole.

Either enhanced automaticity or delayed conduction in the ischemic area may produce simple or complex ventricular premature beats, ventricular tachycardia, or ventricular fibrillation. Sustained ventricular tachycardia and ventricular fibrillation are precipitated by ventricular premature beats that may occur either early or late in diastole, with or without the frequent occurrence of consecutive pairs, trios, or short runs of ventricular tachycardia. Occasionally, supraventricular premature beats may initiate ventricular tachycardia or ventricular fibrillation.[86]

Abnormalities such as hypokalemia or hypomagnesemia may also contribute to ventricular arrhythmia in the early stage of myocardial infarction.[87] Hypokalemia may result from a high level of circulating catecholamines or from previous diuretic therapy.

Primary versus Secondary Arrhythmia

The distinction between primary and secondary ventricular arrhythmia in acute myocardial infarction is an important one. Primary ventricular arrhythmias are those that occur unexpectedly in patients whose infarctions are not so extensive as to produce severe congestive heart failure or cardiogenic shock. Such primary arrhythmias usually occur within the first 24 hours after the onset of infarction. Pallor and sinus tachycardia, which reflect sympathetic overactivity, are particularly frequent among patients with primary ventricular fibrillation. Patients older than 65 years are less susceptible to primary ventricular fibrillation than younger patients.[88] The occurrence of primary ventricular

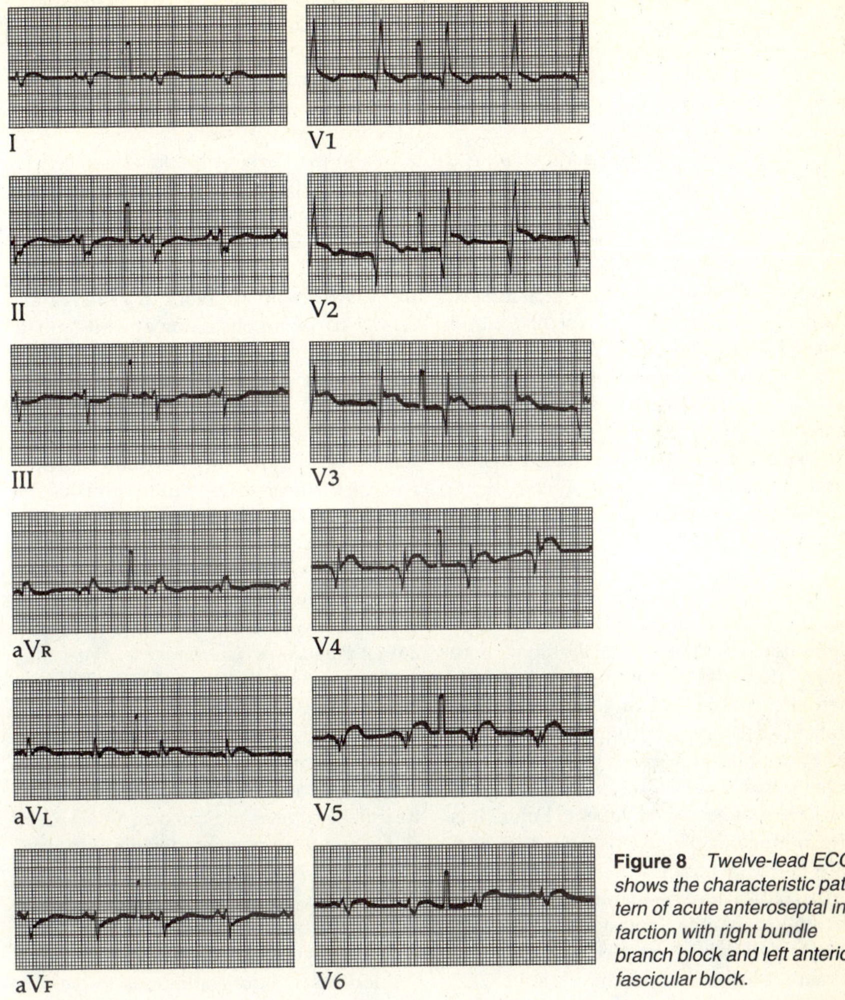

Figure 8 *Twelve-lead ECG shows the characteristic pattern of acute anteroseptal infarction with right bundle branch block and left anterior fascicular block.*

fibrillation has relatively little adverse effect on the long-term prognosis.

Secondary arrhythmias are those that occur after a period of severe congestive heart failure or cardiogenic shock, usually many hours or several days after the onset of infarction. They tend to recur repeatedly and respond poorly to treatment.

Lidocaine Therapy

Lidocaine, which acts to suppress ectopic impulse formation, is the most useful drug for control of ventricular arrhythmias in acute myocardial infarction. The drug must be given by continuous intravenous infusion because it is rapidly removed from the circulating blood by the liver. Therapeutic blood levels are established almost immediately by giving a loading dose of 50 to 100 mg, followed by a continuous infusion of 1 to 4 mg/min. Fluctuations in the blood level that occur during the distribution and equilibration phases may be overcome by giving additional boluses during the first half hour or by using an initial infusion rate higher than 4 mg/min. Another method employs two drip bottles, with a more dilute solution dripping into a concentrated solution, resulting in an exponential decline in the rate of administration with a constant volume of infusion.[89]

The infusion rate of lidocaine should be lowered in the presence of reduced hepatic blood flow, which is expected in patients who are elderly or thin or who have congestive heart failure or other low cardiac output states. Coadministration of propranolol also reduces the clearance rate of lidocaine.[90] Lidocaine toxicity is manifested mainly by central nervous system symptoms, such as drowsiness, confusion, or speech disturbance, which may progress to convulsive seizures in severe cases. Because symptoms of lidocaine toxicity are poorly correlated with blood levels of the drug, clinical observation is the most important method of monitoring the dosage.

Lidocaine is cleared from the blood more slowly after discontinuance of an infusion than after administration of a single dose, probably because the drug that is bound to various organs is released slowly. Because of the slow clearance rate, a lidocaine infusion does not need to be tapered before it is discontinued.

A patient whose ventricular arrhythmia is not controlled by maximum tolerated lidocaine infusions (about 20 percent of cases) is usually best treated with procainamide infusion. A loading dose of 1,000 mg given during a period of one hour, followed by an infusion of about 200 mg/hr, will quickly raise the blood level of the drug to 6 mg/L, which is usually effective. Some patients may require doses and blood levels that are two or three times higher. In patients with renal impairment or severe congestive heart failure, lower doses should be used.

Accelerated Idioventricular Rhythm

The arrhythmia known as accelerated idioventricular rhythm [*see Figure 9*] occurs in a high proportion of patients with acute myocardial infarction. Its occurrence is related to reperfusion of the infarcted area, either spontaneously or as a result of thrombolytic therapy. This arrhythmia is a rhythm of enhanced automaticity and probably arises in the Purkinje branches adjacent to the infarcted area. Thus, its features are intermediate between those of classic junctional rhythms and idioventricular rhythms. Occasionally, it represents ventricular tachycardia with exit block in a ratio of 2:1, 3:1, or 4:1. More often, however, it has the character of an escape rhythm that appears when the sinus rhythm is slow. Thus, each instance of accelerated idioventricular rhythm represents both enhanced automaticity and an escape rhythm; either form of rhythm disturbance may predominate. The escape rhythm characteristically begins with a ventricular beat that has a long coupling interval. Those instances of accelerated idioventricular rhythm that begin with a premature beat may be more appropriately termed slow ventricular tachycardia.

Accelerated idioventricular rhythm does not necessarily require treatment if it does not appear to impair the hemodynamic status or threaten to precipitate ventricular tachycardia or ventricular fibrillation. When treatment appears indicated and the escape rhythm is predominant, atropine or atrial pacing is preferred. When enhanced automaticity predominates, lidocaine is preferable. Accelerated idioventricular rhythm often occurs only in brief runs that could be overlooked without continuous electrocardiographic monitoring.

Cardiac Arrest

Cardiac arrest in patients with acute myocardial infarction is usually caused by ventricular fibrillation, but it may also result from ventricular asystole or from electromechanical dissociation.

When ventricular fibrillation occurs in a patient in a coronary care unit and is observed at its onset, a defibrillation countershock of 200 to 300 joules should be delivered as soon as possible, before other resuscitative procedures are initiated. If un-

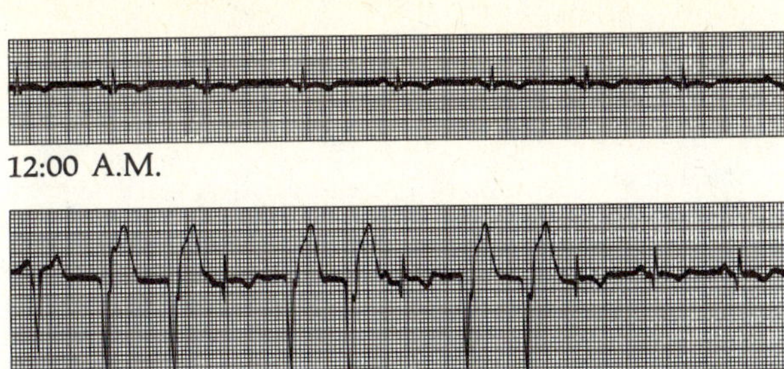

12:00 A.M.

1:25 A.M.

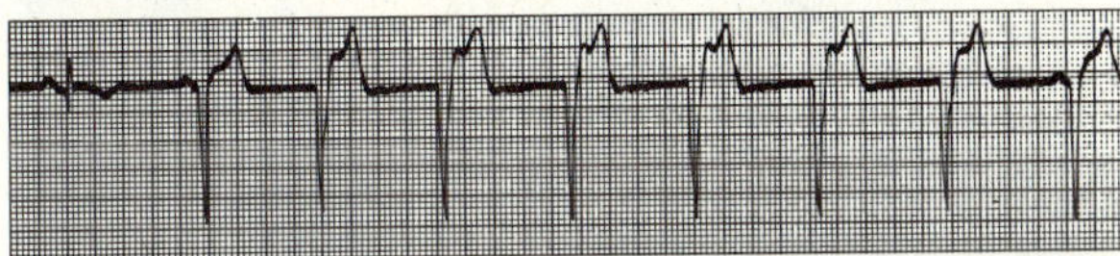

3:00 A.M.

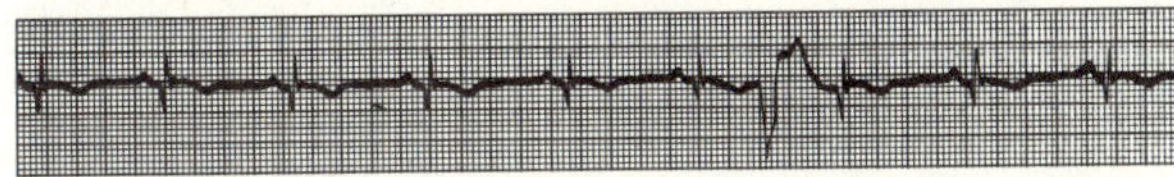

3:30 A.M.

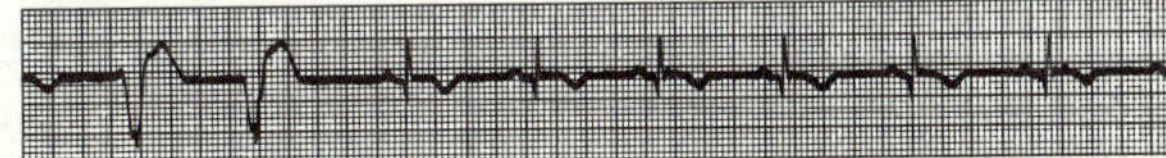

4:15 A.M.

Figure 9   *Enhanced idio-ventricular automaticity is observed in a patient with an acute inferior myocardial infarction. ECGs were made during the eight to 12 hours after onset of symptoms. Idioventricular beats appear, with coupling intervals ranging from 0.40 to 0.64 second. During episodes of sinus bradycardia, there are periods of accelerated idioventricular rhythm, with a cycle length of about 0.84 second.*

successful, the countershock should be repeated immediately. If still unsuccessful, the basic life support protocol should be started (artificial respiration with supplemental oxygen and closed-chest compression). Intravenous or intratracheal epinephrine, 0.5 to 1.0 mg (5 to 10 ml of a 1:10,000 solution), should be administered, and the countershock should be repeated, using 300 to 350 joules.

When cardiac arrest persists for more than five minutes, intravenous administration of sodium bicarbonate may be indicated, depending on the results of arterial blood gas determination. Additional doses of epinephrine should be given every five minutes, and other drugs, such as calcium chloride (5 ml of a 10 percent solution), lidocaine, procainamide, or bretylium, should be given. After sinus rhythm is established, a lidocaine bolus should be given, followed by a continuous infusion.

Complete AV block without a ventricular escape rhythm or with an extremely slow and ineffective ventricular escape rhythm can result in ventricular asystole [*see Figure 7*]. Appropriate management of this condition entails insertion of a temporary transcutaneous or transvenous right ventricular pacemaker as soon as possible. Until pacing is established, it may be possible to initiate heartbeats by lightly thumping the chest wall overlying the heart. Alternatively, the patient may be able to maintain the circulation by coughing repeatedly. If neither of these methods works, the circulation must be maintained by closed-chest compression until pacing is established.

If ventricular asystole occurs as a result of a total cardiac standstill rather than AV block, resuscitation is unlikely to be successful. Epinephrine and bicarbonate should be given immediately and repeated every 10 minutes. Calcium chloride should be given if intravenous or intratracheal epinephrine does not establish a heartbeat. Intracardiac epinephrine and intravenous isoproterenol should be used next. Insertion of a transcutaneous or transvenous pacemaker should be tried, but this approach is unlikely to be successful.

Electromechanical dissociation is simply a severe form of cardiogenic shock in which the heartbeat is mechanically ineffective even though the electrical activation of the heart is intact. It may occur as the primary event in cardiac arrest, but it is more likely to occur when cardiac rupture results in acute severe cardiac tamponade [see Surgically Treatable Complications, Cardiac Rupture and Pseudoaneurysm, below]. Emergency pericardiocentesis, as well as the appropriate basic and advanced cardiac life support protocol, is indicated in patients with acute myocardial infarction who exhibit electromechanical dissociation.

Atrial Arrhythmias

All forms of atrial arrhythmia occur in acute myocardial infarction; atrial premature beats, atrial flutter, and atrial fibrillation are the most common. These arrhythmias are usually seen during the in-hospital phase in patients who have substantial degrees of congestive heart failure. They may reflect atrial stretch caused by an acute rise in atrial pressure resulting from left ventricular failure. Atrial ischemia or infarction is a factor in some cases, especially in those patients in whom atrial fibrillation develops within three hours after onset.[91] Atrial arrhythmias are also associated with pericarditis.

Atrial arrhythmias tend to stop spontaneously. Treatment is urgent when they produce marked hemodynamic disturbance, primarily as a result of a rapid ventricular rate. Administration of digoxin, verapamil, propranolol, or adenosine to slow the ventricular rate and the use of other measures to control congestive heart failure are usually appropriate and effective. Reversion by countershock is indicated in patients with severe hemodynamic impairment. Rapid atrial pacing is an alternative method of reversion and is particularly useful in atrial flutter.

Congestive Heart Failure and Cardiogenic Shock

Assessment of Pump Dysfunction

In patients with acute myocardial infarction, it is useful to distinguish four grades of congestive heart failure, or so-called pump dysfunction, on the basis of either clinical [see Table 1] or hemodynamic criteria. In general, the clinical and hemodynamic criteria correspond rather well, although a larger proportion of patients show abnormalities on hemodynamic studies than on clinical examination. The severity of hemodynamic abnormalities is directly related to the extent of the myocardial infarction, including any previous infarction to which the acute infarction has been added. Mortality in acute myocardial infarction correlates with the reduction in stroke volume and arterial pressure, reflected in the stroke work.

Cardiogenic Shock

Hypotension and a shocklike picture in patients with acute myocardial infarction may occur as manifestations of parasympathetic nervous system overactivity (Jarisch-Bezold reflex) or of intravascular volume depletion resulting from such factors as insufficient fluid intake, sweating, or vomiting. These forms of shock, seen most often during the first 12 hours after onset of infarction, respond readily to simple treatment. The term cardiogenic shock should be restricted to those instances of hypotension and oliguria that remain after relief of severe pain, abatement of excessive vagal activity, replacement of volume deficit, and correction of arrhythmias. Cardiogenic shock in this sense of the term is essentially an advanced form of acute congestive heart failure in which the cardiac output is insufficient to maintain normal arterial pressure or to perfuse the kidneys and other organs adequately. The usual hemodynamic picture is one of low cardiac output, high systemic vascular resistance, low arterial pressure, and high left ventricular filling pressure, with marked pulmonary congestion and arterial hypoxemia. Pulmonary arterial pressure is elevated at least moderately, but right-sided central venous pressure is frequently normal. The spectrum of congestive heart failure in acute myocardial infarction, with cardiogenic shock as its most severe form, has been aptly termed power failure. Such power failure accounts for most of the mortality during the in-hospital phase of acute myocardial infarction. Patients who have cardiogenic shock characteristically show infarction of greater than 40 percent of the left ventricular myocardium. The myocardial damage is usually produced by a combination of old and recent infarction, but sometimes, it is caused exclusively by an extensive acute anterior infarction.

Right Ventricular Infarction

Infarction of the right ventricle occurs frequently in association with acute inferior myocardial infarction, especially in those patients who have a proximal occlusion of the right coronary artery.[92,93] The infarction involves primarily the posterior region of the right ventricle and is associated with infarction of the inferoposterior region of the left ventricle and the posterior portion of the ventricular septum. Because the infarction of the left ventricle is not necessarily extensive, there may be a syndrome of right ventricular failure with little or no evidence of left ventricular failure. Hypotension and a shocklike picture in such cases may result from predominant right ventricular failure, with a low cardiac output, elevated central venous pressure, and a normal left ventricular filling pressure. Right atrial pressure may exceed left atrial pressure, and in patients with an anatomically patent foramen ovale, arterial desaturation may result from right-to-left shunting of blood through this defect.[94]

Management

In patients with heart failure and cardiogenic shock in acute myocardial infarction, it is usually prudent to monitor the therapy with a thermodilution pulmonary artery (Swan-Ganz) catheter and an indwelling radial artery catheter. The principles of medical management of congestive heart failure and cardiogenic shock in acute myocardial infarction are essentially the same as those of acute severe congestive heart failure in general and may be summarized as follows[95]:

1. A diastolic filling pressure appropriate to a damaged left ventricle should be maintained. Such a ventricle has a depressed function curve and usually requires a filling pressure in the range of 15 to 20 mm Hg to produce an adequate stroke volume and cardiac output. Higher levels are associated with aggravation of pulmonary vascular congestion.

2. Vasodilator agents should be used to lower the impedance against which the left ventricle ejects blood in systole. Nitroglycerin infusion produces dilation of veins, systemic arterioles, and coronary arteries and thus plays a unique role in acute myocardial infarction. Nitroglycerin should be given first, and if it is not effective, then sodium nitroprusside can be tried. Sodium nitroprusside is a more selective arteriolar vasodilator and is more suitable for control of severe congestive heart failure.

3. Inotropic support should be provided for the left ventricle.[96] The most useful inotropic agent for treating acute myocardial infarction is dobutamine, which should be infused intravenously at a rate of 2.5 µg/kg/min initially and gradually increased to a usual final dosage of about 10 to 15 µg/kg/min. Digitalis preparations have variable effects but usually are not strikingly beneficial. These agents are most likely to produce some benefit in patients who have a moderate degree of left ventricular failure.[97]

4. Mean arterial pressure should be kept at a level higher than approximately 80 mm Hg to maintain coronary, renal, and cerebral perfusion. It may be necessary to limit or withdraw vasodilator therapy

and to use another vasoconstrictive agent such as norepinephrine, in a dosage of 2 to 8 µg/kg/min, in addition to dobutamine to keep the blood pressure in this range.

5. Renal perfusion should be promoted by the administration of dopamine in a low dosage (5 µg/kg/min).

6. Oxygenation of the arterial blood should be optimized, using tracheal intubation and mechanically assisted ventilation if necessary and diuretic therapy to reduce pulmonary congestion.

In addition, intervention with the intra-aortic balloon pump, coronary angioplasty, coronary artery bypass surgery, left ventricular assist device, or cardiac transplantation should be considered. The circulation can be maintained with devices such as the balloon pump and the assist device, but survival is unlikely unless cardiac function is improved by another intervention.[98] Reperfusion of the infarct region by angioplasty or bypass surgery appears to contribute to survival in cardiogenic shock, although controlled trials have not been carried out.[99] Cardiac transplantation is a last resort that may occasionally be possible.

Surgically Treatable Complications

In contrast to congestive heart failure and cardiogenic shock that are caused simply by extensive infarction, there are several gross anatomic complications of acute myocardial infarction that can also cause congestive heart failure and cardiogenic shock and that are amenable to specific surgical repair.[100]

Ventricular Septal Rupture

Rupture of the ventricular septum occurs in 0.5 to one percent of patients with acute myocardial infarction. One typical pathologic picture is a large acute anteroseptal infarction with rupture of the anterior area of the septum near the apex. Patients with inferior infarcts are more likely to show a complex type of rupture, such as a serpiginous dissection tract.[101,102] The diagnosis is usually made easily from the appearance of a new, loud pansystolic murmur that is loudest at the fourth left parasternal interspace, often with a thrill at that area. The diagnosis, as well as the anatomic details, can usually be confirmed with echocardiography and color Doppler ultrasonography.[103] Determination of the oxygen saturation of blood samples from the right heart chambers, obtained via a Swan-Ganz catheter, also provides confirmation of the diagnosis.

Surgical repair should usually be performed in the acute phase of infarction and is essential when cardiogenic shock or severe congestive heart failure is present.

Mitral Regurgitation

Murmurs of various types suggesting mitral regurgitation are found in a remarkably high proportion of patients with acute myocardial infarction when looked for specifically by frequent examination. These murmurs are presumably caused by transient myocardial dysfunction, particularly of the papillary muscles, and have relatively little significance in most instances. A dramatic complication, however, is acute severe mitral regurgitation from rupture of an infarcted papillary muscle.[104] This complication usually develops in the posterior papillary muscle, or it may affect one of the tips of papillary muscles that are attached to a portion of the chordae tendineae. True rupture of chordae tendineae, however, is not part of ischemic heart disease or myocardial infarction.

Diagnosis is usually easily made on the basis of the sudden appearance of a loud apical pansystolic murmur, often with an associated thrill localized to the apex. Echocardiography will often indicate the presence of a flail mitral leaflet as well as document the presence of mitral regurgitation. Confirmation of the diagnosis may be obtained by recording indirect left atrial pressure with a venous catheter; typically, the systolic V wave is very prominent, reaching 60 to 70 mm Hg in some cases. Acute severe mitral regurgitation may also result from papillary muscle dysfunction without rupture. In these cases, the murmur may be less typical or may vary from time to time, and the diagnosis is more difficult.

Surgery is indicated in acute myocardial infarction with papillary muscle rupture whenever this complication leads to severe pulmonary congestion because the prognosis is then very unfavorable. Usually, mitral valve replacement is necessary.

Left Ventricular Aneurysm

Acute or subacute left ventricular aneurysm that develops within the first few weeks after an acute myocardial infarction is part of a process of ventricular remodeling in which infarcted segments expand and become thinner while normal segments undergo hypertrophy.[71] This process has been called expaneurysm. The location of the aneurysm is usually anterior or anterolateral. Surgical resection during the acute or subacute phase may be indicated in patients who have intractable congestive heart failure, usually with some degree of hypotension, a large aneurysm, and reasonably intact function of the remainder of the left ventricle.[105]

Cardiac Rupture and Pseudoaneurysm

Cardiac rupture occurs in about two to three percent of patients with acute myocardial infarction and accounts for five to 15 percent of the in-hospital mortality. Most typically, it develops three to 10 days after the initial onset, but 30 percent of cases of cardiac rupture occur within the first 24 hours.[106] Cardiac rupture occurs more frequently in patients who are experiencing a first myocardial infarction, particularly in women with hypertension. There is usually little warning before the sudden collapse, which is associated with acute cardiac tamponade and electromechanical dissociation. Occasionally, the rupture occurs subacutely, over a period of hours or days, permitting successful surgical therapy.[107]

One form of limited cardiac rupture leads to formation of a false aneurysm of the left ventricle. It may resemble true aneurysm clinically, or it may present as hemopericardium. This form of rupture is surgically correctable. Hemopericardium may occur in acute myocardial infarction without cardiac rupture, either free or limited. It occurs particularly in cases in which anticoagulants have been used and probably arises because of oozing of blood from areas involved with pericarditis. Echocardiography, especially when performed with Doppler color flow imaging, is useful in distinguishing a pseudoaneurysm, which usually has a narrow neck, from a true aneurysm.[108] Radionuclide angiography may also make this differentiation.

Management of Uncomplicated Cases during Convalescence

Mobilization and Hospital Stay

For patients with uncomplicated acute myocardial infarction, a stay in the coronary care unit of two to three days is usually sufficient. These patients should begin mild leg exercises immediately. They should begin progressive ambulation even before leaving the coronary care unit and should be walking in the hospital corridor after four to five days. They may be safely discharged from the hospital six to 10 days after the acute infarction. Selected patients may be discharged as early as three days after myocardial infarction.[109] Patients with persisting arrhythmias, congestive heart failure, hypotension, or ischemic chest pain require individualized management and longer stays in the coronary care unit and the hospital.

Long-term Prognosis

Patients who are discharged from the hospital after recovery from acute myocardial infarction have a mortality of six to 10 percent in the following year. Most of the deaths are sudden and occur during the first three months. The risk of late death is related primarily to the degree of left ventricular dysfunction, the degree of left ventricular ischemia, and the potential for ventricular arrhythmias. These three factors are interrelated, but each has an independent association with risk. Thus, estimating the patient's long-term prognosis and planning the management requires an evaluation of these three problems before the patient leaves the hospital.[110,111]

Evaluation of Left Ventricular Function

Left ventricular dysfunction may be apparent from the patient's symptoms, or it may be detected by the finding of cardiac enlargement and pulmonary vascular congestion in the plain chest x-ray. More subtle dysfunction may be detected by echocardiography or by radionuclide angiography, either of which may show enlargement of the left ventricle, reduced ejection fraction, or extensive regional abnormality in the systolic wall motion. Patients with an ejection fraction of less than 0.30 have a particularly high late mortality.

Evaluation of Potential Myocardial Ischemia

Patients who are free of angina on light activity in the hospital may experience stress-induced ischemia, which can be shown by an exercise ECG, a myocardial perfusion scan, or ambulatory ECG monitoring. Treadmill exercise testing before hospital discharge after acute myocardial infarction has been shown to be safe in selected uncomplicated cases. Such testing has great value in the many patients who show good exercise performance without precipitation of angina, ST segment depression, or arrhythmia. Their rehabilitation can be rapid and complete, and the psychological support from the test performance is important.

Abnormal treadmill exercise test findings, particularly the inability to raise the arterial pressure during exercise, can be used to predict reinfarction and heart failure. Ischemic ST segment depression helps identify those patients who are likely to have angina and who should probably undergo coronary arteriography to determine whether they are suitable candidates for balloon angioplasty or coronary bypass surgery.

Coronary arteriography in patients who have recovered from a first episode of acute myocardial infarction shows obstruction of coronary arteries in addition to the one responsible for the acute infarction in about two thirds of cases. Older patients or those with angina have multivessel disease more often than younger patients or those without angina. The coronary angiogram alone is helpful in predicting late mortality only in patients whose ejection fraction is moderately but not extremely reduced (i.e., in the range of 0.20 to 0.49).

Non–Q Wave Infarcts

Although patients with non–Q wave infarcts, as a group, have smaller infarcts and lower mortality in the acute phase than those with Q wave infarcts, their long-term prognosis is not significantly different.[112] Patients who demonstrate ST segment depression in the resting ECG during the acute phase of the non–Q wave infarct have a particularly high risk of late reinfarction or death.[113] Patients with non–Q wave infarcts have a higher prevalence of multivessel coronary disease and of severe but nontotal coronary obstructions than a comparable group with Q wave infarcts.[114] Diltiazem reduced the incidence of both reinfarction and angina in one study of patients with non–Q wave infarcts, suggesting that such patients are more likely to have ischemia than patients with Q wave infarcts.[115] Thus, the predischarge treadmill exercise test is particularly important in patients with non–Q wave infarcts because it can aid in selecting those patients who should have coronary arteriography.

Evaluation of Potential Arrhythmia

Ventricular premature complexes (VPCs) are often seen during the convalescent period after acute myocardial infarction. Continuous ambulatory ECGs show a considerably higher incidence of such VPCs than does the clinical examination or the routine bedside ECG monitor. Frequent VPCs or complex VPCs each correlate independently with an increase in the risk of late death.[116,117] Analysis of the signal-averaged ECG for abnormal late QRS potentials, which indicate abnormally slowed conduction in the area of an infarct, can also help assess the risk for late arrhythmia.[118] Electrophysiologic studies that attempt to induce ventricular arrhythmia by electrical stimulation may also be used to predict the risk of later ventricular tachycardia or ventricular fibrillation and to guide antiarrhythmic drug therapy.[119]

Special studies such as continuous ambulatory ECG recordings, signal-averaged ECG, and intracardiac electrophysiologic studies should be reserved for selected patients in whom the suspicion of potential ventricular tachycardia or ventricular fibrillation is high. Although many physicians prescribe antiarrhythmic drugs to reduce the risk of arrhythmia in patients after acute myocardial infarction, it is not known whether such therapy decreases the risk of death. Indeed, a controlled trial indicated that the antiarrhythmic agents flecainide and encainide increased the risk of sudden death in post–myocardial infarction patients who had frequent VPCs [*see Chapter 2*]. Digitalis may also enhance the risk of late arrhythmic complications in such patients.[120]

Management after Hospital Discharge

Rehabilitation

A progressive increase in physical activities aimed at a return to normal function in about two months should be a prime objective in convalescence after acute myocardial infarction. Prevention of psychologically induced invalidism is often the greatest contribution the physician can make in the treatment of this condition. Usually, a program of walking, arranged to suit the particular circumstances, is sufficient. Organized programs of jogging, running, and gymnasium exercise are not routinely indicated but may have value, particularly in young patients who are attempting to lose weight.[121] Sexual relations can be resumed after the patient has become normally ambulatory at home, usually three to four weeks after the acute infarction in uncomplicated cases. Marital sexual activity in middle-aged men typically increases the heart rate to only 120 to 130 beats/min, which is comparable to walking up one flight of steps.

Coronary Risk Factors

A special report of the American Heart Association summarizes available information about the value of general measures in long-term prevention of recurrent myocardial infarction.[122] The most important preventive measure is cessation of smoking. Hypertension, diabetes, and hyperlipidemia should be managed in the same manner as in other patients.

Beta-adrenergic Blocking Drugs

Several studies have indicated that treatment with a beta-adrenergic blocking drug during the first three years after myocardial infarction is associated with a reduced likelihood of mortality. A large-scale trial of propranolol therapy in the United States showed a mortality of seven percent over approximately two years in the treated group, compared with 9.5 percent in the untreated group.[123] Similar results were obtained in studies in Norway and Sweden that employed timolol and metoprolol.[124,125] The mechanism by which beta blockers reduce late mortality after myocardial infarction is uncertain, but the prevention of ventricular arrhythmia by blocking the catecholamine effect on the heart appears likely. The prophylactic value of beta blockers is probably limited to high-risk patients, because in low-risk patients, the side effects of beta blockade may outweigh the benefits. Patients recovering from a first myocardial infarction who have no significant left ventricular dysfunction or ventricular arrhythmia, who have no angina, and who show good performance on a treadmill exercise test can be considered to be at low risk for reinfarction and do not require prophylactic beta antagonists.[126]

Antithrombotic Treatment

Long-term warfarin therapy after acute myocardial infarction has not been recommended routinely in recent years, but it should be considered in patients with atrial fibrillation, previous systemic or venous thromboembolism, severe heart failure, or a left ventricular mural thrombus, especially a thrombus that is relatively large or mobile.[127] The dose of warfarin should be adjusted to prolong the prothrombin time to an INR (international normalized ratio) of 2.0 to 3.0 (1.2 to 1.5 times the control prothrombin time using rabbit-brain thromboplastin). Significant reductions in total mortality, reinfarction, and stroke were observed in a Norwegian study that evaluated the effect of warfarin therapy after acute myocardial infarction. In this study, the target INR was 2.8 to 4.8. Serious bleeding occurred in 0.6 percent of patients per year with this dose of warfarin.[128]

The use of aspirin (in patients who are not taking warfarin) is a matter of individual judgment. Most cardiologists now advise aspirin, in doses ranging from 80 mg to 325 mg daily or on alternate days, if gastrointestinal intolerance is not expected to be a problem. Sulfinpyrazone and dipyridamole are not recommended.

Spontaneous platelet aggregation, as measured in vitro, has been reported to be predictive of coronary events and mortality in low-risk survivors of acute myocardial infarction.[129]

References

1. Circulation 79(suppl I):I-13, 1989
2. Hosp Pract 23(April):87, 1988
3. Circulation 73:233, 1986
4. Ann Intern Med 88:155, 1978
5. Am J Cardiol 64:471, 1989
6. J Am Coll Cardiol 9:964, 1987
7. N Engl J Med 321:1557, 1989
8. Q J Med 64:679, 1987
9. N Engl J Med 311:1144, 1984
10. JAMA 239:2566, 1978
11. Am J Cardiol 60:1182, 1987
12. Arch Emerg Med 3:20, 1986
13. Br Heart J 62:165, 1989
14. Am Heart J 119:642, 1990
15. Am Heart J 118:138, 1989
16. Am Heart J 117:82, 1989
17. J Am Coll Cardiol 12:1156, 1988
18. Am J Med 78:765, 1985
19. Am J Cardiol 65:567, 1990
20. J Am Coll Cardiol 15:801, 1990
21. Arch Intern Med 149:1294, 1989
22. J Chronic Dis 37:369, 1984
23. J Am Coll Cardiol 16:249, 1990
24. Br Heart J 61:9, 1989
25. JAMA 260:2088, 1988
26. Ann Intern Med 106:414, 1987
27. Br Med J 297:497, 1988
28. J Am Coll Cardiol 12 (suppl):85A, 1988
29. Lancet 335:905, 1990
30. Am J Cardiol 59:519, 1987
31. Circulation 79:217, 1989
32. Ann Intern Med 112:529, 1990
33. Lancet 2:871, 1987
34. Lancet 2:349, 1988
35. Lancet 2:525, 1988
36. Lancet 335:427, 1990
37. Annual Scientific Session of the American College of Cardiology, New Orleans, March 22, 1990
38. Med Lett Drugs Ther 32:15, 1990
39. Br Heart J 61:489, 1989
40. Circulation 66:1145, 1982
41. Am Heart J 117:211, 1989
42. Prog Cardiovasc Dis 30:23, 1987
43. Am J Cardiol 65:953, 1990
44. Circulation 81:1457, 1990
45. J Am Coll Cardiol 15:1188, 1990
46. J Am Coll Cardiol 10:970, 1987
47. Ann Intern Med 112:17, 1990
48. N Engl J Med 318:1512, 1585, 1988
49. Ann Intern Med 111:1010, 1989
50. Ann Intern Med 110:957, 1989
51. Am J Cardiol 59:6, 1987
52. Circulation 81:401, 1990
53. Am J Cardiol 59:1, 1987
54. Am J Cardiol 64:1221, 1989
55. J Am Coll Cardiol 14:65, 1989
56. J Am Coll Cardiol 15:534, 1990
57. J Am Coll Cardiol 12(suppl):78A, 1988
57a. N Engl J Med 323:1433, 1990
58. Chest 93(suppl):3S, 1988
59. Ann Intern Med 105:221, 1986
60. Am Heart J 111:1041, 1986
61. Hosp Pract 24:65, 1989
62. AJR 148:247, 1987
63. J Am Coll Cardiol 14:40, 1989
64. JAMA 260:1910, 1988
65. Arch Intern Med 149:2694, 1989
66. N Engl J Med 305:1101, 1981
67. Am J Cardiol 62:679, 1988
68. J Am Coll Cardiol 6:1121, 1985
69. Circulation 74:1365, 1986
70. Prog Cardiovasc Dis 30:73, 1987
71. Circulation 81:1161, 1990
72. Lancet 335:759, 1990
73. Am J Cardiol 65:674, 1990
74. Am J Cardiol 62:310, 1988
75. J Am Coll Cardiol 15:790, 1990
76. Am Heart J 119:73, 1990
77. Circulation 74(suppl III):III-1, 1987
78. Am Heart J 117:86, 1989
79. Circulation 73:294, 1986
80. Am J Cardiol 55:1631, 1985
81. Circulation 75:733, 1987
82. J Am Coll Cardiol 12:589, 1988
83. Am J Cardiol 57:1213, 1986
84. Am Heart J 108:496, 1984
85. Physiol Rev 69:1049, 1989
86. Br Heart J 59:190, 1988
87. Arch Intern Med 147:465, 1987
88. N Engl J Med 317:257, 1987
89. Ann Intern Med 101:632, 1984
90. N Engl J Med 303:373, 1980
91. Circulation 75:146, 1987
92. J Am Coll Cardiol 6:1264, 1985
93. Br Heart J 56:19, 1986
94. J Am Coll Cardiol 5:188, 1985
95. Chest 93(suppl):17S, 1988
96. Chest 93(suppl):22S, 1988
97. Am Heart J 109:63, 1985
98. Am Heart J 111:497, 1986
99. Circulation 74(suppl III):III-11, 1986
100. JAMA 263:1237, 1990
101. Am J Cardiol 54:1201, 1984
102. Circulation 74:45, 1986

103. J Am Coll Cardiol 15:1449, 1990
104. J Am Coll Cardiol 8:558, 1986
105. N Engl J Med 311:1001, 1984
106. Am J Cardiol 62:847, 1988
107. Am Heart J 114:78, 1987
108. J Am Coll Cardiol 12:807, 1988
109. N Engl J Med 318:1083, 1988
110. N Engl J Med 314:161, 1986
111. Ann Intern Med 110:470, 1989
112. J Am Coll Cardiol 15:1208, 1990
113. J Am Coll Cardiol 15:940, 1990
114. N Engl J Med 315:417, 1986
115. Am J Cardiol 60:203, 1987
116. Am J Cardiol 58:1151, 1986
117. J Am Coll Cardiol 10:231, 1987
118. J Am Coll Cardiol 15:1277, 1990
119. Br Heart J 61:410, 1989
120. Am J Cardiol 55:623, 1985
121. J Am Coll Cardiol 15:983, 1990
122. Circulation 65:216A, 1982
123. JAMA 247:1707, 1982
124. N Engl J Med 313:1055, 1985
125. J Am Coll Cardiol 5:1428, 1985
126. Am J Med 76:900, 1984
127. Chest 89(suppl):54S, 1986
128. N Engl J Med 323:147, 1990
129. N Engl J Med 322:1549, 1990

Acknowledgments

Table 3 Adapted from "Early Intervention for Interruption of Acute Myocardial Infarction," by R. E. Genton and B. E. Sobel, in *Modern Concepts of Cardiovascular Disease* 56:35, 1987. Used by permission of the American Heart Association, Inc.

Figures 1–9 Al Miller.

 Diseases of the Pericardium

E. WILLIAM HANCOCK, M.D.

Pericardial disease results from diverse causes, many of which produce responses to injury that are pathologically and clinically similar. These responses most frequently take the form of acute pericarditis, pericardial effusion, or constrictive pericarditis.

Acute Pericarditis

Acute pericarditis that occurs as a primary illness is usually assumed to be caused by viral infection.[1] Because most cases follow a brief and uncomplicated natural course, the syndrome is often termed acute benign pericarditis. Cases resulting from other conditions, such as rheumatic diseases or radiation therapy, often exhibit clinical features that are similar to those of acute benign pericarditis.

Clinical Features and Diagnosis

The clinical diagnosis of acute pericarditis rests primarily on the findings of chest pain, pericardial friction rub, and electrocardiographic changes. The chest pain of acute pericarditis typically develops suddenly and is severe and constant over the anterior chest. The fact that the pain worsens with inspiration is helpful in distinguishing it from the pain of myocardial infarction. Low-grade fever and sinus tachycardia are usually present.

A pericardial friction rub can be detected in most patients if listened for repeatedly during the period when symptoms are acute. Pericardial friction rubs are typically triphasic: systolic and diastolic components are followed in later diastole by a third component associated with atrial contraction.[2]

Electrocardiographic changes are common in most forms of acute pericarditis, particularly those of infectious etiology in which the associated inflammation in the superficial layer of myocardium is prominent. The characteristic change is a diffuse ST segment elevation during the first several days of illness, present in all leads except those in which the positive electrode faces the ventricular cavity rather than the epicardial surface (leads aVr and sometimes III or V1, or both). The diffuseness of the ST segment elevation and the absence of reciprocal ST segment depression in oppositely oriented epicardial leads distinguish the characteristic pattern of acute pericarditis from the pattern seen in acute myocardial infarction. The normal variant pattern of ST segment elevation often complicates the differential diagnosis [*see Figure 1*]. The normal variant pattern is usually distinguished by a normal or slow heart rate and tall T waves relative to the height of the ST segment; furthermore, this pattern remains stable in serial electrocardiograms.[3] Depression of the PR segment, reflecting inflammation of the atrial myocardium, is also seen in acute pericarditis. This feature, which often simulates ST segment elevation, is a separate phenomenon that occurs almost as frequently as true ST segment elevation.

Treatment

Treatment is usually directed toward the relief of symptoms. Analgesic agents, such as codeine in a dosage of 15 to 30 mg orally every four to six hours, often provide adequate relief from pain, which typically subsides considerably after the first day or two. Salicylates in a dosage of 4 to 6 g/day initially or indomethacin in a dosage of 25 mg four times daily is often effective in reducing pericardial inflammation.[4] Adrenal corticosteroids, such as prednisone in an initial dosage of 40 to 60 mg/day, will often greatly relieve symptoms; however, they should be reserved for severe cases unresponsive to other therapy, because symptoms may recur after withdrawal. The dosage of corticosteroid should be reduced as soon as a clinical

a

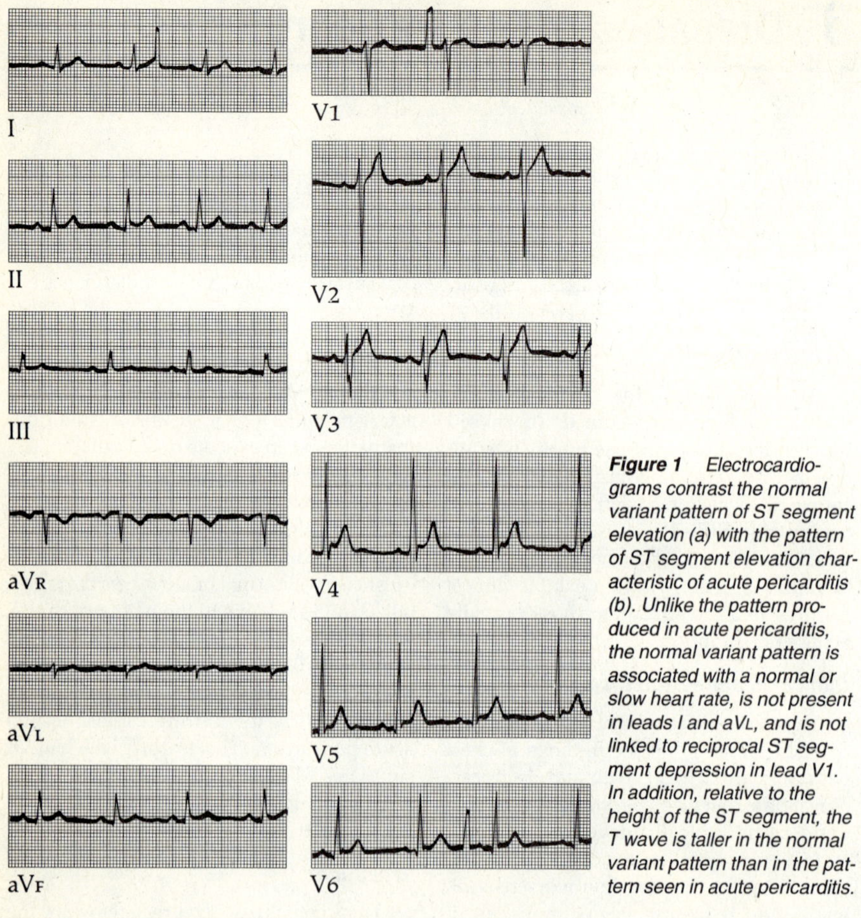

Figure 1   Electrocardiograms contrast the normal variant pattern of ST segment elevation (a) with the pattern of ST segment elevation characteristic of acute pericarditis (b). Unlike the pattern produced in acute pericarditis, the normal variant pattern is associated with a normal or slow heart rate, is not present in leads I and aVL, and is not linked to reciprocal ST segment depression in lead V1. In addition, relative to the height of the ST segment, the T wave is taller in the normal variant pattern than in the pattern seen in acute pericarditis.

response is observed and tapered to zero during a period of two to four weeks.

Other Forms of Acute Pericarditis

Relapsing Pericarditis

Acute pericarditis of any etiology may follow a recurrent or chronic relapsing course in a small number of patients. The basis for the relapse is not known, but it is generally assumed that the patient is experiencing an immunohypersensitivity reaction. In many instances, the symptoms that characterize this syndrome are subjective and are associated with additional subjective complaints, so that assessment and management are difficult.

Progression to Constriction

Acute pericarditis progresses to constrictive pericarditis of a subacute or chronic nature in a few instances. In these cases, the pericarditis may be idiopathic or have a bacterial, viral, rheumatoid, radiation-induced, or uremic origin. Initially, most patients have subacute rather than acute pericarditis; pericardial effusion is present at the onset, usually with some degree of cardiac tamponade. Acute benign pericarditis that is unaccompanied by tamponade or substantial pericardial

b

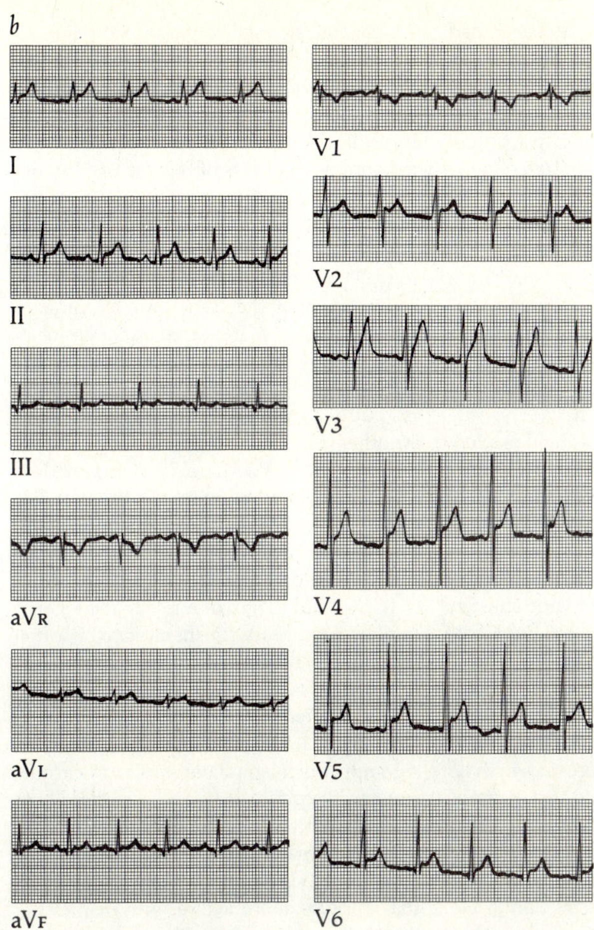

effusion in the acute phase rarely progresses to constrictive pericarditis.

Pericardial Effusion

Fluid may accumulate in the pericardial cavity in virtually all forms of pericardial disease. The fluid may be a transudate, as are the serous cavity effusions that develop in patients with congestive heart failure, overhydration, or hypoproteinemia. More often, however, the pericardial effusion is an exudate, reflecting the presence of pericardial injury. Serosanguineous pericardial fluid is a classic sign in tuberculous and neoplastic diseases, but this type of effusion also occurs frequently in cases of uremic, radiation-induced, and idiopathic pericarditis. Frank blood in the pericardial space may occur in cases of aortic aneurysm or aortic dissection because of leakage or rupture into the pericardial space. Hemopericardium may also be produced by closed or penetrating trauma, rupture of the heart in acute myocardial infarction, perforation of the heart by cardiac catheters, or bleeding caused by coagulation defects. The presence of effused chyle in the pericardial space, or chylopericardium, occurs rarely as a consequence of leakage from the thoracic duct.[5] Any chronic pericardial effusion in which large lipoprotein molecules are reabsorbed less rapidly than any other constituents may lead to cholesterol pericarditis. This syndrome, which is probably nonspecific, develops because unabsorbed lipoprotein molecules are gradually concentrated in the pericardial fluid.[6]

Pathophysiology

The mere presence of pericardial fluid, even in large amounts, is not necessarily clinically significant apart from the fact that such fluid accumulation indicates the existence of an underlying disease. The clinical effects of the effusion itself depend on whether the fluid is under increased pressure and producing cardiac tamponade. No consistent relation exists between the volume of pericardial fluid and the level of intrapericardial pressure. For example, if the effusion develops gradually, the pericardium can stretch enough to accommodate a very large effusion with no significant increase in pressure. However, if the effusion develops acutely, even a small volume of pericardial fluid (100 to 200 ml) may cause cardiac tamponade, as in the case of hemopericardium caused by trauma. As the pericardial fluid pressure rises from its normal value, which is close to that of atmospheric and intrapleural pressures, the right atrial and central venous pressures rise correspondingly. Thus, the central venous pressure reading is an accurate reflection of the intrapericardial pressure and can be used to determine whether cardiac tamponade is present.

As a rule, paradoxic pulse, or a greater than normal inspiratory fall in arterial pressure, is present in patients with cardiac tamponade, although it may not be easy to detect on clinical examination [*see Figure* 2].[7] The value of 10 mm Hg is commonly used to indicate the upper limit of the normal fall in arterial pressure with inspiration; however, 10 mm Hg is an arbitrary value and should not be regarded as a definitive criterion for evaluating the presence of cardiac tamponade. Any degree of paradoxic pulse perceptible by simple palpation of the radial pulse is abnormal.

The physiology of paradoxic pulse remains somewhat of a mystery. It is clear that the inspiratory drop in arterial pressure reflects a selective impairment of diastolic filling of the left ventricle,[8] probably caused by the combined effects of two factors that operate in cardiac tamponade. First, inspiratory filling of the right ventricle is augmented, which limits left ventricular filling (Dornhorst theory). Secondly, blood is sequestered in the lungs and pulmonary veins as a result of impaired transmission of intrapleural pressure changes to the left atrium and the intrapericardial portions of the pulmonary veins (Katz-Gauchat theory). Another factor that contributes to paradoxic pulse in patients with cardiac tamponade is a reduction in volume in all of the cardiac chambers, which magnifies the relative importance of inspiratory changes in intracardiac flow and volume.[9]

Kussmaul's sign, or a rise in the level of venous pressure with inspiration, is often mentioned as a sign of cardiac tamponade; however, it occurs only in cases of tamponade associated with constriction and not in uncomplicated tamponade. Kussmaul's sign appears in some patients with chronic constrictive pericarditis and occasionally in patients with severe congestive heart failure. When making a bedside assessment of Kussmaul's sign, a jugular venous pulsation that appears more active with inspiration may be mistaken for a true rise in mean venous pressure [*see Figure* 2].

Diagnosis

Echocardiography is the most accurate and easily applicable method for the clinical detection of pericardial effusion [*see Figure* 3]. An effusion as small as 20 ml can be detected by echocardiography, and characteristic echocardiographic findings are obtained with effusions larger than 100 ml. Two-dimensional echocardiography has an advantage over M mode echocardiography because it shows the extent and distribution of fluid around the heart [*see Figure* 4]. Computed tomography (CT) is also a highly reliable method for detecting pericardial ef-

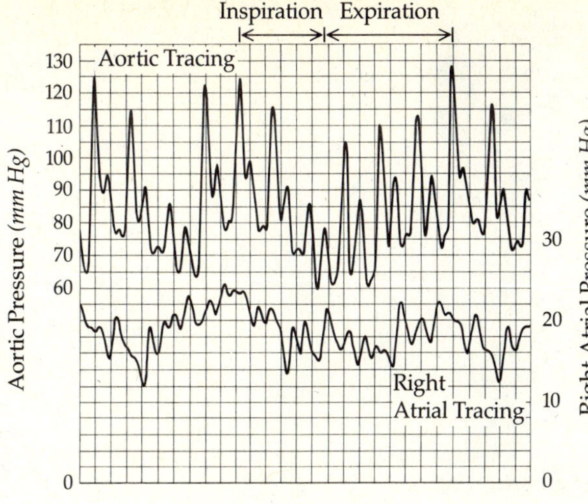

Figure 2 The aortic and right atrial pressures are recorded during quiet breathing in a patient with cardiac tamponade. The marked fall in aortic pressure that occurs with inspiration is a paradoxic pulse. The decrease in aortic pulse pressure, defined as the difference between systolic and diastolic pressures, that accompanies the fall in systolic pressure indicates that a reduction in left ventricular stroke volume occurs with inspiration. Central venous pressure, as indicated by the right atrial pressure, also falls with inspiration.

fusions and pericardial thickening.[10] CT should be used when echocardiography results are inconclusive [*see Figure 5*]. Nuclear magnetic resonance (NMR) provides information similar to that of CT.[11]

Radionuclide scans and angiocardiography detect moderate or large effusions, but these methods are cumbersome. As a rule, clinical examination, electrocardiography, chest roentgenography, and fluoroscopy should not be relied on for the detection of pericardial effusion. The finding of radiolucent fat lines in the lateral chest roentgenogram, however, may be a useful diagnostic

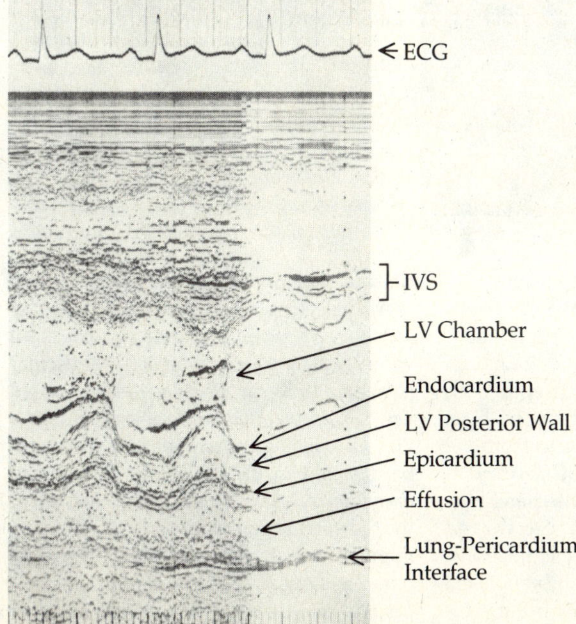

Figure 3 The echocardiogram discloses the presence of pericardial effusion. When the recording sensitivity of the echocardiogram is reduced, as on the right, only the strongest echoes are received. The single strongest echo, from the posterior heart, identifies the lung-pericardium interface. On the left, normal recording sensitivity reveals the interventricular septum (IVS), left ventricular (LV) chamber, and left ventricular posterior wall. In the presence of effusion, the epicardium is separated from the pericardium; the intervening, fluid-filled layer appears as an echo-free space on the echocardiogram.

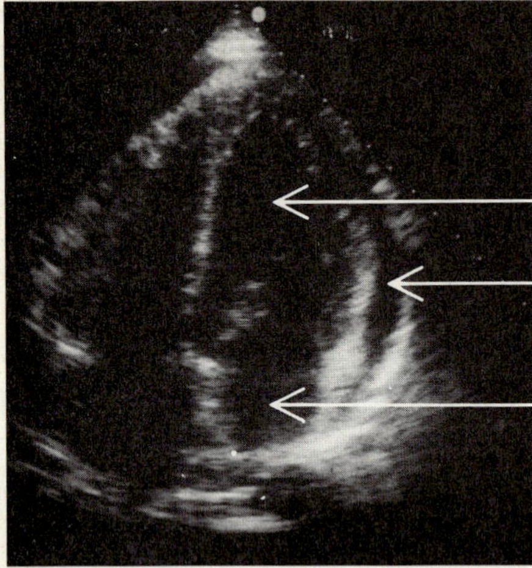

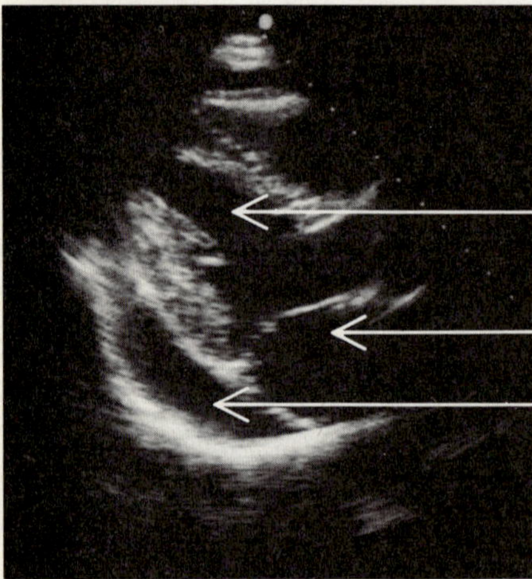

Figure 4 *Pericardial effusion is seen in the 2-D echocardiogram as an echo-free space outside of the cardiac chambers. Two characteristic sites are lateral to the left ventricle in the apical four-chamber view (top) and posterior to the left ventricle in the parasternal long-axis view (bottom).*

clue; such fat lines reflect the presence of a radiolucent layer of epicardial fat between the myocardium and the pericardial fluid.[12]

Electrical alternans, which has long been recognized as an electrocardiographic sign of pericardial effusion, is produced by a beat-to-beat oscillation of the heart from one position to another within the pericardial sac [*see Figure 6*]. Electrical alternans thus indicates that a large effusion is present and the heart is freely mobile; this sign is most common with effusion caused by neoplasm.

The demonstration of pericardial effusion does not in itself indicate cardiac tamponade. Tamponade is usually present if there is electrical alternans. Exaggerated respiratory variation in mitral and tricuspid valvular flow rate and in left ventricular stroke volume can be detected by pulsed Doppler ultrasound recordings [*see Figure 7*].[13] Another sign of tamponade, which can be detected in the echocardiogram, is an early diastolic inward motion of the wall of the right atrium and right ventricle; this sign appears earlier than a marked degree of paradoxic pulse.[14] Loculated pericardial effusions may selectively compress one or more chambers of the heart, producing re-

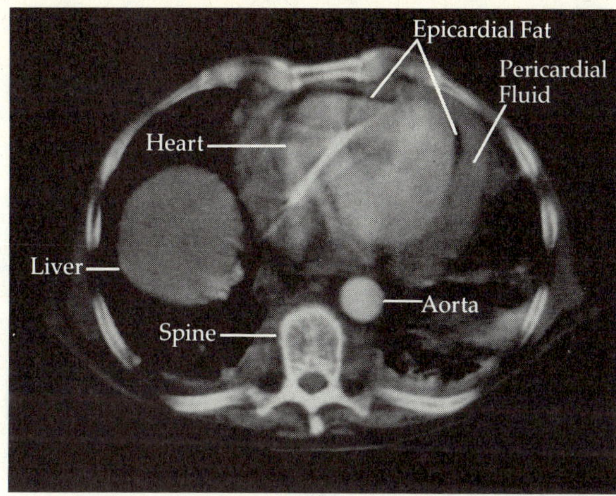

Figure 5 *In a CT scan of the chest of a patient with pericardial effusion, pericardial fluid appears less dense than the heart and is separated from the myocardium by epicardial fat in some areas.*

gional cardiac tamponade; this condition occurs most frequently after chest surgery. The clinical signs of regional tamponade are atypical.[15]

Treatment

Cardiac tamponade may be managed by pericardiocentesis, by surgical pericardiostomy with tube drainage, or by limited or extensive pericardiectomy. Shock caused by acute cardiac tamponade may be reversed by infusing fluid and isoproterenol before decompressing the pericardial fluid.

The most acute forms of cardiac tamponade, particularly those caused by trauma, rupture of an aortic aneurysm or an aortic dissection into the pericardial space, or purulent bacterial pericarditis, generally require prompt surgery.[16] Pericardiocentesis is most valuable in the treatment of subacute forms of pericardial effusion and tamponade, especially in cases caused by neoplasm. One or more pericardiocenteses may often relieve the tamponade and thus eliminate the need for surgery; the precise diagnosis may be revealed by laboratory studies of the aspirated fluid.[17]

Studies of pericardial fluid will probably determine whether purulent pericarditis or secondary neoplastic involvement is the specific diagnosis; similarly, negative bacteriologic and cytologic studies will normally rule out bacterial infection and neoplasm as causes of pericardial effusion. After the presence of fluid has been demonstrated by echocardiography, pericardiocentesis is usually done by the subxiphoid approach with the aid of a monitoring electrocardiogram transmitted from the needle tip. Two-dimensional echocardiography is useful in selecting the optimal site for insertion of the needle used for pericardiocentesis and in guiding the insertion of the needle or catheter in the pericardial space.[18]

When venous pressure is elevated, the pressure in the pericardial space and in the right atrium or a central vein should be measured before and after removal of the fluid to ascertain whether the tamponade has been adequately relieved. A reduction of the intrapericardial pressure to normal levels indicates that the tamponade has been alleviated; elevated right atrial or central venous pressure readings indicate the presence of residual epicardial constrictive pericarditis.[19] Surgical intervention is required for the treatment of both inadequately relieved cardiac tamponade and constrictive pericarditis.

It is often wise to leave an indwelling catheter in the pericardial space after pericardiocentesis has been performed.[20] The

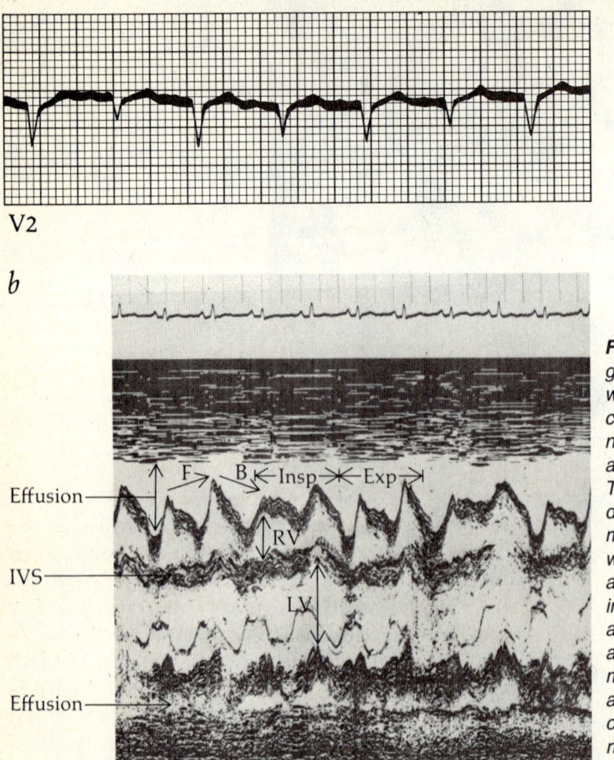

Figure 6   *The electrocardiogram (V2 lead) from a patient with pericardial effusion caused by malignant melanoma reveals a low voltage and electrical alternans (a). The echocardiogram (b) demonstrates that the heart moves forward (F) and backward (B) within the effusion on alternate beats, thus producing the alternation of the QRS axis characteristic of electrical alternans. The heart also moves with inspiration (Insp) and expiration (Exp), which accounts for a change in anterior wall motion with every two cardiac cycles.*

catheter can be used for draining recurrent effusion and instilling drugs, if necessary.

Subxiphoid pericardiostomy, the most widely used surgical method for the relief of cardiac tamponade, is a more reliable therapeutic approach than pericardiocentesis.[21] It may be performed under local anesthesia, and the pleural cavities are not necessarily entered. Pericardiostomy should be employed in all cases in which pericardiocentesis does not adequately relieve the tamponade or in which the effusion reaccumulates rapidly after the procedure. Some surgeons prefer to perform a thoracotomy for resection of varying amounts of the pericardium, particularly for purulent pericarditis, but pericardiectomy is not needed routinely unless constrictive pericarditis is present.[22]

Specific Etiologic Forms of Acute Pericarditis and Pericardial Effusion

Uremic Pericarditis

Acute pericarditis with pericardial effusion can occur in uremic patients who are not on dialysis; its presence indicates a need for dialysis. A possibly different form of acute pericarditis occurs in patients who are on successful chronic dialysis. In these cases, conservative management utilizing more intensive dialysis and nonsteroidal anti-inflammatory drugs, with pericardiocentesis if tamponade is suspected, is usually successful. Most clinicians resort to surgery only in the rare instances of recurrent tamponade or of actual constrictive pericarditis.[23] Uremic pericarditis accompanied by

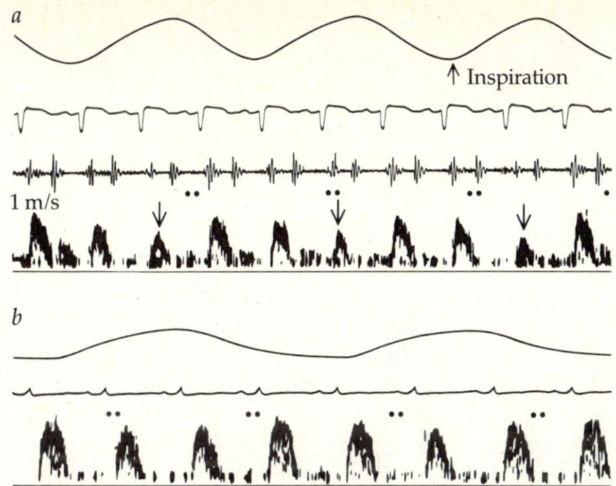

Figure 7 Pulsed Doppler ultrasound recordings of the velocity of blood flow in the aorta in a patient with pericardial effusion reveal significant improvement after pericardiocentesis. Before pericardiocentesis (a), there is notable respiratory variation in the velocity of flow, which correlates with cardiac tamponade and paradoxic pulse (arrow). The variation is greatly decreased after pericardiocentesis (b).

effusion is often associated with fluid overload and left ventricular failure. If left ventricular failure is present, the recognition of cardiac tamponade is difficult, and paradoxic pulse is often absent.[24] Cardiac catheterization in combination with pericardiocentesis is particularly useful in patients who have uremic pericarditis with effusion.

Radiation-induced Pericardial Effusion

Pericardial effusion develops relatively frequently in patients with Hodgkin's disease, in those with other lymphomas, or in individuals with breast carcinoma who survive for prolonged periods after receiving large doses of radiation to the mediastinum.[25] Radiation-induced pericardial effusion may evolve into chronic constrictive pericarditis many years later.

Neoplastic Pericardial Effusion

Pericardial effusion caused by neoplasms can often be managed palliatively with pericardiocentesis, radiotherapy, or chemotherapy. Injection of tetracycline into the pericardial space induces pericardial sclerosis and thus prevents recurrent fluid accumulation. This method is more consistently successful than the instillation of cancer chemotherapeutic agents into the pericardial space. Pericardiostomy can be reserved for those patients who do not respond to tetracycline sclerotherapy.[26]

Purulent Pericarditis

In cases of purulent pericarditis, tamponade is usually present and normally recurs rapidly after pericardiocentesis. Purulent pericarditis nearly always requires surgical drainage of the pericardial space, and often, a pericardiectomy must be performed.[27] However, because antibiotics enter the pericardial cavity in effective concentrations, surgery may not be required in those patients in whom tamponade or constriction does not develop. Active tuberculous pericarditis with effusion is likely to progress to constrictive pericarditis. Antituberculous chemotherapy is usually effective in such cases, but pericardiectomy is also frequently required.[28] The incidence of tuberculous pericarditis and other forms of bacterial pericarditis in the United States is increasing as a result of the acquired immunodeficiency syndrome (AIDS) epidemic.[29]

Drug-induced Pericarditis

Several drugs have been implicated in the etiology of acute pericarditis; these include procainamide, which leads to a lupuslike syndrome, and the antihypertensive drug minoxidil, which has been linked to pericardial effusion.[30]

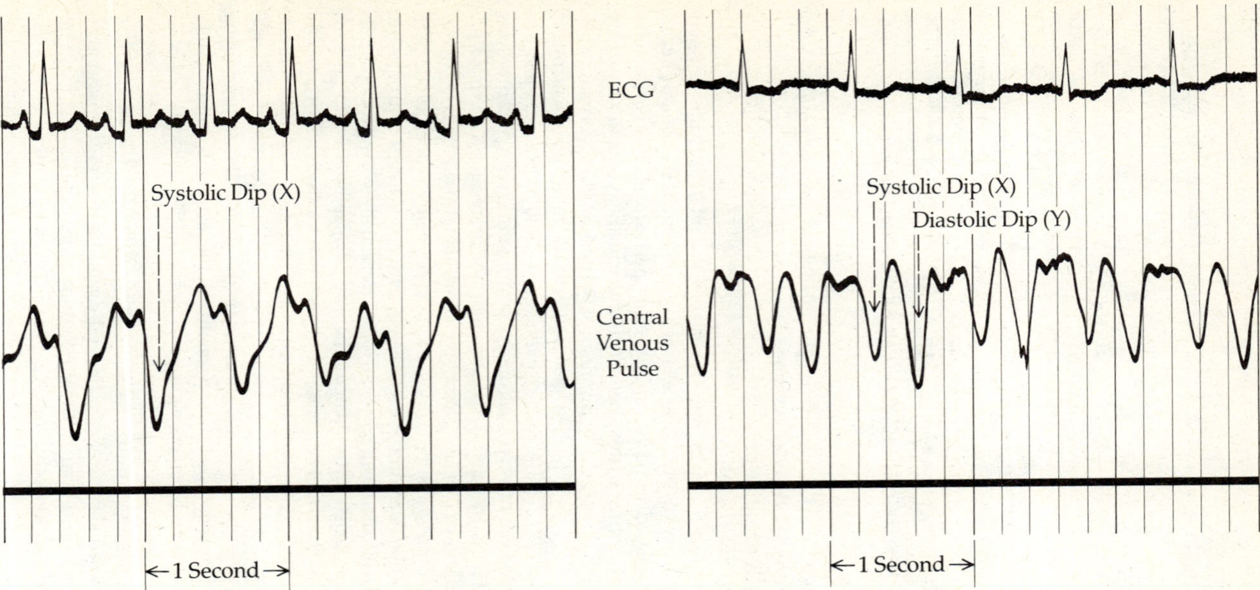

Figure 8 *Differences between the central venous pulse contours characteristic of cardiac tamponade (left) and chronic constrictive pericarditis (right) provide the basis for differential diagnosis. The pressure contour in a patient with pericardial effusion and tamponade has a prominent systolic dip (X) but little or no diastolic deflection. The central venous pulse pattern in a patient with chronic constrictive pericarditis displays an M or W contour consisting of both systolic and diastolic dips (Y), the Y descent being more prominent.*

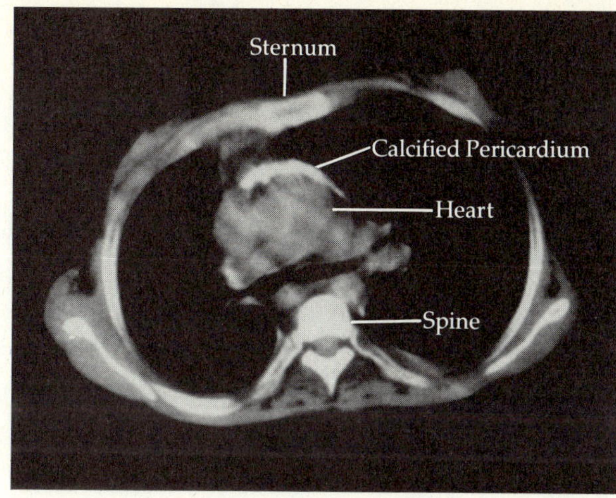

Figure 9 *In this CT scan of the chest of a patient with chronic constrictive pericarditis, the dense layer on the anterior surface of the heart represents thickened and partially calcified pericardium.*

Pericarditis after Cardiac Surgery

The postcardiotomy syndrome presents primarily as an acute pericarditis. A high prevalence of viral infection was observed in one series of patients with the syndrome, most of whom were children.[31] In some cases, cardiac tamponade that was not related to anticoagulation therapy appeared after hospital discharge.[32] Complications resembling the postcardiotomy syndrome have followed epicardial pacemaker implantation.[33]

Constrictive Pericarditis

In the United States, constrictive pericarditis was formerly considered to be primarily a tuberculous lesion; it is still regarded as such in many areas of the world. Most cases now seen in the United States are idiopathic, but cases resulting from exposure to radiation, from rheumatoid arthritis, or from uremia have become more frequent. Previous cardiac surgery, usually coronary artery bypass surgery, has also emerged as an important cause of constrictive pericarditis.[34] Constrictive pericarditis usually appears three to 12 months after the operation but may appear as early as two weeks after surgery and is not necessarily preceded by an unusually severe postcardiotomy reaction. Previous radiotherapy and cardiac surgery each accounted for approximately one third of cases of constrictive pericarditis at Stanford Medical Center during the 1980s.[35]

In the classic form of chronic constrictive pericarditis, fibrous scarring and adhesion of both pericardial layers obliterate the pericardial cavity. The resulting fibrotic lesion has been likened to a rigid shell around the heart. This analogy is particularly apt when there is considerable calcification of the pericardium, a feature seen in long-standing cases. The subacute form of constrictive pericarditis is now more common than the chronic calcific type. In the subacute variant, the constriction is rather fibroelastic and may be produced by fibrous contracture of the visceral pericardial layer (epicardium) alone. The fibroelastic constriction may also act in conjunction with persisting loculated or totally free pericardial effusion; this form is termed effusive-constrictive pericarditis.[19,36]

Pathophysiology

The pathophysiology of constrictive pericarditis is similar to that of tamponade in that both conditions impede diastolic filling of the heart and lead to increased venous pressure and ultimately to reduced cardiac output. Differences exist in the diagnostic signs, however. Paradoxic pulse is a regular feature of cardiac tamponade but may be inconspicuous or absent in constrictive pericarditis. Kussmaul's sign occurs in some patients with constrictive pericarditis but is not seen in patients with pure cardiac tamponade. When tamponade is present, the venous pulse shows a predominant systolic dip, whereas in constrictive pericarditis, the early diastolic dip is the more prominent deflection [*see Figure 8*].

The early diastolic sound (pericardial knock) is heard in constrictive pericarditis but not in tamponade; its presence is directly related to the extent to which ventricular filling is restricted to early diastole.[37]

Diagnosis

Clinical diagnosis of constrictive pericarditis depends on the recognition of elevated venous pressure in a patient who does not have other obvious signs or symptoms of heart disease. Constrictive pericarditis is frequently misdiagnosed for prolonged periods as liver disease or as idiopathic pleural effusion because the physician does not recognize elevated venous pressure in the examination of the neck veins. Echocardiography usually shows evidence of pericardial thickening, but this finding is nonspecific and does not differentiate constrictive pericarditis from non-constrictive adhesive pericarditis. CT is superior to echocardiography for the demonstration of pericardial thickening [*see Figure 9*]; a CT scan that shows a normal pericardial thickness is usually a reliable indication that constrictive pericarditis is not present.

A form of occult constrictive pericarditis exists. In this syndrome, venous pressure and other hemodynamic parameters are normal under usual conditions but show constrictive features after a sudden, large intravenous volume infusion.[38] It is occasionally difficult to distinguish constrictive pericarditis from restrictive cardiomyopathy or cardiac amyloidosis. Results of cardiac catheterization and angiocardiography usually help distinguish the conditions, and myocardial biopsy is also informative.[39]

Treatment

Constrictive pericarditis occasionally reverses spontaneously when it develops as a complication of acute pericarditis.[40] In most instances, however, relief of constrictive pericarditis requires surgical stripping and removal of both layers of the adherent constricting pericardium. This operation is far more difficult to perform than the operation for the relief of pericardial effusion, which requires removal of only the parietal pericardium. The operation must be thorough to obtain a good result. The need for excision of the innermost pericardial layer, however, carries with it the risk of hemorrhage from perforations of the wall of the heart during the stripping procedure. In recent years, cardiopulmonary bypass has been used increasingly to facilitate the stripping procedure. Elevated venous pressure readings should return to normal levels within three months after surgery.[41] Inadequate long-term relief after surgical removal of the pericardium may reflect the presence of associated myocardial disease, particularly in instances of radiation-induced pericarditis.[42,43] In general, however, myocardial function is normal in patients with constrictive pericarditis.

Miscellaneous Pericardial Disorders

Pericardial Cysts

Most pericardial cysts are located near the right cardiophrenic angle and are congenital. They probably arise from mesothelial tissues that failed to fuse with the rest of the pericardium during embryologic development.[44] Large diverticula of the pericardial sac may present a similar picture. Certain pericardial cysts, however, are acquired as a result of previous trauma or pericarditis, whereas others, such as bronchiogenic or teratomatous cysts, have a different origin.

Primary Pericardial Tumors

Primary neoplasms of the pericardium are far less common than secondary involvement of the pericardium by malignant disorders such as lymphoma, leukemia, lung cancer, or breast cancer. The most important primary neoplasm is the mesothelioma.[45] By the time the characteristic signs and symptoms of this tumor (i.e., cough, chest pain, and constriction of the heart) have appeared, it has usually encased the heart extensively.

Congenital Pericardial Defects

Congenital defects of the pericardium may be total or partial. The most frequent defect is absence of the left pericardium. Accentuation of the contours of the left heart border in patients with this disorder produces a characteristic chest roentgenogram.[46] Partial defects of the pericardium rarely lead to herniation and strangulation of the heart.[47] Most pericardial defects are benign anomalies that are important chiefly because they can account for an unusual chest roentgenogram in a healthy person. Echocardiography and CT are helpful in confirming the diagnosis.[48]

References

1. Am J Cardiol 56:623, 1985
2. Am J Cardiol 35:357, 1975
3. Circulation 65:1004, 1982
4. J Am Coll Cardiol 7:300, 1986
5. Arch Intern Med 144:1857, 1984
6. Am J Med 41:235, 1966
7. Circulation 64:633, 1981
8. Heart Disease. Braunwald E, Ed. WB Saunders, Philadelphia, 3rd ed, 1988, p 1484
9. Am J Cardiol 52:159, 1983
10. Ann Intern Med 101:801, 1984
11. Radiology 150:469, 1984
12. JAMA 257:3266, 1987
13. J Am Coll Cardiol 11:1020, 1988
14. Circulation 70:966, 1984
15. J Am Coll Cardiol 10:164, 1987
16. Ann Emerg Med 13:924, 1984
17. Am J Med 65:808, 1978
18. Am J Cardiol 55:476, 1985
19. Circulation 43:183, 1971
20. Am J Cardiol 58:633, 1986
21. JAMA 247:1143, 1982
22. Chest 88:30, 1985
23. Arch Intern Med 144:1317, 1984
24. Circulation 58:265, 1978
25. Prog Cardiovasc Dis 27:173, 1984
26. JAMA 257:1088, 1987
27. Am J Med 56:68, 1975
28. J Am Coll Cardiol 11:724, 1988
29. NY State J Med 86:592, 1986
30. South Med J 76:815, 1983
31. Circulation 62:1151, 1980
32. Circulation 63:1323, 1981
33. Am J Cardiol 45:1088, 1980
34. Br Heart J 51:205, 1984
35. Am Heart J 113:354, 1987
36. Am Heart J 100:917, 1980
37. Am J Cardiol 47:791, 1981
38. Circulation 56:924, 1977
39. Lancet 2:372, 1987
40. Am J Cardiol 59:961, 1987
41. Ann Thorac Surg 29:146, 1980
42. Circulation 72(suppl 2):264, 1985
43. J Thorac Cardiovasc Surg 89:340, 1985
44. AJR 141:292, 1983
45. Cancer 53:377, 1984
46. Circulation 51:183, 1975
47. Am Heart J 100:866, 1980
48. Chest 81:610, 1982

Acknowledgments

Figures 1, 8   Al Miller.

Figure 2   Sally Black.

Figure 6   Al Miller. Electrocardiogram provided by R. J. Noble and echocardiogram provided by N. Weyman, from *Self-Assessment: Electrocardiographic Patterns*, test booklet prepared by R. J. Noble for The Twenty-Sixth Annual Scientific Session of the American College of Cardiology, March 1977.

7 Thromboembolism

EDWARD RUBENSTEIN, M.D.

Incidence, Predisposing Factors, and Pathophysiology

Venous thrombosis and pulmonary embolism are among the leading causes of morbidity and death in hospitalized patients. Predisposing factors include posttraumatic and postoperative immobility (particularly in middle-aged and elderly patients), pregnancy, previous episodes of venous thrombosis, use of oral contraceptives, stroke, neoplasia, obesity (in women), systemic lupus erythematosus, nephrotic syndrome, polycythemia vera, inflammatory bowel disease, homocystinuria, hyperhomocysteinemia, paroxysmal nocturnal hemoglobinuria, shock, and congestive heart failure; other factors that have been shown to predispose to thromboembolism include deficiencies of procoagulants or of inhibitors of the clotting mechanism.

Studies with radioactively labeled fibrinogen reveal venous thrombi in the lower legs of about one fourth of all patients older than 50 years who have undergone routine inguinal herniorrhaphy, in more than one half of all prostatectomy or hip surgery patients, and in about one third of all patients with acute myocardial infarction.[1] Although mortality from pulmonary embolism in hospitalized patients is declining, possibly because of improvements in prevention, diagnosis, and therapy,[2] major pulmonary embolism continues to be underdiagnosed.[3]

Unlike the flat, tightly adherent, relatively small, platelet-dense white thrombi that form on arterial intimae, venous thrombi consist almost entirely of fibrin and enmeshed red blood cells. These red thrombi are large, friable casts of the venous channel with branching arms that extend into tributary veins and a tapering tail. Too often, such thrombi have only a weak proximal attachment to the venous intima, usually at a valve or a bifurcation. Cross sections usually show strata of platelet and white blood cell deposits (the lines of Zahn), indicating that the thrombus formed in flowing blood rather than after death.

Stasis, endothelial damage, and hypercoagulability predispose to venous thrombosis. Procoagulants, such as those that accumulate during surgical or accidental trauma, probably induce thromboses at sites of venous stasis. Injury to the endothelium activates the liquid-clotting mechanism and causes local adherence and aggregation of platelets.

Deficiencies of three endogenous anticoagulants—antithrombin III, protein C, and protein S—have been identified as causes of hypercoagulability. Inadequate activity of any one of these factors leads to recurrent thromboembolic syndromes.

Whether inadequate fibrinolysis is associated with venous thromboembolism is controversial.[4] Impaired synthesis or release of tissue plasminogen activator and increased concentrations of tissue plasminogen activator inhibitor have been identified in patients with recurrent venous thromboembolism,[5] as have quantitative and qualitative abnormalities of plasminogen.[6] Abnormal fibrinogen that is excessively resistant to plasmin has also been reported.[7]

In one study, the prevalence of deficiencies of antithrombin III, protein C, protein S, and plasminogen in patients with venographically proven acute deep venous thrombosis was about eight percent, as compared with two percent in matched control patients without thrombosis.[8] Even though the likelihood of detecting a deficiency of an endogenous anticoagulant increases when the thrombotic disorder is recurrent, is familial, or begins during youth (before age 40), the underlying cause cannot be identified in the vast majority of cases.[8]

Antiphospholipid antibodies, which appear in patients with systemic lupus erythematosus and related disorders, have been found to predispose to thrombosis (both venous and arterial), thrombocytopenia, neurologic disorders, and fetal loss.[9-11]

The use of oral contraceptive agents containing synthetic estrogens, such as ethinyl estradiol, may increase the risk of arterial or venous thrombosis. The effect is dose dependent, and it can be mitigated by lowering the content of the synthetic estrogen.[12] On the other hand, the administration of estrogens in the doses used for postmenopausal replacement therapy does not appear to increase the risk of thromboembolism in the general population.[12,13] An individualized and cautious approach to replacement therapy is appropriate in high-risk patients, especially those who have acquired thromboembolic disease while pregnant or while taking an oral contraceptive.

Venous thrombi that are present below the knees rarely give rise to significant pulmonary emboli, but thrombi that propagate into the iliofemoral system can.[14] The presence of such disorders as congestive heart failure, shock, or malignant disease increases the likelihood that an embolus will result in pulmonary infarction.[15] A complex interplay of mechanisms is involved in thrombus formation [*see Chapter 14*].

Superficial or deep migratory thrombophlebitis or pulmonary embolism sometimes occurs in the apparent absence of predisposing factors. Some studies suggest that there is an increased incidence of underlying neoplasia of the lung, the gastrointestinal tract, the breast, or the uterus in patients with unexplained venous thromboembolism, but other studies do not confirm this association.[16,17] Rarely, recurring and devastating venous and arterial thromboses that are preceded by disseminated intravascular coagulation appear in patients who have neoplasms (Trousseau's syndrome). Immediate and long-term heparinization are required in such patients. Treatment with warfarin is ineffective.[18]

Chemotherapy for stage II breast cancer has been associated with an increased risk of thrombotic disease.[19] Rifampin therapy for hospitalized patients with tuberculosis has been implicated as predisposing to deep venous thrombosis.[20]

Clinical Features and Diagnosis

Venous Thrombosis

Superficial thrombophlebitis is readily recognized by the presence of a tender vein, in which a thrombus can often be palpated, surrounded by an area of erythema, heat, and edema. The presence of fever increases the likelihood of bacterial infection. *Campylobacter fetus* infection should be considered in patients who have unusual presentations, especially phlebitis at puncture sites.[21] Deep venous thrombosis may occur in association with superficial disease, particularly in patients who do not have varicosities, but emboli are rare.[22] In most cases, treatment is conservative: elevation of the affected limb, local heat, and antibiotics for suspected infections. There is an increased risk of cellulitis in the vein-donor leg after coronary artery bypass grafting; the presence of tinea pedis predisposes to this complication.[23]

Deep venous thrombi may be silent and often cannot be detected by bedside examination, even after the diagnosis of pulmonary embolism has been established. Edema, distended veins, localized areas of discoloration, and increased heat and tenderness over venous structures are clues. Conditions that are likely to be mistaken for deep venous thrombosis include rupture of calf muscle fibers (usually found in middle-aged weekend athletes) and dissection or rupture of popliteal synovial cysts (usually found in patients with arthropathy involving the knee). Painful and tender swelling of the lower extremity, associated with overlying cutaneous erythema, has occurred in patients with the acquired immunodeficiency syndrome (AIDS); four of five such patients had Kaposi's sarcoma. This condition mimics venous thrombosis, but venograms are negative.[24]

The most reliable technique for diagnosing deep venous thrombosis is ascending venography. A positive diagnosis can be made if a filling defect is demonstrated, especially if the defect is apparent in more than one view. Preferably, a layer of contrast medium should be seen surrounding part of the defect in at least one projection. Nonfilling of the vein, disordered flow patterns, and abnormal collateral channels cannot be regarded as conclusive. A normal venogram essentially rules out the diagnosis of deep venous thrombosis, but lower extremity venography is negative in about one third of patients in whom the presence of pulmonary embolism has been documented.[25]

Because of the morbidity associated with venography, including possible initiation of venous thrombosis, other screening methods have been advocated. Impedance plethysmography (IPG) and duplex ultrasonography are noninvasive means for detecting deep venous thrombi. The term duplex ultrasonography refers to the combined use of high-resolution, high-frequency ultrasound transducers, which provide assessment of the deep venous system, and pulse-gated Doppler technology. Duplex ultrasonography represents a major diagnostic advance.[26] Venous channels can be well visualized with this technique, and the failure of the lumen to collapse under gentle probe pressure is a criterion for the presence of a thrombus. The thrombus may also give rise to increased intraluminal echoes. The absence of flow, as shown by pulse Doppler ultrasonography, provides corroborative evidence of thrombus. The Doppler signal from erythrocytes can be used to generate a color image, in which blood moving toward the transducer is in one color and blood moving away is in a different color. Flow velocity determines color intensity.

Real-time ultrasonography is still being evaluated. Current data indicate that the sensitivity and the specificity for all deep venous thrombi vary from 78 to 100 percent. The method has significant limitations for the evaluation of deep calf veins and the common iliac veins. On the other hand, it is an effective means of diagnosing thrombi in the popliteal and femoral veins, for which the mean sensitivity is 96 percent and the mean specificity is 99 percent.[27]

Ultrasonography has the distinct advantage of detecting Baker's cysts and hematomas of the calf.

A blinded, retrospective cohort study of patients with objectively confirmed or refuted previous episodes of suspected deep venous thrombosis has shown that the combination of photoplethysmography and venous Doppler ultrasonography can reliably determine the presence or absence of venous valvular incompetence that results from previous proximal deep venous thrombosis.[28] Doppler reflux was found to be specific for previous proximal thrombi. The combination of normal plethysmographic and ultrasonographic results is reliable for the exclusion of such thrombi. An abnormal plethysmographic result with a normal Doppler ultrasonographic result does not reliably confirm or refute the diagnosis.[28]

The current view that calf vein thrombi, unlike iliofemoral thrombi, rarely result in clinically significant pulmonary emboli has led to the formulation of a diagnostic strategy that focuses on the location of the thrombotic process. Because IPG has such a high sensitivity for iliofemoral thrombi (probably greater than 95 percent), it can effectively discriminate between those patients who should receive anticoagulants and those who should not. When the diagnosis of iliofemoral thrombosis is suspected clinically, anticoagulant therapy is given if the test is positive and withheld if the test is negative.[29] Because calf vein thrombi do occasionally propagate into the large proximal veins, serial IPGs have been employed to detect thrombus extension; the use of serial examinations has increased the diagnostic accuracy of this procedure, which may be comparable to that of venography.[30] IPG test results return to normal in almost all patients after nine months; follow-up examinations are therefore helpful for evaluating those with suspected recurrences.[31] Although impedance plethysmography is noninvasive and can be done in an outpatient setting, the inconvenience and cost of serial tests need to be weighed in the decision-making process.

Most patients with acute deep venous thrombosis escape the sequelae of edema, pigmentation, and ulceration. Patency and valvular competency in the distal deep veins suggest a favorable prognosis.[32] Patients in whom the postphlebitic syndrome develops complain of gradually progressive leg pain and swelling, especially after prolonged standing and walking. Physicians may need to perform objective tests in such patients to distinguish sudden exacerbations of symptoms from acute deep venous thrombosis.

Squamous cell and basal cell carcinomas and malignant fibrous histiocytomas are rare complications of chronic ulcerations caused by venous stasis.[33] These neoplasms are potentially curable if recognized early; therefore, biopsy should be considered in the presence of suspicious lesions.

Pulmonary Embolism

Pulmonary emboli may have a very subtle presentation and are easily missed, especially in the elderly. Symptoms include apprehension, hyperventilation, weakness, faintness or syncope, dyspnea, and oppressive substernal pain that is indistinguishable from the pain of myocardial infarction. The triad of cough, hemoptysis, and pleuritic pain signals that embolism has produced infarction, often hours or even days after the embolus first formed.

When the emboli produce pulmonary artery hypertension, the signs of acute cor pulmonale are noted, including distended neck veins, tachycardia, accentuated and split pulmonic closure sound, Kussmaul's sign (distention of the jugular veins on inspiration), and pulsus paradoxus (exaggerated fall in blood pressure with inspiration). Sustained systemic hypotension and signs of shock indicate the presence of a massive pulmonary embolus; if such findings persist after the start of therapy, the prognosis is ominous. Auscultation of the lungs often discloses wheezes. When pulmonary infarction occurs, the signs of consolidation or effusion, temperature of up to 39° C (102.2° F), and rales may be found.

Bland infarction occasionally leads to cavitation, which may be complicated by bacterial superinfection, often with gram-negative organisms. The cavitation occurs quickly and is associated with fever, purulent sputum, and granulocytosis.

Laboratory Findings

If a case of pulmonary embolism begins with substernal pain, continuous electrocardiographic monitoring should be done to exclude acute myocardial infarction. Other tests to confirm the diagnosis and monitor anticoagulation therapy can then be performed.

Blood gases Typically, in pulmonary embolism the arterial P_{O_2} is below 80 mm Hg and the P_{CO_2} is below 40 mm Hg while the patient is breathing room air. The alveolar-arterial oxygen gradient may be either normal or increased.[34] The hyperventilation that follows pulmonary embolism is responsible for the low P_{CO_2} and the associated mild respiratory alkalemia. The blood gas findings must be interpreted cautiously; probably 10 to 15 percent of patients with pulmonary emboli have arterial oxygen tensions greater than 80 mm Hg. Furthermore, there is also a host of other causes of hypoxemia and hypocapnia.

Scintigraphy The diagnostic utility of combined ventilation-perfusion (V/Q) scanning has provoked controversy since its inception. Various criteria have been developed to increase its predictive value.[35,36] A multicenter study involving more than 900 patients, the Prospective Investigation of Pulmonary Embolism Diagnosis (PIOPED), determined the sensitivities and specificities of V/Q scanning for pulmonary embolism as documented by arteriography.[37] Scans were classified as normal or as indicating a high, intermediate, low, or very low probability of pulmonary embolism [see Tables 1 and 2]. Almost all patients with pulmonary embolism had abnormal scans, ranging from low to high probability. Scans were also abnormal in most patients in whom pulmonary embolism was clinically suspected but later excluded. Thus, the sensitivity of scanning is high (98 percent), but the specificity is low (10 percent). High-probability scans were associated with pulmonary embolism in 88 percent of the instances; however, fewer than half of patients with pulmonary embolism had high-probability scans (sensitivity, 41 percent; specificity, 97 percent). Thirty-three percent of the patients who had intermediate-probability scans had pulmonary embolism, and 12 percent of the patients with low-probability scans had pulmonary embolism. Clinicians should be alert to possible pulmonary embolism in patients with low-probability scans; such scans do not rule out the diagnosis.[38] Although it was widely believed that a normal lung scan ruled out the diagnosis, PIOPED

Table 1   PIOPED* Central Scan Interpretation Categories and Criteria

Category	*Scan Pattern*
High probability of pulmonary embolism	Two or more large (>75% of a segment) segmental perfusion defects that lack corresponding ventilation or roentgenographic abnormalities or that are substantially larger than either matching ventilation or chest roentgenographic abnormalities
	Two or more moderate segmental (25%–75% of a segment) perfusion defects without matching ventilation or chest roentgenographic abnormalities and one large mismatched segmental defect
	Four or more moderate segmental perfusion defects without ventilation or chest roentgenographic abnormalities
Intermediate (indeterminate) probability of pulmonary embolism	Does not fall into the categories of normal, very low, low, or high probability
	Borderline high or borderline low probability
	Difficult to categorize as low or high probability
Low probability of pulmonary embolism	Nonsegmental perfusion defects (e.g., very small effusion causing blunting of the costophrenic angle; cardiomegaly; enlarged aorta, hila, and mediastinum; and elevated diaphragm)
	Single moderate mismatched segmental perfusion defect with normal chest roentgenogram
	Any perfusion defect with a substantially larger chest roentgenographic abnormality
	Large or moderate segmental perfusion defects involving no more than four segments in one lung and no more than three segments in one lung region, with matching ventilation defects that are as large as or larger than the perfusion defects and a chest x-ray that either is normal or shows abnormalities that are substantially smaller than the perfusion defects
	More than three small segmental perfusion defects (<25% of a segment) with a normal chest roentgenogram
Very low probability of pulmonary embolism	Three or fewer small segmental perfusion defects with a normal chest roentgenogram
Normal	No perfusion defects present
	Perfusion outlines exactly the shape of the lungs as seen on the chest roentgenogram (hilar and aortic impressions may be seen; chest roentgenogram, ventilation study, or both may be abnormal)

*PIOPED—Prospective Investigation of Pulmonary Embolism Diagnosis

Table 2 Sensitivity and Specificity of PIOPED Scan Category as Indicated by Angiographic Findings

Scan Category	Sensitivity (%)	Specificity (%)
High probability of pulmonary embolism	41	97
High or intermediate probability of pulmonary embolism	82	52
High, intermediate, or low probability of pulmonary embolism	98	10

investigators found that four percent of normal or near-normal scans were associated with pulmonary embolism.

Combining the results of clinical assessment and lung scanning was helpful. When the clinical impression and the scan both indicated a high probability of pulmonary embolism, the condition was present in 96 percent of instances (28 of 29 patients). When the clinical impression and the scan both indicated a low probability, the diagnosis was correctly excluded in 96 percent of cases (86 of 90 patients). Because such concordance between clinical impressions and scan results is not usual, pulmonary arteriography is often required for diagnosis.[39]

Arteriography If the diagnosis remains in doubt, the method of greatest sensitivity and specificity for pulmonary embolism is pulmonary arteriography. Specific findings include filling defects, prunings, and cutoffs. Other findings that suggest pulmonary embolism are oligemia, asymmetric filling, lower-zone delay, and prolonged arterial phase.[40]

Pulmonary arteriography is the reference standard for the diagnosis of pulmonary embolism. However, because of its cost and associated morbidity, it cannot be used in every case of suspected pulmonary embolism.

A decision to treat suspected pulmonary embolism with anticoagulants on the basis of lower extremity studies and ambiguous scintigraphic findings leaves the explanation of the presenting chest complaints in doubt. In some circumstances, arteriography is required to settle the issue. If the embolus is present in large or segmental vessels, selective arteriography is reliable, but the interpretation of lesions involving subsegmental vessels is often problematic.[41]

Intravenous digital subtraction pulmonary arteriography may prove to be an acceptable substitute for the more invasive conventional method in many cases of deep venous thrombosis.[42]

Chest x-ray Nonspecific chest x-ray abnormalities develop in about 45 percent of patients who have angiographically proven emboli.[43] The time it takes for abnormalities to appear ranges from a few hours to a few days, averaging about two days.[44] Infiltrates, pleura-based consolidations, effusions, decreased vascular branches, and the radiologic signs of acute cor pulmonale—dilated hilar arteries, distention of the superior vena cava and the azygos vein, and dilatation of the right side of the heart—are characteristic in patients with deep venous thrombi. Computed tomography detects areas of attenuation not apparent on conventional x-rays, but it adds little to the diagnostic workup.

Electrocardiographic findings ECG changes are usually sought, but they are not likely to be helpful diagnostically except in cases of severe pulmonary embolism in which the hemodynamic disturbance is profound enough to cause acute cor pulmonale. In such cases, any of the following can be found: sinus tachycardia, atrial flutter or fibrillation, peaked P waves, right-axis shift, clockwise rotation, incomplete or complete right bundle branch block, or a deep S_I and a prominent Q_{III} with inversion of T_{III}. The ECG is mainly used to help promptly distinguish between massive pulmonary embolus and acute myocardial infarction.

Serum enzyme changes A delayed, nonspecific elevation of the serum level of lactic dehydrogenase (LDH) isoenzyme 3 occurs in about 80 percent of cases of pulmonary embolism. Serum aspartate aminotransferase (AST, formerly termed SGOT) levels and the myocardial fraction of creatine kinase (CK-MB) tend to remain normal in patients with pulmonary embolism.

A Management Strategy

A prospective, comparative study of 874 consecutive patients with suspected pulmonary embolism has shown that patients with abnormal, but not high-probability, lung scans and negative serial objective tests for proximal venous thrombosis have a good prognosis without anticoagulant therapy.[45]

Prevention

General Measures

Venous stasis should be avoided. Patients who are at high risk for venous thrombosis should exercise their legs by repeatedly flexing and extending their ankles and feet. These exercises empty the veins of the lower leg. The knees should also be frequently flexed and extended. Patients who are in discomfort can usually perform this exercise by sliding their heels back and forth between the foot of the bed and the buttocks.

It is essential to explain these exercises to the patient before the period of expected immobility. A wise practice is to teach the exercises to the patient and other family members the night before an elective surgical procedure is performed, with emphasis on their importance. Family members can then assist with passive exercises during the first hours of drowsiness after the patient returns from the recovery room.

Properly fitted, carefully applied elastic stockings that provide graded compression from ankle to thigh decrease venous stasis and reduce the incidence (from 49 percent to 23 percent) of isotopically diagnosed deep venous thrombosis in patients undergoing major surgery.[46] Such stockings, which need not be custom-made, are safe and effective when applied preoperatively; the protective effect appears to be additive to that of low-dose heparin. Proper fit and positioning are essential; arterial thromboses have occurred when stockings were applied incorrectly.[47] Stockings are inexpensive and, in many situations, the most cost-effective prophylactic measure.[48] The role of external pneumatic calf compression is being assessed.[49] This method has been shown to be useful in patients undergoing neurosurgical procedures or total hip replacement.[50,51]

Evaluating the Patient for Anticoagulation

Before therapy, the risk of anticoagulation should be assessed. Anticoagulants should be used with caution or avoided if there is a history of abnormal bleeding, recent peptic ulcer or esophageal bleeding, corticosteroid therapy, recent intraocular or intracranial bleeding, or recent pericarditis. The patient should be asked about the use of antiplatelet agents (e.g., aspirin and dipyridamole) and nonsteroidal anti-inflammatory agents.

Except in dire emergencies, hemostatic competence should be assessed with complete blood count and description of platelet morphology, platelet count, partial thromboplastin time, prothrombin time, and, in some instances, standardized bleeding time.

Anticoagulation during Pregnancy

Thromboembolic disease in pregnancy creates vexing diagnostic and therapeutic problems. Venous thrombosis is common, and pulmonary embolism is a leading cause of maternal mortality.[52] Evaluating the patient can be difficult because distended, aching, and tender lower extremity veins, varicosities, and edema may occur in the absence of venous thrombosis. Real-time B-mode ultrasonography is insensitive to an isolated iliac vein thrombus (the results of studies with color imaging are awaited), and ascending venography exposes the fetus to radiation. A prospective study of 152 pregnant patients suspected of having deep venous thrombosis has shown that anticoagulation can be safely withheld if serial impedance plethysmograms are normal. False positive results occur during late pregnancy when the patient is examined in the supine position; therefore, the patient should be examined in the lateral decubitus position, and care should be taken to ensure optimal venous filling.[53]

Anticoagulant therapy during pregnancy also poses significant problems. Warfarin crosses the placenta and affects the fetus, in addition to being associated with hemorrhagic complications. An embryopathy (nasal hypoplasia, altered bone growth, and stippled epiphyses) has been clearly attributed to coumarin derivatives; the critical period for exposure appears to be between the sixth week and the 12th week of gestation.[54] The same embryopathy has been observed in a child with a congenital deficiency of multiple vitamin K–dependent procoagulants. This finding suggests that the malformations are the result of impaired posttranslational carboxylation of glutamyl residues of noncoagulant proteins.[55]

Far less common are such serious fetal central nervous system abnormalities as mental retardation, blindness, deafness, spasticity, and seizures. These defects appear to be unrelated to any critical period of exposure and may be associated with warfarin administration during the second and third trimesters. Various congenital ocular abnormalities have also been reported after warfarin therapy.[56] In a series of 418 pregnancies, one sixth of patients treated with coumarin derivatives were delivered of abnormal live-born infants, another sixth of the pregnancies ended in abortion or stillbirth, and two thirds of the patients gave birth to apparently normal infants.[54]

Heparin does not cross the placenta, and the use of this agent during pregnancy may offer advantages over warfarin administration. However, in a series of 135 cases, about one eighth of the pregnancies ended in stillbirth, and one fifth of the mothers gave birth to premature infants, one third of whom died; in two thirds of the cases, neither the infants nor the mothers appeared to suffer any ill effects.[54] In a series of 37 pregnancies in 35 women who were receiving heparin, 25 of the pregnancies were uncomplicated, and premature labor occurred in seven; other problems included retained placenta, premature detachment of the placenta, and minor hematomas. Serious bleeding did not occur, and the treatment did not appear to harm the offspring.[57] A retrospective study of heparin therapy in 77 women, involving 98 pregnancies that were complicated by venous thromboembolism and two pregnancies that were complicated by prosthetic heart valves, found that the rates of prematurity, abortion, stillbirth, neonatal death, and congenital abnormalities were similar to those in the general population. There were two bleeding episodes and no instances of thrombosis.[58]

Adjusted-dose heparin therapy is probably the preferred method of long-term anticoagulation during pregnancy. The dose of heparin, which is administered subcutaneously every 12 hours, is adjusted to maintain the activated partial thromboplastin time (APTT), which is measured six hours after injection, at one and one-half times the control value [*see* Treatment, Long-term Anticoagulation, *below*].[59]

Warfarin appears not to be excreted in human breast milk, and there probably is no significant risk of anticoagulating breast-fed infants in this way.[60]

Specific Preventive Therapy for Venous Thromboembolism

In 1986, the National Conference on Antithrombotic Therapy made the recommendations that follow; whenever possible, these conclusions were based on rigorously controlled investigations.[61] New studies may produce significant modifications of these recommendations.

1. Moderate-risk patients. Preventive therapy for patients judged to be at moderate risk for thromboembolism consists of low-dose heparin (5,000 units subcutaneously every 12 hours) or intermittent pneumatic compression.[61]
2. Neurosurgical procedures, urologic surgery, and major knee surgery. Patients undergoing neurosurgery or urologic or major knee surgery should be treated with intermittent pneumatic compression.[61] A randomized trial has since shown that graduated compression stockings, alone or in combination with intermittent pneumatic compression, reduce the risk of deep venous thrombosis in neurosurgical patients.[50]
3. Elective hip surgery. Patients undergoing elective hip surgery should receive prophylaxis with adjusted-dose heparin to prolong the APTT to a value in the upper half of the normal range or with moderate-dose warfarin to prolong the prothrombin time to 1.2 to 1.5 times the control value (using rabbit-brain thromboplastin).[61] The World Health Organization has introduced a system for international standardization of the prothrombin time, using a unit termed the international normalized ratio (INR).[62] For elective hip surgery, the recommended INR is 2.0 to 3.0. A randomized trial involving 194 patients has shown that postoperative therapy with warfarin (INR, 2.0 to 2.7) or with aspirin (650 mg, in enteric-coated tablets, twice a day) reduces the risk of proximal venous thrombosis or pulmonary embolism.[63]
4. Patients with hip fracture. Patients undergoing surgery for hip fracture should receive prophylactic therapy with moderate-dose warfarin to prolong the prothrombin time to 1.2 to 1.5 times the control value (using rabbit-brain thromboplastin) or to produce an INR of 2.0 to 3.0.[61] Studies have suggested that the administration of warfarin and antithrombin III (AT-III) together with low-dose heparin exerts prophylactic action in patients undergoing total hip arthroplasty.[64,65] A randomized trial involving 310 patients has demonstrated that intermittent pneumatic leg compression reduces the risk of venographically proven deep venous thromboses from 49 percent to 24 percent.[51] Combined plethysmography and ^{125}I-fibrinogen scanning was insensitive in 46 percent of patients with deep venous thrombosis; venography was required to detect thrombosis in these patients.[51]

An analysis of more than 70 randomized trials involving 16,000 patients who had undergone general, elective or traumatic orthopedic, or urologic surgery has demonstrated that the perioperative use of subcutaneous heparin reduced the incidence of pulmonary embolism by one half and the incidence of deep venous thrombosis by two thirds.[66] The high risk of thromboembolism during the first two months after spinal cord injury can be reduced by adjusted-dose heparin therapy, but the risk of bleeding in these patients is high.[67]

Other Preventive Measures

A National Institutes of Health consensus development panel also issued recommendations for preventive therapy in 1986.[68] In addition to the measures already described, the panel recommended the use of gradient elastic stockings, dextran, and dihydroergotamine in combination with heparin. Aspirin was not found to be beneficial. The NIH panel called attention to the need for tailoring prophylactic therapy according to the patient's disease and degree of risk.

Treatment

Deep Venous Thrombosis

Prompt administration of intravenous heparin is indicated for deep venous thrombosis.[69] Heparin works immediately, prevents further thrombus formation, and, in therapeutic doses, prevents the release of serotonin and thromboxane A_2 from platelets adherent to thrombi that embolize to the lungs. These vasoactive substances are suspected mediators of the intense pulmonary arteriolar vasoconstriction that results in sudden and severe pulmonary artery hypertension, acute right-sided hemodynamic failure, and cardiogenic shock; the last disorder, if it is prolonged, is usually fatal. Heparin's rapid action in preventing thrombus propagation and in blocking platelet release is the rationale for its immediate intravenous use.

The half-life of a therapeutic dose of intravenous heparin is usually about 90 minutes, but it varies directly with the size of the dose.[70] Acute pulmonary embolism probably shortens the half-life; renal failure and cirrhosis may lengthen it.[70] Heparin can be given either by intermittent injections into an indwelling intravenous cannula or by pump-driven infusion at a constant rate.

Therapy should begin with an initial priming dose of about 5,000 units of heparin administered as a bolus. Thereafter, most patients require about 1,000 U/hr. The exact effective dosage varies with the patient's weight and is influenced by unknown factors. Heparin requirements tend to be highest during the first three days of therapy. A circadian variation in the effect of heparin on the activated partial thromboplastin time, the thrombin time, and the factor Xa inhibition assay has been described; maximum anticoagulation activity has been observed at night and minimum activity in the morning.[71] The APTT is the test most widely used to monitor the effects of heparin. The end-point prolongation should be 1.5 to 2.0 times the control value. Excellent results have also been obtained by monitoring the whole-blood activated coagulation time (ACT).[72]

Heparin is usually given for seven to 10 days. In one study, a five-day course of heparin was found to be as effective as a 10-day course of the drug.[73] The optimal time to begin oral anticoagulation with warfarin is uncertain. Data suggest that early warfarin therapy, started within three days of initial heparinization, shortens the length of hospitalization and is probably as effective and safe as therapy begun after three days.[74]

Although intravenous administration of heparin is generally preferred, the National Conference on Antithrombotic Therapy also recommended subcutaneous heparin therapy for deep venous thrombosis, and one randomized trial found adjusted-dose subcutaneous heparin (initial dose of 15,000 units, with subsequent doses adjusted to prolong the APTT to 50 to 70 seconds) to be as effective and safe as continuous I.V. therapy.[61,75]

Heparin solutions contain a collection of mucopolysaccharides with molecular weights that range from 2,000 to 40,000 daltons. Only some of these polymers, however, have anticoagulant activity. The lower-molecular-weight molecules appear to be therapeutically potent and safe, and they also display high bioavailability.[76,77] In addition, low-molecular-weight heparin has a longer half-life than conventional heparin.[77] In one double-blind study, fixed-dose low-molecular-weight heparin given once a day subcutaneously was found to be as effective and safe as adjusted-dose heparin given by continuous I.V. infusion in the treatment of proximal vein thrombosis.[77] A similar result was reported in another study, in which subcutaneous low-molecular-weight heparin was given every 12 hours.[78]

Warfarin interferes with the γ-carboxylation of glutamic acid residues in the vitamin K–dependent synthesis of factors II, VII, IX, and X in liver mitochondria.[79] The drug is completely absorbed and is predominantly protein-bound in the plasma (only three percent is free), where its half-life is 42 hours. It is degraded in the liver, and its metabolites, which are inactive, are excreted in the urine and stool.[80] Warfarin will not affect procoagulant proteins already formed in the liver and released into the circulation. The half-life of some of these factors is longer than 24 hours, and several days are usually required to achieve effective anticoagulation. The anticoagulant response to warfarin is increased in the elderly.[81]

Warfarin is administered in a single daily dose, usually 2.5 to 10.0 mg, to prolong the prothrombin time to 1.2 to 1.5 times the control value (using rabbit-brain thromboplastin) or to produce an INR of 2.0 to 3.0.[61] If oral anticoagulants are contraindicated or inconvenient, adjusted-dose subcutaneous heparin can be given every 12 hours in doses that prolong the APTT to 1.5 times the control value at the mid-dosing interval.[61,82]

Long-term Anticoagulation

The proper duration of anticoagulation therapy has not been established. Oral anticoagulation that is continued for a period of three months significantly reduces the rate of recurrence of venous thrombosis.[83] Treatment should be given for longer periods in cases of major pulmonary infarction or recurrence and should probably be continued indefinitely for those patients in whom pulmonary hypertension develops.[84]

The risk of bleeding may be as high as 20 percent during prolonged treatment with previously recommended doses of warfarin. If the dose is reduced so that the prothrombin time (using rabbit-brain thromboplastin) is approximately 15 seconds, or 1.25 times the control value, the bleeding complication rate is reduced to about five percent, and the thromboembolism recurrence rate is only about two percent.[85]

Table 3   Warfarin Antagonists and Potentiators

Antagonists	Potentiators
Vitamin K	Phenylbutazone
Barbiturates	Oxyphenbutazone
Glutethimide	Anabolic steroids
Rifampin	Clofibrate
Cholestyramine (when administered with warfarin)	Aspirin
	Hepatotoxins
	Disulfiram
	Metronidazole
	Cimetidine
	Amiodarone
	Miconazole
	Third-generation cephalosporins
	Tamoxifen

Long-term, self-administered subcutaneous heparin taken in low doses (5,000 units every 12 hours) very rarely causes bleeding, but it appears to be associated with a recurrence rate as high as 47 percent. When the heparin dose is adjusted to maintain the activated partial thromboplastin time (measured six hours after injection) at 1.5 times the control value, the recurrence rate is reduced to about four percent, and the frequency of bleeding is reduced to less than two percent.[85]

An analysis of the cost-effectiveness of the various approaches to long-term anticoagulation indicates that the reduced-dose warfarin regimen is the optimal approach and is preferred by most patients,[59] except during pregnancy, when adjusted-dose heparin therapy is probably safer.

A number of drugs interact significantly with warfarin [*see Table 3*].[80,86] Hereditary resistance to warfarin, transmitted as an autosomal dominant trait, has been well documented; patients who have such resistance may require 10-fold increases in dosage to maintain a therapeutic effect.[87] Warfarin resistance has also been observed in patients who eat excessive quantities of vitamin K–rich vegetables, such as broccoli.[88]

Complications of Anticoagulation Therapy

Major bleeding may occur during heparinization (usually after 48 hours); such bleeding is especially hazardous if it occurs intracranially. The risk of bleeding is dose related and is higher in women, in severely ill patients, in individuals who consume large amounts of alcohol, and in individuals who take heparin and aspirin concurrently. Patients with thrombocytopenia and patients given intramuscular heparin injections are also at increased risk. The action of heparin can be terminated almost immediately by the intravenous injection, milligram for milligram, of protamine sulfate (10,000 units of heparin is equivalent to about a 100 mg dose). Protamine sulfate should be administered by slow intravenous injection, usually lasting for one to three minutes. Adverse reactions to protamine (rash, urticaria, bronchospasm, pulmonary hypertension, hypotension, and death) are more common in diabetic patients who have received protamine insulin and have developed antiprotamine antibodies.[89] In nondiabetic patients, antiprotamine antibodies increase the risk of adverse reactions to protamine, but some nondiabetic patients who have reactions do not carry antiprotamine antibodies.[89]

Bleeding during oral anticoagulation with warfarin should call attention to the possibility of a previously silent lesion, even when there has been excessive depression of the prothrombin complex. When prompt control of the bleeding is required, hemostatic concentrations of factors II, VII, IX, and X can usually be established by the rapid infusion of 500 to 600 ml of plasma, repeated every six hours. Vitamin K_1 is indicated when there is less urgency; it can be given intravenously, intramuscularly, or subcutaneously. The dose varies from 5 to 25 mg, and when it is given intravenously, the infusion rate should not exceed 5 mg/min. Vitamin K_1 should be diluted only with 0.9 percent saline or with five percent dextrose in water or saline. No other substances should be present in the diluent when the agent is given intravenously. A period of resistance to warfarin will occur after the administration of vitamin K_1.

Heparin-induced thrombocytopenia occurs in three to 30 percent of patients receiving therapeutic doses. It is probably more common with bovine lung heparin than with intestinal mucosa heparin and may be dose related. A complement-mediated immune mechanism may be responsible.[90-94] The platelet count may fall within hours after heparin is given, but usually, thrombocytopenia occurs two to eight days later and promptly reverses, often within a day, after the drug is stopped. The platelet count occasionally falls below $50,000/mm^3$. Dangerous hemorrhagic and arterial thrombotic complications may develop; these risks argue for monitoring the platelet count.[93] The incidence of such events with low-dose heparin is unknown but may be less than that with usual therapeutic doses.[95,96] Heparin-dependent immune injury to endothelial cells may play a role in the thrombocytopenia and arterial thromboses.

Rare but serious complications of heparin therapy include anaphylaxis, vertebral fractures secondary to osteoporosis (after prolonged administration), arterial thromboses, and hyperkalemia.[69,97-99] Hyperkalemia, which has been noted in association with low-dose as well as usual-dose therapy, may be the result of heparin-induced hypoaldosteronism. This unusual complication appears more likely to occur in patients who have diabetes mellitus or renal insufficiency. Necrosis of the skin and subcutaneous tissue has been attributed to the use of both heparin and warfarin.[69,100] The predisposition of individuals with the heterozygous form of protein C deficiency to warfarin-induced skin necrosis is well established and has important implications for therapy. A disorder termed the purple toes syndrome is a result of cholesterol microembolization; its relation to anticoagulation is unknown, but it has been attributed to arterially invasive procedures.[101]

Elevations of serum aminotransferase levels occur in most patients who receive heparin, and they frequently reach abnormal values. The increases, of unknown origin, tend to peak after seven days and may decline despite continued treatment.[102] The covert use of warfarin or heparin may cause factitious bleeding.[103,104] Patients are usually young adult members of the health professions or elderly persons previously given anticoagulants.

An interaction between heparin and nitroglycerin is controversial. Intravenous nitroglycerin has been reported to induce heparin resistance; in healthy adults, however, intravenous nitroglycerin (5 mg) given after intravenous heparin (5,000 units) does not influence heparin's effect on the activated partial thromboplastin time or the thrombin time.[105,106]

Massive Venous Occlusion

Total iliofemoral occlusion is a dire emergency. Rapid swelling ensues, followed by intense arterial constriction, pain, cyanosis, infection, and gangrene. The left lower extremity is involved more often than the right, perhaps because the left common iliac vein is vulnerable to occluding pressure from the right iliac artery.

Treatment should be instituted as soon as possible. There are two approaches that are currently being used. The older approach, emergency thrombectomy, is carried out under heparinization. Thrombolytic therapy is an alternative to surgery and should be instituted before heparin is given (see below). Even when treatment is timely, the patient is often left with chronic smoldering venous occlusive disease. Infection is common and necessitates vigorous antimicrobial therapy.

Thrombosis of the inferior vena cava, usually diagnosed by phlebography, has also been diagnosed by CT.[107] Development of caval thrombosis should prompt a search for neoplasm, especially in the kidney.[108]

Pulmonary Embolism

If pulmonary embolism is suspected, an effort should be made to obtain a sample of arterial blood for gas analysis before giving oxygen by nasal cannula at a rate of 6 to 8 L/min. Morphine sulfate, 10 to 15 mg, or meperidine, 50 to 100 mg, should also be given. Intravenous heparinization should be instituted immediately and continued for seven to 10 days. Anticoagulation regimens, using heparin and warfarin, are the same as those used for deep venous thrombosis (see above).

Massive Pulmonary Embolism

Massive pulmonary embolism is life threatening: large emboli occlude the proximal pulmonary arterial circulation, which results in acute cor pulmonale, cyanosis, and shock. The principal consideration in the differential diagnosis is myocardial infarction, which can often be recognized by electrocardiography.

If the electrocardiogram favors the diagnosis of massive pulmonary embolism, large doses of intravenous heparin should

be given, along with morphine and oxygen. If shock persists for more than half an hour despite these measures, the outlook is very poor. Pulmonary arteriography should be performed immediately. If it confirms the presence of massive pulmonary emboli, urgent action is needed. The life of a moribund patient can occasionally be saved by emergency pulmonary embolectomy or by transvenous suction-catheter extraction of emboli.[109] The inferior vena cava is usually interrupted at the conclusion of surgical embolectomy (see below). The other intervention that can be tried is thrombolytic therapy, which has been reported to be associated with prompt reversal of the life-threatening syndrome.[110]

Interruption of the Vena Cava

Caval interruption may be required if repetitive life-threatening pulmonary emboli arise from thrombi below the renal veins despite adequate and prolonged intravenous heparin therapy. A compelling contraindication to anticoagulant treatment, such as recent intracranial injury, may also necessitate interruption of the vena cava. Evaluation of the acute and long-term results of various ligating, plicating, clipping, balloon-occluding, and filtering procedures indicates that these interventions carry significant risks.[111,112] Although the intravascular approach circumvents the hazards of laparotomy, it may result in incisional and retroperitoneal bleeding, penetration of the vein wall, misplacement or dislodgment of the device, and total caval occlusion. Both closed and open procedures may be followed by dependent edema, recurrent thromboses, and pulmonary embolism. A valid study comparing these procedures has not been done.[113] The significance of the high rate of perioperative morbidity and mortality associated with caval interruption is difficult to assess in this high-risk group of patients. The extent to which thrombolytic therapy will replace caval interruption in the management of recurrent pulmonary embolism is unknown.

Inferior vena cava filters are often employed instead of anticoagulants for the treatment of venous thromboembolism in patients with cerebral neoplasms because of concern that these patients are at high risk for anticoagulant-associated complications. However, anticoagulation therapy has been used successfully in patients with primary and metastatic brain tumors.[114]

Prognosis

A multicenter study of 399 patients with pulmonary embolism found that only 2.5 percent died of this disorder.[115] Recurrent pulmonary embolism was recognized in 8.3 percent; of this group, 45 percent died during a one-year follow-up period. Of all patients with pulmonary embolism, 23.8 percent died within one year; these deaths were associated with neoplasm, left-sided congestive heart failure, and chronic lung disease. The most common causes of death in patients with pulmonary embolism were neoplasm (34.7 percent), infection (22.1 percent), and cardiac disease (16.8 percent).[115]

Data suggest that complete resolution occurs in about two thirds of all survivors and partial resolution in about one fourth. Chronic pulmonary arterial occlusion occasionally leads to exercise-induced or sustained pulmonary hypertension and, rarely, to cor pulmonale.[116,117] Perfusion scans may underestimate the severity of the hemodynamic disorder in patients with chronic thromboembolic pulmonary hypertension.[118] Proximal obstructions present as pulmonary emboli, whereas distal obstructions present as pulmonary hypertension. Proximal emboli may be amenable to thromboendarterectomy, and distal disease may respond to vasodilators. Some physicians are reluctant to use pulmonary angiography in patients with pulmonary hypertension and right-sided heart failure, but the procedure was performed safely in a group of 67 such patients, and useful anatomic data were obtained.[119] Long-term anticoagulation should be instituted in patients with chronic pulmonary artery occlusive disease,[83] but the prognosis is often poor. Fiberoptic angioscopy has been used to determine surgical resectability.[120]

Thrombolytic Therapy

Although the risks and benefits of thrombolytic therapy are not entirely clear, this approach is suitable for the management of massive pulmonary embolism, submassive pulmonary embolism with shock, and severe deep venous thrombosis.[121] Three thrombolytic agents are available for intravenous use in the treatment of thromboembolism: urokinase, which is harvested from human fetal kidney cells and cleaves plasminogen to plasmin; streptokinase, which is derived from streptococci and complexes with and activates plasminogen; and recombinant tissue plasminogen activator (rt-PA). These agents may hasten thrombus dissolution, but they also lyse hemostatic fibrin and may cause hemorrhage. In addition, the nonrecombinant agents are pyrogens and potential allergens, especially streptokinase, which has been associated with anaphylaxis. Skin testing for sensitivity to streptokinase is undergoing evaluation.[122,123]

Thrombolytic agents rapidly induce a lytic state after infusion, shown by a decreased level of clottable plasma protein (fibrinogen), the appearance of fibrin-fibrinogen split products, a decrease in the whole-blood euglobulin lysis time, and prolongation of the thrombin time and the reptilase time.

Hemostatic competence before treatment should be assessed with thrombin time, partial thromboplastin time, prothrombin time, fibrinogen level, hematocrit, and platelet count. Some experts also measure the fibrin D dimer level to exclude the presence of disseminated intravascular coagulation [see Chapter 14]. Before therapy is started, the thrombin time and the partial thromboplastin time should be less than twice the normal control values.

The thrombolytic agents are most effective when given as soon as possible (within seven days) after onset of the thromboembolic event. The usual loading dose of streptokinase is 250,000 units given intravenously over a period of 30 minutes, followed by 100,000 U/hr. Urokinase is given in an initial loading dose of 4,400 U/kg (2,000 U/lb) over a 10-minute period, followed by a continuous infusion of 4,400 U/kg/hr (2,000 U/lb/hr) for 12 hours. Recombinant human tissue-type plasminogen activator has been administered to patients with massive pulmonary embolism and shock in a dose of 100 mg infused into a peripheral vein over a period of two to three hours.[124] The optimal duration of thrombolytic therapy in treating pulmonary embolism is uncertain, but urokinase is used for a period of 12 hours and streptokinase for 24 hours. Treatment of deep venous thrombosis has been continued for as long as 72 hours, but a shorter course may be effective; streptokinase is the only thrombolytic agent that has been approved for use in deep venous thrombosis.

Thrombolytic agents and anticoagulants should not be given together. If heparin has been used, the thrombolytic agent should be withheld until the thrombin time is less than twice the normal control value. At the completion of thrombolytic therapy, heparin should be given, provided the thrombin time is less than twice normal.

Suggested contraindications for thrombolytic therapy are based on limited experience. Active internal bleeding and recent stroke (within the past two months) or another active intracranial process are regarded as absolute contraindications. Relative contraindications include recent major surgery (within 10 days), delivery, organ biopsy, and previous puncture of noncompressible vessels; recent serious gastrointestinal bleeding; recent serious trauma; and severe arterial hypertension (systolic $\geq$ 200 mm Hg or diastolic $\geq$ 110 mm Hg). Relative contraindications of a minor nature are recent minor trauma (including cardiopulmonary resuscitation), high likelihood of left heart thrombus (e.g., mitral valve disease with atrial fibrillation), infective endocarditis, hemostatic defects (including those associated with severe hepatic or renal disease), pregnancy, age older than 75 years, and diabetic hemorrhagic retinopathy.[125]

The patient should be kept at bed rest, and vital signs should be monitored frequently. To avoid dislodgment of deep venous thrombi, the blood pressure should not be taken in the lower extremities.

Oozing from injection sites can usually be controlled with local pressure. Arterial blood gas samples should be taken from the upper extremity, followed by digital compression on the puncture site for at least 30 minutes. No other invasive procedures should be performed except for venipunctures with a No. 22 or 23 gauge needle. Major bleeding may require discontinuation of therapy, transfusion of whole blood (preferably fresh) or packed red blood cells together with cryoprecipitate or frozen plasma, and possibly use of ε-aminocaproic acid.

The adult respiratory distress syndrome developed in one patient with massive pulmonary embolism after streptokinase therapy.[126]

Some data suggest that thrombolytic therapy hastens thrombus resolution and preserves the pulmonary microcirculation to a greater extent than heparin treatment.[121,127,128] Results from randomized studies indicate that thrombolysis is achieved 3.7 times more often with streptokinase therapy than with heparin therapy; however, these studies also indicate that major bleeding complications are 2.9 times more common in patients treated with streptokinase than in patients treated with heparin.[129] Because of the risks of thrombolytic therapy, including the estimated one percent risk of cerebral bleeding,[125,130,131] I prefer to use thrombolytic agents only in patients with massive venous occlusion or massive pulmonary embolism. Thrombolytic therapy may also be useful in patients with acute vena caval thrombosis and in patients with renal vein thrombosis, in whom rapid thrombolysis with preservation of renal function can occur after prompt administration of streptokinase or urokinase.[132,133] A central infusion of streptokinase has been used with apparent success in three patients with pulmonary embolism and right atrial thrombi.[134]

The fibrin-selective agent rt-PA has been used to treat proximal venous thrombosis and acute pulmonary embolism.[135-138] In one randomized, controlled trial, this agent appeared to act more rapidly and to be safer than urokinase in the doses employed.[135]

Miscellaneous Thromboembolic Disorders

Chest Wall Thrombi

Thrombosis occasionally arises in the veins of the upper extremities, the anterior chest wall, or the breast (Mondor's disease).[139-141] Sometimes, trauma or stasis is responsible, but the cause is usually not determined. The prognosis is generally good, and supportive therapy is all that is required in most cases.

Mesenteric Vein Thrombosis

Mesenteric vein thrombosis, a rare disorder affecting middle-aged persons, presents with abdominal pain, vomiting, rectal bleeding, and fever. Abdominal examination discloses distention, tenderness, and diminished peristalsis; x-rays may show intestinal obstruction. Leukocytosis and hemoconcentration are typical. Laparotomy reveals small bowel infarction, bloody ascites, and mesenteric vein thrombosis. The mesenteric arteries are normal. Bowel resection is required, after which intravenous heparin is administered. Antithrombin III, protein C, and protein S deficiencies have been reported in some instances; however, the cause is often unknown, and there may be recurrences.[14,142-144]

Hepatic Veno-occlusive Disease

Pyrrolizidine alkaloids found in many plants may cause hepatic veno-occlusive disease. This syndrome is characterized by jaundice, painful hepatomegaly, ascites, and weight gain. In addition to the pyrrolizidines of *Heliotropium*, *Senecio*, and *Crotalaria* species, there are numerous hepatotoxic pyrrolizidine alkaloids in comfrey leaves and roots. Herbal comfrey tea, which is sold in health food stores in the United States, has been implicated in severe perivenular fibrosis.[145]

High-dose chemotherapy, especially with busulfan, has been implicated as the cause of veno-occlusive disease of the liver in one to 20 percent of patients undergoing bone marrow transplantation.[146] Other suspected agents include cyclophosphamide, carmustine (BCNU), and mitoxantrone. Doppler ultrasonography may provide useful diagnostic information.[147]

Antithrombin III Deficiency

Antithrombin III inactivates thrombin (factor IIa) and factors XIIa, XIa, IXa, and Xa. Because its effects are markedly accelerated and potentiated by heparin, AT-III is known as heparin cofactor. AT-III deficiency causes a hypercoagulable state, leading to recurrent thromboses involving the upper and lower extremities and the mesenteric, renal, hepatic, and portal veins as well as the vena cava. Pulmonary embolism occurs in almost half of such episodes, which may appear in early adulthood, either spontaneously or during early pregnancy or after minor trauma or surgery.[148-151]

Familial AT-III deficiency is a serious disorder. It is an autosomal dominant trait that affects males and females equally and is widely distributed throughout the world. A number of different genotypes that can give rise to this deficiency have been identified, and gene deletion has been found in one family.[152] In another variant, the AT-III molecule interacts normally with heparin but fails to bind and inhibit thrombin and factor Xa.[153] Other genetic defects have been identified.[154] Levels of AT-III are usually decreased to 25 to 60 percent of normal. Although many affected individuals are free of clinical problems, thromboembolic disease eventually develops in most cases. Plasma concentrations of AT-III are also diminished after surgery, thromboembolism, or the administration of heparin or estrogens and in some patients with disseminated intravascular coagulation, nephrotic syndrome, vasculitis, stroke, or chronic liver disease. Acquired AT-III deficiency with deep venous thrombosis has occurred in patients with ischemic and ulcerative colitis. Gastrointestinal loss and intravascular consumption of AT-III may account for the syndrome, which abates during remission of the colitis.[155]

Diagnosis of familial AT-III deficiency is based on clinical findings, on individual history and family history, and on AT-III assay. Both immunoassays and functional assays are available. Because immunoassays may not detect some variants, functional assays may be preferable for screening. Because familial AT-III deficiency is rare (one in 2,000 to one in 5,000),[156] probably only a few percent of all patients with thromboembolism have this disorder. Thus, routine use of the assays is debatable, but in high-risk individuals with thromboembolism (the young, those in early pregnancy, or those with a positive family history of spontaneous thrombosis or with thrombosis at an unusual site), assays are indicated both for the patient and for family members. Patients with AT-III levels exceeding 60 percent of normal are not usually predisposed to thrombosis.

Treatment with heparin is ineffective in some patients and may even lower AT-III levels further. AT-III should be infused if there is no response to heparin. Concentrates of the factor have been used for this purpose, but they are not readily available. Fresh frozen plasma is also a source of AT-III, and its administration can reverse heparin insensitivity.[157] AT-III functional activity has been found to persist in whole blood stored at 2° C to 6° C for 42 days.[158] Warfarin should be administered as soon as a thromboembolic episode occurs, and in many cases, it should be continued indefinitely thereafter. One group of investigators performed a literature review to assess the prevalence of thrombosis in AT-III–deficient kindreds and concluded that because of the unsatisfactory quality of the available evidence, no firm recommendations could be made regarding the advisability of lifetime anticoagulation in asymptomatic carriers.[159] Study of a large Canadian kindred with AT-III–Hamilton deficiency indicated that lifelong prophylaxis is not warranted for asymptomatic carriers of that specific defect.[159] The role of thrombolytic therapy in the management of AT-III deficiency and thromboembolism is undetermined.

Danazol administration has produced significant increases in AT-III levels in some patients.[160] The agent may prove useful in preparing patients for surgery or as an alternative to long-term anticoagulation in patients with AT-III deficiency.[161] Preoperative prophylaxis with AT-III concentrate may prevent thromboembolism; dextran has also been used for this purpose.[162]

Protein C Deficiency

Protein C is the precursor of a potent, naturally occurring anticoagulant.[163] It is synthesized in the liver in a process that requires vitamin K. Thrombin converts protein C to a serine protease that inhibits activated coagulation factors V and VIII:C and that stimulates fibrinolysis. Contact of protein C with the endothelial cell surface accelerates its conversion to an active form [*see Chapter 14*].[163,164]

A number of kindreds have been described in which hereditary protein C deficiency was transmitted as an autosomal dominant trait. Individuals who are homozygous for the trait display virtual absence of the anticoagulant and have succumbed to neonatal thromboses.[165] One infant with purpura fulminans was successfully managed with infusions of fresh frozen plasma for eight months; thereafter, the plasma infusions were gradually withdrawn as warfarin therapy was instituted.[162] Heterozygous individuals have variably diminished levels of protein C; most remain asymptomatic, although some experience venous thromboembolism in early adult life.[163,166,167] Protein C deficiencies have been associated with splanchnic venous thrombosis.[168] The thrombotic episodes occur spontaneously or after minor trauma or surgery. One patient with protein C deficiency has had recurrent humeral artery thrombosis.[169] Causes of diminished levels of protein C include liver disease, disseminated intravascular coagulation, and warfarin therapy.[170]

The long-term administration of warfarin to patients deficient in protein C has been thought to reduce the frequency of thrombotic episodes, and withdrawal of the drug has been associated with recurrences.[171] However, because warfarin can induce skin necrosis (see below) and because the synthesis of protein C is a vitamin K–dependent process, optimal treatment may prove to be long-term, adjusted-dose subcutaneous heparin. In one case, danazol restored protein C to nearly normal levels but produced no change in protein C activity.[172]

Several cases of skin necrosis have been reported in individuals with protein C deficiency who were receiving warfarin.[173] Any area of the skin may be involved, but there appears to be a predilection for the skin of the penis. The process begins as painful erythema during the first week of oral anticoagulation and quickly progresses to hemorrhagic necrosis. Because protein C antigen levels fall more rapidly after warfarin administration than the levels of coagulation factors II, IX, and X, it has been proposed that warfarin induces a transient hypercoagulable state in these individuals.[173] Suggested management includes the prompt administration of vitamin K_1 to terminate the action of warfarin and the administration of heparin to treat the original thrombotic disorder. Heparinization followed by modest doses of warfarin may reduce the risk of skin necrosis in those predisposed to this complication.[173] Protein C levels can be assayed in patients given warfarin.[174]

Protein S Deficiency

Protein S is a vitamin K–dependent cofactor for protein C [*see Chapter 14*]. Protein S deficiency is inherited as an autosomal dominant trait. Clinical manifestations of the disorder include superficial and deep venous thromboses and pulmonary embolism. Thromboses have occurred in the axillary, mesenteric, and cerebral veins and often appear spontaneously.[141] Protein S deficiency has been reported in association with the nephrotic syndrome.[175] Long-term oral anticoagulation has been effective in preventing episodes of venous thrombosis.[176] Two adults with partial deficiencies of this cofactor have remained asymptomatic.[177,178]

Hyperhomocysteinemia

The usual cause of homocystinuria is an autosomal recessive hereditary deficiency of cystathionine β-synthase, although defects in absorption or metabolism of vitamin B_{12} and deficiency of 5,10-methylenetetrahydrofolate reductase can also produce this disorder.[179] Cystathionine β-synthase catalyzes the conversion of homocysteine to cystathionine, which is subsequently converted to cysteine. Deficiency of cystathionine β-synthase results in an increased concentration of homocysteine and its dietary precursor, methionine, in blood (hyperhomocysteinemia) and other body fluids. Homozygotes for this disorder exhibit ectopia lentis, osteoporosis, skeletal abnormalities resembling Marfan's syndrome, and arterial and venous thromboses. About two thirds of homozygotes exhibit mental retardation, and about one fourth of homozygotes die before 30 years of age of occlusive vascular disease.[179]

Studies of obligate heterozygotes for the genetic impairment of cystathionine β-synthase (i.e., the parents of a child proved to be homozygous for the disorder) have revealed that such individuals also have significantly higher serum levels of homocysteine after methionine loading than do control subjects.[180] Furthermore, in a study of 123 patients with premature vascular disease, hyperhomocysteinemia has been found to be associated with arteriosclerotic vascular disease in persons younger than 55 years.[180] Hyperhomocysteinemia was present in 42 percent of those with cerebrovascular disease, 28 percent of those with peripheral vascular disease, and 30 percent of those with coronary artery disease.[180] By contrast, in the general population, only an estimated one to two percent of individuals are heterozygous for this disorder. These findings indicate that hyperhomocysteinemia is an independent risk factor for arteriosclerosis. The degree to which the metabolic defect can be ameliorated in some patients by the restriction of dietary methionine and by the administration of pyridoxine, folic acid, and vitamin B_{12} remains to be determined.

Thromboangiitis Obliterans

A rare form of vasculitis called thrombo-angiitis obliterans (Buerger's disease) involves both arteries and veins, especially those of the lower extremities. The incidence of this disorder is much higher in Israel, eastern Europe, Japan, and the Far East than in the United States. An immune mechanism appears to be responsible for some of the pathological features.[181] It usually occurs in young men who are heavy smokers. This occasionally migratory thrombophlebitis is associated with tender areas of erythema. Arterial insufficiency often causes claudication of the foot, Raynaud's phenomenon, and trophic changes. Cerebral, coronary, and visceral vessels can be affected. Patients should be told peremptorily to stop smoking; if they do so, the disease process will usually be arrested.

Fat Embolism

The syndrome of fat embolism appears 12 to 48 hours after long-bone fracture, especially of the femur or tibia, and almost invariably causes respiratory failure.[182] Widespread embolic intravascular fat droplets have also been found at necropsy in the lungs of recipients of bone marrow transplants.[183] The failure may be clinically silent and manifested only by arterial desaturation, or it may be fulminant and progress from tachypnea to the full-blown picture of the adult respiratory distress syndrome.[182,184]

Central nervous system dysfunction is present, especially in association with severe pulmonary insufficiency; it ranges from irritability and restlessness to confusion and, eventually, to coma. Focal neurologic signs and seizures may occur. Urinary incontinence is common, even in alert patients. Transient diabetes insipidus is among the sequelae of fat embolism, many of which are cognitive or neurologic.

Petechiae, especially over the anterior neck, the shoulders, and the chest, occur in at least half of the patients who have clinically evident disease. Retinal streaky hemorrhages and fluffy exudates are presumably the result of microinfarctions. Temperatures of up to 42° C (107.6° F) and tachycardia are often present. Coagulopathies, thrombocytopenia, and acute peptic ulceration are probably related to the other complications of severe trauma, including disseminated intravascular coagulation.

The mechanisms underlying fat embolism formation are imperfectly understood. Increased intramedullary pressure from hemorrhage and swelling at the fracture site may cause embolization of damaged marrow contents.[185] Intrapulmonary lipolysis may release toxic free fatty acids that damage the endothelium.

Uncertainty surrounds the diagnosis, which must be based on clinical data. Even autopsy sometimes fails to resolve the question. The recognition of histologic changes, including the presence of fat in tissues, depends on the time course of the disorder and on the proper processing and staining of sections. Biopsy of petechiae has been used in an attempt to arrive at an antemortem diagnosis of fat embolism.

Management of adult respiratory distress syndrome and immobilization of fractures are the only approaches that have been proved effective in the established fat embolism syndrome. Prophylactic use of corticosteroids for patients at high risk was shown to be effective in one prospective study; the efficacy of corticosteroids for the established syndrome is not known.[186]

Livedo Reticularis and Livedo Vasculitis

Livedo reticularis is a vascular disorder characterized by a reddish-blue mottling of the skin. The discoloration, which often exhibits a fishnet pattern, is usually found on the extremities but can occur on the buttocks or trunk. The pattern probably reflects the geometry of the arterial supply and venous drainage of the skin.

The idiopathic form of livedo reticularis occurs predominantly in young adult and middle-aged women. In these individuals, the mottling tends to be precipitated by stasis or exposure to cold and may be associated with mild tingling or numbness. Occasionally, livedo reticularis is the expression of another disorder. A wide spectrum of underlying diseases has been identified: hyperviscosity syndromes,[187] immune vasculitides,[188,189] endocarditis,[190] thrombocythemia,[191] vascular occlusion by cholesterol emboli[192] or oxalate crystals,[193] and chronic syphilis and tuberculosis.

Livedo reticularis usually causes only minimal symptoms and inconvenience because of its appearance, and treatment is not required. On the other hand, livedo vasculitis, a related but more serious peripheral vascular disorder, is chronic and relapsing and is associated with microvascular occlusions, severe pain, and skin ulcerations, especially of the feet and ankles. Increased platelet adhesiveness and hyperaggregation may play a role in this form of vasculitis.[190,194] There is a disturbingly high incidence of severe and premature cerebrovascular disease in some patients who have livedo vasculitis or extensive livedo reticularis.[195]

Aspirin, dipyridamole, and low-dose heparin have been used to manage livedo vasculitis.[196,197] The effectiveness of such therapy is difficult to assess.

References

1. JAMA 233:970, 1975
2. JAMA 255:2039, 1986
3. Arch Intern Med 148:1425, 1988
4. Arch Intern Med 151:1721, 1991
5. Br Med J 290:1453, 1985
6. Clin Res 31:318A, 1983
7. Blood 62:439, 1983
8. N Engl J Med 323:1512, 1990
9. Medicine (Baltimore) 68:353, 1989
10. Medicine (Baltimore) 68:366, 1989
11. Ann Intern Med 112:682, 1990
12. Am J Med 92:283, 1992
13. Am J Med 92:275, 1992
14. Ann Intern Med 94:439, 1981
15. Am J Med 72:599, 1982
16. Ann Intern Med 96:556, 1982
17. Arch Intern Med 147:1907, 1987
18. Am J Med 79:423, 1985
19. N Engl J Med 318:404, 1988
20. Lancet 2:434, 1989
21. Medicine (Baltimore) 64:244, 1985
22. Br Med J 292:658, 1986
23. Ann Intern Med 97:565, 1982
24. Am J Med 78:317, 1985
25. Ann Intern Med 98:891, 1983
26. Ann Intern Med 111:297, 1989
27. Arch Intern Med 149:1731, 1989
28. Arch Intern Med 149:2255, 1989
29. Ann Intern Med 102:21, 1985
30. N Engl J Med 314:823, 1986
31. Arch Intern Med 148:681, 1988
32. JAMA 250:1289, 1983
33. Br Med J 298:230, 1989
34. Arch Intern Med 148:1617, 1988
35. JAMA 257:3257, 1987
36. Radiology 164:297, 1987
37. JAMA 263:2753, 1990
38. Ann Intern Med 114:142, 1991
39. JAMA 263:2794, 1990
40. Am J Med 75:763, 1983
41. AJR 149:469, 1987
42. Radiology 147:345, 1983
43. N Engl J Med 296:1431, 1977
44. Clin Nucl Med 8:497, 1983
45. Arch Intern Med 149:2549, 1989
46. Br Med J 2:969, 1976
47. Br Med J 295:580, 1987
48. Am J Med 82:889, 1987
49. Ann Surg 206:636, 1987
50. Arch Intern Med 149:679, 1989
51. JAMA 263:2313, 1990
52. Clin Obstet Gynaecol 8:455, 1981
53. Ann Intern Med 112:663, 1990
54. Am J Med 68:122, 1980
55. Am J Hum Genet 41:566, 1987
56. Br J Ophthalmol 64:633, 1980
57. Gynecol Obstet Invest 13:76, 1982
58. Arch Intern Med 149:2233, 1989
59. JAMA 252:235, 1984
60. J Pediatr 103:325, 1983
61. Chest 89(suppl):1S, 1986
62. Br Med J 290:1683, 1985
63. Arch Intern Med 149:771, 1989
64. J Bone Joint Surg 71:321, 1989
65. J Bone Joint Surg 71:327, 1989
66. N Engl J Med 318:1162, 1988
67. JAMA 260:1255, 1988
68. National Institutes of Health Consensus Development Conference Statement. Bethesda, Maryland, March 24–26, 1986
69. N Engl J Med 324:1565, 1991
70. Blood 53:525, 1979
71. Br Med J 290:341, 1985
72. JAMA 250:1413, 1983
73. N Engl J Med 322:1260, 1990
74. Lancet 2:1293, 1986
75. Ann Intern Med 107:441, 1987
76. Ann Intern Med 113:571, 1990
77. N Engl J Med 326:975, 1992
78. Lancet 339:441, 1992
79. N Engl J Med 324:1865, 1991
80. Arch Intern Med 146:581, 1986
81. Ann Intern Med 116:901, 1992
82. N Engl J Med 306:189, 1982
83. Lancet 2:515, 1985
84. Circulation 70:580, 1984
85. Arch Intern Med 143:2061, 1983
86. Br Med J 298:93, 1989
87. Arch Intern Med 145:499, 1985
88. N Engl J Med 308:1229, 1983
89. N Engl J Med 320:886, 1989
90. N Engl J Med 303:902, 1980
91. N Engl J Med 303:788, 1980
92. Thromb Haemost 43:61, 1980
93. Am J Hematol 6:125, 1979
94. JAMA 241:2396, 1979
95. Arch Intern Med 138:1489, 1978
96. Am Heart J 99:816, 1980
97. JAMA 241:2417, 1979
98. JAMA 246:2189, 1981
99. Arch Intern Med 145:1070, 1985
100. Am J Med 85:721, 1988
101. Medicine (Baltimore) 67:389, 1988

102. Ann Intern Med 100:646, 1984
103. Medicine (Baltimore) 55:389, 1976
104. Ann Intern Med 95:592, 1981
105. Arch Intern Med 147:857, 1987
106. Arch Intern Med 150:2117, 1990
107. AJR 131:843, 1978
108. Arch Intern Med 136:799, 1976
109. Ann Surg 195:726, 1982
110. Chest 96:939, 1989
111. J Vasc Surg 6:609, 1987
112. Am Surg 53:580, 1987
113. Am J Med 76:512, 1984
114. Arch Intern Med 147:2177, 1987
115. N Engl J Med 326:1240, 1992
116. Am J Med 69:790, 1980
117. Ann Intern Med 108:425, 1988
118. Chest 93:1180, 1988
119. Ann Intern Med 107:565, 1987
120. Ann Intern Med 103:844, 1985
121. N Engl J Med 318:1512, 1585, 1988
122. JAMA 252:1314, 1984
123. Arch Intern Med 146:305, 1986
124. Am J Med 90:255, 1991
125. National Institutes of Health Consensus Development Conference, April 10–12, 1980. Summary, Vol 3, No 1
126. Chest 83:151, 1983
127. N Engl J Med 306:1268, 1982
128. Arch Intern Med 142:684, 1982
129. Am J Med 76:393, 1984
130. JAMA 253:1777, 1985
131. Arch Intern Med 149:1841, 1989
132. Ann Intern Med 100:237, 1984
133. Am J Med 77:1111, 1984
134. Mayo Clin Proc 63:1181, 1988
135. Lancet 2:293, 1988
136. Br J Surg 74:991, 1987
137. N Engl J Med 319:925, 1988
138. Am J Med 88:235, 1990
139. Obstet Gynecol 58:117, 1981
140. Br Med J 283:265, 1981
141. Acta Chir Scand 149:333, 1983
142. Surg Gynecol Obstet 154:205, 1982
143. Gastroenterology 92:240, 1987
144. Ann Intern Med 106:677, 1987
145. Am J Med 87:97, 1989
146. Ann Intern Med 112:881, 1990
147. Am J Roentgenol 154:721, 1990
148. Lancet 1:1021, 1983
149. Am J Med 74:529, 1983
150. Medicine (Baltimore) 62:209, 1983
151. Surgery 97:242, 1985
152. N Engl J Med 308:1549, 1983
153. J Clin Invest 77:887, 1986
154. Blood 70:1273, 1987
155. Gastroenterology 89:421, 1985
156. Clin Haematol 10:369, 1981
157. Minn Med 61:79, 1978
158. Transfusion 24:57, 1984
159. Ann Intern Med 116:754, 1992
160. Lancet 2:1272, 1984
161. Haemostasis 15:119, 1985
162. Acta Chir Scand 154:179, 1988
163. N Engl J Med 314:1298, 1986
164. Science 235:1348, 1987
165. N Engl J Med 310:559, 1984
166. Pediatrics 81:272, 1988
167. N Engl J Med 317:991, 1987
168. Am J Med 82:1171, 1987
169. Br Med J 289:1285, 1984
170. N Engl J Med 317:1638, 1987
171. Ann Intern Med 104:659, 1986
172. Blood 71:370, 1988
173. Ann Intern Med 100:59, 1984
174. J Clin Invest 77:416, 1986
175. Ann Intern Med 107:42, 1987
176. Br Med J 295:641, 1987
177. N Engl J Med 311:1525, 1984
178. J Clin Invest 74:2082, 1984
179. The Johns Hopkins University Press, Baltimore, 1988, p 988
180. N Engl J Med 324:1149, 1991
181. N Engl J Med 308:1113, 1983
182. American Academy of Orthopedic Surgeons: Instructional Course Lectures 22:38, 1973
183. Lancet 1:715, 1983
184. Chest 79:131, 1981
185. Am J Forensic Med Pathol 3:73, 1982
186. Ann Intern Med 99:438, 1983
187. Br J Dermatol 93:519, 1975
188. J Clin Pathol 32:154, 1979
189. Arch Dermatol 111:188, 1975
190. Am J Med Sci 282:131, 1981
191. Br J Dermatol 95(suppl 14):63, 1976
192. Br J Dermatol 97:93, 1977
193. Arch Dermatol 116:213, 1980
194. J Am Acad Dermatol 7:359, 1982
195. Lancet 1:1263, 1988
196. N Engl J Med 298:281, 1978
197. J Am Acad Dermatol 8:23, 1983

Acknowledgments

Tables 1 and 2 Modified from "Value of the Ventilation/Perfusion Scan in Acute Pulmonary Embolism: Results of the Prospective Investigation of Pulmonary Embolism Diagnosis (PIOPED)," by The PIOPED Investigators, in *Journal of the American Medical Association* 263:2753, 1990. Used by permission.

8 Cardiopulmonary Resuscitation

The updated standards and guidelines proposed by the 1985 National Conference on Cardiopulmonary Resuscitation (CPR) and Emergency Cardiac Care (ECC)[1] are presented here. Because information on drug therapy and life-support devices used in advanced cardiac life support (ACLS) changes so rapidly, we have chosen to follow the recommendations on these topics outlined in various discussions elsewhere in this book [*see Chapters 1, 2, 3, and 5*] rather than those put forth by the national conference. The revised guidelines of the conference regarding basic life support (BLS) include:

1. Recommendations for simplifying instruction of basic life-support procedures to laypersons, by teaching only one-rescuer CPR and by teaching only the head tilt–chin lift method for opening the airway.
2. New recommendations for ventilation in intubated cardiac arrest victims.
3. A decrease in the number of initial ventilations from four quick, full breaths to two breaths lasting about one and one-half seconds each.
4. An increase in the number of chest compressions from 60 to 80 a minute to 80 to 100 a minute.
5. The designation of the Heimlich maneuver as the preferred method for dislodging foreign matter from the airway.
6. Advice on how to avoid disease transmission from CPR training manikins.

Adult Basic Life Support

Basic life support (BLS) is that particular phase of emergency cardiac care that either (1) prevents circulatory or respiratory arrest or insufficiency through prompt recognition and intervention or (2) externally supports the circulation and ventilation of a victim of cardiac or respiratory arrest through cardio-pulmonary resuscitation (CPR). The major objective of performing CPR is to provide oxygen to the brain, heart, and other vital organs until appropriate, definitive medical treatment (advanced cardiac life support) can restore normal heart and ventilatory action. Speed is critical—it is the key to success. The highest hospital discharge rate has been achieved in those patients for whom CPR was initiated within four minutes of the time of the arrest and who, in addition, were provided with advanced cardiac life support measures within eight minutes of their arrest. Early bystander CPR intervention and fast emergency medical system (EMS) response are therefore essential to improve survival rates and for good neurologic recovery rates.

Basic life support includes the teaching of primary and secondary prevention. The basic concept, put forward by the American Heart Association during the past 20 years, that it is possible to prevent and control coronary heart disease, should be reinforced during the teaching of BLS, with an emphasis on so-called prudent heart living and the role of risk-factor modification. The earlier this information is transmitted to the community, the stronger the impact on mortality and morbidity; therefore, efforts must be made to include BLS in the curricula of schools. Cardiopulmonary resuscitation training should include information on danger signals, actions for survival, and entry into the EMS system to help to prevent sudden death in individuals who have sustained myocardial infarctions.

Indications for BLS

Respiratory Arrest

When there is primary respiratory arrest, the heart can continue to pump blood for several minutes, and existing stores of oxy-

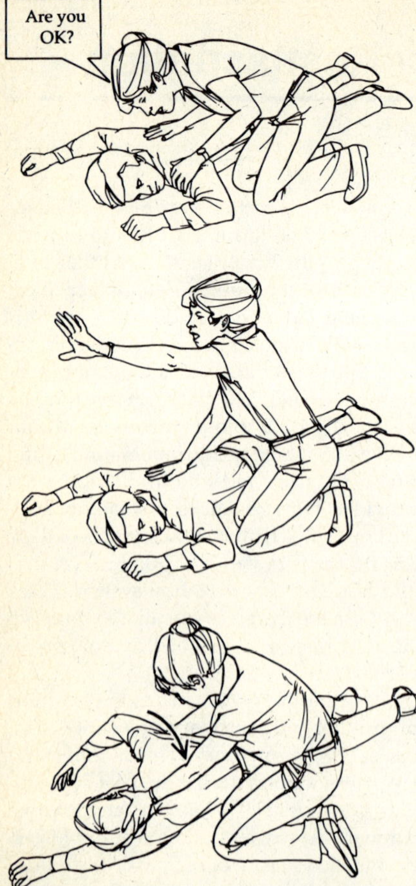

Figure 1 *The initial steps of cardiopulmonary resuscitation involve determining unresponsiveness (top), calling for help (middle), and positioning the victim (bottom).*

gen in the lungs and blood will continue to circulate to the brain and other vital organs. Early intervention for victims in whom respirations have stopped or the airway is obstructed can prevent cardiac arrest. Respiratory arrest can result from drowning, stroke, foreign-body airway obstruction, smoke inhalation, drug overdose, electrocution, suffocation, injuries, myocardial infarction, injury by lightning, and coma of any cause that leads to airway obstruction.

Cardiac Arrest

When there is primary cardiac arrest, oxygen is not circulated, and oxygen stored in the vital organs is depleted in a few seconds. Cardiac arrest can be accompanied by the following electrical phenomena: ventricular fibrillation, ventricular tachycardia, asystole, or electromechanical dissociation.

The Sequence of BLS: Assessment and the Abc's of CPR

The assessment phases of BLS are crucial. No victim should undergo any one of the more intrusive procedures of cardiopulmonary resuscitation (i.e., positioning, opening the airway, rescue breathing, and external chest compression) until the need for it has been established by the appropriate assessment. The importance of assessment should be stressed in the teaching of CPR.

Each of the *ABC*s of CPR, *A*irway, *B*reathing, and *C*irculation, begins with an assessment phase: determine unresponsiveness, determine breathlessness, and determine pulselessness, respectively. Assessment also involves a more subtle, constant process of observing and interacting with the victim.

Airway

Assessment: Determine Unresponsiveness

The rescuer arriving at the scene of the collapsed victim must quickly assess any injury and determine whether the individual is unconscious [*see Figure 1, top*]. If the victim has sustained trauma to the head and neck, the rescuer should move the victim only if absolutely necessary because improper movement may cause paralysis in the victim with a neck injury.

The rescuer should tap or gently shake the victim and shout, "Are you OK?" This precaution will prevent injury from attempted resuscitation of a person who is not truly unconscious.

Call for Help

If the victim does not respond to attempts at arousal, call for help [*see Figure 1,*

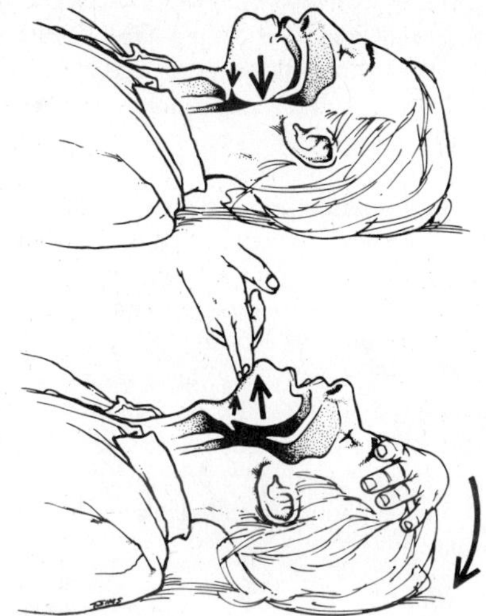

Figure 2 *Airway obstruction can be caused by the tongue or epiglottis (top); obstruction can be relieved by the head tilt–chin lift maneuver (bottom).*

middle]. When someone responds, send that person to activate the EMS system.

Position the Victim

For CPR to be effective, the victim must be supine and on a firm, flat surface [*see Figure 1, bottom*]; even flawlessly performed external chest compressions will produce inadequate blood flow to the brain if the head is positioned higher than the thorax. If the victim is lying face down, the rescuer must roll the victim as a unit so that the head, shoulders, and torso move simultaneously with no twisting. The head and neck should remain in the same plane as the torso, and the body should be moved as a unit. Once the body is supine, the victim's arms should be placed alongside the body. The victim is now appropriately positioned for the next step in CPR.

Rescuer Position

By kneeling at the level of the victim's shoulders, the rescuer can perform rescue breathing and chest compressions, in turn, without moving the knees.

Open Airway

The most important action for successful resuscitation is immediate opening of the airway. In the absence of sufficient muscle tone, the tongue or the epiglottis, or both, will obstruct the pharynx and the larynx, respectively [*see Figure 2, top*]. The tongue is the most common cause of airway obstruction in the unconscious victim. Since the tongue is attached to the lower jaw, moving the lower jaw forward will lift the tongue away from the back of the throat and open the airway. Either the tongue or the epiglottis, or both, may also produce obstruction when negative pressure is created in the airway by inspiratory effort, which causes a valve-type mechanism to occlude the entrance to the trachea.

The rescuer should use the head tilt–chin lift maneuver (see below) to open the airway [*see Figure 2, bottom*]. If foreign material or vomitus is visible in the mouth, it should be removed. Excessive time must not be taken. Liquids or semiliquids should be wiped out with the index and middle fingers, covered by a piece of cloth; solid material should be extracted with a hooked index finger. The mouth can be opened by the so-called crossed-finger technique.

Head tilt–chin lift maneuver Head tilt–chin lift is more effective in opening the airway than the previously recommended head tilt–neck lift. Head tilt is accomplished by placing one hand on the victim's forehead and applying firm, backward pressure with the palm to tilt the head back. To complete the head tilt–chin lift maneuver, place the fingers of the other hand under the bony part of the lower jaw near the chin and lift to bring the chin forward and the teeth almost to occlusion; this maneuver supports the jaw and helps to tilt the head back. The fingers must not press deeply into the soft tissue under the chin, which might obstruct the airway. The thumb should not be used for lifting the chin. The mouth should not be completely closed (unless mouth-to-nose breathing is the technique of choice for that particular victim). When mouth-to-nose ventilation is indicated, the hand that is on the chin can close the mouth by applying increased force. If the victim has loose dentures, head tilt–chin lift maintains their position and makes a mouth-to-mouth seal easier. Dentures should be removed if they cannot be managed in place.

Jaw-thrust maneuver Forward displacement of the mandible can be accomplished by grasping the angles of the victim's lower jaw and lifting with both hands, one on each side, displacing the mandible forward while tilting the head backward. The rescuer's elbows should rest on the surface on which the victim is lying. If the lips close, the lower lip can be retracted with the thumb. If mouth-to-mouth breathing is necessary, the nostrils may be closed by placing the rescuer's cheek tightly against them. This technique is very effective in opening the airway but is very fatiguing and technically difficult.

The jaw-thrust technique without head tilt is the safest first approach to opening the airway of the victim with suspected neck injury because it usually can be accomplished without extending the neck. The head should be carefully supported without tilting it backward or turning it from side to side. If jaw thrust alone is unsuccessful, the head should be tilted backward very slightly.

Recommendations for opening the airway A layperson should learn only one maneuver for opening the airway. The recommended technique must be simple, safe, easily learned, and effective. Because head tilt–chin lift meets these criteria, it should be the method of choice. Professional rescuers (emergency medical technicians and other medical and health care providers) should be trained in both head tilt–chin lift and jaw thrust.

Breathing

Assessment: Determine Breathlessness

To assess the presence or absence of spontaneous breathing, the rescuer should place his or her ear over the victim's mouth and nose while maintaining an open airway [*see Figure 3*]. Then, while observing the victim's chest, the rescuer should (1) *look* for the chest to rise and fall, (2) *listen* for air escaping during exhalation, and (3) *feel* for the flow of air. If the chest does not rise and fall and no air is exhaled, the victim is breathless. This evaluation procedure should take only three to five seconds.

Although the rescuer may notice that the victim is making respiratory efforts, it should be stressed that the airway may still be obstructed, and opening the airway may be all that is needed. If the victim resumes breathing, the rescuer should continue to help to maintain an open airway.

Perform Rescue Breathing

Mouth-to-mouth Rescue breathing using the mouth-to-mouth technique is a quick and effective way of providing the necessary oxygen to the victim's lungs [*see Figure 4, top*]. The rescuer's exhaled air contains sufficient oxygen to supply the victim's needs. Rescue breathing requires that the rescuer inflate the victim's lungs adequately with

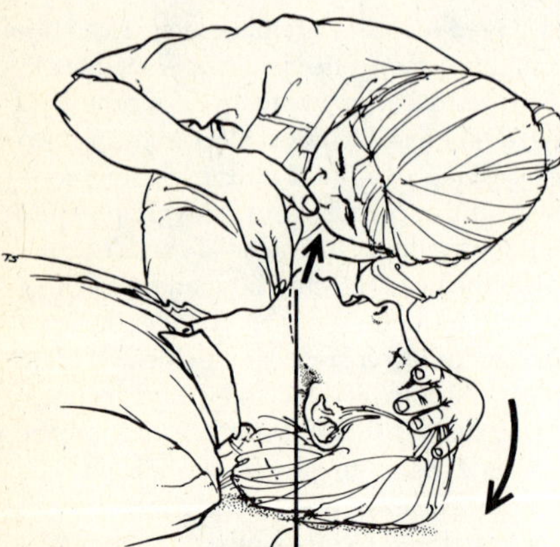

Figure 3 *To determine breathlessness, the rescuer places his or her head over the victim's mouth and looks for the chest to rise and fall, listens for air during exhalation, and feels for the flow of air.*

each breath. Keeping the airway open by the head tilt–chin lift maneuver, the rescuer gently pinches the nose closed using the thumb and index finger of the hand on the forehead, which thereby prevents air from escaping through the victim's nose. The rescuer takes a deep breath and seals his or her lips around the outside of the victim's mouth, which creates an airtight seal; the rescuer then gives two full breaths.

Adequate time for the two breaths (one to one and one-half seconds per breath) should be allowed to provide good chest expansion and decrease the possibility of gastric distention. (Measurements of time per breath given herein are, more precisely, measurements of the victim's inspiratory time.) The rescuer should take a breath after each ventilation, and each individual ventilation should be of sufficient volume to make the chest rise. In most adults, this volume will be 800 ml (0.8 L). Adequate ventilation usually does not need to exceed 1,200 ml (1.2 L). An excess of air and fast inspiratory flow rates are likely to cause pharyngeal pressures that exceed esophageal opening pressures, which allows air to enter the stomach and thus results in gastric distention. Indicators of adequate ventilation are (1) observing the chest rise and fall and (2) hearing and feeling the air escape during exhalation.

If the initial attempt to ventilate the victim is unsuccessful, reposition the victim's head and repeat rescue breathing. Improper chin and head positioning is the most common cause of difficulty with ventilation. If the victim cannot be ventilated after repositioning the head, proceed with foreign-body airway obstruction maneuvers (see below).

Mouth-to-nose This technique is more effective in some cases than mouth-to-mouth [*see Figure 4, middle*]. The technique is recommended when it is impossible to ventilate through the victim's mouth, the mouth cannot be opened (trismus), the mouth is seriously injured, or a tight mouth-to-mouth seal is difficult to achieve. The rescuer keeps the victim's head tilted back with one hand on the forehead and uses the other hand to lift the victim's lower jaw (as in head tilt–chin lift) and close the mouth. The rescuer then takes a deep breath, seals the lips around the victim's nose, and blows into the nose. The rescuer's mouth is then removed, and the victim exhales passively. It may be necessary to open the victim's mouth intermittently or separate the lips (with the thumb) to allow air to be exhaled because nasal obstruction may be present during exhalation.

Mouth-to-stoma Persons who have undergone a laryngectomy (surgical removal of the larynx) have a permanent stoma (opening) that connects the trachea directly to the skin. The stoma can be recognized as an opening at the front base of the neck. When such an individual requires rescue breathing, direct mouth-to-stoma ventilation should be performed [*see Figure 4, bottom*]. The rescuer's mouth is sealed around the stoma, and air is blown into the victim's stoma until the chest rises. When the rescuer's mouth is removed from the stoma, the victim is permitted to exhale passively.

Other persons may have a temporary tracheostomy tube in the trachea. To ventilate these persons, the victim's mouth and nose usually must be sealed by the rescuer's hand or by a tightly fitting face mask to prevent leakage of air when the rescuer blows into the tracheostomy tube. This problem is alleviated when the tracheostomy tube has a cuff that can be inflated.

Recommendations for rescue breathing (1) The four quick initial ventilations formerly recommended in one-rescuer CPR have been changed to two initial breaths of one to one and one-half seconds each. Those ventilations should no longer be given to create a so-called staircase effect. By giving the ventilations with a slower inspiratory flow rate and by avoiding trapping air in the lungs between breaths, the possibility of exceeding the esophageal opening pressure will be lessened. This technique should result in less gastric distention, regurgitation, and aspiration. Also, an equal number of initial and subsequent ventilations should enhance retention by trainees.

(2) In two-rescuer CPR, a pause for ventilations should be allowed after every five external chest compressions. However, such pauses for ventilations (one to one and one-half seconds) decrease the total number of compressions a minute, affecting the blood flow to vital organs; therefore, a faster compression rate than was previously recommended is necessary for adequate blood flow [*see* Recommendations for External Chest Compression, *below*].

Circulation

Assessment: Determine Pulselessness

Cardiac arrest is recognized by pulselessness in the large arteries of the unconscious victim [*see Figure 5*]. The pulse check should take five to 10 seconds, and the carotid artery should be used. It lies in a groove created by the trachea and the large strap muscles of the neck. While maintaining head tilt with one hand on the forehead, the rescuer locates the victim's larynx with two or three fingers of the other hand. The rescuer then slides these fingers into the groove between the trachea and the muscles at the side of the neck where the carotid pulse can be felt. The pulse area must be pressed gently, to avoid compressing the artery. This technique is usually more easily performed on the side near the rescuer. Adequate time should be allowed because the pulse may be slow, irregular, or very weak and rapid. This is the most accessible, reliable, and easily learned technique for locating the pulse in adults and children. The pulse in the carotid artery will persist when more peripheral pulses (e.g., radial) are no longer palpable. For health care professionals or in the hospital setting, determining pulselessness using the femoral pulse is also acceptable; however, this pulse is difficult to locate in a fully clothed patient.

Proper assessment of the victim's condition must be made because performing external chest compressions on a patient who has a pulse may result in serious medical

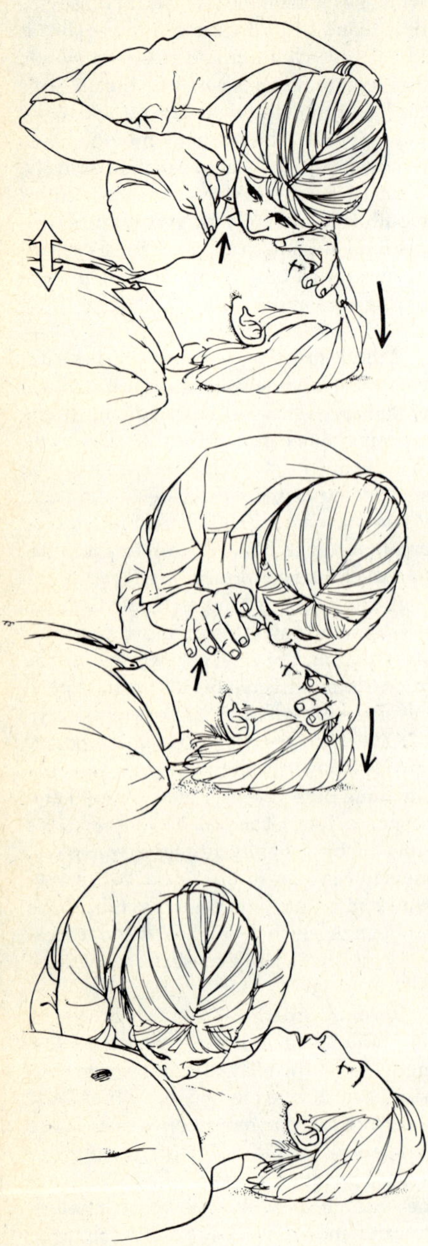

Figure 4   *Three recommended procedures for rescue breathing are mouth-to-mouth (top), mouth-to-nose (middle), and mouth-to-stoma (bottom).*

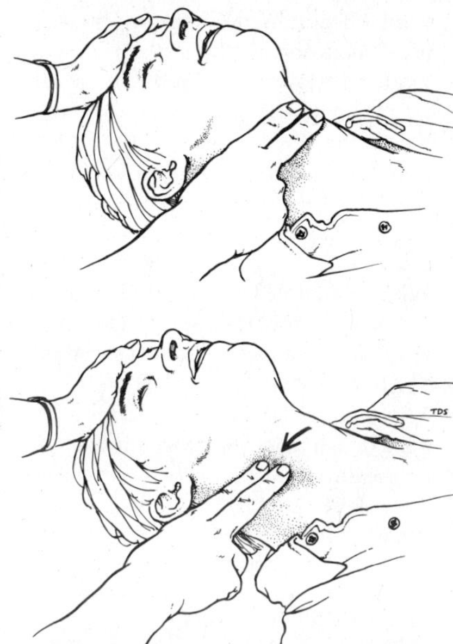

Figure 5 *To determine pulselessness, the rescuer places two or three fingers on the victim's larynx (top); these fingers are then slid into the groove between the trachea and the strap muscles of the neck so that the carotid artery can be palpated (bottom).*

complications. If a pulse is present but there is no breathing, rescue breathing should be initiated at a rate of 12 times a minute (once every five seconds) after two initial breaths of one to one and one-half seconds each.

If no pulse is palpated, the diagnosis of cardiac arrest is confirmed. If not yet done, the EMS system should be activated and external chest compression begun after the initial two breaths.

Activate the EMS System

The EMS system is activated by calling the local emergency telephone number (911, if available). This number should be widely publicized in each community. The person who calls the EMS system should be prepared to give the following information as calmly as possible: (1) where the emergency is (with names of cross streets or roads, if possible), (2) the telephone number from which the call is made, (3) what happened—heart attack, auto accident, etc., (4) how many persons need help, (5) condition of the victim or victims, (6) what aid is being given to the victim or victims, and (7) any other information requested. To ensure that EMS personnel have no more questions, the caller should hang up last.

If no one responds to the call for help and the rescuer is alone, CPR should be performed for about one minute, and then help should be summoned. The decision when to leave the victim to telephone for help is affected by a number of variables, including the possibility of someone else arriving on the scene. If the rescuer is unable to activate the EMS system, the only option is to continue with CPR.

External Chest Compression

Cardiac arrest is recognized by pulselessness in the large arteries of the unconscious, breathless victim. All the *ABC*s of CPR are required in rapid succession to optimize the chances for survival.

The external chest compression technique consists of serial, rhythmic applications of pressure over the lower half of the sternum [*see Figure 6*]. These compressions provide circulation to the heart, lungs, brain, and other organs as a result of a generalized increase in intrathoracic pressure or direct compression of the heart, or both. Blood circulated to the lungs by external chest compressions will receive sufficient oxygen to maintain life when the compressions are accompanied by properly performed rescue breathing.

During cardiac arrest, properly performed external chest compressions can produce systolic blood pressure peaks of more than 100 mm Hg, but the diastolic blood pressure is low; the mean blood pressure in the carotid arteries seldom exceeds 40 mm Hg. The carotid artery blood flow resulting from external chest compressions on a cardiac arrest victim usually is only one fourth to one third of normal.

The patient must be in the horizontal, supine position when external chest compressions are performed. Even during

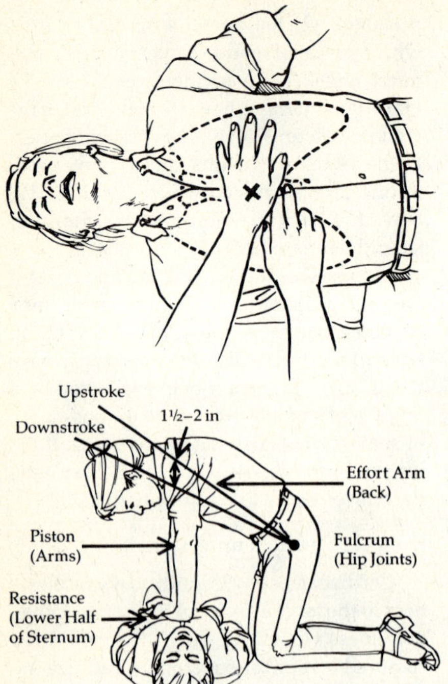

Figure 6   *External chest compression requires proper placement of the hands on the sternum (top) and proper positioning over the victim (bottom). The rescuer's shoulders should be placed directly over the victim's sternum, with the rescuer's elbows in a locked position.*

properly performed external chest compression, blood flow to the brain is reduced. With any elevation of the head above the heart, blood flow to the brain is further reduced or even eliminated. If the victim is in bed, a board, preferably the full width of the bed, should be placed under the back of the patient. Elevation of the lower extremities, while keeping the rest of the body horizontal, may promote venous return and augment artificial circulation during chest compressions.

Proper hand position   Proper hand placement is established by the following guidelines [*see Figure 6, top*]:

1. With the middle and index fingers of the hand nearest the victim's legs, the rescuer locates the lower margin of the victim's rib cage on the side of the victim next to the rescuer.
2. The fingers are then moved up the rib cage to the notch where the ribs meet the sternum in the center of the lower part of the chest.
3. With the middle finger on this notch, the index finger is placed next to the middle finger on the lower end of the sternum.
4. The heel of the hand nearest the patient's head (which had been used on the forehead to maintain head position) is placed on the lower half of the sternum, close to the index finger that is next to the middle finger in the notch. The long axis of the heel of the rescuer's hand should be placed on the long axis of the sternum. This will keep the main force of compression on the sternum and decrease the chance of rib fracture.
5. The first hand is then removed from the notch and placed on top of the hand on the sternum, so that both hands are parallel to each other.
6. The fingers may be either extended or interlaced but must be kept off the chest.
7. Because of the varying sizes and shapes of different persons' hands, an alternative acceptable hand position is to grasp the wrist of the hand on the chest with the hand that has been locating the lower end of the sternum. This technique is helpful for rescuers with arthritic problems of the hands and wrists.

Proper compression techniques   Effective compression is accomplished by attention to the following guidelines [*see Figure 6, bottom*]:

1. The elbows of the rescuer are locked into position, the arms are straightened, and the shoulders are positioned directly over the hands so that the thrust for each external chest compression is straight down on the sternum. If the thrust is other than straight down, the torso has a tendency to

roll, losing part of the force, and the chest compression may be less effective.

2. The sternum must be depressed 1.5 to 2.0 in (3.8 to 5.0 cm) for the normal-sized adult.
3. The external chest compression pressure is released to allow blood to flow into the heart. The pressure must be released completely and the chest allowed to return to its normal position after each compression. The time allowed for release should equal the time required for compression.
4. The hands should not be lifted from the chest or the position changed in any way, lest correct hand position be lost.

Rescue breathing and external chest compression must be combined for effective resuscitation of the cardiopulmonary arrest victim.

Physiology of circulation The technique of closed-chest cardiac massage was well accepted in the early 1960s by professional people and, later, by laypersons. It became known as standard or conventional CPR. It was believed that external chest compression resulted in the direct compression of the heart between the sternum and the spine, with an increase in pressure within the ventricles and a closure of the valves (mitral and tricuspid). This pressure was thought to cause blood to move into the pulmonary artery and the aorta.

In support of this cardiac pump theory are the recent studies that demonstrated higher stroke volume and coronary blood flow with high-impulse (moderate force and brief duration) external chest compressions at high rates. Preliminary studies reported that there are valve motion and cardiac chamber compression during the initial five minutes of external chest compression.

This conventional theory of blood flow during CPR has been challenged by several workers who have advanced the thoracic pump mechanism theory. According to this theory, external chest compression produces a rise in the intrathoracic pressure that is transmitted equally to all intrathoracic vascular structures. Because arteries resist collapse, there is nearly full transmission of pressure from intrathoracic to extrathoracic arteries. Competent venous valves and venous collapse prevent full transmission of pressure to extrathoracic veins. An extrathoracic arteriovenous pressure gradient is produced, which causes blood to flow. This thoracic pump theory is supported by the following observations:

1. In patients with flail chests and who need CPR, arterial pressure does not increase during chest compressions unless the chest is stabilized with a belt, which allows intrathoracic pressure to increase.
2. It has been observed that some patients who sustain a cardiac arrest and are asked to cough vigorously before loss of consciousness are able to remain conscious and that the systolic arterial pressure during coughing is higher than 100 mm Hg. This significant increase in intrathoracic pressure provides blood flow to the brain. The increase in intrathoracic pressure during coughing results from the contraction of the diaphragm, intercostal, and abdominal muscles against a closed glottis.
3. Two-dimensional echocardiography shows that mitral and tricuspid valves remain open during CPR, supporting the concept that the heart is a passive conduit rather than a pump.

Recently, there has been important research in new techniques to improve blood flow during CPR: (1) simultaneous chest compression and ventilation (SCV-CPR), (2) abdominal compression with synchronized ventilation, (3) CPR augmented with military antishock trousers, (4) interposed abdominal compression (IAC-CPR), and (5) continuous abdominal binding. Because many of the proposed techniques require the use of devices (e.g., endotracheal intubation, binders, trousers, and mechanical compressors), they cannot be recommended as BLS techniques. Additionally, more information regarding survival rates, neurologic outcome, and complications is needed before changes in the technique of external chest compressions are recommended.

It is possible that both mechanisms for blood flow play a role during external chest compression. Which one is predominant in a particular victim may depend on several factors, including the size of the heart, ventrodorsal chest diameter, compliance of the chest wall, magnitude of chest compressions, and perhaps, unknown factors.

Recommendations for external chest compression The only change from past practice recommended at this time is an increase in the compression rate. The external chest compression rate should be increased to a minimum of 80 compressions a minute and to 100 a minute if possible. This change is consistent with both the cardiac pump theory and the thoracic pump theory. If the direct compression of the heart is operative, it is clear that a faster rate will increase blood flow. If the increase in intrathoracic pressure is the mechanism of blood flow during CPR, compression with high force and a duration of 50 percent of cycle time will increase flow to the brain and the heart. However, higher compression force and the 50 percent compression duration are very difficult to obtain with a rate of 60 compressions a minute; if the compression rate is increased, the result is an optimal compression-relaxation duration. A faster compression rate will also allow for a pause for ventilation (in two-rescuer CPR), which is now delivered at an inspiratory flow rate slower than previously recommended.

Cough CPR

Self-induced CPR is possible; however, its applications are limited to clinical situations in which the patient has a cardiac monitor, the arrest was recognized before loss of consciousness (usually within 10 to 15 seconds from the cardiac arrest), and the patient has the ability to cough forcefully. The increase in intrathoracic pressure will generate blood flow to the brain to maintain consciousness for a longer period of time.

CPR Performed by One Rescuer

A layperson should learn only one-rescuer CPR. The previously recommended two-rescuer technique is thought to cause too much confusion and to be infrequently used by laypersons in actual rescue situations. Teaching only one-rescuer CPR should result in better retention of skills and, possibly, better performance. One-rescuer CPR is effective in maintaining adequate circulation and ventilation but is more exhausting than two-rescuer CPR. When trained professionals arrive at the scene of an emergency, they will proceed with two-rescuer CPR and advanced cardiac life support, as appropriate for the situation. The lay rescuer is relieved of responsibility at that point.

One-rescuer CPR should be performed as follows:

Airway (1) Assessment: determine unresponsiveness (tap or gently shake and shout), (2) call for help, (3) position the victim, and (4) open the airway by the head tilt–chin lift maneuver.

Breathing Assessment: determine breathlessness. *If the victim is breathing,* (1) monitor breathing, (2) maintain an open airway, and (3) activate the EMS system (if not done previously). *If the victim is not breathing,* perform rescue breathing by giving two initial breaths. If unable to give two breaths, (1) reposition the head and attempt to ventilate again, and (2) if still unsuccessful, perform the foreign-body airway obstruction sequence. If successful, continue to the next step.

Circulation (1) Assessment: determine pulselessness. If pulse is present, continue rescue breathing at 12 times a minute and activate the EMS system. (2) If pulse is absent, activate the EMS system (if not done previously) and continue to the next step. (3) Begin external chest compression: (a) Locate proper hand position. (b) Perform 15 external chest compressions at a rate of 80 to 100 a minute. Count "one and, two and, three and, four and, five and, six and, seven and, eight and, nine and, 10 and, 11 and, 12 and, 13 and, 14 and, 15." (Any mnemonic that accomplishes the same compression rate is acceptable.) (c) Open the airway and deliver two rescue breaths. (d) Locate the proper hand position and begin 15 more compressions at a rate of 80 to 100 a minute. (e) Perform four complete cycles of 15 compressions and two ventilations.

Reassessment After four cycles of compressions and ventilations (15:2 ratio), re-evaluate the patient. (1) Check for return of the carotid pulse (five seconds). If it is absent, resume CPR with two ventilations followed by compressions. If it is present, continue to next step. (2) Check breathing (three to five seconds). If breathing is present, monitor breathing and pulse closely. If breathing is absent, perform rescue breathing at 12 times a minute and monitor pulse closely. (3) If CPR is continued, stop and check for return of pulse and spontaneous breathing every few minutes. Do not interrupt CPR for more than seven seconds, except in special cases.

One-rescuer CPR with entry of a second rescuer When another rescuer is available at the scene, it is recommended that this second rescuer should activate the EMS system (if not done previously) and perform one-rescuer CPR when the first rescuer, who initiated CPR, becomes fatigued.

The following steps are recommended for entry of the second rescuer. The second person should identify himself or herself as a qualified rescuer who is willing to help. If the first rescuer is fatigued and has requested help, the sequence is as follows: (1) The first rescuer stops CPR after two ventilations. (2) The second rescuer kneels down and checks for pulse for five seconds. (3) If there is no pulse, the second rescuer gives two breaths. (4) The second rescuer commences external chest compressions at the recommended rate and ratio for one-person CPR. (5) The first rescuer assesses the adequacy of the second rescuer's ventilations and compressions. This can be done by watching the chest rise during rescue breathing and by checking the pulse during the chest compressions.

CPR Performed by Two Rescuers

All professional rescuers (emergency medicine technicians and medical and health care professionals) should learn both the one-rescuer technique and the two-rescuer coordinated technique, which is less fatiguing. Because this is a two-rescuer technique done by professionals, mouth-to-mask ventilation is an acceptable alternative to mouth-to-mouth ventilation.

One person is positioned at the victim's side and performs external chest compressions, while the other remains at the victim's head, maintains an open airway, monitors the carotid pulse for adequacy of chest compressions, and provides rescue breathing. The compression rate for two-rescuer CPR is 80 to 100 a minute. The compression-ventilation ratio is 5:1, with a pause for ventilation (one to one and one-half seconds). When the compressor becomes fatigued, the rescuers should exchange positions as soon as possible.

Two rescuers should be able to coordinate and perform the following sequences, as appropriate:

1. If CPR is in progress by one rescuer, the logical time for entrance of the two-professionals rescuer team is immediately after the first rescuer has completed a cycle of 15 compressions and two breaths:

   One rescuer moves to the head, opens the airway, and checks for a pulse, while the other member of the team locates the area for external chest compressions and finds the proper hand position. This should take five seconds.

   If there is no pulse, the ventilator gives one breath, and the compressor begins external chest compressions at the rate of 80 to 100 a minute, counting "one and, two and, three and, four and, five."

   At the end of the fifth compression, a pause should be allowed for the ventilation (one to one and one-half seconds a breath). The compression-ventilation ratio for two rescuers is 5:1. The pause for ventilation may be shorter or may be interposed if the victim is intubated, as faster inspiratory flow rates are possible without the problem of gastric distention, regurgitation, and aspiration. After the airway is protected by the placement of an esophageal obturator airway or endotracheal tube, ventilations may be given in an asynchronous mode at a rate of 12 to 15 a minute.

2. If no CPR is in progress and the two rescuers arrive on the scene at the same time, both must determine what needs to be done and start immediately, without wasting time. One rescuer should ensure that the EMS system is activated. If this person leaves the area, the other person should institute one-person CPR.

If both persons are available, one rescuer should go to the head of the victim and proceed as follows: (1) determine unresponsiveness, (2) position the victim, (3) open the airway, (4) check for breathing, (5) if breathing is absent, say "No breathing" and give two ventilations, and (6) check for pulse. If there is no pulse, say "No pulse."

The second rescuer should simultaneously (1) find the location for external chest compressions, (2) assume the proper hand position, and (3) initiate external chest compressions after the first rescuer states "No pulse."

Monitoring the victim The victim's condition must be monitored to assess the effectiveness of the rescue effort. The ventilator assumes this responsibility for monitoring the pulse and breathing, which serves to (1) evaluate the effectiveness of compressions and (2) determine if the victim resumes spontaneous circulation and breathing.

To assess the effectiveness of the partner's external chest compressions, the pulse should be checked during the compressions. To determine if the victim has resumed spontaneous breathing and circulation,

chest compressions must be stopped for five seconds at about the end of the first minute and every few minutes thereafter. When the compressor is fatigued, the rescuers should exchange places.

Management of Foreign-body Airway Obstruction

Causes and Precautions

Upper airway obstruction can cause unconsciousness and cardiopulmonary arrest, but far more often, upper airway obstruction is caused by unconsciousness and cardiopulmonary arrest.

An unconscious patient can develop airway obstruction when the tongue falls backward into the pharynx, obstructing the upper airway. The epiglottis could block the entrance of the airway in unconscious victims. Regurgitation of stomach contents into the pharynx, resulting in an obstructed airway, can occur during a cardiopulmonary arrest or during resuscitative attempts. Head and facial injuries may result in blood clots obstructing the upper airway, particularly in unconscious patients.

The National Safety Council reported that foreign-body airway obstruction accounted for approximately 3,100 deaths in 1984. Management of upper airway obstruction should be taught within the context of BLS because of the associated ventilatory and circulatory problems if the victim becomes unconscious. Any victim, especially a younger victim, who suddenly stops breathing, becomes cyanotic, and falls unconscious for no apparent reason should have foreign-body airway obstruction considered in the differential diagnosis.

Foreign-body obstruction of the airway usually occurs during eating. In adults, meat is the most common cause of obstruction, although a variety of other foods and foreign bodies have been the cause of choking in children and some adults. Common factors associated with choking on food include (1) large, poorly chewed pieces of food, (2) elevated blood alcohol levels, and (3) upper or lower dentures, or both. Obstruction, when

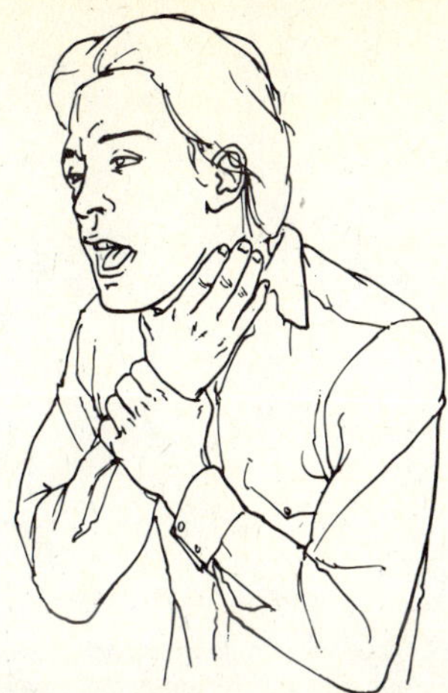

Figure 7　*The universal distress signal for foreign-body airway obstruction involves clutching the neck between thumb and fingers.*

it occurs in restaurants, has been mistaken for a heart attack, giving rise to the name café coronary.

The following precautions may prevent foreign-body airway obstruction: (1) cutting food into small pieces and chewing slowly and thoroughly, especially if one is wearing dentures, (2) avoiding laughing and talking during chewing and swallowing, (3) avoiding excessive intake of alcohol before and during meals, (4) restricting children from walking, running, or playing with food or foreign objects in their mouths, and (5) keeping foreign objects (e.g., marbles, beads, or thumbtacks) away from infants and small children.

Recognition of Foreign-Body Airway Obstruction

Because early recognition of airway obstruction is the key to successful management, it is important to distinguish this emergency from fainting, stroke, heart attack, epilepsy, drug overdose, or other conditions that cause sudden respiratory failure but are managed differently.

Foreign bodies may cause either partial airway obstruction or complete airway obstruction. With partial airway obstruction, the victim may be capable of either good or poor air exchange. With good air exchange, the victim can cough forcefully, although frequently there is wheezing between coughs. As long as good air exchange continues, the victim should be encouraged to persist with spontaneous coughing and breathing efforts. At this point, do not interfere with attempts to expel the foreign body; stay with the victim and monitor these attempts. If partial airway obstruction persists, activate the EMS system.

Poor air exchange may occur initially, or good air exchange may progress to poor air exchange, as indicated by a weak, ineffective cough, high-pitched noise while inhaling, increased respiratory difficulty, and possibly, cyanosis. A partial obstruction with poor air exchange should be managed as if it were a complete airway obstruction.

With complete airway obstruction, the victim is unable to speak, breathe, or cough and may clutch the neck between the thumb and fingers [*see Figure 7*]. (The public should be encouraged to use this sign, the universal distress signal.) Ask the victim if he or she is choking. Movement of air will be absent if complete airway obstruction is present. Oxygen saturation in the blood will decrease rapidly because the obstructed airway prevents entry of air into the lungs. The brain will develop an oxygen deficit resulting in unconsciousness, and death will follow rapidly if prompt action is not taken.

Management of the Obstructed Airway

The Heimlich maneuver (subdiaphragmatic abdominal thrusts) is recommended for relieving foreign-body airway obstruction. (The term abdominal thrust has been used synonymously with the term Heimlich maneuver since 1976. For the sake of uniformity, Heimlich maneuver should be employed, with the more descriptive subdiaphragmatic abdominal thrusts or abdominal thrusts used interchangeably, depending on the circumstance.)

A subdiaphragmatic abdominal thrust, by elevating the diaphragm, can force air from the lungs in sufficient quantity to create an artificial cough intended to move and expel an obstructing foreign body in an airway. Each individual thrust should be administered with the intent of relieving the obstruction. It may be necessary to repeat the thrust six to 10 times to clear the airway. An important consideration during application of the maneuver is possible damage to internal organs, such as rupture or laceration of abdominal or thoracic viscera. The rescuer's hands should never be placed on the xiphoid process of the sternum or on the lower margins of the rib cage. They should be below this area but above the navel and in the midline. Regurgitation may occur as a result of abdominal thrusts. Training and proper performance should minimize these problems.

Heimlich maneuver with victim standing or sitting (conscious) The rescuer should stand behind the victim, wrap his or her arms around the victim's waist, and proceed as follows [*see Figure 8*]: Make a fist with one hand. Place the thumb side of the fist against the victim's abdomen, in the midline slightly above the navel and well below the tip of the xiphoid process. Grasp the fist with the other hand. Press the fist into the victim's abdomen with a quick upward thrust. Each new thrust should be a separate and distinct movement.

Heimlich maneuver with victim lying (unconscious) The victim should be placed in the supine position with the face up [*see Figure 9*]. The rescuer kneels astride the victim's thighs. The rescuer places the heel of one hand against the victim's abdomen, in the midline slightly above the navel and well below the tip of the xiphoid process, and the second hand directly on top of the first. The rescuer presses into the abdomen with a quick upward thrust. If the rescuer is in the correct position, he or she has a natural midabdominal position and is thus unlikely to direct the thrust to the right or left. A rescuer who is too short to reach around the waist of a victim who is conscious can use this technique. The rescuer can use his or her body weight to perform the Heimlich manuever.

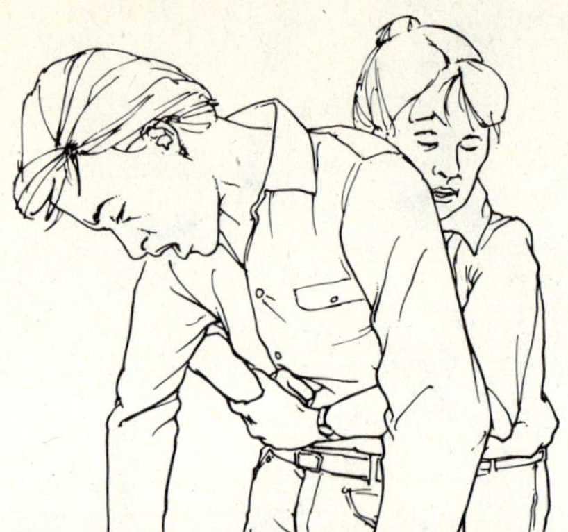

Figure 8 *To administer the Heimlich maneuver to a conscious victim of foreign-body airway obstruction, the rescuer should stand behind the victim, wrap his or her arms around the victim's waist, place a fist against the abdomen (in the midline, slightly above the navel and well below the xiphoid process), grasp the fist with the other hand, and press into the abdomen with a quick upward thrust.*

Finger sweep This maneuver should be used only in the unconscious victim. With the face up, open the victim's mouth by grasping both the tongue and lower jaw between the thumb and fingers and lifting the mandible (tongue-jaw lift). This action draws the tongue away from the back of the throat and away from a foreign body that may be lodged there. This action alone may partially relieve the obstruction. Insert the index finger of the other hand down along the inside of the cheek and deeply into the throat to the base of the tongue. Then, use a hooking action to dislodge the foreign body and maneuver it into the mouth so that it can be removed. It is sometimes necessary to use the index finger to push the foreign body against the opposite side of the throat to dislodge and remove it. Be careful not to force the object deeper into the airway. If the foreign body comes within reach, grasp and remove it.

Self-administered Heimlich maneuver Treatment of one's own complete foreign-body airway obstruction is as follows: make

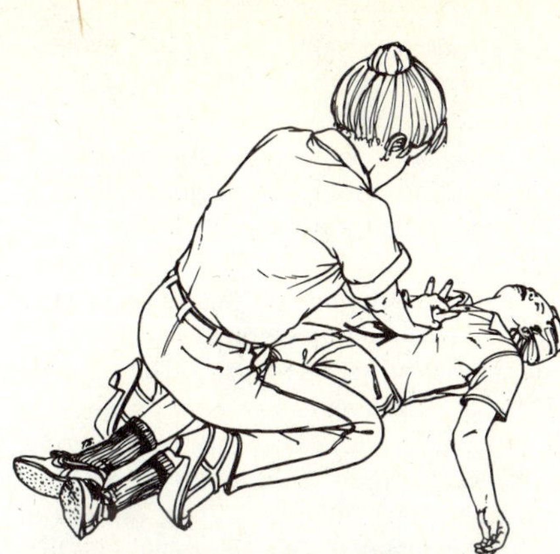

Figure 9 *To administer the Heimlich maneuver to an unconscious victim, the rescuer should kneel astride the victim's thighs, place the heel of one hand on the abdomen (in the midline, slightly above the navel and well below the xiphoid process), place the second hand directly on top of the first, and press into the abdomen with a quick upward thrust.*

a fist with one hand, place the thumb side on the abdomen above the navel and below the xiphoid process, grasp the fist with the other hand, and then press inward and upward toward the diaphragm with a quick motion. If this maneuver is unsuccessful, the victim should press the upper abdomen quickly over any firm surface, such as the back of a chair, the side of a table, or a porch railing. Several thrusts may be needed to clear the airway.

Chest thrusts with victim standing or sitting (conscious) This technique is to be used only in the advanced stages of pregnancy or in the markedly obese victim. The rescuer should stand behind the victim, put his or her arms directly under the victim's armpits, and encircle the victim's chest. The rescuer should place the thumb side of his or her fist on the middle of the breastbone, taking care to avoid the xiphoid process and the margins of the rib cage. The rescuer should then grab his or her fist with the other hand and perform backward thrusts until the foreign body is expelled or the victim becomes unconscious. Each thrust

should be administered with the intent of relieving the obstruction.

Chest thrusts with victim lying (unconscious) This maneuver must be used only in the advanced stages of pregnancy and when the rescuer cannot apply the Heimlich maneuver effectively to the unconscious, markedly obese victim. The rescuer should place the victim on the victim's back and kneel close to the side of the victim's body. The hand position for the application of chest thrusts is the same as that for external heart compressions; for example, in the adult, the heel of the hand is on the lower half of the sternum. Each thrust should be delivered slowly, distinctly, and with the intent of relieving the obstruction.

Recommended sequence for the conscious victim or the victim who becomes unconscious (1) Identify airway obstruction, and ask the victim if he or she is choking. (2) Apply the Heimlich maneuver until the foreign body is expelled or the victim becomes unconscious. (3) Open the mouth of the now unconscious victim, and perform the finger sweep. (4) Open the airway and attempt rescue breathing. (5) If unable to ventilate, perform additional (six to 10) subdiaphragmatic abdominal thrusts. (6) Open the mouth and perform the finger sweep. (7) Attempt to ventilate. (8) Repeat the sequence of Heimlich maneuver, finger sweep, and attempt to ventilate. (9) Persist in these efforts as long as necessary. (10) A second person, if available, should activate the EMS system as soon as possible.

Recommended sequence for the unconscious victim If a rescuer has found an unconscious victim and is unable to ventilate, he or she should reposition the head and try again to ventilate. If this attempt is unsuccessful, subdiaphragmatic abdominal thrusts, followed by the finger sweep, should be performed. If unsuccessful in removing the foreign body, repeat the sequence: thrusts, finger sweep, and attempt to ventilate.

General recommendations (1) The Heimlich maneuver is the recommended technique for the removal of foreign-body airway obstruction in the adult. The use of only this method, which is at least as effective and as safe as any other single method, will simplify training programs and should result in better skills retention. (2) It has previously been recommended that the chest thrust be used only in the markedly obese person and in the advanced stages of pregnancy when there is no room between the enlarging uterus and the rib cage in which to perform the thrusts. There was no evidence reported at the national conference to suggest that this recommendation should not be continued. It is acknowledged that these incidents are rare. Further investigation is necessary. At present, the chest thrust should remain as an alternative for the victim of foreign-body airway obstruction in advanced pregnancy and in the markedly obese person. (3) Data were presented at the conference that suggest that as a single method back blows may not be as effective as the Heimlich maneuver in adults. Because of these data, and in an effort to simplify training, the Heimlich maneuver is the only method recommended at this time. More research is necessary. (4) Under no circumstances should students practice the Heimlich maneuver on each other. (5) The use of devices for relieving foreign-body airway obstruction is restricted to those properly trained in their use and application. The use of devices by persons who are not proficient in their use is unacceptable, and any efforts to support such activity, by legislation or other means, are seen by this conference as a distinct threat to the well-being of patients in need of emergency airway care. The two types of conventional forceps that are acceptable at the present time, but only in the hands of trained persons proficient in their use, are the Kelly clamp and the Magill forceps. Both types of forceps should be used only with direct visualization of the foreign body. Either a laryngoscope or tongue blade and flashlight can be used in order to allow direct visualization.

Warning Signs of Stroke Cerebrovascular disease (stroke) may precipitate conditions requiring rescue breathing, external chest compressions, or both. The lay public and health care professionals should know the early warning signs of stroke, and this information should be included in CPR classes so that prompt, early action can be taken.

Emergency care of the stroke victim should be initiated as soon as warning signs or symptoms are recognized. The warning signs or symptoms of stroke may include (1) paralysis on one or both sides of the body, (2) loss of speech or difficulty in speaking, (3) severe dizziness or stupor, (4) loss of vision, particularly in one eye, and (5) loss of consciousness.

The above-mentioned warning signs of stroke may also be temporary. They may last less than 24 hours and, indeed, often last for only a few minutes. If any of these signs or symptoms occur, a physician should be sought immediately or the EMS system activated, depending on the severity of the symptoms. Similar signs may also be due to alcohol, drugs, insulin reactions, or other diseases, but they may also be warning signs of stroke, even when transient.

Unique Situations

Changing location A victim should not be moved from a cramped or busy location for convenience until effective CPR has been started and the victim has a spontaneous pulse or until help arrives, so that CPR can be performed without interruption.

Stairways In some instances, a victim has to be transported up or down a flight of stairs. It is best to perform CPR effectively at the head or the foot of the stairs and, at a predetermined signal, to interrupt CPR and move as quickly as possible to the next level, where CPR should be resumed. Interruptions should not last longer than 30 seconds and should be avoided if possible.

Litters While transferring a victim into an ambulance or other mobile emergency care unit, CPR should not be interrupted.

Even as the victim is being moved to an ambulance, CPR must continue. With a low-wheeled litter, the rescuer can stand alongside, maintaining the locked-arm position for compression. With a high litter or bed, the rescuer may have to kneel beside the victim on the bed or litter to gain the needed height over the victim's sternum.

Cardiopulmonary resuscitation should not be interrupted for more than seven seconds unless endotracheal intubation is being performed by trained individuals or there are problems with transportation.

Pitfalls and Complications of CPR

If CPR is performed improperly or inadequately, external chest compression and rescue breathing may be ineffective in supporting life. Even properly performed CPR may result in complications.

Rescue Breathing

Techniques for opening the airway should be carefully followed to avoid potential neck and spine complications. The most common reason for inability to ventilate a patient is improper head position.

The major problem associated with excess ventilation volume and fast ventilatory flow rates is gastric distention. Rescue breathing frequently causes distention of the stomach, especially in children. This usually occurs when excessive inflation pressures are used or if the airway is partially or completely obstructed. Gastric distention can be minimized by maintaining an open airway, limiting ventilation volumes to the point at which the chest rises, and not exceeding esophageal opening pressure. Other techniques have been reported to prevent gastric distention:

1. Mouth-to-nose ventilation. Because the nose provides greater resistance to the flow of ventilating gases, it will decrease the pressure of the gases reaching the pharynx.
2. Slow inflation time during ventilation. The slower inspiratory flow rates will produce less pressure in the pharynx and thereby minimize the risk of gastric distention.
3. Cricoid pressure. This technique consists of applying backward pressure on the cricoid cartilage against the cervical vertebra to prevent regurgitation. Cricoid pressure has been found to be effective in preventing regurgitation against esophageal pressure of up to 100 cm of water. This technique should be applied only by health care professionals in two-rescuer CPR situations; its application is simple, but it requires an assistant.

Marked distention of the stomach may promote regurgitation and reduce lung volume by elevation of the diaphragm. If the stomach becomes distended during rescue breathing, recheck and reposition the airway, observe the rise and fall of the chest, and avoid excessive airway pressure. Continue rescue breathing without attempting to expel the stomach contents. Experience has shown that attempting to relieve stomach distention by manual pressure over the victim's upper abdomen is almost certain to cause regurgitation if the stomach is full. If regurgitation does occur, turn the victim's entire body to the side, wipe out the mouth, return the body to the supine position, and continue CPR.

If severe gastric distention results in inadequate ventilation, apply pressure over the epigastrium after placing the victim on his or her side to expel the air from the stomach. This maneuver may be necessary despite the risk of inducing regurgitation and aspiration. The use of suction by trained individuals will minimize aspiration in this situation.

Continuous pressure should not be maintained on the abdomen to help to prevent gastric distention because of the danger of trapping the liver, possibly causing liver rupture. An additional reason to avoid such pressure is the possibility of regurgitation and aspiration of gastric contents.

External Chest Compression

Care should be taken to comply with the recommendations concerning external chest compression techniques. Pulselessness must be established prior to performing compressions. Proper CPR techniques lessen the possibilities of complications resulting from improperly performed compressions.

Even properly performed external chest compression can cause rib fractures in some patients. Other complications that may occur despite proper CPR techniques include fracture of the sternum, separation of the ribs from the sternum, pneumothorax, hemothorax, lung contusions, lacerations of the liver and spleen, and fat emboli. These complications may be minimized by careful attention to details of performance but cannot be entirely prevented. Accordingly, concern for injuries that may result even from properly performed CPR should not impede prompt and energetic application of the technique. The only alternative to timely initiation of effective CPR for the cardiac arrest victim is death.

Improper hand position for external chest compression should be avoided by careful identification of landmarks. Applying pressure too low on the chest may cause the tip of the sternum to cut into the liver and cause internal bleeding.

The rescuer's fingers should not rest on the victim's ribs during compression. Interlocking the fingers of the hands may help to avoid this improper position. Pressure with fingers on the ribs or lateral (sideways) pressure increases the possibility of rib fractures and costochondral separations. Between compressions, the heel of the hand must completely release its pressure but should remain in constant contact with the chest wall over the lower half of the sternum.

Compressions should be smooth, regular, and uninterrupted except for rescue breathing. There should be equal compression and relaxation cycles. Sudden or jerking movements should be avoided. Jabs can increase the possibility of injury to the ribs and internal organs and may decrease the amount of blood circulated by each compression. The lower half of the sternum of an adult must be depressed about 1.5 to 2.0 in (3.8 to 5.0 cm) during chest compres-

sion. Less depth of compression may be ineffective.

Safety in Training for and Providing CPR

Safety in CPR training from the students' and instructors' perspective has gained increased attention. Adherence to the following recommendations should minimize any possible complications for instructors and students during CPR training.

Disease Transmission and CPR Training

The following recommendations for decontaminating manikins used in CPR training were updated in 1983 by members of the Multidisciplinary Ad Hoc Committee for Evaluation of Sanitary Practices in Cardiopulmonary Resuscitation Training. The committee was represented by the American Heart Association (Subcommittee on Emergency Cardiac Care), the American Red Cross (First Aid and CPR Programs), and the Centers for Disease Control (Center for Infectious Diseases and Laboratory Program Office). Instructors should follow these recommendations from the Centers for Disease Control when manikins are used in CPR training.

In past years, the CDC has received numerous inquiries concerning the possible role of cardiopulmonary resuscitation (CPR) training manikins in the transmission of viral hepatitis type B. Recently, inquiries have been received about the potential for transmission of not only hepatitis B but also acquired immunodeficiency syndrome (AIDS), herpesviruses, and various upper and lower respiratory infections (e.g., influenza, infectious mononucleosis, tuberculosis). The use of CPR manikins has increased rapidly because of expanded training programs sponsored by medical and emergency organizations. To date, it is estimated that more than 40 million people have had direct contact with manikins during training courses. In the United States, a number of companies distribute multiple model lines of manikins for training programs in hospitals, police and fire departments, service organizations, lay groups, and schools as part of health, first-aid, and physical education courses. Because practicing with a manikin is an integral part of CPR training, the care and maintenance of the manikins is of utmost importance. Instructors and training agencies rely heavily on manufacturers' recommendations for manikin use and maintenance; these recommendations should be examined closely before purchasing manikins.

The use of CPR training manikins has never been documented as being responsible for an outbreak or even an isolated case of bacterial, fungal, or viral disease. However, manikin surfaces may present a risk of disease transmission under certain circumstances, and these surfaces should be cleaned and disinfected consistently to minimize this risk. Although the major portion of the following discussion was written in 1978 pertaining only to sanitary practices that should be followed to prevent transmission of hepatitis type B, the current revision by the Ad Hoc Committee for Evaluation of Sanitary Practices in Cardiopulmonary Resuscitation Training is applicable to lessening the risks of transmitting a wide variety of infectious diseases.

There are several important infection control considerations in CPR training. First, the act of mouth-to-mouth or mouth-to-nose artificial respiration obviously requires close physical contact, in which a potential rescuer must ignore his or her concerns for personal protection or aesthetic apprehensions to save the life of a victim. Accordingly, in training sessions, students are urged to overcome such hesitations, and they may practice on manikins contaminated by the hands and oral fluids of previous students. This situation becomes especially obvious during the practice of two-rescuer CPR, in which the manikin cannot be adequately cleaned between uses by the two students. Also, the practice of removing upper airway obstruction involves sweeping the back of the manikin throat with a finger, and in this situation, contamination from previous students may be smeared on the manikin face. In practice, there is usually no pause at this point to decontaminate the face before beginning mouth-to-mouth breathing [*see* Recommendations, *below*]. Additionally, the valve mechanisms and lungs in manikin airways invariably become contaminated during use, and if they are not appropriately dismantled and cleaned after class, they may serve as contamination sources for subsequent classes. There is no recognized evidence, however, that the manikin valve mechanisms produce aerosols even when air is forcibly expelled during chest compression exercises.

Some manufacturers have provided protective face shields for manikins to improve hygienic conditions during training sessions, but it is unlikely that such shields would be changed after each use by students learning the two-rescuer resuscitation method. Protective shields and detailed instruction for sanitizing the manikin between uses by students and classes are available from several manufacturers.

When dealing with potential contamination by microorganisms having resistance levels that have not been fully characterized (e.g., human immunodeficiency virus [HIV], hepatitis, and herpesviruses), the manikins pose a difficult disinfection problem. Although there are several intermediate- to high-level disinfectants recommended for use in instances of contamination, such as by hepatitis B virus, the majority would meet with objection because of either material incompatibility with the manikin (e.g., staining or other damage of plastic materials by iodine compounds) or undesirable residues, odors, or toxicities that may affect students (e.g., formaldehyde, glutaraldehyde) when used during the training sessions. Alcohols, quaternary ammonium compounds, and phenolics are not generally recommended, because proper contact times for effective action are difficult to achieve (e.g., alcohols evaporate rapidly) or the compounds are not broad-spectrum agents (e.g., quaternary ammonium compounds have limited action against certain viruses and bacteria).

Recommendations

1. Purchasers of training manikins should thoroughly examine the manufacturers' recommendations and provisions for sanitary practices.

2. Students should be told in advance that the training sessions will involve close physical contact with their fellow students.

3. Students or instructors should not actively participate in training sessions (hands-on training with manikins) if they have dermatologic lesions on hands or in oral or circumoral areas, if they are known to be seropositive for hepatitis B surface antigen (HB$_s$Ag), if they have upper respiratory tract infections, if they have acquired immunodeficiency syndrome (AIDS), or if the student or instructor has reason to believe that he or she has been exposed to or is in the active stage of any infectious process.

4. If more than one CPR manikin is used in a particular training class, students should preferably be assigned in pairs, with each pair having contact with only one manikin. This approach would lessen the possible contamination of several manikins by one individual and therefore limit possible exposure of other class members.

5. All persons responsible for CPR training should be thoroughly familiar with hygienic concepts (e.g., thorough hand washing prior to manikin contact and not eating during class to avoid contaminating manikins with food particles) as well as the procedures for cleaning and maintaining manikins and accessories (e.g., face shields). Manikins should be inspected routinely for signs of physical deterioration, such as cracks or tears in plastic surfaces, which make thorough cleaning difficult or impossible. The clothes and hair of manikins should be washed periodically (e.g., monthly or whenever visibly soiled).

6. During the training of two-rescuer CPR, there is no opportunity to disinfect the manikin between students when the so-called switching procedure is practiced. To limit the potential for disease transmission during this exercise, the student taking over ventilation on the manikin should simulate ventilation instead of blowing into the manikin. This recommendation is consistent with current training recommendations of the American Red Cross and the American Heart Association.

7. Training for the obstructed airway procedure involves the student using his or her finger to sweep foreign matter out of the manikin's mouth. This action could contaminate the student's finger with exhaled moisture and saliva from previous students in the same class or contaminate the manikin with material from the student's finger. When practicing this procedure, the finger sweep should be either simulated or done on a manikin whose airway was decontaminated before the procedure and will be decontaminated after the procedure.

8. Personnel conducting the manikin disassembly and decontamination should wear protective latex gloves and wash their hands after finishing. At the end of each class, the following procedures should be done as soon as possible to avoid drying of contamination on manikin surfaces: (a) disassemble the manikin as directed by manufacturer, (b) as indicated, thoroughly wash all external and internal surfaces (also reusable protective face shields) with warm soapy water and brushes, (c) rinse all surfaces with fresh water, (d) wet all surfaces with a sodium hypochlorite solution having at least 500 ppm of free available chlorine (one-quarter cup of liquid household bleach per gallon of tap water) for 10 minutes (this solution must be made fresh at each class and discarded after each use), and (e) rinse with fresh water and immediately

dry all external and internal surfaces; rinsing with alcohol will aid drying of internal surfaces, and this drying will prevent the survival and growth of bacterial or fungal pathogens if the manikins are stored for periods longer than the day of cleaning.

9. Each time a different student uses the manikin in a training class, the individual protective face shield, if used, should be changed. Between students or after the instructor demonstrates a procedure such as clearing any obstruction from the airway, the face and inside of the mouth of the manikin should be wiped vigorously with clean, absorbent material (e.g., 4 in by 4 in gauze pad) wet with either the hypochlorite solution described in recommendation 8d, above, or with 70 percent alcohol (isopropanol or ethanol). The surfaces should remain wet for at least 30 seconds before they are wiped dry with a second piece of clean, absorbent material.

The committee is somewhat reluctant to recommend use of alcohols in this instance and do so only as an alternative because some persons find the odor of hypochlorite objectionable. Although highly bactericidal, alcohols are not considered to be broad-spectrum agents, and use of alcohols here is recommended primarily as an aid in mechanical cleaning; also, in a short contact period, alcohols may not be effective against bacteria or other pathogens. Nonetheless, in the context of vigorous cleaning with alcohol and absorbent material, little viable microbial contamination is likely after the cleaning procedure.

10. People responsible for the use and maintenance of CPR manikins should be encouraged not to rely totally on the mere presence of a disinfectant to protect them and their students from cross-infection during training programs. Emphasis should be placed on the necessity of thorough physical cleaning (scrubbing, wiping) as the first step in an effective decontamination protocol. Microbial contamination is easily removed from smooth, nonporous surfaces by using disposable cleaning cloths moistened with a detergent solution, and there is no evidence that a soaking procedure alone in a liquid is as effective as the same procedure accompanied by vigorous scrubbing.

11. With specific regard to concerns about potential for hepatitis B and AIDS transmission in CPR training, it has recently been shown that the hepatitis B virus is not as resistant to disinfectant chemicals as it was once thought to be. Current recommendations for strategies dealing with AIDS contamination are the same as those for viral hepatitis B.

In 1985, there was a dramatic increase in the number of inquiries regarding the adequacy of the current recommendation for manikin decontamination in killing the viral agent of the acquired immunodeficiency syndrome (AIDS). Recent studies have shown that the retroviral agent that causes AIDS, human immunodeficiency virus (HIV), which was formerly called human T cell lymphotropic virus type III/lymphadenopathy-associated virus (HTLV-III/LAV), is comparatively delicate and is inactivated in less than 10 minutes at room temperature by a number of disinfectant chemicals, including the recommended agents, alcohol and sodium hypochlorite. Coupled with scrubbing and rinsing with soap and water, the sodium hypochlorite dilution will ensure that HIV, as well as a wide variety of other infectious agents with potential for contaminating manikin surfaces, will be killed. In fact, if the steps in recommendation 8, above, are consistently followed, the students of each class should be presented with manikins having a sanitary quality equal to or better than eating utensils in a properly operated restaurant. A higher level of surface disinfection is not warranted, and the recommended disinfectant chemicals (alcohol and household bleach) are safe, effective, inexpensive, easily obtained, and well tolerated by students, instructors, and manikin surfaces when properly used.

Current research and recommendations for preventing HIV contamination of surfaces has been published. It is emphasized that there is no evidence to date that AIDS is transmitted either by casual personal contact, by indirect contact with inanimate surfaces, or by the airborne route.

The risk of transmission of any infectious disease by manikin practice appears to be low. While an estimated 40 million people in the United States and perhaps 150 million worldwide have been taught mouth-to-mouth breathing on manikins in the past 25 years, there has never been a documented case of transmission of bacterial, fungal, or viral disease by a CPR training manikin. Thus, in the absence of evidence of infectious disease risk, including risk for AIDS, the lifesaving potential of CPR should continue to be vigorously emphasized, and energetic efforts in support of broad-scale CPR training should be continued.

Disease Transmission and Actual Performance of CPR

The vast majority of CPR performed in the United States is done by health care and public safety personnel, many of whom perform mouth-to-mouth ventilation frequently throughout the year on cardiac arrest victims about whom they have little or no medical information. An individual layperson is less likely to be in a situation to perform CPR than are health care personnel. A layperson who performs CPR is most likely to do so in the home (where 70 to 80 percent of cardiac arrests occur), commonly knows the cardiac arrest victim, and often has prior knowledge of the victim's health. There should be no reluctance by the rescuer in this situation to institute CPR.

The greatest concern about the theoretical risk of disease transmission from mouth-to-mouth resuscitation should be directed at individuals who perform CPR frequently, such as health care and public safety personnel and prehospital emergency health care providers.

Providers of prehospital emergency health care include paramedics, emergency medical technicians, law enforcement personnel, firefighters, lifeguards, and others whose jobs might require them to provide first-response medical care. The risk of transmission of infection from infected persons to providers of prehospital emergency health care should be no higher than that for health care workers providing emergency care in the hospital if appropriate precautions are taken to prevent exposure to blood or other body fluids.

No transmission of hepatitis B virus infection during mouth-to-mouth resuscitation has been documented. However, because of the theoretical risk of salivary transmission of HIV during mouth-to-mouth resuscitation, special attention should be given to the use of disposable airway equipment or resuscitation bags and the wearing of gloves when in contact with blood or other body fluids. Resuscitation equipment and devices known or suspected to be contaminated with blood or other body fluids should be used once and disposed of or be thoroughly cleaned and disinfected after each use.[2]

Clear plastic face masks with one-way valves are available for use during mouth-to-mask ventilation. These masks provide diversion of the victim's exhaled gas away from the rescuer and may be used by health care providers and public safety personnel properly trained in their use during two-person rescue, in place of mouth-to-mouth ventilation. The need for and effectiveness of this adjunct in preventing transmission of an infectious disease during mouth-to-mouth ventilation are unknown. If this type of device is to be used as reassurance to the rescuer that a potential risk might be minimized, the rescuer must be adequately trained in its use, especially with respect to making an adequate seal on the face and maintaining a patent airway. Such a device would be applicable only to two-rescuer CPR because it requires two hands to secure a proper face seal and to maintain an open airway. As an additional precaution, the rescuer may elect to wear latex gloves because saliva or blood on the victim's mouth or face may be transferred to the rescuer's hands.

The Physically Challenged CPR Student

The CPR learner who has a disability such as deafness or blindness requires modifications in instructional methods. Many successes have been reported in training and actual resuscitation with and by the physically challenged. Training agencies should use appropriate resources to train the handicapped, modifying BLS courses to meet the needs of this population.

Other populations exist, however, whose handicaps become evident only when they become CPR learners. Due to the nature of the psychomotor skill development during CPR training and the requisite physical exertion, individuals with certain medical conditions and health care problems may not learn the skills of CPR at the same pace as the healthy learner. Furthermore, these same individuals may find the required exertion unsafe in that certain conditions may become aggravated as a result of skills practice.

An estimated 10 percent of all CPR learners will present with some condition or history that may affect their ability to perform CPR. These individuals are generally not considered disabled, because the impairment does not impede performance of daily activities, nor does society consider these learners disabled. Several reports are found in the literature citing specific cases of physical disability among CPR learners.

No single specific solution exists to help these learners to overcome their physical disabilities, except additional practice time and patience. However, additional practice time may contribute to the aggravation of these existing health problems. Instructors must therefore balance practice time with rest periods and observe learners closely for signs of fatigue during actual practice.

Cardiopulmonary resuscitation activity requires physical effort by healthy performers. There are data that suggest that individuals with preexisting conditions may experience aggravation of these problems. Instructors should advise all CPR learners about the level of physical activity and to pace their practice according to individual ability. The following guidelines should be used during CPR training: (1) at the beginning of CPR training, use a liability statement to make an announcement regarding physical activity, (2) identify learners with preexisting medical conditions and other health care problems, (3) observe learners during practice, and when participants appear fatigued, intervene to prevent harm to learners, (4) establish realistic expectations of learners with preexisting conditions, (5) provide alternative practice periods and rest periods that help the impaired learner to achieve personal and course goals while still remaining within the standards, and (6) practice patience.

Pediatric Basic Life Support

Cardiopulmonary resuscitation (CPR) in the pediatric age group should be part of a communitywide effort that smoothly integrates pediatric basic life support (BLS), pediatric advanced life support (ALS), and postresuscitation care. Basic life support is that phase of emergency care that (1) prevents respiratory and circulatory arrest through prompt recognition and intervention or (2) supports or provides ventilation and, if necessary, circulation to a victim, without the use of adjuncts. Except for neonates, the number of children who require resuscitation is small; for best results, therefore, each community must ensure that its EMS personnel are optimally trained and equipped to care for pediatric emergencies. There is evidence that this is not currently the case. It is further recommended that (1) BLS for infants and children be the major focus of courses offered to certain audiences (i.e., parents of young children, day-care personnel, and parents of infants at high risk for sudden infant death), (2) personnel at ALS emergency facilities have demonstrated competence in pediatric BLS and pediatric ALS, and (3) each ALS facility have an ongoing agreement with an identified tertiary pediatric service where postresuscitation care for infants and children can be given in a pediatric intensive care unit under the supervision of trained personnel.

Causes of Cardiopulmonary Arrest

Cardiac arrest in the pediatric age group is rarely primarily of cardiac origin; more commonly, it results from a low oxygen level secondary to respiratory difficulty or arrest. Because the cardiac arrest is the result of a long period of hypoxemia, it is not surprising that outcomes of CPR in children who have suffered a cardiac arrest have been poor. Conversely, the outcome of resuscitation for respiratory arrest, before the development of cardiac arrest, is considerably better. It should be possible to improve the current poor results with an educational program—directed at parents, child-care personnel, and members of the EMS system—that emphasizes prevention, early recognition of the child in distress, and rapid intervention before cardiac arrest occurs.

The major events that may necessitate resuscitation include (1) injuries, (2) suffocation caused by foreign bodies (e.g., toys, foods, plastic covers), (3) smoke inhalation, (4) sudden infant death syndrome, and (5) infections, especially of the respiratory tract. Injuries account for nearly 9,000 pediatric fatalities annually in the United States and represent approximately 44 percent of deaths in children between the ages of one and 14 years. Of these, 45 percent involve motor vehicles; 17 percent involve drowning; and 21 percent involve burns, firearms, or poisoning. In children younger than one year, 41 percent of accidental deaths involve poisons, suffocation, or motor vehicles.

The vast majority of emergency situations requiring CPR are preventable, and special attention must therefore be paid to producing environments for children that are safe and protective without suppressing their need for exploration and discovery. Children should be taught respect for matches and fires, and young children should not be left unsupervised. Toys given to toddlers should be carefully examined for small parts that could be aspirated. Beads, small toys, marbles, and peanuts must be kept away from infants and preschool children. In automobiles, age-appropriate restraints, including infant car seats and seat belts, should be used. Children should be taught to swim, and water safety should be emphasized. It is important to remember that time spent mastering CPR is much less productive than time spent preventing the situation leading to its need.

The Sequence of CPR

Each of the *ABC*s of CPR, *A*irway, *B*reathing, and *C*irculation, begins with an assessment phase: determine unresponsiveness, determine breathlessness, and determine pulselessness, respectively. Assessment also involves a more subtle, constant process of observing and interacting with the victim.

Airway

Determine Unresponsiveness or Respiratory Difficulty

The rescuer must quickly assess the extent of any injury and determine whether the child is unconscious. Special care must be taken if the victim has sustained head or neck trauma, so as not to cause spinal cord injury. Unconsciousness is determined by gently shaking the victim to elicit a response. If the child is struggling to breathe but is conscious, he or she should be transported as rapidly as possible to' an ALS facility. Children will often find the best position for keeping a partially obstructed airway open and should therefore be allowed to maintain the position affording them the greatest comfort.

Call for Help

After determining unresponsiveness or respiratory difficulty, the rescuer should call out for help. If the rescuer is alone and the child is obviously not breathing, CPR should be performed for one minute before calling for help.

Position the Victim

For CPR to be effective, the victim must be lying on his or her back on a firm, flat surface. Great care must be taken in moving a child into this position, especially if there is evidence of head or neck injury. The circum-

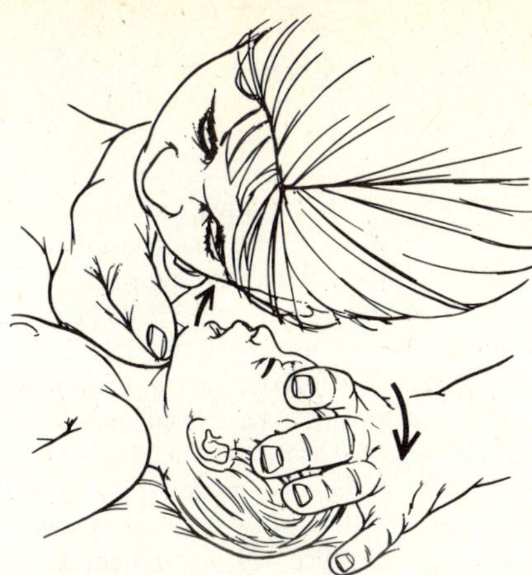

Figure 10 *The recommended technique for opening the airway of a child is the head tilt–chin lift maneuver.*

stances in which the child is found should influence the care that may be needed in positioning him or her. The likelihood of neck, spine, or bone injuries is greater if a child is found unconscious at the scene of an accident—for example, at the base of a tree—than if an infant is found in bed not breathing. The size of the child will also influence how he or she is positioned, but the principle to bear in mind is that the child must be turned as a unit, with firm support of the head and neck so that the head does not roll, twist, or tilt backward or forward.

Open the Airway

The small air passages of an infant or child can easily be obstructed by mucus, blood, vomitus, or in an unconscious victim, the tongue. The tongue is attached to the lower jaw; with loss of consciousness, the muscles relax and the tongue falls back, obstructing the airway. The first maneuver, after determining unconsciousness and turning the victim into the supine position, is to open the airway. This is accomplished by the head tilt–chin lift maneuver. If the child is having respiratory difficulty but is conscious, time should not be wasted on an attempt to open the airway; the child should be transported to an ALS facility as rapidly as possible.

Head tilt–chin lift The rescuer places the hand closest to the child's head on the forehead and tilts the head gently back into a sniffing or neutral position in infants and slightly further back in children [*see Figure 10*]. Some experts believe that overextension of the head closes the trachea in small babies; there are no data that this is so, but because it is unnecessary, overextension is best avoided. The head should not be tilted in suspected neck injury; jaw thrust without head tilt may be used instead.

To augment head tilt, the rescuer lifts the chin with its attached structures, including the tongue, from the airway. The fingers, but not the thumb, of the hand away from the victim's head are placed under the bony part of the lower jaw at the chin, and the chin is lifted upward. So as not to obstruct the airway, care must be exercised not to close the mouth completely or to push on the soft parts of the underchin. Except in cases of suspected neck injury, the rescuer's other hand continues to tilt the head backward.

Jaw thrust The rescuer places two or three fingers under each side of the lower jaw at its angle and lifts the jaw upward [*see Figure 11*]. The rescuer's elbows should rest on the surface on which the victim is lying. Jaw thrust may be accompanied by slight head tilt or can be used alone. Jaw thrust without head tilt is the safest technique for opening the airway when neck injury is suspected.

Breathing

Determine Whether the Victim Is Breathing

If it is unclear whether the victim is breathing, the airway is opened, and while patency is being maintained, the rescuer places his or her ear close to the victim's mouth and nose while *looking* at the chest and abdomen for movement, *listening* for exhaled air, and *feeling* for exhaled air flow [*see Figure 10*]. If the child is breathing, continued patency of the airway must be maintained. If no breathing is detected, the rescuer must breathe for the victim.

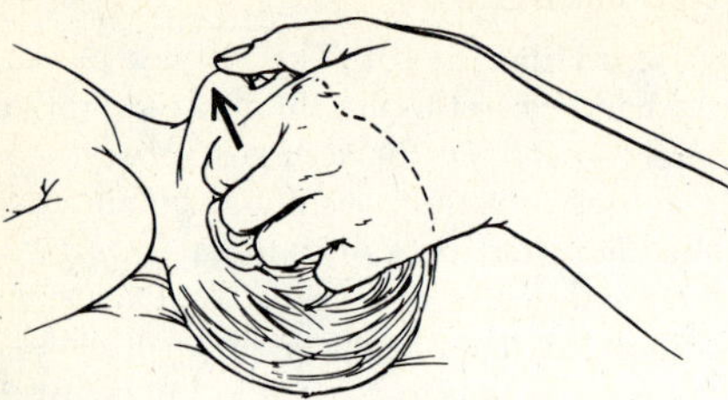

Figure 11 *The jaw-thrust maneuver is the safest technique for opening the airway of a child when neck injury is suspected.*

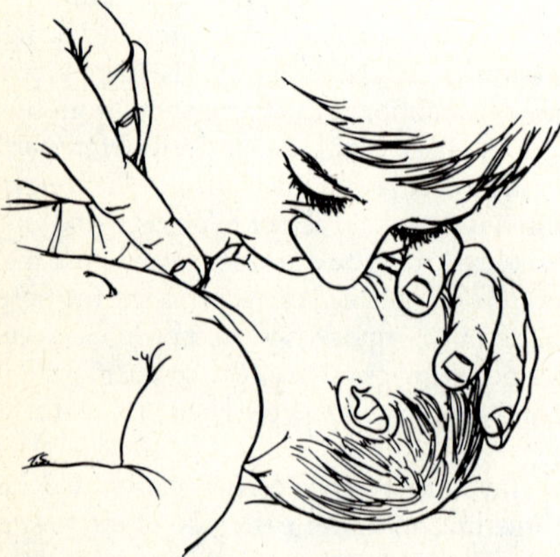

Figure 12 *In rescue breathing for the infant, the rescuer's mouth makes a tight seal with the victim's nose and mouth.*

Breathe for the Victim

If the victim does not breathe after the airway is opened, rescue breathing must be applied to provide the victim's lungs with oxygen. While continuing to maintain patency of the airway, the rescuer takes a breath and makes a seal between his mouth and the mouth, or mouth and nose, of the victim. If the victim is an infant, the rescuer's mouth will make a tight seal with the mouth and nose [*see Figure 12*]. If the victim is larger, the nose is pinched tightly with the fingers of the hand that is maintaining head tilt, and a mouth-to-mouth seal is made [*see Figure 4*]. Two slow breaths (1.0 to 1.5 seconds per breath) are given, with a pause between for the rescuer to take a breath. (Measure-

ments of time per breath given herein are, more precisely, measurements of the victim's inspiratory time.)

The volume of air in an infant's lungs is smaller than that in an adult's lungs, and an infant's air passages are also considerably smaller, with resistance to flow potentially quite high. Because these differences are also relative, it is impossible to make a recommendation about the force or volume of the rescue breaths. The critical points are that (1) rescue breaths are the single most important maneuver in assisting a non-breathing child victim, (2) an appropriate volume is that which will make the chest rise and fall, and (3) by giving the breaths slowly, an adequate volume will be provided at the lowest possible pressure, thereby avoiding gastric distention.

If air enters freely and the chest rises, the airway is clear. If air does not enter freely (i.e., the chest does not rise), the airway is obstructed. Improper opening of the airway is the most common cause of obstruction, and head tilt–chin lift should be adjusted. If a repeated rescue breathing attempt does not allow air to enter freely as evidenced by lack of chest movement, a foreign-body obstruction should be suspected.

Gastric distention Rescue breathing, especially if rapidly applied, can cause gastric distention, which if excessive can interfere with rescue breathing by elevating the diaphragm, thus decreasing lung volume. The incidence of gastric distention can be minimized by limiting the rate of chest inflation and the ventilation volume to the point at which the chest rises, thereby not exceeding the esophageal opening pressure. Attempts at relieving gastric distention by pressure on the abdomen should be avoided because of the danger of aspiration of stomach contents into the lungs.

Gastric decompression should be attempted only if the abdomen is so tense that ventilation is ineffective. In such a situation, the victim's entire body is turned as a unit onto the side, with the head down if possible, before pressure is applied to the abdomen.

Circulation

Check the Pulse

Ineffective or absent cardiac contractions are recognized by the absence of a pulse in a large central artery. In a child older than one year, the carotid is the most central and accessible artery; in an infant younger than one year, the short, chubby neck makes the carotid difficult to palpate, so the brachial artery is recommended instead. The femoral pulse is often used by health professionals in a hospital setting; however, it is recommended that lay rescuers be instructed in locating the carotid and brachial arteries only.

The carotid artery lies on the side of the neck between the windpipe and the strap muscles. While maintaining head tilt with one hand on the forehead, the rescuer locates the victim's Adam's apple with two or three fingers of the other hand. The fingers are then slid into the groove, on the side closest to the rescuer, between the trachea and the neck muscles, and the artery is gently palpated [*see Figure 5*].

The brachial pulse is located on the inside of the upper arm, between the elbow and the shoulder. With the rescuer's thumb on the outside of the arm, the index and middle fingers are pressed gently until the pulse is felt [*see Figure 13*].

When there is a pulse but no breathing, rescue breathing should be initiated and continued until spontaneous breathing resumes. For an infant, the rescue breathing rate should be once every three seconds, or 20 times a minute, and for a child, once every four seconds, or 15 times a minute. If a pulse is not present, a diagnosis of cardiac arrest is made, and chest compressions must be initiated and coordinated with rescue breathing.

Activate the EMS System

If a second rescuer is present or arrives to help, one rescuer should activate the EMS system by calling the local emergency telephone number, which in many communities is 911. If no help is forthcoming, the decision when to leave the victim to telephone is a difficult one and is affected by a number of

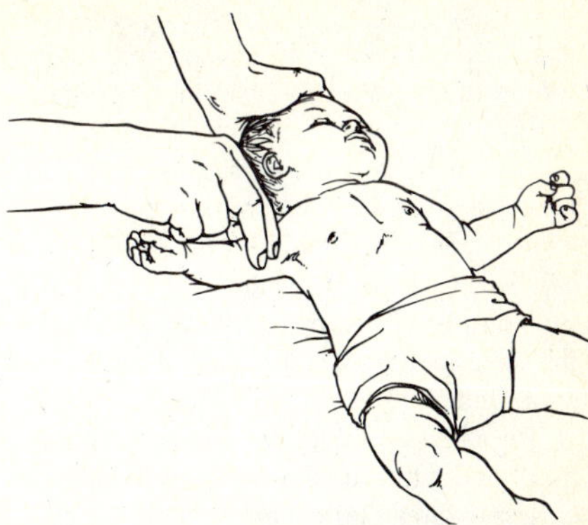

Figure 13 To determine pulselessness in infants younger than one year, the brachial rather than the carotid pulse is located and palpated.

variables, including the probability of someone else arriving on the scene. If the rescuer is unable to activate the EMS system, the only option is to continue CPR.

The rescuer calling the EMS system should give the following information: (1) the location of the emergency, including address and names of streets or landmarks, (2) the telephone number from which the call is being made, (3) what happened (e.g., auto accident, drowning), (4) the number of victims, (5) the condition of the victim or victims, (6) the nature of the aid being given, and (7) any other information requested. To ensure this last item, the caller should hang up last.

Perform Chest Compressions

External chest compression consists of serial, rhythmic compressions of the chest by which blood is circulated to the vital organs (heart, lungs, and brain) to keep them viable until ALS care can be given. Chest compressions must always be accompanied by rescue breathing. The mechanism by which blood is circulated by chest compressions is still a subject of controversy. It is not clear whether blood circulation takes place by a change in the thoracic pressure, by direct compression of the heart, or by both mechanisms [*see* Adult Basic Life Support, Physiology of Circulation, *above*]; however, direct heart compression may be the more important mechanism in the pediatric age group.

For optimal compressions, the child must be in a horizontal, supine position on a hard surface. In an infant, the hard surface can be the palm of the hand not performing the compressions; head tilt is provided by the weight of the head and a slight lift of the shoulders.

Recent evidence has shown that the heart of the infant is lower in relation to the external chest landmarks than was previously thought. In the following recommendations, therefore, the area of compression for infants is lower than in previous standards.

In the infant　(1) An imaginary line between the nipples is located over the breastbone [*see Figure 14*]. (2) The index finger of the hand farther from the infant's head is placed just under the intermammary line where it intersects the sternum. The area of compression is one finger's width below this intersection, at the location of the middle and ring fingers. (3) Using two or three fingers, the breastbone is compressed to a depth of 0.5 to 1.0 in (1.3 to 2.5 cm) at a rate of at least 100 times a minute. (4) At the end of each compression, pressure is released and the sternum is allowed to come to its normal position, without removing the fingers from the sternum. A compression-relaxation rhythm should be developed that has equal time allotted to each phase and is smooth (i.e., without jerky movements).

In the child　(1) The lower margin of the victim's rib cage is located on the side next to the rescuer with the middle and index fingers [*see Figure 15*]. (2) The margin of the rib cage is followed with the middle finger to the notch where the ribs and breastbone meet. (3) With the middle finger on this notch, the index finger is placed next to the middle finger. (4) The heel of the hand is placed next to the index finger, with the long axis of the heel parallel to that of the ster-

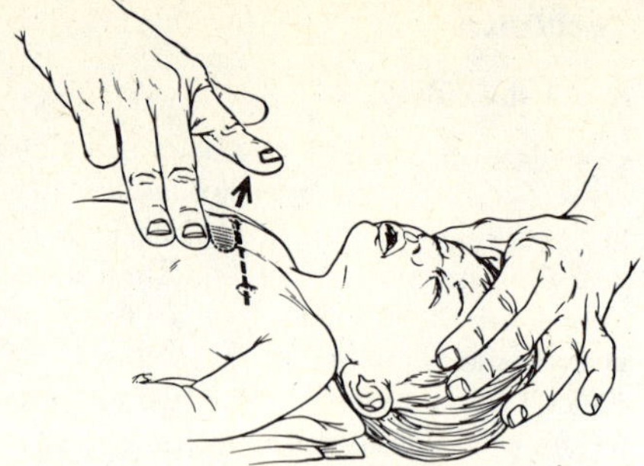

Figure 14　*To position the fingers correctly for chest compression in infants, the rescuer places two or three fingers on the sternum, one finger's width below the imaginary line connecting the nipples.*

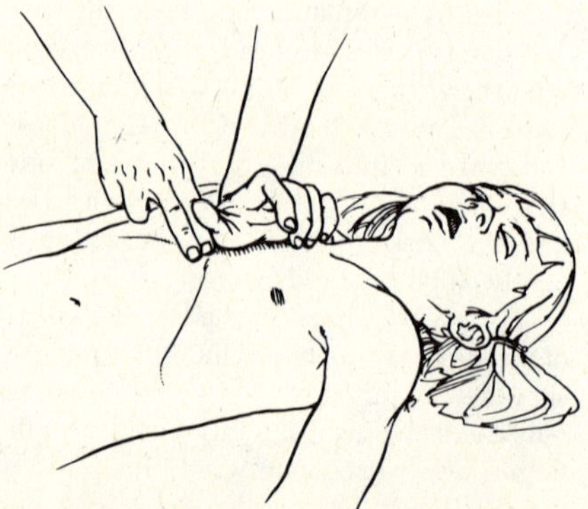

Figure 15　*To locate the proper hand position for chest compression in the child, the rescuer places the heel of the hand on the sternum, two fingers' width above the notch where the ribs and breastbone meet.*

num. (5) The chest is compressed with one hand to a depth of 1.0 to 1.5 in (2.5 to 3.8 cm) at a rate of 80 to 100 times a minute. The fingers should be kept off the ribs. (6) The compressions should be smooth, not jerky; the chest should be allowed to return to its resting position after each compression, but the hand should not be lifted off the chest. Each compression and relaxation phase should be equal in time. (7) If the child is large or older than approximately eight years, the method described for adults should be used [*see* Adult Basic Life Support, *above*].

Coordinate Compressions and Rescue Breathing

External chest compressions must always be accompanied by rescue breathing. At the end of every fifth compression, a pause should be allowed for a ventilation (1.0 to 1.5 seconds per breath). In the infant and child, the 5:1 compression-ventilation ratio is maintained for both one and two rescuers. The two-rescuer technique should be used only by health care professionals. Because compressions must be briefly interrupted to allow for an adequate ventilation, a rate of 80 to 100 compressions a minute is recommended. The infant and child should be reassessed after 10 cycles of compressions and ventilations (approximately one minute) and every few minutes thereafter.

Management of Airway Obstruction

More than 90 percent of deaths from foreign-body aspiration in the pediatric age group occur in children younger than five years, and 65 percent are in infants. The 1985 National Conference noted the marked decline in pediatric deaths from foreign-body aspiration since the last conference. The reason for this decline is not clear. Aspirated materials include foods (e.g., hot dogs, round candies, nuts, and grapes) and other small objects. Foreign-body airway obstruction should be suspected in infants and children experiencing acute respiratory distress associated with coughing, gagging, or stridor (a high-pitched noisy breathing).

Signs and symptoms of airway obstruction may also be due to infections that cause airway swelling, such as epiglottitis and croup. Children with an infectious cause of airway obstruction need prompt attention in an ALS facility, and time should not be wasted in a futile attempt to relieve their obstruction. Attempts at clearing the airway should be considered for (1) a child whose aspiration is witnessed or strongly sus-

pected and (2) an unconscious, nonbreathing child whose airway remains obstructed despite the usual maneuvers to open it. In a witnessed or strongly suspected aspiration, the rescuer should encourage the child to persist with spontaneous coughing and breathing efforts as long as the cough is forceful. Relief of the obstruction should be attempted only if the cough is, or becomes, ineffective or if there is increased respiratory difficulty accompanied by a high-pitched noise while inhaling (stridor), or both. The EMS system should be activated as soon as a second rescuer is available.

The optimal method for relief of foreign-body obstruction remains a matter of controversy, and further data are needed to distinguish opinions and personal experiences from objective facts. If the victim is a child, the Heimlich maneuver is recommended. This maneuver, which increases intrathoracic pressures, creates an artificial cough that forces air and, it is hoped, a foreign body out of the airway. Six to 10 thrusts are repeated in rapid sequence until the foreign body is expelled. However, although the conference recognized the pedagogic value of uniformity, there was concern for potential intra-abdominal injury resulting from subdiaphragmatic abdominal thrusts in infants younger than one year. In this age group, therefore, the combination of back blows and chest thrusts continues to be recommended. Some experts believe that in the infant this combination is an indirect application of the Heimlich maneuver.

Following maneuvers to remove an airway obstruction, the airway is opened using head tilt–chin lift, and if spontaneous breathing is absent, rescue breathing is performed. If the chest does not rise, the head is repositioned, the airway is opened, and rescue breathing is attempted again. If rescue breathing is still unsuccessful (i.e., the chest does not rise), maneuvers to relieve foreign-body obstruction should be repeated.

In the Infant

The infant is straddled over the rescuer's arm, with the head lower than the trunk, and the head is supported by firmly holding the jaw. The rescuer rests his or her forearm on his or her thigh and delivers four back blows forcefully with the heel of the hand between the infant's shoulder blades [*see Figure 16*]. After delivering the back blows, the rescuer places his or her free hand on the infant's back so that the victim is sandwiched between the two hands, one supporting the neck, jaw, and chest, while the other supports the back. While still supporting the head and neck, the infant is turned and placed on the thigh with the head lower than the trunk; then four chest thrusts are performed in the same location as external chest compressions but at a slower rate [*see Figure 16*]. Rescuers whose hands are small may find it physically difficult to perform the back blows and chest thrusts in the described manner, especially if the infant is large. An alternative method is to lay the infant face down on the rescuer's lap, the head lower than the trunk, with the head firmly supported. After the four back blows have been performed, the infant is turned as a unit to the supine position, and the chest thrusts are performed.

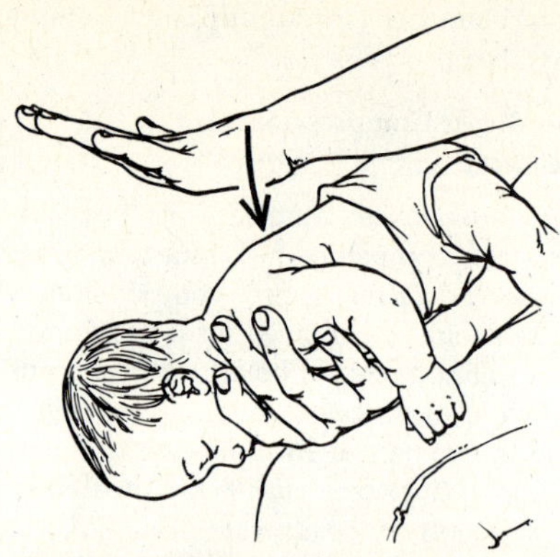

Figure 16   *In infants younger than one year, foreign-body airway obstruction is relieved by back blows alternated with chest compressions, rather than by abdominal thrusts. Back blows are delivered forcefully between the infant's shoulder blades with the heel of the hand.*

In the Child

Heimlich maneuver with victim standing or sitting (conscious)   The rescuer should stand behind the victim and wrap his or her arms around the victim's waist, with one hand made into a fist [*see Figure 17*].

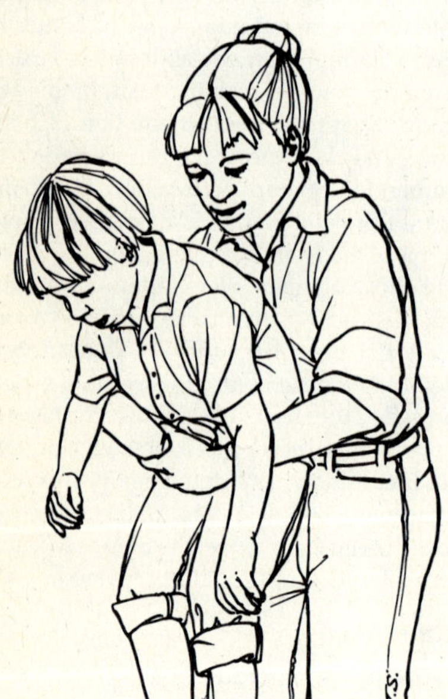

Figure 17   *The Heimlich maneuver for the conscious child older than one year follows the same procedure used for adults. The rescuer should stand behind the victim, wrap his or her arms around the victim's waist, place a fist against the abdomen (in the midline, slightly above the navel and well below the xiphoid process), grasp the fist with the other hand, and press into the abdomen with a quick upward thrust.*

The thumb side of the fist should rest against the victim's abdomen in the midline, slightly above the navel and well below the tip of the xiphoid process. The fist should be grasped by the other hand and pressed into the victim's abdomen with a quick upward thrust. The rescuer's hands should not touch the xiphoid process or the lower margins of the rib cage because of possible damage to internal organs. Each thrust should be a separate and distinct movement.

Heimlich maneuver with victim lying (conscious or unconscious) The rescuer should position the child face up on his or her back and kneel at the child's feet, if the child is on the floor, or stand at the child's feet, if the child is on a table [*see Figure 9*]. (The astride position is not recommended for small children but may be used in the case of a large child.) The rescuer should place the heel of one hand on the child's abdomen in the midline slightly above the navel and well below the rib cage. The other hand should be placed on top of the first and pressed into the abdomen with a quick upward thrust. Care should be exercised to direct the thrusts upward in the midline and not to either side of the abdomen. Several thrusts may be necessary to expel the object. In small children, the maneuver must be applied gently.

Finger Sweep

Blind finger sweeps are to be avoided in infants and children because the foreign body may be pushed back into the airway, causing further obstruction. In the unconscious, nonbreathing victim, following the chest thrusts or subdiaphragmatic abdominal thrusts, the victim's mouth is opened by grasping both the tongue and the lower jaw between the thumb and finger and lifting (tongue-jaw lift). This action draws the tongue away from the back of the throat and may itself partially relieve the obstruction. If the foreign body is visualized, it should be removed.

References

1. JAMA 255:2915, 1986
2. MMWR 34:681, 1985

Acknowledgment

Figures 1 to 17 Reprinted from "Standards and Guidelines for Cardiopulmonary Resuscitation (CPR) and Emergency Cardiac Care (ECC)," in *The Journal of the American Medical Association* 255:2915, 1986. Reproduced with permission. © JAMA, June 6, 1986. American Heart Association.

9 Inflammatory Bowel Disease

GARY M. GRAY, M.D.

Two types of nonspecific inflammatory bowel disease are distinguished on the basis of clinical and pathological findings: ulcerative colitis and Crohn's disease. It is important to consider the two disorders in detail because each has a different prognosis and treatment and because both can be confused with other diseases of the colon or small intestine, including diseases caused by infection or ischemia.

Ulcerative Colitis

Ulcerative colitis is primarily an inflammatory disease affecting the superficial epithelial layer of the rectum and the distal colon, although it may extend proximally to involve the entire colonic mucosa. The cause of the disease is unknown, and remissions and exacerbations are common. In the past, it was believed that the disease might be psychogenic in origin, particularly because many patients were described as having a passive personality with a tendency to suppress personal conflicts. These criteria have not held up in recent years, however, and there are now few proponents of the psychosomatic theory. Ulcerative colitis may actually consist of a group of diseases, each presenting as the colitis syndrome.

There is a definite clustering of the disease within certain ethnic groups. It is two to four times more common among Jews than among non-Jews and four times more common among whites than among non-whites. Ten percent of patients have family members within two generations who also have the disease, and more than one third know of a relative who has the disease.[1] On the basis of routine sigmoidoscopy of a healthy population group, asymptomatic ulcerative colitis appears to occur in four out of 100,000 people.[2] Symptomatic ulcerative colitis usually develops between 25 and 45 years of age. Females are more commonly affected than males. Although the illness occurs less often in the elderly, attacks in patients older than 60 years may be severe, and morbidity and mortality are very high for this group.

Clinical Manifestations

The most common early symptoms of ulcerative colitis are constipation and passage of blood or mucus with the stools. Patients may also report urgency to defecate, followed by passage of only small amounts of blood and mucus. These symptoms may continue for several months, or even years, before the onset of diarrhea or systemic manifestations. Complaints confined to the abdomen and perianal area usually indicate mild or moderate disease. Prominent generalized symptoms, such as fatigue and weight loss, suggest the presence of severe disease.

In general, when a patient first consults a physician, the disease is usually mild. Patients with moderately severe or severe disease are usually referred to major medical centers. Once the pattern of disease has become established, it is important to consider the relative severity of the disease [*see Table 1*] because this factor is closely correlated with the long-term prognosis.

Mild Colitis

The majority of patients with ulcerative colitis have mild disease that is confined to the distal colon and rectum. Subsequent extension of disease to the remainder of the colon occurs in 15 percent of cases. Patients with mild colitis have intermittent diarrhea consisting of three to five stools a day with mild, cramping abdominal pain and no significant extracolonic or systemic manifestations. Physical examination is usually negative, although there may be localized tenderness over the distal colon.

Table 1   Categories of Ulcerative Colitis

	Mild	Moderately Severe	Severe
Proportion of total cases	60%	25%	15%
Site	Distal colon and rectum; progression to remainder of colon in 15% of patients	Usually involves one third to one half of colon; total involvement in 30% of patients	Usually involves entire colon
Diarrhea	Intermittent, 3–5 stools/day, often without cramping pain	>5 stools/day with gross blood and cramping pain	Profuse or constant liquid stools with blood
Fever	Absent	Intermittent (38° C)	38°–40° C
Anorexia and weight loss	Usually absent	Intermittent during exacerbations	Severe and often persistent
Systemic symptoms	Absent	Intermittent fatigue, increased sleep requirement	Extreme fatigue, weakness, prostration
Physical examination	Normal	Tenderness over colon	Distended abdomen, tympany, bowel sounds often absent
Laboratory tests	Usually normal	Mild intermittent anemia, normal serum albumin, elevated serum alkaline phosphatase (25% of patients)	Leukocytosis >20,000/mm^3, moderate to severe anemia, hypoalbuminemia, elevated serum alkaline phosphatase (40% of patients)
Extracolonic complications	Unusual	Relatively common	Common and often severe

Moderately Severe Colitis

Moderately severe disease accounts for 25 percent of ulcerative colitis cases. Patients usually pass more than five stools a day. Stools consist of watery or pasty material with mucus and gross quantities of blood. In most cases, cramping abdominal pain and rectal urgency are present. Intermittent fatigue and an increased requirement for sleep are common. Low-grade fevers and mild weight loss may also occur during exacerbations.

Severe Colitis

The small percentage of patients who have severe colitis experience recurrent exacerbations of disease that lead to hospitalization. Typically, they have temperatures of 38° C (100° F) or higher and profuse, constant, loose, bloody stools. Patients are apathetic and may be prostrate. Anorexia is severe, and if symptoms continue, extensive weight loss can occur. Physical examination may be normal, but a distended abdomen with tympany, absent bowel sounds, and rebound pain on percussion may reflect a fulminant flare of the disease.

Diagnosis

Sigmoidoscopy

When patients present with symptoms suggestive of either type of inflammatory bowel disease, a sigmoidoscopy is crucial for diagnosis [*see Table 2*]. This examination

	Mild	*Moderately Severe*	*Severe*
Risk of colonic cancer	Probably not increased	Precancerous lesions (severe dysplasia) develop in 4% of patients at 15 years, 7% at 20 years, and 13% at 25 years; cancer risk is 3% at 15 years, 5% at 20 years, and 7% at 25 years	Precancerous lesions (severe dysplasia) develop in 4% of patients at 15 years, 7% at 20 years, and 13% at 25 years; cancer risk is 3% at 15 years, 5% at 20 years, and 7% at 25 years
Mortality from acute attack	0.4%	2%	10%–25%
Recommended therapy	1. Diphenoxylate, 1–2 tabs q.i.d.; loperamide, 1 cap q.i.d.; or deodorized tincture of opium, 10–20 gtt in water q.i.d. 2. Sulfasalazine, 4–6 g/day 3. Corticosteroid enemas	1. Use of antidiarrheal agents, sulfasalazine, and corticosteroid enemas as described for mild colitis 2. Intermittent use of prednisone, 40–80 mg/day; if no response in 2 weeks, start trial of ACTH, 40–80 units/day I.M. 3. If systemic symptoms persist after 3 to 4 weeks of corticosteroid or ACTH therapy, add azathioprine or 6-mercaptopurine (50 mg/kg/day)	1. Therapy may be similar to that for moderate colitis; if fulminant colitis, start nasogastric suction and I.V. fluid and electrolytes 2. No antidiarrheal agents 3. Prednisolone, 100 mg/day I.V. (slow continuous drip), or ACTH, 40 units q 12 hr I.V. 4. If toxic megacolon, add ampicillin 4–8 g/day I.V. 5. If drug therapy fails, perform proctocolectomy

may be done either with the rigid 25 cm instrument or with the flexible fiberoptic sigmoidoscope. Because minimal friability can be observed only after vigorous swabbing with a cotton-covered probe via the rigid sigmoidoscope, I prefer to examine patients with the rigid instrument. The patient is placed in the knee-chest position, preferably on a motorized table that allows support of the knees below the level of the abdomen. A preparative enema is not administered, because little solid stool is usually found in the presence of inflammatory bowel disease, and the enema fluid may produce mucosal changes that interfere with interpretation of results. The sigmoidoscope is carefully introduced, and any liquid colonic contents are aspirated. A cotton swab is pressed firmly against the mucosa and rotated 360 degrees to remove adherent mucus and debris and to determine the integrity of the epithelium. Three abnormalities of the mucosa are particularly important: gross ulcerations, which are usually not seen in ulcerative colitis but are common in Crohn's disease; a coarse granular mucosal surface, which usually indicates the presence of microulcerations and scarring; and friability (i.e., the appearance of blood as punctate spots of 1 mm or less in diameter within a few seconds after swabbing). It is useful to grade friability on a scale of 1 to 4, with 1 indicating friability only after swabbing, 2 constituting a trace of spontaneous friability

Table 2   Comparison of Findings by Sigmoidoscopy and Biopsy in Ulcerative Colitis and Crohn's Disease

	Findings	*Ulcerative Colitis*	*Crohn's Disease*
Sigmoidoscopy findings	Granular mucosa	Typical	Common but may be absent
	Friable mucosa	Earliest finding, always present in active disease	Variable
	Ulcerations	Small pits 1 mm in diameter with bleeding from base after cotton swabbing; generalized involvement	Gross (0.5–1.0 cm in diameter or larger) with yellow or gray base; may be stellate in shape; often not associated with friability; spotty involvement with adjacent areas of normal mucosa
Biopsy findings	Ulcerations	Superficial microulcerations with acute inflammatory exudate	Linear ulcers extending into submucosa
	Granulomas	Usually absent	Usually present
	Inflammation	Acute, segmented leukocytes in crypts (crypt abscesses)	Chronic, extensive mono-nuclear cell infiltration

that is markedly aggravated by swabbing, 3 representing moderate spontaneous bleeding from the mucosal surface, and 4 meaning unprovoked bleeding before swabbing. Both friability and granularity are characteristic features of ulcerative colitis, but friability is a much more reliable and reproducible finding. The presence of erythema is not particularly important in the diagnosis of ulcerative colitis, because patients with diarrhea from any cause will show marked erythema, either spontaneously or after cotton swabbing. Patients with chronic ulcerative colitis may have pseudopolyps (nodules of regenerative mucosa) rather than true polyps.

Rectal Biopsy

A punch biopsy specimen can be taken at the 10 to 15 cm level at the time of sigmoidoscopy; a suction biopsy specimen can be taken at higher levels, where punch biopsy might introduce the risk of perforation. Alternatively, smaller biopsy specimens may be safely obtained above the 10 to 15 cm level via the flexible sigmoidoscope. Light microscopy reveals the presence of increased numbers of lymphocytes, plasma cells, and polymorphonuclear leukocytes. The most characteristic signs of ulcerative colitis are atrophy of the mucosal glands and the presence of polymorphonuclear leukocytes in the crypts of Lieberkühn, often called crypt abscesses. Although these histologic abnormalities are distinctive, they are not definitively diagnostic. Crypt abscesses may also develop in patients with Crohn's disease, but penetrating fissures and ulcers involving all layers of the mucosa and evidence of chronic inflammation with granuloma formation are more typical of that disorder. Even though the biopsy specimen is not diagnostic of ulcerative colitis, it is important to obtain a tissue sample at the time of the initial evaluation to determine whether an idiopathic colitis is present. In addition, a sample of colonic contents should be obtained with a cotton swab and then examined immediately for the presence of amebae and cultured for bacteria. Both amebiasis and bacterial infections can produce a colitis that may be indistinguishable from acute ulcerative colitis.

Barium Contrast X-ray

Crohn's disease, when confined to the colon, may mimic ulcerative colitis. Barium contrast x-ray is the most useful means of distinguishing between these two types of inflammatory bowel disease [*see Table 3*]. Other distinguishing features are considered in detail [*see* Crohn's Disease—Granulomatous Ileitis, Colitis, and Ileocolitis, *below*].

It is important to obtain a barium contrast x-ray in patients with a history suggestive of ulcerative colitis because the typical distribution of inflammation and loss of mucosal detail in the distal colon are rarely seen except in inflammatory bowel disease. Although examination of the entire colon by means of colonoscopy is useful for assessing the full extent of the disease and determining whether microscopic epithelial dysplasia is present, in most cases, barium contrast x-ray in combination with routine rectal biopsy and sigmoidoscopy is sufficient to establish a diagnosis. However, because a rectal biopsy will leave a residual defect that may be misinterpreted as a mucosal ulcer when seen on barium contrast x-ray, it is preferable to wait about seven to 10 days after biopsy before obtaining the x-ray. Although haustral markings may be lost from the distal colon in chronic diarrhea regardless of the cause of the diarrhea, the presence of a narrow, foreshortened colon and the loss of redundancy in the rectosigmoid region, coupled with a mottled appearance of the barium and roughening at the barium-mucosa interface, are highly characteristic of the microulcerations of ulcerative colitis. Patients with ulcerative colitis show neither the marked distortion of the bowel wall contour nor the intervening areas of normal mucosa that are characteristic of the extensive submucosal infiltration in Crohn's disease. Furthermore, enteroenteric fistulas and deep spikelike ulcers, although characteristic of Crohn's disease, are unusual in ulcerative colitis.

Colonoscopy

The development of fiberoptic instruments has allowed examination of the co-

Table 3   Comparison of Common Findings by Barium Contrast X-ray in Ulcerative Colitis and Crohn's Disease

Findings on X-ray	Ulcerative Colitis	Crohn's Disease
Loss of haustra	Typical in early distal disease	Present only if disease is extensive
Foreshortening	Typical in chronic disease	Absent
Gross ulcers at mucosal margin	Multiple, about 1 mm in diameter, occasionally "collar button" type	Spikelike or "rose thorn" with deep linear tracts parallel to mucosal surface
Usual site of disease	Rectum and distal colon with direct "stockinglike" extension proximally; dilated featureless ileum (backwash ileitis)	Nodular or stenotic distal ileum and right colon; other segments involved with intervening areas of normal mucosa (skip areas)
Eccentric involvement	Rare	Typical—transmural involvement and mural defect "thumbprinting" on one side only
Fistulas and fissures	Uncommon	Rectocutaneous and enteroenteric are common

lonic surface from the anus to the ileocecal valve. Colonoscopy requires special expertise but is now available in most medical centers. The technique may be particularly useful in patients whose disease is beyond the reach of the sigmoidoscope, especially if mucosal irregularities identified by barium contrast x-ray suggest the possibility of malignant change.

Because barium contrast x-ray may not define the full extent of mucosal disease, some authorities believe that colonoscopy should be performed and multiple mucosal biopsy specimens obtained when a patient is first shown by x-ray to have involvement extending proximal to the rectum and sigmoid colon. In most cases, however, barium contrast x-ray in combination with routine rectal biopsy and sigmoidoscopy provides an accurate assessment. Colonoscopy and multiple mucosal biopsies are indicated in patients who are shown to have mucosal nodules or distortion of the mucosal surface and in patients who have had disease for eight years or longer, when the risk of cancer becomes an important consideration [*see* Cancer, *below*].

Differential Diagnosis

Ulcerative colitis must be distinguished from other diseases that produce bloody diarrhea. Occasionally, local trauma related to the insertion of foreign objects into the rectum can produce a syndrome that mimics colitis. Usually, however, trauma can be distinguished from colitis by the localized pattern of damage seen on sigmoidoscopy. If symptoms of ulcerative colitis have continued for two weeks or longer, other conditions must be considered in the differential diagnosis. These include bacterial gastroenteritis, ischemic colitis, diverticulitis, Crohn's disease, and irritable bowel syndrome.

Patients with bacterial gastroenteritis usually have watery diarrhea, occasionally accompanied by blood. They typically pass little or no bloody mucus and have less tenesmus than individuals with ulcerative colitis. Sigmoidoscopy, however, may not reveal any features that would distinguish the two disorders. Thus, it is important to obtain a bacterial culture before treating patients for idiopathic ulcerative colitis. The invasive bacteria that most commonly cause acute colitis are the *Shigella* species.

Ischemic colitis tends to occur in elderly people. It may progress very rapidly, with catastrophic consequences. Gross blood may be passed, usually without much mucus. Ischemic colitis tends to run a short course leading either to rapid clinical improvement or to progressive deterioration. Special tests such as arteriography are often required to establish the diagnosis. Barium contrast studies tend to show edema and stenosis, findings that are different from those encountered in acute ulcerative colitis but often similar to those seen in Crohn's disease.

Patients with diverticulitis may occasionally pass large quantities of blood. Nonbloody watery diarrhea, however, is more common. Localized tenderness may be present over the sigmoid colon. Sigmoidoscopy usually does not reveal any abnormalities except for the presence of gross blood.

Amebiasis often produces acute colitis with bloody diarrhea, but sigmoidoscopy usually shows visible ulcers that range from several millimeters to more than 1 cm in diameter, and motile amebae can be recovered from fresh stool specimens. The mucosal surface between these ulcers is usually erythematous but is neither granular nor friable.

Watery diarrhea is often a component of the irritable bowel syndrome. However, stools do not contain blood, and sigmoidoscopy reveals only a nonspecific erythema in this disorder.

Therapy

Antidiarrheal Agents

Patients with mild ulcerative colitis usually can obtain appreciable relief by using antidiarrheal agents such as diphenoxylate (Lomotil), loperamide (Imodium), or deodorized tincture of opium [*see Table 1*]. Patients with otherwise mild disease may suffer greatly from abdominal cramping and diarrhea that can be safely treated with appropriate antidiarrheal agents. Physicians are often reluctant to treat these symptoms because they fear that a more severe, fulminant colitis will be precipitated. However, such a complication of antidiarrheal therapy is highly unusual. When diphenoxylate or loperamide is ineffective, deodorized tincture of opium will usually reduce the number of stools. The goal should be reduction of stool frequency to about three a day.

Sulfasalazine

Sulfasalazine is structurally related to both aspirin and the sulfa drugs. It is cleaved in the colon to 5-aminosalicylic acid (5-ASA), the active anti-inflammatory component, and sulfapyridine.[3] Although sulfasalazine is effective when given as the sole drug in patients with mild active colitis, it appears to be more useful in maintaining a remission after an acute episode of ulcerative colitis has been controlled.[4] The drug is started at a low dosage, 0.5 g two times daily (or 8 mg/kg/day). It is then increased over two to four days to a dosage of 0.5 to 1.5 g four times daily (or 50 to 70 mg/kg/day). Many patients obtain excellent prophylaxis at a dosage of 2 g/day. Nausea and epigastric discomfort are common side effects; however, when the dosage is increased gradually and the drug is given in four divided doses, only 10 percent of patients complain of epigastric symptoms. Other side effects include temporary oligospermia with consequent reversible infertility[5] and folate deficiency caused by the inhibition of folate absorption[6] and metabolism.[7] Patients with low serum folate levels may be given 1 mg/day of folic acid while they are taking sulfasalazine. Most specialists believe that patients with ulcerative colitis should continue to take sulfasalazine indefinitely. Not infrequently, withdrawal of maintenance sulfasalazine therapy results in an acute exacerbation of ulcerative colitis within a few weeks.

Sulfasalazine should not be prescribed for patients with acute colitis who have the associated systemic manifestations of anorexia, fatigue, and weight loss. The drug does not reliably produce remission in patients with severe disease, and it often increases gastrointestinal distress and anorexia, which may make the clinical status difficult to evaluate. Rarely, sulfasalazine may even induce an exacerbation of ulcerative colitis.[8] Thus, it is preferable to reserve this drug for maintenance of a remission or for those patients who have mild colonic symptoms.

Olsalazine

Because an appreciable minority of patients receiving sulfasalazine experience troublesome side effects (probably caused by the sulfapyridine component) and because 5-ASA is the active ingredient in the drug, new formulations of 5-ASA that are resistant to absorption in the upper small bowel have been prepared. The most widely tested of these is olsalazine, a diazo-linked dimer of 5-ASA, which is cleaved by bacteria in the lower ileum and colon to yield free 5-ASA. This agent appears to be as effective as sulfasalazine in the prophylaxis of recurrent ulcerative colitis; its effectiveness in the treatment of active colitis is uncertain. One study of more than 100 patients given olsalazine (2 g/day) revealed little evidence that the drug was superior to placebo in the treatment of mild to moderate ulcerative colitis.[9] Other controlled studies showed it to be as effective as sulfasalazine in treating first attacks of ulcerative colitis[10] and in preventing relapses for patients in remission.[11] In patients intolerant of the side effects of sulfasalazine, olsalazine (1.5 to 3.0 g/day) was twice as effective as placebo in producing clinical improvement, although only a minority of patients responded (35 percent versus 16 percent with placebo).[12] Unlike sulfasalazine or free 5-ASA, olsalazine produces diarrhea in about 10 percent of patients, probably by enhancing bicarbonate and sodium chloride secretion[13] and by inhibiting assimilation of carbohydrate and protein nutrients.[14] Olsalazine has now been approved for use in the treatment of ulcerative colitis (dosage, 250 mg four times daily). Because it is relatively expensive (about $2 a day versus about 50 cents a day for sulfasalazine) and, like sulfasalazine, does not play a major role in the treatment of moderately severe or severe ulcerative colitis, its use should probably be restricted to long-term prophylaxis in patients in remission or to treatment of mild active disease in patients intolerant of sulfasalazine.

Azathioprine and 6-Mercaptopurine

Whereas early controlled trials of immunosuppressive agents in patients with ulcerative colitis had yielded conflicting results, these trials involved relatively short-term administration, lasting only a few weeks. More recently, studies focusing on 6-mercaptopurine (6-MP),[15,16] a purine analogue, and azathioprine,[17,18] an active metabolite of 6-MP, indicate that there may be a place for these drugs in the treatment of patients who respond slowly (or not at all) to glucocorticoid therapy. Because they are potentially mutagenic and carcinogenic, they should be given to patients with ulcerative colitis only under special circumstances. Appropriate candidates are elderly, debilitated patients with moderately severe or severe disease or patients who have other serious diseases that would increase the mortality risk of a curative total colectomy; the goal is to produce a remission—or at least a partial remission—that will reduce the risk of colectomy. In such patients, 6-MP (50 µg/day) or azathioprine (50 µg/day; occasionally as much as 100 to 150 µg/day) should be given for a period of at least several months, the principal goal being to reduce and eventually eliminate the steroid therapy. When given in this way, these drugs appear to promote remission in about 50 percent of cases.

Side effects include reversible bone marrow depression, skin lesions (most commonly, aphthous ulcers or warts caused by viral infections), drug-induced hepatitis (about one percent of patients), and pancreatitis (about three percent). Despite the potential for mutagenesis, no increase in the

incidence of cancer has been documented after extensive use of these drugs in inflammatory bowel disease and particularly in chronic rheumatoid arthritis.

Cyclosporine

Cyclosporine, a potent immunosuppressive agent often used to prevent rejection of transplanted organs, has been administered to a few patients with acute, severe ulcerative colitis who did not respond to 10 or more days of intravenous glucocorticoid therapy.[19] Nearly three fourths of these patients improved when given cyclosporine (4 mg/kg/day I.V.) within a few days (mean response time, 5.8 days) and consequently did not have to undergo a total colectomy. When therapy was continued orally (6 to 8 mg/kg/day) for six months, steroids could be discontinued in more than half of those who initially responded. Because of its potentially serious neurosensory, neuromotor, nephrotoxic, and vascular complications,[20] cyclosporine therapy cannot yet be recommended for general use in severe ulcerative colitis but may be chosen in certain special patients with severe disease for whom colectomy would pose an inordinate risk.

Topical Glucocorticoids and 5-ASA

If symptoms continue despite the use of antidiarrheal drugs and sulfasalazine or olsalazine, glucocorticoids should be given by enema. Patients usually find it most convenient to administer the enema on retiring. The capacity to retain enema fluid is increased if the patient lies in the left lateral decubitus position. The use of a water-soluble steroid, such as prednisolone 21-phosphate (20 mg in 100 ml of saline) is preferable. A 100 ml dose of the steroid solution can be administered by means of a volume reservoir (e.g., Volu-Trole) and an intravenous tubing set. Hydrocortisone sodium succinate (100 mg in 100 ml of saline) can also be administered by enema, but this form of steroid is unstable in water solution and therefore must be added to saline at the time of each administration. Commercially available enema preparations of water-insoluble steroids containing cortisone acetate in a methylcellulose vehicle or in vegetable oil may also be useful in the treatment of ulcerative colitis, although controlled clinical trials demonstrating their efficacy are lacking.

Long-term treatment (12 to 34 weeks or longer) with daily enemas containing 5-ASA has been reported to be effective in a high percentage of patients with distal ulcerative colitis who had responded poorly to glucocorticoid therapy.[21] Further studies comparing glucocorticoid enemas with 5-ASA enemas are necessary to determine their relative usefulness.

Systemic Glucocorticoids and Adrenocorticotropic Hormone

Treatment with systemic glucocorticoids or adrenocorticotropic hormone (ACTH) is reserved for patients with moderate to severe ulcerative colitis [*see Table 1*]. Glucocorticoids produce remission in 75 to 90 percent of these patients. In mild disease of the distal colon, glucocorticoid enemas are usually sufficient to induce marked clinical improvement. For patients with active, moderately severe ulcerative colitis who have systemic manifestations or extracolonic complications, steroids should be administered systemically. Prednisone or another highly potent glucocorticoid, such as dexamethasone or prednisolone, is the drug of choice for the initial treatment of patients with moderately severe disease. In most cases, prednisone at a dosage of 40 to 80 mg/day is satisfactory. Patients should be maintained at this dosage level for approximately four weeks. When a remission is obtained, the steroid can be tapered at a rate of 2.5 to 5.0 mg every three days. Because glucocorticoids have not been shown to cure disease or to maintain remission, they should be withdrawn gradually with careful surveillance for an exacerbation. If glucocorticoid therapy does not ameliorate symptoms, a trial of ACTH, administered intramuscularly in a dosage of 40 to 80 U/day, may be worthwhile. The relative merits of systemic glucocorticoid

and ACTH therapy have long been debated, but the two forms of treatment appear to be equally effective when given in amounts producing comparable elevations of plasma cortisol.[22] In practice, it is rarely necessary to use ACTH.

Patients with severe disease must be hospitalized. A nasogastric tube should be inserted and fluids and electrolytes given intravenously to restore extracellular volume and maintain electrolyte balance. Systemic administration of a glucocorticoid, such as prednisolone (100 mg I.V. over a period of 24 hours) or ACTH (40 units I.V. every 12 hours), is essential. A complete remission cannot be expected for seven to 14 days. If the patient is critically ill (e.g., with toxic megacolon), a significant response, with reduction in pulse rate, decrease in fever, and improved sense of well-being, should occur within 96 hours. If there is no response to therapy after that time, proctocolectomy is indicated [*see* Surgery, *below*].

Diet

In mild to moderate ulcerative colitis, there is no need to impose general dietary restrictions. For some patients, however, elimination of milk products often markedly reduces diarrhea. Such patients may be lactase deficient; a failure to digest lactose increases the osmotic load on the colon, thereby aggravating secretory diarrhea.

Psychotherapy

Psychotherapy may be worthwhile in certain patients who have serious psychiatric difficulty, but studies have not shown that it is an essential adjuvant for most patients with ulcerative colitis.

Long-term Prognosis

Although the use of antidiarrheal drugs, sulfasalazine, and glucocorticoids is effective in the vast majority of patients with ulcerative colitis, recurrent disease is very common.[23,24] The prognosis appears to be related, at least in part, to the severity of the clinical syndrome over months or even years. Hence, patients with mild disease typically continue to have mild disease, and systemic manifestations or total involvement of the colon is unusual. On the other hand, patients with moderately severe disease may eventually have extensive symptoms. For these individuals, the five-year mortality is 10 to 20 percent. Patients whose disease begins with a severe attack run a 10 to 40 percent risk of death over a five-year period, and 10 percent of those who die do so at the time of their first attack. Of all patients with ulcerative colitis of any severity, 25 percent will undergo total proctocolectomy within five years of the first attack. Hence, although mild colitis is the most common form of disease and usually responds well to treatment, more severe forms are associated with considerable morbidity and mortality, even when treatment is optimal.

Complications Involving the Colon

Colonic complications of ulcerative colitis include toxic megacolon, perforation, cancer, stricture, and hemorrhage [*see Table 4*].

Toxic Megacolon

Toxic megacolon is a form of fulminant colitis that occurs in one to three percent of all patients with ulcerative colitis.[25] An appreciable proportion (25 to 40 percent) of patients who manifest this complication do so at the time of their first attack. The toxic megacolon of ulcerative colitis should be distinguished from the megacolon seen in enteric infections caused by infection with *Salmonella*,[26] *Shigella*,[27] cytomegalovirus,[28] or *Cryptosporidium*[29]; from that produced as a side effect of the phenothiazine drugs; and from that observed in some patients with pseudo-obstruction. The disorder is manifested by the sudden onset of fever, with temperatures as high as 40° C (104° F), apathy, tachycardia, dehydration, and marked dilatation of the colon. At the onset of systemic symptoms, diarrhea may be minimal, particularly if toxic megacolon develops during a first attack of colitis. Hence, it is important to consider this diagnosis when a patient with no previous history of colitis

Table 4   Complications of Ulcerative Colitis

	Complication	Incidence (%)
Colonic	Toxic megacolon	1–3
	Perforation	3
	Stricture	10
	Severe hemorrhage	4
	Carcinoma	2.5–30
Extracolonic[*]	Skin lesions	
	Erythema nodosum	3
	Pyoderma gangrenosum	0.5
	Aphthous mouth ulcers	10
	Iritis, episcleritis	5–10
	Arthritis	5–10
	Liver lesions	
	Fatty infiltration	40
	Pericholangitis (portal triaditis)	5–10[†]
	Cirrhosis (postnecrotic)	3
	Sclerosing cholangitis	<1
	Bile duct carcinoma	0.5

[*]Extracolonic complications in Crohn's disease are similar in' prevalence to those in ulcerative colitis.

[†]Based on clinical and laboratory abnormalities; a higher incidence (30 to 50 percent) is found on liver biopsy.

presents with what appears to be a severe bacterial infection or gastroenteritis.

Physical examination may reveal marked distention and tympany. If perforation has occurred, there may be marked rebound pain. Abdominal x-ray displays dilatation of loops of the colon to a diameter of at least 7 cm, especially in the transverse and descending portions. In most patients, sigmoidoscopy reveals severe granularity and grade 3+ to 4+ friability caused by severe involvement in the distal colon.

Appropriate supportive therapy is essentially the same as that for severe acute ulcerative colitis—nasogastric suction, intravenous fluid and electrolyte replacement, and restoration of blood volume. Because antidiarrheal agents (opiates and anticholinergics) may precipitate a toxic megacolon, they should be discontinued immediately if the patient is taking them. Intravenous glucocorticoids should be given as described above for acute severe ulcerative colitis. Because of high fever, prostration, and the possibility that perforation with sepsis may occur, it is probably advisable to administer a broad-spectrum antibiotic such as ampicillin (4 to 8 g I.V. every 24 hours). In one study, placing patients in the prone position appeared to be useful in decompressing the colon and decreasing mortality.[30] Decompression via colonoscopy has also been used.[31] Whether decompression of the colon actually aborts an attack of fulminant colitis is uncertain, but these maneuvers are relatively simple and safe. Therapy should be directed toward stabilizing the patient within 48 to 96 hours. Even when maximal medical support is provided, more than half of patients with toxic megacolon will have to undergo total proctocolectomy.[32] With drug and supportive therapy, the mortality for toxic megacolon is 15 to 50 percent. Surgical mortality is comparably high, but the marked increase in mortality that ensues after 48 to 96 hours if medical treatment has not been effective makes total proctocolectomy preferred at that time.

Perforation

Perforation of the diseased colon occurs in three percent of patients with ulcerative colitis. Risk of perforation appears to be higher at the time of the first attack. One third of all patients who die of ulcerative colitis are found to have a colonic perforation. The overall mortality associated with perforation is approximately 50 percent. Peritoneal signs are usually present but may be muted in patients receiving high-dose steroid therapy.

Cancer

Apparently because of the chronic inflammation produced by ulcerative colitis, patients with this disease are at increased risk for colonic cancer. One third of all deaths related to ulcerative colitis are caused by cancer of the colon. Factors favoring the development of colonic cancer in ulcerative colitis are duration of the disease for eight years or longer, involvement of the entire colon, continuous clinical activity, and, possibly, a severe initial attack.[32,33] The cumulative risk of cancer of the colon is substantial, reaching nine percent after 25 years of disease.[34]

Surveillance criteria for cancer in patients with ulcerative colitis have evolved because of the general availability of colonoscopy and biopsy and the emergence of morphological criteria for epithelial dysplasia. In patients at significant risk for colonic cancer (disease of eight or more years' duration with generalized colonic involvement or disease of 15 years' duration that is restricted to the distal colon and rectum[32]), elective colonoscopy should be carried out and biopsy specimens should be obtained at 10 cm intervals along the length of the colon on an annual basis.

Comprehensive surveillance for malignant change in patients with ulcerative colitis has been emphasized because tumors not infrequently originate in more proximal regions of the colon.[35,36] Many pathologists believe that a precancerous condition can be identified by careful analysis of colonic cytologic architecture, particularly in the crypt regions. In high-grade dysplasia, crypt nuclei lose their orderly basal position and become crowded together at varying angles, crypts become branched, and a villuslike configuration of surface epithelium develops.[36] Nearly all colitis patients found to have colonic cancer have epithelial dysplasia in regions remote from the malignant tissue. Dysplasia can be demonstrated by rectal or colonic biopsy in about 25 percent of patients with chronic ulcerative colitis involving the entire colonic mucosa. Severe dysplasia, a precancerous condition, develops in 13 percent of patients after 25 years of disease.[34] Colonic cancer will develop in at least one quarter of patients at high risk for cancer who have high-grade epithelial dysplasia.

When high-grade dysplasia is discovered in a patient who has colitis of eight or more years' duration, performance of an elective colectomy should be considered, particularly if the entire colonic mucosa is involved in the inflammatory process.[36] The Inflammatory Bowel Disease–Dysplasia Morphology Study Group has proposed a standard classification for dysplasia. However, because criteria for dysplasia are still emerging and because many pathologists are not experienced in the evaluation of colonic dysplasia, the presence of high-grade dysplasia should be verified by a second pathologist who is familiar with the current criteria.[36] In addition, for further verification, it is preferable that a second biopsy specimen taken from the same area of the colon also be found to harbor high-grade dysplasia. For patients with extensive colitis of eight or more years' duration who are found to have low-grade dysplasia, a complete colonoscopy should be performed, and biopsy specimens should be taken every 10 cm along the length of the colon as well as from grossly altered areas of mucosa. The finding of high-grade dysplasia in macroscopically normal mucosa or low-grade dysplasia in association with grossly distorted mucosa in such patients constitutes an indication for elective total colectomy.

Stricture

Approximately 10 percent of patients with ulcerative colitis acquire a stricture, usually in the rectosigmoid area. Although stricture can develop in patients with acute disease, it is more often associated with chronic intermittent colitis. There is usually marked fibrosis in the colonic wall, which must be distinguished from scirrhous carcinoma. An elective colectomy is indicated in any patient with chronic ulcerative colitis of eight or more years' duration in whom dysplastic epithelium is found in the area of the narrowing.

Hemorrhage

Massive hemorrhage develops in four percent of ulcerative colitis patients, but it usually can be treated without surgery [*see Chapter 12*].

Extracolonic Complications

Skin Lesions

Erythema nodosum occurs in three percent of patients with inflammatory bowel disease, and pyoderma gangrenosum occurs in approximately 0.5 percent. The pyoderma lesion starts as a purplish-domed boil that is exquisitely tender; it contains a sterile fluid with very few white blood cells. There may be extensive necrosis that can produce scarring on healing. The lesion is most commonly located on the extremities but can arise anywhere. In most cases, the lesion is associated with severe colitis. If recurrent and extensive pyoderma gangrenosum occurs, it may be debilitating. Although colectomy has been performed in an attempt to provide relief, some patients continue to acquire these skin lesions even after total colectomy.

Aphthous Ulcers

Aphthous ulcers, a troublesome but usually not serious complication of ulcerative colitis, occur in approximately 10 percent of patients. There is no specific treatment except for good oral hygiene. A small percentage of patients with aphthous ulcers also manifest oral moniliasis. These patients generally respond to treatment with mycostatin mouthwash.

Iritis

Inflammation of the iris and the conjunctiva occurs in five to 10 percent of patients with ulcerative colitis. Some patients also manifest severe bilateral episcleritis. In a third of patients with iritis, symptoms of the complication precede those of the colitis. In another third, symptoms occur while the patient is in remission from the colon disease. In the remainder of patients, iritis develops while the colitis is active. Most patients with this complication have other manifestations of extracolonic disease, such as arthritis or skin lesions. Because iritis can produce permanent damage, it is often necessary to treat it with prednisone in an intermediate dosage (20 mg/day).

Arthritis

Patients with ulcerative colitis frequently complain of painful joints and monoarticular enlargement with the presence of warmth over involved joints. Erythema is not uncommon. The arthritis tends to be restricted to the large joints, is frequently migratory, and usually presents when the colitis is clinically active. It occurs in approximately five to 10 percent of patients. No residual chronic deformity develops, regardless of the severity of the arthritis. Aspirin (600 mg every six hours) or another nonsteroidal anti-inflammatory drug usually helps reduce arthritic symptoms in these patients, but the main focus of therapy should be on obtaining a remission of the colitis.

Ulcerative colitis patients also appear to acquire ankylosing spondylitis 10 to 20 times more frequently than patients with other chronic diseases. This association can be accounted for by the increased prevalence of histocompatibility antigen HLA-B27 in patients with ulcerative colitis.

Liver Disease

Jaundice develops in about one to three percent of patients with ulcerative colitis. The most common type of liver disease associated with colitis is chronic pericholangitis, or so-called portal triaditis. It appears to be related to the extent of colonic involvement and is manifested clinically in five to 10 percent of colitis patients. Usually, there are no clinical manifestations, but the liver may be moderately enlarged, and the serum alkaline phosphatase level may be two to four times higher than normal, suggesting the presence of biliary tract disease. Another common disorder associated with colitis is fatty infiltration of the liver, which occurs in 40 percent of patients. The incidence of cirrhosis, sclerosing cholangitis, and bile duct carcinoma appears to be greater in patients with colitis than in the general population. Sclerosing cholangitis, although rare, occurs often enough in ulcerative colitis to indicate a definite association.

Surgery

Although partial colectomy and colonic bypass procedures have been carried out in the past, it is risky to remove only a portion of the colon because recurrent disease involving even a few inches of retained rectum or colon may produce serious recurrent inflammation and even death. Hence, if surgery is to be performed, proctocolectomy is the recommended procedure. The mortality associated with elective colectomy is approximately three percent; in the presence of acute severe or fulminant colitis, it is 10 to 15 percent. If there is perforation of the colon with acute colitis, the mortality from emergency colectomy may reach 50 percent.

There are four major indications for proctocolectomy: (1) failure of intensive drug and supportive therapy to manage severe colitis over a period of two to four weeks (the presence of high-grade colonic dysplasia in such patients makes surgery mandatory), (2) lack of response to treatment of toxic megacolon during a 96-hour period, (3) a markedly increased risk of cancer or the presence of a stricture that cannot be distinguished from cancer, and (4) severe, debilitating extracolonic manifestations. On the basis of these indications, it is necessary to recommend total colectomy for approximately 25 percent of patients during the first five years of their disease. Although some chronic postoperative complications are associated with proctocolectomy, removal of the total colon is the only curative treatment for ulcerative colitis.

Although in the past most patients undergoing a total colectomy for ulcerative colitis required an ileostomy and a plastic collection bag on the abdominal wall, alternative approaches are being used increasingly. These approaches include the continent ileostomy, which does not require an external appliance, and particularly the ileal pouch, in which an ileal-anal anastomosis is created to allow direct voluntary delivery of fecal contents. Studies of several hundred patients treated with these procedures have revealed excellent results.[37-42] Most patients pass an average of four to eight partially formed stools a day, and minor anal leakage occurs in nearly 50 percent.[42] Transient small bowel obstruction develops in about 15 percent of patients after the ileal pouch is fashioned, and in half of these patients, surgical revision is required. The major morbidity associated with the ileal reservoir is the development of mucosal inflammation in the pouch, often called pouch ileitis, or pouchitis. Pouchitis occurs in 20 to 30 percent of patients with an ileal reservoir, usually as a late complication (one to two years after surgery). Pouchitis is manifested by fever, nausea, low abdominal pain, increased output of liquid stools (often including blood), and signs of mucosal inflammation (edema, friability, and visible ulcers) on endoscopic examination. The cause is unknown, but stasis and the action of bacterial flora may play contributory roles. Treatment with metronidazole (250 mg, t.i.d.) is usually effective,[43,44] although prednisone in an intermediate dosage (20 mg/day) may be necessary in some patients. Despite the disadvantages of the ileal reservoir with an ileal-anal anastomosis, patients tend to find it highly satisfactory and to prefer it to the conventional ileostomy or the continent ileostomy. A continent ileostomy or an ileal pouch is not recommended for patients in whom Crohn's colitis is the established or tentative diagnosis, because there is a high risk that granulomatous inflammation may develop in the reservoir in such patients.

Crohn's Disease—Granulomatous Ileitis, Colitis, and Ileocolitis

Granulomatous involvement of the terminal ileum (classic Crohn's disease) has been recognized for half a century, but the colitis associated with it was not generally accepted as an entity separate from ulcerative colitis until the early 1960s. It is now generally accepted that classic regional ileitis and granulomatous colitis constitute variations of the same syndrome: granulomatous ileocolitis, now referred to as Crohn's disease. About one half of patients with Crohn's disease have both ileal and colonic involvement; the remainder are equally divided between those with disease restricted to the small intestine and those with disease confined to the colon.

The cause of Crohn's disease is unknown, although clustering in families has been shown. In the United States, the annual incidence of the disease is about two per 100,000 individuals, with a slight predominance among females. The incidence appears to be increasing in the Western world.[45] Crohn's disease is more common among Jews of middle European origin than among non-Jews,[46,47] and it develops in twins and siblings at a much higher rate than predicted by chance.[48] The permissive gene may be recessively inherited with incomplete penetrance.[49]

Crohn's disease usually involves the terminal ileum or colon, but it may manifest as a widespread illness involving any portion of the hollow gut from mouth to anus. There have been increasing reports of granulomatous inflammation occuring in the esophagus, where it causes dysphagia,[50] as well as in the vulva[51-53]; an initial diagnosis of Behçet's syndrome may be made before the onset of the bowel symptoms that point to the correct diagnosis of Crohn's disease.[54]

Crohn's disease is manifested by chronic inflammation of all layers of the bowel. Usually, the disease process can be distinguished from ulcerative colitis both clinically and pathologically. There is a peak incidence at about 30 years of age, with most disease occurring in patients between 20 and 40 years of age. Probably because of the transmural inflammation, there is a tendency for penetrating fistulous tracts to form between the diseased intestinal loops and the adjacent structures, such as the bladder, other segments of bowel, and the skin.

Clinical Manifestations

Unlike ulcerative colitis, which often presents initially as an acute, severe, even fulminant disease, Crohn's disease frequently becomes chronic before the patient sees a physician. The average patient has symptoms for five years before the diagnosis is made. Rather than being acute and fulminating, it is an indolent or so-called smoldering disease. The most common manifestations are pain, mild nonbloody diarrhea, anorexia, and mild anemia. Pain is almost always confined to the lower abdomen and may be aching or cramping in nature; patients may mention that it is similar in quality to a toothache. Mild aching pain is often misinterpreted as being caused by an irritable bowel syndrome. At times, however, pain is so severe that narcotics are required for relief. The development of pain before the onset of change in bowel habits is not uncommon. Children, for example, may complain of pain, develop anorexia, and fail to grow normally before alterations in bowel habits become evident. It is not unusual for patients to complain bitterly of severe generalized fatigue that prevents them from performing ordinary daily activities.

Complications of Crohn's disease may generate major complaints, such as a burning sensation in the eyes or blurred vision caused by iritis, lancinating pain associated with rectocutaneous fistulas, or the burning and urgency of a urinary tract infection related to an enterovesical fistula. Bleeding is unusual early in the course of Crohn's disease but not uncommon after many years.

The patient usually appears chronically ill and may show pallor and weight loss. An abdominal mass, caused by a thickened bowel loop or transmural inflammation, may be palpated in as many as 25 percent of patients. Because the disease tends to penetrate the bowel wall deeply, evidence of inflammation is often found in the perianal area. If the small intestine is extensively involved, there may be evidence of malnutrition: symptoms may include a smooth, reddened tongue, particularly on the lateral and anterior margins; cheilitis; and tetany related to hypocalcemia.

Complications

Rectal fissures, rectocutaneous fistulas, or perirectal abscesses occur in as many as 50 percent of patients at some time during the course of their disease. Extracolonic complications of Crohn's disease, found in one to 10 percent of patients, include arthritis, iritis, erythema nodosum, pyoderma gangrenosum, and aphthous ulcers [*see Table 4 and* Extracolonic Complications, *above*]. Acquired epidermolysis bullosa, a rare, intracutaneous disease that is manifested by subepithelial blistering over points of mechanical trauma, has been described in several patients with inflammatory bowel disease, particularly in those with Crohn's disease.[55,56] A small percentage of patients with Crohn's disease develop a fulminant colitis [*see* Toxic Megacolon, *above*], but this complication is less common in Crohn's disease than it is in ulcerative colitis.

Although development of cancer is much less common in Crohn's disease than in ulcerative colitis, patients with Crohn's disease of 15 years' duration are at increased risk for malignant disease. This increased risk is presumably caused by the persistent chronic inflammation characteristic of the disease. The dysplastic changes described for ulcerative colitis [*see* Cancer, *above*] may signify malignant change; however, surveillance with colonoscopy is less useful in patients with Crohn's disease because the small intestine, involved in at least half of cases of Crohn's disease, can rarely be directly examined and biopsied.

Renal stones containing calcium oxalate are frequently found in patients with Crohn's disease, especially if the ileum is involved.[57,58] Bile acids and fatty acids that escape ileal absorption and pass into the colon facilitate increased colonic absorption of oxalate. Increased oxalate absorption leads to hyperoxaluria and the formation of stones in the renal calyceal system. The elimination of oxalate-containing foods, such as spinach, tomatoes, and rhubarb, along with alkalinization of urine may prevent calculus formation.

The prevalence of gallstones appears to be higher (35 percent) in patients who have more than 100 cm of ileal disease or ileal resection than in those who have minor ileal involvement or resection (12 percent).[59] This higher prevalence may be related to bile salt malabsorption.

Laboratory Evaluation

Patients with Crohn's disease usually have a moderate anemia, which is often caused by several factors, such as iron deficiency, vitamin B_{12} deficiency related to extensive disease of the terminal ileum, or folate deficiency produced by anorexia and consequent poor dietary intake of folic acid or by inhibition of folate absorption by sulfasalazine. Mild leukocytosis (about $10,000/mm^3$) and a decrease in serum albumin caused by its loss through the diseased mucosa are common.

Diagnosis

Sigmoidoscopy

Because Crohn's disease most often affects only the terminal ileum, cecum, and ascending colon, sigmoidoscopic examination is normal in 30 to 50 percent of patients. Yet, sigmoidoscopy often reveals granularity, friability, linear ulceration, and nodule formation in the lower colon in cases in which barium contrast x-rays show disease only in the ileum or ascending colon. It is often stated that the granularity and friability typical of ulcerative colitis are also common in Crohn's disease. Although this may be true in a minority of cases, the sigmoidoscopic findings in Crohn's disease are usually distinctly different from those in ulcerative colitis. In Crohn's disease, there typically is gross ulceration, and the absence of mucosa may be so extensive that the denuded area is much larger than the aperture of the instrument. Thus, the observer may not realize that an ulcer even exists until an abrupt ridge of tissue representing the normal mucosal border appears. The ulcers usually range from several millimeters to 1 cm or more in diameter and may be elliptical, stellate, or linear. They often have sharply defined nonerythematous margins surrounded by intervening areas of normal mucosa. Granularity may be evident, but friability is often minimal compared with that seen in ulcerative colitis [*see Table* 2].

Biopsy

Tissue obtained at surgery and autopsy often reveals chronic inflammatory involvement of the submucosal layers of the bowel wall, manifested mainly by lymphocytic infiltration, with associated lymphoid hyperplasia and formation of noncaseating granulomas [*see Table* 2]. Mucosal biopsy specimens taken at sigmoidoscopy, however, will usually provide tissue only to the level of the muscularis mucosae. Atrophy of the mucosa with lymphoid hyperplasia and granulomas may be seen in only one third to one half of patients with Crohn's disease. Even when surgical specimens demonstrate submucosal inflammation, these histopathologic findings are not specific for Crohn's disease, because chronic inflammation and occasional granuloma formation may occur in ulcerative colitis as well. The biopsy often yields supportive evidence of Crohn's disease, but final differentiation from ulcerative colitis rests heavily on the history, the clinical course, and, in particular, the pattern seen on barium contrast x-ray studies.

Barium Contrast X-ray

A barium contrast x-ray examination is the most important single diagnostic procedure because it frequently reveals the characteristic changes of Crohn's disease. It is important to be aware of the features that distinguish Crohn's disease from ulcerative colitis [*see Table* 3]. Particularly characteristic of Crohn's disease is segmental involvement of two or more areas, most commonly in the ascending colon, and intervening segments of normal mucosa. Because of the transmural involvement, an eccentric, convex defect protruding into the lumen, so-called thumbprinting, is often seen. The ulcers are commonly penetrating, pointed at the base, and similar in configuration to a spike, in contrast to the so-called collar button ulcers encountered in chronic ulcerative colitis. There may be undermining at the ulcer base, with movement of barium into the submucosa in a pattern parallel to the long axis of the colon.

Differential Diagnosis

There are only a few diseases of the colon that resemble Crohn's disease on clinical, radiologic, or sigmoidoscopic examination.

The most important disease that must be differentiated from Crohn's disease is ulcerative colitis [*see Table 5*]. In general, ulcerative colitis is a more acute disease, manifested by bloody diarrhea related to severe superficial ulcerative disease. Crohn's disease, on the other hand, is described as a smoldering chronic disease marked by transmural inflammation and a tendency to fistula formation. At times, it is not possible to separate the diseases completely, but it is important to do so because ulcerative colitis predisposes to cancer in a much higher proportion of patients and because it can be cured by a proctocolectomy. Granulomatous colitis is associated with cancer in only a very small percentage of cases, and recurrence after surgery is common.

Amebic colitis may be associated with inanition, fatigue, fever, and watery diarrhea. Primary involvement is most common in the cecal area, with punched-out ulcers ranging from 2 to 15 mm in diameter. Such ulcers may be seen on colonoscopy or barium enema x-ray or, when the lower colon is involved, on sigmoidoscopy. The diagnosis can be made by careful analysis of the stools for *Entamoeba histolytica*. Presence of infection can be verified by a positive serum hemagglutination test.

At times, diverticulitis may be difficult to distinguish from Crohn's disease. Diverticulitis tends to be a more acute illness, however, and the symptoms and signs are localized to the area of the inflamed diverticulum. Sigmoidoscopy does not usually demonstrate any abnormalities except for the occasional presence of gross blood. Barium contrast x-ray examination or abdominal CT commonly reveals a smooth extramural defect that does not suggest any mucosal alteration. The mere presence of diverticula (i.e., diverticulosis), of course, does not signify the presence of diverticulitis, because asymptomatic diverticulosis is very common, particularly in elderly patients.

Table 5   Comparative Features in Ulcerative Colitis and Crohn's Disease

	Ulcerative Colitis	*Crohn's Disease*
Acute, toxic symptoms	Common in severe disease	Unusual; a "smoldering" disease
Stools	Bloody, watery with mucus	Mushy or watery; gross blood is unusual
Perirectal involvement	Occurs in 10%–20% but is usually self-limiting	Deep fissures, abscesses, or rectocutaneous fistulas in 50%
Sigmoidoscopy	*See Table 2*	
Barium contrast x-ray	*See Table 3*	
Extracolonic complications	Common and similar in both diseases [*see Table 4*]	
Colonic cancer	5% after 10 years; related to continual disease activity and severity	1%; probably not related to extent or duration of disease
Surgical therapy	Total colectomy is curative	Recurrence at anastomosis is very high for ileocolitis and colitis [*see Table 6*]

Ischemic colitis is an acute illness that develops abruptly, producing gross bleeding. Sigmoidoscopic findings are likely to be negative. Barium contrast x-rays display marked edema of the mucosal folds and thumbprinting that is at times difficult to distinguish from that seen in Crohn's disease. The most common sites of involvement, however, are the areas supplied by the terminal branches of the perfusing arterial system—namely, the splenic flexure and the rectosigmoid junction. Usually, ischemic colitis either abates within a day or two or progresses and requires surgery. When rapid improvement occurs, the marked abnormalities seen on barium contrast x-rays may disappear within a few days to a week or so. It is very common, however, for a stricture to develop at the ischemic site; when this occurs, surgery may eventually become necessary.

Intestinal tuberculosis, which most frequently involves the distal ileum and the ascending colon, may be very difficult to distinguish from Crohn's disease. Enteral tuberculosis, however, is no longer common in the Western world, and a negative tuberculin skin test is helpful in eliminating intestinal tuberculosis from the differential diagnosis. Unfortunately, a positive skin test may merely reflect an old, previously healed case of pulmonary tuberculosis. In rare instances, it may be necessary to perform exploratory laparotomy to be certain that intestinal tuberculosis is not present.

Therapy

Treatment of Crohn's disease is similar to that of ulcerative colitis.

Drug Therapy

Patients with systemic symptoms should be treated with antidiarrheal drugs and systemic glucocorticoids in the manner described for moderately severe ulcerative colitis [*see Table 1*]. Controlled clinical trials from the United States[60] and Europe[61] have shown the efficacy of therapy with prednisone (40 to 60 mg/day p.o.) or methylprednisolone (32 to 48 mg/day p.o.) in patients with Crohn's disease. With either regimen, at least 60 percent of patients enter remission within six to eight weeks. Sulfasalazine (4 to 6 g/day in four divided doses) is also effective, but it must be administered for three to four months to produce a remission, and remission is achieved in only about 40 percent of patients. Consequently, the drug should be used mainly in patients who have only troublesome local symptoms such as diarrhea or pain. The combination of prednisone and sulfasalazine is no better than prednisone alone. Patients who present with weight loss or severe symptoms of fatigue, fever, anorexia, and diarrhea should be given prednisone in a high dosage (40 to 80 mg/day p.o.) for four to 12 weeks; the dosage is then gradually tapered by 2.5 mg increments twice a week. Unfortunately, it is often necessary to keep patients on prolonged prednisone therapy at a dosage of 10 to 20 mg/day or higher to maintain the remission.

6-Mercaptopurine (6-MP) and its derivative, azathioprine, have been used for several years in the treatment of Crohn's disease. Although these agents are not as effective as glucocorticoids, they may be useful in some patients with resistant disease because they may permit a reduction of the glucocorticoid dosage and enhance the healing of enterocutaneous fistulas.[15,62] These drugs act slowly, however, and many patients require treatment for three months or longer before a response is obtained. The usual initial dosage for azathioprine is 2 to 3 mg/kg/day given orally in divided doses; for 6-mercaptopurine, the initial oral dosage is 1.5 mg/kg/day. Doses of these drugs should be adjusted to maintain the patient's blood leukocyte count above $4,500/mm^3$ and the platelet count above $100,000/mm^3$.

In a pilot study, intramuscular administration of methotrexate, 25 mg/week for 12 weeks, was effective in 11 to 14 patients with Crohn's disease.[63] Although not all of these patients had been receiving high dosages of steroids immediately before receiving methotrexate, the findings are encouraging and suggest that further clinical trials with this antimetabolite are in order.

Other drugs and therapies, including ampicillin, cromolyn, levamisole, and bacillus Calmette-Guérin (BCG) immunization, have been claimed to be effective in small, uncontrolled studies. None of these agents, however, has been studied systematically and shown to be effective in Crohn's disease; therefore, their use cannot be recommended. Large controlled trials have not shown drug prophylaxis to be useful in patients with Crohn's disease,[60,61] but one small controlled study found that prednisolone in an intermediate dosage (0.25 mg/kg/day) prevented clinical relapse over a period of 18 months.[64] Notably, however, this dosage, equivalent to 22 mg/day for a 70 kg person, is in the therapeutic range for active Crohn's disease; it is therefore questionable whether such a regimen actually constitutes prophylaxis. Preventive measures that are not associated with serious side effects, such as those produced by glucocorticoids, remain to be discovered.

Enteral and Parenteral Nutrition

Because anorexia is common in Crohn's disease, secondary malnutrition and weight loss occur frequently. Hence, repletion of calories, protein, and vitamins is necessary. Supplemental nutrients are available commercially either as an elemental mixture that does not require digestion (e.g., Vivonex, Norwich-Eaton Pharmaceuticals) or as a polymeric liquid preparation (e.g., Isocal, Mead Johnson & Company; Ensure, Ross Laboratories). Generally, the polymeric mixtures are less expensive than the monomeric types and appear to be equally effective in nutritional repletion of Crohn's disease patients. Supplemental nutrients can be administered either by mouth or by small-bore nasoesophageal or nasogastric tube.[65]

Total parenteral nutrition through a superior vena caval catheter [*see Chapter 13*] has been advocated as primary treatment of Crohn's disease.[66,67] This recommendation is not based on controlled clinical trials, however, and most patients who have responded to parenteral nutrition were also treated with glucocorticoids. In certain instances, such as refractory childhood Crohn's disease, when glucocorticoid therapy alone has been unsuccessful, parenteral nutrition may allow patients to resume normal growth. The complication rate of long-term parenteral nutrition is at least 15 percent over a period of several weeks to months. Untoward effects include hyperglycemia, pneumothorax, sepsis, and deficiencies of copper, zinc, and fatty acids. Therefore, parenteral nutrition should be reserved for severely ill patients who do not respond to conventional drug therapy.

Although nutritional repletion with an elemental mixture (e.g., Vivonex) may be useful in an acute attack of Crohn's disease, this form of treatment is expensive, may have to be administered for prolonged periods, and is poorly tolerated by many patients. In general, both parenteral and enteral nutrition should be used as additional supportive measures rather than as primary therapy for Crohn's disease.[68,69]

Surgery

The failure rate of drug therapy is relatively high, as noted above, and such treatment may be even less successful for subsequent attacks. There is no question, however, that surgery plays an important role in the treatment of Crohn's disease. At least 60 percent of patients will require an operation within five years, either because of the failure of other therapy or because of complications such as intra-abdominal fistulas or stricture formation.[45] Unlike ulcerative colitis, which does not recur after total colectomy, Crohn's disease has a very high postoperative recurrence rate: 85 percent within the ensuing three years, as determined by means of endoscopic examination.[70] This rate varies depending on the initial operative procedure used, the site of involvement of the disease, and the age of the patient [*see Table 6*]. When all patients at risk in a given year are considered, including those who have already had one or more operations for Crohn's disease, the cumula-

Table 6   Requirement for Reoperation in Crohn's Disease

	Initial Procedure	Cumulative Reoperation Required	
		Percent of Patients	Years after First Operation
All patients with Crohn's disease	Resection	40	7
	Bypass[*]	55	7
Colitis	Resection	20	5
Ileocolitis	Resection	45	5
All patients with Crohn's disease			
Age at onset <25 years	Resection	55	6
	Bypass	90	12
Age at onset >25 years	Resection	25	6
	Bypass	80	12

[*]Bypass indicates transection of bowel proximal to disease, either with enteroanastomosis beyond distal extent of disease or with proximal diverting ileostomy.

tive recurrence rate is 10 percent a year,[69] and 15 percent of patients undergo surgery each year over a 15-year period.[71] The success rate of surgery for the disease is controversial. The cumulative risk of recurrent disease that requires additional surgical resection is greater than 40 percent 15 years after the initial operation; this risk is highest in patients with disease involving both the ileum and the colon.[72] The high incidence of recurrence and its complications produces considerable morbidity over the years. Caution, therefore, is needed when surgery is being considered for a patient with Crohn's disease. In general, surgery should be considered only when persistent debilitating complications or intractable systemic symptoms occur despite optimal drug therapy. After several years of chronic disease, the possibility of an increased risk of cancer,[73] including lymphoma,[74] must also be considered [*see* Complications, *above*].

References

1. Scand J Gastroenterol Suppl 170:64, 1989
2. Gastroenterology 51:757, 1966
3. Gut 21:632, 1980
4. Gut 5:437, 1964
5. Gut 22:445, 1981
6. N Engl J Med 305:1513, 1981
7. J Clin Invest 61:221, 1978
8. N Engl J Med 306:409, 1982
9. Gut 30:1354, 1989
10. Gut 30:675, 1989
11. Gut 29:835, 1988
12. Gastroenterology 93:1255, 1987
13. Gastroenterology 95:975, 1988
14. Gut 28:346, 1987
15. N Engl J Med 302:981, 1980
16. Am J Gastroenterol 85:717, 1990
17. J Clin Gastroenterol 12:271, 1990
18. Dis Colon Rectum 33:374, 1990
19. Lancet 336:16, 1990
20. Dig Dis Sci 34:1387, 1989
21. Gastroenterology 99:113, 1990
22. Gastroenterology 69:91, 1975
23. Gut 4:309, 1964
24. Gastroenterology 59:598, 1970
25. Medicine (Baltimore) 48:229, 1969
26. Br J Surg 76:796, 1989
27. J R Coll Surg Edinb 32:109, 1987
28. Am J Gastroenterol 84:794, 1989
29. Postgrad Med J 63:1103, 1987
30. J Clin Gastroenterol 10:485, 1988
31. Am J Gastroenterol 82:692, 1987
32. Ann Intern Med 95:642, 1981
33. Br Med J 1:1442, 1966
34. Gut 31:800, 1990
35. Gastroenterology 76:1, 1979
36. Hum Pathol 14:931, 1983
37. World J Surg 4:143, 1980
38. Ann Surg 211:622, 1990
39. Schweiz Med Wochenschr 120:485, 1990

40. Hepatogastroenterology 36:227, 1989
41. Dig Dis Sci 34:1505, 1989
42. Ann Surg 210:268, 1989
43. Int Surg 73:187, 1988
44. J Clin Gastroenterol 5:149, 1983
45. Gastroenterology 68:627, 1975
46. Gastroenterology 97:900, 1989
47. Gastroenterology 96:1016, 1989
48. Hepatogastroenterology 37:81, 1990
49. Am J Med Genet 32:105, 1989
50. J Pediatr Gastroenterol Nutr 7:451, 1988
51. Br J Dermatol 119:87, 1988
52. Pediatr Dermatol 5:103, 1988
53. Am J Gastroenterol 82:1328, 1987
54. Am J Gastroenterol 84:322, 1989
55. JAMA 250:1746, 1983
56. Arch Intern Med 148:1457, 1988
57. Ann Intern Med 79:383, 1973
58. Klin Wochenschr 66:87, 1988
59. Scand J Gastroenterol 22:253, 1987
60. Gastroenterology 77:847, 1979
61. Gastroenterology 86:249, 1984
62. J Clin Gastroenterol 9:654, 1987
63. Ann Intern Med 110:353, 1989
64. J Clin Gastroenterol 10:631, 1988
65. Ann Intern Med 90:63, 1979
66. Lancet 1:122, 1976
67. Med Clin North Am 62:185, 1978
68. Proc Nutr Soc 48:355, 1989
69. Gut 27(suppl 1):76, 1986
70. Med Clin North Am 74:183, 1990
71. N Engl J Med 293:685, 1975
72. N Engl J Med 304:1586, 1981
73. Med Clin North Am 74:189, 1990
74. Histopathology 15:325, 1989

Acknowledgments

Table 6 Data from "Reoperation and Recurrence in Crohn's Colitis and Ileocolitis: Crude and Cumulative Rates," by A. J. Greenstein, D. B. Sachar, B. S. Pasternack, et al. Reprinted by permission from *New England Journal of Medicine* 293:685, 1975.

10 Diseases of the Pancreas

GARY M. GRAY, M.D.

Pancreatitis

Conditions that predispose to pancreatitis include chronic alcoholism, gallstones, hypercalcemia, hyperlipoproteinemia, blunt abdominal trauma, and penetrating peptic ulcer. Predisposition may also be inherited as an autosomal dominant trait. Although the specific pathogenesis is unknown, most of these factors strongly suggest that obstructive disease of the pancreatic ducts may play a crucial role.

Acute Pancreatitis

The vast majority of persons with severe intermittent progressive pancreatitis consume greater than average quantities of alcohol. By the time these individuals develop chronic pancreatitis, they are consuming more than twice as much alcohol (~145 ml/day) as control populations (~40 ml/day).[1] In those who experience a single attack of severe acute pancreatitis, biliary tract disease may be the main contributing cause. Indeed, in up to one third of all persons who develop acute pancreatitis, coexisting cholelithiasis is found[2]; however, only a small fraction of cases involve a stone in the common bile duct that might obstruct the pancreatic duct at the ampulla of Vater. Slow-growing mucinous pancreatic cystadenoma[3] or congenital anomalies such as annular pancreas[4] may produce acute recurrent pancreatitis presumably secondary to intermittent ductular obstruction.

Hereditary pancreatitis is manifested by dilated, saccular ducts, by calcifications in the pancreas, and by a high incidence of carcinoma of the organ. A rare disorder, it has been reported in only a few families.[5] Posterior penetrating peptic ulcer disease may be associated with severe pain typical of acute pancreatitis and may produce elevated serum amylases, but the disease is usually not progressive. Occasionally, infections that involve the pancreas, such as those caused by mumps virus, *Salmonella typhi*, or streptococci, produce an acute suppurative pancreatitis. Mild pancreatitis may sometimes develop in malnourished individuals in response to an abrupt twofold increase in food intake.[6]

Pancreatitis also appears to be associated at times with Type I or V hyperlipoproteinemia.[7] About one fourth of patients with acute pancreatitis have hyperlipoproteinemia, and most of these have a history of severe abdominal pain. When hyperlipemia is associated with acute pancreatitis, the serum triglyceride levels are usually above 1,000 mg/dl. Chylomicronemia and hyperprebetalipoproteinemia are present during acute attacks. Serum cholesterol levels are normal or only slightly elevated. Normalization of serum lipids can prevent subsequent pancreatitis attacks.

A variety of drugs reportedly precipitate acute pancreatitis, but supporting evidence is scant. Azathioprine, thiazides, sulfonamides, furosemide, estrogens, tetracycline, and cytosine arabinoside appear to have been directly associated with episodes of acute pancreatitis[8-10]; data are inconclusive on the capacity of corticosteroids, L-asparaginase, ethacrynic acid, phenformin, and procainamide to produce pancreatic inflammation.[8-11]

Clinical Manifestations

At least 95 percent of persons with acute pancreatitis complain of excruciating midepigastric pain, which within minutes or hours usually radiates directly through to the back. The pain is nonfluctuating and may last for many hours or even days, usually compelling the patient to consult a physician or appear at an emergency room. About 75 to 85 percent of patients experience nausea and vomiting after the pain reaches its maximum, and more than half develop fever, although usually there is no demonstrable infection. Shock and obtundation occur in nearly half of these patients if the episode persists for more than several hours. An ileus often develops in conjunction with signs of hypovolemia.

Physical Examination

The patient is acutely ill with severe pain and a temperature of about 38° C (100.4° F). Apparently because retroperitoneal structures are involved, many patients find that sitting and leaning forward relieves the pain. Breathing may be painful if there is an associated pleural effusion and pleuritis; there may be signs of shock with rapid pulse and cool, moist extremities. The abdomen is frequently distended, and bowel sounds are decreased or absent because of a secondary ileus. Physical examination, however, usually reveals a soft abdomen or only mild voluntary guarding. If severe hemorrhagic pancreatitis has developed, the pain may be excruciating, with marked guarding and even rebound tenderness. In recurrent pancreatitis, a mass may be palpated, indicating the presence of a pseudocyst. Because hypocalcemia may develop, the patient should be observed for signs of tetany. Occasionally, severe hemorrhagic pancreatitis leads to severe hyperglycemia and diabetic coma. A few patients develop mild jaundice as a result of common bile duct compression by the edematous pancreatic head.

Laboratory Findings

The white blood cell count is frequently elevated from 10,000 to 30,000 cells/mm³; the sedimentation rate is increased to 30 mm/hour or more in most patients. The serum bilirubin or alkaline phosphatase may be moderately elevated because of common duct compression or because of an impacted common bile duct stone. The hallmark of pancreatitis is an elevated serum amylase and an increased renal clearance of amylase. Increased amylase may also be caused by cholecystitis, hepatitis, intestinal obstruction, mesenteric thrombosis, parotitis, perforated duodenal ulcer, and a ruptured aortic aneurysm. It is relatively simple clinically to separate these disorders from acute pancreatitis. If there is a pleural effusion or ascites, needle aspiration will reveal a markedly high amylase content. In general, a high amylase concentration may occur in effusions in various diseases, but absence of amylase elevation in such fluids strongly militates against acute pancreatitis.

The amylase to creatinine clearance ratio may also be helpful in the diagnosis of acute pancreatitis. Its measurement requires that amylase and creatinine concentrations be determined simultaneously in serum and urine.[12] The normal ratio of amylase clearance to creatinine clearance is 3.1 ± 1.1 percent; in pancreatitis, the ratio may be as high as 9.8 ± 3.5 percent. Although the ratio has been found to be markedly elevated in common bile duct obstruction associated with pancreatitis, it is not increased in common duct obstruction alone. The mechanism producing the elevated clearance ratios in acute pancreatitis is unknown.

If the measurement of this ratio is to be reliable, the urine specimen must be obtained after intravenous fluids have been given to promote urinary output of at least 30 ml/hr. Because renal clearance of amylase reflects the number of functioning nephrons and depends on the partial tubular reabsorption of the filtered amylase, uremia or acute tubular damage may cause elevated urinary amylase to creatinine clearance ratios in the absence of acute pancreatitis.[13]

Trypsin, an enzyme that originates in the pancreas but is absent from exocrine glands such as the parotid, can now be measured in serum by immunoassay.[14] It may even prove to be more useful than serum amylase in documenting acute pancreatitis because of its probable higher sensitivity and greater specificity. Other than pancreatitis, only chronic renal failure produces an elevated serum trypsin level.

Hyperlipoproteinemia is found in a significant percentage of patients with acute pancreatitis, and serum should be carefully analyzed for lipid and triglyceride concentrations. A triglyceride level of 1,000 mg/dl or more predisposes to pancreatitis. Elevated lipid or triglyceride levels may indicate hyperbetalipoproteinemia or lipoprotein CII deficiency, which is a recessively inherited condition.[15]

Diagnostic Procedures

Abdominal radiography Enhancement of the perirenal fat related to retroperitoeal inflammation in pancreatitis may produce a distinct radiolucent halo around the margin of the left kidney; this renal halo sign can be seen on the plain abdominal radiograph.[16] Upper gastrointestinal x-rays often reveal an abnormal duodenal loop, and it is frequently stated that enlargement of the loop occurs with acute pancreatitis. This finding, however, commonly appears in chronic pancreatitis in which pseudocyst formation produces extrinsic compression of the duodenum. In acute pancreatitis, there tends to be widening of duodenal mucosal folds, with edema and angulation caused by inflammation and encroachment by the inflamed pancreatic head.

Ultrasonic scan A scan may aid in demonstrating an enlarged edematous pancreas by revealing a sonolucent area related to the development of edema or of a pseudocyst, which may develop after repeated episodes of pancreatitis.

Computed tomographic x-ray scan The computed tomographic scan may help estimate the size and shape of the pancreas in acute pancreatitis. The edema associated with acute inflammation often produces enlargement of the pancreatic head, though minimal pancreatic enlargement may elude such detection. A CT scan is warranted only when the diagnosis is equivocal by clinical, laboratory, and ultrasonic parameters.

Differential Diagnosis

To be considered in the differential diagnosis are the diseases that cause severe abdominal pain and those that markedly elevate serum amylase or the renal clearance of amylase. Perforated duodenal ulcer can cause severe abdominal pain that radiates to the back because of involvement of retroperitoneal structures; there may even be an associated acute pancreatitis, usually milder than that seen in primary acute pancreatitis. An acute abdomen with rebound tenderness and extreme involuntary guarding suggests that the ulcer has perforated. An abdominal x-ray series often reveals free air.

Patients with acute cholecystitis may have severe abdominal pain and elevated serum amylase, particularly if the common bile duct passes sludge or stones. As with a perforated duodenal ulcer, there may be secondary pancreatitis, which is usually mild. The definitive diagnosis often must await demonstration of stones in the gallbladder. Several days of inpatient supportive therapy may be required before the two entities can be clearly differentiated. Fortunately, pancreatitis and cholecystitis need not be distinguished in the first few days unless emergency surgery is being contemplated.

Myocardial infarction may cause severe abdominal pain, but serum amylase is usually not increased; characteristic findings establish this diagnosis.

Patients with pneumonia may present with severe epigastric pain associated with fever, but there is usually little else implicating pancreatitis, and the renal amylase clearance is not increased.

Medical and Supportive Therapy

The patient should be placed on nasogastric suction, and fluid and electrolytes should be administered intravenously. Mild cases are sometimes managed without nasogastric suction. Intrapancreatic activation of proteases retained in the blocked ductular system may damage the organ. For this reason, anticholinergic agents as well as glucagon and cimetidine are often used in efforts to reduce pancreatic acinar secretion. Neither anticholinergics nor cimetidine (alone or with glucagon) has produced a better clinical outcome than has nasogastric suction.[17] Preliminary studies with the inhibitory hormone somatostatin have been encouraging, and a multicenter trial is currently in progress.[18]

It is usually necessary to give narcotic analgesics such as meperidine (Demerol), 50 to 100 mg I.M. q 2 to 4 hr. If fever is greater than 38° C or if there is a suggestion of toxicity, which might reflect sepsis, it is advisable to give an antibiotic such as ampicillin (500 mg q 6 hr) or kanamycin (500 mg q 6 hr).

Patients usually recover after a few days to a week; a liquid diet can then be instituted and slowly replaced over a few days by a regular diet.

The mortality associated with an uncomplicated acute attack is relatively low (five percent), given the severity of the disease; the rate associated with suppurative or hemorrhagic acute pancreatitis, however, is 50 to 90 percent. If serum amylase remains elevated for more than five to seven days, there may be obstruction of a major pancreatic duct, partial obstruction of the common bile duct, or a pseudocyst. Ultrasonic examination of the pancreatic area and retrograde cholangiopancreatography should be used to detect a discrete correctable lesion in the head of the pancreas.

The long-term prognosis in acute pancreatitis depends on the inciting cause. Alcoholic pancreatitis frequently leads to chronic disease. Patients with traumatic pancreatitis often experience only a single severe attack without subsequent debility. The pancreatitis associated with hyperlipoproteinemia can be controlled, provided serum triglycerides are maintained close to normal levels. The pancreatitis related to hypercalcemia usually does not recur after surgical treatment of the underlying disease. Similarly, chronic cholelithiasis and passage of common bile duct stones, a benign pancreatic tumor, or a congenital anomaly usually do not progress to chronic pancreatitis if appropriate surgery is performed after the first attack. In a small series of seven patients, surgical treatment of hereditary pancreatitis with a longitudinal pancreatojejunostomy eliminated recurrent episodes of pancreatitis.[19]

Complications

Hypotension and ileus are common complications, which usually improve with supportive therapy. Sometimes, however, hypovolemia proceeds to shock and acute renal failure. Pseudocysts form mainly in patients with alcoholic pancreatitis who have had previous attacks. Usually, the pseudocyst will spontaneously stabilize and decrease in size as the attack of pancreatitis subsides. Pulmonary effusions are usually transitory. Pancreatic ascites may reflect either a torn duct related to traumatic pancreatitis or a pseudocyst that communicates freely with the abdominal cavity.[20] If the effusion persists, it may be necessary surgically to correct the underlying condition.

Nodules of fat necrosis (Weber-Christian syndrome) may develop in areas remote from the pancreas, particularly in the abdominal wall and extremities. They may be painful but require no treatment and usually disappear spontaneously. Diabetic coma, a rare complication, usually occurs only in fulminant or hemorrhagic pancreatitis. Hypocalcemia may be secondary to an increased serum glucagon, which results in stimulation of thyrocalcitonin and decreased bone resorption. If tetany develops, it may be necessary to administer intravenous calcium gluconate. Jaundice, if it occurs, is usually mild and related to duct compression; it rarely lasts more than a few days.

Occasionally, edema, spasm, or even a mass lesion in the region of the transverse or splenic flexure of the colon is seen. Although the presence of a colonic mass should be reevaluated after the pancreatitis has subsided, it usually reflects pancreatic inflammation rather than neoplasm or ischemic bowel disease.

Chronic Pancreatitis

Chronic pancreatitis is seen in three major clinical settings. By far the commonest is that of chronic alcoholism. Ten to 20 percent of alcoholics have developed chronic pancreatitis at autopsy. Alcoholic pancreatitis seems to be prevalent in populations that ingest large amounts of protein and fat. Males are affected five to 10 times more frequently than females, and the average age of onset is 38 years.

The initial attack of alcoholic pancreatitis occurs after several years of intermittent heavy drinking. The average age of the onset of alcoholism is about 25 years; less than 10 years later a series of attacks of pain begin. By the age of 40, calcifications of the pancreas, which reflect the chronicity of the disease, and mild diabetes develop. Steatorrhea often ensues five years later, and the patient's life is usually shortened; a typical age at death is about 50 years. Death, however, may not be directly related to the pancreatitis.

The second predisposing condition is severe biliary tract disease, especially if the common bile duct repetitively passes stones and sludge. In such cases, recurrent acute pancreatitis attacks may transpire, but this complication rarely leads to chronic disease. Once a series of relapsing episodes of pancreatitis has developed, however, correction of the cause may not halt the process.

The third clinical condition, traumatic pancreatitis, is frequently caused by blunt trauma, which may have occurred many years before the apparent onset of recurrent disease and so may have been forgotten by the patient. Typical mishaps are steering wheel injury to the abdomen, a punch to the abdomen, or a fall on a blunt object. Such an episode may tear the main pancreatic duct, leading to pain that occurs weeks later; the development of a pseudocyst is very common. Operative intervention is often helpful.

Hereditary pancreatitis often leads to chronic duct destruction and severe debilitating recurrent pancreatitis. As noted above, longitudinal anastomosis of the dilated ducts to the jejunum may be beneficial.

Pathology

The initial lesion occurs within a lobule; atrophy of the ductal epithelium is common. Plugs of viscous material, which stain as protein, may obstruct ductules[1] and subsequently become calcified. The main pancreatic duct is normal early in the disease but eventually becomes involved as the pancreas becomes shrunken and fibrotic.

Clinical Manifestations

Episodes of severe abdominal pain similar to that in acute pancreatitis develop, although bouts of only moderately severe pain also occur. As the disease becomes established in later years, episodes may persist or recur daily for weeks or months. Very severe pain requiring continuous parenteral narcotics may last two to 14 days. Jaundice develops in 10 percent of patients with chronic disease. Steatorrhea begins when about 80 percent of the pancreas is destroyed. The patient complains of oily stools that are difficult to flush down the toilet. Although hyperglycemia is common, frank diabetic acidosis is unusual, even in advanced disease.

Physical Examination

The patient is usually a thin or emaciated male who appears to be older than his age. He may have tender subcutaneous nodules over the abdomen and extremities which reflect development of fat necrosis, and a friction rub may be heard over the abdomen at the time of acute inflammation. A venous hum may be noted if the splenic vein is compressed by a pseudocyst. Although excessive alcohol use frequently leads to fatty infiltration of the liver, liver enlargement is usually not seen. Often, even massive pseudocysts cannot be palpated because of their retroperitoneal location.

Laboratory Findings

Routine laboratory tests are usually normal. The patient may have a low serum cholesterol related to inanition and poor dietary intake. Serum amylase and renal clearance of amylase are most often normal in recurrent episodes of chronic pancreatitis. Once exocrine secretion becomes markedly reduced so that the level of enzymes entering the duodenum is 10 to 20 percent of normal, gross maldigestion of fat and protein supervenes. Fecal fat excretion may reach 60 to 80 g per day on an 80 to 100 g fat diet (normal is 6 g per day).

Diagnostic Procedures

Abdominal radiography The plain abdominal x-ray may demonstrate calcifications in the area of the pancreas. An upper gastrointestinal x-ray series frequently demonstrates widening of the duodenal loop or an extrinsic pressure defect on the greater curvature of the stomach, related to the development of a pancreatic pseudocyst.

Special serum analysis Serum analysis is usually normal in quiescent chronic pancreatitis; it may be either normal or elevated when there is symptomatic recurrence of the inflammation. In contrast, about 60 percent of patients with established chronic pancreatitis have low levels of serum immunotrypsin. When both trypsin and amylase are expressed as a ratio, more than 80 percent of patients with chronic pancreatitis show a reduction.[14] This ratio may prove useful in identifying asymptomatic chronic pancreatitis, although a decrease in the ratio is also observed in pancreatic carcinoma.

Lactoferrin, a nonenzymatic protein secreted in pancreatic juice, has been found in increased levels in duodenal aspirates in patients with chronic pancreatitis. The determination of the ratio of lactoferrin to the lipase activity in duodenal contents appears to distinguish chronic pancreatitis from other pancreatic diseases such as acute pancreatitis or carcinoma.[21] Although the lactoferrin test offers promise in the evaluation of chronic pancreatitis, more clinical experience is necessary before it can be generally recommended.

Secretin test If it is unclear whether the steatorrhea is caused by a defect in the small intestine or the pancreas, a secretin-cholecystokinin (CCK) test can be carried out. In chronic pancreatitis, the first abnormality is a decrease in the bicarbonate secretion; only later is there a decrease in volume output. In pancreatic carcinoma, however, the bicarbonate secretion is usually normal, but the volume of fluid secreted decreases because of discrete obstruction of large pancreatic ducts.

If the secretin-CCK test is not available, a trial of oral pancreatic enzyme supplements can be administered for two weeks and the fecal fat determined while therapy continues. If the fecal fat excretion is markedly reduced by pancreatic enzyme supplements, then a diagnosis of pancreatic maldigestion is very likely.

Ultrasonography Abdominal ultrasound examination may reveal an enlarged pancreatic head or a dilated ductular system. Ultrasonography is particularly useful in identifying a fluid-filled pseudocyst that may contribute to recurrence by impinging on or obstructing a major pancreatic duct.[22]

Endoscopic retrograde pancreatography Most patients who develop chronic alcoholic pancreatitis do not benefit from surgical exploration and attempts at drainage. Still, it is important to be certain that there is no discrete lesion blocking a major duct of the pancreas. The most fruitful procedure is endoscopic retrograde pancreatography with contrast x-ray study of the pancreatic ductular system. If there is a discrete lesion, then surgical decompression and reestablishment of ductular continuity is the treatment of choice.

In chronic alcoholic pancreatitis, alternating dilated and narrowed duct segments are usually observed. These changes often progress despite abstinence from alcohol.[23] Patients with nonalcoholic chronic pancreatitis may have a lesion obstructing the main pancreatic duct, but secondary generalized ductular changes, as seen in alcoholic pancreatitis, do not usually develop.[23]

Therapy for Chronic Pancreatitis

Although alcohol ingestion is clearly the major cause of chronic pancreatitis, abstinence late in the course of the disease usually does not prevent the relentless recurrent attacks. Pancreatic extracts such as pancreatin (Viokase) or pancrelipase (Pancrease or Cotazym) can be given to improve nutritional status, although most patients are able to maintain a low-normal weight without enzyme supplements. Typical dosages are five to 10 of the 300 mg tablets with each meal. The chronic episodes of severe pain often require regular doses of narcotics. Such therapy may produce a treacherous situation because alcoholic patients are prone to addiction and tend to abuse narcotics.

Surgical therapy may be attempted if the pancreatitis is caused by stones in the common bile duct, a discrete lesion in the head of the pancreas (such as that related to trauma or a benign cyst), or an adenoma. Although the incidence of recurrent attacks of chronic alcoholic pancreatitis has been greatly reduced by various drainage procedures,[24] painful attacks tend to wax and wane spontaneously over the course of many years. Despite reports of surgical success, most experts believe that prevention of recurring pancreatitis can be expected in only a minority of cases. Subtotal pancreatectomy with partial gastrectomy and gastrojejunostomy may sometimes help alleviate episodes of pain; yet even after splanchnicectomy, many patients continue to have acute attacks. Controlled trials measuring the relative efficacy of surgical and medical therapy have not been done.

Pancreatic pseudocysts usually drain spontaneously and only become enlarged at the time of recurrent attacks. Complications from pseudocysts occur in five to 10 percent of cases and require surgical correction or drainage.[25] Indications for operation include infection of a cyst, chronic pleural effusion or pancreatic ascites with direct communication between the cyst and the pleura or the peritoneum,[26] or compression by the cyst of adjacent structures such as the stomach or duodenum. Rupture of pancreatic pseudocysts resulting in sudden death is a rare complication.

Pancreatic Neoplasms

The major neoplasms of the pancreas are endocrinoma, cystadenoma, cystadenocarcinoma, and adenocarcinoma that is of duct origin. Although many potent diagnostic techniques are available, including ultrasonography, CT scanning, endoscopic retrograde cholangiopancreatography, and needle biopsy of the pancreas, the prognosis for pancreatic carcinoma remains dismal.

References

1. Digestion 18:337, 1978
2. Scan J Gastroenterol 16:305, 1981
3. Gastroenterology 79:944, 1980
4. Gastroenterology 77:1109, 1979
5. Ann Intern Med 68:88, 1968
6. J Pediatr 97:441, 1980
7. Am J Med 54:161, 1973
8. Gastroenterology 78:813, 1980
9. Gastroenterology 81:1134, 1981
10. Cancer 49:1384, 1982
11. Gastroenterology 81:799, 1981
12. N Engl J Med 292:325, 1975
13. Gastroenterology 77:86, 1979
14. Scan J Gastroenterol 15:97, 1980
15. N Engl J Med 299:1421, 1978
16. Radiology 142:323, 1982
17. Mayo Clin Proc 56:499, 1981
18. N Engl J Med 303:999, 1980
19. Arch Intern Med 135:558, 1975
20. Medicine (Baltimore) 53:183, 1974
21. Gut 22:350, 1981
22. N Engl J Med 300:590, 1979
23. Gastroenterology 81:884, 1981
24. Ann Surg 194:313, 1981
25. Ann Surg 189:386, 1979
26. Gastroenterology 74:134, 1978

11 Cirrhosis of the Liver

PETER B. GREGORY, M.D.

Cirrhosis is the sequela to a wide variety of chronic, progressive liver diseases. Cirrhosis exists when these processes have so scarred the liver that its normal architecture is disrupted and regenerating nodules of parenchyma appear. The pattern of scarring seldom permits determination of the specific etiology, but associated histologic features may point to the cause. A specific diagnosis generally requires a combination of history, physical findings, laboratory tests, and identification of characteristic histologic features.

In the United States, excess alcohol intake is by far the most common cause of cirrhosis. Chronic hepatitis is often the major etiologic event in other countries.

Clinical Manifestations

Fatigue, malaise, and loss of vigor are common in all forms of cirrhosis, but these nonspecific symptoms are found in almost all acute and chronic liver diseases. Furthermore, no physical abnormality conclusively establishes that the liver is cirrhotic. Characteristic but nondiagnostic findings include palmar erythema (a blotchy, purplish-red lesion over the hypothenar region of the hand) and spider nevi. Other typical findings include gynecomastia, testicular atrophy, and evidence of portal hypertension (splenomegaly, ascites, esophageal varices, and prominence of the veins of the abdominal wall). Other physical abnormalities such as Dupuytren's contracture, xanthelasma, xanthomas, Kayser-Fleischer ring, a bronze discoloration of the skin, or hyperpigmentation are more frequent in specific forms of cirrhosis.

The cirrhotic liver is usually large, and the left lobe is often palpable below the xiphoid process. Only a patient in the advanced inactive stage of disease exhibits a small and shrunken liver. The cirrhotic liver is also firm on palpation and may even feel rock hard when cirrhosis is marked. Occasionally, large regenerative nodules on the surface can be detected on physical examination, but it is impossible to appreciate the fine nodularity of micronodular cirrhosis.

Diagnostic Evaluation

Percutaneous liver biopsy is often the only procedure that can unequivocally establish the presence of cirrhosis.[1] This procedure can be performed safely when there is no history of unusual bleeding following surgery, dental work, or previous biopsies and when tests for coagulation yield normal or only mildly abnormal results. Reasonable guidelines include a prothrombin time no more than two to three seconds beyond the control value, a partial thromboplastin time no more than 10 seconds beyond the control value, a platelet count of at least 50,000/mm^3, and a normal bleeding time. Under exceptional circumstances, the biopsy may be done when clotting abnormalities are more marked. However, vigorous correction of any coagulation abnormality should be undertaken prior to biopsy. Other relative contraindications to biopsy include lack of patient cooperation, ascites, and right lower lobe pneumonia.

Marked distortion of hepatic architecture, with regenerative nodules surrounded by scar tissue, provides definitive evidence of cirrhosis. However, because the percutaneous liver biopsy tends to underestimate the presence of cirrhosis, the condition may be present even though the biopsy is nondiagnostic.

Percutaneous liver biopsy also helps identify the cause of cirrhosis. In particular, bile duct invasion and destruction with associated granulomas suggests the presence of primary biliary cirrhosis; excess iron in bile duct cells and liver cells points to pri-

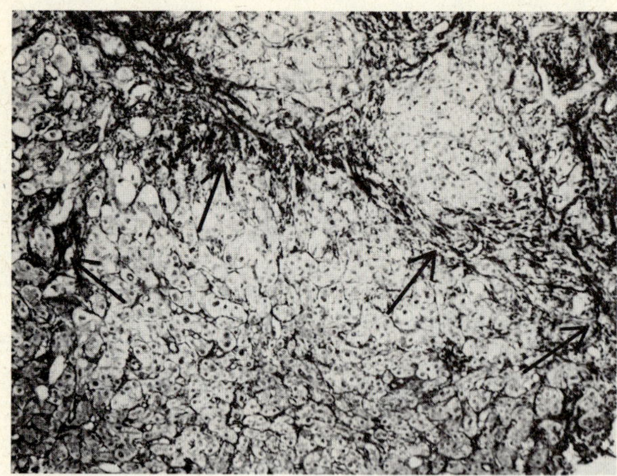

Figure 1 *Alcoholic cirrhosis in the liver of a 58-year-old man produces distortion with scar tissue (arrows) that spreads through the parenchyma and outlines small regenerating nodules.*

mary hemochromatosis; and alcoholic hyalin associated with polymorphonuclear cell reaction indicates alcoholic liver disease.

Depression of serum albumin and a prolonged prothrombin time are characteristic of cirrhosis. Other liver function tests often yield abnormal results. The liver scan is seldom helpful in diagnosing cirrhosis; the most common pattern on scanning is a large liver and a large spleen, a finding consistent with noncirrhotic processes as well as with a wide variety of acute and chronic liver diseases.[2] Technetium-colloid liver scan commonly shows one or more defects in a cirrhotic liver; thus, its utility for detecting the presence of associated metastatic disease or hepatoma is questionable.[3] The CT scan and ultrasonography may also fail to distinguish malignant disease from a regenerative nodule.

Determining hepatic vein wedge pressure can be useful in diagnosing cirrhosis.[4] A catheter is advanced through the vena cava into the hepatic veins and then wedged into a distal small hepatic vein. The pressure recorded corresponds to intrahepatic pressure and indirectly reflects the portal pressure. Under normal circumstances, the wedge pressure is no more than 4 mm Hg greater than the free hepatic vein pressure. When the wedge pressure is normal despite obvious signs of portal hypertension, the

diagnosis of prehepatic venous obstruction must be considered. When the pressure is elevated, the diagnosis of cirrhosis is quite likely.

Although the esophagram is useful in detecting large varices [*see* Complications of Cirrhosis, Varices *below*], it does not detect varices in 30 to 40 percent of cases. If it is critically important to establish the presence of varices, the appropriate test to perform is esophagoscopy.[5]

Arteriography may be helpful when the cause of portal hypertension remains uncertain.[6,7] In the arterial phase, a typical corkscrewing of the hepatic arteries in the cirrhotic liver may be observed; in the venous phase, arteriography indicates patency of the splenic and portal veins. Selective arterial injections can be employed to visualize the renal and mesenteric veins in cases in which shunt surgery is being considered.

Some centers perform splenoportography to visualize the splenic and portal vein radicles. This procedure, which involves puncture of the spleen and injection of dye, does provide direct measurement of the portal vein pressure. Splenoportography, however, is associated with a five percent complication rate and does not allow visualization of the renal and mesenteric veins.

Peritoneoscopy allows visualization of the liver surface and helps to guide a liver

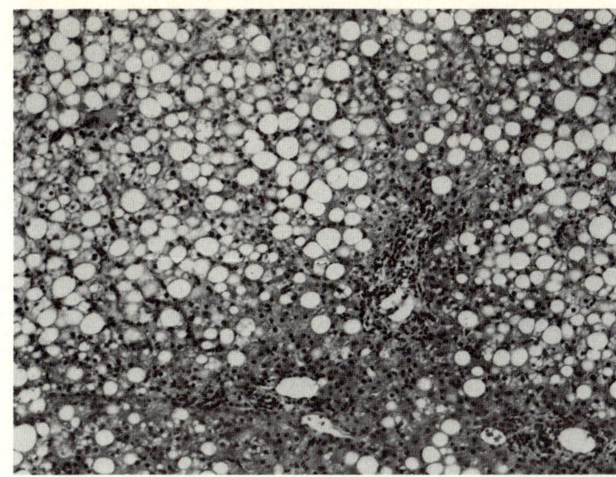

Figure 2 *Marked fatty infiltration (the round white regions) is apparent in the liver cells of a 29-year-old woman who had been drinking heavily for one year. The fatty infiltration usually disappears when alcohol intake ceases.*

biopsy.[8] Peritoneoscopy is particularly useful in investigating the possibility of a superimposed malignant disorder.

Specific Forms of Cirrhosis

Alcoholic Cirrhosis

Synonyms for alcoholic cirrhosis include portal, Laënnec's, nutritional, and micronodular cirrhosis. Because alcohol produces a direct toxic effect on the liver in experimental animals, alcoholic cirrhosis is the most appropriate term.[9,10] Physical examination usually shows the liver to be enlarged, sometimes to a marked degree. A weight of approximately 2,000 g or more at autopsy is not uncommon. Hepatomegaly reflects inflammation, fatty infiltration, and extensive scar formation. The typical histologic picture consists of a weblike scar that separates liver cell cords and surrounds small nodules of liver cells [*see Figure 1*].

Alcoholic cirrhosis is directly attributable to chronic ingestion of large quantities of alcohol. Its development does not require concomitant malnutrition, although this condition is almost invariably present. Malnutrition undoubtedly reflects a substitution of alcohol for normal dietary calories.[11] All persons who drink heavily develop a bland fatty infiltration, which is totally reversible when alcohol ingestion ceases [*see Figure 2*].[12]

Although the development of alcoholic cirrhosis usually requires 10 to 15 years of heavy drinking (i.e., greater than one pint of whiskey daily), the disease can develop rapidly. Fatal alcoholic liver disease has been reported in teenagers. Alcoholic cirrhosis typically progresses as a result of repeated bouts of clinical and subclinical alcoholic hepatitis. Alcoholic hepatitis refers to the pathologic findings of alcoholic hyalin surrounded by polymorphonuclear cell inflammation [*see Figure 3*]. These necrotic lesions are accompanied by collagen formation. In the earliest stages of this process, the lesions are typically found in a pericentral location. When the process is marked, central vein scarring (sclerosing hyaline necrosis) occurs.[13]

An acute clinical syndrome presents in only a minority of cases in which alcoholic hepatitis can be histopathologically demonstrated. This syndrome, which warrants immediate hospitalization, consists of fever of 38° C (100.4° F) or higher, right upper quadrant pain and tenderness, a markedly enlarged liver, leukocytosis, and deep jaundice. Not all features are necessarily evident. The mortality in such cases ranges from 10 to 40 percent. Although the great majority of patients with alcoholic hepatitis demonstrated by biopsy have accompanying cirrhosis, some do not.[14] In half of non-

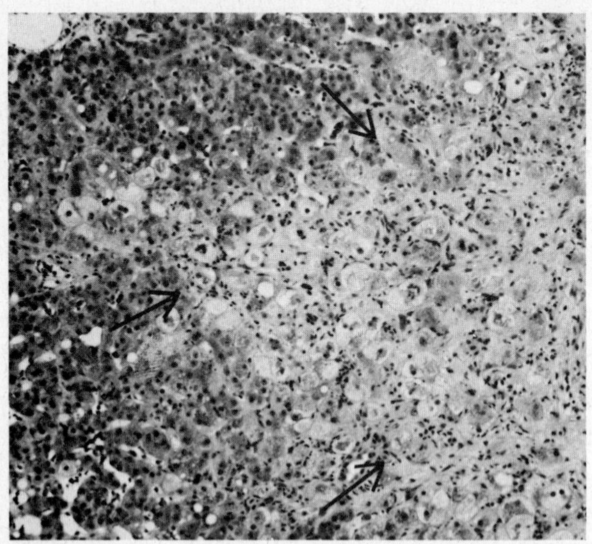

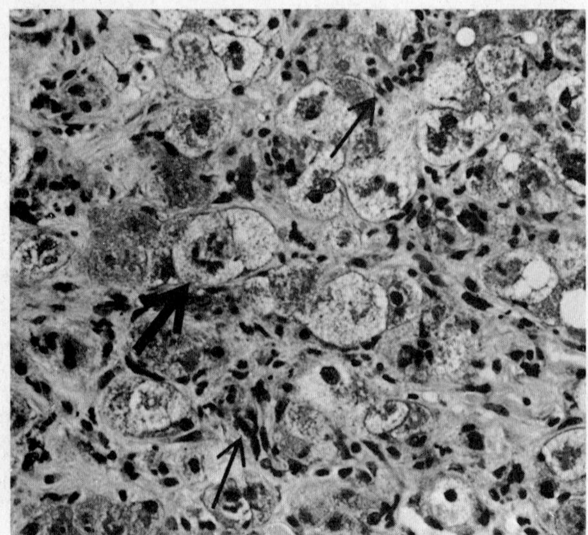

Figure 3   Liver biopsy specimen from a 34-year-old man with a seven-year history of heavy alcohol intake (top) demonstrates a zone of fibrosis, ballooning liver cells, and inflammation (arrows). Higher magnification (bottom) reveals typical alcoholic hyalin (thick arrow) and polymorphonuclear cell inflammatory reaction (thin arrows), which are features of alcoholic hepatitis.

cirrhotic patients, the liver will return to normal after cessation of alcohol; the remainder will develop cirrhosis. Spider angiomas, palmar erythema, splenomegaly, and ascites are common in patients with alcoholic liver disease.

In patients with decompensated alcoholic cirrhosis, the serum bilirubin level is elevated, often markedly (20 to 40 mg/dl). The serum aspartate aminotransferase (SGOT) level is usually elevated, perhaps as high as 200 to 300 IU/l. Characteristically, the aspartate aminotransferase level is more abnormal than the alanine aminotransferase (SGPT) level. Reversal of this relation or the presence of aminotransferase levels greater than 300 IU/l suggests that the diagnosis may not be alcoholic liver disease. The alkaline phosphatase level is often moderately elevated. Reduction of the serum albumin level below 3.5 g/dl and prolongation of the prothrombin time are common.

As the disease progresses, usually in the setting of continued alcohol consumption and poor nutrition, the patient loses muscle mass in the face, neck, shoulders, forearms, and hands. Weight loss usually occurs, although it may be counterbalanced by the accumulation of ascitic fluid. Ascites can be identified most readily by the detection of shifting dullness on physical examination. A fluid wave is pathognomonic for ascites but is apparent only when fluid accumulation is marked. The patient may exhibit a prominent abdominal venous pattern, signaling collateral circulation through the periumbilical vessels. Hepatomegaly is almost invariably present, and splenomegaly is common. Palmar erythema appears, and spider angiomas are usually seen over the face, upper back, arms, and chest. Subcutaneous bleeding often occurs as a result of vitamin deficiencies and a reduction in coagulation factors. Gynecomastia, which may be painful, and testicular atrophy are quite common. Hepatic encephalopathy may be present, and varices, when sought, are usually found.

The only established therapy for patients with alcoholic liver disease is to stop drinking alcohol. Patients with alcoholic cirrhosis who continue to drink seem to have a poorer prognosis than those who stop. The five-year survival rate for patients who drink is less than 40 percent but may reach 60 to 70 percent if abstinence is maintained.[15] Although pessimism abounds, as many as 30 percent of patients with alcoholic liver disease may succeed in abstaining completely.[15] Thus, the emphasis in treatment should be to support patients' efforts to stop drinking. Various rehabilitation units, peer support groups, and psychotherapeutic techniques are currently available.

Several studies have evaluated the efficacy of corticosteroids in patients with decompensated alcoholic liver disease.[14,16-20] These patients had either the histologic finding of alcoholic hepatitis or a consistent clinical syndrome. Corticosteroids were given at a dosage of 40 mg of prednisone daily for three to four weeks. The benefit of therapy is uncertain, but no study has proved corticosteroids to be harmful at this dosage. Corticosteroids increased survival in a predominantly female group of patients who were encephalopathic and who were able to undergo a liver biopsy.[14] Because the vast majority of patients do not fit this profile, however, prednisone cannot be routinely recommended for alcoholic cirrhosis.

Anabolic steroids such as oxandrolone have also been used. Oxandrolone was compared with prednisolone and placebo in a large Veterans Administration cooperative trial[21]; overall survival was not enhanced by either form of steroid treatment.

Propylthiouracil has been advocated on the premise that a hypermetabolic state exists in patients with alcoholic liver disease that increases the susceptibility of the liver cell to injury. Although improvement in liver function was noted with propylthiouracil therapy in one study, this finding could not be confirmed by other investigators.[22,23] Moreover, no beneficial effect on survival has ever been demonstrated. Colchicine has also been used in patients with alcoholic liver disease without evident benefit. Therefore, aside from the cessation of alcohol, therapy should be supportive and aimed at improving nutrition and treating complications.

Postnecrotic Cirrhosis

Postnecrotic cirrhosis is characterized by a shrunken liver containing regenerating nodules of varying size [*see Figure 4*]. The term postnecrotic is unsatisfactory, however, because all cirrhoses occur subsequent to liver cell necrosis. The most common cause of this condition is chronic active hepatitis. For many patients, however, the etiology is uncertain, and the term cryptogenic cirrhosis is applied. In such cases, it seems likely that cryptogenic cirrhosis develops as a sequela to subclinical, slowly progressive, chronic active hepatitis. Rarely, the disease

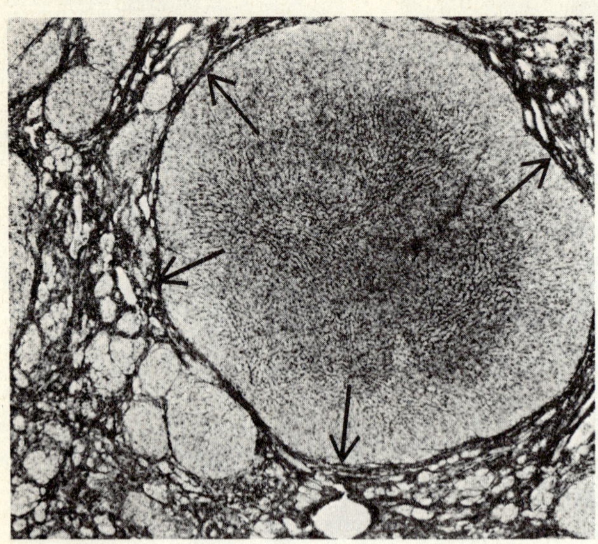

Figure 4   *At the time of splenectomy, a 29-year-old man
also underwent surgical
biopsy of the liver. The liver
was small and grossly nodular, the spleen huge. The
microscopic features typify
postnecrotic cirrhosis: hepatic
cell nodules of varying size
are surrounded by bands of
scar tissue (arrows).*

results from exposure to a toxic agent such as carbon tetrachloride.

Patients with postnecrotic cirrhosis often first seek medical attention for variceal bleeding; the condition is also sometimes discovered during the workup for an enlarged spleen. The distinguishing clinical features of the disorder are its predominance in females and the presence of a small liver, elevated gamma globulin, and occasionally, hepatitis B surface antigen. A small subgroup of patients also have marked abnormalities of alkaline phosphatase and signs and symptoms of cholestasis.[24] In postnecrotic cirrhosis, more often than in any other form of cirrhosis, the percutaneous liver biopsy may appear, misleadingly, to be normal.[25] The most likely explanation is that the biopsy needle has pierced a fibrous band and removed the center of a regenerating nodule, which may be almost normal in appearance.

Postnecrotic cirrhosis apparently progresses insidiously, even when it is seemingly inactive or when the treatment of chronic active hepatitis has been judged successful.[26] The usual cause of death is gastrointestinal bleeding or hepatic failure. About 10 to 15 percent of patients who have postnecrotic cirrhosis develop primary liver cell carcinoma.

When associated hepatitis is active, corticosteroids may be appropriate. However, when cirrhosis is advanced and evidence of hepatitis is minimal, no specific therapy is advocated; treatment must be supportive and aimed at complications.

Primary Biliary Cirrhosis

Primary biliary cirrhosis most often occurs in women between 30 and 50 years of age.[27] The presence of serum autoantibodies, an association with other autoimmune diseases, and the resemblance of the bile duct lesions in primary biliary cirrhosis to those seen in chronic graft versus host disease suggest that immune mechanisms play an important role in the pathogenesis of this disorder.[28] Presenting complaints are fatigue and generalized pruritus. Pruritus may be present for months or years before the individual consults a physician, often for advice about brown-pigmented skin, which is caused in part by chronic scratching. Jaundice may not develop until five to 10 years after the onset of pruritus and systemic symptoms. Some patients experience bone pain, multiple fractures, and vertebral collapse. The usual cause is osteoporosis, which occurs in 20 to 30 percent of patients and which appears to be due to a marked reduction in osteoblast function.[29] Less commonly, osteomalacia is also present. Factors that give rise to the bone abnormalities include malabsorption of calcium and phosphate, altered vitamin D metabolism, cholestyramine therapy, and poor nutrition. Physical examination often reveals xanthelasma, xanthomas, hepatosplenomegaly, hyperpigmentation, and excoriation of the skin. If the disease is advanced, scleral icterus, ascites, and edema will also be present.

Typical laboratory findings include an elevated alkaline phosphatase level (invariably 300 IU/l and often 700 IU/l), a serum cholesterol level greater than 300 mg/dl, and a positive antimitochondrial antibody test (90 to 95 percent of patients).

A moderate number of patients with primary biliary cirrhosis have concomitant disease such as renal tubular acidosis, scleroderma, CREST syndrome, or Sjögren's syndrome. A few familial cases of primary biliary cirrhosis have been reported.

Because primary biliary cirrhosis must be differentiated from cirrhosis occurring secondary to chronic biliary tract disease, the biliary tree should be visualized by transhepatic cholangiography or endoscopic retrograde cholangiopancreatography. At times, surgery may be required to make the differential diagnosis. Carcinoma of the pancreas or biliary tree, common duct stones, postoperative common bile duct stricture, chronic pericholangitis secondary to inflammatory bowel disease, or sclerosing cholangitis can all mimic the clinical and histologic features of primary biliary cirrhosis.

Liver biopsy may reveal bile duct destruction with lymphocytic-plasmacytic infiltration of portal areas, periportal granuloma formation, and portal scarring with linking of portal tracts [see Figure 5]. Ductular proliferation is common. When scarring is extensive, nodule formation, often with retention of the central veins, can be found. Bile stasis is usually periportal and indicates advanced disease.

Unfortunately, histologic changes typical of primary biliary cirrhosis are found in only a minority of cases. In the remainder, histologic features are very similar to those of chronic active hepatitis, and the two diseases are then distinguished based on clinical features and laboratory abnormalities.

The prognosis varies, but the clinical course is generally indolent. Major hepatic dysfunction usually does not occur until very late. The median survival time for symptomatic patients is about 10 years; it is significantly longer for asymptomatic patients.[30,31]

Corticosteroids, azathioprine, penicillamine, and colchicine have been suggested as therapy for patients with primary biliary cirrhosis. Adequate controlled studies of the effects of corticosteroids have not been conducted, but because these drugs may exacerbate the bone disease that occurs so frequently in patients with primary biliary cirrhosis, they should not be used. Two randomized trials of azathioprine therapy have been conducted. In the first trial, azathioprine, given at a dosage of 2 mg/kg/day, did not produce benefit, and side effects occurred in 27 percent of patients.[32] In the second trial, azathioprine, given at a lower dosage of 50 to 100 mg/day, produced a trend toward enhanced survival, but side effects were observed in 11 percent of those treated.[33] Penicillamine, given at dosages of 600 to 1,000 mg/day, was evaluated in five prospective randomized trials.[34-38] In four of these trials, the drug did not enhance survival, and benefit in the fifth was modest. Side effects of penicillamine therapy are common and include nausea, vomiting, alteration in taste, stomatitis, fever, myalgias, arthralgias, lichen planus, proteinuria, and bone marrow aplasia; drug-induced fatalities have been reported. Because azathioprine and penicillamine are of doubtful efficacy in treating primary biliary cirrhosis, the frequent associated side effects weigh against their use. Two randomized clinical trials evaluated the efficacy of colchicine therapy at a dosage of 0.6 mg twice daily. One group reported modest improvement in liver function test results and enhanced survival[39];

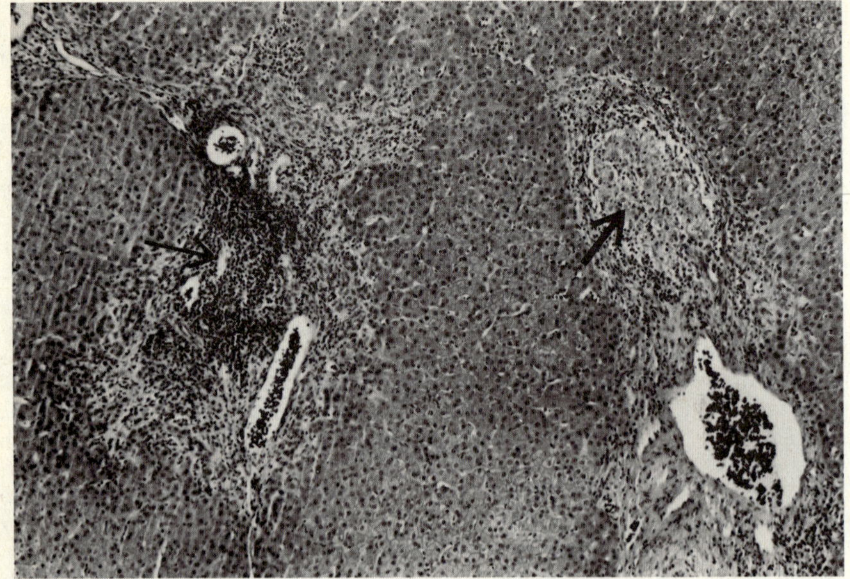

Figure 5   Dense portal inflammatory reaction (thin arrow) and portal granulomas (thick arrow) characterize primary biliary cirrhosis affecting the liver of a 29-year-old woman who underwent a cholecystectomy.

the other trial reported a trend toward improved survival.[40] Because colchicine produced only minor side effects easily controlled by dose reduction and is generally considered safe, its use in primary biliary cirrhosis seems warranted until an equally well-tolerated but more effective treatment is found.

Nonspecific therapy is directed at relieving symptoms during the slow but relentless course of the disease. The anion exchange resin cholestyramine may help to alleviate pruritus. The usual dosage is 4 g given orally three times a day. Some patients find relief at a lower dosage, although others require up to 16 to 20 g/day. Cholestyramine is often poorly tolerated but may be more palatable when taken with meals or mixed in applesauce or juice. Terfenadine is no longer used to treat pruritus in this group of patients, because life-threatening arrhythmias have occurred in patients with liver disease. In small groups of patients with primary biliary cirrhosis, short courses of therapy with rifampin (300 to 450 mg/day in divided doses)[41] or ursodiol (10 to 15 mg/kg/day) have proved effective for pruritus.

Vitamin supplements are recommended. A water-soluble form of vitamin A should be given daily in a dosage of 5,000 units. If the prothrombin time lengthens, vitamin K should be administered in a water-soluble form at a dosage of 5 mg/day. Patients who have osteomalacia should receive an active metabolite of vitamin D, either 25-(OH)D$_3$ (calcifediol) or 1,25-(OH)$_2$D$_3$ (calcitriol). These agents have produced improvement in cases of osteomalacia,[42] but their beneficial effect in osteoporosis, which is a more common complication, is less certain.[43] The usual dosages for symptomatic bone disease are 0.5 to 1.0 µg of 1,25-(OH)$_2$D$_3$ daily or 40 to 120 µg of 25-(OH)D$_3$ daily. Supplemental calcium should also be added at a daily dosage of 1 to 2 g. In addition, I recommend that either 0.25 µg of 1,25-$(OH)_2D_3$ or 20 µg of 25-$(OH)D_3$ be given daily as a prophylactic measure in asymptomatic patients. Serum calcium levels should be monitored during the first few months of vitamin D and calcium therapy.

Hemochromatosis

Hemochromatosis develops when large amounts of iron are deposited in the liver parenchymal cells [*see Figure 6*].[44] The accumulation leads to periportal cell destruction and hepatic scarring, culminating in cirrhosis. The disease occurs 10 times more often in males than in females. Symptoms generally appear between the ages of 40 and 60 in men or after menopause in women. Occasionally, the disease manifests at a much earlier age.

The disease is inherited as an autosomal recessive defect. The affected gene is closely linked to the HLA-A locus on chromosome 6.[45,46] The gene frequency is estimated at 0.056, and as many as three in 1,000 persons may be homozygotes. Heterozygotes may show some abnormalities of iron storage but do not develop clinical disease under normal circumstances. If hereditary hemochromatosis has been confirmed in a patient, HLA typing can be used if necessary to identify normal, heterozygous, and homozygous first-degree relatives.[47]

Iron deposits in the pancreas and heart muscle lead to dysfunction of these organs. When the symptoms of hepatic dysfunction first appear, about half of the patients have diabetes mellitus, 15 percent have congestive heart failure or arrhythmias, and a significant minority have stiffness and joint pain. Impotence, apparently related to pituitary dysfunction, is also common.[48]

In advanced disease, bronze discoloration of the skin secondary to deposition of both melanin and iron appears. The liver is moderately enlarged; splenomegaly is noted in about half of patients. When disease is less advanced, the skin may have normal color, and the liver may be barely palpable. Signs of portal hypertension even-

tually develop in most cases. Primary liver cell cancer occurs in about 15 to 20 percent of patients.

Laboratory analysis reveals an increase in serum iron associated with an 80 to 90 percent saturation of serum transferrin (15 to 47 percent saturation is normal). Serum ferritin is usually elevated as well.[49] An elevated mean linear attenuation coefficient (CT number) on CT scanning of the liver may signal the presence of increased hepatic iron stores.[50] Mild elevations of serum aminotransferase and alkaline phosphatase levels are not uncommon, but jaundice is unusual. The serum albumin level and the prothrombin time remain in the normal range until late in the course.

An elevated serum iron or serum ferritin level is not diagnostic, because these values can be raised in a wide variety of liver diseases marked by hepatic cell death. Elevated serum iron or ferritin is not uncommon in decompensated alcoholic liver disease, acute viral hepatitis, or chronic active hepatitis. Therefore, the diagnosis of hemochromatosis can be established only by liver biopsy.[51] The characteristic finding is a heavy deposit of hemosiderin granules in hepatocytes and bile duct cells. Fibrosis may range from minimal to well-established cirrhosis. At times, primary hemochromatosis is difficult to distinguish from cirrhosis with secondary iron overload. A preponderance of parenchymal iron relative to the amount of scar tissue and the presence of iron in the bile duct cells characterize primary hemochromatosis. Iron overload secondary to underlying cirrhosis usually correlates with an advanced cirrhosis, with relatively less iron, and with sparing of the bile ducts. When excess hepatic iron derives from an exogenous source, such as a series of massive transfusions for chronic hemolytic anemia, iron will be prominent in the Kupffer cells. Tissue obtained from the heart, pancreas, or skin of patients with hemochromatosis will show heavy infiltration of stainable iron.

Early detection and treatment of patients with primary hemochromatosis are essential. The usual therapy is removal of the

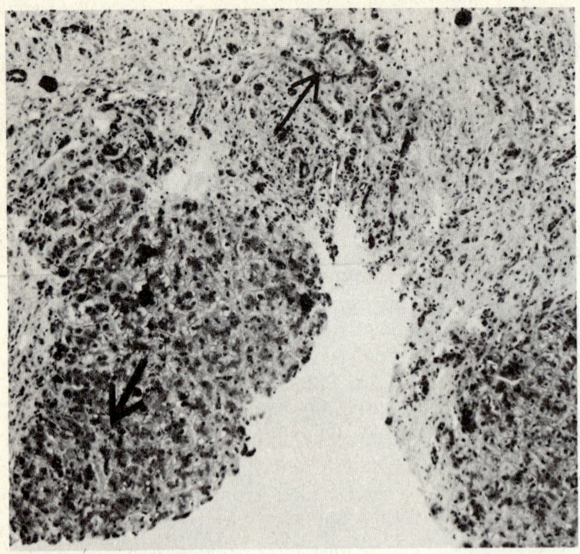

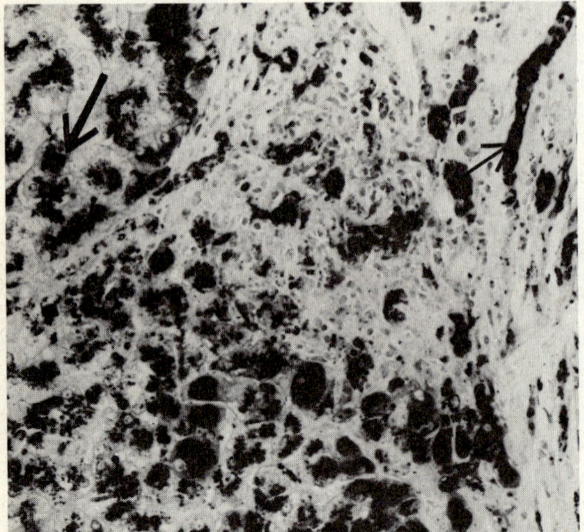

Figure 6 *A percutaneous liver biopsy specimen was taken from a 30-year-old woman with hepatosplenomegaly and amenorrhea of six months' duration. Pigment both in hepatic parenchymal cells (thick arrow) and in bile ductular cells (thin arrow) is apparent (top). The higher-magnification iron stain of the specimen (bottom) confirms the pigment to be iron in both parenchymal cells (thick arrow) and bile ductular cells (thin arrow). This woman with hemochromatosis required removal of 72 units of blood during one and a half years to render her liver free of excess iron.*

excess iron by weekly phlebotomies.[52] Because each pint of blood contains 250 mg of iron, removal of a pint of blood per week will deplete the iron stores in most patients with hemochromatosis in one to two years. Therapy aims for persistently low serum iron levels and absence of stainable iron on liver biopsy. Subsequent phlebotomies can be carried out every two to three months to prevent reaccumulation of iron. If patients are identified prior to developing cirrhosis and total body iron depletion is successfully accomplished, life expectancy approaches normal.[53] Treated patients who have cirrhosis do better than untreated patients but remain at risk of developing primary liver cell cancer years after successful iron depletion. Failure to deplete iron stores after 18 months of treatment is a poor prognostic sign. Signs of liver disease abate in 70 percent of treated patients, but endocrine abnormalities and arthropathy are improved in only 20 percent of those treated.

Repeated phlebotomies are obviously impractical in managing iron overload that results from the therapy for hemolytic anemia. In such patients, deferoxamine, administered subcutaneously at a dosage of 1 to 3 g over 12 hours, produces an average urinary iron loss of 50 mg each day.[54] The addition of ascorbic acid, 500 mg/day orally, may double the rate of urinary iron excretion.

Wilson's Disease

Wilson's disease, or hepatolenticular degeneration, is an autosomal recessive disorder found in about one person per million.[55] In this disorder, the excretion of copper into the bile appears to be defective, leading to an accumulation of excess copper in most body tissues. By 15 years of age, affected individuals have usually experienced symptoms due to either neurologic or hepatic dysfunction. Although Wilson's disease has presented for the first time in individuals as old as 30 years of age, this late an onset is the distinct exception. The first manifestations of the disease in about half of patients are symptoms related to hepatic dysfunction. The hepatic disease is usually a chronic disorder manifested by fatigue, jaundice, spider nevi, ascites, edema, splenomegaly, and variceal hemorrhage. Associated hemolytic anemia is a clue to the diagnosis. Occasionally, the liver disease may mimic severe acute hepatitis and progress to death in a few days to weeks. Neurologic symptoms include tremors, rigidity, gait disturbances and clumsiness, slurring of speech, and personality changes. Hypoparathyroidism has also been observed.[56]

The pathognomonic sign is the Kayser-Fleischer ring, a thin, brown crescent of pigmentation at the periphery of the cornea. Although this feature is usually circumferen-

tial, it may be located only superiorly and inferiorly. Early in the disease, a slit-lamp examination may be required to identify the telltale ring. It may be particularly difficult to detect on routine eye examination in brown-eyed patients.

On first examination, at least 50 percent of patients have hepatosplenomegaly and moderate liver function abnormality. Two distinguishing laboratory findings are depression or absence of serum ceruloplasmin and an increase of urinary copper levels from a normal value of less than 50 µg/day to as high as 1,000 µg/day. In a small percentage of patients with Wilson's disease, serum ceruloplasmin or urinary copper levels may be normal, and Kayser-Fleischer rings may be absent. Hence, it is wise to evaluate all three of these factors because it is likely that at least one will be abnormal. If doubt persists, the ultimate standard is evidence of decreased incorporation of radioactive copper into ceruloplasmin.

Treatment of Wilson's disease requires the administration of penicillamine, a chelating agent that binds copper and promotes the urinary excretion of 1,000 to 3,000 µg of copper per day.[57] The usual dose is 1 g/day. Clinical improvement usually parallels depletion of the tissue copper buildup. Penicillamine therapy is associated with significant side effects—most commonly, nausea and abdominal discomfort immediately after taking the medication. More serious side effects include leukopenia and thrombocytopenia, which may, in a rare case, lead to aplastic anemia. A small percentage of patients develop the nephrotic syndrome. All patients with Wilson's disease should be followed closely with routine urinalyses and blood counts, particularly during the first few months of therapy. Because penicillamine is a pyridoxine antagonist, 50 mg of pyridoxine should be given once each week. If penicillamine cannot be tolerated, oral zinc therapy should be considered. Elemental zinc may be administered in the form of zinc acetate in divided doses on an empty stomach for a total daily dose of 150 mg. Zinc therapy increases fecal copper loss and in-

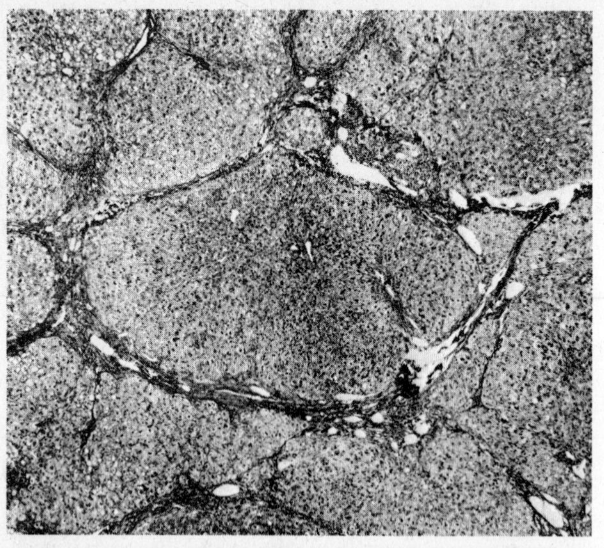

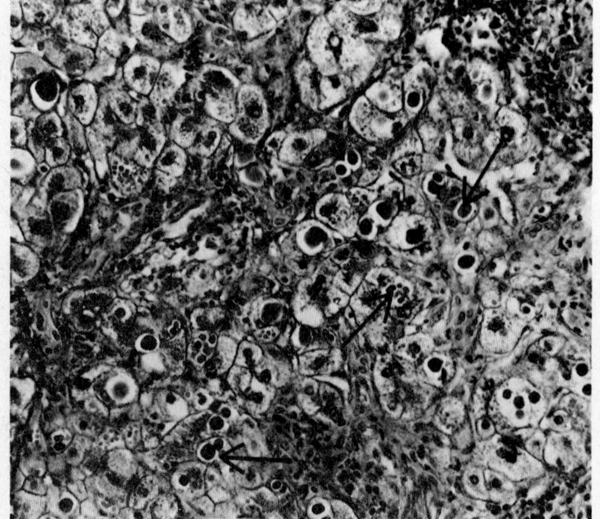

Figure 7 *Nodules of liver tissue surrounded by scar—features of cirrhosis—are seen in a surgical liver biopsy specimen from a 67-year-old man with emphysema and mild hepatomegaly (top). In the high-power view (bottom), multiple round hepatic cell inclusion bodies (arrows) are distinctive for alpha$_1$-antitrypsin globulin deficiency.*

duces a negative copper balance in patients with Wilson's disease.[58] The onset of action is delayed, however, and the long-term efficacy of zinc therapy is unknown.

Alpha$_1$-Antitrypsin Globulin Deficiency

Homozygous alpha$_1$-antitrypsin globulin deficiency is associated with a rare syndrome of progressive cirrhosis.[59] Although originally described in children with juvenile cirrhosis, the combination of alpha$_1$-antitrypsin deficiency and portal cirrhosis has been reported in adults. Adult patients usually have accompanying emphysema.[60] The diagnosis of alpha$_1$-antitrypsin globulin deficiency should always be considered in cases in which the cirrhosis does not have an obvious antecedent.

On first presentation, most patients have moderate hepatomegaly and mild abnormality of liver function. Absence of alpha$_1$-globulin on protein electrophoresis makes the diagnosis very likely. Specific measurements of alpha$_1$-antitrypsin levels in the blood confirm the diagnosis. Genetic variants have been found, reflecting the existence of more than 25 different alleles for the gene that controls production of alpha$_1$-antitrypsin.[59] PiZZ (protease inhibitor type ZZ) is the genotype generally associated with cirrhosis and emphysema. Characteristic periodic acid-Schiff–positive (diastase-resistant) inclusion bodies containing abnormal alpha$_1$-antitrypsin globulin can be seen in the hepatocytes [*see Figure 7*]. No therapy exists for this disorder.

Schistosomiasis

Cirrhosis following schistosome infestation, unusual in the United States, is more common in the Far East, Egypt, and parts of South America.[61] In schistosomiasis, eggs in the portal radicles elicit a granulomatous fibrotic reaction that at times leads either to diffuse periportal fibrosis or to the so-called pipestem fibrosis. The presenting complaint is often acute variceal hemorrhage, and examination reveals prominent hepatosplenomegaly. Stigmata of chronic liver disease are seldom seen. Signs of hepatic insufficiency or hepatic failure appear rarely. Treatment of schistosomiasis is not always satisfactory, particularly in advanced disease.[62]

Cirrhosis Associated with Jejunoileal Bypass

Increased hepatic fat accumulation occurs in virtually all patients during the period of rapid weight loss following jejunoileal bypass surgery.[63] A small number of patients will develop progressive liver disease that is indistinguishable from alcoholic cirrhosis. The liver is usually enlarged, and hepatic function progressively deteriorates.[64,65] The cause of this catastrophic complication is unknown. This syndrome has also been reported to follow gastroplasty.[66] Although scattered reports indicate improvement of liver function following parenteral hyperalimentation, the only certain treatment of progressive liver disease is reanastomosis of the bowel or take-down of the gastroplasty. If this procedure is not done promptly, the liver disease may prove fatal.

Cirrhosis and Fatty Liver

Although there is little evidence that fat accumulation leads to cirrhosis, there have been reports of an idiopathic cirrhosis associated with increased hepatic fat.[67,68] Most of the affected patients were female, middle-aged, and obese; several had diabetes mellitus. A careful history was taken from family, friends, and employers to exclude the possibility of surreptitious drinking. These patients commonly exhibit a quite enlarged liver but only mild functional abnormalities. Stigmata of liver disease are common. The mechanisms of hepatic damage are completely unknown as is the long-term course of the disease. No specific therapy for this form of cirrhosis is available.

Cardiac Cirrhosis

Cardiac cirrhosis has become rare because the introduction of prosthetic valve replacements has allowed correction of valvular disorders. The disease arises after years or even decades of severe right-sided heart failure or tricuspid insufficiency. The histologic picture consists of central scarring with fibrous tissue linking central veins and of the eventual formation of nodules that often contain a portal triad. The liver is usually large, and hepatojugular reflux can frequently be demonstrated. Treatment of cardiac cirrhosis involves correcting the valvular abnormality.

Some patients with Budd-Chiari syndrome (hepatic vein thrombosis) may survive the acute illness and develop a histologic picture of cardiac cirrhosis.[69]

Miscellaneous Cirrhoses

Chronic exposure to arsenic, methotrexate, or excessive amounts of vitamin A can lead to cirrhosis.[70-72] In addition, various diseases unique to children can eventuate in

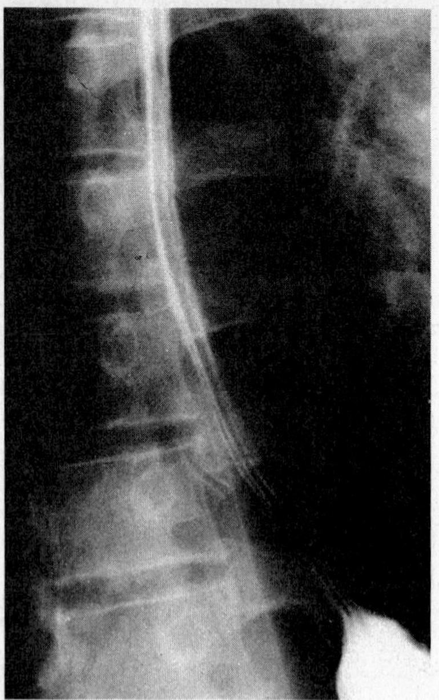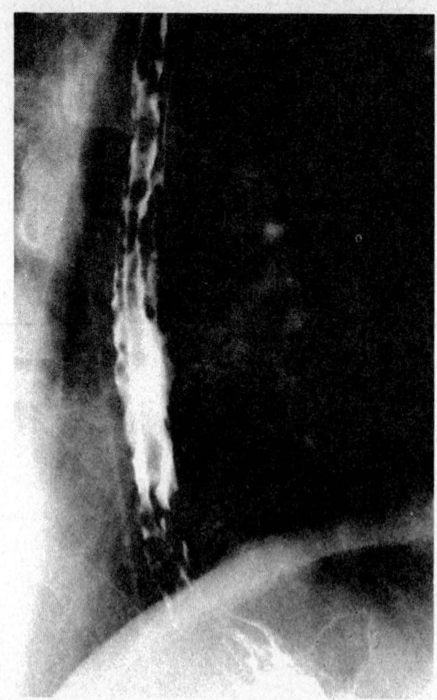

Figure 8　*Esophagram (left) is normal except for a small hiatal hernia; smooth, thin folds outline the distal part of the esophagus. In contrast, multiple irregular nodular densities impinge on the barium column when varices are present (right).*

cirrhosis. The most common of these childhood disorders are cystic fibrosis, glycogen storage disease, biliary atresia, and congenital hepatic fibrosis.[73-75]

Complications of Cirrhosis

Varices

Bleeding varices constitute one of the most serious complications of cirrhosis. Mortality during the acute episode may reach 60 to 70 percent.[76] Many factors associated with decompensated cirrhosis augment this high risk, including general debility, coagulation defects, and hepatic encephalopathy. Recurrent bleeding, common within the first two weeks of the initial episode, also contributes to the high mortality. If the individual survives beyond six weeks, the risk of recurrent bleeding drops sharply and approaches that of cirrhotic patients who have never bled.[77]

Barium contrast x-ray studies or esophagoscopy can identify esophageal varices [*see Figure 8*]. Treatment of esophageal varices entails the usual supportive therapy, infusion of intravenous fluid to restore plasma volume and electrolyte balance, and the administration of blood. When clotting abnormalities are prominent, subcutaneous vitamin K, fresh frozen plasma, and platelets should also be administered [*see Chapter 14*].

If variceal bleeding persists or recurs, insertion of a Sengstaken-Blakemore tube will stop the bleeding, at least temporarily, in more than 90 percent of patients.[78] Many of the difficulties that have been associated with the procedure can be avoided if the patient is monitored in an intensive care unit. Proper procedure requires inserting the tube through either the mouth or the nose, inflating the gastric balloon with 250 to 300 ml of air, and positioning the balloon tightly against the cardioesophageal junction. In most patients, this procedure alone will stop the bleeding. If not, the esophageal balloon must be inflated to a pressure of 30 to 40 mm Hg. It is wise to place a nasogastric suction tube above the balloon to prevent the accumulation of blood and mucus. Because the chance of complications from the Sengstaken-Blakemore tube increases with the length of time the balloon is kept inflated, an attempt should be made to deflate the balloon at 24 hours. If bleeding has stopped, the tube should be removed in another 24 hours.

Intra-arterial vasopressin may temporarily slow or stop bleeding, but it does not improve overall survival, and its administration requires specialized angiographic expertise that is not widely available. Vasopressin administered intravenously in a continuous drip does not appear to be effective.[79]

Propranolol produces a sustained reduction in portal pressure in patients with cirrhosis and might be expected to prevent bleeding from esophageal varices.[80] One study noted a dramatic reduction in episodes of rebleeding and improved two-year survival when propranolol was given in a sufficient dosage to reduce the resting heart rate by 25 percent.[81] However, another study found no decrease in variceal hemorrhage with a similar regimen and further reported that the beta blockade induced by propranolol complicated the resuscitation of bleeding patients.[82] The drug may also precipitate hepatic encephalopathy in susceptible patients.[83] Propranolol must be used with extreme caution even in the well-motivated patient who has recovered from an episode of bleeding from large varices.

Sclerotherapy, the injection of a sclerosing agent into esophageal varices, appears to be effective in the immediate control of variceal bleeding [*see Chapter 12*]. It may also prove to be effective in the long-term control of variceal hemorrhage, particularly in patients with nonalcoholic cirrhosis.[84,85] Whether sclerotherapy enhances survival remains uncertain.[86,87] The sclerosing agent causes severe necrotizing inflammation of the esophageal wall followed by a marked fibrotic reaction.[88] Complications are common and include ulceration, hemorrhage, pleural effusion, stricture, and perforation.

Percutaneous transhepatic obliteration of varices also controls active variceal hemorrhage 70 percent of the time; however, bleeding usually recurs after the use of this procedure.[89]

Recurrent or continued bleeding may indicate a need for a portasystemic shunt. This major operation carries a mortality of approximately 40 percent when performed on an emergency basis.[90] If bleeding can be stopped and surgery performed electively, mortality declines substantially. Although portasystemic shunting procedures do not appear to prolong survival, they do prevent subsequent bleeding. The major problem following surgery is intractable hepatic encephalopathy and hepatic failure.[91] The preferred shunt procedure is the one with which the surgeon is most experienced. In general, a larger shunt is more effective in preventing variceal bleeding but carries a greater risk of inducing severe encephalopathy than a smaller shunt. The smaller shunt is more likely to thrombose and lead to recurrent variceal hemorrhage. A distal splenorenal shunt with concomitant gastroesophageal devascularization selectively decompresses esophageal varices while maintaining mesenteric blood flow to the liver. In most but not all studies, use of the distal splenorenal shunt reduced the incidence of severe encephalopathy as a late complication following surgery, as compared with conventional shunts.[92-94] The procedure is technically difficult; time will reveal if it possesses any long-term advantages.

Emergency portacaval shunts have been compared with sclerotherapy in the treatment of patients with severely decompensated alcoholic liver disease and active variceal hemorrhaging.[95] Although initial transfusion requirements were higher in patients who received shunts, subsequent recurrence of bleeding was much less frequent in these patients than in those who received sclerotherapy. The incidence of encephalopathy was somewhat greater in the group that received shunts, but survival was comparable in the two groups.

Insertion of a prophylactic portasystemic shunt prior to bleeding cannot be recommended for patients with cirrhosis and varices. Several controlled trials have shown that the resultant overall survival of the patient is not improved.[96] Patients with idiopathic portal hypertension or portal vein thrombosis often tolerate shunt surgery quite well.[97]

Ascites

Ascites, a common sequela of many forms of cirrhosis, is usually detected by finding shifting dullness or a fluid wave on physical examination of the abdomen. Occasionally, ascites presents as a right-sided pleural effusion.[98] Portal hypertension, decreased serum albumin with consequent loss of oncotic force within the vascular and interstitial spaces, and renal retention of sodium and water contribute to ascites formation.

Although infectious, pancreatic, or neoplastic causes of ascites are infrequent, they should not be overlooked, because therapy and prognosis differ for each condition.[99] To exclude such possible causes, a small amount of ascitic fluid should be removed from the abdominal cavity using a narrow-gauge needle. The gross appearance of the fluid may suggest an unusual etiology: for instance, cloudy fluid implies an infectious etiology; bloody fluid, a tumor; and milky fluid, a lymphatic obstruction. Laboratory studies of the fluid should include white cell and differential cell counts, protein and amylase determinations, cytology, and culture. In transudative ascites due to cirrhosis, the total protein is less than 2.5 g/dl, the total white cell count is less than $300/mm^3$, the proportion of granulocytes is less than 30 percent, fluid amylase levels are less than serum levels, and both cultures and cytology are negative.

The treatment of uncomplicated ascites in patients with cirrhosis is straightforward. First, any medications that inhibit prostaglandin synthesis should be discontinued because they reduce base-line urine sodium excretion and blunt the natriuretic response to diuretics.[100] Indomethacin and aspirin are the most commonly used prostaglandin inhibitors. After such agents have been withdrawn, salt and water restriction should be instituted. Although extreme sodium and water restriction can be accomplished in the hospital, it is not usually necessary, nor will it be maintained once the patient goes home. A diet in which sodium is restricted to 2 g and water is restricted to 2,000 ml daily is often well tolerated.[101] If dietary restriction and bed rest do not induce diuresis, the medication of choice is spironolactone.[102] Seventy-five percent of hospitalized patients with ascites obtain relief with spironolactone alone. The drug's efficacy in cirrhotic patients with ascites is in marked contrast to its weak diuretic action in patients with salt and water retention from other causes. Because spironolactone inhibits the action of aldosterone, it tends to prevent the renal excretion of potassium—a desirable pharmacologic action in patients with cirrhosis. For this reason, however, use of the agent is not advisable in patients with renal insufficiency. High-dose long-term use produces gynecomastia in 20 to 30 percent of patients.

Spironolactone is given in an initial dosage of 25 mg four times daily. After three to four days, this dosage can be increased to 200 mg/day and again, after a similar interval, to 400 mg/day. If diuresis does not ensue at the highest dose, furosemide at 40 mg/day should be added. Furosemide may be increased by increments of 40 mg/day. Most patients begin to respond before doses reach 120 to 160 mg of furosemide and 400 mg of spironolactone. The aim is to use the lowest possible drug dosages.

The maximum diuresis of ascitic fluid should not exceed 1,000 ml/day.[103] For that reason, daily weight loss in cirrhotic patients should not exceed 1 to 2 lb. A more rapid diuresis, particularly in the patient with little or no peripheral edema, leads to dangerous diminution of intravascular and intracellular fluid volumes.

Complications of diuretic treatment include severe electrolyte abnormalities, encephalopathy, azotemia, and dehydration. Complications are most common when the diuresis has been rapid or when diuretic medication has been continued after the patient has been clinically judged free of excess body fluid.

In about five percent of patients, ascites will not respond to the usual doses of conventional diuretic medication, or diuresis will be achieved only at the expense of renal function. In these patients, insertion of the LeVeen peritoneovenous shunt should be considered.[104] The shunt routes ascitic fluid subcutaneously from the peritoneal cavity to the internal jugular vein via a one-way valve. Refractory ascites may resolve after shunt placement. Because most patients continue to require diuretics, although at lower doses, the shunt may produce benefit by increasing renal blood flow.

Serious complications of the shunt occur in five to 10 percent of patients and may prove fatal; they include bacterial infection of the peritoneum, disseminated intravascular coagulation, and rupture of esophageal varices. In addition, the shunt may clot and require replacement. The shunt should not be inserted in any patient whose ascites can be controlled with diet and medication. It is also inappropriate when the severe ascites can be expected to be short-lived, as is often the case during an episode of alcoholic hepatitis or following portacaval shunt surgery. In general, a patient should not be judged to have refractory ascites until it persists for four to six months. Finally, there is no reason to insert a peritoneovenous shunt unless the patient is severely disabled by chronic ascites.

Before potent diuretics became available, repeated paracenteses were the usual treatment of ascites. This procedure has been abandoned for long-term treatment because of its costs and risks and because diuresis can usually be accomplished with drugs. Paracentesis may still have a place in the initial treatment of patients with recent onset of ascites.[105,106]

Portacaval anastomoses have been performed for refractory ascites but cannot be recommended except in the gravest circumstances, because the procedure is associated with extremely high mortality and morbidity. The insertion of a peritoneovenous shunt is simpler and is generally preferable.

Spontaneous Bacterial Peritonitis

Spontaneous bacterial peritonitis develops in a few patients with cirrhosis and ascites.[107,108] The cirrhosis is usually advanced and active, as manifested by hepatic encephalopathy, esophageal varices, and deep jaundice. The pathogenesis is unknown. Presumably, hematogenous seeding of the ascitic fluid, which functions as an ideal bacterial culture medium, serves as a major route of infection. Cirrhosis undoubtedly facilitates the process by allowing enteric organisms to enter the portal venous stream via the portasystemic collaterals, thus bypassing the major reticuloendothelial system in the liver.

The typical attack of bacterial peritonitis is heralded by fever, peripheral leukocytosis, abdominal pain, hypoactive or absent bowel sounds, and rebound tenderness. Not all patients have all these findings, and some will not have any. Hence, ascitic fluid should be analyzed whenever the condition of a patient with cirrhosis suddenly deteriorates.

The ascitic fluid is often turbid due to leukocytosis and bacterial growth. Leukocyte counts greater than 1,000 cells/mm^3 consisting of more than 85 percent granulocytes are common.[107] Almost all patients have ascitic fluid cell counts greater than 300 cells/mm^3, and more than half of these cells are polymorphonuclear cells. However, not all patients with ascitic fluid leukocytosis have bacterial peritonitis. In practice, it is wise to treat all patients with antibiotics when the clinical picture is suggestive and the ascitic fluid contains more than 500 white blood cells/mm^3.[109] The ultimate criterion for infection is demonstration of organisms either by Gram's stain of the fluid (one fourth of cases) or by culture. Two thirds of the causative organisms are enteric; *Escherichia coli* and *Klebsiella* species are the most common agents. Pneumococci and streptococci are responsible for as many as 20 percent of the cases. In nearly half of cases, blood cultures are positive for the same organism found in the ascitic fluid.

Antibiotic therapy with gentamicin (1.5 mg/kg I.V. q 8 hr) and a second agent such as cefazolin (2 g I.V. q 8 hr) should be given for 10 to 14 days. A reduction in the dosage of both agents should be considered in the setting of renal failure. Patients should be monitored closely and ascitic fluid checked at least once to ensure that the infection is being effectively treated. Despite optimal therapy, 40 to 60 percent of these patients die. Half die as a direct result of the peritonitis; the remainder die of other complications of their severe liver disease.

Hepatorenal Syndrome

The hepatorenal syndrome is defined as a functional renal failure associated with well-established and usually decompensated cirrhosis. When the hepatorenal syndrome develops, the outcome is usually fatal.[110] The typical patient is deeply jaundiced, is obviously moribund, and exhibits tense ascites, hypoalbuminemia and hypoprothrombinemia, and encephalopathy. As liver disease progresses, urine volume and sodium excretion fall, and serum creatinine and blood urea nitrogen increase prior to death. In this setting, renal failure is incidental to the overwhelming liver disease. In perhaps 10 to 20 percent of patients, however, liver disease may be reasonably stable, and progressive renal failure represents the major threat to the patient's life.

The pathogenesis of the hepatorenal syndrome is uncertain, but a reduced renal blood flow and reduced glomerular filtration rate may precede overt renal failure by several months. Paradoxically, these alterations occur in association with increased plasma volume.[111] An increase in blood flow to the renal medulla at the expense of the cortex (intrarenal shunting) occurs as well. Because many patients have associated hypotension and respond poorly to pressor agents, false neurotransmitters have been implicated in the pathogenesis of the hepatorenal syndrome.

Although many diseases can affect the liver and kidney in tandem, a patient's history, oliguria, marked sodium retention, and presence of severe liver disease usually reduce the diagnostic possibilities to two—the hepatorenal syndrome or prerenal azotemia. Because these two causes of renal failure are indistinguishable by common laboratory tests and physical signs, it is imperative that patients be initially treated as though they had prerenal azotemia.[112] Diuretic medication should be discontinued, any blood loss replaced, and the plasma expanded with saline or glucose solutions. These steps should be taken carefully while the central venous pressure is being monitored, and they should be discontinued if diuresis does not commence when central venous pressure has been raised. Once the presence of prerenal azotemia has been excluded by these measures, treatment of the hepatorenal syndrome should be supportive and conservative. Spontaneous reversion of the syndrome, although infrequent, occurs when the liver disease begins to improve.

Reversion of the hepatorenal syndrome after insertion of a peritoneovenous shunt has been reported. The shunt might be considered in the small percentage of patients with prominent renal failure. Life-threatening complications, however, would not be unusual in these patients. Emergency portacaval shunt, corticosteroids, phenoxybenzamine, metaraminol, and methyldopa have all been used without major benefit.

Hepatic Encephalopathy

The diagnosis of hepatic encephalopathy depends on documentation of mental obtundation, asterixis, and fetor hepaticus.[113] Fetor hepaticus is an offensive, mixed feculent-fruity odor of the breath. Asterixis, the irregular flexion of the extremities, is most easily elicited by asking a patient to hold his or her arm horizontally with hands extended at the wrist. The flapping motion caused by intermittent loss of extensor tone clearly marks hepatic encephalopathy, although asterixis may also develop in patients with uremia or severe pulmonary disease. Slowing or flattening of waves on an electroencephalogram verifies encephalopathy.

Hepatic encephalopathy can be roughly classified into four stages. The first stage consists of agitation without accompanying physical findings. Patients in this stage often receive sedatives that promptly deepen the encephalopathy. In the second stage, the patient is moderately obtunded but still responsive, and asterixis can be elicited. The patient in the third stage is stuporous and barely responsive. In the fourth stage, the patient sinks into deep coma. In the third and fourth stages, asterixis may be absent.

The cause of hepatic encephalopathy is undoubtedly multifactorial. Elevated concentrations of blood ammonia, short-chain fatty acids, false neurotransmitters, and certain amino acids have all been incriminated in the genesis of this syndrome.[114] Both the shunting of blood around the liver, as a consequence of portal hypertension, and poor function of the diseased liver contribute to the pathogenesis. In addition, the central nervous system of the patient with cirrhosis appears to be very sensitive to the sedative effects of endogenous products and exogenous medications.

In most instances of hepatic encephalopathy, a precipitating cause can be identified.[115] Initiating events include gastrointestinal bleeding, electrolyte abnormalities, acid-base disorders, hypoxia, CO_2 retention, infection, or the injudicious use of diuretics, sedatives, or other medications.

The most important aspect of therapy is removal or correction of precipitating causes. The medication chart should be scrupulously searched for sedatives, which should be discontinued. Once these measures have been undertaken, standard therapy for hepatic encephalopathy includes dietary protein restriction and neomycin and lactulose administration. The usual approach restricts dietary protein to 40 to 60 g/day. Long-term restriction to much less than 60 g/day will result in protein malnutrition.

The drug of choice, lactulose, is a disaccharide that travels undigested to the colon, where it undergoes bacterial degradation to two- and three-carbon acids that reduce the intraluminal pH and produce diarrhea. The usual dosage is 30 ml three or four times a day. The mechanism of action of lactulose is uncertain. Apparently, the reduced stool pH causes ammonia to be protonated to its ionic form (NH_4), which is poorly absorbed and is excreted in the stool.

Lactulose has proved as effective as neomycin in the treatment of chronic or recurrent hepatic encephalopathy. Approximately 80 percent of patients respond to one of these drugs.[116] In certain patients, neomycin may be effective when lactulose is not. The usual dosage of neomycin is 1 g given orally every six hours; it may be increased to as much as 12 g/day. Although neomycin is poorly absorbed from the intestine, ototoxicity and renal damage have occurred. Because lactulose is less toxic than neomycin, it should be tried first. Although it might appear theoretically that neomycin would interfere with lactulose, evidence indicates that the two drugs may act synergistically.

Lactulose and neomycin are effective in chronic or recurrent encephalopathy, but their benefit is less certain in the encephalopathy that accompanies acute overwhelming hepatic disease. A few patients may develop refractory chronic encephalopathy, often as a consequence of portasystemic shunting.

Gallstones

The incidence of gallstones is increased in patients with cirrhosis, possibly because of the elevated bilirubin load generated by chronic hemolytic anemia and hypersplenism.[117] Hence, the possibility of a common duct stone should be considered in a patient with cirrhosis and jaundice. Fortunately, this complication is unusual because the detection of choledocholithiasis in a patient with decompensated cirrhosis may be very difficult. Ultrasonography simply and accurately detects dilated ducts more than 90 percent of the time.[118] This procedure should be done promptly whenever common duct stones are suspected. An intravenous cholangiogram is useless because the common duct cannot be visualized in a patient with liver disease and jaundice. If it is necessary to exclude bile duct disease conclusively, percutaneous transhepatic cholangiography or endoscopic retrograde cholangiography should be considered.[119] The best approach would be to withhold these procedures unless the suspicion of choledocholithiasis is high.

Peptic Ulcer

Peptic ulcer occurs more commonly in patients with cirrhosis than in the general population. The diagnosis should be considered if abdominal pain or upper gastrointestinal bleeding develops.

Because of the importance of differentiating a bleeding peptic ulcer from bleeding esophageal varices, it is usually necessary to perform upper gastrointestinal endoscopy when gross gastrointestinal bleeding develops [see Chapter 12].

Hypoxia

Hypoxia is frequent in patients with advanced cirrhosis, and Po_2 values of 60 to 70 mm Hg are not uncommon in these patients. Ascites impairs ventilation, and pulmonary angiomas may be responsible for right-to-left shunting of blood.[120] Because many cirrhotic patients both drink and smoke, chronic obstructive pulmonary disease often complicates the picture.

Primary Liver Cell Cancer

Primary liver cell cancer develops in five to 20 percent of patients with cirrhosis. Untreated, the disease follows a rapidly progressive course.

References

1. N Engl J Med 283:582, 1970
2. Am J Dig Dis 21:655, 1976
3. Ann Intern Med 69:283, 1968
4. Am J Med 49:649, 1970
5. Arch Surg 107:133, 1973
6. Radiol Clin North Am 8:147, 1970
7. Gastroenterology 71:1083, 1976
9. N Engl J Med 298:888, 1978
10. N Engl J Med 290:128, 1974
11. N Engl J Med 288:356, 1973
12. N Engl J Med 278:869, 1968
13. Ann Intern Med 70:497, 1969
14. Ann Intern Med 74:311, 1971
15. Am J Med 44:406, 1968
16. N Engl J Med 284:1350, 1971
17. Ann Intern Med 79:625, 1973
18. Gastroenterology 74:169, 1978
19. Gastroenterology 75:193, 1978
20. Gastroenterology 78:524, 1980
21. N Engl J Med 311:1464, 1984
22. Gastroenterology 76:105, 1979
23. Gastroenterology 83:925, 1982
24. Gut 4:223, 1963
25. Arch Intern Med 139:667, 1979
26. Gastroenterology 78:1153, 1980
27. N Engl J Med 289:674, 1973
28. Ann Intern Med 99:500, 1983
29. Ann Intern Med 103:855, 1985
30. N Engl J Med 308:1, 1983
31. Gastroenterology 89:267, 1985
32. Gastroenterology 70:656, 1976
33. Gastroenterology 89:1084, 1985
34. Lancet 1:1275, 1981
35. N Engl J Med 306:319, 1982
36. N Engl J Med 312:1011, 1985
37. Hepatology 5:1139, 1985
38. Gut 26:114, 1985
39. Hepatology 5:968, 1985
40. Hepatology 5:967, 1985
41. Gastroenterology 94:488, 1988
42. Gastroenterology 78:512, 1980
43. Gastroenterology 83:97, 1982
44. Medicine (Baltimore) 34:381, 1955
45. N Engl J Med 297:1017, 1977
46. N Engl J Med 301:175, 1979
47. Ann Intern Med 101:707, 1984
48. Lancet 2:298, 1972
49. Lancet 1:533, 1979
50. Gastroenterology 84:209, 1983
51. Am J Med 44:837, 1968
52. Q J Med 38:1, 1969
53. N Engl J Med 313:1256, 1985
54. N Engl J Med 297:418, 1977
55. Medicine (Baltimore) 54:113, 1975
56. N Engl J Med 309:873, 1983
57. Ann Intern Med 75:57, 1971
58. Ann Intern Med 99:314, 1983
59. N Engl J Med 314:736, 1986
60. Gastroenterology 65:284, 1973
61. Ann Intern Med 62:1113, 1965
62. Ann NY Acad Sci 160:602, 1969
63. N Engl J Med 290:296, 1974
64. Arch Surg 110:332, 1975
65. Gastroenterology 63:872, 1972
66. Gastroenterology 85:722, 1983
67. Am J Med 67:811, 1979
68. Gastroenterology 77:A27, 1979
69. Medicine (Baltimore) 61:199, 1982
70. Gastroenterology 66:86, 1974
71. N Engl J Med 291:435, 1974
72. Br Med J 1:654, 1972
73. Gastroenterology 70:645, 1976
74. Am J Dis Child 116:271, 1968
75. Gut 19:514, 1978
76. Am J Med 26:228, 1959
77. Gastroenterology 82:968, 1982
78. Gastroenterology 61:291, 1971
79. Ann Intern Med 96:565, 1982
80. Hepatology 2:523, 1982
81. Hepatology 4:355, 1984
82. N Engl J Med 309:1539, 1983
83. Br Med J 287:585, 1983
84. Hepatology 5:827, 1985
85. N Engl J Med 311:1594, 1984
86. Lancet 2:1328, 1983
87. Hepatology 5:584, 1985
88. Ann Intern Med 98:900, 1983
89. Gastroenterology 85:146, 1983
90. N Engl J Med 295:24, 80, 1976
91. Ann Surg 174:672, 1971
92. N Engl J Med 295:1089, 1976
93. Hepatology 1:151, 1981
94. Gastroenterology 88:424, 1985
95. N Engl J Med 311:1589, 1984
96. Medicine (Baltimore) 51:27, 1972
97. Ann Intern Med 66:41, 1967
98. Gastroenterology 88:188, 1985

99. Am J Med Sci 143:1, 1912
100. Hepatology 3:50, 1983
101. Gut 19:549, 1978
102. Gastroenterology 73:534, 1977
103. N Engl J Med 282:1391, 1970
104. Ann Surg 180:580, 1974
105. Lancet 1:611, 1985
106. Hepatology 5:403, 1985
107. Am J Med 64:592, 1978
108. Med Clin North Am 59:963, 1975
109. Gastroenterology 70:455, 1976
110. Ann Intern Med 60:353, 1964
111. Ann Intern Med 66:307, 1967
112. Gastroenterology 65:321, 1973
113. Metabolic and Toxic Diseases of the Nervous System. Williams & Wilkins, Baltimore, 1953, p 198
114. N Engl J Med 313:865, 1985
115. N Engl J Med 259:1145, 1958
116. Gastroenterology 72:573, 1977
117. Gastroenterology 63:112, 1972
118. Ann Intern Med 89:61, 1978
119. Gastroenterology 71:439, 1976
120. Trans Assoc Am Physicians 88:202, 1975

Acknowledgment

Figure 8 Radiographs courtesy of Malcolm Anderson, M.D., Department of Radiology, Stanford University School of Medicine.

12 Gastrointestinal Bleeding

GARY M. GRAY, M.D.
HARVEY S. YOUNG, M.D.

Clinical Manifestations and Differential Diagnosis

Gastrointestinal bleeding is responsible for two percent of all medical and surgical hospital admissions in the United States.[1] Of the approximately 85,000 patients admitted to hospitals each year with this problem, many are emergency cases, and 10 to 20 percent undergo surgery to control bleeding. Overall mortality is high—about eight percent[2]—despite the use of such reliable diagnostic procedures as fiberoptic endoscopy and selective mesenteric arteriography.

Although the exact location of hemorrhage is often difficult to document, most patients who present with gross gastrointestinal bleeding are found to have bleeding at the level of the duodenum or proximal to it.

Patients with acute severe gastrointestinal hemorrhage experience symptoms and signs of hypotension if the blood loss is about 1,500 ml (or about 25 percent of the total blood volume), particularly if the loss has occurred within minutes to a few hours. Impaired vision and light-headedness usually occur when the systolic blood pressure falls below 100 mm Hg and the pulse rate is greater than 100 beats/min. Such symptoms are particularly apparent when patients rise from the sitting or recumbent position. Other early signs include a sense of uneasiness or anxiety; cold, sweaty extremities; and syncope when the patient is in an upright position. Patients frequently report that they have passed very dark or black stools hours or a day or two before a hypotensive episode. Although the passage of black stools usually indicates that bleeding has occurred from a site above the level of the cecum, the degree of blackening is also dependent on the length of time the blood remains in the gut. It is well known, for example, that a cecal lesion such as carcinoma can produce melena and that very rapidly bleeding peptic ulcers may lead to the passage of grossly bloody or mahogany-colored stools.

There are several causes of upper gastrointestinal bleeding, which vary according to the hospital population [*see Table 1*]. Peptic ulcer continues to be the most common cause; erosive gastritis and esophageal lesions, such as erosive esophagitis and varices, are also significant causes of hemorrhage.[3]

Only a few conditions commonly lead to severe gastrointestinal bleeding; therefore, it is worthwhile to consider some of the symptoms and signs that help distinguish among the possible causes of this disorder. A history of epigastric pain that precedes the passage of black stools by one to two weeks suggests peptic ulcer disease. Weight loss, anorexia, and chronic anemia may antedate acute bleeding from gastric carcinoma. Recurrent retching just before hematemesis may be reported by more than half of the patients with a Mallory-Weiss tear at the esophagogastric junction. Sudden or gross hematemesis in patients who have ingested large quantities

Table 1 Causes of Upper Gastrointestinal Bleeding

Cause	Patients (%)
Duodenal ulcer	27
Erosive gastritis	23
Varices	14
Esophagitis	13
Gastric ulcer	8
Mallory-Weiss tear	7
No diagnosis	5
Bowel infarct	3

Note: see reference 3.

of ethanol for an extended period or who are taking regular doses of aspirin or other non-steroidal anti-inflammatory agents should alert the physician to possible hemorrhagic gastritis. Lower abdominal cramping pain, fever, and bloody diarrhea are common in diverticulitis. Painless hematochezia is usually associated with bleeding from colonic angiodysplasia or tumors.

Physical examination may disclose no abnormalities if bleeding is moderate. Brisk hemorrhage usually causes apprehension, tachycardia, and orthostatic hypotension, and the extremities become cool and moist. Although less prominent in the hypovolemic patient, ascites and the stigmata of liver disease (e.g., spider angiomas and palmar erythema) may be seen in the patient with variceal bleeding. Mucous membrane, cutaneous, or other bleeding may reflect impaired procoagulant synthesis by a diseased liver or the presence of other hemostatic disorders. Supraclavicular lymphadenopathy may be noted in patients with gastric carcinoma. Bowel sounds are usually hyperactive because of the presence of blood; the presence of an ileus may indicate that intestinal infarction has occurred.

Laboratory Analysis

Most patients with symptoms of hypotension have a hematocrit of less than 30 percent. The hematocrit may be normal, however, early in the course of massive acute arterial or variceal bleeding because of insufficient time for equilibration of plasma volume. In rapid and severe upper gastrointestinal bleeding, the blood urea nitrogen (BUN) level is usually greater than 40 mg/dl because of the absorbed nitrogen load from blood in the small intestine. Colonic bleeding does not usually lead to a rise in the BUN level. Because the plasma creatinine level is usually normal in gastrointestinal bleeding, the ratio of plasma concentration of urea to plasma concentration of creatinine may be particularly useful in localizing the source of bleeding to the upper or lower gastrointestinal tract. When the patient is first seen at the hospital, the serum urea nitrogen to cre-

atinine concentration ratio is almost always greater than 25 (values of each expressed as mg/dl) in upper gastrointestinal bleeding and less than 25 (mean, about 15) in colonic bleeding, even when the estimated blood loss is only one to two units.[4] Hypovolemic shock secondary to massive bleeding may produce centrilobular liver necrosis, reflected by a rise in the levels of alanine aminotransferase (ALT, formerly termed SGPT) and aspartate aminotransferase (AST, formerly termed SGOT) to 10 times normal or greater. Other liver function tests are usually normal.

Approach to the Patient with Acute Gastrointestinal Bleeding

Most gastrointestinal bleeding is self-limited; as a result, almost all patients (80 to 90 percent) who are treated conservatively cease bleeding within 24 to 48 hours. However, prompt and appropriate fluid replacement is essential to prevent the development of complications from acute hypovolemia. Careful attention should be given to identifying the small group of patients with gastrointestinal bleeding who are likely to continue bleeding or to experience recurrent bleeding after admission so that appropriate diagnostic and therapeutic plans can be formulated.

Supportive Therapy

Immediate attention should be given to assessing the degree of hypovolemia. Although the blood pressure and pulse rate may be normal when the patient is reclining, a pulse rate increase of 10 to 20 beats/min and a decrease in systolic pressure of 10 to 20 mm Hg when the patient sits upright suggest that a significant loss of blood has occurred.

Intravenous fluid replacement should begin immediately with a large-bore catheter via an arm vein. Thereafter, it is usually advisable to install a central venous catheter so that fluids and blood can be administered rapidly; the catheter can also be used to monitor the central venous pressure. A nasogastric tube should be passed to the 50 cm level and its position in the patient's stomach verified by auscultation during air insufflation. If the patient's hematocrit is less than 30 percent, blood replacement should begin as soon as possible. It is advisable to give isotonic saline and then to administer red blood cells. Dilutional thrombocytopenia may ensue after massive transfusion. Replacement of platelets or other blood components may be required.

After the patient's condition has been stabilized through the use of supportive therapy, diazepam can be administered in a dosage of 5 mg intramuscularly every six hours if severe anxiety persists.

Surgical Consultation

Surgical consultation should be obtained early. When the surgeon and the physician follow the course of the patient's condition, no time is lost in making the joint decision that is required if surgical treatment eventually becomes necessary.

Diagnostic Procedures in Upper Gastrointestinal Bleeding

Endoscopy is the diagnostic procedure of choice in patients with upper gastrointestinal bleeding. It can be accomplished rapidly and usually yields the correct diagnosis with relatively low morbidity when performed by an experienced individual. However, the information provided by the routine performance of immediate diagnostic endoscopy has no effect on the amount of blood replacement, the length of hospital stay, the requirement for surgery, or mortality.[3,5-7] In the majority of patients whose bleeding is self-limited, endoscopy should be performed electively after the patients are stabilized. This approach will further minimize the associated risks of the procedure.[8,9]

However, patients who bleed continuously or massively despite supportive therapy should undergo emergency endoscopy to identify the site of the lesion and to aid in formulating definitive therapy [*see Figure 1*]. Urgent endoscopy is particularly useful when the major clinical diagnosis being considered is a disease that is likely to cause continuous, severe bleeding or recurrent bleeding and for which specific endoscopic or surgical therapy is likely to halt the blood loss. For instance, esophageal varices should be treated immediately because they are associated with a high risk of continued bleeding and death. In addition, patients who have massive and continuous bleeding and are suspected of having peptic ulcers may be candidates for urgent endoscopic therapy. Before performing endoscopy in these emergency settings, especially when endoscopic therapy is contemplated, endotracheal intubation should be considered to prevent aspiration during the procedure.

If no blood is seen in the stomach or duodenum by endoscopy despite brisk blood loss in stools or if hemorrhage is so massive that the bleeding site cannot be located, selective mesenteric arteriography will detect the lesion in a high percentage of patients. This technique is successful, however, only when bleeding is from a discrete site and occurs at a rate of at least 2 to 5 ml/min. After the catheter has been positioned in the mesenteric artery and the bleeding site has been defined, vasopressin then can be administered intra-arterially through the indwelling catheter. Alternatively, the artery can be embolized with particulate agents. Intra-arterial infusion of vasopressin has frequently proved to be effective in controlling the bleeding, at least temporarily, and it is a good alternative to total gastrectomy in hemorrhagic gastritis, which is associated with a high mortality.

Therapy for Upper Gastrointestinal Bleeding

Pharmacological Therapy

Intravenous administration of H_2-receptor blockers has been commonly used for the initial resuscitation of patients with upper gastrointestinal bleeding. However, acid suppression does not effectively change the natural course of acute upper gastrointestinal bleeding. Despite the ability of acid neutralization to prevent clot lysis by gastric juices in vitro, administration of antacid or intravenous infusion of H_2-receptor block-

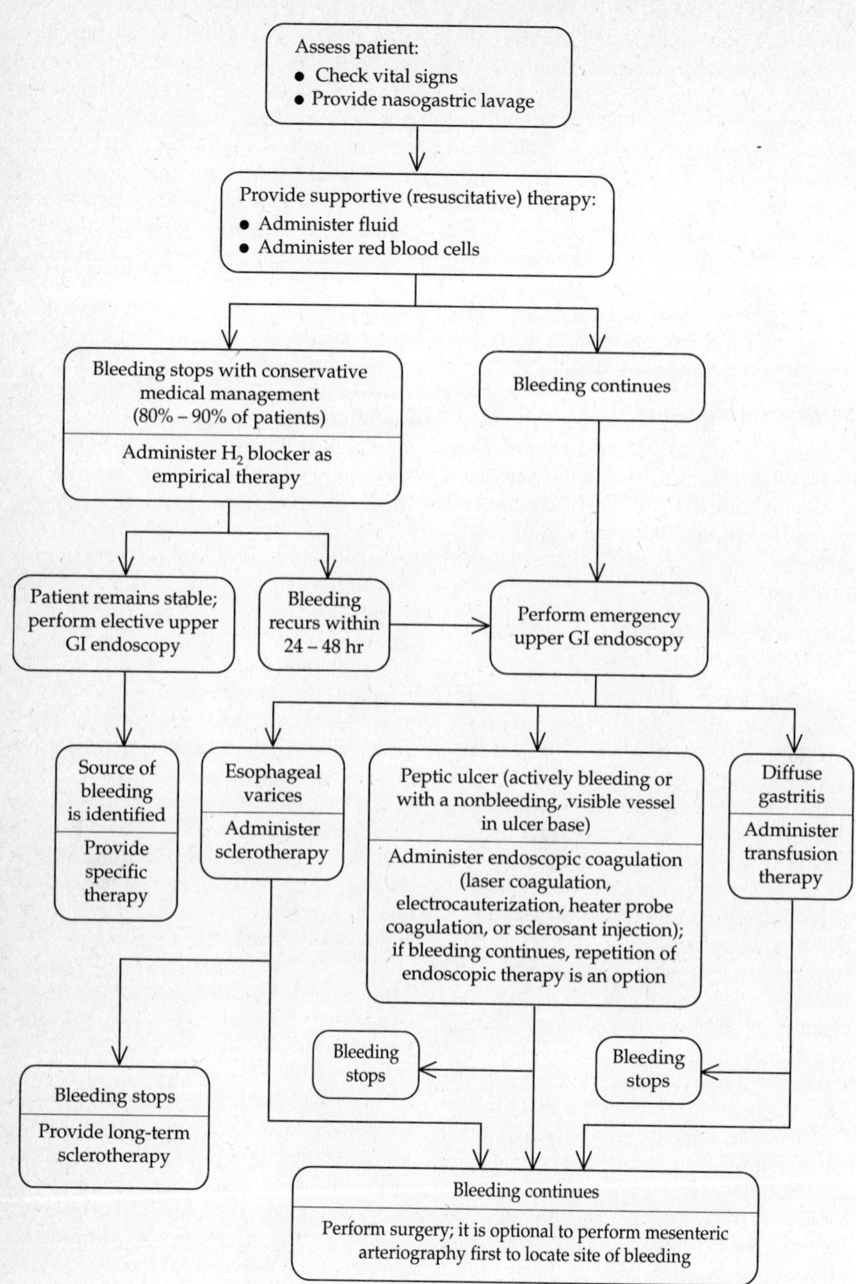

Figure 1 *This flowchart depicts the diagnosis and management of a patient with upper gastrointestinal tract bleeding.*

ers does not lower the incidence of recurrent bleeding in patients with bleeding peptic ulcers.[10,11] It is possible that these regimens do not lower the gastric acidity enough. Omeprazole, an H^+-K^+–ATPase inhibitor that can produce near total acid suppression, may prevent recurrent bleeding; however, controlled trials are needed.

The vasoconstrictive hormone vasopressin has been used to control gastrointestinal bleeding. Early clinical studies suggested that it was effective, especially for treatment of esophageal varices.[12,13] However, a well-controlled trial of intravenous vasopressin versus placebo showed that vasopressin did not control the bleeding or improve the prognosis.[14] This finding also negates the validity of trials that compared the efficacy of other drugs with that of vasopressin. Intravenous somatostatin and other peptides, as well as synthetic prostaglandins and tranexamic acid, also do not control bleeding.[15-17]

Endoscopic Therapy

Several endoscopic techniques can provide effective low-morbidity therapy for certain discrete and localized upper gastrointestinal bleeding lesions. Clinical trials indicate that acute bleeding from peptic ulcers, esophageal varices, and angiodysplastic lesions can be controlled by one or more therapeutic endoscopic techniques. For patients with bleeding peptic ulcers, endoscopic coagulation therapy is indicated only when active bleeding is seen during endoscopy or when a visible vessel (a red, blue, or black protuberance in the ulcer bed, representing a sentinel clot over a disrupted artery) is found in the ulcer base. An ulcer with an actively bleeding vessel or a nonbleeding visible vessel is associated with a 50 to 80 percent rebleeding rate; rebleeding rate for an ulcer with a clean base is five percent.[18,19]

The efficacy of endoscopic laser therapy for bleeding peptic ulcers has been studied since the mid-1970s. The argon laser was initially the laser of choice; however, conflicting results regarding its efficacy were reported from controlled trials.[20,21] In addition, its shallow tissue penetration was found to be inadequate for coagulating bleeding vessels that were covered with blood clots. The neodymium-yttrium-aluminum-garnet (Nd-YAG) laser initially replaced the argon laser in endoscopic laser therapy. Several studies have shown that the Nd-YAG laser is able to achieve immediate hemostasis in bleeding ulcers, and it prevents rebleeding.[22-27] These studies also indicate that a trend toward reducing the number of blood transfusions, decreasing the need for emergency surgery, and lowering mortality have occurred. In experienced hands, complications are rare. Perforation or exacerbation of bleeding by the laser may occur in about one percent of patients. However, because of poor portability, technical difficulties in using the instrument, and expense, the Nd-YAG laser has mostly been replaced by newer and less expensive techniques for endoscopic hemostasis.

Electrocauterization and Heater Probe Coagulation

Two thermotherapeutic endoscopic modalities have become standard endoscopic tools in the treatment of upper gastrointestinal bleeding. The bipolar or multipolar probe and the heater probe appear to achieve hemostasis in 80 to 90 percent of patients in uncontrolled studies. In several controlled studies, the multipolar instrument, which electrocoagulates by use of current flow among six different electrodes on the tip of the probe, was effective in controlling bleeding and in reducing the need for blood transfusions and surgery.[28-30] The multipolar probe was as effective as the Nd-YAG laser in one controlled trial.[31] The heater probe, which coagulates tissue at high local temperatures, was more effective than the Nd-YAG laser in producing hemostasis.[32,33] These electrocoagulation probes do not seem to impair ulcer healing. However, perforations induced by these probes have been reported in about three percent of patients. Because they are compact, portable, and much less expensive, these two probes have replaced the laser as the frontline endoscopic tool for hemostasis. However, additional in vitro and in vivo studies are under way to standardize several important technical parameters, such as power settings and tamponade force.

Injection Therapy

Endoscopic injection of epinephrine or a variety of sclerosants such as ethanol and polidocanol into a bleeding ulcer has been shown to be efficacious for acute hemostasis. Several controlled trials reported the efficacy of injection therapy in reducing the requirement for blood transfusions and the need for emergency surgery in these high-risk patients.[34,35] Injection therapy is as effective as the Nd-YAG laser and the multipolar and heater probes.[36-38] Its complication rate may also be lower than these other techniques. Injection therapy is now the least expensive and technically the easiest endoscopic hemostatic technique. It will very likely become the most widely used endoscopic therapy for hemostasis.

Sclerotherapy for Esophageal Varices

Bleeding from esophageal varices, which can be devastating, appears to be amenable to treatment by endoscopic sclerotherapy. This technique was initially described in 1939 but was refined and re-emerged as an effective therapy for bleeding esophageal varices in the 1980s. Several different compounds, such as morrhuate sodium, sodium tetradecyl sulfate, and ethanolamine oleate, are currently used in the United States as sclerosing agents. In Europe, polidocanol is the most commonly used agent. These agents are probably equally efficacious and safe. They are injected into or around the variceal channels with a No. 25 gauge needle through the endoscope's biopsy channel.

Emergency sclerotherapy was effective in controlling the acute bleeding episode in 74 to 91 percent of patients with bleeding esophageal varices, whereas balloon tamponade was effective in only 42 to 55 percent.[39,40] Also, the magnitude and frequency of rebleeding were lower when sclerotherapy was compared with tamponade or medical

therapy alone.[39-43] However, sclerotherapy is not effective for treating bleeding gastric varices unless they are located within 2 cm below the gastroesophageal junction.

A short course of sclerotherapy with two to three treatment sessions in the few days after the initial bleeding incident will not improve the long-term survival of patients with bleeding esophageal varices.[44,45] In patients presenting with severe liver disease, both sclerotherapy and emergency shunt surgery are associated with an acute mortality of about 50 percent.[46] The long-term efficacy of sclerotherapy will not be apparent until all the variceal channels are obliterated. It usually takes four to six outpatient sclerotherapy sessions during a period of approximately three months to achieve this goal. Several controlled trials have reported significant reduction in recurrent variceal bleeding in patients who underwent long-term sclerotherapy (rebleeding rate of 30 to 40 percent) compared with those who were followed medically (rebleeding rate of 60 to 75 percent).[39,42,45,47,48] The effect of sclerotherapy on the long-term survival of patients with varices is still controversial. Meta-analysis of all the reported controlled trial data suggests that sclerotherapy might improve survival in the treated patients by 25 percent.[49]

Endoscopic sclerotherapy is a fairly safe procedure. About half of the patients may experience transient dysphagia, substernal chest pain, and fever in the first 48 hours after sclerotherapy.[50,51] Superficial ulcerations at the injection sites probably occur in all patients undergoing sclerotherapy. This result reflects the natural course of the therapy, which induces fibrosis at the injection sites.[52] However, deep ulceration with necrosis and significant hemorrhage from these ulcers may occur in about 10 percent of patients.[50] Esophageal perforation immediately after the procedure is rare with the flexible fiberoptic endoscope but may occur in two to four percent of patients with the rigid endoscope.[53] Delayed perforation from transmural necrosis had been reported, but the actual incidence of this complication is unknown.[50]

Strictures at the injection sites, which usually respond to simple dilatation,[54] develop in about 15 percent of patients. Other very rare complications, such as pericarditis, clinically significant pleural effusion, adult respiratory distress syndrome (ARDS), brain abscess, and spinal artery occlusion, have been reported.[50,51,55-57] Overall, clinically significant complications occur in only 10 to 15 percent of patients undergoing sclerotherapy. This rate compares favorably with the rate of complications associated with the alternative therapy, decompressive shunt surgery, in patients with bleeding esophageal varices.

Prognosis and Complications

Regardless of the cause of the upper gastrointestinal bleeding, recurrent hemorrhage occurs in five to 30 percent of patients after definitive surgery.[58-61] When surgery is required for control of hemorrhage, the mortality is similar to that for medical supportive therapy for massive bleeding.[62] Because surgery has not been shown to be prophylactic against subsequent bleeding episodes, it should be reserved for those patients who lose more than six units of blood in 24 hours despite optimal support and in whom appropriate therapeutic endoscopy is unsuccessful.

Nongastrointestinal complications are related principally to severe hypotension and shock. Oliguria may occur because of inadequate renal perfusion and may be followed by acute tubular necrosis. Other conditions produced by marked decrease in blood flow include mesenteric insufficiency and infarction, acute hepatic necrosis, and myocardial ischemia and infarction. All of these complications are more likely to occur in elderly patients with arteriosclerotic vascular disease.

Bleeding in the Small Intestine

Although uncommon, bleeding from sites in the distal duodenum to the lower ileum may be indolent and difficult to localize. Angiodysplasia is believed to be the major source of bleeding in the small intestine; Meckel's diverticulum and benign tumors are also frequently responsible for bleeding. These lesions can be localized usually by arteriography or exploratory surgery with intraoperative enteroscopy or, occasionally, by barium contrast x-ray of the small intestine.[63]

Other techniques used to localize a bleeding site or a potentially bleeding lesion, especially when the bleeding is relatively slow, are red cell scintigraphy[64] and intestinal intubation with a small-diameter plastic tube fitted with a terminal weight. During intubation, the patient is fed a liquid diet, and the tube is aspirated hourly as it is propelled by peristalsis through the small intestine. When gross blood is first identified, the tube can be taped to the face of the patient; a Gastrograffin x-ray contrast study is performed to localize the bleeding lesion before surgery. Small bowel endoscopy using a pediatric colonoscope or an enteroscope may be able to identify small bowel bleeding lesions in one third of patients with chronic gastrointestinal bleeding of obscure origin.[65,66]

Lower Gastrointestinal Bleeding

Bleeding from the colon is much less frequent than from the stomach or duodenum. It is important to realize, however, that blood loss from the colon, with the passage of red blood and clots, may be very abrupt. The most important diagnoses to consider are perirectal disease such as hemorrhoids or fissure, acute diverticulitis, and tumor. In addition to the same supportive therapy as that used for upper gastrointestinal bleeding, sigmoidoscopy should be done as soon as the patient is stabilized [*see Figure 2*]. A suction device and an ample supply of cotton swabs should be available so that the blood can be evacuated and the site of the bleeding lesion identified. Before concluding that the acute bleeding arises from a site above the 25 cm reach of the sigmoidoscope, the physician should take great care that blood has been removed from the mucosa and that any fresh blood appearing within the field arises from a site beyond the instrument rather than from the margins of the field. Brisk bleeding from internal hemor-

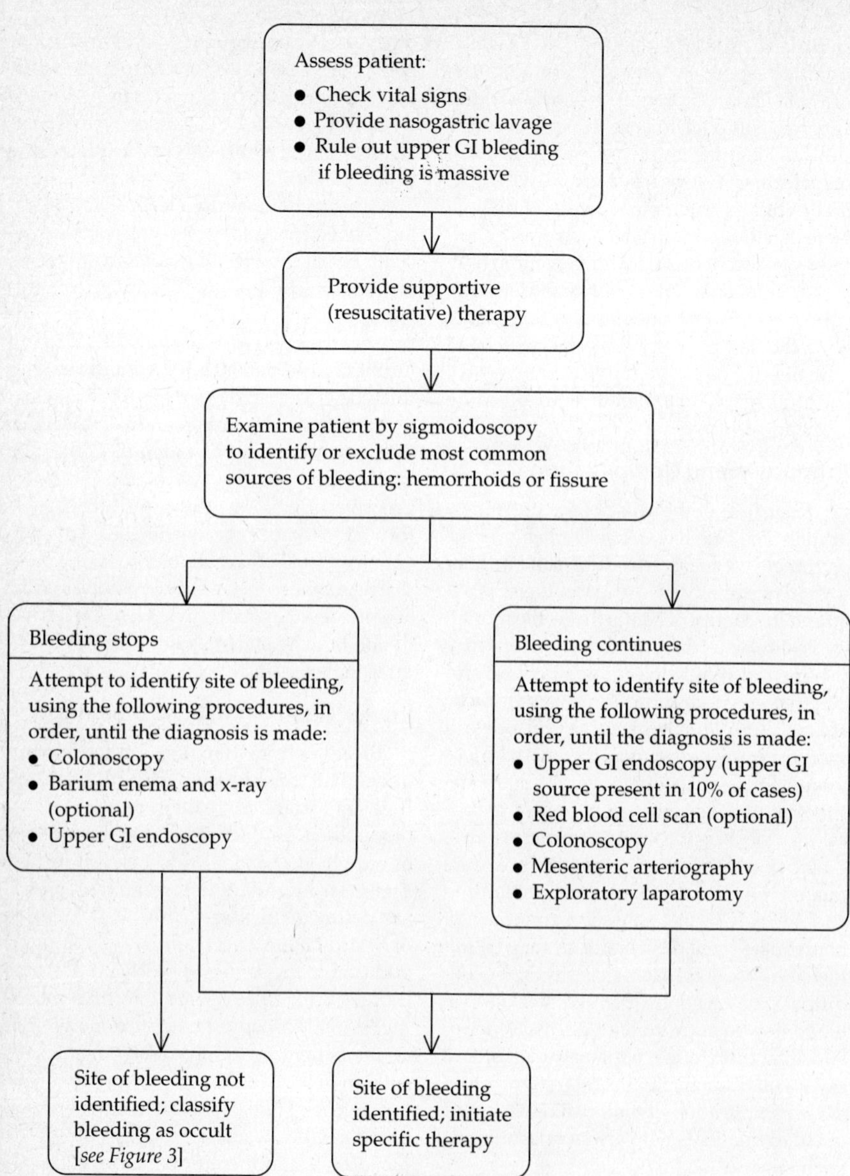

Figure 2   *This flowchart depicts the diagnosis of a patient with lower gastrointestinal tract bleeding.*

rhoids may result in retrograde blood flow along the exterior of the sigmoidoscope; the blood from rectal hemorrhoids can appear at the periphery of the field even when the instrument has been inserted to a distance of 25 cm.

The other important diagnostic proce- dure to consider in severe lower gastrointestinal bleeding is selective mesenteric arteriography, which may be particularly helpful when a bleeding diverticulum or a vascular lesion is present. Embolic therapy may be possible if the bleeding lesion is identified. Colonoscopy is feasible if bleeding is moderate; polyethylene glycol electrolyte solution (e.g., Colyte or GoLYTELY) can be given orally to flush out residual blood and clots.[67] Unfortunately, continuous brisk bleeding usually obviates colonoscopy.

Chronic and Recurrent Gastrointestinal Bleeding from an Unknown Source

Chronic gastrointestinal bleeding from an obscure source has been reported in five percent of all patients with gastrointestinal hemorrhage. The cause of bleeding is not determined in almost half of these patients despite vigorous and laborious testing. Special procedures to localize the lesion may be necessary in patients who hemorrhage repeatedly. Bleeding is often occult; the only manifestations are iron deficiency anemia and positive chemical analysis for blood in stools (i.e., guaiac test or Hemoccult test). Studies of healthy persons who were 40 to 50 years of age revealed that 2.0 to 3.5 percent had positive Hemoccult tests when given a low-meat diet; about 30 percent of those with positive Hemoccult tests had neoplasms (20 percent had benign polyps), and eight to 10 percent had carcinomas.[68,69] Unfortunately, a reduction in mortality from colon cancer has not yet been established despite identification by occult blood-screening techniques of asymptomatic colonic neoplasms.[70] The Hemoccult test may be falsely negative under certain circumstances: if the specimen has dried before analysis, if the patient is taking oral ascorbic acid during the collection period, or if gastrointestinal transport is slow enough to permit hemoglobin degradation. The HemoQuant test (available from Smith Kline Bioscience Laboratories, King of Prussia, Pennsylvania), which is a more sensitive and quantitative method for detecting fecal blood, is now available.[71] Because samples must be sent to the manufacturer's laboratory, it is uncertain whether the HemoQuant test will be practical to use in screening for occult gastrointestinal bleeding.

Because of the possibility of an underlying serious disease such as colonic neoplasm, thorough diagnostic study is required in patients with unexplained bleeding [*see Figure 3*]. Patients should have a thorough colonoscopy followed by upper gastrointestinal endoscopy if no lesion is found. Identification of a lesion at any step of this procedure should be followed by appropriate medical or surgical therapy. Colonoscopy may disclose the probable source of bleeding in as many as 40 percent of such cases.[72] If the bleeding source is still not idenfified, several less invasive procedures should be considered. A small bowel enteroclysis study should be performed to

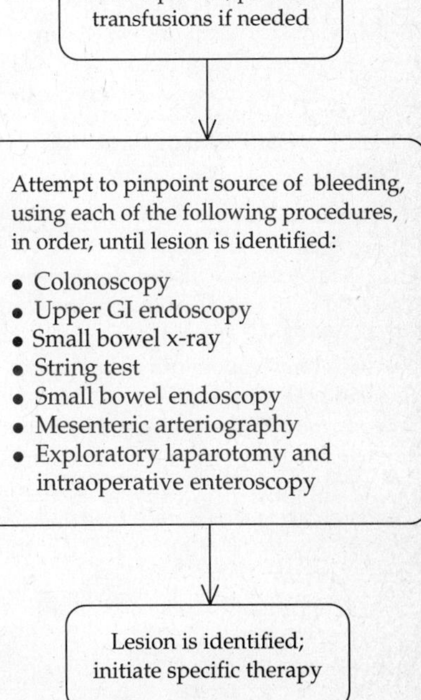

Figure 3 *This flowchart depicts the diagnosis of a patient with chronic occult gastrointestinal tract bleeding.*

rule out rare tumors in the small intestines. As previously mentioned, small bowel angiodysplasia is the most common lesion found in these patients, and small bowel endoscopy may be able to locate 33 percent of these lesions. Intestinal-colonic intubation with a small-diameter plastic tube may be useful when conventional evaluation is unrevealing or when it is important to document that a benign lesion (e.g., a diverticulum) is the true source of bleeding. Another useful diagnostic technique is a modified string test employing a gelatin capsule that has a string wound within its interior.[73] A short length of the string is pulled out and taped to the cheek, and then the patient swallows the capsule. It quickly passes through the esophagus and stomach and into the small intestine. The presence and location of blood stains are noted.

For those patients who require multiple transfusions and in whom the source of bleeding is not identified by less invasive procedures, mesenteric arteriography should be the next step. Exploratory laparotomy with intraoperative enteroscopy will be needed if arteriography is also unrevealing.

Prevention of Gastrointestinal Bleeding

Patients in intensive care units are at especially high risk for gastroduodenal bleeding caused by erosive disease that appears to be related to the stress of their acute illness. Administration of antacids via a nasogastric tube with hourly monitoring of gastric contents and maintenance of pH at 3.5 has been shown to reduce bleeding from 24 percent in the untreated control group to only four percent in those given antacid.[74] This therapy requires an appreciable effort by the medical personnel, and evidence is now emerging that other prophylactic treatments are also effective and can be administered more efficiently. Sucralfate, 1 g crushed and administered in saline via a nasogastric tube every six hours,[75] and cimetidine, 300 mg given intravenously in a priming dose followed by continuous infusion of 37.5 to 50.0 mg/hr, appear to be efficacious in preventing bleeding and gastroduodenal erosions.[76,77] Prostaglandin analogues such as enprostil appear to protect the gastric mucosa against aspirin-induced damage.[78,79] It is not yet known whether these analogues will decrease the incidence of gastrointestinal hemorrhage in chronic users of nonsteroidal anti-inflammatory agents.

When given in doses that reduce the heart rate by 25 percent, propranolol has been demonstrated to be effective in decreasing episodes of variceal bleeding in patients with cirrhosis who had previously experienced upper gastrointestinal bleeding.[80,81] However, subsequent studies produced conflicting results.[82,83] More information is needed on propranolol and other drugs that may prevent recurrent variceal bleeding in patients with cirrhosis before such agents can be recommended.

For cirrhotic patients with esophageal varices who have not bled in the past, prophylactic shunt surgery to prevent the first episode of variceal bleeding is contraindicated.[84] Despite encouraging results reported by German researchers,[85-87] prophylactic sclerotherapy was found to be detrimental in other studies.[89-91] Prophylactic sclerotherapy cannot be recommended at the present time. However, prophylactic therapy with propranolol appears to be promising for these patients.[92-94] Further studies are needed.

References

1. N Engl J Med 290:1158, 1974
2. Br Med J 2:7, 1970
3. Dig Dis Sci 26(suppl):65, 1981
4. Lancet 1:1064, 1986
5. Am J Gastroenterol 61:282, 1974
6. Am J Surg 140:284, 1980
7. N Engl J Med 304:925, 1981
8. Dig Dis Sci 26(suppl):47, 1981

9. Dig Dis Sci 26(suppl):55, 1981
10. N Engl J Med 313:660, 1985
11. Am J Med 76:361, 1984
12. Ann Surg 186:369, 1977
13. Gastroenterology 77:540, 1979
14. Ann Intern Med 96:565, 1982
15. Gastroenterology 97:568, 1989
16. Gastroenterology 88:1550, 1985
17. N Engl J Med 308:1571, 1983
18. Gastroenterology 90:595, 1986
19. N Engl J Med 305:915, 1981
20. Gut 22:228, 1981
21. Gastroenterology 90:595, 1986
22. Lancet 1:1113, 1986
23. Endoscopy 18(suppl 2):46, 1986
24. Gastroenterology 83:410, 1982
25. Br Med J 286:345, 1983
26. Scand J Gastroenterology 16:633, 1981
27. N Engl J Med 316:1618, 1987
28. Gastroenterology 90:1508, 1986
29. Ann Intern Med 110:510, 1989
30. Lancet 1:464, 1986
31. Gastrointest Endosc 33:199, 1987
32. Gastrointest Endosc 31:175, 1985
33. Gastroenterology 98:1239, 1990
34. Lancet 2:1292, 1987
35. Br Med J 296:1631, 1988
36. Lancet 1:1164, 1989
37. Gastroenterology 99:1303, 1990
38. Gastroenterology 100:33, 1991
39. Br J Surg 69:76, 1982
40. Hepatology 5:580, 1985
41. Surg Gynecol Obstet 167:331, 1988
42. Acta Chir Scand 151:449, 1985
43. Hepatology 9:274, 1989
44. JAMA 255:497, 1986
45. N Engl J Med 311:1594, 1984
46. N Engl J Med 316:11, 1987
47. Hepatology 5:584, 1985
48. Hepatology 5:827, 1985
49. Gastroenterology 96:1087, 1989
50. Am J Gastro 82:823, 1987
51. Ann Intern Med 100:608, 1984
52. Am J Gastro 80:595, 1985
53. Ann Surg 208:175, 1988
54. Gastrointest Endosc 32:202, 1986
55. Gastroenterology 85:693, 1983
56. Dig Dis Sci 30:29, 1985
57. Hepatology 4:950, 1984
58. N Engl J Med 259:201, 1958
59. Q J Med 39:539, 1970
60. Ann Surg 174:672, 1971
61. Ann Surg 174:76, 1971
62. Ann Surg 162:550, 1965
63. Br Med J 288:1663, 1984
64. JAMA 247:789, 1982
65. Gastroenterology 94:1117, 1988
66. Gastrointest Endosc 36:337, 1990
67. Gastroenterology 95:1569, 1988
68. Advances in Cancer Control: Epidemiology and Research. CA 32:100, 1982
69. Advances in Cancer Control: Epidemiology and Research. Alan R Liss, Inc, New York, 1984, p 283
70. Gastroenterology 88:820, 1985
71. N Engl J Med 312:1422, 1985
72. Lancet 1:1350, 1978
73. Gut 15:492, 1974
74. N Engl J Med 298:1041, 1978
75. Am J Surg 148:809, 1984
76. Ann Intern Med 103:173, 1985
77. Gastroenterology 89:532, 1985
78. Gastroenterology 88:382, 1985
79. Lancet 2:1277, 1988
80. N Engl J Med 305:1371, 1981
81. Hepatology 4:355, 1984
82. N Engl J Med 309:1539, 1983
83. Hepatology 6:1239, 1986
84. Medicine (Baltimore) 51:27, 1972
85. Endoscopy 14:4, 1982
86. Lancet 1:773, 1985
87. Hepatology 8:1495, 1988
88. Endoscopy 18:40, 1986
89. N Engl J Med 324:1779, 1991
90. N Engl J Med 318:814, 1988
91. N Engl J Med 319:8, 1988
92. N Engl J Med 317:856, 1987
93. Hepatology 8:1, 1988
94. Hepatology 8:1, 1988

Acknowledgments

Table 1   Adapted from "Upper Gastrointestinal Bleeding: Accuracy of Clinical Diagnosis and Prognosis," by P. B. Gregory, C. M. Knauer, M. R. Fogel, et al, in *Digestive Diseases and Sciences* 26(suppl):65, 1981. Used by permission of Plenum Publishing Corporation.

Figures 1 through 3   Janet Betries.

13 Enteral and Parenteral Nutrition In Hospital Patients

DOUGLAS W. WILMORE, M.D.
JOANNE H. VAN WOERT, M.D.

Between 30 and 50 percent of patients in major hospitals are significantly malnourished. Nutritional support services help identify these patients and utilize various techniques of nutritional supplementation for patients who have increased requirements for energy and protein. Decisions concerning the provision of specialized feedings may require as much deliberation, data review, and consultation as decisions concerning surgery, chemotherapy, or dialysis.

Identifying the Patient at Risk for Malnutrition

Assessment of a patient's nutritional status may be difficult because the majority of methods are indirect and the accuracy of traditional markers has been questioned. The initial clinical impression often provides the best assessment. After a thorough history has been taken, including a review of daily food intake and weight loss, and a careful physical examination has been performed, protein-calorie malnutrition may be diagnosed or specific micronutrient deficiencies identified.

Extent of Weight Loss

The most important information to be learned from the history is the rate and degree of weight loss. Short-term loss of more than 10 percent of usual body weight may compromise the patient because undernutrition alters normal gastrointestinal and cardiovascular functions, responses to infection, and wound healing. Weight loss of 35 to 50 percent is life threatening in the non-obese. Loss of body mass has been associated with operative mortality and morbidity. Rapid weight loss tends to be more detrimental than gradual weight loss.

Rapid loss indicates a high degree of metabolic stress, a markedly deficient intake of calories and probably of other essential nutrients, or a combination of these two conditions. Patients with 10 percent or greater loss of body weight should be considered for nutritional support. However, patients with normal body composition who do not have increased metabolic requirements will be able to tolerate five to seven days of inadequate feeding without nutritional intervention.

Traditional Markers of Malnutrition

Traditional markers of malnutrition, including immune function tests and measurement of serum protein levels, have not consistently identified patients at risk for undernutrition. Total peripheral lymphocyte count and skin-test response to common antigens reflect immune status in critically ill patients. These measurements have identified depressed immunity in malnourished individuals, and both may return to normal after nutritional repletion. These indices, however, are not specific for nutritional deficiencies and are directly affected by a variety of disease processes, including cancer, and by treatments such as steroid or radiation therapy. The difficulty in relying on delayed-type hypersensitivity skin tests as an indicator of nutritional repletion is that a state of immune anergy may resolve as the disease process abates even though nutritional support remains inadequate.[1] Therefore, although malnutrition can be correlated with infection, the use of nonspecific immunologic markers in hospitalized patients does not identify specific nutritional deficiencies. These tests may, however, correlate in a general manner with the patient's prognosis; for example, a skin-test–negative individual who converts to skin-test–positive with nutritional support has a high probability of surviving an infectious disease process.

The serum albumin concentration is a useful indicator of the level of hepatic protein synthesis and is a marker for protein-calorie malnutrition. A low serum albumin level correlates with an increased length of hospital stay and an adverse prognosis.[2,3] This measurement, however, does not provide a completely reliable guide to nutritional status, because it is also influenced by changes in the size of the albumin compartment. Such compartmental changes have been observed in patients who have undergone surgery and in those with cancer, renal insufficiency, or third-space (i.e., extracellular space) fluid sequestration. In septic patients, both serum albumin and transferrin levels tend to be decreased because of a redistribution of serum proteins, regardless of whether the patient is malnourished.[1] It has also been shown that serum albumin and transferrin levels have paradoxically fallen in patients receiving intravenous nutrition who appeared to be improving clinically.[4] Serum transferrin has a shorter half-life than albumin, and it may be a sensitive indicator of hepatic protein synthesis and nutritional status. However, serum transferrin levels may be altered by disease processes because transferrin is an acute-phase reactant.

In a patient who is receiving a creatinine-free diet and who has normal renal function, a 24-hour urinary creatinine determination correlates well with muscle mass. Creatinine phosphate, which is located in skeletal muscle, is the primary source of creatinine. Calculation of the creatinine height index (CHI) will yield a number that corrects for the height of the patient and that can be compared with normal control values.[5] It is more accurate to express creatinine excretion in terms of height than in terms of weight because variations in body weight can occur with changes in hydration.

Various methods of analyzing body composition have been suggested as ways of measuring nutritional status. The objectives are to define lean body mass and to detect changes occurring with illness or therapy. If exact quantities of body fat and protein can be determined, the values can be compared with standardized population norms. However, most methods of determining body composition do not directly measure these body compartments, and they are predicated on physiologic assumptions that may be inappropriate in the diseased state. Thus, traditional techniques for measuring body composition may predict lean body mass in healthy adults, but the measurements obtained in malnourished patients are less reliable predictors.

Anthropometric measurements, such as triceps skin-fold thickness and midarm circumference, correlate roughly with body composition. Variations in compressibility of the specific tissue, edema, and differences between investigators make the interpretation of these measurements difficult.[6,7] Low sensitivity and lack of specificity suggest that anthropometric parameters are of minimal value both in assessing nutritional status and in monitoring changes in status in response to feeding.[8]

Body compositional analyses, such as isotopic dilution methods, hydrostatic weighing, and electrical impedance techniques, have attempted to quantify total body fat on the basis of the measurement of total body water, which assumes that the hydration coefficient of lean tissue (ml H_2O/100 g tissue) is constant. However, this coefficient has been shown to vary from 0.67 in healthy adults to as high as 0.85 in patients with advanced anasarca.[9]

Total body potassium can be estimated by whole body counting. Because body potassium is proportional to body protein, measurement of total body potassium gives an estimate of lean body mass.[10] However, to determine the lean body mass from the total body potassium, it must be assumed that the potassium concentration in the intracellular water is constant and that the ratio of total body potassium to lean body mass decreases linearly over time in both males and females. Because neither of these assumptions is strictly correct, the total body potassium does not provide an accurate assessment of lean body mass unless correction is made for sex and age.[10]

The most direct method for assessing lean body mass is to measure total body nitrogen using neutron activation analysis. A beam of fast neutrons is generated and captured by target atoms, leading to the creation of unstable isotopes. Energy is measured as the isotopes emit gamma rays and decay to a stable form. Spectrographic analysis identifies the element on the basis of the spectral energy, and the energy intensity corresponds to the element's abundance.[11] Neutron activation analysis of samples has been used to assess changes in total body nitrogen in patients undergoing aortic repair, in those with gastrointestinal disease receiving parenteral nutrition, and in patients in septic shock.[12-14] The use of neutron activation is limited by its cost and requirement for skilled technologists.

Determining Nutritional Requirements

Nutritional therapy should be goal directed. Depending on the patient's status, the goal may be to diminish the rate of weight loss and body protein breakdown, to maintain body weight and protein stores, or to increase body weight and protein mass.

These general goals must be integrated into overall patient care. Practical considerations such as fluid restriction, intravenous access, presence of bloodstream infection, concomitant use of catabolic drugs, disuse of the skeletal muscle mass, and the patient's previous nutritional status may impede efforts to deliver an ideal level of nutritional support or to achieve a specific clinical goal.

Total energy requirements are governed by several factors, including basal metabolic rate (BMR), measured in kilocalories (kcal)/day; the specific dynamic action of ingested food; and energy expenditure during activity. In hospitalized patients, the BMR is the greatest contributor to energy expenditure.[15] Although BMR is mainly determined by age, sex, temperature, and body

mass, disease processes may have a significant influence.

Patients generally fall into one of three metabolic categories: healthy persons with normal metabolic rates, depleted individuals who are hypometabolic, and stressed individuals who are hypermetabolic. Patients with a normal BMR usually are those undergoing diagnostic evaluation or an elective procedure who have no associated stress (i.e., infection, fever, or therapeutic complications).

Depleted patients without superimposed stress have a reduced body mass and have adapted metabolically to starvation. These persons have usually been undernourished because of (1) psychological or organic central nervous system dysfunction, leading to reduced food intake, (2) benign or malignant obstructive lesions of the esophagus or stomach that prevent enteral feedings, or (3) severe malabsorption. Even when the metabolic rate is estimated on the basis of present weight, it is usually below predicted normal levels for these patients.

Hypermetabolism causes an increase in the BMR ranging from five to 100 percent above predicted normal values. Such elevations are associated with infection, severe injury, major burns, and cancer. The BMR increases by about 15 percent in cancer patients, but this elevation varies greatly and is probably influenced by tumor burden and the proliferative state of the cancer. Hypermetabolic states may also be associated with tissue destruction caused by marked hemolysis, exfoliative dermatitis, or irradiation; chronic obstructive lung disease, which causes increased work of breathing; or cardiac failure, which causes increased cardiopulmonary work. Nutritional support should be considered for patients with increased metabolic requirements, especially when the weight loss approaches 10 percent of the body weight before illness. Anabolism is difficult, if not impossible, to achieve in the presence of the accelerated catabolic drives and complex clinical circumstances that arise in patients with acute renal, cardiac, or respiratory failure, possibly complicated by sepsis. Protein synthesis and tissue anabolism occur after resolution of the disease process. Provision of nutritional maintenance requirements should be the major goal in most of these complex clinical situations. Finally, patients with severe nutritional depletion who lack major catabolic drives should be repleted if nutritional rehabilitation is consistent with overall clinical goals.

Energy requirements should be assessed on the basis of a patient's predicted BMR. The degree of stress imposed by a disease process is then estimated and added to this basal value. If anabolism is the desired goal, then 1,000 kcal/day should be added to the maintenance diet, leading to a weight gain of approximately 1 kg/wk [*see Table 1*].

Once the energy requirements of a patient have been determined, protein needs can be estimated. The major factors that influence nitrogen retention include total energy intake, nitrogen intake, and the metabolic state of the patient. The relation between energy and nitrogen requirements varies in the three categories of patients: those with a normal metabolism, depleted patients, or hypermetabolic individuals. Normal or depleted individuals have extremely efficient protein-conserving mechanisms and can achieve a positive nitrogen balance when as little as seven to eight percent of the total energy requirements is administered in the form of protein. Such individuals can therefore conserve protein efficiently at a calorie-nitrogen ratio of approximately 300:1 to 350:1. Hypermetabolic patients are markedly inefficient at utilizing nitrogen and hence require more dietary protein. In critically ill patients who have normal renal function, the protein intake should constitute about 15 to 20 percent of total caloric requirements; such a diet would provide a calorie-nitrogen ratio for optimal protein efficiency of approximately 150:1.

Once the patient's total caloric demands have been predicted, the amount of protein needed to achieve nitrogen equilibrium can be determined as a percentage of the total energy required [*see Table 1*]. Providing more protein usually allows a more positive nitrogen balance, but this increased nitrogen load may also be associated with a rise in blood urea nitrogen (BUN) and increased urinary excretion of urea nitrogen.

Minerals, Trace Elements, and Vitamins

The major minerals—sodium, potassium, calcium, phosphorus, magnesium, iron, and their various salts—constitute most of the inorganic material in the body and account for three to four percent of body weight. Physiologic trace elements, such as zinc, copper, manganese, and chromium, constitute less than 0.01 percent of body mass but play an important role because they are essential cofactors in biochemical reactions.

Iron

Dietary sources of iron include myoglobin in meat and inorganic iron in plants. Iron (mainly Fe^{3+}) absorption is stimulated by gastric acidity and is further promoted by weak organic acids, such as ascorbic acid. Other sources of iron include nuts, fortified cereals, and egg yolks. In patients in whom iron deficiency develops, oral administration of ferrous sulfate, 300 mg once daily, should be initiated and increased to three times a day if tolerated.

For those who are unable to tolerate oral supplementation, the parenteral route should be considered. Intramuscular iron should be avoided because of soft tissue discomfort and ecchymoses. Intravenous iron (iron dextran) should be used with caution. A test dose of 0.5 ml must precede the supplementation dose because systemic reactions such as fever, flushing, and anaphylaxis have occurred with the use of parenteral iron. Parenteral iron cannot be triple mixed (i.e., mixed with fat, carbohydrate, and protein).

Septic patients should not receive supplemental iron. Bacterial virulence has been enhanced by parenteral injection of iron into septic experimental hosts. This phenomenon has been reported for a variety of bacteria, including *Escherichia coli, Neisseria meningitidis, N. gonorrhoeae,* and *Klebsiella pneumoniae.*[16-19] Pathogens sequester iron either by producing chelating agents or by metabolizing heme-containing compounds.

Table 1 Estimation of Energy and Protein Requirements

FORMULAS FOR DETERMINATIONS

Daily energy requirement for weight maintenance = normal BMR[a] × stress factor[b] × 1.25[c]

Daily energy requirement for weight gain = maintenance energy +1,000 kcal[d]

Daily protein requirement for patients in intensive care (g/day) = (daily energy requirement ÷ 150) × 6.25

Daily protein requirement for minimally depleted patients or those with simple resting starvation (g/day) = (daily energy requirement ÷ 300) × 6.25

TERMS IN PRECEDING FORMULAS

a. Normal BMR (usually 1,500–1,800 kcal/day) can be determined utilizing standard nomograms or formulas. The approximate values of the basal metabolic rate for adults of average size are given below.

Body Weight (kg)	50	55	60	65	70	75	80
Normal BMR kcal/day)	1,316	1,411	1,509	1,602	1,694	1,784	1,872

b. Stress factor is the term used to correct the normal BMR for the effects of a disease process.

Condition	*Stress Factor*
Mild starvation	0.85–1.00
Postoperative recovery (no complications)	1.00–1.05
Cancer[*]	1.10–1.45
Peritonitis[*]	1.05–1.25
Severe infection or multiple trauma[*]	1.30–1.55

[*]Proportional to the extent of the disease.

c. The basal caloric requirements of the stressed patient are adjusted upward an additional 20%–25% for hospital activity and the stress associated with treatment. This adjustment is unnecessary for patients on ventilators who are paralyzed or heavily sedated.

d. If anabolism and weight gain are the goals, an additional 1,000 kcal/day may be added to maintenance requirements to provide for a weight gain of approximately 1 kg (2 lb)/wk. Weight maintenance, not weight gain, should be the primary objective in most critically ill patients.

Physiologic Trace Elements

Serum measurements do not accurately reflect tissue stores of many of the physiologic trace elements. Compartmental shifts occurring secondary to sepsis may lead to increased serum copper and decreased serum zinc concentrations. In addition, the reduced levels of circulating trace element binding proteins encountered in some disease states may change serum concentrations of these ions to a degree suggestive of deficiency. For example, albumin is the major zinc-binding protein; a low serum zinc level (normal range, 7.6 to 23 μmol/L) may be measured if the serum albumin level (normal range, 35 to 55 g/L) has decreased.[20] In addition, elevation of the ceruloplasmin level occurs after estrogen therapy and leads to elevation of the serum copper concentration (normal range, 16 to 31 μmol/L).[21]

In contrast, plasma selenium levels have been shown to be accurate indices of selenium stores.[22] Fluxes in plasma selenium appear to occur more rapidly with altered selenium intake when compared with changes in whole blood or erythrocyte levels. Therefore, plasma selenium levels may be useful for monitoring short-term changes in selenium stores in patients receiving total parenteral nutrition.[22] In a patient in whom the selenium status is still unclear after the plasma selenium levels have been determined, the selenium-dependent glutathione peroxidase activity can be measured.[23]

Adequate amounts of minerals and trace elements are usually provided in most oral diets or prepared feeding formulas. In addition to supplements that provide major minerals, a parenteral mix of trace elements (commonly containing zinc, copper, manganese, and chromium) is also available for addition to intravenous fluids. Most trace element deficiencies occur during long-term total intravenous feeding. Administration of minerals and trace elements is essential for repletion of body tissues during long-term parenteral maintenance [*see Table 2*].[24]

Copper The body of a healthy adult contains 100 to 150 mg of copper. The richest dietary sources are crustaceans, shellfish, and organ meat. Most of the tissue copper is located in the liver, where it is associated with copper-binding proteins and metalloenzymes.[25] More than 90 percent of the copper circulating in the plasma is bound to ceruloplasmin. Copper plays an integral role in the function of metalloenzymes and metallothioneins.[25] Deficiency of copper can occur with prolonged diarrhea or fluid losses from stomach fistulas. Deficiency clinically manifests itself as an anemia accompanied by leukopenia and neutropenia. Because the major route of copper elimination is the bile, patients with cholestasis and impaired biliary excretion of the metal should have their copper intake reduced by 0.15 mg/day; the total parenteral nutrition solution should be copper free.[20]

Table 2 Trace Element Requirements

Trace Element	Suggested Daily I.V. Intake
Zinc	2.5 – 4.0 mg
Selenium	40 – 80 µg
Chromium	10 – 20 µg
Copper	300 – 500 µg
Manganese	150 – 800 µg

Chromium Spices, brewer's yeast, meat, dairy products, and eggs are good sources of chromium. There is a paucity of reported cases of chromium deficiency. Patients receiving home parenteral nutrition appear to be the population at risk if their oral intake is poor.[25] Chromium requirements may be increased by the administration of high concentrations of dextrose, which enhances urinary excretion of chromium.[26]

Manganese Manganese is present in nuts, dried fruit, cereals, tea, noodles, and prunes[27]; Mn^{2+} is a necessary cofactor for certain biosynthetic enzymes (glycosyltransferases) and enzymes functional in cellular energetics (mitochondrial superoxide dismutases); it is also necessary for the action of vitamin K in blood-clotting mechanisms.[28,29] Because manganese is excreted by the biliary tract, it should be eliminated from parenteral nutrition regimens if cholestasis or biliary obstruction occurs.

Selenium Sources of selenium include grains, seafood, and muscle meats. Plant content of selenium varies with the soil content. Selenium serves as an antioxidant because it is an integral component of glutathione peroxidase, which catalyzes the degradation of peroxides. Selenium deficiency is a feature of Keshan disease, which has been described in Chinese children in whom cardiomyopathy developed.[30] Selenium deficiency has also been reported in an American patient with an enterocutaneous fistula complicating multiple gastrointestinal operations for small bowel diverticulosis. Cardiomyopathy developed in the patient after two years of total parenteral nutrition.[31] An inverse correlation has been noted between plasma selenium levels and duration of total parenteral nutrition. It appears that 40 µg of selenium added daily to the parenteral solution is adequate to prevent selenium deficiency in patients receiving home parenteral nutrition.

Zinc Abundant sources of zinc include muscle meats and seafood. Zinc is an integral component of more than 100 enzymes, including DNA polymerase and RNA polymerase.[20,32] Adequate zinc has been shown to be important for growth. Measurement of zinc losses that occur with increased stool, urine, and fistula volume is essential to predict needs.[33] Zinc deficiency may be prevalent among patients with large-volume stool or fistula output.[33-35] Urinary zinc losses are increased during catabolic states.[33] Clinical manifestations of zinc deficiency include an eczematoid, erythematous rash, which commonly involves the nasolabial folds, perineum, and extensor surfaces.

Vitamins

Patients usually receive more than an adequate quantity of vitamins, which serve as cofactors in biochemical reactions. Vitamins are classified as either fat soluble or water soluble. Fat-soluble vitamins (vitamins A, D, E, and K) are stored in the body in limited amounts. In contrast, water-soluble vitamins (vitamin B complex and vitamin C) are not stored in appreciable reserve quantities and must therefore be given to prevent depletion. Any excesses are usually excreted in the urine. Vitamin requirements are usually satisfied by a balanced diet. Oral supplements may be given when necessary. Parenteral mixtures containing both fat- and water-soluble vitamins are available for intravenous supplementation. However, vitamin K is not included in most adult formulations

so as to avoid complications in patients receiving warfarin. For patients who are not receiving anticoagulants, parenteral vitamin K_1 should be given in a dosage of 2 to 4 mg/wk.[36]

Delivery Techniques and Available Diets

Although the regular house diet in most hospitals provides adequate calories and protein, a critically ill patient is frequently unable or unwilling to consume such a diet. Likewise, the usual clear- or full-liquid diets often ordered for patients in preparation for various tests or procedures have inadequate caloric and protein contents. Additional calories (750 to 1,500 kcal/day) may be provided by nutritional supplements given between meals. In addition, juices or other calorie-containing fluids should be used to administer medication when liquids are employed for this purpose. The nursing staff should be instructed as to the caloric goal of an individual patient. The dietitian should follow the progress of the patient by taking daily calorie counts and should supplement intake from the food tray if necessary to achieve the desired goal.

Enteral Tube Feedings

Patients with a functional gastrointestinal tract who are unable to sustain maintenance nutrition because of anorexia, nausea, or oropharyngeal obstruction are best nourished by enteral tube feedings. Available nasogastric feeding tubes are small (No. 8 to No. 10) and soft and may be mercury-weighted at the tip to facilitate passage. A stylet may be inserted to add to the rigidity of the tube if required for placement in the stomach. Because of their small size and soft composition, the tubes are well tolerated; many patients learn to pass the tubes themselves and manage tube feedings successfully on an outpatient basis.

If a permanent feeding tube is required, it is preferable to perform a gastrostomy; the stomach can then serve as a reservoir, allowing delivery of large quantities of nourishment. A feeding gastrostomy is most often used in patients with head and neck cancer who have severe oropharyngeal obstruction, in those who have had strokes, or in patients with long-standing dysphagia. A feeding gastrostomy can be placed with the aid of local or regional anesthesia. However, percutaneous endoscopic gastrostomy is preferred to operative gastrostomy because the former can be performed with a minimal degree of sedation.

A nasojejunal feeding tube is indicated in the presence of gastroesophageal reflux, severe gastritis, or extensive gastric resection—that is, in conditions that eliminate the stomach as a reservoir. Because these tubes are more difficult to position, placement is aided by fluoroscopic visualization and directed by a guide wire. A feeding jejunostomy can also be done with the patient under local anesthesia or during an operative procedure such as a gastrectomy or a pancreatectomy.

A wide variety of tube-feeding formulas, either complete diets or supplements, are available [*see Table 3*]. The majority of these are lactose free. Formulas have also been designed for patients with dietary restrictions associated with renal or hepatic failure. Carbohydrate, fat, and protein are present in these formulas as intact nutrients, in partially digested (hydrolyzed) forms, or as elemental compounds. Formulas containing predigested components tend to have a higher osmolality and should be avoided in patients with a propensity toward diarrhea. Intact proteins may be isolated from their original source (e.g., casein from milk) and partially digested by treating the protein source with enzymes or acid. Supplemental amino acids are added to provide a full nutritional complement of all essential amino acids. Some formulas are composed entirely of elemental amino acids, but they are quite expensive. Dipeptides and tripeptides may be absorbed more efficiently than the elemental amino acids by patients who have diseased small bowels.

Carbohydrate, the major energy source in all enteral formulas, may be present as naturally occurring nutrients, such as starches or polysaccharides, or as a simple sugar, such as glucose. The carbohydrate content will determine the taste (sweetness) and osmotic load (complex sugars produce a lower osmotic load than simple sugars). Fat may be provided in the form of food fats (butterfat) or oils (vegetable, soy, corn, or safflower). Digestion and absorption of all fats proceed via a series of complex steps, and hence, low-fat formulas should be selected for patients with complex gastrointestinal diseases. Medium-chain triglycerides (MCT) in the form of MCT oil, a distillate of coconut oil, are absorbed directly into the portal circulation and do not require the action of bile salts and pancreatic lipase for digestion. MCT oil is therefore an ideal caloric source for patients with fat malabsorption, but it should be given cautiously, as excess administration will cause crampy abdominal pain, diarrhea, or both. Moreover, MCT oil does not provide essential fatty acids. Commercially available complete nutritional formulas contain vitamins and minerals, and when they are fed in volumes sufficient to deliver adequate calories, they meet or exceed the recommended requirements for normal individuals. Not all tube-feeding products are complete diets: some are supplements, and others provide a single nutrient or are designed for use in a single disease. Therefore, some formulas will not provide all nutritional requirements if given alone.

Tube-feeding solutions are started as dilute formulas (one-half to three-quarter strength) and administered slowly so as to assess patient tolerance. Gastric feedings can be given continuously or by intermittent bolus. Ultimately, patients are able to tolerate 200 to 400 ml of feeding solution every two hours. Patients receiving gastrostomy feedings should remain elevated at a 30° angle for one hour after each feeding to avoid aspiration. The residual gastric volume is determined immediately before feeding, and if aspirates exceed 100 ml, feedings are withheld or reduced. In contrast to gastrostomy feedings, jejunal feedings are always given continuously and are usually limited to 100 to 125 ml/hr. This procedure allows gradual absorption of nutrients and

Table 3 Some Available Nutritional Supplements and Defined Diets

Type of Diet and Major Ingredients	Brand Name	Caloric Density (kcal/ml)	Carbo-hydrate (g/L)	Fat (g/L)	Protein (g/L)	Osmolality (mOsm/ kg H₂O)	Sodium (mEq/L)	Potassium (mEq/L)
Intact Nutrient Formula — Calcium and sodium caseinates, soy protein isolates, soy or corn oil, corn syrup solids, sucrose	Enrich	1.10	159.0	37.0	39.0	480	37.0	40.0
	Ensure	1.06	145.0	37.2	37.2	450	32.2	32.5
	Ensure HN	1.06	128.0	32.0	40.0	470	40.0	40.0
	Ensure Plus	1.50	200.0	53.3	55.0	600	46.1	48.6
	Ensure Plus HN	1.50	182.0	45.0	57.0	650	51.0	47.0
	Entrition	1.00	135.0	35.0	35.0	300	30.5	30.7
	Impact	1.00	132.0	28.0	56.0	375	43.0	39.0
	Isocal*	1.06	130.0	44.0	34.2	300	23.1	33.8
	Isocal HCN†	2.00	225.0	91.0	75.0	690	35.0	36.0
	Isotein HN	1.20	156.0	34.0	68.0	300	27.0	27.4
	Magnacal	2.00	250.0	80.0	70.0	590	43.5	32.0
	Newtrition	1.06	160.0	40.0	60.0	300	30.0	30.0
	Osmolite†	1.06	145.0	38.5	37.2	300	23.5	27.1
	Osmolite HN†	1.06	141.0	37.0	44.0	310	40.0	40.0
	Pulmocare	1.50	105.0	92.0	62.4	490	56.9	48.7
	Resource Instant	1.06	145.0	37.2	37.2	450	36.8	40.0
	Sustacal HC	1.50	190.0	58.0	61.0	650	36.0	38.0
	Sustacal Liquid	1.01	136.0	24.8	61.2	625	40.5	65.6
	Traumacal†	1.50	142.0	68.0	82.0	550	52.0	36.0
	Travasorb	1.05	144.0	37.0	37.0	450	32.0	32.5
	TwoCal HN	2.00	217.0	90.0	83.5	700	46.0	59.0

*Contains glucose oligosaccharides. †Contains MCT oil. ‡Contains lactose.

Table 3   (continued)

	Type of Diet and Major Ingredients	Brand Name	Caloric Density (kcal/ml)	Carbo-hydrate (g/L)	Fat (g/L)	Protein (g/L)	Osmolality (mOsm/ kg H$_2$O)	Sodium (mEq/L)	Potassium (mEq/L)
Intact Nutrient Formula (continued)	Egg white solids, soy oil, maltodextrin, sucrose	Citrotein	0.70	121.0	1.7	40.0	495	30.0	17.0
		Isotein HN	1.20	156.0	34.0	68.0	300	29.0	22.0
		Precision HN†	1.05	216.0	1.3	43.9	557	42.7	23.3
		Precison Isotonic†	0.96	144.0	30.1	28.8	300	33.4	24.6
		Precision LR†	1.11	248.0	1.6	26.3	525	30.5	22.4
	Milk derivatives	Meritene Liquid‡	1.00	115.0	33.3	60.0	560	39.9	42.6
		Meritene Powder‡	1.07	119.0	34.6	69.2	690	41.8	75.8
		Sustacal Powder‡	1.01	136.0	24.8	61.2	625	40.5	65.6
	Medium-chain triglycerides (MCT), lactalbumin, caseinate, corn syrup solids	Portagen	1.00	114.8	47.8	35.0	136	20.4	32.0
		Travasorb MCT	1.00	123.0	33.0	49.2	250	15.2	44.5
Blenderized- Food Diet	Meat, vegetable, and fruit purees; corn oil; sucrose	Compleat-B‡	1.07	128.0	42.7	42.7	405	55.1	35.8
		Compleat- Modified Formula	1.07	141.0	37.0	43.0	300	29.1	35.8
		Vitaneed	1.00	125.0	40.0	35.0	375	21.7	32.0

*Contains glucose oligosaccharides.   †Contains MCT oil.   ‡Contains lactose.

Table 3   (continued)

Type of Diet and Major Ingredients		Brand Name	Caloric Density (kcal/ml)	Carbo-hydrate (g/L)	Fat (g/L)	Protein (g/L)	Osmolality (mOsm/ kg H$_2$O)	Potassium (mEq/L)	Sodium (mEq/L)	Fiber 9/1,000 cal
Fiber Formula	Soy, polysaccharide	Enrich	1.10	143.3	33.9	36.2	480	39.4	33.5	13.0
		Jevity	1.06	143.6	34.8	42.0	310	37.7	38.1	13.6
		Newpack Isofiber	1.20	133.3	30.8	41.7	310	32.0	36.0	11.6
		Profiber	1.00	132.0	40.0	40.0	300	32.0	32.0	12.0
		Sustacal with Fiber	1.06	133.0	33.2	43.0	450	33.8	29.5	6.0
Hydrolized Diet	Partially hydrolyzed proteins, MCT oil, corn syrup solids, sucrose	Criticare HN	1.06	202.0	3.1	35.0	650	31.0	25.0	
		Peptamen	1.00	127.0	39.0	40.0	260	16.0	22.0	
		Pepti-2000	1.00	189.0	10.0	40.0	490	29.0	30.0	
		Reabilan	1.00	131.5	39.0	31.5	350	32.0	30.4	
		Travasorb STD*	1.00	190.0	14.0	30.0	450	30.0	40.0	
		Travasorb HN*	1.00	175.0	13.4	45.0	450	29.9	40.0	
		Vital HN	1.00	188.0	10.8	41.7	460	29.8	16.7	
Purified Diet	Crystalline amino acids, glucose, oligosaccharides, safflower oil	Stresstein	1.20	173.0	27.0	69.0	910	29.0	29.0	
		Tolerex	1.00	226.0	1.5	20.6	550	30.0	20.4	
		TraumAid HBC	1.00	166.0	7.4	56.0	760	30.0	23.0	
		Vivonex TEN	1.00	206.0	2.8	38.0	630	20.0	20.0	

*Contains glucose oligosaccharides.   †Contains MCT oil.   ‡Contains lactose.

avoids depositing a bolus of hypertonic solution in the small intestine, which might cause cramping, diarrhea, and subsequent dehydration. Diarrhea is the most common complication of tube feeding in hospitalized patients. It occurs in approximately 60 percent of critically ill patients receiving tube feeding [*see Figure 1*].[37]

Peripheral Vein Infusions

If a patient cannot tolerate enteral nutrition, intravenous nutrition should be considered. Solutions of dextrose, amino acids, and fat emulsions can be infused safely through peripheral veins, but the requirement for isotonicity limits the quantity of calories that can be delivered by this route. The relatively low calorie intake provided by peripheral vein feedings, 1,200 to 2,300 kcal/day in 2,500 to 3,000 ml of fluid volume, limits their use to the following:

1. Weight maintenance in patients who are not hypermetabolic—that is, whose basal expenditure does not exceed 1,800 to 2,000 kcal/day.
2. A preliminary feeding before catheter insertion in patients requiring central venous feedings.
3. A supplement when enteral feedings are limited by gastrointestinal dysfunction.

The 2.5 to 3.0 L of fluid required to administer sufficient calories by peripheral vein feeding often limits use of this technique in patients with renal or congestive heart failure.

A peripheral vein solution that provides 286 kcal and 4.63 g of nitrogen (N) per liter can be prepared by mixing 500 ml of 10 percent dextrose with 500 ml of a 5.5 percent amino acid solution. Additional nonprotein calories are provided by fat emulsions. The dextrose–amino acid solution should be infused through a large-bore peripheral vein, and the infusion catheter should be changed every 48 hours to avoid thrombophlebitis.

Fat emulsions should be infused simultaneously with the dextrose and amino acid solution in a piggyback manner. Blood sampling should be avoided during this process because the associated hyperlipidemia will interfere with many serum measurements. Some antibiotics, other chemotherapeutic agents, blood, and blood products may be administered via the catheter utilized for peripheral vein feedings. Before and after infusion of other parenteral solutions, the dextrose and amino acid solution and the fat emulsion should be temporarily discontinued and the line flushed with normal saline.

Patients receiving peripheral vein feedings should be weighed daily and accurate intake and output records maintained. Initially, serum electrolytes, BUN, and glucose should be monitored three times each week, and liver function tests and calcium, phosphorus, magnesium, and triglyceride levels should be determined weekly if the patient is clinically stable. Mechanical and septic complications are uncommon. The risk of thrombophlebitis and phlebothrombosis can be minimized by using a large peripheral vein, by changing the catheter site every two days, and by adhering to strict aseptic technique during catheter insertion.

Fluid imbalances and electrolyte disturbances are similar to those seen in patients receiving standard intravenous solutions and can be corrected by altering the quantity of infusate or by adding or deleting appropriate electrolytes.

Hyperglycemia and glucosuria are rarely observed unless the patient is diabetic. Occasionally, the BUN is mildly elevated in patients receiving peripheral vein feedings. In the absence of renal failure, this finding usually indicates dehydration. BUN may also be increased when large quantities of amino acids are given without concomitant administration of appropriate nonprotein calories. The BUN elevation is corrected by increasing the volume of additional protein-free I.V. fluid or the amount of nonprotein calories.

Fat Emulsions

Fat provides more energy per unit weight (9 kcal/g) than does either carbohydrate (3.4 kcal/g) or protein (4 kcal/g). Fat is given in the form of an emulsion in which chylomi-

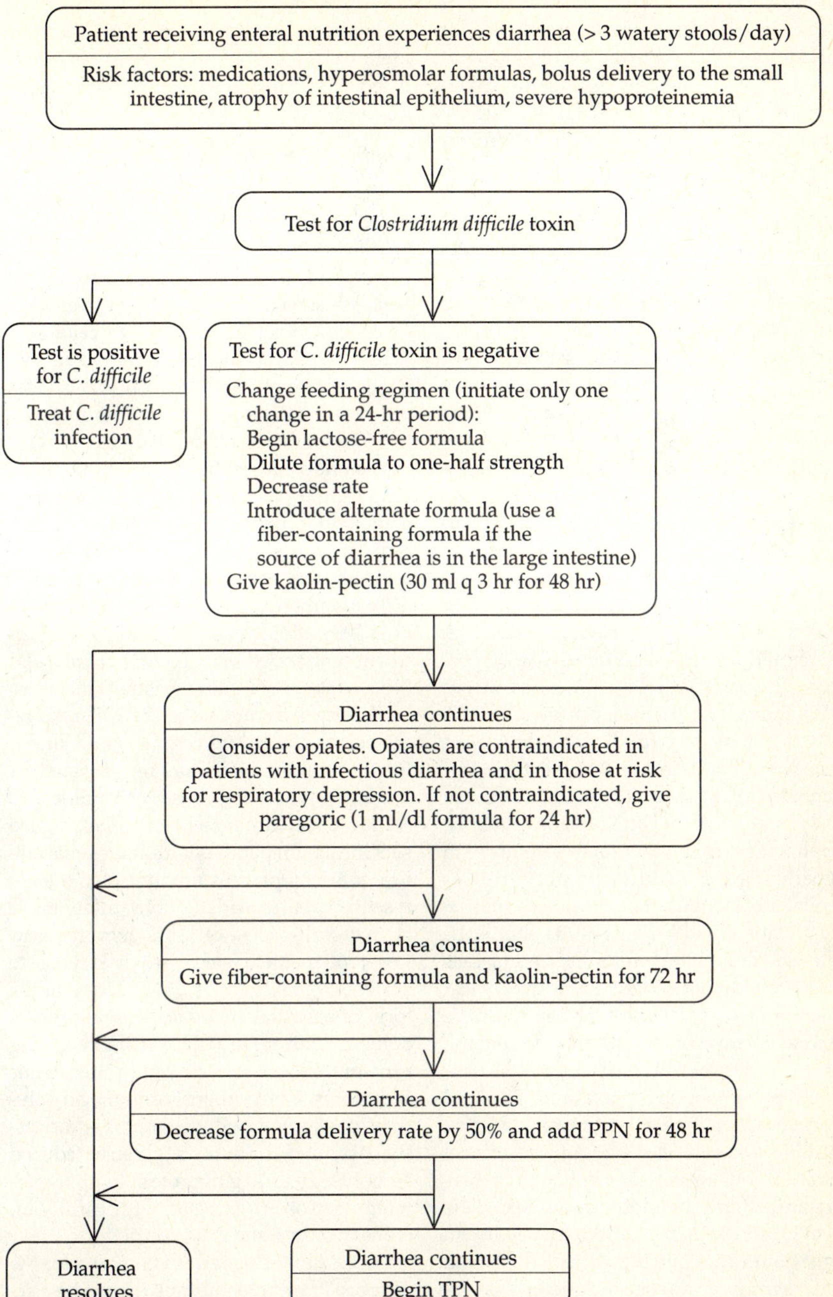

Figure 1 *Flowchart outlines an approach to the management of diarrhea in tube-fed patients.*

cron-size particles are dispersed; the fat particles are cleared from the bloodstream in a manner similar to that of the chylomicrons. Fat emulsions provide essential fatty acids and may also serve as a nonprotein caloric source. When fat emulsion is used as a major source of calories during parenteral nutrition, positive nitrogen balance and weight gain may be achieved in both adults and children.

The body can synthesize most long-chain fatty acids, but two essential polyunsaturated fatty acids cannot be synthesized—linoleic and linolenic acid. Fatty acid deficiency can be prevented by supplying at least four to 10 percent of daily caloric requirements as essential fatty acids.[38] This goal may be accomplished in patients receiving intravenous nutrition by giving two to three 500 ml bottles of 10 percent fat emulsion each week.

A 10 percent fat emulsion provides 1.1 kcal/ml (one 500 ml bottle yields 550 kcal); a 20 percent emulsion provides 2 kcal/ml. Fat should constitute no more than 60 percent of the nonprotein calories; adult patients should not receive more than 2.0 to 2.5 g fat/kg body weight/day. Fat emulsions have a high caloric density, but their low osmolarity (280 mOsm/L) permits delivery by peripheral vein. Fat emulsions must be given with extreme caution to patients with hyperlipidemia, adult respiratory distress syndrome, hepatic failure, or coagulopathies. Patients with pancreatitis should be able to tolerate intravenous lipid emulsions unless the baseline triglyceride level is elevated or increases while fat is being administered. Because of their phosphate content, fat emulsions should also be used with caution in patients with renal failure. To avoid most complications of fat emulsion administration, a baseline fasting triglyceride level should be obtained before initiation of therapy and should be monitored weekly; the weekly serum sample should be drawn eight hours after infusion. Because elevated plasma triglyceride concentrations often develop in patients with gram-negative infection and hepatic dysfunction, more frequent monitoring is essential whenever such patients receive fat emulsions. If the triglyceride level is elevated, the quantity of fat infused should be reduced or the fat emulsion discontinued.

Central Vein Infusions

Hypertonic solutions containing concentrated glucose as the major caloric source may be infused through a catheter in the superior vena cava. This technique is indicated for patients who require long-term (more than seven days) intravenous support with calorically dense solutions (1 kcal/ml). Central vein infusion provides 2,000 to 3,000 kcal and all other essential nutrients to patients needing 2 to 3 L of intravenous fluid daily.

Central vein solutions are formulated in the hospital pharmacy. These solutions are commonly combinations of 500 ml of 50 percent dextrose with 500 ml of 8.5 percent amino acid solution. The final preparation contains 250 g of carbohydrate and 7.15 g of N, providing 1,000 kcal/L. Minerals, vitamins, and electrolytes are added as required [*see Table 4*].

Because of volume restrictions that must be observed in patients with renal, respiratory, or cardiac failure, central vein solutions for these individuals may be prepared by mixing 70 percent dextrose with amino acid solutions. One amino acid formula designed specifically for patients with acute renal failure is a 5.25 percent mixture of the eight essential amino acids (Nephramine, made by Kendall-McGaw). This hypercaloric, low-protein diet, which provides 1,000 to 2,500 kcal/day and 2 to 5 g N/day in the form of essential amino acids, will prevent patients with renal failure from becoming protein deficient and may alleviate uremic symptoms. Conventional amino acid solutions containing both essential and nonessential amino acids may be given in reduced amounts (20 to 40 g of protein) with hypertonic dextrose to patients with cardiopulmonary failure and fluid restriction.

Access to the superior vena cava for the purpose of intravenous nutrition is best accomplished by percutaneous cannulation of the subclavian vein.[39] A secondary but acceptable route is catheterization of a jugular

Table 4 Contents of One Liter of Standard Parenteral Nutrition Solution

Component	Standard Central Vein Solution	Standard Peripheral Vein Solution
Amino acids	42.5 g (7.15 g N)	27.5 g (4.63 g N)
Dextrose	250 g	50 g
Sodium	35 mEq	30 mEq
Potassium	30 mEq	30 mEq
Magnesium	5 mEq	5 mEq
Calcium	4.7 mEq	4.7 mEq
Phosphate	15 mM	5 mM
Acetate	67.5 mEq	48 mEq
Chloride	35 mEq	34 mEq
MVI-12 (10 ml)*		
Vitamin C	100 mg	100 mg
Vitamin A	3,300 U	3,300 U
Ergocalciferol	200 U	200 U
Thiamine (B1)	3 mg	3 mg
Riboflavin (B2)	3.6 mg	3.6 mg
Pyridoxine (B6)	4 mg	4 mg
Niacinamide	40 mg	40 mg
Dexpanthenol	15 mg	15 mg
2-Tocopheryl (E)	10 U	10 U
Biotin	60 µg	60 µg
Folic acid	400 µg	400 µg
Cyanocobalamin (B12)	5 µg	5 µg
Phytonadione (vitamin K)†	10 mg	10 mg
mOsm	1,970	655
Total kcal	1,029	286
kcal/N	119	37

*Administered once daily in a volume of 1 L.
†Administered weekly.

vein. Catheterization should be performed only by a physician experienced with this procedure, using strict aseptic technique. Percutaneous venipuncture of a central vein should not be attempted when platelet counts are below 50,000/mm^3 or when bleeding time is prolonged. In such instances, patients should be transfused with platelets or fresh plasma (or components) before catheter insertion. Alternatively, a jugular vein cutdown could be performed. After venipuncture, a chest roentgenogram is obtained to confirm the position of the catheter tip in the superior vena cava. The catheter is considered inviolate and is used solely as a route of administration for the hypertonic nutrient solution.[39] Some have advocated use of central venous lines for multiple purposes, such as nutrient administration, blood drawing, central venous pressure monitoring, and administration of antibiotics and other chemotherapeutic agents. The reported rates of localized catheter infection and sepsis in these instances, however, are unacceptably high and preclude such injudicious use of central venous lines. In addition, a strict hospital protocol outlining care of the catheter entrance site and other aspects of nutrient fluid administration is essential. A parenteral nutrition team optimizes nutrient delivery and minimizes complications.

Patients receiving central vein feedings should be weighed daily and accurate intake and output records maintained. The urine glucose is monitored every six hours or more frequently if indicated. Persistent glucosuria indicates hyperglycemia and may be associated with concomitant osmotic diuresis and dehydration. Sustained glucosuria should be followed by blood glucose determinations. Hyperglycemia should be treated by administering regular insulin or, if persistent, by diminishing the rate of glucose infusion.

Weight gain may reflect substantial positive energy balance or fluid retention. An intake of 7,000 kcal in excess of metabolic requirements should produce an increase of approximately 1 kg in body weight, a safe weekly weight gain. By estimating metabolic requirements and subtracting this value from caloric intake, energy balance can be determined. Agreement between this estimate and actual weight gain provides assurance that the increase in body weight is not the result of fluid retention.

Protein anabolism, as reflected by nitrogen balance studies, should be verified during nutritional repletion. Although total body nitrogen is most accurately measured by neutron activation, this technique is limited by its cost and the need for skilled technicians. An estimate of nitrogen equilibrium can be more readily obtained by measuring urinary urea nitrogen. The urinary urea nitrogen concentration in grams per liter multiplied by the total volume of urine output a day (L/24 hr) yields the total number of grams of urea nitrogen excreted in that 24-hour period. Because urea contains only approximately 80 percent of the nitrogen excreted in urine, the value for the 24-hour urinary urea nitrogen must be increased by an additional 20 percent. This quantity and an additional 2 g/day are added to the value for the urinary urea nitrogen to account for nonurea nitrogen, stool, and integumentary losses. Total nitrogen loss is then subtracted from total nitrogen intake; the difference is an estimate of nitrogen balance [*see Table 5*].

If nitrogen balance has not been achieved by the method of nutritional support in use, then protein and caloric intake should be increased to attain positive nitrogen balance.

Complications

Complications of central vein infusion may be mechanical, septic, or metabolic. Mechanical complications can be minimized by using proper technique during catheter insertion and by appropriate monitoring of the patient during the postinsertion period. Many mechanical complications may be recognized or avoided by obtaining a chest x-ray immediately before infusing the hypertonic nutrient solution. It has been suggested that the use of Silastic catheters reduces the incidence of subclavian and superior vena caval thrombosis.

The most serious complication associated with use of central venous catheters is sepsis. It has been estimated to occur in three to seven percent of patients in whom catheters have been used to deliver total parenteral nutrition.[40] Primary catheter sepsis is clinically defined as the symptoms and signs of infection, including a febrile episode, associated with an indwelling catheter that is identified as the source of infection. Cultures should be obtained from the catheter tip and the peripheral blood. In primary catheter sepsis, cultures of the catheter tip

will yield more than 10^3 organisms.[41] Secondary catheter sepsis is associated with an infectious focus located outside the catheter that leads to bacteremia and seeds the catheter. The most common organisms associated with catheter sepsis are *Staphylococcus epidermidis*, *S. aureus*, *K. pneumoniae*, and *Candida albicans*.[15]

Catheter-related infections can be minimized by adhering to strict protocols for catheter insertion and maintenance. A team of nutritional support nurses can ensure line care by daily surveillance. It is essential that those performing central venous catheterization have adequate expertise or seek experienced supervision. Every 48 to 72 hours, the catheter dressing should be changed, the site should be inspected and cleansed with an alcohol and acetone swab, Betadine ointment should be applied, and a new sterile dressing should be put in place. Because platelets are crucial components in the early response to bleeding, percutaneous insertion of a central venous catheter should be delayed if the platelet count is less than $50,000/\mu l$ or the bleeding time is prolonged beyond seven minutes. If these hematologic abnormalities exist, treatment with platelets or fresh frozen plasma should be considered before the procedure.

After the line is placed, at least one port should be reserved for the sole purpose of infusing parenteral nutrients. Measuring blood pressure, obtaining blood samples, and infusing medications via the designated total parenteral nutrition port must be avoided so as to minimize the risk of sepsis. The risk may also be decreased by maintaining the dextrose concentration at less than 15 percent if the catheter tip lies within the iliac vein or the inferior vena cava.

When septicemia is suspected, blood cultures should be obtained from the peripheral blood and the catheter. In addition, a complete blood count with a white cell differential count, a chest x-ray, and a urinalysis should be obtained. If peripheral blood cultures are negative, the catheter may be changed over a guide wire and the catheter tip cultured. In contrast, if blood cultures are

---

Table 5   Calculation of Nitrogen Balance in a Patient Receiving Parenteral Nutrition

EXAMPLE

A 24-year-old woman with lower extremity lymphedema and cellulitis is receiving 2 L of central vein parenteral nutrition daily; she is also consuming 25 g of protein orally daily. Her urine urea nitrogen (UUN) is 500 mg/dl, and she is voiding 2,500 ml/day. Is she in positive nitrogen balance?

CALCULATION

Nitrogen balance = N intake – N output

$$\text{N output (g/day)} = \frac{\text{UUN (mg/dl)} \times \text{urine volume (L/day)}}{100} + 20\% \text{ of total UUN} + 2 \text{ g/day}$$

N intake: I.V. = 14 g N (2 L central vein solution)

        p.o. = 4 g N (25 g protein/6.25)

        Thus, I.V. N (14 g) + p.o. N (4 g) = 18 g/day total N intake

N output: Urine volume = 2.5 L/day

        UUN = 500 mg/dl

$$\text{Thus, N output} = \frac{500 \text{ mg/dl} \times 2.5 \text{ L/Day}}{100} + 20\% \text{ of total UUN} + 2 \text{ g/day}$$

$$= 12.5 \text{ g/day} + 20\% \,(12.5 \text{ g/day}) + 2 \text{ g/day}$$
$$= 17 \text{ g/day}$$

NITROGEN BALANCE

N balance = 18 g/day (N intake) – 17 g/day (N output) = 1 g/day
    Thus, this patient is in positive nitrogen balance, retaining approximately 1 g/day.

---

positive, the catheter should be removed to avoid complications associated with a contaminated indwelling catheter. If there is a positive culture from the catheter exit site, purulent drainage around the site, or evidence of hypotension, the line should be removed and replaced by a new percutaneous insertion. A positive blood culture for *C. albicans* in a patient who is under intensive care necessitates removal of the catheter and consideration of treatment with amphotericin B.

Patients requiring long-term nutritional support usually have either a Hickman or a Broviac catheter tunneled to the right atrium and anchored subcutaneously with a Dacron cuff. The incidence of catheter sepsis may be as high as 30 percent in patients with Hickman catheters and is most commonly associated with *S. epidermidis* infection.[42-45] It has been suggested that many of these infections may be cured without catheter removal. In contrast, *S. aureus*, which tends to be a more virulent organism, is less frequently associated with the Hickman catheter; nine percent of cases are attributable to *S. aureus*, compared with 39 percent that are attributable to *S. epidermidis*.[42-47]

Infectious complications associated with long-term indwelling catheters include exit-site infections, tunnel infections, and catheter-related bacteremias without local signs of inflammation. An exit-site infection is implied by erythema, purulence, or induration located within 2 cm of the skin exit site of the catheter.[46] A tunnel infection is defined as erythema, tenderness, or induration along the subcutaneous track of the Hickman catheter that extends more than 2 cm from the exit site. A retrospective review of Hickman catheter–related *S. aureus* bacteremias used these definitions to assess optimal methods of treatment. Because only 18 percent of Hickman catheter–associated *S. aureus* bacteremias and only 10 percent of cases with exit-site infections resolve without catheter removal, it has been recommended that early catheter removal should be considered except in cases with an established noncatheter source of infection and cases without catheter-related physical signs (i.e., purulence or induration) in which the blood culture colony counts are less than 1/ml.[46]

In addition to the type of catheter, different nutritional formulas may also be associated with different rates of sepsis. A study of neonates in two intensive care units indicated that those who received intravenous lipid emulsion were at significantly greater risk for staphylococcal coagulase–negative bacteremia (5.8 times) than control subjects.[48] The lipid was infused via Teflon peripheral venous catheters. Various strains of staphylococci produce a mucoid substance that enhances the growth of colonies on the surface of a synthetic polymer that is a catheter component.[49] It has been proposed that the mucoid layer may act as a barrier, protecting the bacteria from phagocytosis and inhibiting the action of antibiotics.[50]

Immunosuppressed critically ill patients receiving multiple broad-spectrum antibiotics are also at risk for *Candida* septicemia. Most episodes of candidemia related to an indwelling catheter resolve after catheter removal. Repeated positive *C. albicans* blood cultures that occur after catheter removal indicate persistent infection, requiring treatment with amphotericin B. An ophthalmologist should examine the eyegrounds of patients with proven candidemia to exclude the possibility of metastatic *Candida* ophthalmitis.

A wide variety of metabolic complications may occur during parenteral feeding; they are minimized by frequent monitoring [*see Table 6*] and appropriate adjustment of the nutrients in the infusate [*see Table 7*].

Modified Parenteral Solutions for Special Needs

Renal Failure

Metabolic studies in patients with acute and chronic renal failure have focused on the quantity and quality of dietary protein ad-

ministered. Although urea can serve as a nonprotein source of nitrogen for synthesis of nonessential amino acids, it may do so only during severe protein depletion when adequate carbohydrate calories are provided. These findings led to an attempt to lower the level of BUN in patients with acute and chronic renal failure by limiting intake of nonessential amino acids. In this therapy, protein of high biologic value is given along with adequate calories, primarily in the form of carbohydrate. When enteral feeding is not feasible, a central venous infusion containing a higher concentration of essential amino acids than standard solutions (e.g., Renamin in a hypertonic dextrose solution) can provide the protein and calories needed for support of the body cell mass. This therapy permits gradual lowering of BUN during protein administration; it maintains reduction of serum potassium, phosphate, and magnesium concentrations; it may improve the rate of recovery of renal function in acute renal failure; and it decreases the frequency of dialysis. If marked volume restriction is needed, 70 percent glucose can be used in the nutrient mix and extra calories can be given as 20 percent fat emulsion. Thus, 1,100 to 2,900 kcal, an amount generally sufficient to achieve nutritional maintenance, can be given in a volume of 1,000 to 1,500 ml.

When uremic symptoms are reversed or BUN is lowered below 100 mg/dl, the protein intake is gradually liberalized. A standard amino acid solution is substituted for the essential amino acid mixture, and both essential and nonessential amino acids are given with hypertonic glucose to provide approximately 20 g N/day. (This solution is prepared by mixing 250 ml of an 8.5 percent amino acid solution with 500 ml of 70 percent glucose.) As acute renal failure resolves or the factors that accelerated protein catabolism (sepsis or injury) are successfully treated, additional amino acids are administered. In general, the protein intake is liberalized in a stepwise manner as BUN falls; the quantity of protein administered should not elevate BUN above 100 mg/dl. As soon as oral intake is possible, tube-feeding formu-

Table 6 Variables to Be Monitored during Intravenous Alimentation and Suggested Frequency of Monitoring

Variables	Suggested Monitoring Frequency	
	First Week	*Later*
Energy Balance		
Weight	Daily	Daily
Metabolic Variables		
Blood measurements		
Plasma electrolytes (Na^+, K^+, Cl^-)	Daily	3 × weekly
Blood urea nitrogen	3 × weekly	2 × weekly
Plasma osmolarity*	Daily	3 × weekly
Plasma total calcium and inorganic phosphorus	3 × weekly	2 × weekly
Blood glucose	Daily	3 × weekly
Plasma aminotransferases	3 × weekly	2 × weekly
Plasma total protein and fractions	2 × weekly	Weekly
Blood acid-base status	As indicated	As indicated
Hemoglobin	Weekly	Weekly
Magnesium	2 × weekly	Weekly
Triglycerides	Weekly	Weekly
Urine measurements		
Glucose	4–6 × daily	2 × daily
Specific gravity or osmolarity	2–4 × daily	Daily
General measurements		
Volume of infusate	Daily	Daily
Oral intake (if any)	Daily	Daily
Urinary output	Daily	Daily
Prevention and Detection of Infection		
Clinical observations (activity, vital signs, integument)	Daily	Daily
WBC and differential counts	As indicated	As indicated
Cultures	As indicated	As indicated

*May be predicted from 2 × Na concentration (mEq/L) + [blood glucose (mg/dl) ÷ 18].

las of similar composition are prepared and administered.

Hepatic Disease and Hepatic Failure

Hepatic disease is usually associated with varying degrees of malnutrition. For example, persons who have subclinical hepatic disease may show no evidence of nutritional deficiencies. On the other hand jaundiced patients with ascites often have overt signs and symptoms of malnutrition and specific vitamin deficiencies. Patients with acute hepatitis may have no nutritional deficiency at the onset of their disease, but individuals with prolonged illness are usually wasted.

Liver disease leads to failure of protein synthesis, amino acid imbalance, failure to store vitamins A and B_{12}, and hepatic accumulation of triglyceride fat, which may contribute to functional and morphological alterations in the liver. Most patients with

Table 7 Metabolic Complications of Total Parenteral Nutrition

Problems	*Possible Causes*	*Solutions*
Glucose		
Hyperglycemia, glycosuria, osmotic diuresis, hyperosmolar nonketotic dehydration and coma	Excessive total dose or rate of infusion of glucose; inadequate endogenous insulin; increased glucocorticoids; sepsis	Reduce amount of glucose infused; increase insulin; administer a portion of calories as fat emulsion
Ketoacidosis in diabetes mellitus	Inadequate endogenous insulin response; inadequate exogenous insulin therapy	Give insulin; reduce glucose input
Postinfusion (rebound) hypoglycemia	Persistence of endogenous insulin production secondary to prolonged stimulation of islet cells by high-carbohydrate infusion	Administer 5%–10% glucose before infusate is discontinued
Fat		
Pyrogenic reaction	Fat emulsion, other solutions	Exclude other causes of fever
Altered coagulation	Hyperlipidemia	Restudy after fat has cleared bloodstream
Hypertriglyceridemia	Rapid infusion, decreased clearance	Decrease rate of infusion; allow clearance before blood tests
Impaired liver function test results	May be caused by fat emulsion or by an underlying disease process	Exclude other causes of hepatic dysfunction
Cyanosis	Altered pulmonary diffusion capacity	Discontinue fat infusion
Essential fatty acid deficiency	Inadequate essential fatty acid administration	Administer essential fatty acids in the form of one 500 ml bottle of fat emulsion every 2–3 days
Amino Acids		
Hyperchloremic metabolic acidosis	Excessive chloride and monohydrochloride content of crystalline amino acid solutions	Administer Na^+ and K^+ as acetate or lactate salts
Serum amino acid imbalance	Unphysiologic amino acid profile of the nutrient solution; differential amino acid utilization with various disorders	Use experimental solutions if indicated
Hyperammonemia	Excessive ammonia in protein hydrolysate solutions; deficiency of arginine, ornithine, aspartic acid, or glutamic acid, or a combination of these deficiencies in amino acid solutions; primary hepatic disorder	Reduce amino acid intake
Prerenal azotemia	Excessive amino acid infusion with inadequate calorie administration	Reduce amino acid intake; increase glucose calories

Table 7 (continued)

Problems	Possible Causes	Solutions
Calcium and Phosphorus		
Hypophosphatemia	Inadequate phosphorus administration; redistribution of serum phosphorus into cells, bones, or both	Administer phosphorus (20 mEq potassium dihydrogen phosphate/1,000 I.V. calories); evaluate antacid or calcium administration, or both
Hypocalcemia	Inadequate calcium administration; reciprocal response to phosphorus repletion without simultaneous calcium infusion; hypoalbuminemia	Administer calcium
Hypercalcemia	Excessive calcium administration with or without high doses of albumin; excessive vitamin D administration	Decrease calcium or vitamin D
Vitamin D deficiency; hypervitaminosis D	Inadequate or excessive vitamin D	Alter vitamin D administration
Miscellaneous		
Hypokalemia	Potassium intake inadequate relative to increased requirements for protein anabolism; diuresis	Alter nutrient administration
Hyperkalemia	Excessive potassium administration, especially in metabolic acidosis; renal failure	Alter nutrient administration
Hypomagnesemia	Inadequate magnesium administration relative to increased requirements for protein anabolism and glucose metabolism; cisplatin administration	Alter nutrient administration
Hypermagnesemia	Excessive magnesium administration; renal failure	Alter nutrient administration
Anemia	Iron deficiency; folic acid deficiency; vitamin B_{12} deficiency; copper deficiency; other deficiencies	Alter nutrient administration
Bleeding	Vitamin K deficiency	Alter nutrient administration
Hypervitaminosis A	Excessive vitamin A administration	Alter nutrient administration
Elevations in SGOT, SGPT, and serum alkaline phosphatase levels	Enzyme induction secondary to amino acid imbalance or to excessive deposition of glycogen or fat, or both, in the liver	Reevaluate status of patient

alcoholic cirrhosis have a low serum albumin concentration, an abnormality attributed to depressed hepatic synthesis and reduced dietary intake of protein.

Patients with chronic liver disease have elevated levels of aromatic amino acids (phenylalanine, tyrosine, and tryptophan) and low levels of branched-chain amino acids (leucine, isoleucine, and valine). These alterations are thought to occur because of increased protein degradation; portasystemic venous shunting; increased plasma insulin and glucagon; and dietary deficiency of protein, appropriate calories, or both. These alterations in the plasma amino acid pattern are not unique to alcoholic cirrhosis; they are observed in patients with other forms of liver disease or catabolic illnesses, such as sepsis or injury.

Most stable patients with chronic liver disease can tolerate dietary protein at a rate of 1 g/kg/day. In acute alcoholic hepatitis, malnutrition may be profound because of anorexia and vomiting. Standard amino acid solutions administered via a peripheral vein appear to be well tolerated in such patients, and their use has been associated with increased survival.[51]

The nutritional support of patients who have chronic liver disease and encephalopathy remains controversial. It appears that cirrhotic patients have greater tolerance for parenterally administered amino acids than for similar amounts of protein given orally. Hepatic encephalopathy related to protein intake often occurs when intravenous intake exceeds 20 to 40 g of protein a day. Encephalopathy may also occur when a catabolic event, such as an operation or an infection, accelerates net protein catabolism.

Intravenous or oral feedings rich in branched-chain amino acids are said to improve nutrition in chronic liver disease and to exert anticatabolic effects on protein degradation, thus sparing muscle protein.[52] Moreover, alterations in central nervous system function have been related to abnormalities in the plasma amino acid profile. A causal relationship between encephalopathy and derangements in plasma amino acid concentrations has been hypothesized on the basis of the theory that branched-chain amino acids compete with the aromatic amino acids for penetration of the blood-brain barrier. For example, brain serotonin concentration is determined not only by the plasma concentration of tryptophan but also by the ratio of the concentration of this aro-

matic amino acid to other plasma amino acids, such as tyrosine, phenylalanine, leucine, isoleucine, and valine.[53] In addition, an increased plasma concentration of phenylalanine may alter the transport of amino acids that are precursors for the synthesis of brain dopamine and catecholamines.[54] Thus, the levels of neurotransmitters in the brains of patients with liver failure may be determined in part by the abnormal concentration of amino acids in their plasma.

Attempts to normalize the plasma amino acid pattern and reverse the hepatic coma in encephalopathic cirrhotics by infusing specialized mixtures high in branched-chain amino acids and low in aromatic amino acids (Heptamine) along with additional calories have produced variable results.[55] A recent meta-analysis of a series of studies of patients treated with branched-chain amino acid–enriched total parenteral nutrition suggested that these solutions may have improved the mental status of encephalopathic patients, but no conclusion could be drawn regarding effects on morbidity or mortality.[55] In addition, administration of standard amino acid mixtures has been compared with administration of branched-chain–fortified mixtures in chronic encephalopathic patients.[56] The usual amino acid mixtures were as effective as the specialized solutions. Thus, the efficacy of solutions rich in branched-chain amino acids remains uncertain. Furthermore, these specialized solutions are about six to 10 times costlier than natural protein or standard amino acid mixtures. It is not clear whether these solutions allow the administration of moderate quantities of dietary protein without causing progression of neurologic sequelae. Further study is required to assess the benefits of and define indications for the use of these expensive mixtures.

Cardiac Failure

Patients with stage III or stage IV cardiac failure are frequently cachectic, and those who undergo long-term rehabilitative therapy, surgery, or both frequently require prolonged hospitalization and vigorous intensive care. Because gastrointestinal dysfunction is a problem in these individuals, a concentrated solution of amino acids and hypertonic dextrose (a solution similar to the fluid used for renal failure) may be required to provide maximum calories within a limited volume. In addition, 20 percent fat emulsion may be infused to provide additional energy.

Respiratory Insufficiency

Many feeding formulas that provide enteral or parenteral nutrition in critically ill patients contain large carbohydrate loads. The glucose is oxidized to carbon dioxide, which is excreted via the lungs. The relation between carbon dioxide excretion and oxygen consumption is referred to as the respiratory quotient (RQ). The RQ is defined as the ratio of CO_2 produced and expired divided by the quantity of O_2 consumed. RQ changes as combustion of body fuel is altered. For example, the RQ for oxidation of carbohydrate is 1.0, that for fat is 0.7, and that for a mixed diet is approximately 0.85. Production of CO_2 increases as the amount of infused glucose increases; the RQ exceeds 1.0 when lipogenesis occurs. In patients with normal ventilatory function, the effect of the infusion on the RQ is not a major consideration in selecting substrates for nutritional support; however, in patients with compromised ventilation, increasing CO_2 production may precipitate respiratory failure, or it may delay or prevent weaning from a ventilator.[57]

Thus, in patients with respiratory insufficiency, maintenance caloric requirements must be defined more precisely. When a patient is being weaned from a ventilator, caloric intake is stabilized at maintenance levels. If weaning is hindered by CO_2 retention, the carbohydrate load is reduced to provide about 60 to 70 percent of the maintenance caloric requirements as glucose and 30 to 40 percent of requirements as fat emulsion.

Cancer

Dietary studies have demonstrated that hospitalized patients with severe illnesses consume inadequate essential nutrients when allowed an ad-lib diet from food trays. Patients with malignant disorders also fail to maintain energy balance; in the hospital setting, they consume nutrients below the recommended dietary allowance even for persons whose metabolism is normal.[58] Inadequate nutrient intake is particularly significant among cancer patients because they have caloric and protein requirements greater than those of normal individuals.

Hypercatabolism coupled with inadequate nutrient intake over prolonged periods is one indication for nutritional intervention. Such support should be integrated into the overall treatment program of the patient and, in general, should be provided only when antineoplastic therapy is given.

The effects of short-term parenteral nutrition in patients undergoing chemotherapy have been studied. Such treatment maintains body weight and improves nitrogen retention, but these benefits have not been translated into diminished morbidity or mortality.[59] No study has convincingly demonstrated decreased toxicity of chemotherapy regimens or more rapid return of white cells or platelets when intravenous nutritional support is used instead of ad-lib feeding alone.

Complex, multimodality antineoplastic therapy, however, may cause such profound anorexia and gastrointestinal toxicity that prolonged nutritional support is essential. For example, patients undergoing bone marrow transplantation for hematologic disorders often require nutritional support for two months or more. The period of combination drug therapy, total body irradiation, and graft versus host disease is often characterized by deterioration of gastrointestinal function. Oral intake or tube feedings accentuate diarrhea, which approaches 5 L/day in some patients. Starvation of normal persons usually leads to death in 60 to 70 days. Thus, these patients would not survive the complications of malnutrition during their prolonged treatment if intravenous nutrients were not provided. However, there is no evidence to support the routine use of parenteral or enteral nutrition in patients undergoing chemotherapy. One meta-analysis pooled the results of 12 randomized, controlled trials to summarize the effect of parenteral feedings on outcome.[60] Mortality in patients receiving parenteral nutrition was 19 percent greater than in control patients. Furthermore, the probability of a complete or partial response to chemotherapy was 32 percent greater in the control patients than in those given parenteral nutrition.[60] The use of total parenteral nutrition was associated with a fourfold increased risk of infection.[60] It should be noted that the majority of patients reviewed in these trials were not significantly malnourished. Because it has been suggested that patients who are severely malnourished may benefit from nutritional support, further analysis of supplemental feeding must be done in significantly depleted patients before nutritional support is excluded from treatment regimens of cancer patients.[61]

Combined therapies are becoming more common, and chemotherapy or radiation therapy is often given before surgical extirpation of a tumor. To maintain the patient in the best possible nutritional state before operation, enteral or parenteral nutrition is often provided, usually on an outpatient basis. This approach is particularly effective for patients with cancer of the head, neck, or esophagus. Such adjuvant nutritional support is based on the results of controlled trials[62] and retrospective observations[63] suggesting that adequate preoperative feeding reduces morbidity and mortality in selected patient groups.

All methods of nutritional support are applicable for use in patients with cancer, including ad-lib oral diet with supplements, tube feedings, and peripheral vein nutrition. If central vein infusion is being considered, it is preferable to insert the catheter before hematologic changes, such as reduced numbers of platelets or altered clotting factors, occur as a sequel to chemotherapy or radiation treatment. With some advanced treatment protocols, operative insertion of an indwelling central venous catheter should be performed before initiation of therapy. When proper hospital protocols for catheter care are observed and administration of the nutrient solutions is under the direction of a nutritional support team, the prevalence of infection resulting from the use of central venous catheters in patients with cancer is no higher than that in the general hospital population.

Perioperative Nutrition

The benefits of perioperative feeding should be estimated in terms of the prospects for reducing morbidity, mortality, and length of hospital stay and minimizing postoperative complications. Preoperative feeding may benefit a select group of severely malnourished patients; however, few data exist to help the clinician with guidelines for preoperative or postoperative feeding.[61]

Preoperative

Two controlled studies of patients receiving enteral nutrition have demonstrated a shorter length of hospital stay and fewer postoperative complications than in control patients receiving a routine hospital diet. There was a lower incidence of wound infections, anastomotic leakage, and liver or renal failure in patients who were tube fed for 10 to 21 days preoperatively than in control patients, who received an oral diet.[64,65]

Six studies have evaluated the use of parenteral nutrition before surgery. Three of these studies failed to show any benefit of preoperative total parenteral nutrition, whereas three others did suggest some advantages.

The study most strongly supportive of preoperative parenteral nutrition reviewed results in 125 patients with gastrointestinal cancer.[62] Total parenteral nutrition was infused for 10 days preoperatively and continued postoperatively until oral intake was resumed. Patients who received total parenteral nutrition had a lower mortality than control patients, who received a standard diet (five percent versus 19 percent, respectively); the former group also had a lower incidence of major complications (17 percent versus 32 percent).[62] Preliminary analyses of data from 460 patients after noncardiac thoracotomy or major laparotomy suggest that preoperative parenteral feeding offers benefit to only the most severely malnourished patients.[61] Patients in this multicenter trial were classified as malnourished on the basis of the subjective global assessment or the nutrition risk index [*see Table 8*].[61] Fewer than five percent of patients in this Veterans Administration study were classified as severely malnourished; they appeared to benefit from seven to 15 days of preoperative feeding, as evidenced by a lower rate of noninfectious complications, such as venous or pulmonary thromboses or impaired wound healing, as compared with control patients. There was no overall difference in mortality between control patients and patients given preoperative total parenteral nutrition who underwent major abdominal or thoracic procedures. The severely malnourished patients given total parenteral nutrition had a lower complication rate than those who did not receive such therapy. By contrast, the moderately malnourished patients who received total parenteral nutrition had an increased rate of infectious complications compared with other moderately malnourished patients who did not receive such preoperative feeding.[61]

Neither enteral nor parenteral feeding preoperatively has a significant effect on mortality or morbidity of patients undergoing surgery. It may be beneficial to postpone surgery to give severely malnourished patients 10 days of preoperative nutritional support, as suggested by the lower rate of noninfectious complications noted in the VA multi-institutional trial. Enteral nutrition is less expensive than parenteral nutrition and helps maintain mucosal integrity and function and should therefore be the first mode of therapy attempted when preoperative supplemental nutrition is indicated.

Postoperative

Nine controlled trials examined the use of postoperative feeding via the enteral route. Diagnoses included gastrointestinal cancer, hip fractures, and critical illnesses. Beneficial effects of postoperative nutritional supplementation included decreased length of hospital stay and duration of intravenous feeding, although these benefits were less common among the critically ill patients.[46,66,67] In cases in which enteral nutrition was initiated immediately after surgery, before clinical evidence of restored gastrointestinal function, adverse complications prolonging the hospital stay were noted.[68] It is safe to institute parenteral nutrition via a jejunal tube a few hours after surgery; this is in contrast to gastric enteral nutrition, which should be deferred until there is clinical evidence that gastrointestinal function has returned.

Few trials have assessed the efficacy of postoperative feeding with parenteral nutrition. Of five controlled trials, only two demonstrated beneficial effects on outcome, such as improved wound healing, decreased hospital stay, and decreased side effects with chemotherapy.[69,70] The duration of postoperative feeding ranged from five to 18 days and averaged 11 days.

In four studies that compared enteral postoperative nutrition with parenteral postoperative nutrition, there was no evidence of decreased morbidity or mortality with either feeding route.[71-74] Cost savings were

---

Table 8   Calculation of
Nutrition Risk Index

Nutrition risk index = (15.9 × serum albumin level) + (0.417 × %usual body weight)

%Usual body weight = current body weight ÷ usual body weight

Combination of weight loss + hypoalbuminemia that will produce nutrition risk index values of less than 83.5*:

%Usual Body Weight	Albumin (mg/dl)
100	< 2.78
90	< 3.02
80	< 3.31

*A nutrition risk index value less than 83.5 signals a need for 10 to 15 days of preoperative parenteral nutrition.

noted for patients given enteral nutrition.[74] Postoperative parenteral nutrition should be reserved for those patients who were severely malnourished before surgery or who cannot tolerate postoperative enteral nutrition for more than 10 days.

Home Nutritional Support

Specialized nutritional support is often required for patients who have chronic disease or for those undergoing long-term rehabilitation. To facilitate return to a more normal way of life and to minimize costs, home nutritional support is indicated for selected individuals. Such support can be combined with long-term intravenous hydration therapy or parenteral antibiotic administration. Weeks, if not months, of nutritional repletion are often required to produce a substantial alteration in body composition; a regimen of home self-care capitalizes on the combined anabolic effects of long-term nutritional support and exercise to optimize the rebuilding of skeletal muscle mass. The costs of home support are approximately one fourth those of in-hospital treatment. Government and third-party insurers whose reimbursement structures limit payments for in-hospital support often encourage the use of these less expensive outpatient services. In the years ahead, the need for home nutritional support will continue to grow.

Patient Selection

Candidates for home feeding are usually first seen during a hospital stay. Initiation and training generally require hospitalization and intensive patient interaction with a nutritional support service team, although occasionally, selected patients can be instructed on an outpatient basis in nasogastric tube feeding techniques. The patient's pathological processes must be stable before he or she can be discharged from the hospital. In addition to nutritional support, patients may have other specialized needs, including intravenous antibiotics, daily fluid and electrolyte management requiring varying quantities of salt and water, frequent

plasma and blood chemistry determinations, wound care, and pulmonary and physical therapy. Most of these needs can be met in the home setting.

Long-term parenteral nutrition is usually required in patients whose disease produces temporary or permanent loss of the absorptive surface area of the small intestine. Home parenteral nutrition may be indicated in those with bowel infarction or other pathological conditions resulting in the short bowel syndrome, inflammatory bowel disease with multiple fistulas, malabsorption associated with radiation enteritis or scleroderma, carcinoma of the bowel or abdominal cavity that results in chronic obstruction or intestinal dysfunction, or diarrhea and malabsorption associated with aggressive chemotherapy or abdominal radiation. In contrast, patients requiring home enteral feedings have an adequate small bowel absorptive surface area but usually have an anatomic or physiologic defect that prevents nutrient ingestion. Such patients include those with cancer of the head and neck, anatomic lesions of the upper gastrointestinal tract that preclude oral intake of nutrients, or neurologic or skeletal muscle disorders that prevent swallowing. In all cases, nutritional support must be an essential part of the overall long-term therapeutic plan in order to justify the time, personnel efforts, and costs of initiating home feeding.

When patients in stable condition are referred for home parenteral nutrition, they must have the intellectual capacity and motivation to master the self-care techniques involved. An appropriate, supportive home environment also assures health care providers that sophisticated methods of nutrient administration can be safely and effectively initiated, maintained, and monitored in the home setting.

Routes of Access

Once it has been decided to discharge a patient on home nutrition, an access route must be provided. A nasogastric or nasojejunal tube, a gastrostomy, or a feeding jejunostomy may be used for enteral feedings. If an individual requires a laparotomy during the course of hospitalization, a feeding gastrostomy or a jejunostomy can be performed at the same time, provided that nutritional assessment and home planning have been initiated in the preoperative period. A percutaneous gastrostomy can be performed with or without the aid of endoscopy in patients who do not require a laparotomy; this procedure minimizes the morbidity and mortality associated with operative gastrostomy. If small bowel feedings are indicated, a small feeding catheter can usually be guided into the upper jejunum under fluoroscopic visualization by introducing the feeding tube through an established gastrostomy stoma. Alternatively, a nasojejunal feeding tube may be inserted in patients in whom gastroesophageal reflux prevents gastric feedings.

When intravenous feedings are required, a semipermanent Silastic feeding catheter should be used. The catheter is introduced into the venous system of the upper body, and the distal tip is positioned in the superior vena cava or the right atrium. The proximal end of the catheter is tunneled beneath the skin to the lower anterior chest and is exited over the lower sternum. Because this site can be seen by the patient, daily cleaning and the application of dressings are made easier. The catheter can usually be inserted in less than an hour with local anesthesia.

Initiation of Home Nutritional Support

The patient has usually been exposed to specialized feeding techniques during hospitalization and has gained some familiarity with the use of bags, tubes, and infusion pumps. However, to ensure safety, five to 10 days of instruction may be required before discharge. The patient or family members must master the nursing functions associated with the array of feeding procedures, including preparation of solutions, addition of medications, attachment of feeding catheters and tubes, control of infusion pumps, care of the intravenous catheter, and the use of sterile technique. The individual must be able to monitor the effects of feedings and be able to recognize the signs and symptoms of metabolic or infectious complications. During the last several days of hospitalization, the patient, family members, or both should perform these tasks but with nurses available should problems arise. During the first week at home, a visiting nurse often is scheduled to assist in this self-care process.

Most patients tolerate a regimen of cyclic feedings. The nutrient formula is infused over 12 to 16 hours, usually during the course of the night so that the patient can be detached from the infusion devices during the day. Cyclic feedings should be initiated in the hospital; activities such as tests and exercise rehabilitation can be scheduled during the day when the patient is not being fed.

Follow-up

Follow-up outpatient care is most intensive during the first several weeks after hospital discharge. A visiting nurse and social worker should see the patient at home between outpatient appointments. Frequent telephone conversations are educational for the patient and serve to reinforce solutions to problems that might arise. Blood should be collected during outpatient visits for chemical and electrolyte determinations, especially when fluid and electrolyte balance is a major concern. Blood data form the basis for periodic formula adjustments, which are communicated by the physician to the manufacturing pharmacy or to the patient. If indicated, blood should be evaluated for the more subtle changes associated with vitamin and trace element deficiencies. Many patients who are sustained by home parenteral nutrition for more than four months have deficiency syndromes associated with inadequate administration of calcium, magnesium, zinc, chromium, copper, aluminum, or selenium. It is essential that health care providers have knowledge of the metabolism of these elements so that significant deficiency states do not arise. Throughout the period of home care, the patient should monitor body weight and gastrointestinal losses.

Overall therapeutic goals will vary because of the wide variety of disease processes associated with home nutritional support. Some patients may be weaned from parenteral or enteral feedings after several months. Some may require only supplemental intravenous feedings associated with oral food intake. In others, progression of disease may necessitate rehospitalization. In some patients with the short bowel syndrome, adaptation of the small intestine may never be adequate, and intravenous nutrition may be a lifelong necessity.

Reimbursement

At present, Medicare and Medicaid regulations state that a patient is eligible for coverage of home nutritional therapy if the individual requires such support for at least three months or for the duration of his or her life. Regulations vary among insurance carriers, and a specific company should be consulted to determine whether a particular patient is covered for home therapy. Most carriers have been willing to provide for health care in the home and accept all eligible patients for reimbursement.

Support of the Severely or Terminally Ill

Health care providers working with home nutritional support services are frequently requested to see patients with severe or terminal disease, particularly those with metastatic cancer. In general, nutrition is a method of supportive care and is not a treatment per se. Therefore, nutritional support must be integrated into the overall therapeutic plan.

If nutrition is impaired because of poor enteral intake or severe diarrhea associated with aggressive antineoplastic treatment programs and there is a reasonable chance of cure or significant palliation of disease, nutritional support is essential to prevent the complications associated with malnutrition. However, when no other therapeutic options exist, a program of home feeding is rarely justified as the sole mode of therapy. Exceptions to the rule include patients with very slow growing tumors in the abdominal cavity that cause intestinal obstruction but allow the patient to function for long peri-

ods. We have initiated home nutritional support for such individuals if, in our judgment, they will require such therapy for at least three months.

An alternative approach to the terminally ill patient is to prescribe intravenous fluid for purposes of hydration; such support also provides some nutritional supplementation. Moreover, most patients will report an improved sense of well-being after infusion of intravenous fluids, and this provides an alternate route for the administration of pain medication.

Innovations in Nutritional Support

A positive nitrogen balance is required for growth and optimal immune function. Under normal physiologic and nutritional conditions, this balance is assured through adequate protein and caloric intake and unimpaired utilization. In severely ill patients and patients who have undergone gastrointestinal surgery, there is a need to counter nitrogen losses resulting from protein catabolism, excessive excretion, and malabsorption [*see Table 5*].

Recent clinical studies of the effects of growth hormone, the dibasic amino acid arginine, and glutamine, which has been deemed a conditionally essential amino acid under conditions of stress, suggest that these biochemical ingredients may be useful promoters of nitrogen balance or may at least have a nitrogen-sparing effect when used as nutritional supplements in the critically ill.[74-82] Other clinical benefits may be obtained by their use, but the impact of supplementary growth hormone, arginine, and glutamine on morbidity, quality of life, and mortality requires further study.

Growth Hormone

In addition to its anabolic effects (promotion of amino acid uptake by cells with increased synthesis of body protein and mineral retention), growth hormone stimulates lipolysis and release of free fatty acids. The release of this endogenous fuel may be an alternative energy source when the hormone is combined with hypocaloric feedings. Growth hormone combined with such feedings may be used to preserve protein stores in critically ill patients whose adipose stores, when adequate, can be mobilized for fuel.[78-80,82-86]

Combined with prednisone, growth hormone may prevent glucocorticoid-stimulated catabolism and may thus be helpful to patients receiving chronic steroid therapy.[82] Accelerated wound healing and a low rate of sepsis after commencement of growth hormone treatment in severely ill patients has been reported.[81]

Supplemental growth hormone has been shown to enhance the cytotoxic activity of natural killer cells in humans with growth hormone hyposecretion.[87,88] Patients deficient in these cells may be less able to combat viral infections. In animal models, natural killer cells have demonstrated a role in immune surveillance against both the establishment of primary tumors and the control of metastases.[89]

Because it is not known whether growth hormone stimulates neoplastic growth, its use should be avoided in patients with malignant disorders. Potential side effects mandating cautious use of the hormone in diabetics and patients with a propensity toward fluid retention include hyperglycemia and enhanced sodium retention at the renal tubule.[90]

Arginine

Arginine, given in heavy doses (30 g of arginine HCl daily) to patients undergoing cholecystectomy, has been reported to reduce nitrogen excretion.[77] In addition, cancer patients undergoing major surgery achieved a more rapid positive nitrogen balance if their diet was supplemented with 25 g of arginine daily, as compared with control patients receiving an isonitrogenous glycine supplement.[91]

Arginine appears to enhance immune function in both animals and humans. Peripheral blood lymphocytes from healthy human males demonstrated, in vitro, an increased activity of natural killer cells and lymphokine-activated killer cells with increasing concentrations of arginine.[92]

Supplemental parenteral or enteral arginine has been shown to stimulate secretion of growth hormone, insulin, and prolactin in humans.[93-100] Because arginine potentiates the release of several pituitary hormones, it can be hypothesized that the beneficial effects of pharmacological doses of the amino acid on protein synthesis, wound healing, and immune function may be mediated via a pituitary messenger such as growth hormone.

Glutamine

Several studies have demonstrated decreased muscle glutamine loss and improved nitrogen balance in postoperative patients receiving glutamine-supplemented total parenteral nutrition as compared with those receiving standard formulas. Nitrogen balance was also shown to be preserved in catabolic bone marrow transplant patients who received glutamine-enriched total parenteral nutrition.[74,85,101-103]

Glutamine appears to benefit patients under stress from injury or infection. Thus, it has been suggested that glutamine may have a primary role in preserving gut integrity and immune competence. Glutamine-enriched total parenteral nutrition has been reported to attenuate villous atrophy of the small bowel, which is a complication of standard parenteral nutrition.[75,76] The combination of subcutaneous injections of epidermal growth factor and parenteral nutrition enriched with glutamine has been reported to have a synergistic effect on the thickness of the small bowel mucosa.[104] Immune function is impaired after major injury, and a decrease in T cell activity has been noted after extensive burns.[105,106] Plasma glutamine concentrations have been reported to be 58 percent lower than normal in burn patients.[107] The incidence of positive microbial cultures and clinical infection has been reported as lower in critically ill patients given glutamine-enriched feedings.[108]

Cautious administration of glutamine is advised in patients with hepatic encephalopathy and hyperammonemia (glutamine is metabolized to glutamate and ammonia).

Glutamine-enriched nutritional solutions may be contraindicated in patients with renal failure who have decreased ability to metabolize glutamine in the distal tubules.[109]

References

1. Modern Nutrition in Health and Disease. Lea & Febiger, Philadelphia, 1988, p 1306
2. Ann Surg 199:299, 1984
3. Mayo Clin Proc 57:181, 1982
4. Ann Intern Med 101:303, 1984
5. Am J Clin Nutr 29:1359, 1976
6. Am J Clin Nutr 34:1944, 1981
7. Body-Composition Assessments in Youth and Adults. Ross Laboratories, Columbus, Ohio, 1985, p 5
8. Surgery 88:17, 1980
9. Am J Clin Nutr 32:630, 1979
10. J Lab Clin Med 105:305, 1985
11. Am J Clin Nutr 46:537, 1987
12. Aust N Z J Surg 60:209, 1990
13. Am J Clin Nutr 35(suppl 5):1117, 1982
14. Body-Composition Assessments in Youth and Adults. Ross Laboratories, Columbus, Ohio, 1985, p 65
15. Scientific American, Inc, New York, 1989, Sect II, Chapter 10, p 3
16. Immunology 15:581, 1968
17. Infect Immun 24:545, 1979
18. Immunology 12:1313, 1975
19. J Med Microbiol 12:17, 1979
20. Digestion 16:87, 1977
21. J Clin Pathol 19:498, 1966
22. JPEN 10:545, 1986
23. Nutr International 1986
24. Am J Clin Nutr 49:573, 1989
25. Nutrition in the 1980's: Constraints on Our Knowledge. Alan Liss, New York, 1981, p 99
26. Am J Clin Nutr 30:531, 1977
27. Manual of Nutritional Therapeutics. Little, Brown & Co, Boston, 1983, p 53
28. Arch Biochem Biophys 133:22, 1969
29. J Biol Chem 248:3582, 1973
30. Chin Med J 92:477, 1979
31. N Engl J Med 304:1210, 1981
32. Philos Trans R Soc Lond (Biol) 294:185, 1981
33. Gastroenterology 76:458, 1979
34. Dig Dis Sci 26:865, 1981
35. Gastroenterology 78:272, 1980
36. JPEN 258, 1979
37. Crit Care Med 11:7, 1983
38. Fat Emulsions in Parenteral Nutrition. American Medical Association, Chicago, 1976
39. Total Parenteral Nutrition. Little, Brown & Co, Boston, 1976
40. Am J Med 85:307, 1988
41. N Engl J Med 296:1305, 1977
42. Medicine (Baltimore) 63:189, 1984
43. Cancer 59:1358, 1987
44. Aust N Z J Med 16:211, 1986
45. Am J Surg 149:627, 1985
46. Am J Med 89:137, 1990
47. Cancer 52:2342, 1983
48. N Engl J Med 323:301, 1990
49. N Engl J Med 323:339, 1990
50. J Pediatr 116:497, 1990
51. Am J Gastroenterol 72:535, 1979
52. J Clin Invest 56:1250, 1975
53. J Neurochem 30:1531, 1978
54. Lancet 2:772, 1979
55. Gastroenterology 97:1033, 1989
56. Ann Surg 197:288, 1983
57. JAMA 243:1444, 1980
58. Cancer Res 37:2359, 1977
59. Am J Med 74:40, 1983
60. Ann Intern Med 107:195, 1987
61. Am J Clin Nutr 47(suppl 2):366, 1988
62. Lancet 1:68, 1982
63. Ann Surg 196:203, 1982
64. Indian J Med Res 80:339, 1984
65. Br J Surg 73:716, 1986
66. Am Surg 47:393, 1981
67. Br Med J 1:293, 1979
68. Br J Surg 72:458, 1985
69. Lancet 1:788, 1978
70. Br J Surg 70:267, 1983
71. Gastroenterology 77:652, 1979
72. Clin Nutr 3:35, 1984
73. Am J Surg 149:106, 1985
74. Lancet 1:231, 1989
75. Surg Forum 37:56, 1986
76. J Surg Res 44:506, 1988
77. Biom Express 29:312, 1978
78. Acta Chir Scand 122:1, 1961
79. Ann Surg 166:739, 1967
80. Surg Gynecol Obstet 138:875, 1971
81. JPEN 14:574, 1990
82. J Clin Invest 86:265, 1990
83. Acta Endocrinol 51:943, 1960
84. Metabolism 22:589, 1973
85. Surgery 100:188, 1986
86. Ann Surg 210:513, 1989
87. Metabolism 38:193, 1988
88. Metabolism 39:1320, 1990
89. Int Arch Allergy Appl Immunol 67:169, 1982
90. Endocrinology. WB Saunders Co, Philadelphia, 1989, p 318
91. Ann Surg 208:512, 1988
92. Lancet 337:645, 1991
93. Lancet 2:668, 1965
94. Acta Endocrinol (Copenh) 99:18, 1982
95. Curr Med Res Opin 7:475, 1981
96. J Clin Endocrinol Metab 25:1140, 1965
97. N Engl J Med 276:434, 1967
98. J Clin Endocrinol Metab 37:641, 1973
99. Lancet 2:28, 1968
100. J Clin Invest 45:1487, 1966
101. Ann Surg 209:455, 1989
102. Metabolism 38(8 suppl 1):63, 1989
103. JPEN 14(suppl 4):137s, 1990
104. Surgery 104:358, 1988
105. Immunol Today 9:253, 1988
106. Surg Forum 37:93, 1986
107. Lancet 336:523, 1990
108. Ann Surg 214: 385, 1991
109. N Engl J Med 306:1013, 1982

Acknowledgments

Table 3 The authors thank Lorrie S. Young for her assistance in revising this table.

Figure 1 Janet Betries.

14 Disorders of Hemostasis and Coagulation

STANLEY L. SCHRIER, M.D.

The Hemostasis Scheme

Normal Hemostatic Mechanisms

When a blood vessel wall breaks, the hemostatic response must be quick, localized, and carefully controlled. The break in the endothelium exposes flowing blood to underlying collagen, microfibrils, and the basement membrane. Platelets adhere to the wound site in a highly ordered two-step reaction. First, a platelet pseudopod comes in contact with the subendothelium. The platelet then changes shape and spreads along the damaged area in such a way as to expose a large amount of platelet plasma membrane to the subendothelium.[1] Adhesion leads to platelet activation. In this process, the platelet plasma membrane expresses new receptors, some of the existing receptors undergo a conformational change that alters their function, and the platelet releases materials stored in its granules. Some of these stored substances, such as ADP, induce passing platelets to aggregate, become activated, and release their contents, whereas others, such as thromboxane A_2, produce vasoconstriction. These reactions increase the size of the platelet plug at the vascular break.

While aggregation is in progress, tissue under the site of the vascular injury leaks tissue factor and additional ADP. Tissue factor released by damaged cells interacts with and activates Factor VII to VIIa, thereby initiating the extrinsic pathway of coagulation. Factor VIIa directly converts Factor X to Xa [see Table 1 and Figure 1]; thus, the extrinsic system appears to generate small amounts of thrombin (Factor IIa) rapidly, which causes platelets to undergo release and aggregation. Thrombin further amplifies the coagulation scheme by activating Factors V and VIII.

The disrupted vascular surface also initiates contact activation by activating Hageman factor (Factor XII), which in a complex scheme of interactions triggers the intrinsic coagulation pathway and the kinin pathway [see Figures 2 and 3].[2] Factor XII may also be subject to complement modulation.

These mechanisms bring about localized adhesion and aggregation of platelets to form a hemostatic plug. The intrinsic system, though relatively slow, is quantitatively very important. Fibrin and thrombin interact with platelets to fuse the platelet plug. The actomyosin contractile system of the platelet causes clot retraction, converting a weak meshwork into a firm, tightly woven clot. Finally, injury-induced vessel constriction reduces the size of the vascular defect and slows blood flow.

If the autoamplification properties of coagulation were uncontrolled, each significant hemorrhage would result in generalized coagulation and permanent occlusion of vessels. Coagulation, however, is modulated by a number of mechanisms: dilution of procoagulants in flowing blood; removal of particulate matter and activated factors through the reticuloendothelial system, especially in the liver; and antagonism of the activated procoagulants by circulating inhibitors.

Inhibitors of Coagulation

The most important of the inhibitors of coagulation are antithrombin III–heparin cofactor and protein C. Antithrombin III (AT-III) antagonizes the action of the serine protease procoagulants, Factors XIIa, XIa, IXa, Xa, and IIa, by forming stoichiometric complexes with them. Heparin binds to lysyl residues on AT-III, producing a conformational change that makes the active site on AT-III more accessible to the serine protease

Table 1   Plasma Procoagulants in Humans

Factor	Concentration in Normal Plasma (µg/ml)	Biologic Half-life (hr)
I Fibrinogen	2,500–3,500	95–120
II Prothrombin	100	65–90
V Proaccelerin	10	15–24
VII Proconvertin	0.5	4–6
VIII Antihemophilic factor (AHF)	15	10–12
IX Christmas factor	3	18–30
X Stuart-Prower factor	10	40–60
XI Plasma thromboplastin antecedent (PTA)	< 5	45–60
XII Hageman factor	< 5	50–70
XIII Fibrin-stabilizing factor (FSF)	20	72–120

procoagulants.[3] This action of heparin enhances thrombin inactivation by 750-fold and Factor Xa inactivation to an even greater degree. Heparan sulfate proteoglycans on the luminal surfaces of endothelial cells appear to activate AT-III in a manner identical to that of administered heparin.[3] These proteoglycans are intercalated into the plasma membrane of endothelial cells with the protein moiety inserting into the membrane core while the polysaccharide moiety, which is analogous to heparin, protrudes from the cell surface into the bloodstream.[3] Activated factors such as Xa, however, are protected from degradation by AT-III when they are bound to platelets.[4]

Protein C is a vitamin K–dependent anticoagulant synthesized in the liver. On activation, protein C is converted to a serine protease that destroys Factors Va and VIIIa, the two major procoagulants that are not inactivated by AT-III. Thus, these two control mechanisms, AT-III and protein C, seem to have evolved to modulate all procoagulant activity, and even a modest congenital reduction in either anticoagulant leads to a hypercoagulable state [*see* Hypercoagulable States, *below*].[5] Activated protein C also destroys the inhibitors of tissue plasminogen activator (t-PA), allowing t-PA to activate plasminogen.[6] Thus, these actions of protein C serve to terminate coagulation and set the stage for clot lysis.

Protein C activation is carefully controlled and proceeds in a complicated manner [*see Figure 4*], requiring thrombin and thrombomodulin, a factor that is present on endothelial cells. Activation of the protein C system can be determined by measuring the cleavage product of protein C—that is, protein C activation peptide [*see Figure 4*]. Full activation of protein C seems to require the action of another vitamin K–dependent enzyme, termed protein S.[6] In vitro studies have shown that protein C and protein S form a complex on phospholipid vesicles that enhances the inactivation of Factor Va by activated protein C (protein Ca). It has thus been proposed that protein S enhances the activity of protein Ca by interacting with the phospholipid core of platelets or with the plasma membranes of endothelial cells or other cells. The protein C–protein S system also appears to provide a link between hemostasis and inflammation. For example, the exposure of endothelial cells in vitro to interleukin-1 (IL-1) decreases thrombomodulin levels to about 33 percent of control levels and protein C–protein S function to less than 10 percent of control values.[7]

Plasma Procoagulants

All of the plasma procoagulants except von Willebrand factor (vWF, also termed vWF:Ag)[8] are synthesized in the liver [*see Table 1*]. Of these, the factors whose synthese

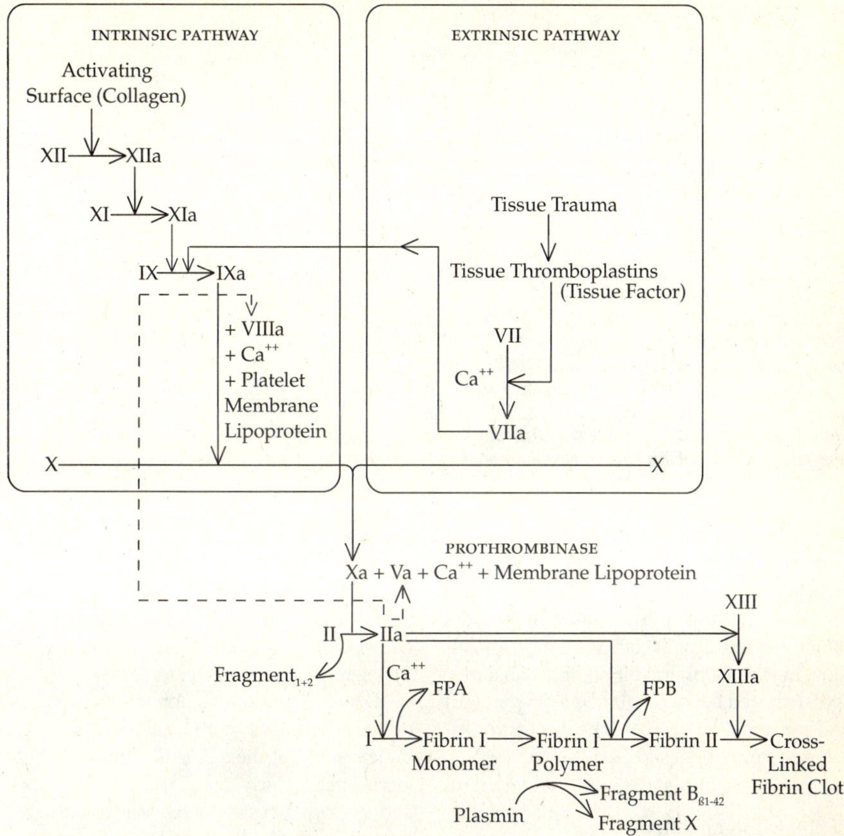

Figure 1 *In the traditional view of coagulation, the intrinsic and extrinsic coagulation pathways converge at the step where Factor X is activated. The enzyme activity formed by the complex of Xa, Va, Ca^{++}, and platelet and endothelial cell membrane lipoprotein has been termed prothrombinase. The activation of fibrinogen (Factor I) to fibrin monomer generates the peptide fragment fibrinopeptide A (FPA). The conversion of fibrin I polymer to fibrin II yields fibrinopeptide B (FPB). Plasmin and thrombin (IIa) compete with each other to attack fibrin I polymer. Further thrombin action leads to the production of the cross-linked fibrin clot, whereas plasmin action generates fragment X and fragment B_{1-42}. Activated factors are indicated by the letter a. Dotted lines indicate that thrombin (Factor IIa) enhances the activity of the other factors.*

is dependent on vitamin K are Factors II, VII, IX, and X. Factor VIII circulates as part of a Factor VIII–vWF complex that has two major components. The smaller part contains the procoagulant activity termed Factor VIII:C and its related antigen, Factor VIII:CAg (now termed Factor VIII:Ag). Factors VIII:C and VIII:Ag are deficient or defective in classical hemophilia A. The molecular weight of Factor VIII:C is approximately 285,000 daltons.[9] The larger moiety of the complex is von Willebrand factor. This protein functions as a carrier for Factor VIII:C and may protect this factor from proteolytic degradation. The major role of vWF, however, is to promote the adhesion of platelets to subendothelial surfaces, particularly at high wall shear rates.[9-11] This protein,

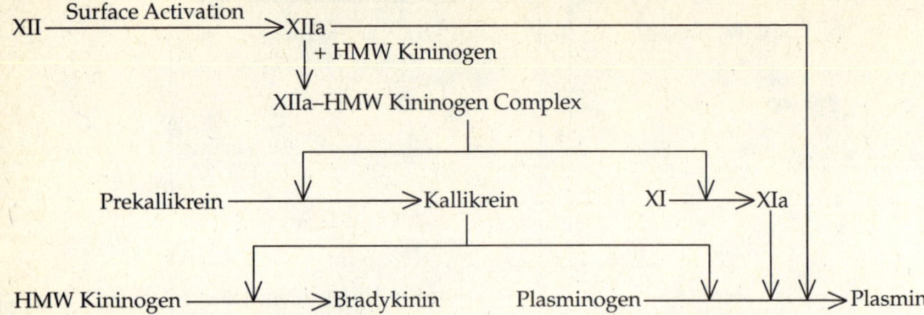

Figure 2 *Activation of Factor XII, or Hageman factor, by exposure to vascular basement membranes or other surfaces initiates the kinin-forming pathway. On activation, Factor XIIa forms a complex with high molecular weight (HMW) kininogen. This complex stimulates the conversion of prekallikrein to kallikrein and activates Factor XI to XIa. Kallikrein then cleaves HMW kininogen to form bradykinin, a peptide that acts as a powerful vasodilator and also increases vascular permeability. Kallikrein and activated Factors XI and XII can convert plasminogen to the fibrinolytic enzyme plasmin, but the in vivo relevance of this sequence has not been established.*

which is synthesized in megakaryocytes and endothelial cells, exists as a series of multimers of a 270,000 dalton subunit.[12] These high molecular weight multimers range in size from 500,000 to 20 million daltons. In the peripheral blood, this substance is distributed between platelets (25 percent) and plasma (75 percent). The largest multimers of von Willebrand factor probably play the major role in platelet adhesion.[11]

Pathway Interactions

Hemostasis has formerly been portrayed as a series of separate, minimally interacting sequences in which platelets, the extrinsic system, and the intrinsic system each perform assigned roles. It now appears, however, that important interactions occur among the components of the hemostatic mechanism.[13] For example, the addition of activated platelets vastly enhances the rate of interaction between Factors Xa and II. This interaction apparently takes place on the platelet membrane, and Factor V seems to be the platelet membrane binding site for Factor Xa.[14] AT-III–heparin cofactor readily attacks and inactivates Factor Xa when the latter is in solution but not when it is bound to the platelet membrane. Factor VIIa in vitro can activate Factor IX, establishing a potentially important link between the in-

trinsic and extrinsic systems.[14] The existence of this alternative pathway to Factor IX activation may account for the contrast between the relative mildness of Factor XI deficiency hemophilia and the severity of Factor IX deficiency [*see Figure 1*].

These various interactions support a view of hemostasis as a more localized process in which many of the steps take place on surfaces—particularly on platelet membranes and damaged vessel walls. Many of the receptors formerly thought to exist only on platelets have now been found on endothelial cells, and it appears likely that damaged endothelial cell surfaces can participate in hemostasis.[15] Consequently, the hemostatic process is more precisely confined to the wound area, the rate of reaction at the appropriate site is markedly enhanced, and spread of the process beyond the wound site is limited.

The interactions outlined are most relevant to the formation and degradation of fibrin-rich red thrombi, which form in veins under conditions of stasis. By contrast, white thrombi, which form on damaged arterial subendothelium, are composed mainly of aggregated platelets.

Fibrinolytic System

Both contact activation and tissue damage set off the fibrinolytic system. After he-

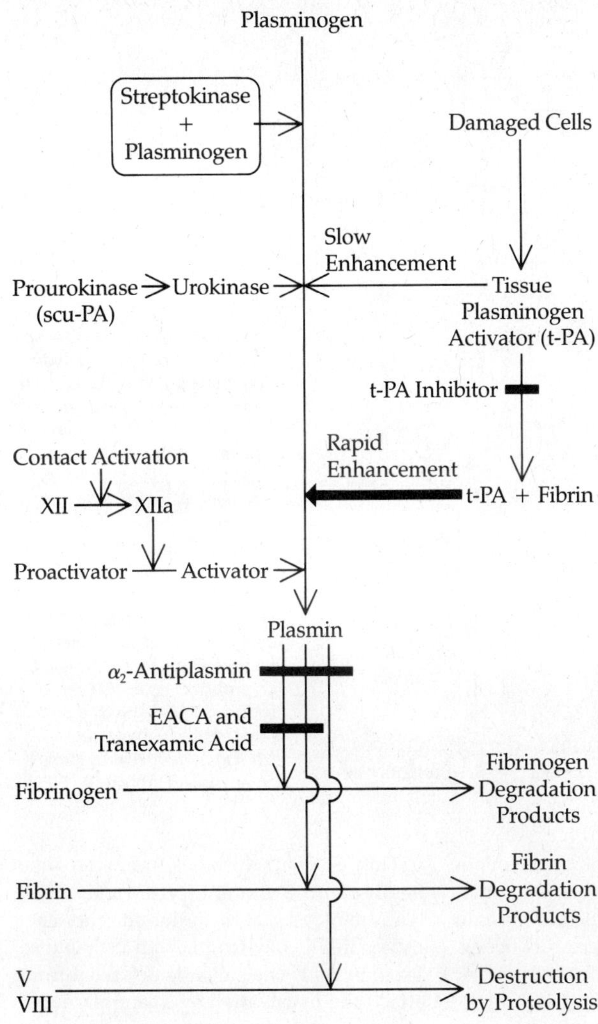

Figure 3 *Diagram depicts normal fibrinolysis and the pharmacologic agents that can be used to modulate this process. The fibrinolytic system is activated primarily by tissue plasminogen activator (t-PA), which is provided by damaged cells in the blood vessel wall. t-PA can produce either slow enhancement of fibrinolysis or, when combined with fibrin, rapid enhancement of this process. The effect of t-PA on fibrinolysis can be blocked by t-PA inhibitor. Streptokinase (which forms a complex with plasminogen), urokinase, and prourokinase (also termed single-chain urokinase-type plasminogen activator, or scu-PA) all activate plasminogen and can be used therapeutically to enhance fibrinolysis. ε-Aminocaproic acid (EACA) and tranexamic acid block fibrinolysis by inhibiting the binding of plasminogen and plasmin to fibrin.*

mostasis has been achieved, the clot must be lysed to restore blood flow. Tissue damage results in the release of an activator of fibrinolysis, tissue plasminogen activator [*see Figures 2 and 3*], a serine protease that is synthesized in endothelial cells and is found in almost all tissues. After t-PA has been released into the circulation, it can be detected as vascular plasminogen activator (v-PA). Plasma inhibitors of t-PA help to maintain a balance between hemostasis and fibrinolysis.[16,17] There are three types of such inhibitors: plasma activator inhibitor-1 (PAI-1), which is derived from endothelial cells; PAI-2, which is found in placental cells; and protease nexin-I.

Tissue plasminogen activator seeks and binds to fibrin, a process that greatly enhances the activation of t-PA. Plasminogen, the substrate for t-PA, circulates in plasma at a concentration of 20 mg/dl. This molecule has an unusual structure consisting of five triple-loop elements termed kringles. Each kringle contains a lysine binding site,

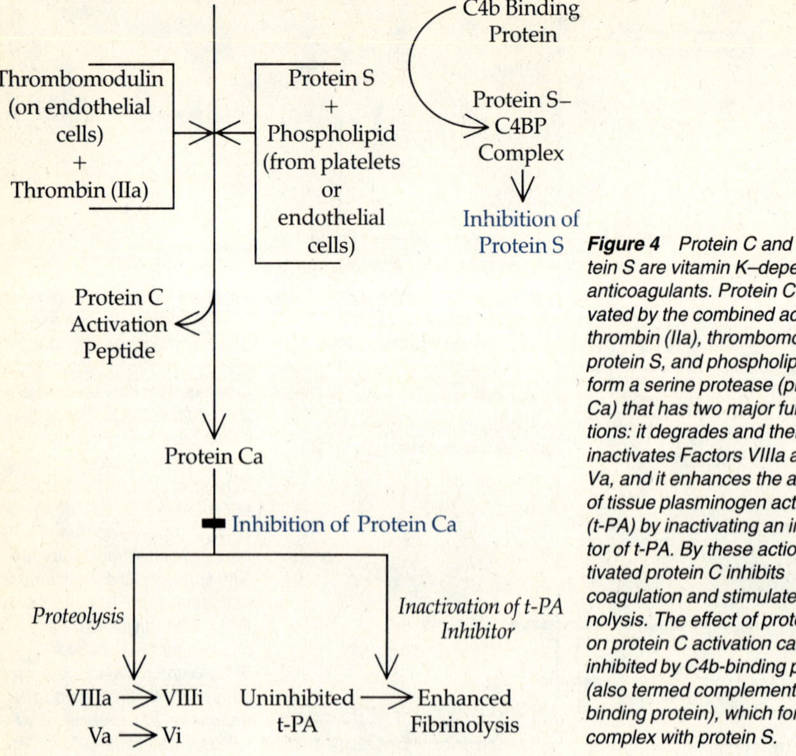

Figure 4   *Protein C and protein S are vitamin K–dependent anticoagulants. Protein C is activated by the combined action of thrombin (IIa), thrombomodulin, protein S, and phospholipid to form a serine protease (protein Ca) that has two major functions: it degrades and thereby inactivates Factors VIIIa and Va, and it enhances the action of tissue plasminogen activator (t-PA) by inactivating an inhibitor of t-PA. By these actions, activated protein C inhibits coagulation and stimulates fibrinolysis. The effect of protein S on protein C activation can be inhibited by C4b-binding protein (also termed complement-binding protein), which forms a complex with protein S.*

which controls the interaction of plasminogen with fibrin and with the plasmin inhibitor α_2-antiplasmin (also termed α_2-plasmin inhibitor). The antifibrinolytic agents tranexamic acid and ε-aminocaproic acid (EACA) bind to these lysine sites on the kringle, interfering with the binding of plasminogen and plasmin to fibrin. Thus, under normal circumstances, plasminogen and t-PA bind to sites on fibrin, forming a trimolecular complex in which the activated t-PA converts adjacent plasminogen into plasmin [see Figure 3]. Plasmin then dissolves the clot, restoring vessel patency.

Plasmin is a proteolytic enzyme of broad action that, if uncontrolled, will attack fibrinogen, Factors VIII and V, complement, and proinsulin, in addition to lysing fibrin. The presence of α_2-antiplasmin in plasma prevents such runaway hyperplasminemia.

α_2-Antiplasmin, which belongs to the same family of proteins as antitrypsin and AT-III, binds to plasmin at the lysine site and inactivates it. Thus, when plasmin is bound to fibrin by its lysine site, it is protected from attack and inactivation by α_2-antiplasmin.[16] The fibrinolytic system can thereby cause localized clot lysis without inducing generalized hyperplasminemia and attendant unregulated proteolysis.

Tissue plasminogen activator shows great promise as a therapeutic clot-lysing agent because its lytic effect is confined to the clot. A form of t-PA prepared by recombinant DNA techniques received FDA approval in 1987 for use immediately after an acute myocardial infarction in an effort to prevent permanent heart damage. The agent should not be administered to patients at risk for hemorrhaging. Unlike t-PA, the fibrinolytic agents streptokinase and urokinase [*see Figure 3*] have a low affinity for fibrin, and they can activate circulating plasminogen directly, causing hyperplasminemia. This side effect accounts for the incidence of significant hemorrhage in patients treated with these agents.[18]

Two other substances also show promise as therapeutic clot-lysing agents because of their ability to home to the clot and initiate local thrombolysis. Prourokinase, or single-chain urokinase-type plasminogen activator (scu-PA), may be useful as a fibrin-specific thrombolytic agent. Because the plasma inhibitor of this agent is inactivated by fibrin, prourokinase is free to act at the clot surface.[16] Similar specificity has been achieved with a streptokinase-plasminogen complex that has been selectively acylated at its proteolytic site. The fibrin binding site remains free to act only on fibrin within a clot.[16] The duration of action of such fibrinolytic compounds can be varied by substituting different acylated side chains.[16]

Platelets and Platelet Function

Platelets are derived from megakaryocytes, which arise from pluripotent myeloid stem cells. Platelet production appears to be controlled by a thrombopoietin that is involved in the final maturation of the megakaryocyte. Another factor, megakaryocyte colony-stimulating activity (Meg-CSA), appears to control cell proliferation and may determine which of the undifferentiated stem cells mature into megakaryocytes.[19] Megakaryocytes undergo endomitosis, in which nuclear divisions occur without cell division and are followed by nuclear fusion, to yield a cell with a chromosomal content of 8n, 16n, or 32n. In response to an unknown signal, the megakaryocyte cytoplasm changes into a series of thin, cylindrical strands, which then develop a beaded appearance. These constrictions along the tubelike protrusions become more pronounced, and eventually, the strands fragment into pieces of megakaryocytes that have the approximate dimensions of platelets.[20] Megakaryocyte volume correlates with ploidy and cytoplasmic maturity; the largest megakaryocytes produce the greatest number of platelets.

Large platelets called megathrombocytes are seen in the peripheral blood in thrombocytopenic states, especially in idiopathic thrombocytopenic purpura (ITP). There is much debate about whether or not megathrombocytes are young platelets. Some very large platelets that are seen in patients recovering from immune thrombocytopenia may be incompletely separated, beaded strands derived from rapidly maturing megakaryocytes.[21] The presence of such so-called proplatelets could account for the increase in mean platelet volume that occurs during response to, or recovery from, acute thrombocytopenia.

Platelets entering the circulation survive about 8.5 to 10 days and have a half-life of about four days. Approximately 30 to 40 percent of the platelets are present in a splenic pool that can freely exchange with the circulation.[22] When the need for platelets arises, production can increase sevenfold to eightfold. Because there is no marrow pool of platelets waiting to be released, increasing requirements for platelets must be met by increased synthesis. Megakaryocyte maturation time does not appear to be shortened, but megakaryocyte volume may increase under circumstances of platelet need. Presumably, an enhanced influx of committed cells from the proliferating stem cell pool, and perhaps an increase in megakaryocytic volume, brings about an increased number of platelets.

The platelet is a highly evolved, specialized structure. The platelet glycoprotein Ib (GPIb) is the molecule on activated platelets that binds the larger multimers of von Willebrand factor; this glycoprotein is absent in Bernard-Soulier syndrome.[11,23] Platelet adhesion to the subendothelium in the presence of a high shear rate probably depends on a bridging action by vWF between the subendothelium and the GPIb of activated platelets.[11,23] Two other platelet glycoproteins, GPIIb and GPIIIa, exist as a calcium-dependent heterodimer, termed GPIIb/IIIa, in the platelet plasma membrane. On platelet activation, these dimers form aggregates. The glycoprotein GPIIIa contains a major platelet antigen termed Pl[A1] (now termed Zw[a]).[12] GPIIb/IIIa is absent from the platelets of patients with Glanzmann's thrombasthenia. When the platelet is activated by ADP or perhaps thrombin, GPIIb/IIIa apparently forms the platelet receptor for fibrinogen, which then induces platelet aggregation. In addition, a glycoprotein termed thrombospondin[24] that is released from alpha granules may act as the endogenous platelet ligand, forming a complex with fibrinogen and thereby stabilizing the platelet aggregates. Platelet aggregation that occurs at high shear rates appears to require an interaction between the larger von Willebrand factor multimers and both GPIb and GPIIb/IIIa.[25,26]

After adhering to the subendothelium, the platelet changes from a disk to a sphere and begins to release its granular contents. In addition to thrombospondin, the alpha granules contain von Willebrand factor, fibrinogen, fibronectin, high molecular weight kininogen, platelet factor 4 (PF4), albumin, β-thromboglobulin, histidine-rich glycoprotein, platelet-derived growth factor (PDGF), and transforming growth factor-β (TGF-β). PDGF acts as a chemoattractant for fibroblasts and stimulates their growth. TGF-β causes a rapid angiogenic and fibrogenic response and can control the response of cells to other growth factors.[27] PF4 is an antiheparin. Its strongly cationic structure may facilitate binding to the vessel wall, where it may partially neutralize the electrostatic repulsion that limits cell contact. The dense granules carry calcium, pyrophosphate, serotonin, ADP, and ATP. Lysosomes, which contain the acid hydrolases, are also present in platelets.[11]

When appropriate concentrations of ADP are added to citrated platelets in vitro, there is a wave of aggregation, followed momentarily by a second wave. The second wave of aggregation is stimulated by the substances released from the platelets involved in the initial ADP-induced aggregation [see Figure 5].[28]

The mechanisms underlying both release and aggregation appear to depend on the formation of cyclic endoperoxides [see Figure 6]. The enzyme phospholipase A₂ initiates this process by catalyzing the formation of arachidonic acid, a precursor of cyclic endoperoxides, from platelet phospholipids. Thrombin, however, can induce platelet release at a concentration lower than that required to activate phospholipase A₂, which indicates that release can probably also proceed by an alternate pathway. Both cyclic endoperoxides and thromboxane A₂ are potent inducers of release and aggregation. Because cyclic AMP (cAMP) blocks the production of arachidonate from platelet phospholipids,[29,30] elevation of cAMP levels by prostaglandin E₁ (PGE₁) synthesis, by increased adenyl cyclase activity, or by decreased phosphodiesterase activity inhibits aggregation and release.

Clot retraction is mediated by platelet actomyosin, which on platelet activation attaches to the cytosolic extension of GPIIb/IIIa. Platelets help to maintain the integrity of small vessels, and in thrombocytopenic states, red blood cells seem to leak through vessel walls. Platelets play a key role in hemostasis by providing specific surface features that are used by the intrinsic and extrinsic systems of coagulation.[4]

Endothelial cells in culture produce a unique prostaglandin, PGI2 or prostacyclin, by metabolizing the cyclic endoperoxide PGH₂. Prostacyclin is a potent inhibitor of platelet aggregation and a very potent vasodilator. It probably plays an important role in preventing thrombus formation. The potent platelet aggregator and vasoconstrictor thromboxane A₂ is also formed from PGH₂ in platelets [see Figure 6]. Therefore, the synthesis of prostacyclin and thromboxane A₂, compounds that have opposing effects on platelets and vessel walls, proceeds by remarkably similar pathways.[31]

Coagulation Tests and Their Use

Tests of Procoagulants

A few coagulation tests can provide effective screening of procoagulant function. Most of these tests are based on measure-

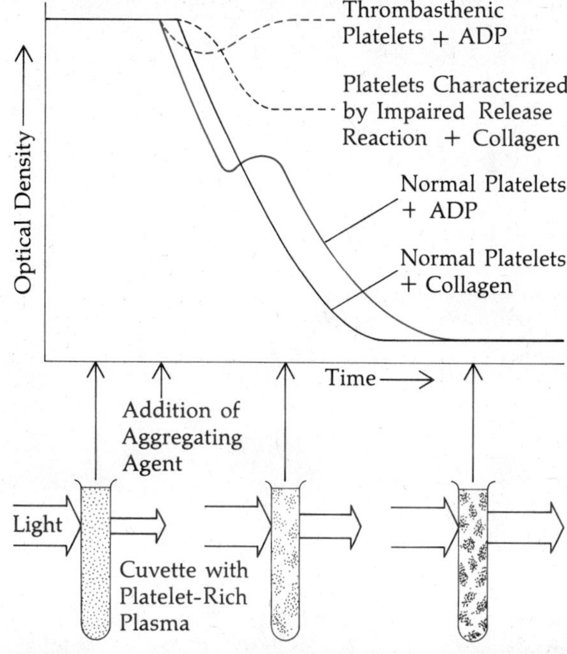

Figure 5 *The platelet aggregation test measures the amount of light absorbed by a cuvette of stirred, platelet-rich plasma. After the addition of an agent such as ADP, collagen, or epinephrine, light absorption changes with time, as shown by a characteristic curve. Aggregation with ADP is reduced in thrombasthenic platelets (dotted colored line) as compared with normal platelets (solid colored line). Second-wave aggregation is normally caused by ADP. Collagen induces the release reaction, which then leads to aggregation of normal platelets (solid black curve). Platelets that have defects involving the release mechanism will show impaired collagen aggregation (black dotted line).*

ments of the time required to form fibrin strands, which can be detected by either optical or electric devices. In each case, unusual prolongation of a test time may represent an abnormally low factor concentration [*see Table 1*], the presence of a biologically inactive factor or factors, or the presence of inhibitors.

Partial thromboplastin time (PTT) The PTT tests the intrinsic coagulation system [*see Figure 1*]. Kaolin, which provides a foreign surface, is added to whole plasma six minutes prior to the test to provide maximal surface activation of Factors XII and XI. Cephalin, a platelet lipid surrogate, is then added to the plasma, and the time required to produce fibrin is recorded. The values for a normal PTT vary in different laboratories but generally range from 25 to 39 seconds. This broad normal range makes it impractical to express the PTT in terms of percent of a normal value. Because the normal prothrombin time is 10 seconds and the time required to form a clot on addition of opti-

mal amounts of thrombin to plasma is six seconds, it is clear that much of the PTT is devoted to the sequence preceding Factor X activation [*see Figure 1*]. The PTT is most sensitive to abnormalities and deficiencies in the sequence of procoagulant activations that occur prior to Factor X activation.

Quick's one-stage prothrombin time (PT) The PT is a test of the extrinsic system. Tissue factor is added to whole plasma, and the resulting fibrin is normally measured in nine to 10 seconds. The PT is usually reported in seconds, but time-activity curves based on commercial standards can also be used to express the PT as the percent of a normal plasma pool response. A third reporting method expresses the result as a ratio related to a normal control value. Thus, a ratio of 2 would be reported if the patient had a prothrombin time of 20 seconds and the control value was 10 seconds. To circumvent the difficulties arising from different laboratory techniques and reporting methods, it has been proposed that all labora-

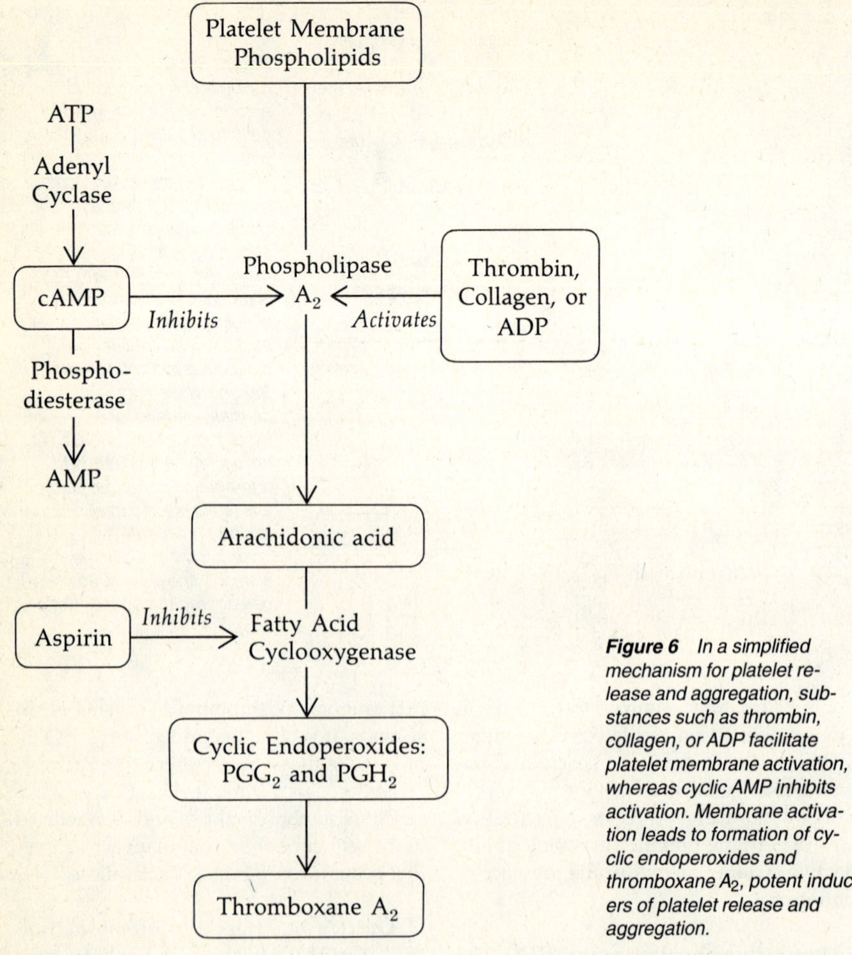

Figure 6 *In a simplified mechanism for platelet release and aggregation, substances such as thrombin, collagen, or ADP facilitate platelet membrane activation, whereas cyclic AMP inhibits activation. Membrane activation leads to formation of cyclic endoperoxides and thromboxane A₂, potent inducers of platelet release and aggregation.*

tories use a United Kingdom source of human thromboplastin and report their results as the international normalized ratio (INR).

The PT can detect deficiencies in Factors I, II, V, VII, and X. Antagonists of the extrinsic coagulation system, including heparin-activated antithrombin III or fibrin degradation products, can prolong the PT.

Prothrombin and proconvertin time (P and P) The P and P is not widely available, but it is very useful for investigating an abnormality detected in the PT. In the P and P,

plasma is diluted $1:10$, thereby decreasing the effects of heparin or fibrin degradation products. Sources of Factors I and V are added to the reaction; hence, the P and P is sensitive to deficiencies of Factors II, VII, and X.

If the PT and the P and P are equally prolonged, there is probably a deficiency of Factor II, VII, or X. If the PT is more prolonged than the P and P, Factors I and V are probably abnormal or inhibitors of the conversion of fibrinogen to fibrin are present. Such inhibitors include fibrin degradation products or heparin-activated antithrombin

III. The P and P is reported both in seconds and as percent of normal.

Thrombin time (TT) The TT is used to test abnormalities affecting the conversion of fibrinogen to fibrin. When optimal amounts of thrombin are added to plasma, fibrin appears in five to six seconds. Because thrombin is such a powerful enzyme, it can overwhelm inhibitors in vitro. If, however, dilutions of thrombin are added to plasma until the normal TT becomes about 16 seconds, inhibitors of fibrinogen-fibrin conversion, such as fibrin degradation products or AT-III–heparin cofactor, can distinctly prolong the TT. Patients with dysfibrinogenemia and paraproteinemias may also have prolonged thrombin times.

Reptilase time (RT) Reptilase is a thrombinlike enzyme that converts fibrinogen to fibrin but is not affected by the antithrombin III–heparin complex. RT is also affected less than the thrombin time by the presence of fibrin-fibrinogen degradation products. The effect of dysfibrinogenemic states on the RT, however, is more pronounced than on the thrombin time. A long thrombin time and normal RT suggest heparin effect.[32] Some clinical laboratories use commercially available adsorption columns that remove heparin to determine if an abnormal test result is caused by this anticoagulant.

Tests of thrombin action Because thrombin plays a key role in coagulation by affecting platelets, fibrinogen, and Factors V, VIII, and XIII, tests have been designed to measure thrombin action. Thrombin acts primarily on fibrinogen by splitting off two molecules each of the fibrinopeptides A and B, leaving one molecule of the fibrin monomer. Attempts to measure the circulating monomer using the ethanol gelation test or the plasma protamine paracoagulation test (PPP) generally have not been successful. A radioimmunoassay for fibrinopeptide A has been described as an index of recent thrombin action. This test can be used to assess thrombin activity in a syringe. Measurements of fibrinopeptide A may provide an effective index of thrombin generation or thrombin activity.[33]

Fibrinogen Fibrinogen, or Factor I, is present in amounts that can be measured chemically, and the results are generally reported in terms of mg/dl.

Fibrin-fibrinogen degradation products The fibrinolytic system is activated by the same factors that initiate coagulation [*see Figures 1 and 3*]. Plasmin attacks both fibrinogen and fibrin, producing fibrin-fibrinogen split products (FDP or FSP), which can be detected by a variety of techniques. A common method used to detect FDP is to measure immunologically identifiable fibrinogen and fibrin in serum. A high titer of fibrin degradation products does not prove that extensive hyperplasminemia, as occurs in disseminated intravascular coagulation (DIC), is present, because extensive injuries or inflammatory disease may also elevate FDP. A more accurate test for split products detects fibrin D dimer, a fragment that is released by the plasmin-mediated degradation of fully polymerized fibrin. Because intravascular coagulation generates fully polymerized fibrin, detection of the fibrin D dimer indicates that intravascular coagulation, followed by plasmin action, has occurred. Plasmin cleavage of fibrinogen or soluble fibrin monomer in cases of primary fibrinolysis does not yield the D dimer [*see Figure 1*].[3]

Factor XIII Factor XIII can be assayed by measuring the solubility of a clot in urea. Because only a few percent of the normal amount of Factor XIII can give a normal result, this test should not be used if the patient has been transfused within the previous two to three weeks.

Plasminogen, plasmin action, and α_2-antiplasmin tests The activation of the plasminogen-plasmin system can be inferred from the findings of a long thrombin time, a low fibrinogen level, and a raised level of fibrin degradation products. Another crude test used to measure plasminogen-plasmin activation is the euglobulin lysis time. In this test, a variant of the clot lysis time, the inhibitors of fibrinolysis have been substantially removed so as to shorten the time required to complete the assay.

It is now possible to measure plasmin and the specific plasmin inhibitor α_2-antiplasmin directly. During extensive thrombosis and fibrinolysis, plasminogen is consumed as it binds to fibrin and is activated by the several plasminogen activators [*see Figure 3*]. If utilization exceeds production, plasminogen levels fall. In primary fibrinolysis, the elevated levels of circulating plasmin are opposed by α_2-antiplasmin. This inhibitor inactivates plasmin by forming a stable inert complex with it, and if the level of hyperplasminemia exceeds the level of α_2-antiplasmin production, the plasma level of the inhibitor will fall. Therefore, low levels of α_2-antiplasmin usually signal hyperplasminemia. Another test of plasmin action, available thus far only in research laboratories, detects the presence in plasma of the peptide fragment $B_{\beta1-42}$ [*see Figure 1*], which is formed by the proteolytic action of plasmin on soluble fibrin polymer.[3]

Tests of Platelets and of Platelet Function

Peripheral smear evaluation Examination of the peripheral smear provides quick, definitive information. On a well-stained normal smear, there will be eight to 12 platelets per high-power (1,000×) magnification field, corresponding to a normal platelet count of 150,000 to 300,000/mm³. The peripheral smear can be examined to determine the extent of platelet granularity and whether megathrombocytes are present.

Bleeding time A carefully performed, standardized bleeding time provides useful information about platelet count and platelet function. A spring-loaded device that is generally available can be used to make a standard incision under a standard head of capillary pressure. The bleeding time is usu-

ally normal at platelet counts greater than 100,000/mm³ and is prolonged in an inverse linear fashion when related to lower counts. A prolonged bleeding time at a platelet count greater than 100,000 indicates impaired platelet function.

Clot retraction Clot retraction is a crude method that can be used to evaluate the function of the platelet contractile mechanism.

Platelet factor 3 There are cumbersome methods for assaying platelet factor 3, the lipid made available by the platelets for coagulation at the point of interaction of Factors IXa, VIII, and X and at the point of interaction of Factors Xa, V, and II [*see Figure 1*]. The test is rarely clinically useful.

Platelet aggregometry Platelet aggregometers are simple devices for recording the transmission of light through a suspension of platelets. When platelets aggregate, light passes through the suspension more readily. To test aggregation, dilute concentrations of ADP are added to citrated platelet-rich plasma. Addition of epinephrine or collagen causes second-wave aggregation, reflecting the induction of the release reaction and indicating the status of the platelet nucleotide stores [*see Figure 5*]. Ristocetin aggregates platelets in the presence of a plasma factor lacking in many patients with von Willebrand's disease.

Tests of Inhibitors of Hemostasis

Antithrombin III Both bioassays and immunoassays are available for assessing AT-III activity.[34] It is important to have two types of assays because some patients who appear to have normal levels of AT-III by immunologic tests are shown to have abnormal AT-III levels when the factor is measured by functional assays.

Protein C and protein S Both functional and immunologic methods are now commercially available for measuring these vitamin K–dependent modulators of coagulation. Both types of tests are useful, especially for the evaluation of protein S deficiency.[6] Protein C and protein S levels can be measured even in patients who have liver disease or who are taking warfarin. If notified in advance, a laboratory can report the level of protein C or protein S relative to the level of either prothrombin or Factor X, accurately determined by the enzyme-linked immunosorbent assay (ELISA). If the protein C or protein S level is depressed as a result of liver disease or the ingestion of a vitamin K antagonist such as warfarin, then the ratio of either of these anticoagulants to prothrombin or Factor X will be about 1; however, if the patient has an underlying deficiency of protein C or S, the ratio will be considerably less than 1.

Approach to the Patient with a Hemorrhagic or Thrombotic Disorder

Clinical clues guide the diagnosis. It is critical to distinguish hereditary hemorrhagic disorders from acquired disorders. Therefore, questions about bleeding at circumcision, bleeding after surgery, and especially bleeding during dental extractions are helpful. Absence of significant bleeding at the time of removal of impacted wisdom teeth is strong evidence against congenital hemorrhagic disorders. Petechial bleeding suggests thrombocytopenia or vascular disorders and is apt to occur on the lower legs or on the buccal membranes. Mucosal bleeding can result from thrombocytopenia or warfarin overdose. Deep tissue bleeding, typically in the form of hemarthroses, is seen in hemophiliacs. Aspirin can significantly impair hemostasis by inhibiting platelet cyclooxygenase [*see Figure 6*]. A problem arises in identifying aspirin as the cause of a hemorrhagic disorder because several hundred formulations contain aspirin, but very often, the name of the preparation provides no clue as to its aspirin content.

In patients with thrombotic disorders, the history should focus on smoking habits and hypertension, as well as thromboses after childbirth, surgery, and orthopedic procedures. Other important clinical clues to the diagnosis include a history of use of estrogen-containing oral contraceptives, a family history of recurrent venous thromboembolism, or thromboembolism beginning in youth. An atypical site of thrombosis suggests the existence of an underlying hypercoagulable state. Hepatic vein thrombosis, mesenteric vein thrombosis, or skin necrosis following the administration of warfarin should prompt a search for a hypercoagulable disorder; spontaneous axillary vein thrombosis may also indicate the presence of such a state [*see* Hypercoagulable States, *below*].

Decreased Platelet Count—Thrombocytopenia

Thrombocytopenia may be caused by abnormal platelet production, accelerated platelet removal resulting from immunologic or nonimmunologic mechanisms, sequestration of platelets in the spleen, or combinations of these mechanisms.

The clinical presentation of thrombocytopenia varies depending on such factors as the presence or absence of pancytopenia and the etiology of the disorder. The hallmark of thrombocytopenia is petechiae, which reflect bleeding probably at the level of the capillary or postcapillary venule. Petechiae usually occur at sites of increased intravascular pressure. For example, they develop over the lower extremities, presumably because of the elevated hydrostatic pressure in the veins of the legs; they appear on the oral mucosa of the cheeks because the masseters generate enormous force on the mucosa during chewing; and they are found at sites where constricting items of clothing, such as brassiere straps, produce an increase in intravascular pressure.

If the platelet count is very low, purpura, mucosal bleeding, and even deep tissue bleeding may also be seen. There is no sharp threshold level of platelets above which patients can be considered safe from thrombocytopenic bleeding. Generally, patients with idiopathic thrombocytopenic purpura bleed less at a given platelet level than patients with aplastic anemia. Measurements of mean platelet volume using automated blood cell counters have clarified this matter. Patients with severe thrombocytopenia (i.e., a platelet level < 20,000/mm^3) who have a low platelet volume (< 6.4 femtoliters per platelet) bleed significantly more than patients with larger platelet volumes. Larger platelets are released into the circulation when platelets are being rapidly regenerated, as would occur in ITP or during recovery from marrow suppression. Presumably, the larger platelets play a more effective role in hemostasis because they are more active metabolically.[35] Elderly patients and patients with other illnesses bleed more than young patients and patients with thrombocytopenia alone. An associated disorder, such as liver dysfunction or connective tissue disease, increases the risk of serious bleeding. Petechiae or purpura alone is rarely a cause for significant clinical concern. Occasionally, vaginal bleeding from ITP can be severe, but the principal hazard is intracranial hemorrhage, and this overriding concern directs therapy.

Consideration of the common clinical causes of thrombocytopenia [*see Table 2*] provides a framework for differential diagnosis. The patient should be questioned about history of drug use (including intravenous substance abuse), about patterns of sexual activity, and about transfusion history; the patient should also be examined for evidence of anemia, neutropenic infection, connective tissue disease, lymphoma, or an immunocompromised state. The evaluation of spleen size merits special attention. The peripheral smear quickly establishes the presence of thrombocytopenia, reveals platelet morphologic abnormalities, and indicates whether polychromatophilia, neutropenia, lymphopenia, spherocytosis, blasts, or fragmented microangiopathic erythrocytes are present. The platelet count, complete blood count, and reticulocyte count confirm the extent of thrombocytopenia, indicate the rate of red blood cell regeneration if anemia is present, and reveal any white blood cell abnormalities. The mean platelet volume, as determined by automated blood cell counters, may provide an additional clue to the cause of the thrombocytopenia. Low platelet volumes (< 6.4 femtoliters) suggest poor production, whereas larger volumes indicate rapid platelet regeneration or dysplastic platelet production.[35] A marrow aspiration with or without Jamshidi biopsy is critical for differential diagnosis.

Platelet Production Defects

The finding of a hypoplastic marrow in which the total cellularity is reduced with a concomitant decrease in megakaryocytes implies aplastic anemia. Drug toxicity should be investigated. A marrow that is fibrosed or infiltrated with leukemic or other malignant cells represents the syndrome of pancytopenia from infiltrated marrow.

A marrow biopsy showing normal cellularity and normal maturation of the erythroid and myeloid precursors with decreased numbers of apparently normal megakaryocytes suggests that the patient has ingested a drug, such as ethanol, that specifically affects the committed megakaryocytic progenitor cells or precursor cells in that line.[19,36-39] Ethanol also produces ineffective megakaryopoiesis.[19] Whether gold has general pancytopenic effects or selectively depresses megakaryocytic lines is unclear. Drug ingestion can also cause thrombocytopenia by increasing platelet removal, in which case, the number of megakaryocytes may be increased.

In vitamin B_{12} deficiency and folate deficiency, all three marrow lines are affected. Consequently, besides megaloblastic ineffective erythropoiesis, affected patients also have ineffective megakaryopoiesis, and their marrow smear shows many large hyperlobated megakaryocytes. Some myeloproliferative disorders are characterized by ineffective megakaryopoiesis with bizarre binucleate megakaryocytes.

Management

If an offending agent is identified, it should be discontinued. Dimercaprol (BAL in Oil) has been used to treat gold-induced thrombocytopenia but with only occasional

Table 2 Causes of Thrombocytopenia

Type	Disorder	Cause
Platelet production abnormalities	Marrow aplasia or hypoplasia, pancytopenia	Radiation Drug-induced: cytotoxic or other drugs Idiopathic
	Marrow infiltration, pancytopenia	Cancer Fibrosis
	Selective impairment of platelet production	Drug-induced: gold, sulfonamides, ethanol, thiazides, phenylbutazone, trimethoprim-sulfamethoxazole Infections: childhood rubella ? Heatstroke
	Ineffective megakaryopoiesis	Vitamin B_{12} deficiency Folic acid deficiency Myeloproliferative diseases Alcohol abuse
	Congenital or acquired platelet production deficiencies	—
Accelerated platelet removal	Immune destruction	Autoantibodies: idiopathic thrombocytopenic purpura (ITP), systemic lupus erythematosus, certain lymphomas, ITP associated with Coombs'-positive hemolytic anemia (Evans' syndrome) Proved drug antibodies: quinidine, quinine Infections: infectious mononucleosis, malaria, gram-negative septicemia, ? varicella Suspected drug antibodies: thiazide diuretics, aminosalicylic acid, acetaminophen, diazepam, sulfisoxazole, phenytoin, heparin[38] Posttransfusion purpura
	Nonimmunologic removal	Disseminated intravascular coagulation, preeclampsia, vasculitis Microangiopathic hemolytic anemia, severe vascular injury, hemolytic-uremic syndrome, thrombotic thrombocytopenic purpura Drug-induced: ristocetin, ? heparin Platelet washout by massive transfusion with stored blood Giant hemangiomas ? Gram-negative septicemia
Platelet sequestration	Hypersplenism	Enlarged spleen (holds 50% to 80% of platelets, instead of normal capacity of 20% to 30%; exchange with circulating platelets is possible)

reports of objective benefit. Specific replacement is required for deficiencies of vitamin B_{12} and folate.

When the thrombocytopenia is causing significant bleeding, platelet replacement will be required until the situation can be aided by other forms of therapy. Each unit of transfused random-donor platelet concentrate raises the platelet count by about $10,000/mm^3/m^2$ of body surface area. Therefore, the administration of five or six platelet packs should increase the platelet count by about 40,000 to $50,000/mm^3$. Half of the transfused platelets will still be circulating in about 24 hours. Such platelet transfusion, given two or three times a week, should be continued to prevent bleeding until the situation improves or until the patient becomes platelet alloimmunized. Continuous administration of prednisone in daily dosages of 20 to 30 mg has been advocated to maintain vascular integrity, but in view of the unproved efficacy and undesirable side effects of corticosteroids, it is questionable whether they should be used.

Accelerated Platelet Removal Due to Immune Destruction

When a patient has thrombocytopenia despite an abundance of normal megakaryocytes in the marrow, it is likely that the mechanism of the disorder is accelerated platelet removal. Such tests as ^{51}Cr-tagged platelet survival or other platelet kinetic measurements, if available, can document the rate of platelet loss. Normally, platelets survive for 10 days and have a half-life of about four days; in accelerated removal states, such as ITP, the platelet half-life may be as short as 30 to 60 minutes. The platelet count will then reflect the balance achieved between accelerated platelet removal and compensatory megakaryopoiesis, which can increase to approximately sevenfold its normal value.

Platelet survival studies are not generally available and are not usually required to determine whether accelerated platelet removal is occurring. In cases in which the mechanism of thrombocytopenia is in doubt, infusion of random-donor platelets can be used as a diagnostic and therapeutic procedure. When accelerated platelet removal is responsible for the thrombocytopenia, transfusion with six platelet packs only slightly elevates the platelet count, which then returns to base-line values in less than 24 hours. This therapeutic test becomes unreliable, however, if the patient has been previously platelet alloimmunized by blood or platelet transfusions or by multiple pregnancies.

When accelerated removal appears to be the cause of the patient's thrombocytopenia, a rapid differential diagnosis should be made [*see Table* 2]. A history of drug use is critical, as is a history of systemic lupus erythematosus, lymphoma, or Coombs'-positive acquired hemolytic anemia. Similarly, infections such as septicemia, varicella, infectious mononucleosis, or infection with human immunodeficiency virus (HIV) may be etiologically important. Concurrent abnormalities of procoagulant tests indicate disseminated intravascular coagulation, whereas evidence of intravascular hemolysis with microangiopathic red blood cells suggests vascular injury, as may occur in thrombotic thrombocytopenic purpura or the hemolytic-uremic syndrome.

Idiopathic Thrombocytopenic Purpura/Autoimmune Thrombocytopenic Purpura (ITP/ATP)

Pathophysiology In 1951, in an attempt to determine the basis for idiopathic thrombocytopenic purpura, the American hematologist William Harrington infused himself with plasma from a patient with this disorder. The fact that severe thrombocytopenia subsequently developed strongly suggested that a circulating destructive antiplatelet factor was involved. The observation that mothers with ITP frequently delivered thrombocytopenic babies also tended to support this hypothesis. Subsequent studies[40] have shown that about 90 percent of patients diagnosed as having ITP have increased amounts of immunoglobulins bound to their platelets, so-called platelet-associated IgG (PA-IgG).[41] The platelet IgG level corresponds directly to the severity of the thrombocytopenia.[41] Although accelerated platelet destruction is the key pathophysiologic event in ITP, depressed platelet production contributes to the severity of the thrombocytopenia in many patients.[42]

Most often, the immunoglobulin on the platelet membrane is IgG, but when the antibody density is sufficiently great, complement may be fixed as well. Occasionally, IgA and IgM antibodies are also found. IgG1 is the most common IgG subclass found on ITP/ATP platelets, but IgG2, IgG3, and IgG4 also occur; subclass IgG3 produces more severe disease. These antibodies are not adsorbed as an immune complex onto the platelet surface, where binding to the platelet Fc sites would occur, but rather are fixed to the platelet membrane by their Fab portions and appear to be directed against platelet membrane antigens.

Circulating immune complexes occur frequently in idiopathic thrombocytopenic purpura[43] and may reflect the binding of antiplatelet antibody to solubilized platelet antigens. Such immune complexes may then bind to the platelet Fc receptors. Binding of immune complexes to platelets may exert no pathologic effect, may enhance macrophagic attack, or may even be the major mechanism inducing the macrophagic attack and destruction of the coated platelets. Circulating immune complexes are common in patients with ITP who are at risk for the acquired immunodeficiency syndrome (AIDS). In addition, many of these patients have a circulating IgG that has anti-F(ab')₂ activity. The significance of these findings is unknown.[44]

These antiplatelet antibodies may also be present in the serum, but they are not always detected in serum assays, perhaps because such assays are technically difficult to perform or because the antibody has such great avidity for platelets that little is left free in solution in the serum. Not all ITP/ATP antibodies are directed against the same antigen; however, the antigens must be shared by most platelets because most ITP antibodies react with most normal platelets. Platelets from patients with Glanzmann's thrombasthenia are deficient in glycoprotein IIb/IIIa. The fact that some ITP antibodies react poorly with such platelets implies that glycoprotein IIb/IIIa may be part of the antigen system that binds PA-IgG. In one study, the antiplatelet antibody in homosexual men with ITP was found to be bound via its F(ab')₂ site to a unique 25,000 dalton platelet membrane antigen, but the function of this antigen is unknown.[45]

Although the antiplatelet antibody is made predominantly in splenic lymphoid cells, it is also synthesized by marrow lymphocytes, a finding that partially accounts for the complex effects of splenectomy. PA-IgG causes the affected platelet to be trapped and destroyed extravascularly in the monocyte-macrophage system. This system recognizes either the Fc portion of the bound antibody or C3b if complement is also fixed. Splenic macrophages are most active in platelet removal and destruction because normally more than one third of the platelets are located in the spleen, splenic blood flow is slow, and the antiplatelet antibody is made locally.[43,46] Hepatic macrophages can also remove antibody-coated platelets but do so only in severe disease.[47]

Idiopathic thrombocytopenic purpura is therefore characterized primarily by rapid platelet destruction. The marrow responds to the thrombocytopenia, particularly when severe, by increasing platelet production. Measurements indicate, however, that the marrow may only increase platelet production by 2.3- to 5.0-fold instead of mounting the theoretical maximal sevenfold increase.[43] It appears that the same antiplatelet antibodies also react with megakaryocyte antigens, which presumably resemble the platelet antigen. This antigen-antibody reaction could hamper megakaryopoiesis and thus partially explain the suboptimal marrow response. In fact, there have been reports of patients with apparent ITP who had no identifiable megakaryocytes in their marrow.[48] In such cases, the antiplatelet antibody inhibited the growth of megakaryocyte colony-forming units.[49]

There may be a genetic predisposition for the development of idiopathic thrombocytopenic purpura, but HLA studies have not yet resolved this issue. Certainly, the finding of ITP in both members of a pair of monozygotic twins suggests a genetic basis for the disease.[50]

Most often, the platelets produced in idiopathic thrombocytopenic purpura are large and very active metabolically; they are also effective in controlling the bleeding time.[46,51] On occasion, however, platelets in patients with idiopathic thrombocytopenic purpura are reported to function abnormally. A patient with ITP who has a platelet count of 50,000 to 100,000/mm^3 and clinical bleeding will probably show a prolonged bleeding time, which indicates the presence of a platelet functional abnormality. In one study, the platelets of three patients with such clinical findings showed abnormal aggregation and disturbances in the metabolism of arachidonic acid to thromboxane A_2.[46,52] Studies of other patients with ITP and abnormal platelets revealed the presence of autoantibodies directed against platelet membrane component GPIb or GPIIb/IIIa that inhibited platelet adhesion or aggregation.[41]

Occasionally, apparent clinical remissions occur in patients who have idiopathic thrombocytopenic purpura. At such times, platelet counts return to normal despite continued accelerated platelet removal.[51] This situation, which is termed compensated thrombolysis, can be compared conceptually with compensated hemolysis. Its existence probably explains the spontaneous remissions and exacerbations that characterize the clinical course of the chronic disorder. When platelets are being removed at an accelerated rate, even a minor variation in platelet production, perhaps caused by drugs or by certain viral infections, can precipitate a clinical relapse. Also, the enhanced function of monocytes during viral infections can further accelerate platelet removal, thereby accounting for such relapses.[43] Similarly, infection may enhance the production of platelet autoantibody by causing polyclonal B cell activation.[41]

Diagnosis Idiopathic thrombocytopenic purpura/autoimmune thrombocytopenic purpura typically appears in young women, but other groups can also be affected. The AIDS epidemic has had a major effect on the prevalence of this disease. In some communities, the prevalence of ITP in young women has been superseded by its occurrence in male patients who are seropositive for HIV infection. Such patients include hemophiliacs who are dependent on transfusions, homosexuals, and intravenous drug abusers.[53,54] There is no relevant history of drug ingestion. Infectious mononucleosis may contribute to autoimmune platelet destruction, and it is important to look for clinical evidence of this disorder.[46] Graves' disease and Hashimoto's thyroiditis are also associated with ITP/ATP.[55,56] Some investigators even recommend doing thyroid function tests on all patients with ITP to avoid performing a splenectomy on a patient with undiagnosed hyperthyroidism.

Uterine bleeding may be extensive in affected women. Blood blisters in the mouth indicate severe thrombocytopenia. Retinal hemorrhages are uncommon. All patients should receive a careful neurologic assessment because of the possibility of central nervous system bleeding.

The spleen is not palpable in classic uncomplicated idiopathic thrombocytopenic purpura. The presence of a palpable spleen raises the possibility that systemic lupus erythematosus, lymphoma, Evans' syndrome, infectious mononucleosis, or hypersplenism may be the source of the thrombocytopenia.

The peripheral smear shows no abnormalities of white cells or red cells unless mucosal bleeding has been significant enough to produce iron deficiency; the few platelets that are present are large and well granulated. The marrow shows abundant megakaryocytes, many of which are young; erythroid and myeloid precursors remain normal. The results of tests for systemic lupus erythematosus are negative.

Platelet-associated immunoglobulin G levels are elevated, but they are also elevated in other forms of thrombocytopenic purpura. The usefulness of tests for PA-IgG in the diagnosis of ITP is a matter of considerable debate. Although the sensitivity of the various tests is about 90 percent, their specificity is only about 25 percent.[41] Therefore, several authorities do not consider the PA-IgG test to be clinically useful.[41,57] Other investigators, however, believe that careful measurement of PA-IgG can distinguish between immune and nonimmune thrombocytopenia.[58] Tests of PA-IgG are usually not needed, because the diagnosis of ITP is often straightforward: clinically significant thrombocytopenia despite normal to increased numbers of normal-appearing megakaryocytes in the marrow in the absence of the characteristic clinical findings (see above).[57] It is in those cases in which the diagnosis of ITP may be in question that the test for PA-IgG becomes less discriminatory.

Acute idiopathic thrombocytopenic purpura is usually confined to children and young adults and is frequently preceded by a viral illness. Permanent spontaneous remission occurs in less than three months. Chronic idiopathic thrombocytopenic purpura, the usual adult variety, refers to disease that persists for more than three months. Although spontaneous remissions and relapses do occur in chronic idiopathic thrombocytopenic purpura, long-term spontaneous remissions are uncommon.

Management Idiopathic thrombocytopenic purpura is a relatively benign disorder that has a mortality of approximately one to five percent; most deaths result from intracranial bleeding.[43,46] The therapeutic approach varies depending on whether the patient presents with petechiae alone, with moderate mucosal bleeding, or with severe mucosal or central nervous system bleeding. Different modalities may also be required to manage patients who have refractory ITP or ITP in pregnancy.

Presentation with petechiae alone (dry purpura) Patients with petechiae alone do not require active therapy. They may be followed and simply alerted to report any mucosal bleeding or crops of new petechiae so that therapy can be instituted immediately if their condition should deteriorate. Bacterial or viral infection may provoke a relapse by causing macrophagic activation, megakaryocytic suppression, or enhancement of B cell activity.[41] Avoidance of aspirin is advised.

Presentation with moderate mucosal bleeding (wet purpura) Therapy for patients with moderate mucosal bleeding is begun with corticosteroids—for example, prednisone at a daily dosage of 60 to 100 mg in divided doses. Unless bleeding is severe, the patient need not be hospitalized and may rest at home. Heavy physical activity, particularly any activity that involves the Valsalva maneuver, should be avoided so as not to increase intracranial pressure. The avoidance of aspirin and other antiplatelet agents should be emphasized. If required, red blood cell transfusions can be given, but it is rarely necessary to transfuse platelets in such cases.

Corticosteroids interfere with the macrophagic attack on platelets and eventually reduce the amount of antiplatelet antibody produced by splenic and marrow lymphoid cells. The platelet count usually rises several days to two to three weeks following the start of therapy. When the platelet count reaches normal levels, the corticosteroids can be tapered over a three- to four-week period. Although some investigators have reported complete, long-term remissions with corticosteroid therapy alone in up to 20 percent of cases,[43,46] we have rarely seen such responses at Stanford University Hospital.

Splenectomy is indicated when the platelet count begins to fall again. The procedure produces long-standing remission in 65 to 80 percent of patients with ITP.[43,46,59] It is best to resume corticosteroids prior to splenectomy so that the patient will have a platelet count of at least 30,000 to 50,000/mm^3 at the time of surgery. The platelet count usually begins to rise on the first postoperative day, often overshooting normal values by the second week. Although there are conflicting reports in the literature, I do not believe that measurements of the splenic sequestration of radioisotope-labeled platelets can accurately predict the success or failure of splenectomy. The effectiveness of splenectomy depends not only on the elimination of the unique filtering trap of the spleen but also on the removal of the pool of splenic lymphoid cells that are a major source of the antiplatelet antibody.[60]

If the patient is elderly or frail and hence may not withstand splenectomy, one can try to control the disease by administering the minimum amount of corticosteroids required to raise the platelet count to 30,000 to 50,000/mm^3, a level above which severe bleeding rarely occurs. Alternatively, one can administer 1 to 2 mg of vincristine intravenously at five- to seven-day intervals. If a response is to occur, it will develop in approximately three to six weeks; thus, prolonging vincristine therapy beyond this point is inadvisable. Even when a response to vincristine does occur, it is frequently transient. It may be preferable to administer vincristine or vinblastine by slow infusion rather than by bolus injection so that when the few remaining immunoglobulin-coated platelets take up the drug and are engulfed by macrophages the macrophages will be killed. In this approach, vincristine, 0.02 mg/kg, or vinblastine, 0.1 mg/kg, is dissolved in 500 to 1,000 ml of isotonic saline and administered via a constant infusion pump over a period of six to eight hours. The I.V. bag and tubing are covered with aluminum foil to prevent degradation of the drugs by ultraviolet light. These treatments can be repeated every five to 10 days, and one drug can be substituted for the other depending on the development of toxicity: neurotoxicity for vincristine; myelosuppression with leukopenia for vinblastine. Although prolonged infusion is attractive in principle, it can present logistical problems when adapted to an ambulatory care program.[61] Because patients with idiopathic thrombocytopenic purpura who are classified as therapeutic failures generally do well clinically, the role of such potentially dangerous agents as cyclophosphamide or azathioprine in the management of such cases remains questionable.

Danazol has also been used in chronic ITP. It can either be given alone or together with a corticosteroid to permit a reduction in the dosage of the latter. The usual dosage of danazol is 200 mg three to four times daily (10 to 15 mg/kg/day p.o.). Responses, if they occur, usually do not develop until after two to three months of therapy. Danazol's beneficial effect may result from a reduction in the number of Fc receptors on monocytes. Vinblastine may have a similar action. Such an effect would impair the ability of monocytes and perhaps of macrophages to ingest IgG-coated platelets.[41,62]

Administration of pneumococcal vaccine to splenectomized patients is common clinical practice. However, this vaccine has reportedly caused relapses of ITP when given to patients who were in remission.[63] One approach to this problem is to withhold the vaccine and monitor the patient carefully for signs of pneumococcal infection. What is probably a preferable course, however, is to administer the vaccine prior to surgery.[46]

Presentation with severe mucosal or central nervous system bleeding Severe mucosal or central nervous system bleeding is a true medical emergency requiring hospitalization. The patient should be placed on a unit that can provide an appropriate level of care. Red cells are transfused as required, and prednisone is administered immediately, beginning with a 100 mg dose and then continuing at a level of 25 mg every six hours. Platelets are transfused in the hope that they will have some effect during their brief circulation, even though they are destroyed along with the patient's own platelets and do not produce a measurable increase in the platelet count. The proper amount of platelets to transfuse is unknown, but the administration of from six to 20 units of random-donor platelets every six to 12 hours appears reasonable.[64] It is my custom to administer 2 mg of vincristine intravenously by continuous infusion over six hours if the logistics can be arranged[61] and to repeat the dose in five days if the platelet count has not begun to rise. There are no data to support vincristine use in such circumstances, but the risks of this therapy are quite small in relation to the potential benefits. When severe uterine bleeding is occurring, a single 25 mg dose of conjugated estrogen can be given intravenously to control the hemorrhage, after which a splenectomy can be performed.

In cases of severe, uncontrollable hemorrhage from the gastrointestinal tract or through the vagina, emergency splenectomy may be indicated. The patient is given 100 mg of methylprednisolone intravenously, followed by six units of random-donor platelets as the surgery is begun. Another six units of platelets are transfused after the surgeon divides the splenic pedicle. Corticosteroids are maintained at levels of 60 to 100 mg of prednisolone or prednisone daily until the platelet count begins to return to normal. Alternative approaches besides emergency splenectomy can also be considered (see below).

If central nervous system hemorrhage is suspected, a lumbar puncture can be performed using a No. 20 needle; the procedure should be done carefully because of the presence of severe thrombocytopenia. If the clinical findings suggest the possibility or probability of evolving central nervous system hemorrhage, a CT scan may be considered to confirm the diagnosis. The decision whether to perform a CT scan is clearly debatable, but it is my practice to resist transferring the patient off the unit for such a procedure because withdrawal of meticulous monitoring and therapy at this time could have disastrous consequences.

When impending or existing CNS hemorrhage or uncontrolled hemorrhage from another site is strongly suspected, the physician has several therapeutic choices: emergency splenectomy (see above), therapeutic plasmapheresis, or the intravenous administration of high-dose human gamma globulin. Although there are no controlled studies comparing these three modalities, I would first try intravenous human IgG, which has produced transient reversals of thrombocytopenia. The IgG is usually infused in a daily dosage of 18 to 25 g over a 30- to 60-minute period; the total recommended dose over a period of four to five days is 1.0 to 1.5 g/kg.[65,66] Another group administers intravenous IgG in daily dosages as high as 0.8 g/kg for five days. Such a high dosage of IgG, which is more than 10 times the amount of IgG synthesized daily, produces a temporary response in approximately five to seven days.[67] In an emergency, intravenous IgG can be administered in a dose of 0.4 g/kg and a bolus of eight to 10 units of random-donor platelets added when the infusion is complete.[68] The platelet transfusion following the I.V. IgG produces a greater and more durable increase in the platelet count. The I.V. IgG may produce reticuloendothelial blockade by swamping the IgG-Fc sites on the monocyte-macrophages.[41]

At times, high-dose IgG administration produces a long-lasting remission, but the explanation for this event is unclear. Although it is very expensive, the infusion of high-dose IgG appears to control hemorrhage in some cases, particularly in young patients with ITP. A splenectomy can then be carried out later under more stable conditions.

There have been anecdotal reports of success with therapeutic plasmapheresis, an alternative or supplementary approach if high-dose IgG is ineffective. Pheresis may be more useful in managing the severe hemorrhage in acute idiopathic thrombocytopenic purpura[69] than in treating recurrent hemorrhage in chronic ITP. Because plasmapheresis is most effective at removing large immune complexes, this technique is better suited for the therapy for thrombocytopenia caused by immune complex disease than that caused by platelet autoantibody attack.[46]

Refractory ITP A patient who, following splenectomy and corticosteroid therapy, remains severely thrombocytopenic or who goes into remission but later relapses and fails to respond to high doses of prednisone is said to have refractory idiopathic thrombocytopenic purpura. Because few patients with chronic thrombocytopenic disease experience serious hemorrhage when their platelet counts are higher than 30,000/mm^3, it is often prudent to accept an incomplete response and not proceed to more toxic forms of management.[70] If, however, the platelet count is very low or if there is clinically significant bleeding, further intervention is necessary. Immunosuppressive agents are then administered, generally in the following sequence:

1. Intravenous vincristine, 1 to 2 mg/wk, is administered for three to six weeks. Vincristine may also stimulate megakaryocyte production. Alternatively, vinblastine can be given in a dose of 0.1 mg/kg. Either vincristine or vinblastine can be administered as a bolus or as a six- to eight-hour continuous I.V. infusion.[61]

2. If vincristine administered along with prednisone does not maintain the splenectomized patient's platelet count at 50,000 to 100,000/mm^3, azathioprine should be started at a daily dosage of 100 to 150 mg. The complete blood count and platelet count should be monitored for three to six weeks. This regimen occasionally produces a prednisone-sparing effect, after which the dose of prednisone can be tapered. The dose of azathioprine can then be tapered as well.

3. Alternatively, or if azathioprine does not work, cyclophosphamide is added at a daily dosage of 100 to 150 mg and continued daily for three to six weeks. The response to this agent may be similar to that following azathioprine. Cyclophosphamide and azathioprine should be used with caution. Both agents are myelosuppressive, and both have been associated with the subsequent development of histiocytic lymphoma and acute myeloid leukemia. If continued administration of prednisone is necessary, an alternate-day program can be instituted in an effort to reduce the effects of hypercorticism.

4. Danazol, given in a daily dosage of 400 to 800 mg over a two- to three-month period, has been reported to be beneficial in some cases.[62,71] Some responses have been reported in patients who have received much lower doses of the drug (50 mg/day).[72]

In the refractory splenectomized patient, it is important to check for the continued presence of Howell-Jolly bodies, which appear in the red blood cells after splenectomy. The disappearance of Howell-Jolly bodies suggests the presence of a remaining accessory spleen or a regenerated spleen. Such accessory spleens have in fact been found in patients whose red blood cells contained persistent Howell-Jolly bodies.[73] Three of five such patients showed a favorable platelet response after undergoing a second splenectomy to remove the accessory spleens. Therefore, if warranted by the clinical situation, a search for an accessory spleen should probably be carried out in refractory splenectomized patients who continue to have Howell-Jolly bodies in peripheral red blood cells. The spleen scan is performed using either ^{99m}Tc- or ^{51}Cr-labeled red blood cells.[73]

Rarely, patients with ITP have no detectable marrow megakaryocytes, because the antiplatelet antibody cross-reacts with antigens on megakaryocytes, causing suppression of megakaryocyte growth and development. In such cases, the diagnosis is difficult, and myelodysplastic syndrome always needs to be excluded. One patient with this disorder responded after about 30 days to cyclophosphamide, given in a daily dosage of 50 to 100 mg p.o.[48] In another study, the patient responded first to extensive plasmapheresis and subsequently to I.V. vinblastine.[49]

The management of ITP in AIDS-related conditions (ARC) presents special problems. Because HIV attacks and destroys cells governing immunocompetence, the use of immunosuppressive agents in such cases may be hazardous. Patients with ARC who have ITP are often aware of this difficulty and may be reluctant to accept therapy with immunosuppressive agents. In cases in which the drop in the platelet count is modest, no therapy is needed. When the thrombocytopenia is severe, a short course of prednisone can be administered, followed by splenectomy. This approach has produced a good response in several cases without inducing severe infectious complications.[53,54,74]

ITP in pregnancy If thrombocytopenia appears for the first time during pregnancy, the initial differential diagnosis must include preeclampsia as well as the other usual causes of this disorder [*see Table 2*]. Once the diagnosis of ITP is made, the therapeutic choices are limited because splenectomy may cause spontaneous abortion and immunosuppressive agents may damage the developing fetal organs. Hence, corticosteroids remain the major therapeutic modality. In cases of severe thrombocytopenic hemorrhage, however, I would use all of the available therapies to protect the life and well-being of the mother.

Because the antiplatelet autoantibody in ITP has broad specificity and is almost always an IgG, it can cross the placenta and produce thrombocytopenia in the fetus. During a vaginal delivery, the pressure applied to the head of a thrombocytopenic fetus may induce an intracranial hemorrhage. Concern about this occurrence had led many experts to recommend early cesarean sections in women with a history of ITP or active disease. It is difficult to estimate the frequency of perinatal deaths occurring among mothers with ITP; the mortality among neonates born to such mothers has been reported as seven percent.[75]

Although they help to minimize fetal morbidity, cesarean sections can cause significant bleeding in the thrombocytopenic mother.[75] In an effort to limit the frequency of the procedure in such cases, attempts have been made to correlate neonatal thrombocytopenia with maternal platelet counts and with levels of maternal PA-IgG; however, these factors have not proved to be reliable predictors.[76] The level of antiplatelet antibody in maternal plasma, however, did show a strong correlation with neonatal platelet counts[76] and thus could be used as a marker to select patients for cesarean section.

Some investigators[75,77] have found that administration of prednisone at a daily dosage of 20 mg for 10 to 14 days before delivery raises neonatal platelet counts and produces a reasonably good neonatal prognosis, presumably because the corticosteroids cross the placenta and exert a therapeutic effect on the fetus. Such maternal prednisone administration, however, does not always benefit the neonate.[76]

Pending studies to resolve these issues further, the following appears to represent a reasonable approach. If assays for serum or plasma antiplatelet IgG are available, they may be used to guide selection of patients for delivery by cesarean section. If not, I would treat all mothers with a history of ITP or active ITP with prednisone or prednisolone at a daily dosage of 20 to 30 mg, starting two weeks before the anticipated date of delivery. During delivery, attempts should be made to obtain samples of fetal scalp venous blood as soon as possible for platelet counts.[78] If the neonatal platelet count is 50,000/mm^3 or lower, vaginal delivery should be interrupted and a cesarean section performed. If the child is thrombocytopenic after delivery, he or she should receive prednisone in a daily dosage of approximately 2 mg/kg.

Secondary Thrombocytopenic Purpura

Patients with systemic lupus erythematosus, Hodgkin's disease, or non-Hodgkin's lymphoma can present with a clinical picture identical to that seen in idiopathic thrombocytopenic purpura. The diagnostic approach and therapy are the same as in ITP.

The so-called ITP syndrome in these conditions may be complicated by other manifestations of the primary disorder. The spleen may be large, and splenic sequestration may be enhanced. In patients with lymphoma, the marrow may be infiltrated with malignant cells, and antineoplastic or immunosuppressive therapy may further reduce megakaryocytic compensatory activity. Several patients with the ITP syndrome have elevated PA-IgG levels similar to those seen in patients with ITP.[79] Patients with systemic lupus erythematosus or lymphoma may have Evans' syndrome, an association of ITP with autoimmune hemolytic anemia. The management of Evans' syndrome is the same as that for ITP and autoimmune hemolytic anemia.

The ITP syndrome associated with Hodgkin's disease may occur in patients who show absolutely no activity of their previously diagnosed and treated malignant disorder. This pattern contrasts with that observed for cases of autoimmune hemolytic anemia associated with Hodgkin's disease. In the latter, the onset and exacerbation of hemolysis appear to coincide with the exacerbation of the underlying disease.

An immune-mediated cause of platelet destruction and thrombocytopenia has been reported in patients with solid tumors in whom disseminated intravascular coagulation has been ruled out.[80] The thrombocytopenia in these patients resembles ITP in that marrow megakaryocytes and PA-IgG are increased, platelet survival is short, and the platelet number rises after corticosteroid therapy. It is not clear that the tumor is playing a causative role; these cases may simply represent coincidental occurrences of two diseases.[81] Diagnosis and management are similar to that for ITP.

Posttransfusion Purpura

Posttransfusion purpura [*see* Surgical Mishap versus Systemic Disorder, Frequent Causes of Postoperative Hemorrhage, *below*] may occur from two to 10 days after a transfusion of whole blood or of components containing platelets. Almost all of the affected patients are women, usually older than 40 years. The platelet count is typically very low, less than 10,000 /mm^3, and there are abundant marrow megakaryocytes. Such disorders as septic thrombocytopenia, DIC, and heparin-induced ITP must be considered in the differential diagnosis. Hemorrhage can be severe, and the thrombocytopenia usually lasts for about four weeks, but cases in which the thrombocytopenia and bleeding have persisted for as long as 120 days have been reported.

The pathophysiology of this disorder is obscure. In most cases, the patient has previously been exposed to platelet alloantigens during pregnancy or delivery or as a result of a transfusion. Tests reveal that most patients have antibodies to the platelet antigen Zw^a, an antigen that is present on the platelets of 90 percent of normal individuals. Patients in whom posttransfusion purpura develops are almost universally Zw^a negative. It is therefore difficult to comprehend how an alloantibody directed against an antigen present on random-donor platelets (or platelet fragments in RBC suspensions) results in destruction of the patient's autologous platelets, which do not express the antigen. Attempts to treat the disorder by transfusing patients with Zw^a-negative platelets have failed.

There are no controlled clinical trials evaluating therapy for posttransfusion purpura, but in such cases, it would be reasonable to administer I.V. IgG in a dosage of 0.4 to 0.8 g/kg over 30 to 60 minutes, followed by the transfusion of eight to 12 units of random-donor platelets. This approach is based on the hope that the reticuloendothelial system blockade induced by the I.V. IgG will allow the transfused platelets to survive long enough to produce a hemostatic effect.[82] Another therapy, which is probably less effective than this approach, involves the administration of prednisone in an initial daily dosage of 2 mg/kg and proceeding up to massive doses until there is a response. If there is no response and the condition is life-threatening, therapeutic plasmapheresis may be useful.[83]

Drug-Induced Immune Platelet Destruction

The clinical picture of drug-induced immune platelet destruction is indistinguishable from that of idiopathic thrombocytopenic purpura, although blood blisters in the mouth may be seen more frequently. Systemic symptoms may be present. The history of drug intake must be pursued aggressively.

The bone marrow shows abundant megakaryocytes. Drug inhibition of clot retraction has been proposed as a test, but it is difficult to perform and frequently gives a false negative result. Special laboratories can detect the presence of antidrug antibodies.

Quinidine and quinine purpura The pathogenetic antibodies in cases of quinidine or quinine purpura develop as early as 12 days after exposure to the offending agent.[84] The antibodies bind to the platelet at their Fab sites (the antigen recognition locus).[85] One hypothesis proposes that platelets coated with the drug express an unstable neoantigen, which is then stabilized by binding to the antibody. Because the drug is required for the continued expression of the hypothetical neoantigen, the antibody appears to be drug dependent.[86]

Obviously, the agent, quinidine or quinine, should be withdrawn. Neither corticosteroid therapy nor emergency splenectomy is of documented benefit in quinidine or quinine purpura. Plasmapheresis to remove drug and antibody would appear to be a logical treatment, but there are no systematic studies of its effectiveness. Transfused platelets are removed as rapidly as the recipient's own platelets. Nevertheless, platelet transfusion may be attempted to control life-threatening bleeding.

Controlled studies are not yet available, but our practice is to treat profound quinidine-induced thrombocytopenia associated with bleeding by administering prednisone in a daily dosage of 100 mg and infusing I.V. IgG in a dose of 0.4 to 0.8 g/kg over a period of one hour. On completion of the infusion, 10 to 12 units of random-donor platelets are given. Our group has had good results with this approach in three cases.

Heparin thrombocytopenia There are probably two types of heparin-induced thrombocytopenia. A mild form occurs within four days of heparin administration in about five percent of cases.[87,88] There is a modest, nonprogressive drop in the platelet count that requires no intervention.[88] The more severe form of heparin thrombocytopenia produces clinically significant platelet reduction, often to less than $50,000/mm^3$,

that is associated with thromboembolism, particularly arterial thromboembolism.[87,88] A heparin-dependent IgG antiplatelet autoantibody appears to be responsible for this severe form of thrombocytopenia. In vitro studies have shown that this antibody can produce extensive aggregation of normal platelets in the presence of heparin.[88] Presumably, the formation of such aggregates in vivo is responsible for both the drop in the platelet count and the development of arterial thrombosis. In some patients with heparin thrombocytopenia, antibodies develop that react with the heparin bound to endothelial cells or with the heparan sulfate that is synthesized there. Thus, these patients have a double lesion: heparin-induced, immune-mediated endothelial cell injury combined with heparin-induced platelet aggregation.[89]

Management of heparin thrombocytopenia can be extremely difficult, particularly if arterial thrombosis has occurred. An attempt can be made to change the type of heparin, particularly if the bovine preparation has been used. If such a change does not prove beneficial, the heparin must be withdrawn. Aspirin may be useful in preventing platelet aggregation, and some investigators recommend the intravenous administration of 500 mg of six percent dextran. The problem of heparin-induced arterial thrombosis can be avoided by starting warfarin therapy at the same time as heparinization. The heparin thrombocytopenia associated with arterial thrombosis usually does not occur until after four to six days of therapy; by this time, warfarin should be producing its therapeutic effect, and the heparin can be safely stopped [*see Chapter 7*].

Gold thrombocytopenia Gold thrombocytopenia probably should be considered as another example of drug-induced immune platelet destruction, although there is no evidence of a drug–antidrug antibody reaction as exists for quinidine and quinine thrombocytopenia. Nevertheless, gold salt therapy for rheumatoid arthritis produces thrombocytopenia in one to three percent of patients. The condition is characterized by increased marrow megakaryocytes, shortened platelet survival, and the occasional presence of platelet antibodies. Most patients respond to therapy with 60 mg of prednisone daily. The usefulness of dimercaprol as a gold-chelating agent has not been established. Patients who are not responding to corticosteroid therapy appear to benefit from splenectomy.[90]

Accelerated Removal of Platelets by Nonimmunologic Mechanisms

There are several possible nonimmunologic mechanisms that could account for the removal of sufficient numbers of platelets to cause significant thrombocytopenia. Abnormalities of vessel walls or damage to endothelial cells could induce intense platelet activation; the appearance in plasma of platelet-activating factors or agglutinating agents could cause significant platelet clumping; and increased thrombin levels in the plasma either locally or systemically could produce intravascular coagulation with platelet consumption as well as intense platelet activation and aggregation.

The distinction between nonimmunologic and immunologic forms of platelet destruction is highly arbitrary, and considerable overlap exists. For example, the level of PA-IgG is increased in several of these conditions. Such a finding may reflect the binding of immune complexes to platelet Fc receptors, which need not implicate a primary immunologic mechanism.

Several of the conditions placed in this category are uncommon, but they are described in some detail because they can be rapidly fatal unless effective therapy is begun promptly.

Thrombotic Thrombocytopenic Purpura and Adult Hemolytic-Uremic Syndrome

Clinical features and diagnosis The term thrombotic thrombocytopenic purpura (TTP) probably does not denote a single, coherent clinical entity. Rather, it seems to encompass a group of clinical syndromes in which some primary event damages the walls of small vessels, leading to the appearance of the five major manifestations of TTP: (1) severe hemolytic anemia associated with a very high serum lactic dehydrogenase (LDH) level and a blood smear showing the schistocytes and helmet cells that characterize microangiopathic hemolysis, (2) moderate to severe thrombocytopenia with increased marrow megakaryocytes, shortened platelet survival, and elevation of serum β-thromboglobulin, which indicates intravascular platelet destruction or activation, (3) fever, occasionally quite high, (4) prominent CNS signs and symptoms that usually begin with transient agitation, headache, and disorientation but often progress explosively to hemiparesis, aphasia, seizures, focal deficits, coma, and death, and (5) renal disease, which is usually mild and produces moderate elevations of serum creatinine and urine protein. Other less common clinical features include severe hepatic failure; occasional ischemic infarcts of skin, bowel, or bone; and congestive heart failure with cardiac arrhythmias. The disorder usually appears between 10 and 40 years of age, has a peak occurrence at age 25, and very rarely occurs in persons older than 50 years; it shows a slight predominance in females.[91,92] A variant of this disorder appears in the postpartum period, and the CNS manifestations may initially be confused with postpartum depression, with tragic results.

The adult form of hemolytic-uremic syndrome (HUS) could be part of the same clinical spectrum as TTP, or it may represent a different disorder. Common features of thrombotic thrombocytopenic purpura and hemolytic-uremic syndrome include microangiopathic hemolysis, thrombocytopenia, and the presence of platelet aggregates and platelet fibrin thrombi in the small vessels.[93] HUS, however, tends to occur in younger patients and shows such striking variations in severity and local incidence that its appearance has occasionally suggested the occurrence of an epidemic. Renal involvement is uniformly severe in HUS, whereas CNS disease is less prominent than in TTP. Because the management of TTP and adult

HUS is quite similar, the two disorders will be considered together.

Both TTP and HUS need to be differentiated from systemic lupus erythematosus and from Evans' syndrome. The finding of microangiopathic hemolysis combined with a significant neutrophilic leukocytosis and a direct Coombs'-negative test (direct antiglobulin test) strongly suggests TTP or HUS. Coagulation tests usually reveal no significant abnormalities, and the serum LDH and β-thromboglobulin levels are elevated. A marrow biopsy, done to evaluate megakaryocyte number and morphology, may show the characteristic, but not pathognomonic, platelet hyaline thrombi surrounded by fibrin that occur primarily in small arteries and arterioles.[94] Gingival biopsy does not appear to aid significantly in the diagnosis.[94,95]

The complexity of TTP/HUS is emphasized by the fact that aggressive management with plasma exchange may produce such a long-standing remission in some patients that they appear to be cured of this life-threatening illness. Other patients, who do not appear clinically different, relapse months or years after such therapy. This observation suggests that there may be chronic and acute forms of TTP/HUS.

Several circumstances may predispose to the development of thrombotic thrombocytopenic purpura or the hemolytic-uremic syndrome. Adult HUS has been anecdotally reported to develop after normal delivery,[96] placental abruption, or preeclampsia; in patients who have a retained placenta; and even in association with the use of oral contraceptives.[97] One case of TTP seemed to develop as a complication of Legionnaires' disease.[98] TTP/HUS has been reported in patients with cancer; some of these patients had been treated with mitomycin, and the role of this agent is suspect.[99,100]

Pathophysiology Two mechanisms, which are not mutually exclusive, have been proposed to account for TTP/HUS.[93] One hypothesis postulates that the primary mechanism is the release of a factor that agglutinates platelets or stimulates them to aggregate. The platelet clumps would then occlude and damage arterioles and perhaps produce distal ischemic effects. Subsequent adherence of more platelets would contribute to further vascular damage, thrombocytopenia, and microangiopathic hemolysis. The second hypothesis suggests that the primary defect is extensive arteriolar endothelial damage. Subsequent platelet activation, adherence, occlusion, and fibrin strand formation would then lead to thrombocytopenia and microangiopathic hemolysis.

Some authors have reported that serum from patients with thrombotic thrombocytopenic purpura contains an IgG antibody that is cytotoxic for human endothelial cells in culture.[101] Other reports have documented the presence of a platelet-agglutinating factor in the plasma of patients with TTP.[101,102]

One study indicates that in the chronic relapsing form of TTP, the Factor VIII–von Willebrand factor complex exists in the form of unusually large multimers.[103] The circulating Factor VIII–vWF complex normally has several functions, including Factor VIII coagulant properties and ristocetin cofactor–aggregating activity. The large multimers found in patients with TTP might cause platelets to aggregate in the presence of naturally occurring substances with ristocetinlike properties. In contrast to their normal mechanism of action, the vWF multimers in the serum of patients with TTP do not cause aggregation by binding to platelet membrane GPIb.[104] In the patients studied, the levels of these excessively large multimers rose during remission and fell during relapse; these findings suggest that the multimers were consumed in the process of producing platelet aggregates.[103] Perhaps patients with chronic relapsing TTP are unable to produce normal-sized multimers. Events such as pregnancy or infection may then precipitate the release of ristocetinlike substances that could induce intravascular platelet aggregation. The presence of large multimers, which would be effectively removed by plasma exchange, could account for the previously unexplained benefits of this technique in TTP/HUS. The occasional benefits described following infusion of normal plasma may be from proteolytic enzymes that degrade the large multimers to normal size.[102] A platelet-aggregating immune complex has been identified in cases of cancer-related TTP/HUS.[100]

Some investigators found that patients with TTP completely lack the plasminogen activator that is normally present in the vascular intima. Thus, the clot lysis that would normally occur is absent in TTP, perhaps explaining the buildup and even propagation of thrombi in this disorder.[105]

Two products of endoperoxide metabolism, thromboxane A_2 and prostacyclin, play important roles in platelet function: thromboxane A_2 is a very potent aggregating agent [*see Figure 6*], and prostacyclin is a very effective antiaggregating agent. Hence, attempts have been made to identify abnormalities of endoperoxide metabolism in TTP, but there has been no conclusive evidence of such abnormalities.[106,107]

The difficulty in distinguishing between immunologic and nonimmunologic mechanisms of thrombocytopenia is illustrated in TTP. Although intravascular platelet destruction appears to result from such nonimmunologic mechanisms as endothelial damage or platelet aggregation, some patients with TTP also reportedly have elevated PA-IgG levels.[46] Hence, this antibody assay cannot be used to differentiate between TTP and ITP.

Disseminated intravascular coagulation is no longer regarded as a mechanism of TTP/HUS.

Management A large number of agents have been used in the treatment of TTP. The variety of approaches reflects the explosive nature of TTP (most patients have died within 10 days of diagnosis) and its high mortality (60 to 80 percent). Classical clinical trials have not yet been undertaken. Corticosteroids are given to control vascular inflammation, and dipyridamole, aspirin, sulfinpyrazone, and dextrans are used to block platelet aggregation. (Heparin was used formerly, when it was thought that disseminated intravascular coagulation might be involved in TTP.) Plasma infusion and plasma exchange techniques have now been introduced and have led to a substantial improvement in response, producing long-lasting clinical remissions and sharply reducing mortality. Plasma exchange may remove substances that are injurious to endothelial cells or that cause platelet clumping. Plasma infusion may supply a deficient inhibitor or provide a substance that degrades large Factor VIII–vWF multimers to their normal size.[108]

The therapeutic proposals to be outlined reflect my current practice in the management of TTP/HUS. The patient's CNS status is critical in determining the intensity of therapy. Useful additional data include serial evaluation of LDH, β-thromboglobulin (if available), peripheral blood smear, and reticulocyte count. Therapy is begun with 60 mg of prednisone daily in divided doses, 0.3 g of aspirin every 12 hours, and 100 mg of dipyridamole every six hours. Some investigators have expressed considerable enthusiasm for administering vincristine in a dosage of 2 mg intravenously over four hours and repeating this dose at four- to seven-day intervals if there has been no improvement.[109,110] Because the toxicity of vincristine is not great, I would add it to the program pending further evaluation.

If the thrombocytopenia is moderate and the patient has no neurologic impairment, a simple plasma infusion can be tried. The suggested dosage is a single plasma volume (2,500 to 3,000 ml, or about 45 ml/kg, or 10 to 12 units of fresh frozen plasma) over the first 24 hours and then three units of fresh frozen plasma daily.[111] If the patient manifests even the slightest evidence of confusion or neurologic deterioration or if the platelet counts fall or the LDH soars, intense plasmapheresis should be initiated. A single volume of plasma is removed and replaced with compatible fresh frozen plasma. The effects of plasma exchange must be meticulously monitored to ensure that electrolytes, plasma proteins, and procoagulants remain at normal levels. Although there have been isolated reports of patients who have responded to plasma infusion alone, intensive plasmapheresis combined with plasma infusion should be used in severely affected patients.

Because pheresis tends to lower further the platelet count in a patient who is already thrombocytopenic, the problem of platelet replacement transfusion arises. Some authors have observed that platelet infusion in TTP may lead to exacerbation of the disease.[112] Others use platelet transfusions as required,[113] which is also our practice. The optimal amount and frequency of plasmapheresis and of plasma replacement have not been established. If the patient's condition begins to show improvement, we continue the program. If the patient's condition continues to deteriorate, the pheresis program is intensified to double-volume removal with plasma exchange (5,000 to 6,000 ml/day, or approximately 80 ml/kg/day). Once therapeutic benefit has been achieved, as measured by restoration of normal CNS function, by rising platelet counts, and by falling LDH levels, the intensity and frequency of plasma exchange can be reduced, shifting to single-volume plasma exchanges, first three times and then twice weekly. Corticosteroids can then be tapered, aspirin can be reduced to 0.3 g daily and then 0.3 g every other day, and finally, dipyridamole can be reduced and withdrawn.

Microangiopathy may persist for weeks or months after all other evidence of disease has subsided. Some patients have remained in complete clinical remission for years, which suggests they had an acute, self-limited attack precipitated by a particular event. By contrast, other patients who have apparently identical manifestations have relapsed in months or years and therefore appear to have a chronic relapsing form of TTP.

Splenectomy has been highly recommended by several experienced clinicians,[114] and we have had one remarkable success with this approach. However, there have also been several failures that were complicated by the effects of splenectomy in an already difficult clinical situation, and thus, we do not routinely employ splenectomy in patients with TTP.

The infusion of the antiplatelet agent dextran has been advocated.[114] The usefulness of prostacyclin remains to be determined.[106] The same modalities employed in TTP have also been used in the therapy for HUS, along with hemodialysis for renal failure[115] and medical management for hypertension.

Disseminated Intravascular Coagulation

Intense activation of the coagulation mechanism leads to hyperthrombinemia with platelet activation, intravascular coagulation, and platelet removal. Disseminated intravascular coagulation, which represents another nonimmunologic mechanism of thrombocytopenia, is discussed in greater detail later [*see* Acquired Hemorrhagic Disorders, Disseminated Intravascular Coagulation, *below*].

Thrombocytopenia Induced by Infection

Severe viral, bacterial, fungal, or parasitic infection can produce DIC and, consequently, thrombocytopenia; however, mechanisms other than DIC may also cause infection-associated thrombocytopenia.

Viral infections Viral infections such as dengue fever and congenital rubella can directly damage the megakaryocytes.[116] Varicella can cause a form of thrombocytopenia that has the characteristics of an immune reaction: increased numbers of megakaryocytes, no evidence of DIC, and the presence of PA-IgG or PA-IgM.[117] Usually, no therapy is required.

The acute thrombocytopenia in infectious mononucleosis is probably immune mediated, as shown by the increase in marrow megakaryocytes, the rise in PA-IgG, and the favorable response to corticosteroids. At times, the thrombocytopenia is severe, but as noted, it responds to corticosteroids.[116]

Bacterial septicemia Patients who have severe gram-negative septicemia and platelet counts lower than 50,000/mm^3 have evidence of DIC.[116] However, many patients who have both gram-negative and gram-positive septicemia and platelet counts between 50,000 and 150,000/mm³ have no signs of DIC. An immunologic mechanism may be involved in these cases because the patients' PA-IgG levels are often elevated, and the degree of elevation correlates with the severity of the thrombocytopenia.

The key to controlling the thrombocytopenia is establishing appropriate therapy for the infection. If DIC is present, it should be managed as described [*see* Acquired Hemorrhagic Disorders, Disseminated Intravascular Coagulation, *below*] with careful control of hypotension and blood volume. If clinically significant thrombocytopenia that has not been caused by DIC is present, platelet transfusion should be given as required to prevent hemorrhage.

Protozoan infection Thrombocytopenia is common in malaria,[116] although DIC is rare. Platelet survival is short, and PA-IgG has been found to be elevated. The IgG antibody appears to bind via its Fab portion to a platelet membrane antigen.[118] Platelets have receptors for malarial antigens, and during parasitemia, these antigens bind to the platelet surface. Antimalarial IgG antibodies produced during the immune response to infection then attack the antigens that are bound to the platelets. If the patient is severely thrombocytopenic and has no evidence of DIC, platelets should be transfused.

Thrombocytopenia during Pregnancy and Peripartum Period

In addition to hypertension, proteinuria, and evidence of pathologic changes in the kidneys, liver, central nervous system, and placenta, approximately 15 percent of patients with preeclampsia have moderate thrombocytopenia. Only a minority of patients with preeclampsia and thrombocytopenia demonstrate laboratory evidence of DIC.

The megakaryocyte level is increased, platelet survival is somewhat shortened, and the β-thromboglobulin level is elevated.

Some patients with preeclampsia and thrombocytopenia also have microangiopathic hemolysis, which suggests that damaged vessels containing fibrin strands are destroying red blood cells and platelets. Increased levels of PA-IgG in some patients indicate the possibility of an immunologic or an immune complex–mediated mechanism. Intense vasospasm that causes endothelial damage and leads to platelet activation, adherence, and destruction may also play a role.

Management consists of prenatal care for preeclampsia and efforts to detect thrombocytopenia as early as possible. Thrombocytopenia first noticed at the time of delivery can pose special problems. The differential diagnosis in such cases includes preeclampsia as well as acute ITP; if the patient has the latter disorder, neonatal thrombocytopenia is also a concern. In such circumstances, an accurate differential diagnosis may be impossible. If thrombocytopenia is severe, it may be necessary to start corticosteroids and infuse platelets and thereafter manage the delivery in such a way as to minimize the risks of neonatal thrombocytopenia (see above).[119]

About five percent of women have platelet counts lower than 136,000/mm³ during the prenatal and postpartum period and are thus considered to be thrombocytopenic. The platelet count usually returns to normal within one week after delivery, and there are no serious clinical consequences. Some of these thrombocytopenic women have elevated PA-IgG levels, but more often, the level of platelet-associated C3 is elevated. The cause of the thrombocytopenia in such patients is unclear.[120]

Thrombocytopenia in Hypothermia

Thrombocytopenia can occasionally occur during the hypothermia induced during cardiac surgery. Hypothermia in the elderly apparently can also cause thrombocytopenia; platelet levels as low as 30,000/mm³ have been reported in such cases.[121] The mechanisms proposed to account for the thrombocytopenia include DIC and hepatic and splenic sequestration. After the patient's body temperature has been restored to normal levels, the platelet count spontaneously returns to normal over a period of one to two weeks.

Platelet Washout and Vascular Bed Abnormalities

Perioperative platelet washout formerly was a frequent cause of nonimmune thrombocytopenia. Patients who had brisk bleeding during surgery and were transfused with stored whole blood developed thrombocytopenia after they had received about 10 units of stored blood. In effect, the patients had undergone an exchange transfusion with blood that contained nonviable platelets. The disorder develops rapidly because there are no reserve platelet stores in the marrow. The platelet count is low; the PT, PTT, and TT are normal.

Platelet washout can be avoided by using four units of properly stored platelets for every four units of red blood cells transfused during surgery. If platelet washout does occur, transfusion of six to eight platelet packs will generally correct the situation.

Platelets may also be removed by an abnormal vascular bed. In giant hemangiomas, there is sluggish blood flow through improperly endothelialized channels. These surfaces may produce low-grade disseminated intravascular coagulation. Gram-negative septicemia with endotoxemia can cause transient acute thrombocytopenia, presumably by causing platelets to adhere to damaged endothelium.

Platelet Sequestration

The third major mechanism of thrombocytopenia is platelet sequestration. Relatively modest thrombocytopenia with platelet counts on the order of 40,000 to 80,000/mm^3 is seen in patients with marked splenomegaly. Clinically significant hemorrhage rarely occurs unless a coexistent hemorrhagic disorder is present, as might occur in severe liver disease with congestive splenomegaly. There may be associated anemia and leukopenia.

The platelet sequestration appears to be a consequence of enlargement of the splenic vascular bed. Normally, 20 to 30 percent of circulating platelets are reversibly sequestered in the splenic vascular bed, and these platelets presumably exchange with platelets in the circulation. In hypersplenism, 50 to 80 percent of the total platelet mass may be sequestered in the spleen.[22]

The platelet survival time is slightly shortened, to about two and one-half days, but marrow platelet output increases to only one and one-half to two times normal.[51] The failure of the marrow to mount a maximum response offers some clues to the mechanism determining the adequacy of platelet production. The mechanism apparently is not a counter that measures concentration of platelets per unit volume but rather a sensor that responds to the total platelet mass or to the metabolic products of platelet mass. Certain diseases cause a hypersplenism that can either produce or contribute to thrombocytopenia [*see Table 3*].

Management is directed toward the primary disease. Splenectomy is rarely justified on the basis of thrombocytopenic hemorrhage alone.

Table 3 Diseases Causing Hypersplenism and Thrombocytopenia

Congestive splenomegaly	Hepatic cirrhosis
	Portal vein obstruction
	Congestive heart failure
Infiltrative diseases	Gaucher's disease, other reticuloendothelioses
	Lymphoma, myeloproliferative diseases
Infections or inflammatory responses	Tuberculosis, other granulomatoses (e.g., sarcoidosis)
	Connective tissue diseases, vasculitis
Hyperplastic responses	Chronic hemolysis, sickle–hemoglobin C disease, hereditary spherocytosis, autoimmune hemolytic anemia

Platelet Function Disorders

The clue to the existence of a platelet function defect is the finding of clinical hemorrhage in the presence of a prolonged bleeding time and a platelet count higher than 100,000/mm^3. Petechiae are rare. Platelet morphology and, rarely, crude tests of platelet function, such as clot retraction, may be abnormal [*see Table 4*].

Hereditary Abnormalities

Platelet Membrane Disorders

Hereditary abnormalities of platelet membrane function are rare. In Bernard-Soulier syndrome, giant platelets are seen on the peripheral smear. The bleeding time is prolonged, and moderate thrombocytopenia is present. Fatal hemorrhage, usually from mucosal surfaces, can occur. The defect, an absence of platelet glycoprotein Ib, the von Willebrand factor binding site of the activated platelet, causes impaired platelet adhesion to wound surfaces. In addition, because ristocetin-induced platelet agglutination depends on the binding of vWF to GPIb, such agglutination is also abnormal and is not corrected by the addition of normal plasma containing von Willebrand factor.[11] Acute hemorrhage can be managed by transfusing normal random-donor platelets; if frequent transfusions are required, platelets should be obtained from a sibling or another donor who has been HLA matched to the patient.

Fatal hemorrhage from mucosal surfaces has also been observed in Glanzmann's thrombasthenia, a rare autosomal recessive

Table 4 Classification of Platelet Function Disorders

Type	Characteristic	Cause
Congenital	Membrane abnormalities	Bernard-Soulier disease: impaired adhesion; absence of membrane glycoprotein Ib Thrombasthenia: impaired aggregation, normal adhesion; absence of membrane glycoprotein IIb/IIIa
	Granule abnormalities	Gray platelet syndrome: absence of alpha granules impairs platelet adhesion and platelet-supported coagulation Dense granule deficiency: decline in the dense granule content of ADP impairs ADP-mediated reactions
	Deficiency of a plasma factor	Von Willebrand's disease: factor deficiency interferes with platelet adhesion in vessels with high wall shear rates
Acquired	Production of abnormal platelets with storage pool defects	Myeloproliferative diseases (chronic myelocytic leukemia, polycythemia vera, essential thrombocythemia, acute myeloblastic leukemia)
	Modification of normal platelets	Association with uremia, liver disease, or macroglobulinemia and other dysproteinemias Drug-induced: aspirin and other nonsteroidal anti-inflammatory agents, dextran, antibiotics (carbenicillin, penicillin, moxalactam), ?antihistamines, ?psychoactive agents

disorder. Platelet morphology and platelet count are normal in patients with this disorder, but the bleeding time is long. Because the critically important glycoprotein IIb/IIIa that forms the platelet binding site for fibrinogen is absent, the platelets do not undergo ADP- or collagen-induced platelet aggregation. Ristocetin-induced agglutination, however, is normal.[11] The binding of fibronectin and vWF to thrombasthenic platelets is also defective, presumably because these factors also have a binding site somewhere on the GPIIb/IIIa complex.[122] Acute hemorrhage is treated as in Bernard-Soulier syndrome.

Platelet Granule Disorders

Gray platelet and dense granule deficiency syndromes Patients with the gray platelet syndrome, a rare disorder, have mucosal bleeding, ecchymoses, and petechiae. Moderate thrombocytopenia is present, and the bleeding time is prolonged. The platelets are larger than normal and appear agranular because of the absence of alpha granules. Because the alpha granular contents are severely reduced, platelet adhesion and platelet-supported coagulation are deficient. Platelet aggregation with collagen is abnormal. Bleeding episodes should be treated by infusion of normal platelets.[11]

Another rare disorder, the dense granule deficiency syndrome, is characterized by mucosal bleeding associated with a normal platelet count, normal platelet morphology, and variable prolongation of the bleeding time. Platelet aggregation with ADP and collagen are abnormal. The decrease in the dense granular contents of ADP impairs ADP-mediated events. Hemorrhage is treated by platelet transfusion.[11]

An alternative therapy for patients with primary platelet disorders such as the gray platelet and dense granule deficiency syndromes who require surgery is treatment with 1-desamino-8-D-arginine vasopressin (DDAVP), 0.3 µg/kg in saline, given just before surgery and 12 to 24 hours later if the bleeding again becomes prolonged. DDAVP

may exert its effect by releasing vWF multimers from endothelial cells.[123]

Von Willebrand's Disease

Because von Willebrand's disease is caused by a deficiency of a plasma factor, the von Willebrand factor, it will be discussed under the hereditary coagulation disorders [*see* Hereditary Coagulation Disorders, *below*]. vWF does, however, mediate platelet adhesion to subendothelial surfaces, and so von Willebrand disease can also be regarded as a hereditary disorder of platelet function [*see Table 4*].

Acquired Abnormalities

Myeloproliferative Diseases

Platelet function abnormalities occur in the myeloproliferative diseases: chronic myeloid leukemia, polycythemia vera, essential thrombocythemia, and acute leukemia. The platelet count in chronic myeloproliferative disorders is often very high, but the bleeding time may be prolonged, and clinical bleeding may appear as mucosal hemorrhage and hematomas. The abnormality resembles an acquired storage pool defect. Megakaryocytes often are abnormal with separated nuclei; the peripheral blood platelets are large and may be degranulated.

Management of acute hemorrhage consists of transfusion of normal platelets to bring the level of normal platelets up to 50,000/mm^3. The patient's defective platelets are unable to undergo the release reaction, although they may still be able to aggregate reasonably well. The normal transfused platelets undergo the release reaction, providing ADP that can induce aggregation of the patient's abnormal platelets. Transfusion of about six platelet packs is required if a coexistent thrombocytopenia is not present.

Uremia

A prolonged bleeding time associated with clinical bleeding despite a normal platelet count has been well documented in uremia, but the cause remains obscure.

Hemodialysis, to remove the presumed inhibitory products, or platelet infusions were formerly used to manage spontaneous uremic bleeding or to prepare a uremic patient for surgery. The observation that infusion of 10 units of cryoprecipitate can control severe uremic hemorrhage and shorten bleeding time, however, has led to a new approach to this disorder.[124] It has now been shown that DDAVP, a nonvasoconstricting analogue of vasopressin, is also effective in controlling uremic bleeding.[125] DDAVP has been used to treat mild vWF disease and mild hemophilia because it causes stored Factor VIII–vWF to be released from endothelial cells into the plasma. The intravenous infusion of DDAVP, 0.3 µg/kg in 50 ml of saline over a 30-minute period, shortens the bleeding time of uremic patients within one hour of its administration. DDAVP infusion produces an increase in plasma vWF activity and particularly in the larger multimers of vWF (see below). Elevation of the level of such large multimers may enhance platelet adhesion in uremic patients even though such patients typically have normal or high endogenous levels of vWF activity.

The hematocrit should probably be maintained above 30 percent in bleeding uremic patients because the bleeding time is more prolonged when the hematocrit is lower than 26.[126] If a uremic patient has clinically significant bleeding with a long bleeding time or requires surgery, the bleeding may be controlled by the use of conjugated estrogens. In one study, the administration of conjugated estrogen (Premarin) orally or intravenously in a daily dosage of 10 to 15 mg for approximately 10 days shortened the bleeding time after two to six days and stopped clinically significant bleeding. The bleeding time remained shorter than the base-line bleeding time for three to 10 days after Premarin was withdrawn.[127] In a confirmatory study, given another conjugated estrogen, Emopremarin, in a daily dosage of 0.6 mg/kg I.V. for five consecutive days, also shortened the bleeding time, usually within six hours after the initial infusion.

The mechanism of estrogen action is unknown, but it appears that estrogen therapy can help to control uremic hemorrhage in defined circumstances, and it avoids the use of blood products that carry the risk of infection. Because the onset of the beneficial effect of estrogens occurs after six hours, DDAVP or cryoprecipitate should be used to obtain immediate hemostasis in cases of acute and severe uremic bleeding. Infusion of conjugated estrogens should be started at the same time to achieve a more prolonged effect.[128]

Liver Disease

In addition to hypersplenism and defective procoagulant synthesis, there is evidence that low-grade DIC occurs continually in severe liver disease. Impaired clearance of plasminogen activators may further contribute to high plasma levels of fibrin-fibrinogen degradation products. These products may interfere with platelet function and fibrin polymerization, and their level correlates with clinical hemorrhage in severe hepatic cirrhosis. Therapy for this condition must be directed against the primary disease.

Macroglobulinemia and Other Dysproteinemias

The presence of high concentrations of viscous proteins produces complicated effects on the entire hemostatic mechanism. The proteins appear to coat platelets and interfere with adhesion and perhaps with aggregation. Instances have been reported in which the abnormal serum protein interacted with and coated collagen, thereby interfering with platelet-collagen interaction. Management is directed at the primary disease, but if hyperviscosity and bleeding are significant, prompt plasmapheresis may be required to lower the level of abnormal protein and to correct the bleeding disorder.

Drug-Induced Disorders

Aspirin and other nonsteroidal anti-inflammatory agents Ingestion of 0.6 g of aspirin prolongs the template bleeding time by two to three minutes in normal subjects.

The platelets are irreversibly affected. Cyclic endoperoxides and thromboxane A_2 are potent inducers of platelet release and aggregation [*see Figure 6*]. Aspirin acetylates and irreversibly inhibits the cyclooxygenase that catalyzes the synthesis of the endoperoxides.[29,30] Some apparently normal subjects display marked sensitivity to the action of aspirin, so that their bleeding times are very much prolonged and they have severe clinical hemorrhage, particularly during or after surgery or trauma. These patients may have a mild form of storage pool disease.

Uremic patients are especially sensitive to bleeding induced by aspirin. A small dose of aspirin ($100 \, mg/m^2$ p.o.) does not prolong the bleeding time of normal individuals but produces a significant prolongation, often as much as 15 minutes, in uremic patients.[129] The mechanism by which aspirin prolongs the bleeding time in uremia is unknown, but it appears to depend on a pathway that does not involve cyclooxygenase inhibition.[130] The combination of alcohol and aspirin is also dangerous because of its ability to prolong the bleeding time.

Aspirin-induced hemorrhage is diagnosed by determining that an acquired platelet function defect exists (a platelet count $> 100,000/mm^3$, prolonged bleeding time, and no history of hemorrhage) and then seeking evidence of aspirin ingestion. Because some 300 compounds on the market contain aspirin, a negative history should be supplemented by the following tests: a serum salicylate level; addition of ferric chloride to the urine, which turns a blue-black color if salicylate is present; and, the best method, detection of an abnormal collagen aggregation pattern that reverts to normal in seven days, which is typical of aspirin ingestion.

Platelets modified by aspirin can aggregate when exposed to ADP but do not undergo the release reaction. Therefore, management of acute aspirin-induced hemorrhage involves the transfusion of enough normal platelets to increase the platelet count by $50,000/mm^3$. The transfused platelets undergo the release reaction, after which the platelets modified by aspirin can aggregate. Usually, six units of platelet concentrate are required, and the administration can be repeated daily or on alternate days until bleeding stops or until the majority of the patient's platelets are no longer modified. Because aspirin acetylates platelets irreversibly, the hemostatic compromise might last for four to five days after the aspirin has been discontinued.

If the patient needs analgesia, acetaminophen or codeine can be used because neither prolongs the bleeding time. If the patient still requires high doses of salicylates, as in the therapy for rheumatoid arthritis, sodium salicylate is preferred because it modifies the platelets only slightly.

Alcohol In addition to producing thrombocytopenia by suppressing platelet production, alcohol consumption can also cause platelet functional defects.[131] The bleeding time is prolonged in chronic alcoholics even when the platelet count is normal. In vitro studies have shown that alcohol impairs platelet aggregation and thromboxane A_2 release. Platelet function returns to normal after two to three weeks of abstinence.

Dextrans The 40,000 MW form of dextran is readily excreted, but the 70,000 MW dextran may persist in the circulation for three days and interfere with platelet surface action. In addition to a prolonged bleeding time, patients given the 70,000 MW dextran show evidence of red blood cell aggregation. Management involves support until the dextran is excreted. Transfused platelets are affected by the dextran in plasma.

Antibiotics Carbenicillin and ticarcillin can inhibit platelet aggregation and contribute to a bleeding disorder, as can massive doses of penicillin. Massive doses of penicillin prolong the bleeding time and impair collagen- and ristocetin-induced platelet aggregation. The clinical situation is particularly disconcerting when a platelet function defect that adds to the hemorrhage develops in a pancytopenic patient being treated for septicemia. Discontinuing the antibiotics or reducing the dose is a reasonable maneuver.[132]

Moxalactam, a β-lactam antibiotic with a structure similar to that of carbenicillin, can cause hemorrhage by several apparently different mechanisms.[133] This third-generation cephalosporin can cause a platelet functional disorder after three to five days of therapy at a daily dosage of 4 g or more. This disorder is characterized by a long bleeding time and a normal platelet count. Moxalactam presumably binds to a site on the platelet membrane that interferes with the development of the ADP-induced lectin required for platelet aggregation. If a moxalactam-related bleeding disorder is diagnosed, the drug should be withdrawn. Concomitant use of moxalactam and nonsteroidal anti-inflammatory agents that inhibit platelet cyclooxygenase should be avoided because these two classes of inhibitors may have additive and potentially disastrous effects on platelet function.

Many of the other third-generation cephalosporins minimally prolong the bleeding time; the acylureidopenicillins seem to be safer than either carbenicillin or moxalactam. However, there appears to be some variation in response from individual to individual. Therefore, if bleeding develops in a patient being treated with one of these agents, a template bleeding time and platelet count should be done; if the bleeding time is prolonged, in the absence of other possible causes, the antibiotic should be withdrawn pending resolution of the matter.[134] Some of these antibiotics also produce bleeding by interfering with vitamin K–dependent function.

A rare ITP-like syndrome has also been described following moxalactam administration. After the diagnosis has been established and moxalactam has been withdrawn, corticosteroids should be begun if warranted by evidence of clinical bleeding.

Miscellaneous agents A wide variety of other agents—antihistamines, adrenergic blocking agents (phentolamine), antidepressants (imipramine)—can modify platelet function, but it is not clear that these agents cause clinical hemorrhage.

Thrombocytosis and Thrombocythemia

An elevated platelet count, that is, higher than $500,000/mm^3$, can occur in response to a variety of clinical disorders and is referred to as reactive thrombocytosis [*see Table 5*]. In reactive thrombocytosis, tests of platelet function, including the bleeding time and measurements of platelet adhesion and aggregation, are generally normal, and patients do not experience increased incidence of hemorrhage or thromboembolism even when the platelet count exceeds $1,000,000/mm^3$.[135]

In contrast, the platelet count can be increased autonomously in the myeloproliferative disorders: chronic myeloid leukemia, agnogenic myeloid metaplasia with myelofibrosis, polycythemia vera, and essential thrombocythemia.[136] In essential thrombocythemia, the number of colony-forming units–megakaryocyte (CFU-Meg) in the marrow is increased. Just as the colony-forming units–erythroid (CFU_E) in patients with polycythemia vera can grow without added erythropoietin, some of the CFU-Meg in essential thrombocythemia can grow without the addition of conditioned media.[137]

The platelet count can vary from 1,000,000 to $3,000,000/mm^3$ or more, and tests of platelet function, including the bleeding time, are frequently abnormal [*see Platelet Function Disorders, above*] [*see Chapter 15*]. Some of these patients appear to show an enhanced propensity for hemorrhage and thromboembolism. No distinct

---

Table 5   Causes of Reactive Thrombocytosis

Acute trauma, surgery, blood loss, chronic iron deficiency

Splenectomy for hemolytic anemia

Infections: osteomyelitis, tuberculosis

Inflammatory disease: rheumatoid arthritis, chronic ulcerative colitis, vasculitis

Cancer: carcinoma, Hodgkin's disease

Rebound after alcohol-induced suppression of platelet production

level of thrombocytosis correlates well with clinical manifestations. In one patient who was followed, the platelet count remained at 14,000,000/mm³ for three years, but there were no other abnormal signs or symptoms. In polycythemia vera, thromboembolic complications can generally be explained by the increased red blood cell mass, but in the other myeloproliferative diseases, the poorly functioning platelets evidently predispose to hemorrhage and, paradoxically, to thrombosis. Neither platelet number nor measurements of platelet function predict the degree of thrombosis or hemorrhage. Platelet lipoxygenase activity is always normal in patients with reactive thrombocytosis, but it is deficient in some patients with the thrombocythemia of myeloproliferative disorders. Curiously, these thrombocythemic patients were much more likely to have bleeding complications (67 percent of patients) rather than thrombotic events (13 percent of patients).[138,139]

Clinically, the hemorrhagic signs include mucosal (particularly gastrointestinal) bleeding, hematomas, and ecchymoses. There may be splenic vein thrombosis, portal or mesenteric vein thrombosis, and recurrent deep vein thrombosis with or without pulmonary embolism. Arterial thrombosis is less common. In thrombocythemia, the key problem is defective platelet function, although the absolute increase in platelet numbers may play an additional, though poorly defined, role. Some investigators believe that chemotherapy could suppress the more dysplastic megakaryocyte clones, thereby allowing the more normally differentiated clones to deliver platelets.

Management

Patients with essential thrombocythemia and polycythemia vera may have debilitating erythromelalgia (burning and itching of the fingers and toes) that can progress to ischemic acrocyanosis.[140] This symptom complex appears to be caused by occlusion and inflammation of arterioles by platelet aggregates. Aspirin or indomethacin produces relief within hours. Aspirin given at a dosage of 0.3 to 0.6 g every other day can produce lasting benefit.

The Polycythemia Vera Study Group has proposed criteria for the diagnosis of essential thrombocythemia.[141] Such criteria consist of a platelet count higher than 600,000/mm³ and exclusion of other possible causes such as another myeloproliferative disorder or reactive thrombocytosis. Findings that would indicate the presence of another underlying disorder include an elevated hemoglobin level and red blood cell mass, evidence of iron deficiency, the presence of the Philadelphia chromosome on cytogenetic analysis (chronic myeloid leukemia), and extensive marrow fibrosis (agnogenic myeloid metaplasia).

The key to the management of thrombocythemia is to recognize that there is no specific platelet level that is predictive of either hemorrhage or thrombosis and that either complication is uncommon even in patients with platelet counts of 1,000,000/mm³.[135] One series revealed that even when hemorrhage did occur it often developed in patients who were concomitantly receiving aspirin or corticosteroids. In a patient with essential thrombocythemia who has clinically significant hemorrhage or thrombosis, good control of the platelet count can be achieved with melphalan, given in a daily oral dosage of 10 mg for five days and then 2 mg daily thereafter; the dose can be adjusted as required.[141] Busulfan, given in two-week courses, can also produce good reductions in the platelet count.[142] There are no satisfactory studies, however, of the overall benefit of alkylator therapy in essential thrombocythemia. Because the incidence of hemorrhage and thrombosis in such patients is low,[135] the potential benefit of this treatment must be balanced against the enhanced risk of acute leukemia, another malignant disorder, or myelofibrosis developing.[141-143] Perhaps oral hydroxyurea, 15 mg/kg/day with adjustments in the dosage as needed, can lower the platelet count without causing a second malignant disorder.[141] Hydroxyurea therapy requires careful monitoring of the blood count; the long-term consequences of this approach are unknown.

A very common and vexing problem is choosing appropriate therapy for a patient who has a very high platelet count (> 1,000,000/mm³) caused by a chronic myeloproliferative disease but who does not have compelling signs of hemorrhage or thrombosis and is either asymptomatic or has nonspecific symptoms such as weakness, malaise, or mild headache. My own preference in such cases, supported in part by another study,[144] is to refrain from using cytotoxic agents unless there is clear evidence of hemorrhage or thrombosis and to counsel patients to avoid aspirin and other anti-inflammatory agents that may induce hemorrhage. If recurrent thromboembolism then develops, an attempt should be made to lower the platelet count with hydroxyurea. Low-dosage aspirin (300 mg q.o.d.) should also be given. High-dosage aspirin causes hemorrhage in polycythemia vera patients with thrombocythemia.[141] In cases of recurrent thrombocythemic hemorrhage, hydroxyurea therapy can be tried if there is time. If the bleeding is severe, however, transfusion with six to 10 units of normal platelets may be required to correct defective platelet function. If the patient is experiencing thromboembolism or uncontrollable hemorrhage, the platelet count can be rapidly lowered to a level of about 400,000/mm³ by plateletpheresis. Some authorities suggest that boluses of nitrogen mustard be used in this situation. However, because the platelet life span is about 10 days, a substantial reduction in the platelet count will not be achieved for several days even if megakaryopoiesis is totally ablated immediately after nitrogen mustard administration. For example, in a patient who has a platelet count of 3,000,000/mm³, the count will still be as high as about 2,500,000/mm³ the day after nitrogen mustard administration.

Vascular Purpuras

Vascular purpuras are a very heterogeneous group of disorders [*see Table 6*] that are usually characterized by cutaneous hemorrhage, occasionally associated with mucosal bleeding. The leakage occurs from terminal arterioles, capillaries, and postcapillary venules.[145] The results of tests of platelet number and function and tests of procoagulant function are normal.

Hereditary Hemorrhagic Telangiectasia

Hereditary hemorrhagic telangiectasia is transmitted as an autosomal dominant trait and is manifested clinically as epistaxis or gastrointestinal bleeding. Physical examination reveals telangiectases on finger pads, buccal mucosa, the tongue, and lip borders. There may be arteriovenous shunts in the liver and lungs. Coagulation tests are normal, although some platelet function tests may be abnormal. Management is difficult and often involves devising methods for obtaining nasal tamponade—it should be remembered that rebleeding usually occurs when a nasal pack that has been left in place for more than 24 hours is removed. Gastrointestinal bleeding is managed by the use of iron preparations when possible; this circumstance is unique in that it may require the administration of intravenous iron. Estrogen therapy has been proposed, but no real benefit has been shown.

Scurvy

Vitamin C is required for the normal metabolism of collagen, folate, and perhaps iron. The patient with scurvy suffers primarily from impaired collagen synthesis. The lack of proper collagen support for the microvasculature leads to perifollicular hemorrhages, bleeding gums, and even deep tissue hematomas. Presumably, similar collagen defects lead to the so-called corkscrew hair and hyperkeratosis associated with this disorder.[146,147] The characteristic clinical picture in a malnourished person suggests the diagnosis. Plasma or buffy coat levels of ascorbic acid are low, and other vitamin deficiencies are usually present as well. Effective therapy consists of 1 g of ascorbic acid daily in divided doses.

Corticosteroid Excess

Corticosteroid excess, whether from endogenous or exogenous causes, produces

Table 6 Classification of the Vascular Purpuras

Type	Causes
Direct damage to the endothelium	Infections: rickettsioses, infections associated with endotoxin production Toxins: snake venoms ? Immune complex diseases
Damage to supporting structures that decreases the mechanical strength of the microvasculature	Scurvy Amyloidosis Hereditary connective tissue disorders: Ehlers-Danlos syndrome, Marfan's syndrome, pseudoxanthoma elasticum Hereditary hemorrhagic telangiectasia Senile purpura Adrenal cortisol excess
Leukocytoclastic vasculitis	Rheumatic diseases: systemic lupus erythematosus, polyarteritis nodosa, Wegener's granulomatosis Idiopathic immune complex diseases: Waldenström's macroglobulinemia, cryoglobulinemia, hepatitis B, Schönlein-Henoch purpura, drug-induced disease (e.g., by sulfonamides)
Damage to the microvasculature by emboli	Fat embolization Cholesterol embolization Hemostasis Leukostasis Septic and bland emboli from heart valves: subacute bacterial endocarditis (SBE)
Miscellaneous	Autoerythrocyte purpura Psychogenic purpura

cutaneous hemorrhages, probably because of corticosteroid-induced catabolism of protein in vascular supportive tissues.

Amyloidosis

Amyloidosis can present with subcutaneous ecchymoses that have a predilection for the neck and upper chest. Biopsy of the site shows the amyloid, which by its infiltration may weaken the vessel walls or interfere with surface activation of platelets or procoagulants, or both.

Leukocytoclastic Vasculitis

The purpuric lesions in patients with leukocytoclastic vasculitis may be raised (palpable purpura). On biopsy, these lesions may show mast cell degranulation and, when stained appropriately, immune complex deposition. Presumably, the immune complexes provide the chemotactic stimulation that leads to the congregation of neutrophils. Damage to the microvasculature is caused by the complement attack complex and by the release of the contents of the neutrophil granules. This inflammatory component produces the palpable purpura.[148]

The classic example of vasculitis is Schönlein-Henoch purpura (allergic purpura, anaphylactoid purpura), which is more common in children than in adults. The disease consists of raised purpuric lesions that itch or bite, subcutaneous edema, polyarthritis, gastrointestinal symptoms including bleeding, and acute glomerulonephritis. Polyclonal hypergammaglobulinemia and cryoglobulinemia may also be present.[149] Biopsy examination of the purpuric lesion shows acute vasculitis with red blood cells passing through the vessel walls. Immunofluorescent stains show deposition of IgA and complement components and, less frequently, IgG and IgM. The search for drugs or other allergens has generally been unrewarding. Treatment is based on bed rest and the avoidance of aspirin and phenacetin. Uncontrolled trials with corticosteroids, azathioprine, and cyclophosphamide for the management of the acute nephritis have provided no evidence of benefit.[150]

Drug reactions can produce a vasculitic purpura with crops of raised, pruritic purpuric lesions. Antihistamines and corticosteroids have been used to treat the eruption, with no clear indication of benefit.

Senile Purpura

Patients with senile purpura have cutaneous hemorrhages on the dorsum of the hand, the wrist, and the upper arms and occasionally on the calves. Serious bleeding does not occur; no treatment is required. Presumably, this condition represents an age-dependent deterioration of the vascular supportive tissue.

Autoerythrocyte Purpura

Autoerythrocyte purpura is a rare and bizarre disorder that occurs almost exclusively in middle-aged women. Patients have painful, occasionally huge, subcutaneous hematomas, sometimes associated with systemic symptoms. The disorder distinctly impairs the quality of the patient's life. Psychiatric evaluation generally reveals patterns of suppressed rage. Although some studies have indicated the disorder is factitious, self-mutilation cannot be demonstrated in many cases. The name derives from the observation that the painful ecchymoses could be reproduced if the patient's own red cells were injected subcutaneously. Management with corticosteroids, antihistamines, chloroquine, low-allergen diets, and psychotherapy has been ineffective.

Damage to the Microvasculature due to Emboli

DIC and TTP can cause localized vaso-occlusions leading to microvascular damage and leakage of red blood cells. Similar damage can be caused by emboli that arise from infected heart valves. Fat embolism may complicate fractures of the long bones and pelvis. The syndrome consists of fever, confusion, and petechiae or purpura, or both, over the neck, chest, face, and axillae. Cholesterol embolism can also cause petechiae, usually over the lower extremities. It typically occurs in a patient with severe atherosclerosis who has recently undergone an invasive procedure involving the abdominal aorta or renal arteries. Biopsy of the purpura shows cholesterol crystals when an appropriate stain is used.

Hereditary Coagulation Disorders

The coagulation disorders appear clinically as either spontaneous hemorrhage or excessive hemorrhage after trauma or surgery. The history usually indicates whether the disorder is congenital or acquired. The hereditary disorders are characterized by appearance in early life and by the presence of a single abnormality that can account for the entire clinical picture.[151]

Von Willebrand's Disease

Von Willebrand's disease (vWD), which may be the most common hereditary procoagulant disorder, is caused by a deficient or defective plasma von Willebrand factor. An epidemiologic study conducted in Italy found that 0.5 to 1.0 percent of the children tested met the criteria for classic heterozygous type I von Willebrand's disease.[152] Insights into the structure and function of the Factor VIII–vWF complex have yielded a much clearer understanding of the pathophysiology of the related diseases von Willebrand's disease and classic hemophilia A. The Factor VIII–vWF complex has two major components: the Factor VIII procoagulant activity (VIII:C) and vWF [*see* The Hemostasis Scheme, Plasma Procoagulants, *above*]. vWF is now defined as the antigen that is absent in severe von Willebrand's disease, and it can be measured using immunologic techniques.[8] The genes coding for Factor VIII procoagulant activity are on the X chromosome, whereas those coding for vWF are on autosomes.

The main function of vWF is to mediate platelet adhesion to wound surfaces in vessels that have relatively high wall shear rates.[9,10] The release of vWF from the Weibel-Palade bodies in endothelial cells is induced by the presence of fibrin.[153] The larger multimers of vWF (i.e., those in the 12,000 kd range) are probably most effective in promoting the adhesion of activated platelets, possibly by bridging from the platelet GPIb receptor to the subendothelium.[11] vWF can also bind to glycoprotein IIb/IIIa[154] and apparently serves as a carrier for VIII:C, thereby protecting this factor against proteolysis. A test for vWF is based on the ability of ristocetin to activate GPIb in vitro.[23] In this test, platelet agglutination, which is correlated with the level of vWF, is measured after the addition of ristocetin; this property of vWF is termed ristocetin cofactor activity (VIIIR:RC, or VIIIR:RCo). The in vivo analogue of ristocetin-induced platelet agglutination is not known.

At low wall shear rates, the presence of vWF appears to be less critical, perhaps because under these conditions, the platelets have sufficient time to contact and spread on subendothelial surfaces; however, at high wall shear rates, contact is brief, and vWF is required to mediate adhesion.[1,11,23] In von Willebrand's disease, the bleeding time shows a good, but not perfect, correlation with the level of ristocetin-induced platelet agglutination and with the level of the factor that controls the retention of platelets to a glass bead column.[9,155]

Several variants of von Willebrand's disease have been distinguished. Type I vWD is an autosomal dominant trait that usually appears in the heterozygous form. Patients with classic type I vWD have a lifelong history of mild to moderate bleeding, typically from mucosal surfaces. Often, however, patients are unaware of a bleeding disorder until they undergo surgery or experience trauma, in which case bleeding may be severe. The diagnosis is suggested by the history and the finding of a prolonged bleeding time despite a platelet count that exceeds $100,000/mm^3$. The PTT may be slightly prolonged or normal. A finding of similarly depressed levels of VIII:C, vWF, and ristocetin-induced platelet agglutination (with values of five to 40 percent of normal for each) confirms the diagnosis. Patients with such manifestations are usually heterozygotes. In type I vWD, multimers of all sizes are present.[156] The rare homozygous or doubly heterozygous form of type I vWD is marked by severe hemorrhage, a long PTT, and VIII:C levels of less than five percent. vWF is undetectable.

Type II von Willebrand's disease is characterized by a decrease in the larger, physiologically important multimers. Crossed immunoelectrophoresis of vWF reveals the decrease or absence of the larger, slowly moving multimers and confirms the diagnosis.[11,157] Two subtypes have been described. In type IIa, formation of the largest multimers is hindered, probably because of an abnormality in the vWF molecule. In type IIB, there are small and intermediate-sized multimers, but the very largest multimers are defective and probably reduced in number because they bind excessively to platelets. Ristocetin sensitivity is increased.

A platelet form of von Willebrand's disease, termed pseudo-vWD, has been described in which excessive binding of normal plasma vWF to unstimulated abnormal platelets induces platelet aggregation. This interaction may explain the intermittent thrombocytopenia and depletion of the larger vWF multimers observed in patients with this disorder.[158,159]

Von Willebrand's disease has traditionally been treated by cryoprecipitate infusion because this approach supplies the larger vWF multimers, which are missing from the purified Factor VIII concentrates. A curious, unexplained finding is that after cryoprecipitate infusion in a patient with von Willebrand's disease vWF declines with a half-life (T) of about 12 hours, whereas Factor VIII:C activity rises and peaks after eight to 24 hours. Hence, the usual problem in management is not raising the VIII:C level but rather elevating the level of vWF that influences platelet adhesion. After approximately 10 bags of cryoprecipitate (1,000 to 1,250 units of Factor VIII:C) have been infused, potential improvement can be monitored by measuring the template bleeding time or the level of ristocetin cofactor activity. This therapy can then be repeated every 12 hours until clinical bleeding is controlled. Aspirin must be avoided.

DDAVP has also been shown to be effective in the management of traumatic bleeding in some patients with von Willebrand's disease. DDAVP given intravenously at a dose of 0.3 μg/kg over a 15- to 30-minute period causes the release of VIII:C and vWF from endothelial cell stores.[160] As long as the patient's level of vWF is greater than five percent, DDAVP infusion will significantly raise the level of vWF, and it will occasionally shorten the bleeding time. The injection can be repeated in several hours. Patients with the milder forms of von Willebrand's disease can also be prepared for general abdominal surgery using DDAVP infusion.[161] The rise in vWF achieved by DDAVP has a half-life of about eight hours, and in many patients, repeat injections elicited new bursts of VIII:C and vWF.[160] Because there is considerable individual variation in the response to DDAVP, an infusion of this agent may not produce uniform benefit. It is probably a good practice to determine the response pattern of new patients with mild to moderate von Willebrand's disease by infusing DDAVP and following the change in VIII:C, vWF, and the bleeding time. DDAVP is effective in type I and type IIA von Willebrand's disease,[162] but it should not be used in type IIB disease, because it causes thrombocytopenia in this variant. Because DDAVP seems to enhance fibrinolysis by causing the release of plasminogen activators [see Figure 3], concurrent administration of oral ε-aminocaproic acid, 4 g every four hours (24 g/day), may be advisable,

particularly in circumstances in which local fibrinolysis can be anticipated, such as dental extraction.[162]

The side effects of DDAVP at a dosage of 0.3 μg/kg over a 15- to 30-minute period are mild, consisting of water retention, flushing, tachycardia, and headache. vWF activity tends to rise during pregnancy and may even reach low normal levels, thus aiding management.

Hemophilia A

Hemophilia A, a rare condition that affects one in 10,000 males, is the most studied example of a hereditary hemorrhagic disorder. It is characterized by a deficient or defective Factor VII:C. Because the gene for Factor VIII coagulant activity is carried on the X chromosome, the disease is manifested in hemizygous males [see Figure 7]. All of the daughters of a hemophiliac male will be carriers, whereas half of the sons of a mother who carries the hemophilia trait will be hemophiliac, and half of her daughters will be carriers.

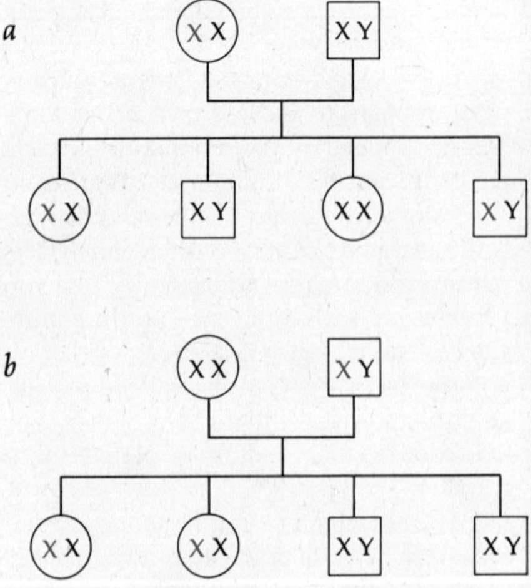

Figure 7 *The patterns of inheritance in hemophilia A are shown diagrammatically. The affected X chromosome is shown in color. Circles designate females; squares designate males. In a, the mother is a carrier of the chromosome. In b, the father is a hemophiliac.*

Most patients with classic hemophilia A show parallel decreases in Factors VIII:C and VIII:Ag and thus are either deficient in Factor VIII procoagulant molecules or else have molecules so defective that human antibodies fail to recognize them. About 10 percent of patients with hemophilia have very low levels of VIII:C but have normal VIII:Ag levels and appear to have synthesized a biologically defective molecule. Cloning of Factor VIII:C from several human patients with hemophilia A has revealed substantial variation in the underlying genetic abnormality. All patients with hemophilia A have normal levels of vWF. Women who are carriers[9] can be recognized [*see Figure 7*] because their VIII:C level is about half of normal, whereas their vWF level is normal. The ratio of VIII:C to vWF for carriers is thus 0.5.

Families appear to be affected to varying degrees, and the clinical severity of hemophilia A correlates with the measured levels of Factor VIII coagulant activity [*see Table 7*].

Diagnosis is made by the clinical picture, family history (positive in three quarters of the cases), and the Factor VIII coagulant activity level. A classic family history and a normal bleeding time rule out von Willebrand's disease in most cases.

General Management Principles for Hemophilia

The psychosocial aspects of hemophilia are complex because of parental concerns and guilt. A child is often absent from school, is prone to crippling deformities, and runs a risk of drug addiction because of the occasionally severe pain.

Factor VIII concentrates have proved effective in controlling spontaneous and traumatic hemorrhage in severe hemophiliacs. In the early 1980s, many hemophiliacs with severe disease were treated with prophylactic programs based on the self-administration of Factor VIII concentrate three times weekly at home. Such programs seemed to allow a severe hemophiliac to lead a more normal life even though the concentrates were associated with a high probability of infection with hepatitis B or non-A, non-B hepatitis.[163] An even more serious problem with this approach emerged with the discovery that the lyophilized Factor VIII concentrates, which were made from pooled plasma samples from as many as 20,000 individual donors,[164] were heavily contaminated with human immunodeficiency virus, the virus that causes AIDS [*see Chapter 18*]. By the mid-1980s, at least 75 percent of Factor VIII concentrate recipients in the United

Table 7   Correlation of Factor VIII Coagulant Activity Level with the Severity of Bleeding in Hemophiliacs

Plasma Level of Factor VIII Coagulant Activity (%)	Bleeding Patterns
<1	Presentation in first year of life, occasionally with bleeding at time of circumcision; spontaneous hemarthrosis and deep tissue bleeding
1–5	Presentation in childhood with hemorrhage after trauma; spontaneous hemarthrosis is rare
5–20	May present in childhood with hemorrhage after trauma, surgery, or dental extraction
20–50	May be undetected until adult life when major trauma or surgery results in severe hemorrhage

States and Western Europe had developed antibodies to HIV.[165-168]

The contamination of Factor VIII concentrates with HIV has had a profound effect on severe hemophiliacs who now must carefully weigh the various therapeutic options. Fortunately, heat treatment of the concentrates seems to kill the AIDS virus in most cases while preserving much of the coagulant action of Factor VIII.[163] As of March 1987, seroconversion had occurred in several hemophiliac patients who had received unscreened, heat-treated factor concentrates. No cases of seroconversion had occurred, however, in patients who received donor-screened, heat-treated concentrates, which are the recommended form of replacement therapy.[169]

It is not known what proportion of HIV-infected hemophiliacs will eventually progress to clinical AIDS. Some of these patients have already progressed to AIDS-related ITP, a particularly troublesome complication of hemophilia.[164] Sexually active infected hemophiliacs are also at risk for spreading HIV infection.[170-172]

Dental prophylaxis is critically important because hemophilia almost always causes complications if dental surgery is required. Drugs that interfere with platelet function, such as aspirin, must be avoided because they cause serious bleeding.

Genetic counseling should be part of the management program. Because of the difficult life severe hemophiliacs lead, many women would opt to terminate pregnancy if they were certain of their carrier status or knew that their fetus was affected.[173] There are several strategies for detecting carriers. One case is obvious: a daughter of a hemophiliac father is an obligatory carrier [*see Figure 7*]. A method for detecting carriers in other cases involves measuring the ratio of Factor VIII:C–vWF antigen: this ratio is about 0.5 in carriers, [166,174] but the error rate for this test is 10 to 17 percent.[175]

A method that uses restriction fragment length polymorphisms (RFLPs) within the Factor VIII:C gene to identify carriers in sporadic cases[173,175] is reported to have an accuracy as high as 96 percent.[176] These molecular probes for RFLPs are now being used to determine the status of the fetus. Measurement of fetal plasma for Factor VIII:C and vWF antigen and for Factor VIII antigen can only be obtained by fetoscopy at 18 to 21 weeks, which is relatively late in gestation. In addition, fetoscopy at this stage is associated with a six percent incidence of spontaneous abortion.[177] Fetal tissue for DNA analysis can be obtained more safely by amniocentesis by the 12th week of gestation[177] and by chorionic villus sampling, which is usually performed between the eighth and 12th week of gestation.[176,177] Specific amplification of genomic sequences by an enzymatic method markedly improves the sensitivity of these techniques.[178]

Management of Acute Hemorrhage

Deep tissue bleeding, hemarthrosis, and hematuria are the common forms of clinical bleeding in hemophilia A. Retroperitoneal hemorrhage, bleeding about the mouth, tongue, or neck that impairs the airway, and intracranial hemorrhage all pose acute threats to life. Both ultrasonography[179] and computed tomography can be used to identify retroperitoneal and intramuscular hematomas. Therapy is based on the location and extent of bleeding.

Principles of Replacement Therapy

A plasma procoagulant level of 100 percent means that there is one unit of procoagulant per milliliter of plasma. Most persons have 40 ml of plasma per kilogram of body weight. Thus, by determining a patient's plasma volume and procoagulant level, one can calculate the required amount of Factor VIII replacement. For example, in the case of a 60 kg boy who has an uncomplicated hemarthrosis of the knee and a baseline Factor VIII of less than one percent, raising the Factor VIII level to about 25 percent (0.25 units/ml) for two to three days should suffice. This patient has a plasma volume of 60 kg × 40 ml/kg, or 2,400 ml; he will need 0.25 units/ml × 2,400 ml, or 600 units of Factor VIII as an initial bolus. Another way of making this calculation is based on the fact that the infusion of one unit of Factor VIII:C per kilogram increases Factor VIII:C levels by two percent, or 0.02 units/ml. In the example cited, an increase of 25 percent (0.25 units/ml) would require $(25 \times 60) \div 2$, or 750 units of Factor VIII:C.[180]

The desired amount of Factor VIII can be administered as six to eight cryoprecipitate bags (there are about 100 units per bag) or as heat-treated lyophilized concentrate, for which the number of units is indicated on the label. The initial half-life of Factor VIII:C during the equilibration stage is only about four hours,[180] but the biologic half-life after equilibration is 12 hours. Therefore, about one half of the initial loading dose is given after the first six hours and then every 12 hours as long as is needed to control the hemorrhage. For the treatment of hemarthrosis, the Factor VIII level should be maintained for two to three days. A controlled trial determined that the correct dose for most acute hemarthroses of knee, ankle, and elbow was 14 units of Factor VIII:C per kilogram, or about 1,000 units of Factor VIII for an adult weighing 70 kg. This infusion should raise the Factor VIII:C level by 28 to 36 percent. For more serious deep tissue bleeding, such as retroperitoneal hemorrhage or bleeding into the soft palate, the Factor VIII:C level should be raised to 0.5 units/ml (50 percent).

Elective Surgery and Dental Extraction

Dental work should be performed by a dentist experienced in the treatment of hemophiliacs. Before dental extraction, Factor VIII is given to raise the level to 50 percent, and the fibrinolytic inhibitor EACA is administered as an intravenous bolus in a dosage of 0.1 g/kg. EACA is continued orally at a dosage of 0.1 g/kg every six hours for 10 days after the dental work. Usually, further administration of Factor VIII is not required.

Prior to elective surgery, the Factor VIII:C level should be raised to 50 to 100 percent (0.5 to 1.0 units/ml) and then maintained above 50 percent for the next 10 to 14 days.[180,181] Maintaining a higher concentration of Factor VIII:C does not reduce the frequency of hemorrhage.[181] The amount of Factor VIII:C concentrate required can be reduced if it is administered as a continuous infusion rather than as boluses, partly because continuous infusion keeps the factor at a plasma level above that at which bleeding may occur.[181]

Because Factor VIII:C has now been cloned, recombinant Factor VIII:C may become available in the future and should be free of the hepatitis and AIDS viruses. Because of the current danger of transmitting viral infections with the biologic preparations, alternative means of treating hemophiliacs have been sought.

One study reported that the attenuated anabolic steroid danazol given at a dosage of 200 mg three times a day increased the plasma Factor VIII:C concentration,[182] particularly in moderate hemophiliacs, to a level sufficient to produce a fivefold decrease in hemorrhagic episodes.[183] Three other studies, however, have found that danazol produced either no increase or only a minimal increase in the level of Factor VIII:C and caused an increase in bleeding, presumably because of its ability to enhance fibrinolysis.[184-186] Therefore, I do not recommend treating hemophiliacs with danazol until this situation has been clarified.

DDAVP can be used to treat acute traumatic hemorrhage in mild or moderate hemophiliacs and even to prepare such patients for minor surgery.[160,161] DDAVP, which appears to cause the release of Factor VIII:C from endothelial cell stores,[160-162,180] cannot be used repeatedly over many days, because such stores become depleted. Thus, in the preoperative preparation of mild to moderate hemophiliacs, DDAVP can be alternated with Factor VIII:C concentrates.[180] DDAVP is infused at a dosage of 0.3 µg/kg in 50 ml of saline over 15 to 30 minutes and produces a prompt increase in Factor VIII:C. The biologic half-life of the released Factor VIII:C is 11 to 12 hours.[160,180] Because DDAVP also releases tissue plasminogen activator [*see Figure 3*], concomitant administration of either EACA, in a dosage of 4 g orally every four hours, or tranexamic acid, 1.5 g orally three times a day, is recommended.

Management of an Inhibitor

Ten percent of hemophiliacs develop an antibody inhibitor against Factor VIII and hence do not achieve the anticipated Factor VIII levels after infusion. Assays for Factor VIII inhibitors should be performed at regular intervals in all patients who have severe hemophilia.

Hemorrhage that occurs in such a circumstance can be life-threatening and should be met by a hierarchy of responses. For severe but not life-threatening bleeds (i.e., not intracranial) in a patient who has an inhibitor titer of less than five Bethesda units and who is not a vigorous antibody responder, a large amount of Factor VIII concentrate should be administered in an attempt to overwhelm the antibody. The amount of Factor VIII concentrate to be given is about 40 units/kg plus an additional 20 units/kg for each Bethesda unit of inhibitor.[180] Thus, a patient with an inhibitor titer of five Bethesda units would receive 40 units/kg + 5 × 20 units/kg, or 140 units/kg. The postinfusion level of Factor VIII:C must be measured to determine if the anticipated end point, 0.3 units/ml of plasma,[187] has been achieved.

For patients with more serious hemorrhage or for those with less severe hemorrhage but high levels of inhibitor against human Factor VIII, porcine Factor VIII:C (Hyate:C) concentrates may be the treatment of choice. The recommended doses are 20 to 50 units/kg porcine Factor VIII:C for moderate hemorrhage or for hemorrhage occurring in patients with an inhibitor titer of less than five Bethesda units; 50 to 100 units/kg for more severe hemorrhage or hemorrhage that occurs in patients who have an inhibitor titer of five to 50 Bethesda units; and 100 units/kg for those with inhibitor titers greater than 50 Bethesda units. Measurement of the inhibitor titer against porcine Factor VIII:C provides useful information: if the titer is greater than 13 Old Oxford units, the administration of porcine

Factor VIII:C will produce no therapeutic benefit.[188,189]

Occasionally, aggressive plasmapheresis can be used to reduce the level of inhibitor against human Factor VIII,[190] followed by the administration of Factor VIII:C concentrates. This procedure, however, is cumbersome to use in a hemophiliac patient who has a potentially life-threatening or crippling hemorrhage. Prothrombin complex concentrates (PCC) such as Proplex or Konyne have been used to treat patients with high titers of inhibitors on the grounds that the factors present in such concentrates might circumvent the Factor VIII:C deficiency. A controlled trial established the efficacy of Konyne or Proplex, administered as a single dose of 75 units/kg, in the management of hemarthrosis.[191]

The use of activated prothrombin complex concentrates (APCC) such as Anti-inhibitor Coagulant Complex (Autoplex) has been introduced in the hope that the activated IXa or VIIa present in these preparations might prove effective in establishing hemostasis[192]; the APCC was administered in a dose of approximately 75 units/kg. In some controlled clinical trials, the APCCs achieved slightly better results than the PCCs,[193,194] but distressing failures have also been reported.[195]

Other Hereditary Hemorrhagic Disorders

Factor IX Deficiency

Factor IX deficiency (Christmas disease, hemophilia B) is a sex-linked disorder that is clinically indistinguishable from hemophilia A. Diagnosis requires a Factor IX assay. The management principles are the same as those for hemophilia A. Factor IX is replaced with fresh frozen plasma or, during dire emergencies, with prothrombin complex concentrates. The level of Factor IX needed to control hemostasis in patients with hemophilia B is somewhat lower than the level of Factor VIII:C required for the treatment of hemophilia A, about 0.15 to 0.20 units/ml in contrast to 0.3 to 0.5 units/ml. Factor IX is a smaller molecule than Factor VIII:C and is distributed in the albumin space. In making replacement calculations, it is assumed that one unit of Factor IX per kilogram will increase the plasma level by one percent, or by 0.01 units/ml. Factor IX has a biphasic half-life, and plasma levels of this factor can be maintained by infusing the concentrate every 24 hours during an acute bleeding episode in a patient with hemophilia B. Patients with hemophilia B are at risk for acquiring HIV infection from transfusion of Factor IX concentrate[163]; the utility of danazol in such patients is controversial.[184-186]

There are variants of Christmas disease that are characterized by differing amounts of cross-reactive procoagulant relative to biologic activity.[151] Gene cloning techniques can now detect the Factor IX deficiency carrier state and permit accurate genetic counseling.[196-198]

Mild Factor VII Deficiency

Occasionally, preoperative screening tests reveal that a patient has a mildly prolonged prothrombin time in the absence of liver disease, poor diet, or antibiotic administration. Some of these patients can be shown to be heterozygous for Factor VII deficiency states, as confirmed by family testing and by measuring the Factor VII antigen level in plasma.[199] Therapy is not required unless major surgery is contemplated, in which case Factor VII can be supplied in the form of prothrombin complex concentrates or fresh frozen plasma.

Fibrinolytic Abnormalities

Two congenital hemorrhagic disorders have been ascribed to abnormalities of fibrinolysis [*see Figure 3*].[200] Deficiency of α_2-antiplasmin, the major plasmin inhibitor, has led to uncontrolled plasmin activity with consequent hemorrhage.[200] Enhanced fibrinolytic activity has also been linked to another hemorrhagic disorder that occurs after trauma. An excess of circulating plasminogen activator leading to the breakdown of fibrinogen and fibrin has been implicated in this disorder. Treatment of both types of fibrinolytic abnormalities consists of the antifibrinolytic agent tranexamic acid, 1.5 g given orally three times a day [*see Figure 3*].[201] An intravenous infusion of 50 mg/kg of tranexamic acid is given as prophylaxis for dental work. Antifibrinolytic agents such as EACA and tranexamic acid block the binding and interaction of plasminogen and plasmin with fibrin.[200]

The remaining hereditary coagulation disorders occur rarely [*see Table 8*].

Acquired Hemorrhagic Disorders

In addition to the hereditary coagulation disorders, several acquired disorders have also been identified that can lead to generalized hemorrhage [*see Table 9*].

Vitamin K Deficiency

A vitamin K–dependent carboxylase in the liver synthesizes γ-carboxyglutamic acid, which is required for the biologic function of Factors II, VII, IX, and X.[202,203] In the absence of vitamin K, an abnormal Factor II, or prothrombin, that lacks γ-carboxyglutamic residues is synthesized.[204] Specific immunoassays performed in patients with vitamin K deficiency reveal a sharp decrease in normal prothrombin and a concomitant increase in the abnormal des-γ-carboxyprothrombin. The same molecular derangement occurs with Factors X, IX, and VII.

Deficiency of vitamin K occurs in severe malnutrition, intestinal malabsorption, and obstructive jaundice [*see Table 9*]. In obstructive jaundice, bile salts, which are necessary for the emulsification and absorption of the fat-soluble vitamins (vitamins A, D, E, and K), cannot enter the intestine. Chronic ingestion of oral antibiotics appears to suppress vitamin K production by intestinal organisms. The antimicrobial moxalactam is particularly effective in suppressing the intestinal bacterial flora that provide vitamin K. The effect of this agent is especially marked in patients who, because of their illness, are unable to consume a full, nourishing diet [*see Platelet Function Disorders, Drug-Induced Disorders, above*]. Deficiency of vitamin K results in decrease of biologic

Table 8　Hereditary Hemorrhagic Disorders Not Involving Factor VIII

Deficient Factor	Inheritance	Type of Bleeding	Assays	Treatment
Factor IX (Christmas disease, PTC deficiency, hemophilia B)	Sex-linked	Identical to that in Factor VIII deficiency	Long PTT Specific assay	Fresh frozen plasma or, rarely, Factor IX concentrates (Proplex) Biologic half-life is 20–24 hr
Factor XI (PTA deficiency)	Autosomal recessive	Less severe than that in hemophilia A or B	Long PTT Specific assay	Fresh frozen plasma Biologic half-life is 60 hr
Factor XII (Hageman trait)	Autosomal recessive	None	Long PTT Specific assay	None
Factor V (parahemophilia)	Autosomal recessive	Postoperative and spontaneous bleeding	Long PTT, PT Normal P and P Specific assay	Fresh frozen plasma Biologic half-life is 60 hr
Factor X (Stuart-Prower)	Autosomal recessive (only homozygotes bleed)	Epistaxis, hemarthrosis, ecchymoses, menorrhagia	Long PT, PTT, P and P Specific assay	Fresh frozen plasma Biologic half-life is 48 hr
Factor VII (proconvertin)	Autosomal recessive (only homozygotes bleed)	Epistaxis, hemarthrosis, ecchymoses, menorrhagia	Long PT, P and P Normal PTT Specific assay	Fresh frozen plasma Biologic half-life is 4–6 hr
Factor II (prothrombin)	Autosomal recessive	Epistaxis, hemarthrosis, ecchymoses, menorrhagia	Long PT, P and P Specific assay	Fresh frozen plasma Biologic half-life is 4–6 hr

Table 8   (continued)

Deficient Factor	Inheritance	Type of Bleeding	Assays	Treatment
Factor I (fibrinogen)	Autosomal recessive	Variable, deep tissue hemorrhage	Long PT Low fibrinogen level	Cryoprecipitate: each bag contains 400–500 mg fibrinogen; 100 mg/dl required for hemostasis; Biologic half-life is 100 hr
Factor XIII (FSF)	Not clear	Umbilical bleeding, posttraumatic and late postoperative bleeding Wound heals slowly with keloid formation	Clot solubility in 5 M urea	Fresh frozen plasma Biologic half-life is 120 hr

Table 9   Acquired Generalized Hemorrhagic Disorders
Deficiency of vitamin K: low intake, impaired absorption of vitamin K, antimicrobial inhibition of the gut flora that provide vitamin K
Drug-induced hemorrhage: heparin, warfarin (also, anticoagulant abuse by patient)
Dysproteinemias: myeloma, macroglobulinemia
Disseminated intravascular coagulation
Severe hepatic disease
Circulating inhibitors of coagulation
Primary fibrinolysis

activity in Factors II, VII, IX, and X. Patients with cancer who receive a combination of cefoperazone and mezlocillin seem particularly prone to hypoprothrombinemia.[205] The combination of cefoxitin and azlocillin has produced similar hypoprothrombinemia.[206] Mucosal bleeding and ecchymoses occur if the procoagulant levels fall below 10 to 15 percent of normal.

The diagnosis can be made if the prothrombin and proconvertin time and the prothrombin time are prolonged, the partial thromboplastin time is normal or slightly prolonged, and the fibrinogen level is normal. Therapy with vitamin K analogues, using a dosage of 10 to 25 mg of oral phytonadione daily for two to three days or using parenteral phytonadione in obstructive jaundice, usually reverses the abnormality in about six to 24 hours. However, if the antimicrobial agent has a side chain similar to that of warfarin, it may take as long as 36 hours before therapy restores prothrombin values to normal.[206] If the patient has severe bleeding, delay may be dangerous, and he or she should be treated with fresh frozen plasma (see above) to restore procoagulant levels to at least 30 percent of normal [*see* Hereditary Coagulation Disorders, Principles of Replacement Therapy, *above*]. About three units (three bags) of fresh frozen plasma are usually required in such cases.

Drug-Induced Hemorrhage

In warfarin overdose, the precipitating event is a misadministered dose of warfarin or the simultaneous ingestion of an agent that potentiates the anticoagulant action of warfarin. Mucosal bleeding, ecchymosis, or subserosal bleeding into the gut wall is the usual pattern. The PT and P and P are prolonged. If hemorrhage is significant, treatment calculated to restore procoagulant levels to 30 percent of normal must be started with fresh frozen plasma. If there is no urgency, oral phytonadione may be given as described (see above). As expected, warfarin use is associated with a decrease in native prothrombin and a concomitant increase in the level of the abnormal des-γ-carboxyprothrombin, which does not clot.[204] Surreptitious warfarin use can be identified by a serum warfarin assay, available at special laboratories.

Heparin overdose may not be obvious. It causes subcutaneous hemorrhages and deep tissue hematomas. The PTT, PT, and TT are vastly prolonged, but the reptilase time is normal. Intravenous protamine at a dose of 1 mg/100 units of administered heparin terminates the disorder. Because the half-life for the disappearance of protamine is faster than that for heparin, a heparin rebound may occur, requiring a second administration of protamine.

Dysproteinemias

The abnormal proteins associated with myeloma and macroglobulinemia can interfere with platelet function and cause clinical bleeding. These proteins or the underlying disease can cause abnormalities in the coagulation tests as well. Both IgG and IgA myeloma proteins can cause prolonged thrombin times without clinical hemorrhage. Deficiencies of Factor V occur sometimes with IgA myeloma. IgA and IgM dysproteinemias can cause hemorrhage by reducing Factor VIII activity.

Management is directed at the primary disease. Plasmapheresis rapidly corrects the defects by abruptly lowering the level of abnormal protein.[207]

Disseminated Intravascular Coagulation

The entire coagulation scheme, whether initiated by the extrinsic pathway or by the intrinsic pathway, is finely tuned to culminate in a burst of thrombin activity (Factor IIa) at the point of the vascular insult. By its catalytic actions on platelets and Factors I, V, VIII, and XIII, thrombin causes focused hemostatic activity at the site of the injury, inducing platelet changes and leading to the deposition of cross-linked fibrin to form the hemostatic plug. Under normal conditions, the deleterious effects of uncontrolled intravascular coagulation (mostly uncontrolled thrombin action) are modulated by the dilutional effects of blood flow, by circulating antithrombins, by removal of particulates and activated factors by the reticuloendothelial cells in the liver, by antiplasmin, and by the factors that down-regulate hemostasis—AT-III and the protein C and protein S systems.

These carefully controlled mechanisms can be overwhelmed under the following circumstances:

1. Massive tissue damage, liberating huge amounts of tissue thromboplastic materials, causing extensive activation of the extrinsic system [*see Figure 1*].
2. Extensive alteration of the vascular endothelium, which exposes significant amounts of the intrinsic procoagulants to subendothelial initiators.
3. Shock, associated with reduced blood flow and loss of the beneficial effects of hemodilution.
4. Impaired hepatic perfusion or function, which causes inadequate hepatic removal of circulating particulates and activated procoagulants.

There are many different circumstances that can cause DIC [*see Table 10*]. In each case, massive activation of hemostatic mechanisms overwhelms the inhibitor mechanisms [*see Figure 8*]. This runaway hemostasis and the physiologic responses to it lead to circular propagation of the unfolding disaster. Massive coagulation depletes

Table 10 Causes of Disseminated Intravascular Coagulation (DIC)

Events that initiate DIC	Massive tissue destruction	Tumor products
		Crash injury, complicated and extensive surgery, severe intracranial damage
		Retained conception products, placental abruption, amniotic fluid embolism
		Certain snake bites
		Hemolytic transfusion reaction (usually ABO mismatch)
		Acute promyelocytic leukemia
		Burn injuries
	Extensive destruction of endothelial surfaces, exposure to foreign surfaces	Vasculitis (meningococcemia or, occasionally, gram-negative septicemia)
		Heatstroke, malignant hyperthermia
		Extensive pump-oxygenation (repair of aortic aneurysm)
		?Eclampsia and preeclampsia
		Giant hemangiomas (Kasabach-Merritt syndrome)
		Immune complexes (? postvaricella purpura gangrenosa)
		Certain snake bites
Events that complicate and propagate DIC	Shock	
	Complement pathway activation	

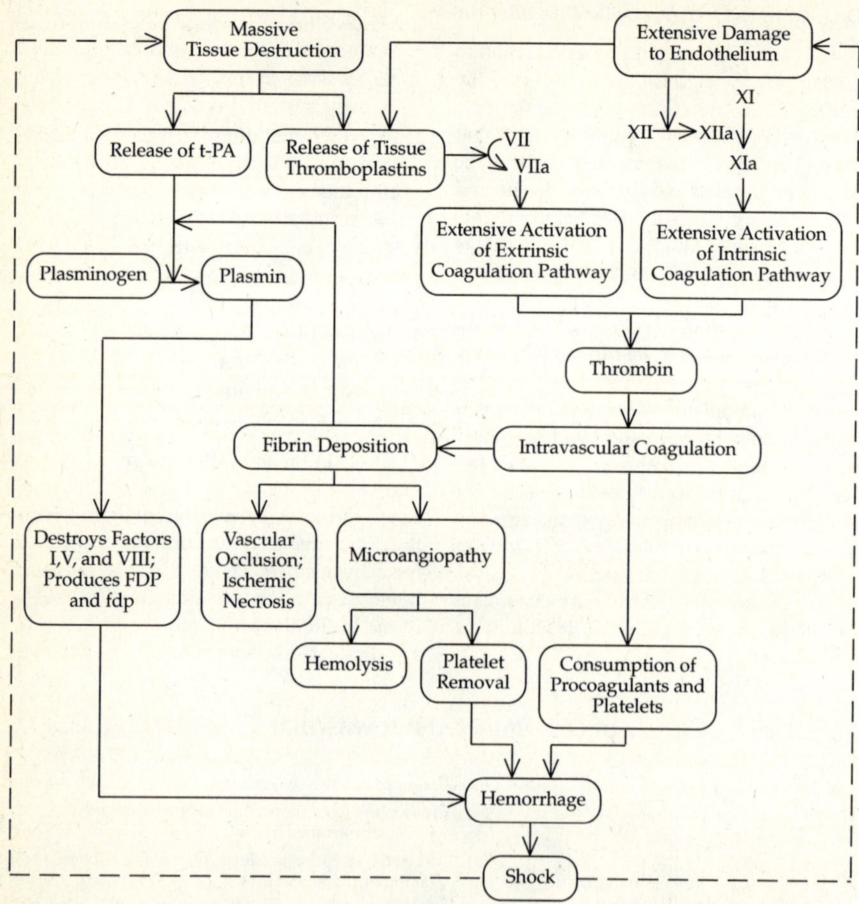

Figure 8 *Flowchart depicts the sequence of interacting events that occurs in disseminated intravascular coagulation, a process that is initiated by massive tissue destruction and extensive damage to the endothelium. Either of these events can generate sufficient thrombin to overwhelm the modulating effects of AT-III and the protein C and protein S systems. The autocatalytic-enhancing role of thrombin intensifies the situation by activating procoagulants and platelets, ultimately producing uncontrolled intravascular coagulation and fibrinolysis associated with the generation of fibrin and fibrinogen degradation products (FDP and fdp). Affected patients can present clinically with hemolysis or thrombosis, or both, depending on the balance achieved between procoagulant activation and procoagulant depletion coupled with the actions of plasmin.*

procoagulants and platelets, causing bleeding. The uncontrolled generation of thrombin results in thromboses in the arterial and venous beds, leading to ischemic infarction and necrosis that intensify the damage and further activate the hemostatic system. Tissue damage and the deposition of fibrin [*see*

Figure 3] result in the release and activation of plasminogen activators and the generation of plasmin in amounts that overwhelm its inhibitor, α_2-antiplasmin. Plasmin degrades Factors VIII, V, and I and produces fibrin-fibrinogen degradation products; these substances, as well as the products of incompletely polymerized fibrin, impair platelet function and normal fibrin polymerization [*see Figure 1*].

Endotoxin released during gram-negative septicemia enhances the expression of tissue factor, thereby accelerating procoagulant activation [*see Figure 1*] while suppressing thrombomodulin expression [*see Figure 4*]. These actions down-regulate the protein S–protein C system, further promoting the tendency to DIC.[208]

DIC has also been observed in patients with solitary or multiple hemangiomas associated with thrombocytopenia (Kasabach-Merritt syndrome). Platelets and fibrinogen are consumed in these tumors—where fibrinolysis appears to be enhanced[209]—and such consumption can lead to hemorrhage and death. The DIC associated with such tumors is presumably initiated by prolonged contact of abnormal neoplastic endothelial cells with blood in areas of vascular stasis.

Certain snake bites can also produce DIC; several mechanisms have been identified. For example, Russell's viper venom contains a powerful procoagulant that can produce almost instantaneous defibrination. The venom also contains a highly lethal nephrotoxin as well as hemorrhagins that damage vascular endothelium and cause platelet abnormalities.[210]

The consequences of disseminated intravascular coagulation depend on its cause and the rapidity with which the initiating event is propagated. If the activation occurs slowly, an excess of activated products is produced, predisposing to thrombosis. The clinical situation consists of vascular infarctions or of venous thrombosis. This condition is sometimes known as compensated, or chronic, DIC. If the reaction is brisk and explosive, the clinical picture is dominated by intravascular coagulation; depletion of platelets and the procoagulant Factors I, II, V, VIII, and XIII (and perhaps Factor VII); and the production by plasmin action of fibrin degradation products, which further interfere with hemostasis. The clinical consequence is hemorrhage surrounding wound sites, intravenous lines, and catheters, as well as bleeding into deep tissues. The intravascular fibrin strands produce microangiopathic hemolytic anemia.

Diagnosis

Microangiopathic red blood cells on smear and a platelet count that is low and continues to fall despite adequate numbers of marrow megakaryocytes suggest the diagnosis. Because of procoagulant depletion, the PTT, PT, P and P, and fibrinogen tests are abnormal. Because fibrin degradation products interfere with fibrin polymerization and produce unclottable complexes, the thrombin time is also prolonged. The level of fibrin degradation products is elevated. Tests of the fibrinolytic system, such as the euglobulin lysis time, show enhanced fibrinolytic activity, and plasminogen levels are low. Measurement of plasminogen, and to a lesser extent of protein C levels, may provide additional laboratory corroboration of DIC.[211] DIC can be distinguished from the rare disorder of primary fibrinolysis by means of the fibrin D dimer test. This test detects the polymerized fibrin fragments that occur in DIC but not in primary fibrinolysis. There is another experimental method that can distinguish between an excess of normal fibrin polymerization, as occurs in DIC, and the plasmin-mediated destruction of soluble or partially polymerized fibrin [*see Figure 1*]. Measurement of the ratio of fibrinopeptide B (FPB), which is derived from fibrin polymerization, to the peptide fragment $B_{\beta1-42}$, which is a product of plasmin attack, will help to determine whether DIC or fibrinolysis is the major event.[3]

Repetition at regular intervals of the coagulation tests listed earlier is critically important because repeated tests provide a kinetic parameter that greatly aids in diagnosis. For example, a patient with aggressive vasculitis or acute graft rejection might have a high fibrinogen level and a high platelet count because of the inflammatory component of the underlying disease. A single determination, however, may show a normal fibrinogen level and a normal platelet count and thus would be misleading in this patient because values were probably substantially higher several hours earlier. Levels of procoagulants and platelets that are falling faster than would be predicted based on their biologic half-life indicate that rapid removal (and probably consumption) is in progress. Similarly, if attempted replacement yields results substantially below those calculated, brisk consumption is probably occurring.

Management

Management must be directed at the primary disease to switch off the initiating event. This approach may involve chemotherapeutic attack on a tumor, treatment of infection, or emptying the uterus when complications of pregnancy have been initiatory. Hemodynamic support is essential. The use of plasminogen-plasmin inhibitors such as EACA or aprotinin should be avoided: these agents block the fibrinolytic system and hence may cause the continued accretion of multiple thrombi and lead to extensive vascular infarction. Infusion of fibrinogen alone adds fuel to the fire because plasmin will convert the newly added fibrinogen to fibrinogen degradation products, which will further interfere with coagulation. Cardiopulmonary support and attention to the primary disorder usually suffice.

The critical question is when, if ever, to use heparin, which directly antagonizes thrombin by its specific interaction with antithrombin III.[212] Treatment with heparin is not justified on the basis of abnormal coagulation tests alone. If, however, there is life-threatening hemorrhage with wound oozing, deep tissue hemorrhage, or bleeding into body cavities, and if a distinct clinical maneuver can also be directed at the basic disease with a reasonable chance of control in two or three days, then heparinization can be considered. It should be emphasized that with the possible exception of the DIC associated with acute promyelocytic leukemia or other forms of AML [*see Chapter 15*] there is no clear-cut evidence supporting the use of heparin. My own practice is to avoid using heparin except for the specific circumstances noted.

There are no randomized clinical trials on which to base the dose of heparin in DIC. Therapy can begin with 500 units/hr of heparin given intravenously by constant infusion pump with or without an initial intravenous bolus of 500 to 1,000 units. After the heparin has been infused for two hours, procoagulant replacement behind the heparin shield can be started. Two to three units of fresh frozen plasma can be given if the patient's cardiovascular system will tolerate the volume load. This dose will supply 500 to 750 units of procoagulants and antithrombin III–heparin cofactor. Four to eight units of platelets can also be added. The use of proplex, a concentrate of Factors II, VII, IX, and X, should be avoided because it contains activated factors that enhance intravascular coagulation.

Once heparin has been started, the prothrombin time, partial thromboplastin time, and thrombin time tests become uninterpretable. It is useful to follow tests of fibrin degradation products (particularly fibrin D dimer), quantitative fibrinogen measurements, and the platelet count at six- to 12-hour intervals. Fibrin degradation products are cleared more rapidly than platelets are produced or than fibrinogen is synthesized. Therefore, a favorable result is usually heralded by a fall in fibrin degradation products and a stable level of platelets and fibrinogen. Subsequent replacement is gauged on the basis of these test results. If the fibrinogen level is very low, cryoprecipitate can be used as a source of fibrinogen replacement. Each bag of cryoprecipitate provides approximately 400 mg of fibrinogen and 80 to 100 units of Factor VIII. If clinical hemorrhage continues and the test results do not show improvement, then the constant infusion of heparin can be increased to between 750 and 1,000 units/hr. After clinical hemorrhage ceases and the patient's condition is stable, the heparin dose should be reduced in a stepwise fashion and the test results monitored until the heparin can be stopped.[213]

Management of the DIC associated with solitary or multiple hemangiomas presents particular problems. When the hemangiomas are localized, they can be excised; occasionally, they show a good response to local irradiation. Attempts to control the DIC using heparin, corticosteroids, aspirin, sulfinpyrazine, estrogens, and dipyridamole have not been successful.[209] However, infusion of cryoprecipitate, 10 bags daily for three days, together with 36 g of EACA daily (twice the usual recommended dosage) produced an excellent response in one case.[209] Presumably, the cryoprecipitate repleted the deficient fibrinogen sufficiently to allow local thrombosis to occur in the hemangiomas; the simultaneous administration of EACA then prevented lysis of these clots. Subsequently, procoagulant and platelet levels improved substantially.[209]

The key to successful management of DIC associated with certain snake bites is identification of the snake and prompt administration of appropriate antivenin.

Primary Fibrinolysis

Cases of generalized primary fibrinolysis are rare, and many of the early reports of primary fibrinolysis probably represented secondary fibrinolysis associated with DIC [see Figures 3 and 8]. As noted, primary fibrinolysis can be distinguished from DIC by using the fibrin D dimer test, which detects the degradation products of polymerized fibrin that occur in DIC. The measurement of the fragment $B_{\beta 1-42}$, a specific product of the plasmin attack on soluble fibrin complexes,[3] may provide a new method for detecting hyperplasminemia.

Snake envenomation may produce afibrinogenemia by two different mechanisms. In one mechanism, extensive tissue destruction caused by the lipases and proteases in venom triggers DIC, depleting fibrinogen levels. Other forms of envenomation, for example, that caused by a western diamondback rattlesnake, *Crotalus atrox*, release endogenous plasminogen activator, thereby inducing primary fibrinogenolysis and afibrinogenemia [see Figure 3].[214]

Postprostatectomy hematuria may constitute a true example of hemorrhage caused by localized fibrinolysis. The high concentration of urokinase in the urine in this condition causes plasminogen to be converted to plasmin [see Figure 3] with resulting clot lysis. If other causes of persistent postoperative hematuria can be ruled out, the condition can be treated with a dose of 0.1 g/kg of oral or intravenous ε-aminocaproic acid. The dose is repeated every six hours until hemorrhage is controlled.[215] Local instillation of EACA by urethral catheter is also effective.

Severe Hepatic Disease

Patients with severe liver disease may suffer life-threatening hemorrhage caused by extensive impairment of their hemostatic mechanisms [see Table 11]. In addition to bleeding varices, gastritis, and peptic ulcer, clinical hemorrhage includes mucosal hemorrhage and tissue bleeding.

Patients with cirrhosis have decreased amounts of normal prothrombin and increased levels of abnormal fibrinogen.[204] Platelet survival is distinctly shortened, and platelet splenic sequestration is increased. Most cirrhotic patients have normal platelet function, as indicated by a normal bleeding time and normal platelet aggregation studies. Fibrinogen turnover is shortened, but the fibrinogen level is usually maintained in the normal range. Fibrin-fibrinogen degradation products are not increased. Plasminogen survival is shortened in cirrhosis, and

Table 11 Hemostatic Abnormalities in Severe Liver Disease

Platelets

Thrombocytopenia
    Ethanol-induced production defect
    Hypersplenism
    Low-grade platelet consumption

Procoagulants

Significant deficiency of Factors II, VII, V, IX, X, and protein C

Consumption of fibrinogen and plasminogen

the plasminogen levels fall.[216] The best screening tests for this disorder include the prothrombin time, prothrombin and proconvertin time, platelet count, and bleeding time.

Replacement is accomplished by administering about 1,000 ml of fresh frozen plasma and platelets as required. Prothrombin complex concentrates should not be used, because they do not contain Factor V and are likely to be contaminated with hepatitis B. Such concentrates also contain activated products that the damaged liver cannot effectively remove and thus may increase the risk of DIC.

Circulating Inhibitors (Anticoagulants)

In addition to the circulating antibody inhibitors seen in severe hemophilias A and B, clinical hemorrhage is occasionally caused by circulating inhibitors of coagulation that seem to appear spontaneously. One type of inhibitor is directed against specific factors such as Factor VIII. This type occurs in rheumatoid diseases, in immunologic diseases, and during the postpartum period.

The clinical features of mucosal hemorrhages, hematomas, and ecchymoses call for coagulation testing. If an inhibitor is present, the partial thromboplastin time, prothrombin time, or thrombin time will be selectively prolonged depending on the inhibitor's site of action. Failure to correct the abnormal test result by mixing equal parts of the patient's plasma and normal plasma strongly suggests that an inhibitor is indeed present. Special coagulation laboratories are equipped to detect inhibitors, to identify their substrate, and to quantify their activity.

The hemorrhage may be clinically life-threatening. Attempts at replacement are usually not successful, because the inhibitor inactivates the replaced procoagulant. Occasionally, however, massive procoagulant replacement can overwhelm the inhibitor. It may be possible to remove the inhibitor by plasmapheresis. Some reports suggest that azathioprine, 100 to 150 mg/day, or cyclophosphamide, 100 to 150 mg/day, with or without added prednisone at 60 mg/day, may reduce the inhibitor level.[217]

Surprisingly, high-dose intravenous IgG can produce long-lasting benefits in nonhemophiliac patients with autoantibodies to Factor VIII:C.[218,219] Patients have been treated with I.V. IgG in a daily dosage of 0.4 g/kg for five consecutive days[218] or in a daily dosage of 0.5 g/kg for eight consecutive days.[219] The infusion produced a decrease in the inhibitor level and an increase in the Factor VIII:C level, and this response seems to have been maintained. Hemophiliac patients who had the alloantibody inhibitor of Factor VIII:C did not respond to this therapy. Such pooled preparations of I.V. IgG contain anti-idiotypic antibodies that can react with and inactivate the autoantibody to Factor VIII:C found in the patients' plasma.[220]

Lupus Anticoagulant

Another type of inhibitor is termed the SLE-like inhibitor, or lupus anticoagulant, because it was first identified in patients with systemic lupus erythematosus and its appearance correlates with the appearance of the biologic false positive Wassermann reaction for syphilis in such patients. The clinician should be alerted to the possible presence of such an inhibitor when a patient who does not have a significant hemorrhagic disorder has a markedly prolonged PTT. In one study, 33 percent of patients with this disorder also had a prolonged prothrombin time, and 25 percent had a prolonged thrombin time.[221] A mixing study performed using a patient's plasma and normal plasma will show immediate prolongation of the PTT.

The lupus anticoagulant appears to be directed against the cephalin added as a surrogate source of the phospholipid component of the prothrombinase complex in the partial thromboplastin time [see Figure 1]. If washed platelets are substituted for the added phospholipid, the PTT usually becomes normal in patients with the lupus anticoagulant.[221] Thus, the lupus anticoagulant, which is found in patients with many types of disorders besides SLE, is actually an in vitro phenomenon.

The lupus anticoagulant is an antibody that displays significant heterogeneity, occurring as polyclonal IgM or IgG[222] and occasionally as monoclonal IgM.[221] Unless persons with this inhibitor also have another abnormality affecting the hemostatic mechanism, they do not have a hemorrhagic disorder, and there is no need to restrict the use of invasive tests in such cases.[223] On the contrary, such patients appear to be especially prone to the development of thromboembolism, particularly following surgery. For the most part, these embolic episodes involve venous thromboses, but arterial thromboses (transient ischemic attacks and axillary and iliofemoral artery occlusions) also occur.[221,224] Chronic treatment with chlorpromazine may lead to the appearance of the lupus anticoagulant; the frequency of its occurrence correlates with the total dose and the duration of chlorpromazine therapy.[225] Many patients with AIDS also have the lupus anticoagulant,[222] which usually appears during opportunistic infection and then disappears with clinical resolution. Because of the heterogeneity of the lupus anticoagulant antibody, it is not surprising that the presence of this antibody is associated with a variety of clinical pictures.[221,222]

The lupus anticoagulant itself may not be the cause of the coagulopathy seen in patients who carry this factor. Rather, venous and cerebral thrombosis is strongly correlated with the titer of the anticardiolipin antibodies that are frequently associated with the lupus anticoagulant.[226] There are several classes of these antibodies, of which the best known is the factor responsible for precipitation in the Venereal Disease Research Laboratory (VDRL) test for syphilis. These anticardiolipin antibodies are highly correlated with a syndrome of recurrent arterial and venous thromboses, pulmonary hypertension, and thrombocytopenia, as well as recurrent abortion.[227]

Patients with the lupus anticoagulant who have experienced repeated abortion have been treated during a subsequent pregnancy with 40 to 50 mg of prednisone and 81 mg of aspirin daily, generally beginning by the eighth week of gestation, to prevent thrombosis in the decidual and placental vessels. This therapy lowered the PTT and inhibited thromboxane generation [*see Figure 6*]; five of eight patients treated with this combination gave birth to live infants.[228] It is not yet clear whether the lupus anticoagulant measurement, the anticardiolipin antibody measurement, or another measurement will correlate best with fetal loss and thrombosis.[229]

Chronic Expanding Hematomas

Occasionally, hematomas develop following surgery or trauma and in the absence of a hemostatic abnormality. Such lesions may continue to expand because of their size and inflammatory properties. It is important to recognize the possibility of a chronic expanding hematoma because the lesion can be removed surgically.[230]

Bleeding after Cardiopulmonary Bypass

Patients who undergo heart surgery with cardiopulmonary bypass frequently have intraoperative and postoperative episodes of life-threatening hemorrhage in the absence of procoagulant consumption or heparin overdose.[231] There appears to be an acquired platelet function disorder, perhaps caused by contact between the platelets and the oxygenator apparatus. The hemorrhage in such cases is associated with a long bleeding time and frequently responds to platelet transfusions. Such transfusions, however, are costly and time-consuming and carry the danger of transmitting hepatitis, AIDS, and other viral infections. In one study,[232] patients undergoing coronary artery bypass grafting were treated with 0.3 µg/kg DDAVP in 50 ml, administered intravenously over 15 minutes after cardiopulmonary bypass had been concluded and after the heparin effect had been reversed by protamine. An approximately 40 percent reduction in postoperative blood loss was associated with a rise in the plasma level of von Willebrand factor. It is possible that this increased level of vWF compensated for a platelet function defect. A similar reduction in blood loss was achieved by the administration of DDAVP to patients undergoing Harrington rod spinal fusion surgery.[233]

Hypercoagulable States

Most cases of thrombosis are caused by a local event such as vessel wall damage (resulting from atherosclerosis or vasculitis) or stasis, but a rheologic problem may also predispose to thrombosis. For example, the elevated hematocrit in polycythemia vera can slow blood flow, and the rigid undeformable erythrocytes present in such hemoglobinopathies as sickle cell disease or hemoglobin C disease can induce thrombosis in the lungs or in the microcirculation. Thrombosis may occur in chronic myeloproliferative diseases in association with a significantly elevated platelet count, yet it is difficult to show a correlation between thrombotic events and the platelet count, platelet function abnormality, or spontaneous level of platelet aggregation.[136] The presence of an underlying hemostatic abnormality is suggested by a family history of thrombosis or the appearance of recurrent thrombosis or thrombosis in atypical sites in otherwise healthy, young persons [*see Table 12*].

Antithrombin III Deficiency

Antithrombin III deficiency, which may be either hereditary or acquired, impairs inactivation of the activated procoagulants Factors Xa and IIa, which leads to enhanced thrombosis [*see Chapter 7*].[34] AT-III appears to inactivate Factors XIIa, XIa, IXa, and Xa by forming a stable stoichiometric complex with each of these factors, which is the same mechanism by which AT-III inactivates thrombin. AT-III is present in sufficient amounts in plasma to inactivate all the thrombin formed in a given plasma volume, but it does so slowly unless it is activated by cell membrane heparans or administered heparin.[234] Normal levels of AT-III activated by naturally occurring heparans exert a steady modulating effect in hemostasis by neutralizing

<table>
<tr><td colspan="1" align="center">Table 12   Causes of the
Hypercoagulable State</td></tr>
<tr><td>
Antithrombin III deficiency
Abnormalities of fibrinolysis
Protein C and protein S deficiencies
Drug administration: oral contraceptives, heparin
Dysfibrinogenemia
Trousseau's syndrome
Presence of the lupus anticoagulant
Homocystinuria
</td></tr>
</table>

excess Factor Xa. Patients with hereditary AT-III deficiency have an increased incidence of venous thrombosis[234]; rarely, arterial thrombosis may occur.[235] Mesenteric vein thrombosis is a typical finding.

There is usually a family history of recurrent thrombosis, generally beginning in youth and often associated with surgery or trauma. Pregnancy and the use of oral contraceptives increase the risk of thromboses in AT-III–deficient patients.[234] The tendency to thrombosis increases with advancing age, so that by age 50 only 10 percent of affected patients are free of symptoms.[34] Patients with this deficiency have a surprisingly modest reduction in AT-III; values measured by both bioassay and an immunoassay range between 25 and 60 percent of normal. Generally, the disorder is diagnosed when a high index of suspicion leads to the ordering of both a bioassay and an immunoassay for AT-III.

Patients with AT-III deficiency probably require lifelong therapy with oral warfarin-type anticoagulants, which usually raise AT-III levels toward normal. An acute episode of thrombosis must be treated with heparin. Because the deficiency of AT-III may render heparin relatively ineffective, the physician should be alert to heparin resistance that is manifested by minimal prolongation of the PTT after the administration of therapeutic doses of heparin, that is, 15 units/kg/hr I.V. following an initial bolus of 5,000 units I.V. If heparin resistance occurs, AT-III should be administered along with heparin either in the form of AT-III concentrates or as fresh frozen plasma. (The AT-III concentrate has not yet been cleared by the FDA for general distribution, but it can be obtained from Cutter Laboratories, Berkeley, California, as an investigational new drug [IND] for compassionate use.)

Two methods have been proposed for calculating the appropriate amount of AT-III to administer to a patient with AT-III deficiency. According to one method of calculation,[234] 0.67 units/kg of AT-III is administered for each desired one percent increase in the AT-III plasma level. For example, to restore AT-III levels to normal in a 70 kg patient with an AT-III level of 40 percent, it is necessary to administer [(100−40)×0.67 units/kg×70 kg], or about 2,800 units of concentrate (or 2,800 ml of fresh frozen plasma). A second method of calculation involves the administration of 50 IU/kg I.V. over a 20-minute period. Because such a volume of fresh frozen plasma would produce vascular overload, the use of AT-III concentrates is preferable.[236] Because the half-life of AT-III is 17.5 to 26.5 hours,[234] AT-III infusions (in a dosage of 35 to 40 units/kg) should be repeated at 24-hour intervals.[236] The heparin dose should be adjusted to achieve a 1.5-fold prolongation of the PTT, and warfarin should be started simultaneously. Warfarin has been the mainstay of chronic therapy for patients with AT-III deficiency and recurrent thromboembolism, but danazol may eventually prove to be the preferred form of therapy for this disorder. Danazol, in an oral dosage of 200 mg two to three times a day, increases AT-III levels and thereby prevents thromboembolism without requiring frequent testing of the PT.[236]

Acquired AT-III deficiency may occur in patients given intravenous heparin for more than three days, in DIC, in severe liver disease, in the nephrotic syndrome, and following asparaginase therapy.[34]

Heparin Cofactor II Deficiency

AT-III accounts for most of the antithrombin activity of plasma, but another clotting inhibitor, called heparin cofactor II, interacts with heparin to inactivate thrombin. This cofactor does not affect the other serine proteases (Factors IXa, XIa, and Xa). Heparin cofactor II requires about 10 times more heparin than AT-III for its activation, and it can also be activated by dermatan sulfate. When activated, it forms a stable complex with thrombin and thereby inactivates it.[237,238]

Hereditary deficiency of cofactor II leads to a hypercoagulable state. Affected family members have about half the normal value of this cofactor and experience both arterial and venous thromboses.[237,238] Acquired deficiency of heparin cofactor II occurs in DIC and severe liver disease, but the pathophysiologic role of the deficiency in these conditions has not been determined.[239]

Protein C and Protein S Deficiency

Deficient or defective protein C or protein S [see Figure 4] results in the loss of the ability to inactivate excess Factor VIIIa and Factor Va and to maintain an appropriate fibrinolytic response.[3,6] Protein C, in conjunction with protein S, inactivates a plasminogen activator inhibitor.[240] Protein C levels are low in patients with DIC and liver disease, probably because the activation of hemostasis consumes this factor.[241]

Homozygous protein C deficiency causes lethal thrombosis in infancy.[242] Heterozygous deficiency of protein C probably occurs with a prevalence of one in 200 to one in 300. The blood levels of protein C in patients with the heterozygous deficiency overlap the lower range of normal values. Many heterozygotes and individuals with low normal values of protein C have no history of thrombosis.[243] Other heterozygotes, however, exhibit a definite tendency to venous thrombosis even though their protein C levels are in the 40 to 50 percent range.[244,245] Cerebral venous thrombosis presumably accounts for cases of cerebral hemorrhagic infarction that occur in young adults with this deficiency.[246] Warfarin-induced skin necrosis is associated with deficiency of protein C.[247]

Oral warfarin anticoagulants are the treatment of choice for preventing thrombosis even though they lower protein C levels still further. Because the half-life of protein C is only six to seven hours,[6] much shorter than that of prothrombin, Factor X, or Factor IX [*see Table 1*], a period of enhanced hypercoagulability follows initiation of warfarin therapy in patients with protein C deficiency. Skin necrosis during warfarin therapy suggests the presence of protein C deficiency. Heparin should be given along with warfarin during the initiation of anticoagulation in such patients [*see Chapter 7*], and the heparin can subsequently be withdrawn.

Deficiency of protein S [*see Figure 4*] also leads to venous thrombosis, including mesenteric vein thrombosis.[247-250] Pregnancy and the use of oral contraceptives lower the protein S level, which may account for some cases of thromboembolism that occur under such circumstances.[251] Protein S deficiency also occurs in patients with the nephrotic syndrome and is partially caused by the selective loss of protein S in the urine. This deficiency may contribute to the thromboembolic episodes observed in such patients.[252]

Assays for protein C and protein S are available in research laboratories.

Abnormalities of Fibrinolysis

Several cases of structurally abnormal plasminogens have been described in patients with recurrent thrombosis. The plasminogens were biologically nonfunctional [*see Figure 3*], presumably leading to inadequate fibrinolytic activity and enhanced thrombosis. Patients with hypoplasminogenemia have also been described.[247] The diagnosis of dysplasminogenemia and hypoplasminogenemia can be established by finding low plasminogen activity (> 50 percent of normal). Patients with dysplasminogenemia have normal levels of immunologically identifiable plasminogen.[247] Patients respond to treatment with warfarin.[200]

An additional cause of the hypercoagulable state is deficient or defective action of plasminogen activators. In such cases, local hemostasis is unopposed by adequate fibrinolysis. Defective fibrinolysis may be an important factor in some cases of recurrent thromboembolism.[253] One study that examined 100 consecutive patients with deep venous thrombosis and pulmonary embolism found that 11 patients released very low levels of t-PA during a standard venous occlusion. In an additional 22 patients, fibrinolysis was defective because the t-PA that was released in normal amounts was inactivated by an excess of t-PA inhibitor.[253] Assays for t-PA and t-PA inhibitor are currently available only in research laboratories, but the findings of this study indicate a need for programs that either increase local t-PA release or block a local excess of t-PA inhibitors.

Dysfibrinogenemia

One case of congenital dysfibrinogenemia has been associated with thrombotic disease. Although the clots that formed in patients with this disorder were defective, they could not be removed, because they were very rigid and resistant to plasmin-mediated lysis. Such conventional laboratory assays as the thrombin time and the reptilase time should be prolonged, but tests performed in a research laboratory are required to make the diagnosis. Incomplete fibrin polymerization should result in a positive test for fibrin degradation products.[247] Therapy with warfarin seems to be beneficial.[254]

Homocystinuria

Homocystinuria is a hereditary disorder characterized by an inability to metabolize homocysteine normally. Because of this defect, the plasma level of homocysteine rises to the point at which it interferes with collagen cross-linking, which eventually causes endothelial and subendothelial damage. This vascular damage leads to arterial and venous thrombosis and perhaps accelerated atherosclerosis.

The diagnosis should be suspected in cases of recurrent thromboembolism in young persons, particularly when the condition is associated with mental retardation and ectopia lentis. The diagnosis can be confirmed using a urine screening test.[247] Treatment with pyridoxine may be useful in addition to anticoagulant therapy.

Drug Administration

Certain drugs have a propensity for causing thrombosis. Oral estrogen-containing contraceptives seem to increase the risk of thromboembolic disease.[255] The explanation for this association is unknown, but women who take oral contraceptives have lower AT-III and protein S levels, elevated Hageman factor (Factor XII) levels, and paradoxically enhanced fibrinolytic activity.

Heparin-associated thrombosis can be a devastating event that occurs in a patient who requires anticoagulation therapy and that is usually associated with heparin-induced thrombocytopenia [*see* Decreased Platelet Count—Thrombocytopenia, Heparin Thrombocytopenia, *above*].[256,257]

Patients who are receiving cyclosporine following transplantation of a kidney from a cadaver donor show an increased incidence of venous thromboembolism.[258] Cyclosporine may also cause a variant of the hemolyticuremic syndrome, but it is not clear that the two thrombotic abnormalities associated with cyclosporine use are related.

Trousseau's Syndrome

Some patients with cancer have an increased propensity for the development of recurrent migratory thromboembolism, an association that has been termed Trousseau's syndrome. It appears that the underlying pathophysiologic event is a chronic subclinical form of DIC and that the activated procoagulants generated in DIC lead to enhanced thrombosis.[259] Overt DIC in such patients is uncommon,[260] but when it occurs, continuous treatment with heparin is required to prevent recurrent episodes of venous and arterial thrombosis. Warfarin is probably ineffective in this setting.[261] Laboratory findings may show low fibrinogen and platelet levels, prolonged prothrombin times, and increased levels of fibrin-fibrinogen degradation products. The key to management is diagnosis and treatment of the underlying tumor, which should lead to control of the DIC. Because the subclinical DIC is associated with thrombosis, however, it is reasonable to institute heparin therapy pending definitive treatment of the tumor.

In my experience, Trousseau's syndrome presents a very difficult and frustrating clinical situation because the neoplasm is often occult and is not identified despite an aggressive search. The deep venous thromboembolism continues to recur despite use of full and controlled doses of warfarin, supplemented with aspirin or sulfinpyrazone. Continuous I.V. heparin or subcutaneous heparin given every 12 hours may be helpful.[261] Ultimately, the tumor often manifests itself explosively and does not respond to the usual therapies.

Lupus Anticoagulant

Patients with the lupus anticoagulant [*see* Acquired Hemorrhagic Disorders, Circulating Inhibitors (Anticoagulants), *above*] have a paradoxically increased incidence of thrombosis, the cause of which is unclear.[262] In one case, the SLE inhibitor inhibited the thrombin-thrombomodulin activation of protein C to protein Ca, establishing a hypercoagulable state.[263]

Patients who have the lupus anticoagulant and who require surgery should be managed with minidose prophylactic heparin or related antithrombotic programs. Patients who have the lupus anticoagulant and established deep vein thrombosis are difficult to treat because the PTT is already greatly prolonged and the PT may also be prolonged. The lupus anticoagulant exhibits a slight association with decreased prothrombin levels and a more frequent association with thrombocytopenia [*see* Acquired Hemorrhagic Disorders, Lupus Anticoagulant, *above*]. Fixed dosage schedules of heparin can be used in an attempt to control the thrombosis; oral warfarin is instituted later, and the P and P time can then be very helpful in adjusting the dosage [*see* Chapter 7].

Surgical Mishap versus Systemic Disorder

Serious hemorrhage during or after surgery is a complicated clinical problem requiring rapid diagnosis and prompt intervention.

If the patient is bleeding only in the operative area, it may be difficult to decide whether or not there is a systemic hemorrhagic disorder. A revealing clue to a systemic malfunction is bleeding at multiple sites, particularly areas other than the surgical wound. Bleeding around a catheter, from venipuncture sites, and from venous cutdowns is highly indicative of a hemorrhagic disorder.

Rapid assessment of the total clinical setting is imperative. Does the patient have underlying renal, hepatic, or malignant disease? Has the surgery required pump bypass techniques or the induction of hypothermia, or has the patient been in shock or hyperthermic? How many units of blood and blood products have been given and over what period of time? Were baseline screening procoagulant tests obtained prior to surgery, and is the patient's frozen plasma still available?

Prompt resolution inevitably requires carefully done coagulation tests including partial thromboplastin time, Quick's one-stage prothrombin time, thrombin time, fibrinogen assay, measurement of fibrin-fibrinogen degradation products, fibrin D dimer test, a platelet count, a well-stained blood smear for evaluation of platelet morphology, and bleeding time (preferably done by a modified Ivy template method). This battery of tests should be performed immediately. More specialized studies can be obtained if there is evidence of a specific disorder.

Frequent Causes of Postoperative Hemorrhage

Platelet-Related Causes

Platelet washout Whenever a small or average-sized patient has been rapidly transfused with eight or more units of blood, there is danger of thrombocytopenic hemorrhage from platelet washout [*see* Decreased Platelet Count—Thrombocytopenia, Platelet Washout and Vascular Bed Abnormalities, *above*].

Immunologic forms of acute thrombocytopenia (posttransfusion purpura) Rarely, devastating acute thrombocytopenia occurs after transfusions of whole blood or components containing platelets. In certain instances, it has been shown that the recipient mounts an antibody response against an antigen called Zw^a (formerly termed Pl^{A1}) on the donor platelets.[264] The patient's own platelets are also affected, even though they lack Zw^a, leading to the development of acute immunologic thrombocytopenic purpura. The mechanism of this reaction is poorly understood.

Corticosteroids administered at the usual doses, splenectomy, and platelet transfusions are usually ineffective. Corticosteroid therapy, from standard dosages up to 2 g methylprednisolone a day for three days, has been proposed.[265] Plasmapheresis has also been used in an attempt to remove the antibody.[266] The current therapy of choice, however, is the infusion of I.V. IgG in a dosage of 0.4 to 0.8 g/kg over a period of 60 minutes, followed by the administration of about 10 to 12 units of random-donor platelets. Without intervention, the platelet count returns to normal over a period of about two weeks.

Platelet function disorders If surgery has required a prolonged pump bypass procedure or if the patient's blood has been in intimate contact with any of a variety of prostheses, postoperative bleeding may occur as a result of a qualitative platelet disorder [*see* Platelet Function Disorders *and* Acquired Hemorrhagic Disorders, Bleeding after Cardiopulmonary Bypass, *above*].

Platelets that have had sustained contact with foreign surfaces may have undergone partial release and discharged substantial amounts of their granular material. Although they can still aggregate, the ability of such platelets to undergo the release reaction is subsequently impaired. This platelet dysfunction is characterized by prolonged bleeding time, the finding of degranulated platelets on a well-stained smear, and a relatively normal platelet count. Such conditions as acute or chronic renal disease and, in some circumstances, acute hepatic disorders may also cause functional defects in platelets.

Dysfunctional platelets will not undergo the release reaction; if, however, appropriate aggregating materials are present, the damaged platelets can aggregate and contribute to the formation of a hemostatic plug. It is therefore necessary to add a threshold number of normal platelets, which can adhere and undergo the release reaction. Transfusion of about four to six units of platelets should raise the platelet count by 30,000 to 40,000/mm^3 and should control bleeding. If the patient has a platelet function defect related to acute uremia, prompt hemodialysis may be needed to control the hemorrhage [*see* Platelet Function Disorders, Uremia, *above*].

Procoagulant-Related Causes of Perioperative Hemorrhage

Heparin Heparin is frequently used during surgery for bypass procedures; it is also employed to keep intravenous lines open. Heparin is customarily neutralized after a surgical procedure by the infusion of protamine. Because heparin is inactivated by enzymes in the liver and excreted by the kidneys, damage to either of these organs results in prolonged heparin activity.

A diagnosis of hemorrhage caused by inadvertent anticoagulation with heparin is suggested by prolonged PTT, PT, and TT in conjunction with a normal reptilase time, bleeding time, and platelet count.

The intravenous administration of protamine in a dosage of 50 mg every one to two hours should return the TT and PTT to normal and stanch the bleeding.

Disseminated intravascular coagulation DIC is a disastrous clotting sequence that usually follows extensive trauma, shock, or surgical repair [*see* Acquired Hemorrhagic Disorders, Disseminated Intravascular Coagulation, *above*].

Impaired hepatic function The liver is the site of synthesis of all of the pro-

coagulants except vWF. The reticuloendothelial cells of the liver remove the particulate and other thromboplastic materials that may circulate in patients who experience shock or trauma. Serious damage to the liver is usually associated with a deficiency of procoagulants and a degree of DIC.

Because multiple factors are depleted, the key diagnostic distinction is between DIC and procoagulant deficiency caused by hepatic disease. The situation is further complicated by the fact that severe liver disease may produce some degree of DIC, which can be of varying clinical importance. Finding a normal TT is helpful because it rules out both heparin effect and the action of the fibrin-fibrinogen degradation products that are produced in DIC. A normal fibrinogen assay also weighs against a diagnosis of DIC, and a normal platelet count is distinctly unusual in this disorder. Replacement should be carried out with fresh frozen plasma.

Undiagnosed hemophilia and von Willebrand's disease Hemophilia and von Willebrand's disease may cause hemorrhage during surgery. The bleeding is usually severe but is confined to the site of the wound.

If the patient has mild or moderate hemophilia and has received extensive transfusions of blood and blood products, he or she may not bleed in the immediate postoperative period but may rebleed two or three days after the surgical procedure, when the procoagulant levels, which had been transiently elevated by the transfusions, have fallen [*see* Hereditary Coagulation Disorders, Hemophilia, *above*].

Von Willebrand's disease may be difficult to diagnose during the postoperative period. In this disorder, Factor VIII coagulant activity is low, but the patient can use substances present in fresh frozen plasma to make biologically active Factor VIII. The rise in this factor is sustained over 18 to 36 hours. Therefore, if the patient has received plasma, the PTT and Factor VIII assay may be normal, and the bleeding time may or may not be prolonged. A ristocetin test may be helpful in this case. For classic Factor VIII deficiency, the patient should be given infusions of cryoprecipitate or Factor VIII concentrate [*see* Hereditary Coagulation Disorders, Principles of Replacement Therapy, *above*]. The management of von Willebrand's disease may present more difficult problems than the management of hemophilia.

Primary Fibrinolysis

Occasionally, primary fibrinolysis must be considered in the differential diagnosis of disseminated intravascular coagulation, particularly in a patient who has had surgery for prostatic cancer and now shows evidence of clot lysis [*see Figure 3*]. Fibrinolysis usually occurs as a response to the stimulus of DIC. Primary fibrinolysis, however, may occur in acute promyelocytic leukemia [*see Chapter 15*] and in other circumstances in which t-PA action is enhanced or unimpeded. The fibrin D dimer test is useful in distinguishing DIC from primary fibrinolysis. Because the D dimer fragment is produced only from fully polymerized fibrin, its presence signals DIC. EACA can be used cautiously in the treatment of fibrinolysis in the case of urogenital surgery [*see* Acquired Hemorrhagic Disorders, Primary Fibrinolysis, *above*]. There are also anecdotal reports of benefit from ε-aminocaproic acid in the treatment of postoperative hemorrhage in children who have congenital heart disease and show evidence of fibrinolysis.

False Abnormalities in Procoagulant Test Results

Occasionally, coagulation test values, particularly the PTT and TT, are markedly prolonged postoperatively. Examination of the patient may or may not reveal significant hemorrhage. At this point, the method used to collect the blood sample should be investigated.[267] Patients with significant postoperative hemorrhage may be in shock and frequently have indwelling intravenous catheters. The test sample may have been obtained from an intravenous catheter kept open with low concentrations of heparin. Furthermore, the blood may have been diluted with saline solutions or glucose solutions, or both. The blood sample may have clotted during collection. A prolonged thrombin time that can be corrected by the addition of protamine is evidence of heparin contamination. Glucose solutions mixed with blood cause erythrocyte deformation on blood smears. These problems can be avoided by obtaining blood samples directly from a vein.[267]

Tests are costly and fallible, and the question of whether or not to employ screening coagulation tests before surgery invariably arises.[268] The importance of the history is emphasized by studies showing that the PTT cannot be used as a general screening test to predict which patients will experience hemorrhage; however, the PTT does have predictive value when used in patients who are selected by the history to be at high risk for bleeding.[269] One recommended preoperative procedure to follow in such cases is:

1. Ask specifically if there is a history of bleeding in the family or if the patient has ever bled excessively during surgery or dental extractions.

2. Order a panel of tests that includes bleeding time, a platelet count, examination of platelets on peripheral smear, PTT, PT, and an estimate of the fibrinogen concentration.

3. Freeze a tube of plasma to save for 24 hours after surgery. Therefore, if the patient bleeds, preoperative as well as postoperative specimens can be tested. This approach greatly facilitates the discovery of previously undiagnosed hemophilia or von Willebrand's disease.

References

1. J Lab Clin Med 102:551, 1983
2. J Clin Invest 73:1249, 1984
3. Hosp Pract 21(March):131, 1986
4. J Clin Invest 71:1383, 1983
5. Blood 70:343, 1987
6. N Engl J Med 314:1298, 1986
7. Science 235:1348, 1987
8. Blood 67:1554, 1986
9. Blood 58:1, 1981
10. Br J Haematol 54:1, 1983
11. N Engl J Med 311:1084, 1984
12. Blood 70:605, 1987
13. Annu Rev Med 29:41, 1978
14. Proc Natl Acad Sci USA 74:5260, 1977
15. Trends in Biochemical Sciences 12:229, 1987
16. Blood 67:1529, 1986
17. Blood 69:381, 1987
18. Br Med J 1:927, 1977
19. Br J Haematol 62:333, 1986
20. Blood Cells 9:407, 1983
21. Blood 69:522, 1987
22. Am J Hematol 23:231, 1986
23. Blood 61:99, 1983
24. J Clin Invest 70:542, 1982
25. J Clin Invest 78:1456, 1986
26. Blood 69:625, 1987
27. J Clin Invest 78:329, 1986
28. N Engl J Med 293:531, 580, 1975
29. J Clin Invest 59:449, 1977
30. Series Haematologica 8:50, 1976
31. Science 196:1072, 1977
32. Br J Haematol 21:43, 1971
33. N Engl J Med 295:428, 1976
34. Lancet 1:1021, 1983
35. Br Med J 285:397, 1982
36. Semin Hematol 10:183, 1973
37. Semin Hematol 10:311, 1973
38. Drug-induced Blood Disorders. Blackwell Scientific Publications, Oxford, 1975
39. Br J Haematol 62:345, 1986
40. N Engl J Med 292:230, 1975
41. Hosp Pract 20(June):95, 1985
42. J Clin Invest 80:33, 1987
43. N Engl J Med 304:1135, 1981
44. J Clin Invest 77:1756, 1986
45. N Engl J Med 313:1375, 1985
46. Semin Thromb Hemost 8:83, 1982
47. Blood 55:730, 1980
48. Am J Med 81:139, 1986
49. N Engl J Med 312:1170, 1985
50. N Engl J Med 307:1495, 1982
51. Hemostasis Manual, 2nd ed. FA Davis Co, Philadelphia, 1974
52. Blood 58:326, 1981
53. Ann Intern Med 103:542, 1985
54. Ann Intern Med 102:737, 1985
55. Arch Intern Med 142:1460, 1982
56. Ann Intern Med 94:27, 1981
57. N Engl J Med 316:211, 1987
58. Blood 69:278, 1987
59. Surg Gynecol Obstet 164:225, 1987
60. Br Med J 282:1497, 1981
61. Ann Intern Med 100:192, 1984
62. N Engl J Med 316:503, 1987
63. JAMA 245:369, 1981
64. Am J Med 80:1051, 1986
65. N Engl J Med 306:1254, 1982
66. Lancet 1:84, 1983
67. Blood 60(suppl 1):190a, 1982
68. Ann Intern Med 104:808, 1986
69. Transfusion 21:291, 1981
70. Am J Med 69:690, 1980
71. N Engl J Med 308:1396, 1983
72. Ann Intern Med 107:177, 1987
73. Am J Med 69:430, 1980
74. Br J Haematol 66:491, 1987
75. Obstet Gynecol 51:590, 1978
76. N Engl J Med 306:836, 1982
77. N Engl J Med 305:936, 1981
78. Am J Obstet Gynecol 136:495, 1980
79. Blood 53:545, 1979
80. Ann Intern Med 98:926, 1983
81. Br J Haematol 51:17, 1982
82. Br J Haematol 64:419, 1986
83. Br J Haematol 50:599, 1982
84. Am J Med 79:253, 1985
85. J Clin Invest 79:912, 1987
86. J Clin Invest 75:310, 1985
87. Ann Intern Med 100:535, 1984
88. Br J Haematol 64:347, 1986
89. N Engl J Med 316:581, 1987
90. Ann Intern Med 95:178, 1981
91. Medicine (Baltimore) 60:413, 1981
92. JAMA 246:1243, 1981
93. Semin Thromb Hemost 8:186, 1982
94. JAMA 241:1709, 1979
95. Ann Intern Med 89:501, 1978
96. JAMA 242:173, 1979
97. Arch Intern Med 140:353, 1980
98. Arch Intern Med 142:2275, 1982
99. Blood 60(suppl 1):185a, 1982
100. Arch Intern Med 143:1617, 1983
101. Blood 60:1030, 1982
102. N Engl J Med 307:1447, 1982
103. N Engl J Med 307:1432, 1982
104. Blood 69:924, 1987
105. JAMA 247:3119, 1982
106. Semin Thromb Hemost 7:43, 1981
107. Br Med J 283:1351, 1981
108. Semin Thromb Hemost 7:1, 1981
109. JAMA 247:1433, 1982
110. Blood 60(suppl 1):186a, 1982
111. Semin Thromb Hemost 7:9, 1981
112. JAMA 246:1931, 1981
113. Semin Thromb Hemost 7:15, 1981
114. Blood 56:302, 1980
115. Br Med J 285:1304, 1982
116. Semin Thromb Hemost 8:217, 1982
117. Am J Hematol 7:255, 1979
118. J Clin Invest 71:832, 1983
119. Semin Thromb Hemost 8:234, 1982
120. Am J Hematol 21:397, 1986
121. Br Med J 291:23, 1985
122. Annu Rev Med 37:179, 1986
123. Am J Hematol 24:215, 1987
124. N Engl J Med 303:1318, 1980
125. N Engl J Med 308:8, 1983
126. Br J Haematol 59:139, 1985
127. Lancet 2:887, 1984
128. N Engl J Med 315:731, 1986
129. Lancet 2:414, 1986
130. J Clin Invest 79:1788, 1987
131. Br Med J 293:715, 1986
132. Lancet 1:510, 1983
133. JAMA 249:69, 1983
134. Ann Intern Med 105:924, 1986
135. Am J Hematol 20:365, 1985
136. Arch Intern Med 122:18, 1968
137. Am J Hematol 24:23, 1987
138. N Engl J Med 306:381, 1982
139. Semin Hematol 14:409, 1977
140. Ann Intern Med 102:466, 1985
141. Semin Hematol 23:177, 1986
142. Br J Haematol 62:229, 1986
143. Blood 63:51, 1984
144. Br J Haematol 50:157, 1982
145. Semin Thromb Hemost 10:173, 1984
146. Semin Hematol 13:211, 1976
147. West J Med 133:485, 1980
148. Semin Thromb Hemost 10:196, 1984
149. West J Med 140:60, 1984
150. Br Med J 1:190, 1977
151. Human Blood Coagulation, Hemostasis and Thrombosis. Blackwell Scientific Publications, Oxford, 1972, p 210
152. Blood 69:454, 1987
153. J Clin Invest 79:117, 1987
154. Annu Rev Med 37:157, 1986
155. Blood 61:27, 1983
156. Blood 70:895, 1987
157. Ann Intern Med 94:47, 1981
158. J Clin Invest 72:1532, 1983
159. Blood 63:226, 1984
160. Br J Haematol 47:283, 1981
161. Lancet 2:774, 1983
162. Ann Intern Med 103:6, 1985
163. Lancet 2:255, 1986
164. J Lab Clin Med 103:653, 1984
165. MMWR 31:365, 1982
166. JAMA 253:3409, 1985
167. Ann Intern Med 102:476, 1985
168. JAMA 256:3205, 1986
169. MMWR 36:121, 1987
170. Ann Intern Med 102:623, 1985

171. JAMA 256:3200, 1986
172. Ann Intern Med 105:886, 1986
173. Nature 314:674, 1985
174. Blood 67:1560, 1986
175. Lancet 1:148, 1986
176. N Engl J Med 312:682, 1985
177. Lancet 1:1407, 1985
178. N Engl J Med 317:985, 1987
179. Lancet 1:872, 1977
180. Clin Haematol 14:489, 1985
181. JAMA 253:1279, 1985
182. N Engl J Med 308:1393, 1983
183. JAMA 253:1151, 1985
184. JAMA 253:1154, 1985
185. Br J Haematol 64:493, 1986
186. Blood 68:673, 1986
187. JAMA 251:68, 1984
188. Blood 63:31, 1984
189. Br J Haematol 58:641, 1984
190. Br Med J 281:1388, 1980
191. N Engl J Med 303:421, 1980
192. Blood 56:978, 1980
193. N Engl J Med 305:717, 1981
194. Blood 62:1135, 1983
195. JAMA 251:67, 1984
196. Lancet 1:242, 1984
197. Lancet 1:239, 1984
198. Blood 67:1508, 1986
199. Am J Hematol 24:37, 1987
200. Semin Thromb Hemost 10:42, 1984
201. Blood 61:267, 1983
202. N Engl J Med 296:624, 1977
203. N Engl J Med 310:1458, 1984
204. N Engl J Med 305:242, 1981
205. Arch Intern Med 146:1397, 1986
206. Ann Intern Med 105:924, 1986
207. Blood 35:695, 1970
208. J Clin Invest 79:124, 1987
209. N Engl J Med 313:309, 1985
210. Lancet 2:1259, 1985
211. Arch Intern Med 146:1997, 1986
212. N Engl J Med 292:146, 1975
213. N Engl J Med 283:686, 1970
214. Blood 63:1, 1984
215. Lancet 1:232, 1966
216. J Lab Clin Med 99:217, 1982
217. Progress in Hemostasis and Thrombosis. Grune & Stratton, Inc, New York, 1972, p 75
218. Lancet 2:765, 1984
219. Lancet 1:273, 1985
220. Proc Natl Acad Sci USA 84:828, 1987
221. Am J Hematol 19:265, 1985
222. Ann Intern Med 104:175, 1986
223. JAMA 256:491, 1986
224. Arch Intern Med 144:510, 1984
225. Ann Intern Med 91:194, 1979
226. Lancet 2:1211, 1983
227. Lancet 1:912, 1985
228. N Engl J Med 313:1322, 1985
229. N Engl J Med 313:1348, 1985
230. JAMA 244:2441, 1980
231. N Engl J Med 314:1446, 1986
232. N Engl J Med 314:1402, 1986
233. Ann Intern Med 107:446, 1987
234. Medicine (Baltimore) 62:209, 1983
235. JAMA 245:1759, 1981
236. Am J Hematol 21:215, 1986
237. Lancet 2:414, 1985
238. Lancet 2:413, 1985
239. Blood 66:769, 1985
240. Blood 69:231, 1987
241. Blood 60:261, 1982
242. N Engl J Med 310:559, 1984
243. N Engl J Med 317:991, 1987
244. Blood 62:1155, 1983
245. N Engl J Med 310:588, 1984
246. Br Med J 290:350, 1985
247. Am J Hematol 21:419, 1986
248. N Engl J Med 311:1525, 1984
249. Gastroenterology 92:240, 1987
250. Ann Intern Med 106:677, 1987
251. Blood 69:692, 1987
252. Ann Intern Med 107:42, 1987
253. Br Med J 290:1453, 1985
254. Blood 62:439, 1983
255. J Lab Clin Med 96:762, 1980
256. Ann Intern Med 99:637, 1983
257. Ann Intern Med 100:535, 1984
258. Lancet 1:999, 1985
259. Medicine (Baltimore) 56:1, 1977
260. Blood 62:14, 1983
261. Am J Med 79:423, 1985
262. Br Med J 287:1021, 1983
263. Blood 62(suppl 1):299a, 1983
264. Am J Hematol 1:339, 1976
265. Br Med J 1:436, 1975
266. N Engl J Med 291:1163, 1974
267. Arch Intern Med 146:2165, 1986
268. Blood 61:229, 1983
269. JAMA 256:750, 1986

Acknowledgments

Figure 1   Dana Burns. Adapted from "The Pathophysiology of the Prethrombotic State in Humans: Insights Gained from Studies Using Markers of Hemostatic System Activation," by K. A. Bauer and R. D. Rosenberg, in *Blood* 70(2):343, 1987. Used by permission.

Figure 2   Hank Iken.

Figures 3, 4   Dana Burns.

Figures 6, 7   Dana Burns.

Figure 8   Al Miller.

Figure 9   Dana Burns.

15 The Leukemias and the Myeloproliferative Disorders

STANLEY L. SCHRIER, M.D.

Biology of the Leukemias

Leukemia can be defined as the proliferation of a clone of abnormal hematopoietic cells that typically has certain characteristics: (1) poor responsiveness to normal regulatory mechanisms, (2) a diminished capacity for normal cell differentiation, (3) the ability to expand at the expense of normal myeloid or lymphoid lines, and (4) the ability to suppress or impair normal myeloid or lymphoid cell growth. Leukemias are named and grouped according to the kind of hematopoietic cell that is primarily involved. Myeloid leukemias affect the descendants of myeloid stem cells, whereas lymphocytic leukemias involve abnormalities in the lymphoid cell line. Leukemias can be acute or chronic or may take intermediate and variable forms. Without treatment, even the chronic disorders may be fatal.

In characterizing the growth characteristics of any cell line in vivo or in vitro, specific terms are used to define cell and tissue kinetic parameters. Microscopic examination is used to determine the number of cells in mitosis. The capacity to incorporate tritiated thymidine (^{3}H-TdR) into the nucleus defines the labeling index.

It was once thought that quick, uncontrolled cell division explained the rapid increase in tumor mass in patients with leukemia. However, normal myeloblasts have a generation time of 24 to 48 hours, whereas leukemic myeloblasts have a generation time of 15 to 60 hours. Furthermore, the growth fraction of leukemic myeloblasts at the time of diagnosis is frequently as low as five to seven percent. The key difference seems to lie in the fact that normal myeloid cells follow a fixed developmental sequence and can undergo cell division only up to the myelocyte stage, after which they differenti-ate, circulate, and die.[1] Many leukemic cells drop out of the normal cell cycle and, in varying degrees, remain almost indefinitely capable of cell division. The result is an expanding mass of cells that do not die in an orderly sequence and that retain the capacity for further growth. These cells are in a prolonged G_1 phase, sometimes called G_0. Leukemic blasts may leave the marrow, circulate, settle in organs, divide, and then re-enter the circulation.[2]

The pathophysiology of the leukemias, particularly the acute leukemias, relates almost directly to the impact of the expanding cell number. The growing cell population infiltrates the marrow and renders the patient functionally aplastic, leading to death by infection or hemorrhage. One to 2 kg of acute leukemic cells, which consists of 1 to 2 $\times 10^{12}$ cells, appears to be sufficient to cause death. The volume occupied by this number of cells would be on the order of 1.7 L, which is also the total marrow volume of an average adult. Because the diagnosis of leukemia cannot usually be made unless the cellular tumor burden is 10^9 cells, it is apparent that only 10 tumor cell doublings (2^{10} equals a 1,000-fold increase) separate the smallest detectable number from a potentially lethal cell number. When a patient is said to be in complete remission in acute leukemia, it means only that the leukemic cells are not clinically detectable and that their number must therefore be less than 10^9. Leukemic cells can also infiltrate organs other than the bone marrow, chiefly the liver, spleen, lymph nodes, and meninges and cause organ dysfunction.

Oncogenesis

The etiology of the leukemias is being elucidated by advances in cytogenetics and molecular biology that are starting to integrate seemingly disparate pieces of information: some animal leukemias and at least one human leukemia (adult T cell leukemia) are caused by RNA tumor viruses[3]; human leukemias can occur after exposure to ionizing radiation[4,5]; agents such as chloramphenicol, phenylbutazone, and benzene can produce marrow hypoplasia, and leukemia subsequently develops in a significant number of patients who survive the pancytopenic episode[6-8]; and in some clinical settings, therapy with alkylating agents is associated with an incidence of leukemia greater than 10 percent.[9-12] It now appears that specific cytogenetic abnormalities are present in many, if not most, of the leukemias [*see Table 1*].[13]

The common thread linking all these apparently unrelated observations is the oncogene, a gene that can mediate carcinogenesis. Oncogenes are present in the normal genome and probably function in cellular growth or differentiation, or both. Presumably, in their usual place in the chromosome, oncogenes are flanked by regions that control their subsequent action. However, after exposure to insults that produce chromosomal aberrations or to the action of RNA retroviruses that alter the oncogene or its context, the oncogene is released from feedback restraint. It may replicate many times and ultimately may induce the uncontrolled growth of a clone of cells that descends from the cell that suffered the initial alteration. Many additional factors will probably be found to be involved in the etiology of leukemias, including genetic predisposition or resistance as well as the immune response to an emerging malignant clone. In addition, newer forms of therapy may play an important etiologic role. For example, there are reports of acute lymphoblastic leukemia (ALL) occurring in children who have been treated with recombinant growth hormone.[14]

Identification and Diagnosis of the Leukemias

The diagnosis of leukemia still rests on cytologic and morphologic grounds. The diagnosis is established by two findings: abnormal cells in the peripheral blood and the presence in marrow of an infiltrate of abnormal cells replacing normal marrow elements. A pathognomonic feature in some cases of acute myeloblastic leukemia (AML) is the finding of Auer rods, or abnormal primary granules, in the myeloblasts. Biopsy of the liver, spleen, lymph nodes, or skin lesions can also yield the diagnosis in patients with leukemia.

The appearance of a leukemic hiatus is evidence of acute myeloid leukemia or of progression of a chronic myeloproliferative disorder to a more aggressive form of leukemia. In such cases, the peripheral smear does not show an orderly progression of maturing granulocytic precursors, as it does in standard chronic myelocytic leukemia (CML) (i.e., one percent myeloblasts, three percent promyelocytes, 10 percent myelocytes, 20 percent metamyelocytes, and 67 percent neutrophils and band forms). Instead, the smear may show the hiatus (i.e., myeloblasts and neutrophils with few intermediate forms). One interpretation is that a new clone, which is incapable of further maturation, exists in the marrow.

Although standard morphologic techniques relying on Romanovsky's stains or hematoxylin-eosin stains are of limited use in classifying the several forms of leukemia, the distinctions made are clinically important for choosing appropriate therapy. Other techniques, such as immunophenotyping with monoclonal antibodies, cytogenetic analysis, and analysis of gene rearrangements, are being used to supplement standard cytologic analysis in the diagnosis of leukemia and in the detection of small numbers of residual leukemic cells in patients who have apparently undergone complete remission. The malignant cell in the acute leukemias is often a primitive undifferentiated cell, and the leukemic marker may merely indicate reversion to a more primitive growth pattern rather than the derivation of the leukemic cell line.

Cytochemical Tests

The French-American-British (FAB) group analyzed patients with acute leukemia

Table 1 Some Cytogenetic Abnormalities Observed in the Leukemias

	Karyotypic Abnormality	*Clinical Picture*	*French-American-British (FAB) Correlation*
Myeloid Leukemias	t(8;21)	Acute myeloblastic leukemia	M_2
	t(15;17)	Acute promyelocytic leukemia	M_3
	t/del(11)	Acute myeloblastic or acute monocytic leukemia	M_{5a}
	inv/del(16)	Acute myelomonocytic leukemia	M_4Eo
	t(9;22)	Chronic myeloid leukemia Acute myeloblastic leukemia (rarely) Acute lymphocytic leukemia [*see* t(9;22), *below*]	—
	t(6;9)	Acute myeloblastic or acute myelomonocytic leukemia with basophilia	M_2 or M_4
	inv(3)	Acute myeloblastic leukemia with thrombocytosis	—
	Trisomy 8	Acute myeloblastic leukemia Myelodysplastic syndrome	—
	Loss of chromosome 5 or 7	Acute myeloblastic leukemia, including therapy-related form Myelodysplastic syndrome, including therapy-related form	—
	7q⁻	Acute myeloblastic leukemia, including therapy-related form Myelodysplastic syndrome, including therapy-related form	—
	5q⁻	Acute myeloblastic leukemia Myelodysplastic syndrome (5q⁻ syndrome)	—
Lymphoid Leukemias	t(8;14), t(2;8), or t(8;22)	Acute lymphocytic leukemia–Burkitt's leukemia	L_3
	t(9;22)	Acute lymphocytic leukemia [*see* t(9;22), *above*]	L_1 or L_2
	Trisomy 12	Chronic lymphocytic leukemia	—

Note: see reference 95.

using Romanovsky's-stained smears of bone marrow aspirates for overall morphologic differentiation, myeloperoxidase or Sudan black B staining to detect myeloid cells, and naphthol ASD chloroacetate esterase (NASDA) reaction with sodium fluoride inhibition to identify monocytes.[15,16] Acute leukemic cells of myeloid origin are generally myeloperoxidase positive. Seven subgroups of acute myeloid leukemia, M_1 through M_7, have been identified. For a disorder to be classified as an acute myeloid leukemia in the FAB system, blasts must constitute more than 30 percent and erythroid precursors less than 50 percent of all nucleated marrow cells; the exception to this general rule is the M_6 variant, in which there is extensive proliferation of immature erythroid precursors. The M_7 subgroup identifies patients with acute megakaryoblastic leukemia. Usually, the marrow is fibrotic and cannot be aspirated in such cases, and thus, cytochemical staining of marrow cells cannot be used to define this subgroup. Identification of M_7 requires peripheral blood studies using electron microscopy to show the unique platelet peroxidase activity or polyclonal or monoclonal antibody assays to identify Factor VIII–related antigen reactivity (platelet von Willebrand factor) or platelet glycoprotein IIb/IIIa.[17,18] Acute leukemic cells of lymphoid origin are myeloperoxidase negative; three subgroups have been established, L_1 through L_3 [see Table 2].

Cell Surface Markers

Immunophenotyping using monoclonal antibodies to T and B cell markers and to myeloid antigens is helpful in the diagnosis of leukemias. Mature B cells are characterized by the presence of surface membrane immunoglobulin (SmIg), whereas their progenitors, which are termed pre–B cells, have no SmIg but contain cytoplasmic μ heavy chains ($C\mu$). Different maturational stages of B cells ranging from the most primitive to the most differentiated, or plasma cells, can now be distinguished by means of monoclonal antibodies that recognize different cell surface antigens. Similarly, there are monoclonal antibodies that can be used to identify all T cells, helper-inducer or suppressor subsets of T cells, and mature and immature T cells. Monoclonal antibodies have been generated that can identify specific antigens on differentiating myeloid cells, monocytes, platelets, and erythrocyte progenitors [see Table 3].[19]

Other Cellular Markers

Terminal deoxynucleotidyl transferase (TdT) is an enzyme that does not occur in normal peripheral lymphocytes of T or B cell origin or in myeloid cells. High values are found, however, in normal thymus tissue, in human T cell lymphoblastoid cell lines, in malignant blasts in some cases of blast crisis in chronic myeloid leukemia, and in the lymphoblasts of most patients with childhood acute lymphocytic leukemia.[20]

For reasons that are not clear, the activity of some intracellular enzymes varies in some forms of acute lymphoblastic leukemia. Adenosine deaminase is high in a T cell variant (T-ALL), and 5'-nucleotidase and purine nucleoside phosphorylase are low in T-ALL.[19]

High levels of the serum enzyme lysozyme (muramidase) indicate the presence of monocytic or myelomonocytic leukemias.

Genetic Markers

Cytogenetic analysis is proving to be increasingly useful for diagnosis and for assessing prognosis [see Table 1]. Molecular probes for the immunoglobulin genes and the T cell receptor genes have been developed that can aid in identifying the origin of leukemic cells. As a B cell matures, it rearranges its variable, diversity, and joining (VDJ) genes to produce a specific immunoglobulin. During maturation, these rearrangements occur in an orderly sequence: the heavy chains rearrange first, then the κ light chains, and finally, the λ light chains. All B cells that arise from a single clone have a unique rearrangement of immunoglobulin genes. When a monoclonal, or malignant, expansion of B lineage cells has occurred and the malignant cells account for one percent or more of the total lymphocyte population, the specific immunoglobulin gene rearrangement can be detected by a molecular probe. Such probes can thus be used to determine whether a lymphocytic expansion is clonal (i.e., neoplastic) and whether it is of B cell origin.[19,21] T cell receptor genes are similarly rearranged during differentiation, and clonality can be probed to identify malignant expansion of T lineage cells.[22-26]

Table 2 French-American-British (FAB) Classification of Acute Leukemias

	Class	Description	Staining Reaction		
			Myeloperoxidase	Naphthol ASD Chloroacetate Esterase (NASDA)	NASDA with Sodium Fluoride Inhibition
Myeloid	M_1	Acute myeloblastic leukemia without maturation	> 3% positive cells	> 3% positive cells	> 3% positive cells
	M_2	Acute myeloblastic leukemia with maturation	> 50% positive cells	> 25% positive cells	> 25% positive cells
	M_3	Acute hypergranular promyelocytic leukemia	> 50% positive cells	> 25% positive cells	> 25% positive cells
	M_4	Acute myelomonocytic leukemia (well differentiated) With abnormal marrow eosinophils (M_4Eo)	> 25% positive cells	> 50% positive cells	3%–25% positive cells
	M_5	Acute monocytic leukemia (poorly differentiated) More than 80 percent monoblasts (M_{5a}) More than 20 percent promonocytes and monocytes (M_{5b})	≤ 3% positive cells	> 50% positive cells	≤ 3% positive cells
	M_6	Erythroleukemia	No reaction	≤ 3% positive cells	≤ 3% positive cells
	M_7	Acute megakaryoblastic leukemia	No reaction	Variable number of positive cells	Variable inhibition
Lymphocytic	L_1	Acute lymphocytic leukemia (common childhood variant— homogeneous population)	No reaction	≤ 3% positive cells	≤ 3% positive cells
	L_2	Acute lymphocytic leukemia (common adult variant— heterogeneous population)	No reaction	≤ 3% positive cells	≤ 3% positive cells
	L_3	Burkitt's cell type	No reaction	≤ 3% positive cells	≤ 3% positive cells

Note: see reference 15.

Molecular probes offer an advantage over karyotypic analysis in that they can be used to study the cytogenetics of cells that are not undergoing mitosis. For example, an area termed the breakpoint cluster region (*bcr*) has been identified at the site on chromo- some 22 where the reciprocal translocation with chromosome 9 occurs in CML. By prob- ing for clonal expansion of leukemic cells that express the *bcr* gene, the equivalent of the 9;22 translocation can be identified. The use of the polymerase chain reaction to pro-

Table 3 Immunophenotyping of Acute Leukemia

Type of Leukemia	Monoclonal Antibody That Gives a Positive Reaction
Acute myeloblastic, acute promyelocytic, acute myelomono- cytic, and acute monocytic leukemia (M_1–M_5)	Anti-CD13 (anti–My-7) Anti-CD14 (anti–My-4) Anti-CD34 (anti–My-10) Anti-CD33 (anti–My-9)
Erythroleukemia (M_6)	Anti–glycophorin A Anti-spectrin
Acute megakaryo- blastic leukemia (M_7)	Anti–platelet GPIIb/IIIa Anti–platelet GPIb
Acute lymphocytic leukemia (CALLA type)	Anti-CD10 (anti- CALLA)
Acute lymphocytic leukemia (T cell type)	Anti-CD5 (anti–Leu-1 or OKT1) Anti-CD3 (anti–Leu-4 or OKT3) Anti-CD2 (anti-T11 or anti–Leu-5)
Acute lymphocytic leukemia (B cell type)	Anti-CD19 (anti-B4) Anti-CD20 (anti-B1)
Acute lymphocytic leukemia (Burkitt's leukemia type)	SmIg (surface membrane immunoglobulin) Anti-CD19 Anti-CD20

Note: see reference 95.

duce DNA amplification greatly increases the sensitivity of this test and should permit detection of one cell in a million carrying the *bcr* leukemic marker.

Growth Patterns

The clonal growth patterns of granulo- cytic progenitor cells have been studied in the leukemias. Leukemic marrow cells from patients with acute or chronic lymphocytic leukemia do not grow in agar culture. Acute myeloblastic leukemic cells either grow poorly or show patterns of abortive colony formation called cluster formations. It has been proposed that the size of the clusters has prognostic value. In chronic myelocytic leukemia, clonal growth is frequently ex- cessive early in the disease but decreases as the disease evolves. Density gradient sepa- ration reveals that the leukemic colony- forming cells in chronic myelocytic leukemia and other myeloproliferative dis- orders are lighter than normal granulocytic progenitor cells.[27]

Principles of Management

Management of some of the leukemias is shifting from attempts to induce com- plete remission to attempts to produce cure. In the acute leukemias and in chronic my- eloid leukemia, a cure is possible if the tech- nical knowledge is matched by the proper circumstances and by the patient's willing- ness to undertake aggressive and hazard- ous programs. Such programs include chemotherapeutic intensification programs or bone marrow transplantation in the acute leukemias and marrow transplanta- tion in chronic myeloid leukemia. These therapies, which may increase the patient's risk of mortality, are administered at rela- tively few specialized centers. Therefore, in designing management programs for pa- tients with leukemia, one must attempt to arrive at a definitive diagnosis using clini- cal information, classical morphology, cy- tochemistry, cytogenetics, molecular biology, and cell surface marker analysis. One must then determine if it is feasible to attempt a cure given the nature of the ill- ness, the therapy that will be required, the age and general condition of the patient, and the patient's attitude after being appro- priately informed about the program. If cure is deemed unfeasible for systemic dis- ease, therapy with cytotoxic agents is ad- ministered to reduce the total tumor mass and to improve organ function and quality of life.

Chemotherapy

Many treatment schedules have several phases. There is an induction phase, in which the tumor mass is treated aggressively to reduce or obliterate the clinically detectable leukemic cell burden, that is, to induce clinical remission. A second phase, called consolidation or cytoreduction, frequently follows, in which the leukemic cells that probably have survived induction (10^8 to 10^9 cells) are further reduced by one or more courses of additional chemotherapy. A third stage of therapy that is sometimes used seeks to destroy the residual leukemic cells or to reduce their number to a level below which they can no longer repopulate tissues; this phase is achieved by administering intensive courses of combinations of agents while the patient is in complete clinical remission. Patients in remission can tolerate larger doses of chemotherapy because their marrow function is essentially normal. Early and late intensification programs cause marrow hypoplasia and usually require hospitalization. Evidence regarding their efficacy has been mixed: the extended complete remissions reported by some investigators have not been reproduced by others. Maintenance therapy is instituted later to keep any residual leukemic cells from growing.[28] The role of maintenance therapy in several forms of leukemia is also being challenged and re-evaluated.

The designing of drug schedules to take advantage of cell cycle kinetics at different parts of the treatment period seems theoretically promising but thus far has proved to be only modestly helpful.[29] Apparently, at the time of diagnosis, most of the leukemic blasts are in a prolonged G_1 or G_0 phase and thus cannot be affected by cell cycle–specific agents.

Chemotherapeutic programs work by killing only a given fraction of cells in a population; therefore, the higher the tumor cell burden, the more difficult the job. Because the leukemia causes functional marrow aplasia and because the drugs that are used are predominantly myelosuppres-sive, infection and hemorrhage are limiting clinical problems.

Combinations of agents can sometimes cause synergistic leukemic blast destruction without killing an equal number of normal cells. If selective agents are available, the job is much easier. In ALL, prednisone, vincristine, and L-asparaginase exhibit selective toxicity for leukemic lymphoblasts. In contrast, no selectively acting agents are available for AML; treatment for this condition probably causes parallel death of normal and leukemic blasts.

An alternative approach currently under investigation is the use of agents that could induce immature leukemic cells to undergo terminal differentiation so that they no longer divide and eventually die. Agents tested thus far include cytarabine given in low dosages and vitamin A derivatives such as retinoic acid, but their efficacy has not yet been proved.

Another approach involves the administration of biologic response modifiers such as the interferons, which are being used to treat such disorders as chronic myeloid leukemia and hairy-cell leukemia.

Disease that is causing severe local problems can be managed with localized forms of therapy. For example, central nervous system disease can be treated by craniospinal irradiation, by intrathecal methotrexate or cytarabine, or by combinations of irradiation and intrathecal chemotherapy.

Hyperuricemia is a common problem; the expanded cell turnover produces a uric acid load, which can cause urate nephropathy and gouty arthritis if it is not handled properly.[30]

It is important to maintain or improve the nutritional status of patients undergoing chemotherapy. Supplementary feedings may be required to prevent development of hypoalbuminemia and loss of immunocompetence and to support optimal regeneration of stem cells.

Bone Marrow Transplantation

Transplantation of bone marrow is a recognized modality for the treatment of aplastic anemia and has been used experimentally to treat β thalassemia major. At present, however, it is employed most frequently in the management of malignant disorders, particularly the acute leukemias and chronic myeloid leukemia.[31]

The purpose of bone marrow transplantation is to restore to the bone marrow the functions of normally proliferating stem cells. In the case of allogeneic transplantation for leukemia, a graft versus leukemic cell effect is also desired. The donor can be the patient (for autologous transplantation), the patient's identical twin (for isogeneic, or syngeneic, transplantation), or a histocompatible donor (for allogeneic transplantation), usually a sibling. Determination of histocompatibility involves matching the donor and recipient at their HLA-A, -B, -C, and -D loci. A given patient has a 30 to 40 percent chance of having a histocompatible sibling donor. However, a histocompatible donor is not a perfect transplantation match. Such a donor is simply compatible at the major histocompatibility loci; minor incompatibilities remain, and allogeneic grafts are regularly rejected unless the immune responses of the recipient are modified.[32-34]

To perform the transplant, approximately 750 ml of marrow suspension (a volume required to administer 3×10^8 cells/kg to the recipient) must be obtained from the donor's posterior and anterior iliac crests. The marrow particles are broken up by passage through sterile stainless steel screens, and the suspension is then administered to the recipient intravenously. The stem cells circulate through the peripheral blood and then home to the marrow cavity.

In preparation for allogeneic (but not autologous or syngeneic) marrow grafts, the host's immune responses must be altered to avoid rejection of the infused cells. If the purpose of the graft is simply to restore marrow function, as in the treatment of severe aplastic anemia, such immunosuppressive therapy may consist solely of high dosages of cyclophosphamide (50 mg/kg I.V. daily for four days). The marrow cells are infused 36 to 48 hours after the last dose

of immunosuppressive drug. Experimental programs using other drugs or total lymphoid irradiation are also being tested for this purpose. If the goals of the transplantation are to restore marrow function and to achieve very long lasting complete remission or even cure after radical destruction of leukemic cells, preparation usually consists of 1,000 cGy (1,000 rads) of total body irradiation, either alone or combined with immunosuppressive or cytotoxic drugs such as cyclophosphamide, carmustine, cytarabine, etoposide, and daunorubicin.[35,36]

The clinical course after allogeneic grafting is very complex. There may be failure of engraftment, particularly if the number of stem cells infused is too low. The graft may take initially and then be rejected. In any case, because of the immunosuppressive and myelosuppressive effects of the pre-transplantation conditioning program, the patient will need erythrocyte transfusions and prophylactic platelet transfusions to prevent hemorrhage. Neutropenia and immunosuppression leave the patient extraordinarily vulnerable to a wide variety of infections. Techniques designed to reduce the frequency of infections include several forms of isolation, special food handling, administration of oral nonabsorbable antibiotics, and avoidance of granulocyte transfusions from donors who are positive for cytomegalovirus.[37]

Engraftment usually becomes apparent after two to four weeks; it is marked first by a rise in circulating granulocytes and later by an increase in the platelet count. Because allogeneic grafts contain immunocompetent[38] cells as well as marrow stem cells, the engrafted cells may mount an attack against the host. Such graft versus host disease (GVHD) occurs in about half of cases.[39]

Two forms of GVHD are recognized: acute and chronic. In acute GVHD, abnormalities in immune function are accompanied by liver disease, skin rash, and an intestinal disorder characterized by very severe diarrhea. The immunodeficiency enhances susceptibility to opportunistic infections. Combinations of methotrexate, cyclosporine, and prednisone are generally used for prophylaxis for the first 100 post-graft days. Other methods of prophylaxis include the use of either antithymocyte globulin or monoclonal antibodies directed against specific T cell subsets. Some investigators have tried to remove the T cells that produce GVHD from the donor marrow by treating the marrow with monoclonal antibodies that destroy these T cells. These techniques have reduced the incidence of GVHD, but their use has been associated with an increased frequency of graft failure and leukemic relapse. Chronic GVHD resembles primary systemic sclerosis or mixed connective tissue disease and is characterized by skin contractures and involvement of the liver and intestines. Treatment with azathioprine and corticosteriods may be helpful, but mortality is still high. Overall, about 20 percent of the patients in whom either acute or chronic GVHD develops will die. This consideration limits the utility of allogeneic marrow grafting. GVHD tends to be more severe in older patients. Many centers will not attempt allogeneic marrow grafting for the treatment of leukemia in patients who are older than 50 years.

A devastating form of interstitial pneumonitis may develop in patients with GVHD who have particularly severe immunosuppression. Often, there is also evidence of pulmonary infection caused by cytomegalovirus (CMV). Both ganciclovir and CMV immune globulin seem to be effective for CMV interstitial pneumonitis.

Autologous marrow transplantation is used in the management of solid tumors,[40] lymphomas, and the acute leukemias. This approach permits the administration of very intensive chemotherapy with subsequent marrow rescue. In a patient with acute leukemia who does not have a compatible donor, chemotherapy is first administered to achieve a complete clinical remission. At this time, the patient's marrow is harvested, and the residual (but invisible) leukemic stem cells are killed by a method that does not destroy normal, nonleukemic, pluripotent stem cells. The purged marrow is then

reinfused into the patient. One method that has achieved some success in purging lymphoblastic leukemic cells from remission marrow involves the use of monoclonal antibodies plus complement.[41] Either single monoclonal antibodies or panels of such antibodies that recognize the common acute lymphoblastic leukemia antigen (CALLA) or other antigens[19] expressed by immature B cells have been employed [*see Table 3*]. An alternative approach that has been used for the treatment of AML consists of incubating autologous remission marrow with 4-hydroperoxycyclophosphamide, an alkylating agent that appears to kill leukemic stem cells without destroying normal pluripotent hematopoietic stem cells. Preliminary results indicate that very long remissions can be achieved in almost half of selected patients who are treated with this method.[42]

Bone marrow transplantation requires special training and support facilities. The procedures are much more difficult than those used for classic AML induction, even though the hypoplastic period is similar. The immunosuppression required for prophylaxis of GVHD in allogeneic transplants is vastly greater, and the added complications if GVHD does develop dramatically increase the difficulties in management.

Myeloproliferative Disorders

The term myeloproliferative was proposed by Dameshek, who noticed that exuberant marrow proliferation of granulocytes, erythroid elements, megakaryocytes, osteoblasts, and fibroblasts characterized diseases such as chronic myelocytic leukemia, agnogenic myeloid metaplasia, polycythemia vera, essential thrombocythemia, acute myeloblastic leukemia, and erythroleukemia (Di Guglielmo's disease). The chronic disorders—chronic myelocytic leukemia, agnogenic myeloid metaplasia, polycythemia vera, and essential thrombocythemia—tended to evolve to blast crisis, a disorder resembling acute myeloblastic leukemia. Furthermore, there were seemingly regular interconversions within the group, so that polycythemia vera tended to evolve into a disease resembling agnogenic myeloid metaplasia.[43] However, the unity of these disorders under the concept of myeloproliferation has been challenged.[20,44] For example, more than 90 percent of patients with chronic myeloid leukemia display a specific cytogenetic abnormality, the 9;22 translocation that produces the Philadelphia chromosome (Ph[1]). Patients with polycythemia vera, agnogenic myeloid metaplasia, and essential thrombocythemia, however, rarely, if ever, show this cytogenetic pattern.

Measurements of glucose-6-phosphate dehydrogenase (G6PD) isoenzymes (Gd[A], Gd[B], Gd[A]-) in heterozygous women have helped clarify the situation by demonstrating that several of the disorders share a similar clonal growth pattern. This technique has shown a common pattern in the peripheral blood cells of G6PD-heterozygous patients with polycythemia vera, chronic myeloid leukemia, agnogenic myeloid metaplasia, and essential thrombocythemia.[45] In a patient with a myeloproliferative disorder, circulating erythrocytes, granulocytes, and platelets, as well as monocytes and macrophages, display only a single G6PD isoenzyme, whereas cultured skin and marrow fibroblasts show approximately equal amounts of two isoenzymes, generally Gd[A] and Gd[B]. Therefore, all of the peripheral blood cells probably descend from the same malignant clone, whereas skin and marrow fibroblasts probably arise from a variety of normal clones. This finding means that the marrow fibrosis seen in patients with these diseases is probably reactive and not part of the malignant hematopoietic clonal proliferation.

Furthermore, when G6PD-heterozygous patients with a chronic myeloproliferative disorder are treated and enter clinical remission, the peripheral blood cells still display only the single malignant clonal G6PD marker. Thus, traditional chemotherapy for chronic myeloproliferative disease does not suppress the malignant clone and allow normal clones to grow. Instead, therapy induces the malignant clone to be more responsive to regulatory mechanisms. The chronic myeloproliferative disorders may arise from a mutation in a single pluripotent stem cell, and the different clinical syndromes probably reflect variable responses of the malignant clone to regulatory mechanisms.[46]

Chronic Myeloproliferative Disorders

Essential Thrombocythemia

Essential thrombocythemia is a clinical syndrome characterized by repeated spontaneous hemorrhages or thromboembolic episodes that are associated with a significant increase in the number of circulating platelets [*see Chapter 14*].

Agnogenic Myeloid Metaplasia

Diagnosis

Agnogenic myeloid metaplasia usually appears in elderly persons. The patient seeks medical consultation when he or she becomes aware of a massively enlarged spleen or is troubled by symptoms of hypermetabolic and hematologic abnormalities, particularly anemia. Clinical findings[47] include weight loss resulting from hypermetabolism; hyperuricemia accompanied by gouty arthritis or urate nephropathy; massive hepatosplenomegaly that is usually caused by extensive extramedullary hematopoiesis; lymphadenopathy caused by extramedullary hematopoiesis; and occasionally, an expanded plasma volume resulting in edema, pleural effusion, and ascites. Additional clinical findings are a leukoerythroblastic peripheral smear showing tailed distorted red cells, nucleated red cells, giant platelets, and immature myeloid cells, including myeloblasts; osteosclerosis on x-ray examination; bone marrow that cannot be aspirated; and a marrow biopsy that shows fibrosis,[48] increased numbers of megakaryocytes, and myelopoiesis with a shift to the left in the differential count. The platelet and white blood cell counts can be high, low, or normal.

Anemia is common and is caused by a combination of hemodilution resulting from expanded plasma volume, enhanced destruction of red blood cells in the spleen, erythroid hypoplasia in fibrotic marrow, and ineffective erythropoiesis in an enlarged spleen or in fibrotic marrow. The bleeding time may be long even when platelet counts are normal or elevated, indicating a platelet functional disorder. The neutrophil alkaline phosphatase score is high. Rarely, extramedullary hematopoiesis may cause portal hypertension with bleeding esophageal varices; masses of hematopoietic tissue may also cause spinal cord compression.

A condition to be excluded in the differential diagnosis is disseminated carcinoma that involves the bone marrow and produces a leukoerythroblastic smear.[49] The history and the presence of carcinoma cells in the marrow biopsy specimen usually resolve the question. On occasion, it has been thought that tuberculosis or other granulomatous diseases can produce a condition similar to agnogenic myeloid metaplasia, but the clinical evidence is not convincing.[50] The conditions other than agnogenic myeloid metaplasia that can cause myelofibrosis become clinically apparent in less than four months. In one large series, hairy-cell leukemia (HCL) was frequently misdiagnosed as agnogenic myeloid metaplasia. HCL can present with an infiltrated, unaspiratable marrow containing increased amounts of reticulin, but unlike the bone marrow in patients with agnogenic myeloid metaplasia, bone marrow in HCL does not demonstrate evidence of myeloproliferation.[51]

Chronic myelocytic leukemia usually does not produce a leukoerythroblastic smear; other distinguishing features of CML include infiltration of marrow with a predominantly granulocytic line, the presence of the Ph[1] chromosome in more than 90 percent of cases, and a low neutrophil alkaline phosphatase score.

Agnogenic myeloid metaplasia is probably a stem cell disorder in which the abnormal clone differentiates into granulocytes, red cells, and platelets. The marrow fibrosis is probably a secondary phenomenon because the fibroblasts do not share either the karyotypic or enzymatic markers of the abnormal clone.[52]

Management

Management must be directed toward solving the significant clinical problems. Poor survival is heralded by unexplained fever, weight loss, night sweats, anemia, and thrombocytopenia.[51] Prognosis is not affected by such factors as the number of immature myeloid cells in the peripheral blood, the size of the liver or spleen, or the degree of marrow cellularity or fibrosis. If the patient is anemic because of a production defect, therapy with androgens, 150 mg/day of oral oxymetholone or an equivalent drug, may produce an expansion of red cell mass in two months. The side effects are cholestatic hepatitis in 15 percent of cases, fluid retention, and virilization in females.

If the patient has symptoms relating to the enlarged spleen (early satiation, an inability to bend, or pleural pain because of splenic infarction), therapy with busulfan, 2 to 4 mg/day given for a period of several weeks or months, may reduce the size of the spleen (or liver). Generally, however, such therapy causes unacceptable anemia, neutropenia, or thrombocytopenia. Hydroxyurea, given orally in a dosage of 20 to 30 mg/kg/day, may also decrease the size of the spleen or liver, but blood counts must be carefully monitored with this therapy. Small doses of local x-ray therapy—a total of 200 to 500 cGy (200 to 500 rads)—can occasionally reduce the size of the spleen, but in agnogenic myeloid metaplasia, this treatment may cause deleterious effects on nonirradiated tissue and significant pancytopenia, and the beneficial effects are only short-lived.[53]

Splenectomy can be done, but it is hazardous in elderly patients, and postsplenectomy rebound thrombocythemia may cause hemorrhage or thrombosis, or both. Concern has been expressed that splenectomy removes the only residual functional marrow in patients with agnogenic myeloid metaplasia. In this disease, however, the spleen is probably a poor site for effective hematopoiesis. Splenectomy produces a satisfactory response in cases of hemolytic anemia as well as in cases of thrombocytopenia if there are residual marrow megakaryocytes. Prophylactic splenectomy is not justified, however; one large series demonstrated that at least half of the patients with agnogenic myeloid metaplasia never required this procedure.[51]

Hypermetabolic symptoms, such as sweating, low-grade fever, and weight loss, occasionally respond to low dosages of busulfan, 1 to 2 mg/day or even less, administered in conjunction with careful monitoring of blood counts. Hydroxyurea, given orally in a dosage of 20 to 30 mg/kg/day, may also be useful in controlling these symptoms. Hyperuricemia is managed with 100 mg of allopurinol, given three times daily with a minimum of 3 L/day of fluid. Thrombocythemia accompanied by hemorrhage is occasionally a problem; it is probably related to the associated platelet function disorder. Acute hemorrhage can be managed by transfusing six units of platelets daily until bleeding stops. Associated thrombocythemic thrombosis, if it occurs, is more difficult to manage. Antiplatelet agents can be tried, such as 0.6 g of aspirin twice daily. Treatment with smaller doses of aspirin, such as 80 to 160 mg/day, has also been suggested, but this approach has not been subjected to rigorous testing. Interferon-alpha, given in a dosage similar to that used for chronic myeloid leukemia (see below), has been reported to lower the platelet count and may also shrink an enlarged spleen.[53-56] Plateletpheresis has been used to lower the platelet count temporarily, but there has been no clear proof of benefit in the associated thromboembolism of thrombocythemia. Chemotherapy with busulfan can reduce the degree of myelofibrosis without altering the number of megakaryocytes; this effect appears to weigh against the theory that the myelofibrosis is caused by platelet-derived growth factor released by the abnormally proliferating megakaryocytes.[57]

Agnogenic myeloid metaplasia is usually a chronic disease, but eventually, it may enter an aggressive phase, which occurs in 10 to 25 percent of patients with agnogenic myeloid metaplasia, reminiscent of blast crisis in chronic myelocytic leukemia (see below). The aggressive phase is marked by enlarging organs, the appearance of blasts and the occasional appearance of a leukemic hiatus in the peripheral smear, progressive anemia, and thrombocytopenia. Management of the aggressive phase, which occurs in 10 to 25 percent of patients with agnogenic myeloid metaplasia, is very unsatisfactory.[58]

There are patients with variants of myeloproliferation that cannot be readily classified as agnogenic myeloid metaplasia, polycythemia vera, or subacute myeloid leukemia. These patients have variable degrees of hepatosplenomegaly, and myeloid and erythroid proliferation in the marrow may be extensive. Myelofibrosis may be present, and the course may range from chronic to aggressive. Such disorders are termed unclassified myeloproliferative diseases and are managed according to the principles that have been outlined for agnogenic myeloid metaplasia.

Chronic Myeloid Leukemia

Chronic myeloid leukemia, which is also termed chronic myelocytic leukemia and chronic granulocytic leukemia, is a clonal disorder in which the leukemic stem cell gives rise to red cells, neutrophils, eosinophils, basophils, monocyte-macrophages, platelets,[59] T cells, and probably, B cells.[60] Three stages of the disease are generally recognized: a chronic stable phase, an accelerated phase, and a blast crisis phase.

Almost all cases of CML are characterized by the presence of the Ph^1 chromosome, which is produced by a reciprocal translocation between chromosomes 9 and 22; the shortened chromosome 22, or Ph^1, can be easily detected using cytogenetic techniques. The important part of the translocation involves the juxtaposition of the *c-abl* oncogene from chromosome 9 with the breakpoint cluster region, or *bcr*, gene on chromosome 22.[61,62] The juxtaposed genes encode a chimeric *bcr*/*c-abl* mRNA, and this abnormal mRNA is produced even in the cells of CML patients who do not have a cytogenetically detectable Ph^1 chromosome.[63] The protein product of this mRNA has an unusual tyrosine kinase activity.[64-66]

Although five to 10 percent of cases of CML were formerly classified as Ph[1] negative, it now appears that Ph[1]-negative CML is extremely rare, if it occurs at all. As noted previously, molecular probes revealed the presence of the 9;22 translocation in some CML patients who had been identified as Ph[1] negative on the basis of cytogenetic studies. In addition, the analysis of 25 presumed cases of Ph[1]-negative CML in one study led to a reclassification of all but one of these cases as another myeloproliferative disease, particularly one of the myelodysplastic syndromes [see Intermediate Forms of Myeloid Disease, below].[67] An interesting finding in this study, which also examined 50 patients with Ph[1]-positive CML, was that all the patients who had the Philadelphia chromosome also had peripheral blood basophilia (i.e., ≥ 250 basophils/mm^3).

Chronic Phase

The initial symptoms of CML relate to hypermetabolism and splenomegaly. The patient experiences weight loss but is rarely febrile, and the spleen and liver are enlarged. There is usually moderate anemia, with few nucleated red cells on the peripheral smear. Platelets may be large on the smear, and the platelet count can be high, low, or normal. The white blood cell count is usually very high—ranging from 50,000 to 300,000/mm^3—and there is an orderly progression from myeloblasts through neutrophils. The granulocytic elements are not grossly abnormal morphologically, and the neutrophil alkaline phosphatase score is low. The marrow is hypercellular, and leftshifted granulopoiesis is evident. The increase in cell mass is caused by delayed maturation, so there is decreased senescence and deferred cell death. Granulocyte production is probably slightly increased. Megakaryocytes in the bone marrow may be increased, normal, or decreased in number, and erythropoiesis is usually decreased.

Accelerated Phase

After a period during which the disease appears to remain stable, the spleen and liver begin to enlarge, and there is progressive anemia and thrombocytopenia. The patient may complain of bone pain, fever, night sweats, and weight loss. The peripheral blood may show eosinophilia, basophilia, immature myeloid cells, or a leukemic hiatus. The appearance of extramedullary involvement of lymph nodes, bone, skin, and soft tissue indicates accelerated disease.[68] Therapy that had been working appears to become less effective.[59,61] There is no sharp demarcation between this phase and the subsequent blast phase.

Blast Phase

In the blast phase, fever, bone pain, and organomegaly become more prominent, and anemia and thrombocytopenia grow more severe. The peripheral blast count increases, and cytogenetic studies may reveal duplication of the Ph[1] chromosome, trisomy 8, or other chromosomal changes.[59,61,65] Perhaps one fourth to one third of patients in this phase of CML experience a lymphoid blast crisis in which the blast cells have a lymphoid morphologic appearance, do not stain with myeloperoxidase, and are positive for such lymphoid markers as TdT and the common acute lymphoblastic leukemia antigen.

Management of the Chronic Phase

Hyperuricemia is common and must be controlled with allopurinol, given in a dosage of 300 mg/day. High leukocyte counts may occasionally result in intravascular leukocyte thrombi and aggregates that lodge in the pulmonary, cerebral, and retinal vasculature, producing obstruction, hemorrhage, and infarction. Leukopheresis will acutely lower the white blood cell count, and intravenous daunorubicin or doxorubicin in a dose of 60 mg/m^2 will cause a rapid fall in the white blood cell count during a period of 36 hours.[69] The patient must be hydrated and must be receiving allopurinol during this period.

Traditionally, therapy for the chronic phase of CML has involved the administration of busulfan, but allogeneic bone marrow transplantation is probably now the treatment of choice for patients with CML who are younger than 50 years and have a histocompatible donor (see below). For those patients who are not candidates for marrow transplantation, busulfan therapy is initiated at a dosage of 4 to 6 mg/day while allopurinol is started; allopurinol therapy is continued while the patient is receiving busulfan. The white blood cell count continues to increase initially because busulfan, a weak alkylator, does not begin to produce an effect for about two weeks. After two weeks, the white blood cell count falls, the spleen and liver decrease in size, and the hemoglobin and platelet count return toward normal. Busulfan treatment can be stopped if the white blood cell count falls to 10,000 to 20,000/mm^3; the effects will continue for two weeks after the drug is withdrawn. The initial response in chronic myelocytic leukemia is gratifying from a clinical point of view. The marrow, however, remains hypercellular with granulocytic elements, and the Ph[1] marker persists, so the improvement is actually only a partial remission marked by reduction in tumor burden and improved cell differentiation. The patient feels much improved and may resume a schedule of full activity.

Busulfan is a treacherous agent that seems to have selective capacities for destroying stem cells. It can cause irreversible marrow aplasia and death. Prescriptions for busulfan should be written for the exact amount required until the next visit and blood count.[70] The efficacy of maintenance therapy in chronic myelocytic leukemia is unproved. Eventually, the white blood cell count rises again, organs enlarge, and the cycle is repeated. The white blood cell count in this disorder accurately reflects total tumor mass, and chemotherapy is generally restarted when the count approaches 30,000 to 50,000/mm^3.

Other agents, such as mercaptopurine and melphalan, have not shown any clearcut advantage over busulfan. Some investigators believe that hydroxyurea therapy can delay the appearance of blast crisis; this

agent can be initiated in a daily oral dosage of 20 to 30 mg/kg, and the dose can be adjusted according to its effect on blood counts and organ size. In my experience, daily hydroxyurea therapy requires weekly or semiweekly monitoring of blood counts. There have been no randomized trials that have directly compared busulfan with hydroxyurea therapy, but the median survival reported for patients treated with either agent is the same.[71]

Induction therapy has been tried, as used in the treatment of acute myeloblastic leukemia, with the aim of producing a complete remission and clearing of the Ph[1] chromosome marker. Although this result was achieved in a few patients, it was short-lived[72,73] and associated with substantial myelosuppressive toxicity. Early splenectomy is not recommended as a routine procedure in CML.[74]

Treatment with human recombinant interferon-alpha produced a clinical response in 80 percent of patients in the stable phase of CML in one study, and this response was accompanied in some cases by a suppression of the Ph[1] chromosome.[75] During an induction phase, 5 million units/m^2 of interferon were given daily intramuscularly. The dosage was adjusted downward if performance status declined or if neurologic symptoms or abnormalities of hepatic or renal function developed, and it was adjusted upward if cytoreduction was not achieved. Improvement occurred during a period of three to six months, and responding patients were maintained on 2.5 to 10 million units/m^2 of interferon given intramuscularly on alternate days.[75,76] The use of interferon for the treatment of CML has not yet been approved by the Food and Drug Administration.[71]

Despite the availability of several chemotherapeutic programs, the overall result of efforts to manage CML in the chronic stable phase has been disappointing; for 40 years, the median duration of survival has remained at three to four years. Therefore, there was good reason to attempt allogeneic marrow transplantation in the chronic stable phase,[35] which has been done using total body irradiation combined with large doses of cyclophosphamide, either alone or in conjunction with busulfan or daunorubicin. The results have been gratifying thus far: disease-free survival among a group of patients followed for seven to 12 years is almost 65 percent.[77,78] Therefore, at least for patients younger than 50 years with CML who have an HLA-identical sib donor, marrow transplantation currently offers the best prospect for long-term survival and health.[79,80]

Management of the Accelerated and Blast Phases

The dosage of hydroxyurea may be increased or bolus therapy with busulfan may be tried when CML enters an accelerated phase, but the response is generally unsatisfactory. Bone marrow transplantation is much less effective in the accelerated or blast crisis phase of CML than in the stable phase.[77-79] However, 15 to 20 percent of patients who receive allogeneic transplants in the accelerated or blast crisis phase may achieve long-term survival.

In general, patients in myeloid blast crisis respond poorly to chemotherapy.[81] However, alternate-day treatment with plicamycin combined with daily administration of hydroxyurea is occasionally helpful because this approach can improve the red and white blood cell counts and reduce fever and splenomegaly. Plicamycin is given in a dosage of 25 μg/kg I.V. during a period of two to four hours on alternate days for three weeks. The dosage of oral hydroxyurea depends on the white blood cell count: 4 g/day is given if the count is greater than 100,000/mm^3; 3 g/day at white blood cell counts of 75,000 to 100,000/mm^3; 2 g/day at 50,000 to 75,000/mm^3; 1.5 g/day at 30,000 to 50,000/mm^3; 1 g/day at 15,000 to 30,000/mm^3; and 0.5 g/day at 7,500 to 15,000/mm^3. No hydroxyurea is given if the white blood cell count is less than 7,500/mm^3. After this combination therapy has been administered for three weeks and if a response has been achieved, a maintenance program is instituted. This program consists of plicamycin,

25 μg/kg I.V., one to three times weekly combined with hydroxyurea in a daily dosage adjusted according to the white blood cell count (see above). Toxic effects of plicamycin include thrombocytopenia, decrease in the serum calcium level, nausea and vomiting, and abnormal levels of the liver enzymes alanine and aspartate aminotransferase.[82] More aggressive forms of therapy, such as high-dose cytarabine combined with mitoxantrone, do not improve the prognosis in patients in myeloid blast crisis and are extremely toxic.[83]

For those patients who clearly have a lymphoblastic crisis, intensive chemotherapy with high doses of vincristine and prednisone may produce a therapeutic response. Lymphoblasts can be identified by morphologic techniques, by their reaction with monoclonal antibody to CALLA, by assays for TdT,[84] or by their presence as a clone of cells that has identical rearrangements of their immunoglobulin genes.[85] Therapy, which lasts between 14 and 21 days, consists of vincristine, 2 mg/m^2/wk given intravenously (maximum single dose of 2 mg), and prednisone, 60 mg/m^2/day orally.[70] If combined therapy with vincristine and prednisone reduces the blast count and decreases organomegaly, the patient can then be switched to a full ALL protocol [*see* Acute Lymphoblastic Leukemia, *below*].[81] Combination chemotherapy with vincristine, doxorubicin, and dexamethasone (the VAD regimen) [*see Chapter 16*] has also been used for patients with lymphoid or undifferentiated CML in blast crisis.[86] This approach was of limited value in patients with lymphoid blast crisis but of no benefit in patients with undifferentiated blast crisis.

Chronic Eosinophilic Leukemia

Eosinophilic leukemia is a malignant myeloproliferative disorder that usually can be distinguished from the hypereosinophilic syndromes. In some cases, in vitro colony growth patterns and karyotypes indicate the clonal and neoplastic nature of eosinophilic leukemia.[87,88]

Acute Myeloid Leukemias

The acute myeloid leukemias are among the most aggressive malignant diseases of humans; if left untreated, they can cause death within 40 to 100 days from the time of diagnosis.[89] Varying forms—acute monoblastic leukemia, acute myelomonocytic leukemia, acute granulocytic leukemia, acute erythroleukemia (M_6), acute megakaryoblastic leukemia (M_7), and acute myelomonoblastic leukemia—are included in this discussion.[90]

There is a distinct increase in the incidence of acute myeloid leukemia that appears to be the result of therapy for malignant disease. Hodgkin's disease, particularly when treated with radiation and MOPP (mechlorethamine, vincristine, procarbazine, and prednisone) chemotherapy, is followed after several years by the appearance of subacute and acute forms of myelocytic and myelomonocytic leukemia in about five percent of cases (see below).[11] Alkylator therapy for multiple myeloma, Waldenström's macroglobulinemia, and ovarian cancer[91] also increases the incidence of acute myeloid leukemia, which is often preceded by a sideroblastic or erythroleukemic phase.

Acute Myeloblastic Leukemia

Diagnosis

Acute myeloblastic leukemia, also termed acute nonlymphoblastic leukemia (ANLL), may progress relatively gradually, and the prodrome of weakness, bleeding, and fever accompanied by infections usually lasts for several days to a few weeks. Physical examination after onset often reveals petechiae and sternal tenderness and, occasionally, adenopathy, splenomegaly, and hepatomegaly. Testicular, cutaneous, and meningeal involvement may also be evident. In patients with monoblastic morphology, leukemic cells often infiltrate the skin, gums, perianal area, and central nervous system and meninges. Although fever has been said to accompany acute leukemia, fever in such cases is typically caused by infection.[92]

The diagnosis is established by bone marrow examination, which reveals a myeloblastic infiltrate that completely replaces all normal elements. Because of such total marrow replacement, patients are subject to anemia, thrombocytopenic hemorrhage, and neutropenic infection. A febrile neutrophilic dermatosis termed Sweet's syndrome can occur in this setting. It is characterized by red, painful skin plaques, and a skin biopsy shows an infiltrate consisting of mature neutrophils (not blasts). This lesion responds quickly to treatment with systemic corticosteroids.[93]

Cytogenetic analysis and immunophenotyping [*see Tables 1, 2, and 3*] complement standard morphologic examination of marrow aspirate and biopsy specimens and can provide additional clinical and prognostic information. This combined approach has revealed the existence of several syndromes of acute myeloblastic leukemia[94]; the more common variants will be discussed (see below). One variant of M_4 myelomonocytic leukemia [*see Table 2*] is characterized by abnormal marrow eosinophils and is associated with inversion, deletion, or translocation of chromosome 16. A correct diagnosis of this variant, which has been termed $M_4Eo/inv(16)$,[95] is important because the likelihood of a sustained complete remission is good despite an unusually high frequency of central nervous system disease. Another AML variant that can have an M_4 phenotype is associated with inversion of chromosome 3 and abnormal megakaryocytes; generally, the platelet count is still relatively high at the time of clinical presentation in such cases. An M_2 variant of AML that is associated with the 6;9 translocation is characterized by a striking marrow basophilia. Auer rods are frequently seen in the myeloblasts of patients with an M_2 variant associated with the 8;21 translocation; approximately 20 percent of such patients have chloromas and splenomegaly.

Treatment

The nature of the disorder must be explained to the patient, who must decide whether or not to undergo induction [*see* General Psychosocial Principles for Management of Patients with Leukemia, *below*]. This is not a trivial decision: induction therapy for AML requires more than one month of hospitalization, generating costs as high as $100,000. For 20 to 30 days of that period, the patient will be aplastic and will suffer from fever caused by repeated and occasionally painful infections, initially caused by bacteria and then by fungi. The patient will be isolated in a protective environment; regular platelet and red blood cell transfusions will certainly be required.[96]

If a standard induction program is used, there is a 65 to 85 percent chance of achieving complete remission.[97] Patients older than 60 years and perhaps even those older than 50 years have lower complete remission rates and a shorter duration of continuous complete remission. The less satisfactory response in older individuals is significant because about half of all new cases of AML occur in patients older than 60 years.[98] In some series, the duration of complete remission ranges from 16 to 24 months, and about 20 to 25 percent of patients in this group are in stable first complete remission after three years. After five to seven years, perhaps 10 to 20 percent of patients will still be alive and will have no evidence of leukemic relapse. The relapse curve does not appear to reach a plateau, indicating no further relapses (a so-called cure), until the eighth year of remission.[99,100]

Patients in complete remission are clinically well. The physical examination, the complete blood count, and the bone marrow are normal. These and other observations led to the hypothesis that during complete remission the leukemic clone is suppressed and incapable of differentiation, leaving normal clones free to multiply, differentiate, and repopulate the marrow. However, at least two studies have shown that the malignant clone persists in the bone marrow of patients who appear to be in complete remission.[101-103] This finding requires reconsideration of the concept of complete remission. It also has important theoretical

implications for the planning of autologous marrow transplantation in so-called complete remission AML and for the therapeutic use of agents that promote differentiation [*see* Principles of Management, Chemotherapy, *above*].

Acute myeloblastic leukemia inductions probably should be done only in institutions that are experienced in this treatment. Factors to be considered include the requirements for platelets and perhaps granulocytes, the difficulties associated with maintaining uninfected vascular access, and the continuing problem of recurrent infections.[104] Because only 10 to 20 percent of patients achieve disease-free survival at five to seven years with currently available chemotherapy regimens, programs relying on allogeneic and autologous bone marrow transplantation have been extensively evaluated.[99,105,106] The risk of leukemic relapse is much lower in patients who are treated with allogeneic bone marrow transplantation than in those who receive standard chemotherapy. However, comparison of survival data for the two groups yields less clear-cut results because approximately 20 to 30 percent of patients receiving allogeneic bone marrow transplantation die of complications of the procedure within the first year.[107-109] Because an approach that combines standard chemotherapy and bone marrow transplantation may improve survival for certain patients with AML, a therapeutic program using these two modalities has been initiated at Stanford. In this approach, patients younger than 50 years receive a standard induction program. On achieving complete remission, they are offered either allogeneic bone marrow transplantation if they have a fully matched sibling donor or autologous bone marrow transplantation with 4-hydroperoxycyclophosphamide (4-HC) purging of the marrow if they do not. Patients who are older than 50 years receive only induction chemotherapy.

The induction program at Stanford is a variant of the standard program, in which daunorubicin is given for three days and cytarabine (Ara-C) and 6-thioguanine are administered for seven days (3/7 DAT) [*see*

Table 4]. When complete remission is established, consolidation is carried out with high-dose cytarabine in all patients. Intensification programs are then carried out in those patients who are not eligible for bone marrow transplantation; eligible patients are prepared for either allogeneic or autologous bone marrow transplantation. Virtually every induction is complicated by fever; initial episodes are assumed to be caused by bacterial sepsis and are treated with intravenous antimicrobials while cultures are being obtained. Subsequently, other types of infections may develop, including *Staphylococcus epidermidis* infection of the Hickman catheter site; herpetic infections of the mouth or esophagus; *Candida* infection of the esophagus, liver, spleen, or blood; or pulmonary aspergillosis.

Although some disagreement exists, it is best to avoid concurrent administration of amphotericin B (for fungal infection) and granulocyte transfusion because the combination may cause sudden pulmonary infiltration, respiratory failure, and even death.[110]

Gonadal function in men apparently returns to normal after standard AML induction therapy.[111]

Meningeal leukemia in adults is less common in acute myeloblastic leukemia (seven percent of cases) than in acute lymphocytic leukemia (40 percent of cases). Because meningeal leukemia does occur in a few patients, it is important to be aware of the neurologic complications.[112] When it has occurred, therapy with intrathecal methotrexate, 12 mg/m^2 (maximum, 12 mg) twice weekly, until the CSF is normal, has proved to be effective. Administration of dilute solutions in large volumes seems to potentiate the antileukemic effect and to reduce drug toxicity.[113,114] Methotrexate should be diluted in saline so that there is about 1 mg of methotrexate per milliliter of saline. In such circumstances, it is probably useful to install an Ommaya reservoir. When it becomes necessary to treat meningeal leukemia aggressively with intrathecal methotrexate, drug-induced neurotoxicity can be avoided by measuring CSF levels of methotrexate.[115]

Chloromatous masses can occur in acute myeloblastic leukemia at the time of presentation or as the first manifestation of the disease. It is not clear if the appearance of chloromatous masses is a poor prognostic sign.[116]

Leukostasis can occur when the blast count rises substantially above 50,000/mm^3 and is common when it exceeds 200,000/mm^3. Blast thrombi and aggregates cause vascular obstruction accompanied by hemorrhage and infarction in the cerebral and pulmonary vasculatures.[117] Patients with very high blast counts should not receive erythrocyte transfusions that raise hemoglobin levels to more than 10 g/dl, because the added viscosity may cause cerebral leukostasis and death.[118]

To reduce the blast count acutely, leukopheresis followed by a single intravenous injection of daunorubicin or doxorubicin in a dose of 60 mg/m^2 can be used.[119] The high uric acid level that results must be managed with allopurinol therapy. To prevent cerebral leukostasis in patients with high blast counts, some researchers recommend emergency x-ray therapy to the cranium, given as a single dose of 400 cGy (400 rads).

Variants of Acute Myeloblastic Leukemia

Therapy-Related Acute Myeloblastic Leukemia

A disorder similar to acute myeloblastic leukemia may develop several years after the administration of alkylating agents or radiation, or both, in the treatment of another cancer. This disorder, which has been termed therapy-related acute myeloblastic leukemia (t-AML), or therapy-related acute nonlymphocytic leukemia (t-ANLL), is generally preceded by a myelodysplastic syndrome that is characterized by cytopenias or refractory anemia with ringed sideroblasts (see below). In one series of Hodgkin's disease patients who were treated with alkylating agents, the incidence of t-AML reached 13 percent at 10 years, after which no further cases were reported.[120] In another series, no new cases of t-AML occurred after 11 years.[121] This variant is frequently associated with deletion of all or a part of chromosome 5 or 7 [*see Table 1*].[94,95,122]

Therapy-related acute myeloblastic leukemia does not respond well to chemotherapy: only 20 to 40 percent of patients achieve a complete remission,[123] and even in such cases, the remission is short (median duration, five months).[124,125] If the patient is less than 50 years of age and has a matched sibling donor, allogeneic bone marrow transplantation should be considered because it has produced satisfactory disease-free survival in some cases.[126] Therapeutic decisions regarding this disorder require careful analysis of the risk-benefit ratio, evaluation of the initial disease that required the previous therapy, and consideration of the patient's age and willingness to undergo further difficult therapy.

Acute Promyelocytic Leukemia

Almost all cases of acute promyelocytic leukemia (APL), designated M_3 in the FAB classification, show the 15;17 translocation [*see Table 1*]. Patients with this variant are at increased risk for disseminated intravascular coagulation (DIC), which causes a markedly enhanced disposition to hemorrhage. Petechial bleeding and hemorrhage occur at the marrow aspiration and intravenous infusion sites, accompanied by central nervous system hemorrhage and bleeding into the neck and paratracheal areas, which can cause sudden death. The clinical and laboratory evidence of DIC is readily detectable [*see Chapter 14*]. It is thought that the malignant promyelocyte releases tissue factor from its granules or from its plasma membrane when it is destroyed and that a bolus of this substance can initiate disseminated intravascular coagulation. Because the severity of the coagulopathy is closely correlated with the decrease in the α_2-plasmin inhibitor (α_2-PI), it appears that the substances released from APL cells may also stimulate the fibrinolytic system directly [*see Chapter 14*]. In patients who bleed, the α_2-PI is less than 30 percent of normal, which

suggests that this factor is consumed in counteracting free circulating plasmin.[127] If DIC is present, it is treated with continuous intravenous heparin infused at a rate of 250 to 500 units/hr and aggressive platelet replacement, with the aim of keeping the platelet count higher than $50,000/mm^3$; the dose of heparin is titered by following the level of fibrinogen and fibrin-fibrinogen degradation products.[128] If the patient continues to bleed, the antifibrinolytic agent ε-aminocaproic acid (EACA) may be added cautiously (0.5 g/hr) to the heparin infusion. Measurements of plasmin and α_2-PI, if available, can aid in deciding when to add EACA. Induction is begun at the same time as efforts to control DIC.

Because destruction of a large amount of tumor all at once could lead to uncontrollable disseminated intravascular coagulation and fibrinolysis, the APL induction is initiated more gently than the standard AML induction. It begins with appropriate testing for DIC and fibrinolysis and meticulous platelet support (see above). In APL induction, daunorubicin is not begun on the first day of the cycle as in AML induction [*see Table 4*] but rather is delayed until the last three days of the initial seven-day cycle. Furthermore, several studies indicate that unlike the case with AML, a complete remission can be achieved in APL without producing total marrow aplasia.[128,129]

Acute Megakaryoblastic Leukemia

Acute megakaryoblastic leukemia,[17,18] designated M_7 in the FAB classification, is a newly characterized disorder that probably encompasses many cases that were previously diagnosed as acute myelofibrosis. The diagnosis of M_7 is based on cytochemical analysis of peripheral blood because the marrow is frequently fibrotic and unaspiratable [*see Table 2*]. Patients have pancytopenia, myelofibrosis, and a bone marrow infiltrate that is probably composed of megakaryoblasts. Splenomegaly is absent, and there is little evidence of either peripheral blood leukoerythroblastosis or extramedullary hematopoiesis.

Table 4   Protocol for Treatment of Acute Myeloblastic Leukemia

Stage of Treatment	Conditions	Regimen*	Schedule
Induction			
Initial therapy	All patients, except high-risk patients 60 years of age or older	D	Days 1–3
	Patients 60 years of age or older at high risk (i.e., WBC > 40,000/mm^3, t-AML)	D	Days 1, 2
	All patients	C_1, T	Days 1–7
	Patients with peripheral blasts on day 8	C_1, T	Days 8, 9
Bone marrow aspiration and biopsy	All patients	—	Day 10
Modification (begins on day 12)	Biopsy results:		
	Group 1—gross leukemic infiltrate (marrow > 50% cellular, mostly blasts)	D C1, T	Days 12, 13 Days 12–15
	Group 2—moderate leukemic infiltrate (marrow 25%–50% cellular, mostly blasts)	D C2, T	Day 12 Days 12–14
	Group 3—minimal leukemic infiltrate (marrow < 25% cellular)	C1, T	Days 12–14
	Group 4—no leukemic infiltrate, no blasts	None	—
Repeat bone marrow biopsy (2 days after completion of additional chemotherapy)	Patients in groups 1–3	—	Day 16 or 17
Additional modification (begins after repeat biopsy specimen is processed)	Some improvement in findings on repeat biopsy but leukemic infiltrate still present	Treat as after biopsy done on day 10	
Salvage (begins after repeat biopsy specimen is processed)	No improvement in findings on repeat biopsy		
	Patients who can tolerate mitoxantrone	M, E_1	Days 1–5
	Patients not eligible for mitoxantrone	C_2, E_1	Days 1–5

Table 4 (continued)

Stage of Treatment	Conditions	Regimen*	Schedule
Consolidation (begins 2–4 wk after complete remission is achieved)	All patients in complete remission	C_3	Days 1–3
First intensification	Patients in complete remission who are not eligible for bone marrow transplantation (begins 3 months after day 1 of consolidation)	D C_1, T	Days 1–3 Days 1–7
Second intensification	Patients in complete remission who are not eligible for bone marrow transplantation (begins 4 months after day 1 of first intensification)	C_3	Days 1–4

Bone marrow transplant preparation (within 6 months after consolidation)	Patients 50 years of age or younger in complete remission
	With histocompatible donor
	  Allogeneic bone marrow transplantation
	
	Without histocompatible donor
	  Autologous bone marrow transplantation
		
		FTBI
		E_2
		
		B
		E_2
			
			Day 1
			Day 1
			
			Days 1–4
			Day 1

Note: studies during induction include daily complete blood cell counts, platelet counts, and determination of electrolytes, BUN, and creatinine levels; semiweekly liver function tests; and weekly chest x-rays. Before administration of chemotherapy, patients are given allopurinol, 300 mg/day (except for those with a drug allergy), which is stopped on day 7 if the risk of urate nephropathy has passed. Urine may be alkalinized and urine flow increased if indicated. Provision must be made for antiemetics. Induction chemotherapy should be initiated without undue delay after admission to the hospital. For individuals with cardiac dysfunction or those who have received a cumulative anthracycline dose that precludes further anthracycline therapy, high-dose cytarabine (3 g/m^2 q 24 hr for 5 days) is substituted for daunorubicin during the initial induction and subsequently as necessary.

*Regimens are abbreviated as follows:

B—Busulfan, 16 mg/kg p.o. over 96 hr
C_1—Cytarabine, 100 mg/m^2 I.V. over 30 min q 12 hr
C_2—Cytarabine, 3 g/m^2 I.V. over 2 hr q 24 hr
C_3—Cytarabine, 1 g/m^2 I.V. over 2 hr q 24 hr
D—Daunorubicin, 60 mg/m^2 I.V., side arm into running I.V., over 15–20 min

E_1—Etoposide, 100 mg/m^2 I.V. over 30 min q 24 hr
E_2—Etoposide, 60 mg/kg I.V. over 4 hr
M—Mitoxantrone, 10 mg/m^2 I.V. over 15 min q 24 hr
T—Thioguanine, 100 mg/m^2 p.o. q 12 hr
FTBI—Fractionated total body irradiation, 1,320 cGY (1,320 rads)

One case of acute myelofibrosis has occurred after cytotoxic therapy, and another was reported after a combination of cytotoxic and radiation therapy.[130] Induction similar to that used for acute myeloblastic leukemia has been attempted; however, the therapeutic response has generally been poor. Allogeneic transplantation has produced long-standing remission.

Acute Erythroleukemia

Acute erythroleukemia, also termed acute erythremic myelosis, is a variant of acute myeloblastic leukemia. It appears either as a spontaneous disorder, usually in elderly patients, or as a presumed consequence of alkylator therapy, as may occur after melphalan therapy for multiple myeloma [*see Chapter 16*]. Patients have anemia caused by ineffective erythropoiesis and pancytopenia. Acute erythroleukemia is the M_6 variety in the FAB classification of AML [*see Table 2*]. Patients are usually treated with AML induction programs. Complete remission was attained in six of 14 patients in one study.[131]

Biphenotypic and Hybrid Acute Leukemias

The leukemic cells of some patients demonstrate both lymphoid and myeloid features by standard cytochemical methods and immunophenotyping techniques. Several different terms have been used to describe such leukemias, including biphenotypic, hybrid, biclonal, and bilineal. The variant in which individual malignant cells display both lymphoid and myeloid markers is termed biphenotypic leukemia. In another variant, referred to as hybrid acute leukemia, the leukemic blasts are heterogeneous, with some displaying myeloid markers and others displaying lymphoid markers. The terms bilineal and biclonal have also been applied to this variant.[132] Cytogenetic analysis may show the 4;11 translocation in some patients with biphenotypic leukemia.[94] The prognosis for patients with either biphenotypic or hybrid acute leukemia is poor. Even when such patients achieve a complete remission, often in response to the induction program used for acute lymphoblastic leukemia, the duration of the remission is short.

Intermediate Forms of Myeloid Disease

Several clinical designations—subacute myeloid leukemia, chronic myelomonocytic leukemia, chronic erythremic myelosis, myelodysplastic syndromes, preleukemia (hematopoietic dysplasia), and smoldering myeloid leukemia—can be considered together.[133] Patients with these disorders have a clinical picture that falls somewhere between the better-defined entities of chronic myeloid leukemia and acute myeloid leukemia. The patients are usually men in their 60s and 70s, and their clinical problems relate to the presence of isolated or multiple cytopenias and the associated cellular dysfunction. There may be a relatively long prodromal period.

The peripheral smear contains hypogranulated neutrophils that occasionally show the pseudo–Pelger-Huet anomaly (bilobed neutrophils appearing as juvenile neutrophils). In addition, there may be blasts in the peripheral smear as well as a leukemic hiatus. Erythrocyte morphology may be normal, or there may be impressive hypochromia and giant macrocytes. The platelet count is frequently decreased, and the platelets are usually large and have decreased granulation. Marrow may be hypercellular but is usually normocellular and even occasionally hypocellular; in any case, physical replacement of the marrow does not account for the pancytopenia. Abnormalities in the development of one to three cell lines include poor granulocytic development, the presence of dwarfed bilobed megakaryocytes, and occasionally, ringed sideroblasts in conjunction with multiple nucleated giant normoblasts. The number of mast cells in marrow may be increased.[134] Careful search usually reveals the presence of clumps of atypical myeloblasts and promyelocytes. The serum lysozyme level may also be increased.

The FAB group has proposed a classification for the myelodysplastic syndromes [*see Table 5*],[135] but its utility remains to be determined. There are several problems with this scheme. For example, the distinction between refractory anemia with excess blasts in transformation (RAEB-Tr) and erythroleukemia, or M_6, depends in part on the ability to distinguish between a level of 20 to 30 percent blasts and a level of more than 30 percent blasts in the marrow aspirate. The bone marrow morphologic features used to distinguish the five classes of myelodysplasia are seen only on the aspirate and do not have a counterpart in bone marrow biopsies.[136] Biopsies, on the other hand, can reveal whether clumps of myeloblasts are present, a finding that may have diagnostic and prognostic importance.[137] A further deficiency with this proposed classification is the fact that the five subtypes have only two general outcomes: patients with refractory anemia (RA) or refractory anemia with ringed sideroblasts (RARS) have median survival rates of 64 and 71 months, respectively, whereas patients with refractory anemia with excess blasts (RAEB), refractory anemia with excess blasts in transformation, or chronic myelomonocytic leukemia (CMML) have median survival rates of seven, five, and eight months, respectively.[138] One study involving 336 patients found that it was not possible to distinguish clearly between acute leukemia and myelodysplastic syndrome on the basis of a specific proportion of marrow blasts. Not surprisingly, however, the higher the percentage of marrow blasts, the shorter the patient survival.[139]

Cytogenetic studies have shown that chromosomal abnormalities occur more fre-

Table 5 FAB Classification of Myelodysplastic Syndromes

Condition	Peripheral Blood Findings	Characteristics of Bone Marrow Aspirate
Refractory anemia (RA)	Reticulocytopenia, variable dyserythropoiesis; <1% blasts; neutropenia, thrombocytopenia, and dysgranulopoiesis are rare	Ranges from normal to hypercellular with erythroid hyperplasia or dyserythropoiesis, or both; <5% blasts; normal granulopoiesis and megakaryopoiesis
Refractory anemia with ringed sideroblasts (RARS) (acquired idiopathic sideroblastic anemia—AISA)	Same as those in RA	Same as those in RA, but ringed sideroblasts account for more than 15% of the nucleated cells
Refractory anemia with excess blasts (RAEB)	Cytopenia and dysplasia of two to three cell lines; dysgranulopoiesis is common; <5% blasts	Hypercellular; variable granulocytic and erythroid hyperplasia along with dysgranulopoiesis, dyserythropoiesis, and dysmegakaryopoiesis; ringed sideroblasts may be seen; 5%–20% blasts; granulocytes mature to promyelocyte stage and beyond
Refractory anemia with excess blasts in transformation (RAEB-Tr)	Similar to those in RAEB but with ≥5% blasts	Similar to those in RAEB but with 20%–30% blasts or the presence of Auer rods
Chronic myelomonocytic leukemia (CMML)	Monocytes >1,000/mm^3 with or without dysgranulopoiesis; <5% blasts	Similar to those in RAEB but may show an increase in monocytic precursors with <5% blasts

quently in RAEB, RAEB-Tr, and CMML, which are the more overtly leukemic syndromes. Similarities and differences have been observed between the cytogenetic abnormalities in the myelodysplastic syndromes and those in AML, AML variants, and CML. Trisomy 8 is fairly common in the myelodysplastic syndromes, as is the loss of chromosomes 5, 7, and Y; however, none of the patients with these syndromes have had the AML patterns of t(8;21) or t(15;17) [*see Table 1*].[140]

The 5q⁻ syndrome, a relatively uncommon myelodysplastic disorder marked by the loss of a piece of the long arm of chromosome 5, is associated with a fairly typical clinical picture consisting of increased numbers of abnormal and dwarf megakaryocytes in the marrow, macro-ovalocytic anemia with abnormally shaped red blood cells, and normal to elevated platelet counts. The bone marrow displays features similar to that of patients with RA, RARS, or RAEB [*see Table 5*]. Because the q portion of chromosome 5 contains the genes for granulocyte-macrophage colony-stimulating factor (GM-CSF), macrophage colony-stimulating factor (M-CSF), interleukin-3 (IL-3), the platelet-derived growth factor (PDGF) receptor, and other growth factors and their receptors,[141] it has been suggested that the loss of one or more of these controlling genes somehow leads to this myelodysplastic variant.

The frequency of myelodysplastic syndromes is increasing because treatment-associated leukemias[9-12] are on the rise and because such disorders typically evolve first into a myelodysplastic clinical picture that is often associated with deletion of chromosomes 5 and 7.[142,143] The combined clinical picture is sometimes referred to as the t-MDS/t-ANLL syndrome because of the regularity of the pattern of evolution. Although therapy with alkylating agents is the common denominator in treatment-associated leukemias, one study indicates that melphalan may be a more potent leukemogen than cyclophosphamide.[144] Another study suggests that treatment with procarbazine or the nitrosoureas may be more leukemogenic than cyclophosphamide therapy.[145]

The clinical course of myelodysplastic syndromes is marked by hemorrhage and infection. The median survival is only 1.5 months for patients in whom either a rising white blood cell count or a falling platelet count develops.[146] Most of the patients die during this stage of the disease, before their condition transforms into a more obvious form of acute myeloblastic leukemia, an event that occurs in 10 to 40 percent of patients. Evidence of a clonal abnormality in the myeloid stem cell was observed in one patient in whom the myelodysplastic syndrome evolved into AML.[147]

Management

Hemolytic anemia, an uncommon manifestation of the myelodysplastic syndromes, occasionally responds to prednisone in a dosage of 30 to 50 mg/day, but this therapy carries the hazard of infection. Danazol given in a dosage of 600 mg/day for a period of several months alleviated thrombocytopenia and hemolysis in three patients with myelodysplastic syndromes.[148] This approach needs to be examined in a large-scale study, however, because danazol is expensive and produces significant side effects, including virilization in women, mood alteration, and hepatic dysfunction. Antimetabolites, such as mercaptopurine and hydroxyurea, have been used to control systemic symptoms, organomegaly, and elevated white blood cell counts.

Most patients with myelodysplastic syndromes are elderly, but for the very few patients with one of these disorders who are younger than 54 years and who have a histocompatible donor, allogeneic bone marrow transplantation offers the best chance for a normal life.[142,149,150]

One group of investigators has aggressively treated patients with a deteriorating myelodysplastic syndrome using AML protocols. Patients older than 50 years responded poorly, and only 25 percent entered complete remission. In the patients who were younger than 50 years, 86 percent entered complete remission, but the duration of the remission appeared to be short.[151]

Treatment attempts are being made using agents that enhance cellular differentiation, in the hope that the abnormal cells will mature and then die, thus reducing their effect on normal marrow and marrow elements. Retinoic acid derivatives can raise the neutrophil level in patients with myelodysplastic syndromes, but they do not produce a beneficial effect on the overall morphology of marrow cells or the platelet count, nor do they reduce the red blood cell transfusion requirements.[152] Therapy with low dosages of cytarabine (10 mg/m^2 s.c. q 12 hr for 15 to 25 days) has produced conflicting results. In addition, this treatment approach usually requires that patients be hospitalized because it produces severe pancytopenia.[142,153]

Hematopoietic growth factors are also being used to enhance differentiation and maturation of the abnormal marrow cells and thereby ameliorate the effects of the cytopenias associated with the myelodysplastic syndrome. However, because the malignant cells in this syndrome require hematopoietic growth factors to proliferate in vitro, there is concern that administration of growth factors will cause this disorder to convert to a more aggressive disease, such as acute myeloblastic leukemia. In one study,[154] GM-CSF increased the level of white blood cells, including neutrophils, but did not produce a sustained increase in platelets or reticulocytes or significantly reduce the transfusion requirement in patients with the myelodysplastic syndrome. In some patients, the proportion of marrow leukemic blasts increased, raising the concern that GM-CSF might cause disproportionate stimulation of the leukemic clone. However, another growth factor, granulocyte colony-stimulating factor (G-CSF), seems to produce significant increases in the white blood cells, including neutrophils, without stimulating the leukemic blast clones.[155] The role of G-CSF in the myelodysplastic syndrome is to be tested in a phase III controlled trial. Neither GM-CSF nor G-

CSF is currently available for routine clinical use.

Chronic and Subacute Leukemias of B Cell Origin

The lymphocytic leukemias include an acute form—which is termed acute lymphoblastic leukemia [*see* Acute Lymphoblastic Leukemia, *below*]—as well as several chronic and subacute forms. There is now reliable evidence indicating that the chronic and subacute leukemias should be subdivided further according to whether they are of B or T cell origin because a close correlation has frequently been observed between the lineage of a leukemia and its biologic behavior.

Chronic Lymphocytic Leukemia

Pathophysiology

Chronic lymphocytic leukemia (CLL) is a malignant clonal disorder of relatively mature lymphocytes, predominantly B cells; however, a malignant disorder of T cells (T-CLL) accounts for about five percent of cases. In CLL, the abnormal clone either replaces normal B cells or inhibits their growth and maturation, depressing immunoglobulin levels and impairing humoral immunity. By detecting the G6PD clonal marker, one research group appears to have demonstrated clonal origin for B cells from two CLL patients. Peripheral blood erythrocytes, platelets, granulocytes, and T cells, however, displayed two G6PD types, indicating that these cells arose from heterogeneous precursors.[156] A cytogenetic abnormality, trisomy 12, has been identified in the malignant B cells of about 50 percent of patients with CLL[157]; abnormalities of chromosome 14 are also observed but somewhat less frequently than trisomy 12. CLL cells typically have a low level of SmIg and therefore display only weak surface immunofluorescence.

The malignant lymphocytes apparently survive for prolonged periods and recirculate from blood to bone marrow to lymph nodes and back to blood again. In some cases, the abnormal lymphocytes respond poorly to mitogenic stimulation by phytohemagglutinin. About 25 percent of patients with CLL have hypogammaglobulinemia, and as many as 10 percent have hypergammaglobulinemia. Both conditions presumably reflect abnormal B cell function. About five percent of patients have a monoclonal gammopathy,[158] typically an IgM gammopathy, that resembles the gammopathy produced in Waldenström's macroglobulinemia [*see Chapter 16*]. IgM production in patients with chronic lymphocytic leukemia, however, usually does not reach a level likely to cause viscosity problems.

Patients with chronic lymphocytic leukemia have a low but distinct incidence of autoimmune hemolytic anemia and a similar incidence of immune thrombocytopenic purpura, but the autoantibodies that cause these disorders are not derived from the malignant B cell clone.[157] Second cancers occur relatively frequently in patients with CLL.

Clinical Manifestations

Patients who have CLL present with a wide spectrum of signs and symptoms that parallel the very wide variation in the course of the disease. Patients may be discovered on routine examination to have an absolute mature lymphocytosis of 15,000/mm^3 or more, even up to 10 times that number. Routine physical examination may turn up generalized nontender adenopathy and moderate splenomegaly. Conversely, patients may have profound pancytopenia, impressive nodal enlargement, organomegaly, and recurrent infections.

The clinical course is largely determined by the extent of infiltration of marrow and the degree of replacement of normal elements, which produces functional aplasia and peripheral pancytopenia. The neutropenia and impaired humoral immunity lead to susceptibility to recurrent infections. Autoimmune hemolytic anemia and equivalent conditions, as well as hypersplenism, can contribute to the pancytopenia. Anemia and thrombocytopenia may be ominous prognostic signs. Nodal enlargement may obstruct ureters, but otherwise, it rarely causes problems. Systemic symptoms are

not usually present in patients with chronic lymphocytic leukemia. In contrast to the situation in chronic myeloid leukemia, blast crisis in chronic lymphocytic leukemia occurs very rarely.[159]

Occasionally, in the later stages of CLL, fever, night sweats, weight loss, and rapidly enlarging masses in nodal and extranodal sites may occur. The peripheral blood may show immature lymphocytes with nucleoli. This transformation, which resembles diffuse large cell lymphoma, is termed Richter's syndrome.[157] The syndrome responds poorly even to the aggressive programs used for the treatment of diffuse large cell lymphoma. Some investigators distinguish between a Richter's transformation characterized by minimal lymphoid immaturity in the peripheral blood and a prolymphocytic transformation (see below) marked by a distinct population of immature cells in the peripheral blood.[160]

Diagnosis

The diagnosis of chronic lymphocytic leukemia is established by absolute lymphocytosis on the peripheral smear, a lymphocytic infiltrate in the bone marrow, and a lymph node biopsy specimen showing the pattern of diffuse well-differentiated lymphoma. Serum protein electrophoresis and quantitative immunoglobulin determinations frequently show panhypogammaglobulinemia and, rarely, a small IgM M protein spike. Care must be exercised in interpreting bone marrow aspirates because lymphoid nodules are normally present. A chronic lymphocytic leukemic infiltrate, however, will consistently show marrow replacement of several spicules. A Jamshidi needle biopsy will also demonstrate the extent of architectural disruption by invading lymphocytes. It is not clear that there are clinical differences between CLL and diffuse well-differentiated lymphoma.[161] Immunophenotypic analysis of peripheral blood or bone marrow, or both, generally shows a proliferation of B cells that display low-level fluorescence when stained for surface membrane immunoglobulin. The proliferation is shown to be clonal by the fact that the cells stain only with either κ or λ light-chain reagents. Immunoglobulin gene rearrangement studies also show evidence of clonal expansion.

Staging

Several staging systems for CLL have been proposed based on the concept that the major prognostic factors are the number of involved nodal areas, the extent of hepatosplenomegaly, the pattern of marrow replacement, and the degree of anemia and thrombocytopenia.[162,163] In the Rai classification,[164] stage 0 represents an absolute lymphocytosis of 15,000/mm^3 or more in the peripheral blood and 40 percent lymphocytosis in the marrow; stage I indicates lymphocytosis with enlarged lymph nodes; stage II encompasses lymphocytosis with enlargement of either the liver or spleen, or both; stage III consists of lymphocytosis with a hemoglobin concentration of less than 11 g/dl; and stage IV consists of lymphocytosis with a platelet count of less than 100,000/mm^3. Stage 0 is thought to predict long-term survival on the order of 10 years, whereas most patients with either stage III or stage IV disease die in less than four years.

The Binet classification[165] reduces the number of stages of CLL from five to three and considers clinical enlargement of five specific areas—spleen, liver, and lymph nodes (either unilateral or bilateral) of the axillary, cervical, and inguinal regions—in addition to the degree of anemia and thrombocytopenia. Patients in group A have no anemia or thrombocytopenia and less than three areas of lymphoid enlargement. Patients in group B also have normal hemoglobin and platelet levels but have three or more areas of lymphoid enlargement. Patients are classified as stage C when they have either a hemoglobin level of less than 10 g/dl or a platelet level of less than 100,000/mm^3, or both, regardless of the number of areas of lymphoid involvement. Stage C patients have the poorest prognosis.

A classification that is based in part on marrow histology has also been proposed.[166] This scheme distinguishes two types of mar-

row infiltration patterns, diffuse and nodular; those patients who have a poor prognosis, corresponding to that of Rai stage III/IV or Binet stage C patients, have a diffusely and densely infiltrated marrow.

Analysis of relatively large series of patients with CLL indicates that other factors may also significantly affect the prognosis. The level of serum immunoglobulins appears to be important because survival is reduced in patients who have gamma-globulin values less than 700 mg/ml. The IgA and, to a lesser extent, the IgG levels appear to correlate most closely with the prognosis.[167] Another study found that a peripheral blood lymphocyte level in excess of 60,000/mm^3 indicated a poor outlook.[168] It is likely that these factors will be important components of future staging systems.

Management

The syndromes of autoimmune hemolytic anemia and immune thrombocytopenic purpura are treated as they would be in patients without chronic lymphocytic leukemia [*see Chapter 14*]. Recurrent infection may require repeated antibiotic intervention, particularly if the patient has chronic urinary tract infections or a disease such as bronchiectasis. It has been shown in controlled trials that patients with recurrent infections associated with hypogammaglobulinemia (i.e., IgG levels less than 400 to 640 mg/dl)[169] have fewer infections if they are treated with intravenous IgG in a dosage of 0.4 g/kg every three weeks.[169,170] Leukostasis is very rare in chronic lymphocytic leukemia even in the presence of very high white blood cell counts. Local disease can be treated with local palliative irradiation.

Difficulty arises in deciding whether to treat a patient with progressive nodal and organ enlargement and pancytopenia that appears to be worsening as a result of progressive marrow infiltration. In contrast to the situation in chronic myeloid leukemia, the white blood cell count in chronic lymphocytic leukemia is not an accurate indicator of the extent of the disease. Studies of therapy for chronic lymphocytic leukemia have been difficult to evaluate because apparently similar cases seem to have had markedly different clinical courses, lasting from several months to more than 15 years.

Because the available therapies are all myelosuppressive and because they thus compound the preexisting pancytopenia and impaired humoral immunity, the preferred strategy is to withhold systemic therapy until there are symptoms and signs of progressive pancytopenia. Some good results have been reported with total body irradiation, but a trial of mediastinal irradiation indicated that such therapy has very serious pancytopenic side effects.[171] Corticosteroids do not destroy chronic lymphocytic leukemic lymphocytes but merely redistribute them from nodes into the peripheral blood. Thus, alkylators have until recently been the mainstay of therapy in single-drug programs. Therapy consists of 0.1 mg/kg/day of chlorambucil or 2.0 mg/kg/day of cyclophosphamide. The drug is given carefully, and blood counts, lymph nodes, and organ size are monitored during the course of therapy. Chlorambucil can also be given every two weeks, starting with a single oral dose of 0.4 mg/kg and progressing by 0.1 mg/kg stepwise increments to the point of myelotoxicity.

A group of French investigators has conducted a unique randomized clinical trial in patients with CLL.[172] Binet stage A patients were randomized to receive either no therapy or a daily course of oral chlorambucil, 0.1 mg/kg for an indefinite period. The study found that chlorambucil therapy was actually harmful for stage A patients.[173] Stage B patients were randomized to receive either daily chlorambucil or CVP (i.e., cyclophosphamide, 300 mg/m^2/day orally on days one through five; vincristine, 1.0 mg/m^2 I.V. on day one; and prednisone, 40 mg/m^2/day orally in four divided doses on days one through five—the cycle is repeated monthly); the two-year survival for the two groups was the same (83 percent). Unfortunately, because there was no stage B group that did not receive therapy, the possibility that stage B patients may not require sys-

temic therapy was not tested. Stage C patients were randomized to receive either CVP or CHOP, which is the same as the CVP regimen but with the addition of doxorubicin, 25 mg/m^2 given intravenously on day one of each monthly cycle. For the stage C patients, the two regimens produced significant differences in survival: at two years, 77 percent of the patients who received CHOP were alive, in contrast to only 44 percent of the CVP group.

Pentostatin, a nucleoside analogue that inhibits adenosine deaminase, has been tested in stage B and C patients, and about 25 to 30 percent of patients have had a good response. Despite the drug's T cell suppressive effect, no infectious complications have occurred. The role of pentostatin in the management of CLL is not clear.[174] Because there is concern that pentostatin may produce long-lasting immunologic or other impairment, it has not yet been released by the FDA. Fludarabine, another agent that has not yet been released by the FDA, also appears to be able to produce beneficial responses in chronic lymphocytic leukemia.[175]

Splenectomy may occasionally have a role in the management of chronic lymphocytic leukemia. The indications for this procedure are painful splenomegaly, profound anemia with an increasingly burdensome transfusion requirement, and clinically significant thrombocytopenia. In carefully selected circumstances, splenectomy can produce clinical improvement; however, the procedure has an associated morbidity of about 20 percent, has a mortality of about five percent, and does not prolong survival.[176]

Chronic Lymphosarcoma Cell Leukemia

The cells in chronic lymphosarcoma cell leukemia are larger than those in CLL, and their nucleoli are usually easily discernible. The peripheral blood smear of patients with this disease occasionally shows many small cleaved lymphocytes. This condition is the leukemic phase of follicular or diffuse lymphomas. The clinical course does not appear to differ from that of patients with chronic lymphocytic leukemia, and I manage these patients as if they had CLL (see above).

Prolymphocytic Leukemia

Prolymphocytic leukemia is a rare variant characterized by systemic symptoms, massive splenomegaly, and large lymphocytes. The leukocyte count is characteristically very high, usually greater than $100,000/mm^3$,[157] and the cells express much more SmIg than do CLL cells. If a peripheral blood prolymphocyte level of more than 55 percent is used as a criterion for defining prolymphocytic leukemia, a distinct group of patients can be identified who show the more typical clinical picture of massive splenomegaly and pronounced elevation of the leukocyte count.[177]

Splenectomy combined with chemotherapy using the CHOP regimen (see above) or a similar program may be useful.

Hairy-Cell Leukemia (Leukemic Reticuloendotheliosis)

The malignant cell in hairy-cell leukemia is usually a B cell that infiltrates and replaces the marrow and infiltrates the spleen, causing splenomegaly.[178] The combination of marrow replacement and splenomegaly causes pancytopenia (including monocytopenia). The morphology on the peripheral smear, on the bone marrow biopsy specimen, and on the spleen biopsy specimen is reasonably characteristic. A positive test for tartrate-resistant acid phosphatase activity is helpful but not pathognomonic.

Infections that are presumably caused by neutropenia are the most serious complications; atypical mycobacterial infections may occur with higher than normal frequency.[179] Vasculitis can occur in the setting of hairy-cell leukemia, usually in association with infection. The vasculitis in patients with this disorder may respond to treatment with interferon-alpha.[180,181]

Splenectomy to correct the pancytopenia had been the mainstay of therapy for hairy-cell leukemia. Now, however, several studies have shown that recombinant inter-

feron-alpha produces a beneficial effect that appears to be long lasting in 75 to 90 percent of patients with this disease; even patients who had not been splenectomized responded to interferon-alpha.[182,183] In a common regimen, interferon-alpha is self-administered by the patient three times weekly for at least six months in a dosage of 2 million units/m^2 subcutaneously or intramuscularly (the latter route is used only if platelets and bleeding time are normal). In another schedule, interferon-alpha is self-administered in a dosage of 3 million units/day for eight weeks.[184]

The usual side effects are flulike symptoms, but some patients show extreme fatigue and weight loss, neurologic symptoms such as diminution of attention span, and elevated aspartate aminotransferase (SGOT) and alanine aminotransferase (SGPT) levels. Beneficial effects include reduction of hepatomegaly and splenomegaly, the disappearance of hairy cells from the marrow, and the restoration of blood counts to normal. If patients relapse after interferon-alpha is withdrawn, improvement can usually be restored by reinstituting therapy. Interferon-alpha generally induces a partial remission, but pentostatin can produce a complete and seemingly long lasting remission.[185,186] In a preliminary study, the administration of G-CSF to neutropenic patients with hairy-cell leukemia resulted in significant increases in the absolute neutrophil count.[187]

Chronic and Subacute Leukemias of T Cell Origin

Although chronic lymphocytic leukemia, prolymphocytic leukemia, and hairy-cell leukemia predominantly involve B cells, T cell variants of each of these disorders have been described. T cell CLL accounts for about five percent of cases of CLL and does not differ significantly from the B cell variant except for an increased frequency of skin involvement.[157] T cell prolymphocytic leukemia does not differ clinically from the B cell variant. T cell hairy-cell leukemia is a rare variant that has been linked to human T cell lymphotropic virus type II (HTLV-II) infection.[157]

Cutaneous T Cell Lymphoma/Leukemia (Sézary Syndrome and Mycosis Fungoides)

Cutaneous T cell lymphoma/leukemia (CTCL) is a chronic disorder of helper-inducer T cells. When the peripheral blood contains many lymphoid cells with buttock-shaped or cerebriform nuclei, the disorder is termed the Sézary syndrome. Skin disease is present in almost all cases. When the disorder is confined to the skin, it is managed locally, and excellent results have been achieved using total skin electron-beam therapy.[188] However, when more than 20 percent of the lymphocytes that are present on the peripheral blood smear are of the abnormal Sézary type, the patients have a poorer prognosis.[189]

Adult T Cell Leukemia/Lymphoma

A rapidly fatal syndrome known as adult T cell leukemia/lymphoma (ATLL), which produces high leukocyte counts, hepatosplenomegaly, lymphadenopathy, skin lesions, and hypercalcemia, has been described in Japan, the West Indies, and the southeastern United States. The malignant cells are thought to be mature helper-inducer T cells. A human retrovirus, which has been termed human T cell lymphotropic virus type I (HTLV-I), has been isolated from several cell cultures from patients, one of whom had cutaneous T cell lymphoma. Patients with ATLL have antibodies to HTLV-I.[190]

Patients in the United States usually present with various cutaneous lesions or with hypercalcemia manifested by malaise, nausea, confusion, thirst, and polyuria. Elevated serum alkaline phosphatase levels, abnormal bone scans, and lytic lesions visible on roentgenograms indicate that accelerated bone turnover is the likely cause of hypercalcemia. Surprisingly, there is little tumor involvement of bone at the sites of destruction, suggesting that the bone destruction represents a form of paraneoplastic activation of osteoclasts. Circulating malignant cells that have lobulated nuclei and are similar to those in the Sézary syndrome are usually found. Although peripheral lymphadenopathy is common, mediastinal adenopathy does not occur, and thus, ATLL can be distinguished from T cell ALL or lymphoblastic lymphoma. Opportunistic infection caused by agents such as *Pneumocystis carinii* and cytomegalovirus is common, as is central nervous system disease.

The diagnosis can be made by skin biopsy, by lymph node biopsy that shows diffuse lymphoma, or by examination of the peripheral blood. Intensive combination chemotherapy using the CHOP regimen or a similar program may produce temporary improvement.[3] The major indicators of a poor prognosis are unsatisfactory performance status, high levels of lactic dehydrogenase (LDH), and a leukemic picture.[191]

Lymphocytosis of Large Granular Lymphocytes

Lymphocytosis of large granular lymphocytes (LGLs), also termed T γ-lymphoproliferative disorder, or leukemia of LGL, is a newly described entity marked by the presence of azurophilic granules in some peripheral lymphocytes. Studies of rearrangements of T cell receptor genes reveal that the disorder may arise from a malignant clonal expansion in some cases. Immunophenotyping studies indicate that the LGLs may be suppressor-cytotoxic T cells, and they occasionally express natural killer cell and antibody-dependent cell-mediated cytotoxic activity.[192]

The clinical picture is variable, but patients typically present with frequent infections or bleeding. The peripheral blood shows a lymphocytosis of LGLs of more than $3,000/mm^3$ and neutropenia, thrombocytopenia, or evidence of hemolysis.[192,193] The spleen may be palpably enlarged, and the marrow can either be normal or show focal collections of lymphocytes. The marrow replacement is never so extensive that it would account for the presenting cytopenia. Antineutrophil and antiplatelet antibodies apparently are responsible for the neutropenia and thrombocytopenia [*see Chapter 14*], and a Coombs'-positive hemolytic anemia has also been described. Some patients have high serum titers of rheumatoid factor. Perhaps some cases that have been classified as atypical Felty's syndrome have actually been caused by lymphocytosis of LGLs. In one case, it appeared that infection with the retrovirus HTLV-I produced a clonal expansion of large granular lymphocytes associated with a clinical picture similar to that of chronic T γ–lymphoproliferative disease. The infected cells presumably released lymphokines that in turn produced the syndrome of pure red cell aplasia.[194]

No studies on therapy for this disorder have been reported; in the few cases that we have seen at Stanford, we have focused on the management of the immune cytopenia.

Possible T Cell Clonal Disorders

Histiocytic Medullary Reticulosis

The rare disorder histiocytic medullary reticulosis resembles leukemia in that it produces high fever, organomegaly, and frequently, pancytopenia. The marrow is infiltrated by large macrophagic cells that ingest erythrocytes and platelets. It appears that in at least some cases of histiocytic medullary reticulosis the patient has an underlying T cell lymphoma whose clonal origin has been confirmed by the rearrangement of the gene encoding the T cell receptor β chain.[195,196] It appears that the lymphoma may secrete lymphokines that activate and recruit clonally normal monocytes and macrophages to the site of involvement, thereby generating the characteristic morphologic appearance of histiocytic medullary reticulosis. Some patients respond briefly to treatment with the CHOP regimen,[197] but results generally are poor. There are no controlled studies.

Angioimmunoblastic Lymphadenopathy

Angioimmunoblastic lymphadenopathy involves a proliferation of lymphoid cells that may be either benign or malignant. Patients present with fever, skin rashes, lymphadenopathy, hypergammaglobulinemia, splenomegaly, autoimmune hemolytic anemia, and thrombocytopenia. This clinical picture is consistent with B cell proliferation and was initially thought to indicate a B cell clonal disorder. Rearrangement of immunoglobulin genes has been detected in some patients, and this finding supports the idea that angioimmunoblastic lymphadenopathy is a B cell clonal disorder. However, evidence of rearrangement of the T cell receptor β chain gene, which indicates the presence of a T cell clonal disorder, has been observed in other patients.[196,198] Immunophenotyping of involved nodes in patients with angioimmunoblastic lymphadenopathy frequently shows a T cell phenotype.

Acute Lymphoblastic Leukemia

Acute lymphoblastic leukemia is less common than acute myeloblastic leukemia in adults; ALL accounts for 10 to 15 percent of cases of acute leukemia in adults. ALL has been subdivided on the basis of immunologic and enzymatic markers into several variants [*see Table 3*]: the common variant (cALL), a pre–B cell form (pre–B-ALL), a mature B cell variant (B-ALL), and a T cell variant (T-ALL). These subclasses can have therapeutic implications, but the unified therapeutic program (see below) is based on the assumption that adult acute lymphoblastic leukemia is always a high-risk disease.[199]

The pathophysiology of the disease and its clinical manifestations are not very different from those of AML, except that the incidence of CNS disease is higher in ALL.[113,200,201] It is crucial to make the morphologic distinction between AML and ALL because there are no tumor-specific agents for the treatment of acute myeloblastic leukemia, whereas L-asparaginase, vincristine, and prednisone specifically attack leukemic lymphoblasts. Poor prognostic signs include a peripheral blood blast count greater than $20,000/mm^3$, relatively advanced age (i.e., older than 30 years), Burkitt's (L_3) leukemia,[202] CALLA immunophenotype, the 9;22 translocation or evidence of the ALL variation of the *bcr* rearrangement, and the requirement of more than four weeks to achieve complete remission.[201,203]

Emerging results have raised hopes that aggressive forms of chemotherapy may produce long-lasting disease-free remissions and even cure. Treatment consists of a four-drug induction program followed by CNS prophylaxis and sequential courses of intensive cytoreductive therapy. The results of chemotherapy reported in two series[201,203] and unpublished findings from the University of California at San Francisco, the City of Hope in Duarte, California, and the Stanford cooperative group were strikingly similar. In each of the three series, disease-free survival was found to reach a plateau after about five years, and it appears that approximately 35 percent of patients may be cured. The protocol that was used at Stanford produced a complete remission in almost 95 percent of patients.[204] This protocol has now been modified [*see Table 6*] in an effort to achieve a greater disease-free survival and to allow for a comparison between chemotherapy and allogeneic bone marrow transplantation in patients younger than 45 years who have matched donors. The results of allogeneic bone marrow transplantation in patients with ALL are not sufficiently clear, and additional studies are required before firm recommendations can be made.[205] Autologous bone marrow transplantation with marrow purging by use of monoclonal antibodies has also been proposed, but the role of this procedure in ALL has not been clearly established.[206,207]

Induction chemotherapy for ALL severely depresses reproductive gonadal function but does not impair endocrine gonadal function in male patients. Chemotherapy for ALL produced no impairment in either reproductive or gonadal function in females.[208]

General Psychosocial Principles for Management of Patients with Leukemia

The physician who assumes primary care for patients with leukemia learns that there are serious difficulties in responding to the emotional needs of the patient and family.

Certain suggestions may prove helpful. Open discussions with the patient and family are useful, but no one other than the patient should be the recipient of direct medical information. Basically, you, the physician, are called on to educate the patient about the natural history of the disease and its consequences.

After the patient knows and understands the prognosis, you should offer reassurance that you will remain the treating physician even if he or she decides to discontinue aggressive chemotherapy. Before the first induction, you know more about the process than the patient does. At the time of reinduction, however, the patient has had firsthand experience in living through the treatment.

It is good to let the patient know that control of pain is important to you and that you are willing to use potent drugs to render the patient free of pain. A corollary of this proposal is that you can tell the patient that you do have the means to control pain if he or she desires it but that the drugs may produce grogginess.

Even after hours of explanation and discussion with the patient and family, nurses or the patient's friends may tell you that the patient says you do not talk enough to him or her. There is no need to feel goaded. Dying patients and their families often cannot evaluate information, acknowledge receipt of information, or decide on the appropriateness of time expenditure. It is reasonable to assume that multiple exposure and reexplanation will be required. The patient and family should be asked to make written lists of their questions, which you should respond to as simply and directly as you can.

After taking a firm position on therapy, the patient may abruptly reverse that position. It is the patient's life, and it is the patient's right to make these changes, although he or she has had no previous experience with making such decisions.

You may hear from friends, relatives, psychiatrists, ministers, or nurses that the patient wants you to stop therapy and let death arrive. Often, this information does not accu-

Table 6 Protocol for Treatment of Acute Lymphoblastic Leukemia

Stage of Treatment	Conditions	Regimen*	Schedule
Induction (phase I) Initial therapy	All patients	D_1	Days 1–3
		V	Days 1, 8, 15, 22
		P	Days 1–28
		A	Days 17–28
Bone marrow biopsy	All patients	—	Day 21
Evaluate biopsy results	Residual leukemia seen on marrow biopsy	D_1	Days 23, 24
		V	Days 29, 36
		P	Days 29–42
Repeat bone marrow biopsy	Patients with residual leukemia in marrow biopsy on day 21		Day 43
Induction (phase II) Extended therapy	Patients in complete remission; phase II begins on day 29 if marrow biopsy on day 21 is clear or begins on day 43 if induction needs to be prolonged because of residual leukemia (phase II induction should be postponed until WBC > 3,000/mm^3)	Cyc	Days 1, 14, 28
		Cyt	Days 1–4, 8–11, 16–19, 22–25
		Mr_1	Days 1–28
		Mt_1	Days 1, 8, 15, 22
		L	Days 2–4, 9–11, 16–18, 23–25
Prophylactic cranial irradiation	Patients in complete remission who are not candidates for allogeneic bone marrow transplantation and who do not have CNS leukemia	I	Days 29+
Consolidation	Patients in complete remission who are not candidates for allogeneic bone marrow transplantation		
Treatment 1	Begins 4 wk after completion of phase II chemotherapy; it should be postponed until WBC > 3,000/mm^3 in patients with slow hematologic recovery	Cyt, Ten	Days 1–5
Treatment 2	Begins 4 wk after start of treatment 1 or when WBC > 3,000/mm^3 in patients with slow hematologic recovery	Same as treatment 1	Same as treatment 1
Treatment 3	Begins 4 wk after start of treatment 2 or when WBC > 3,000/mm^3 in patients with slow hematologic recovery. Patients who have received a cumulative dose of daunorubicin ≥ 300 mg/m^2 should undergo a resting and exercise multiple gated acquisition (MUGA) scan before start of treatment 3; those who have an ejection fraction < 45% or no increase after exercise should not receive the drug	Dex	Days 1–28
		V, D_2	Days 1, 8, 15, 22
		Cyc	Day 29
		Cyt	Days 31–34, 38–41
		T	Days 29–42
Treatment 4	Begins 2 months after start of treatment 3 or when WBC > 3,000/mm^3 in patients with slow hematologic recovery	Same as treatment 1	Same as treatment 1

Table 6   (continued)

Stage of Treatment	Conditions	Regimen*	Schedule
Treatment 5	Begins 28 days after start of treatment 4 or when WBC > 3,000/mm^3 in patients with slow hematologic recovery	Same as treatment 1	Same as treatment 1
Maintenance	Begins as soon as consolidation ends and is continued for 30 months from the date of complete remission; drug doses are adjusted to maintain the granulocyte level at 1,500–4,000/mm^3	Mr$_2$ Mt$_2$	Daily Weekly
Allogeneic bone marrow transplantation	Patients in first complete remission after phase II of induction who have an HLA-identical sibling are eligible; patients must have good to excellent performance status (Karnofsky score > 80), creatinine level < 2 mg/dl, and a bilirubin level < 2 mg/dl and must be HIV seronegative. Any sibling 60 years of age or younger who is histocompatible with the patient will be considered as a possible donor.	—	—

Note: patients should receive allopurinol, 300 mg p.o., q.d., for days 1 through 7 of induction. Vigorous intravenous fluid administration is recommended, such as five percent dextrose in half-normal saline at 150 ml/m^2/hr, as tolerated. If CNS leukemia is present, an Ommaya reservoir should be placed during phase I induction in patients who will not undergo marrow transplantation. Methotrexate, 12 mg intrathecally or intraventricularly, should be given twice weekly until blasts are not present in the spinal fluid. Leucovorin, 5 mg p.o., q.d., should be given for 3 consecutive days after each administration of methotrexate if WBC is < 3,000/mm^3. Cranial irradiation in a dose of 2,400 cGy (2,400 rads) should then be administered. Once the leukemia in the CNS is in remission, methotrexate, 12 mg intrathecally or intraventricularly, should be given once a week for 4 wk and then once a month for 1 yr.

During the consolidation phase, every effort should be made to initiate each course of treatment on time. If unavoidable delays occur between consolidation courses, maintenance therapy should be administered to all patients with WBC > 3,000/mm^3. Female patients of reproductive age with platelet counts <50,000/mm^3 should receive anovulatory therapy such as norethindrone acetate, 10 mg p.o., q.d. Complete blood cell counts should generally be obtained at least twice weekly and chemistry panels once weekly during consolidation cycles, and both should be obtained at least monthly during maintenance. Chest x-rays should be obtained at least every 6 months during consolidation and maintenance therapy.

Patients who are eligible for bone marrow transplantation should undergo the procedure as soon as possible after documentation of complete remission and, in all cases, should receive the transplant within 2 months after complete remission. Patients who have an HLA-identical sibling donor but who do not meet the criteria for transplantation or who refuse to undergo the procedure should receive consolidation and maintenance chemotherapy; however, they will still be considered in the transplant cohort for analysis. A signed informed consent form is required from recipients and donors who are approved by the institutional review board.

*Regimens are abbreviated as follows:

A—L-Asparaginase, 10,000 units I.V. or I.M. q.d.
Cyc—Cyclophosphamide, 650 mg/m^2 I.V. q.d.
Cyt—Cytarabine, 75 mg/m^2 I.V. over 1 hr q.d.
D$_1$—Daunorubicin, 60 mg/m^2 I.V. q.d.
D$_2$—Daunorubicin, 25 mg/m^2 I.V. q.d.
Dex—Dexamethasone, 10 mg/m^2 p.o., q.d.
I—Cranial irradiation, 1,800 cGy total, in 9 divided doses over 2 to 3 wk
L—Leucovorin, 5 mg p.o., q.d.

Mr$_1$—Mercaptopurine, 60 mg/m^2 p.o., q.d.
Mr$_2$—Mercaptopurine, 75 mg/m^2 p.o., q.d.
Mt$_1$—Methotrexate, 12 mg intrathecally
Mt$_2$—Methotrexate, 20 mg/m^2 p.o. or I.V. once weekly
P—Prednisone, 60 mg/m^2 p.o., q.d., in 3 divided doses over 2 wk
T—Thioguanine, 60 mg/m^2 p.o., q.d.
Ten—Teniposide, 60 mg/m^2 I.V. q.d.
V—Vincristine, 1.4 mg/m^2 I.V. (maximum dose, 2.0 mg)

rately reflect the patient's wishes. The patient may be floating these ideas as trial balloons. It is best to talk directly to the patient to see whether these wishes emerge explicitly.

Patients do not die on schedule. It is best not to assume or to let the family assume that because you and the patient have decided to stop aggressive chemotherapy, antibiotics, or transfusions the patient will accommodatingly die in a short time. Everyone must be prepared for the cantankerous ability of the body to survive despite withdrawal of support. It is wise to provide no schedules or dates for the patient or the family.

I have encountered a number of cases in which after all reasonable therapeutic options had failed, the patients did not accept the recommendation that therapy be withdrawn and that future efforts be focused on maintaining comfort and quality time with family and friends. In these cases, the patients pushed for more aggressive therapy even when it was pointed out that none was available and that there were no experimental trials that could be pursued. This situation is the converse of the widespread view that in such circumstances the physician often insists on pursuing more demanding therapy while the patient wishes to stop. It has been suggested that better counseling and rapport with the patient can avoid this situation, but in my experience, that is not always the case.

The patient has rights that must be acknowledged. Even if care is compromised, it is the patient's illness, and he or she does have the right to make certain decisions.

References

1. Cancer 30:1572, 1972
2. Nature 208:1281, 1965
3. N Engl J Med 309:257, 1983
4. Series Haematologica 7:2:192, 1974
5. N Engl J Med 315:828, 1986
6. Series Haematologica 7:2:211, 1974
7. Am J Med 52:160, 1972
8. Lancet 2:934, 1987
9. Annu Rev Med 24:75, 1973
10. N Engl J Med 307:1416, 1982
11. J Clin Oncol 4:821, 1986
12. J Clin Oncol 4:830, 1986
13. West J Med 143:825, 1985
14. Lancet 1:1159, 1988
15. Ann Intern Med 87:740, 1977
16. Br J Haematol 33:451, 1976
17. Ann Intern Med 103:460, 1985
18. Ann Intern Med 103:450, 1985
19. Blood 68:1, 1986
20. Lancet 2:1058, 1976
21. N Engl J Med 309:1593, 1983
22. N Engl J Med 313:529, 1985
23. N Engl J Med 313:776, 1985
24. N Engl J Med 313:534, 1985
25. N Engl J Med 315:509, 1986
26. Blood 73:1402, 1989
27. Am J Med 61:878, 1976
28. Br Med J 4:156, 1974
29. Cancer 50:250, 1982
30. Br Med J 4:216, 1974
31. Blood 62:941, 1983
32. Am J Clin Pathol 72:887, 1979
33. Blood Disorders 6:69, 1980
34. Cancer 49:1963, 1982
35. Cancer Treat Rep 68:145, 1984
36. Cancer 50:1449, 1982
37. Ann Intern Med 96:149, 1982
38. N Engl J Med 320:1655, 1989
39. Br Med J 285:1226, 1982
40. Am J Med 71:973, 1981
41. N Engl J Med 315:186, 1986
42. N Engl J Med 315:141, 1986
43. DM (October):52, 1970
44. Proc Soc Exp Biol Med 147:305, 1974
45. Blood 58:916, 1981
46. Br J Haematol 38:299, 1978
47. Johns Hopkins Med J 132:253, 1973
48. Br J Haematol 16:75, 1969
49. Cancer 63:1539, 1989
50. JAMA 178:1169, 1961
51. Medicine (Baltimore) 62:353, 1983
52. Clin Res 24:439A, 1976
53. Br J Haematol 69:295, 1988
54. Blood 72 (suppl):200a, 1988
55. Lancet 1:634, 1989
56. Am J Med 86:554, 1989
57. Lancet 1:497, 1985
58. Medicine (Baltimore) 50:357, 1971
59. N Engl J Med 304:1201, 1981
60. J Clin Invest 75:1080, 1985
61. West J Med 144:338, 1986
62. N Engl J Med 313:1429, 1985
63. Br J Haematol 60:395, 1985
64. Ann Intern Med 104:671, 1986
65. Lancet 2:666, 1986
66. N Engl J Med 319:990, 1988
67. Br J Haematol 60:457, 1985
68. Cancer 59:297, 1987
69. Br J Haematol 56:661, 1984
70. Br Med J 4:460, 1974
71. Semin Hematol 25:62, 1988
72. J Clin Oncol 3:192, 1985
73. J Clin Oncol 3:135, 1985
74. Cancer 54:333, 1984
75. N Engl J Med 314:1065, 1986
76. Br J Haematol 64:87, 1986
77. Blood 73:861, 1989
78. Ann Intern Med 108:806, 1988
79. Ann Intern Med 104:155, 1986
80. N Engl J Med 314:202, 1986
81. Semin Hematol 23(suppl 1):20, 1986
82. N Engl J Med 315:1433, 1986
83. Cancer 62:672, 1988
84. N Engl J Med 298:812, 1978
85. N Engl J Med 309:1118, 1983
86. Cancer 60:1708, 1987
87. Br J Haematol 62:659, 1986
88. Cancer 55:2395, 1985
89. Arch Intern Med 136:1375, 1976
90. Blood 44:1, 1974
91. Cancer 41:444, 1978
92. Clin Haematol 5:2:227, 1976
93. J Clin Oncol 6:1887, 1988
94. Ann Intern Med 107:748, 1987
95. Br J Haematol 68:487, 1988
96. Hosp Pract 24:93, 1989
97. Am J Med 72:963, 1982
98. Cancer 63:1055, 1989
99. J Clin Oncol 7:326, 1989
100. Br J Haematol 71:189, 1989
101. N Engl J Med 315:15, 1986
102. N Engl J Med 315:56, 1986
103. N Engl J Med 317:468, 1987
104. Cancer 53:411, 1984
105. J Clin Oncol 6:1532, 1988
106. Br J Haematol 72:859, 1989
107. Br J Haematol 72:57, 1989
108. Br J Haematol 72:1, 1989
109. Lancet 1:1119, 1989
110. Blood 54(suppl 1):130a, 1979
111. Br Med J 287:1093, 1983
112. Cancer 33:863, 1974

113. West J Med 121:1, 1974
114. N Engl J Med 291:75, 127, 1974
115. Cancer 56:632, 1985
116. Arch Intern Med 108:864, 1961
117. Medicine (Baltimore) 53:463, 1974
118. Br Med J 1:1169, 1978
119. Blood 60:279, 1982
120. Lancet 2:83, 1987
121. N Engl J Med 316:710, 1987
122. Blood 73:263, 1989
123. Blood 69:1551, 1987
124. Blood 72:1333, 1988
125. Br J Haematol 72:45, 1989
126. J Clin Oncol 6:1558, 1988
127. Blood 66(suppl 1):211a, 1985
128. Am J Med 80:789, 1986
129. Blood 66(suppl 1):209a, 1985
130. Cancer 43:1211, 1979
131. Cancer 51:1795, 1983
132. Br J Haematol 65:261, 1987
133. Blood 61:1035, 1983
134. Am J Clin Pathol 75:34, 1981
135. Br J Haematol 51:189, 1982
136. Br J Haematol 57:423, 1984
137. Br J Haematol 59:659, 1985
138. Cancer 56:553, 1985
139. Cancer 60:3029, 1987
140. Mayo Clin Proc 60:507, 1985
141. Blood 70:1705, 1987
142. Ann Intern Med 103:136, 1985
143. J Clin Oncol 4:325, 1986
144. Ann Intern Med 105:360, 1986
145. J Clin Oncol 4:1748, 1986
146. Am J Med 66:959, 1979
147. Br J Haematol 63:609, 1986
148. Ann Intern Med 103:58, 1985
149. Ann Intern Med 100:689, 1984
150. Br J Haematol 69:29, 1988
151. Br J Haematol 63:477, 1986
152. J Clin Oncol 4:589, 1986
153. Lancet 2:717, 1987
154. Blood 73:31, 1989
155. Ann Intern Med 110:976, 1989
156. Lancet 2:444, 1978
157. Ann Intern Med 103:101, 1985
158. Arch Intern Med 147:1614, 1987
159. Br Med J 4:23, 1973
160. Cancer 57:75, 1986
161. Clin Haematol 6:141, 1977
162. Ann Intern Med 110:236, 1989
163. Am J Hematol 31:26, 1989
164. Blood 46:219, 1975
165. Br J Haematol 48:365, 1981
166. Br J Haematol 51:1, 1982
167. Cancer 61:279, 1988
168. J Clin Oncol 5:398, 1987
169. Blood 73:366, 1989
170. N Engl J Med 319:902, 1988
171. Am J Med 61:892, 1976
172. Lancet 1:1346, 1986
173. Blood 72(suppl):191a, 1988
174. B. J Clin Oncol 7:433, 1989
175. Blood 74:19, 1989
176. Cancer 59:340, 1987
177. Br J Haematol 63:377, 1986
178. Clin Haematol 6:245, 1977
179. Am J Med 80:891, 1986
180. Arch Intern Med 147:660, 1987
181. Am J Hematol 30:261, 1989
182. Cancer 57:1678, 1986
183. Am J Med 80:1111, 1986
184. Am J Med 80:351, 1986
185. J Clin Oncol 7:156, 1989
186. J Clin Oncol 7:168, 1989
187. Ann Intern Med 109:789, 1988
188. J Clin Oncol 4:1094, 1986
189. Ann Intern Med 109:372, 1988
190. West J Med 150:557, 1989
191. J Clin Oncol 6:1088, 1988
192. Arch Intern Med 146:1201, 1986
193. Ann Intern Med 102:169, 1985
194. J Clin Invest 81:538, 1988
195. Am J Med 75:741, 1983
196. Lancet 1:249, 1989
197. Cancer 39:1011, 1977
198. Ann Intern Med 108:575, 1988
199. Blood 73:265, 1989
200. Blood 72:1784, 1988
201. Blood 71:123, 1988
202. Br J Haematol 71:371, 1989
203. J Clin Oncol 6:1014, 1988
204. Blood 69:1242, 1987
205. Lancet 1:786, 1987
206. Br J Haematol 69:35, 1988
207. N Engl J Med 317:461, 1987
208. J Clin Oncol 6:588, 1988

Acknowledgments

Tables 1 and 3   Data from "Morphologic, Immunologic and Cytogenetic (MIC) Working Classification of the Acute Myeloid Leukaemias," by the Second MIC Cooperative Study Group, in *British Journal of Haematology* 68:487, 1988. Used by permission.

Table 2   Data from "Classification of Acute Leukemia," by H. R. Gralnick, D.A.G. Galton, D. Catovsky, et al, in *Annals of Internal Medicine* 87:740, 1977. Used by permission.

Table 5 Data from "Proposals for the Classification of the Myelodysplastic Syndromes," by J. M. Bennett, D. Catovsky, M. T. Daniel, et al, in *British Journal of Haematology* 51:189, 1982. Used by permission.

16 Plasma Cell Myeloma and Related Serum Protein Disorders

STANLEY L. SCHRIER, M.D.

Multiple Myeloma

Plasma cell myeloma, also termed multiple myeloma or myelomatosis, is a malignant neoplasm characterized by the poorly controlled growth of a single clone of plasma cells, which are immunoglobulin-secreting cells derived from B lymphocytes. Malignant plasma cells appear to grow relatively slowly and have a doubling time of two to four months. It is likely that the event that causes malignant transformation occurs approximately four to six years before the myeloma cell line displaces normal plasma cell clones and the disease becomes clinically apparent.

Electron microscopic studies reveal that malignant plasma cells are megaloblastic, with mature cytoplasms and immature nuclei.[1] Such cells frequently have chromosomal abnormalities, but they are not characteristic.

The synthesis of light and heavy chains by the plasma cell is normally synchronized so that only complete immunoglobulin molecules are secreted. The laboratory and clinical abnormalities observed in patients with multiple myeloma or one of the other plasma cell disorders vary depending on the particular molecule being secreted by the malignant clone. If the malignant clone retains the capacity to produce complete immunoglobulin molecules, the classic M protein spike will be observed on serum electrophoresis. M proteins are monoclonal immunoglobulins consisting of a single light-chain type and a single heavy-chain class. Because the plasma cell clone is committed to producing a fixed antibody combining site but not a particular heavy-chain class, a single malignant clone can secrete two different M proteins, such as IgM and IgG. In fact, several cases of such so-called double myeloma have been reported.

It has been suggested that the M protein represents an antibody response to an unknown antigen, but this hypothesis has not been proved. Isolated reports have described M proteins that have antibody function against bacterial products, phosphorylcholine, serum protein, purine or pyrimidine nucleotides, or nitrophenyl haptens.

If the malignant clone produces κ or λ light chains in excess of heavy chains, these light chains appear as monomers or dimers predominantly in urine and in low concentrations in serum and are termed Bence Jones proteins. If the clone completely loses its capacity to make heavy chains, the multiple myeloma may be characterized by hypogammaglobulinemia with Bence Jones proteinemia and proteinuria. Panhypogammaglobulinemia develops when the malignant clone cannot synthesize either heavy or light chains.

Production of more heavy chains than light chains results in one of the heavy-chain diseases: γ, α, or μ. Primary amyloidosis, which is marked by the accumulation of amyloid protein deposits in various tissues, may be a variant of plasma cell myeloma [see Amyloidosis, *below*]. The amyloid deposits usually consist of portions of immunoglobulin light chains.

Pathophysiology

In multiple myeloma, the production of normal immunoglobulins is suppressed, as if the malignant plasma cells had replaced normal-functioning B cells. Precise measurements of B cell levels reveal a severe B cell deficiency, even among myeloma patients who have not been treated.[2] In some patients, the B cells are functionally abnormal and cannot undergo normal maturation.[3] Lymphocytes bearing the myeloma-specific surface immunoglobulin idiotypic marker have been identified in patients with myeloma[4,5]; in some patients, the circulating lymphocytes also express plasma cell antigens.[6] These observations indicate that the precursor lymphocytes of malignant plasma cells have serious abnormalities that partially account for the impaired humoral response in patients with multiple myeloma.

A number of metabolic characteristics of myeloma cells appear to correlate with disease severity. Flow cytometric measurements indicate that myeloma cells have more RNA than normal marrow cells. The lower the RNA content of the malignant cells, the more aggressive the myeloma. It appears that the myeloma cells with a lower RNA content are less well differentiated, grow more aggressively, and respond less well to chemotherapy. The DNA content of myeloma cells is another important factor; patients with hypodiploidy respond poorly to chemotherapy.[7] Myeloma cells in culture produce the lymphokines interleukin-1 (IL-1), tumor necrosis factor-α (TNF-α), interleukin-5 (IL-5), interleukin-6 (IL-6), and tumor necrosis factor-β (TNF-β, or lymphotoxin).[7-9] Receptors for IL-5 and IL-6 are also found on myeloma cells,[7] which suggests that IL-5 and IL-6 may control myeloma growth by autocrine and paracrine mechanisms. In one study, the serum level of IL-6 correlated with myeloma disease activity.[9] The kinetics of myeloma growth have also been evaluated by using tritiated thymidine to measure the labeling index of plasma cells. At the time of diagnosis, the labeling index is usually only about one percent, but this value can be considerably higher on relapse.[9,10]

Consequences of Tumor Infiltration

Because plasma cells reside in bone marrow, myeloma infiltration frequently replaces the normal marrow elements, causing peripheral pancytopenia. Replacement by myeloma is occasionally so extensive that plasmablasts appear in the peripheral blood, resulting in plasma cell leukemia. Such replacement, however, is not the only mechanism that produces pancytopenia in myeloma patients. A large study of bone marrow biopsies in myeloma patients revealed that hypoplasia of normal hematopoietic elements occurred relatively frequently in the absence of total marrow replacement by myeloma.[11]

Bone is eroded diffusely or in the form of tumors called plasmacytomas. The axial skeleton is frequently involved, and the destruction produces painful fractures and vertebral collapse. Osteopenia or lytic lesions without osteoblastic activity are typical in multiple myeloma, but osteoblastic lesions have rarely been reported. Because only osteoblastic lesions are associated with an elevated alkaline phosphatase level, it is not surprising that the serum alkaline phosphatase is usually normal. Bone resorption seems to be caused by cytokines, although it is not clear whether lymphotoxin, IL-1, TNF, or an unidentified cytokine plays the major role.[7,12,13] Bone destruction leads to the breakdown of collagen, a major component of the bone matrix, and releases compounds such as hydroxyproline. The measurement of urinary hydroxyproline excretion has been proposed as an assay for myelomatous bone destruction.[14]

Extension of a plasmacytoma into the spinal canal produces extradural compression and eventually even cord transection.

Extramedullary sites of infiltration with malignant plasma cells include the liver, spleen, subcutaneous tissues, gastrointestinal tract, and lymph nodes; myelomatous pleural effusions have also been observed.[15] Malignant plasma cells have a curious predilection for the nasopharynx and paranasal sinuses. Extramedullary plasmacytoma of the nasopharynx is characterized by slow local progression and a minimal tendency to disseminate as myelomatosis; it may constitute a variant of multiple myeloma.[16]

Bone destruction and resorption mobilize large amounts of calcium. Hypercalcemia, nausea, somnolence, and coma will occur when the kidney cannot excrete this calcium load. Hypercalcemia in myeloma patients is frequently complicated by a low serum albumin level, which leads to a higher concentration of unbound ionized calcium in the serum. Renal impairment (see below) reduces the ability of the kidney to clear the calcium load. Hypercalcemia itself causes renal impairment and, if left untreated, will lead to a vicious circle of rising calcium levels and increased renal damage.

Renal disease is common in multiple myeloma. In addition to hypercalcemia, causes of renal disease include the deposition of light chains in the tubules (myeloma kidney), plasma cell infiltration, amyloidosis, glomerulosclerosis, pyelonephritis, and hyperviscosity.[17] It is likely that light chains are toxic to the tubules. Some researchers believe that the characteristic tubular casts are a consequence and not the cause of myeloma kidney. The idea that the isoelectric point (pI) of the protein determines its nephrotoxicity is currently not supported.[18] β_2-Microglobulin (β_2M), the light chain of class I histocompatibility antigens present on the surface of nucleated cells, is released when such cells are broken down, and it is then excreted through the kidneys. Because serum levels of β_2M appear to correlate directly with levels of disease activity, an assay for this protein can help in assessing the extent of myeloma cell breakdown and renal functional impairment.[19,20]

Symptoms Referable to Abnormal Protein

Hyperviscosity IgG myeloma occasionally produces hyperviscosity (perhaps most often when IgG3 and IgG4 are the abnormal proteins[21]), but IgA myeloma and Waldenström's macroglobulinemia (an IgM disorder) do so more regularly [*see* Other Variants of Plasma Cell Malignancy, Waldenström's Macroglobulinemia, *below*]. Viscosity is related to the concentration of the abnormal protein (termed a paraprotein), to the paraprotein's specific characteristics, such as molecular asymmetry, and to its ability to form aggregates or polymers.[21] Some IgA and IgM myeloma proteins cause enhanced viscosity because they can interact with red blood cells, causing extensive aggregation of erythrocytes and leading to widespread circulatory disturbances.[22]

In some patients, the abnormal protein precipitates during exposure to cold, a condition termed monoclonal cryoglobulinemia; such patients experience vascular obstruction in acral structures.

Occasionally, paraprotein crystals cause tissue dysfunction. Crystals of light chains have been observed in the corneas of patients with myeloma,[23] and such crystal deposition has occasionally been associated with obstructive vasculitis.[24]

Myeloma protein interactions Perhaps the most important myeloma protein interaction is the strong association of protein abnormality in the urine with renal disease. About 70 percent of patients with myelomatous proteinuria have renal disease characterized by casts in the tubules and atrophy of the renal tubular cells, perhaps caused by a toxic reaction to the abnormal light chains.[17] Occasionally, myeloma is associated with renal tubular acidosis. Because the radiopaque dyes used in intravenous pyelography may cause the myeloma protein to precipitate, dehydration should be avoided if this procedure is required. I have seen two patients with myeloma rendered permanently anephric after intravenous pyelography; the physician was evaluating deteriorating renal function and had not considered myeloma in the differential diagnosis.

Inactivation of plasma procoagulants (factors I, II, VIII, and XI) by the myeloma protein may lead to bleeding disorders. The protein may also prolong the bleeding time by interfering with platelet function. Coating of red blood cells by the protein produces rouleaux, autoagglutination, and, occasionally, hemolysis. Accumulation of the myeloma protein may lead to an expansion of the plasma water with pseudohyponatremia. Cationic M proteins cause a decrease in the anion gap.

Some myeloma M proteins impair granulocytic migration, which can be measured by the skin-window assay and by the timed appearance of a cellular exudate. Denatured

Table 1   Initial Workup of Multiple Myeloma

Hematologic studies	Complete blood count
	Platelet count
	Reticulocyte count
	Bleeding time
	Partial thromboplastin time
	Prothrombin time
	Direct Coombs' test
Blood chemistry studies	Blood urea nitrogen
	Creatine clearance
	Serum calcium
	Serum uric acid
	Serum protein electrophoresis
	Quantitative immunoglobulins
	Lactic dehydrogenase
	β_2-Microglobulin
	Serum viscosity
	Immunoelectrophoresis
Urine studies	Quantitative 24-hr protein
	Urine protein electrophoresis
	Urine immunoelectrophoresis (if indicated)
Radiologic and imaging studies	Metastatic survey, including skull and chest x-rays and x-rays of the long bones
	Computed tomography
	Magnetic resonance imaging of spine (if indicated)

light chains deposited in endothelium, smooth muscle, skin, and salivary glands produce a clinical picture of primary amyloidosis. Rarely, myeloma proteins bind calcium, which may contribute to the development of hypercalcemia.

Peripheral neuropathy occurs in less than one percent of myeloma cases[25] and may be associated with elevated CSF protein levels. Biopsy samples of affected nerves may show segmentary demyelination, perhaps caused by the M protein.[26]

Other Consequences of Plasma Cell Malignancy

In active multiple myeloma, the peripheral blood B cell population is decreased. Because of this deficiency of normal circulating B cells, insufficient quantities of antibody may be produced in response to antigenic stimulation, and polyclonal serum levels of IgG, IgA, and IgM may be decreased. Other abnormalities in patients with multiple myeloma include neutropenia caused by myeloma invasion of marrow or by chemotherapy, poor antibody response to antigenic challenge, increased immunoglobulin turnover, cellular anergy, impaired migration of neutrophils to wound sites, and decreased opsonic activity.[27] Because of their impaired immune responses, myeloma patients have an increased susceptibility to infection. The serum albumin level is frequently reduced, but the nephrotic syndrome with associated albuminuria rarely occurs in patients with multiple myeloma in the absence of concurrent amyloidosis.

Diagnosis

The diagnosis of multiple myeloma is frequently suggested by a report of elevated serum protein levels on a chemistry screening panel. The patient's presenting complaints may arise from bone destruction associated with pathologic fractures, pancytopenia, azotemia, or hypercalcemia, or they may reflect the characteristics of the paraprotein being secreted (see above). Hypercalcemia is suggested by nausea, vomiting, somnolence, azotemia, thirst, or polyuria [*see Chapter 37*].

Accurate diagnosis of myeloma is based on a combination of morphologic findings, radiologic studies, and protein and other chemical measurements [*see Table 1*]. One group has outlined useful criteria for the diagnosis of myeloma [*see Table 2*]. When analyzing the results of protein and other chemical measurements, it is important to bear in mind the existence of rare forms of myeloma in which the malignant plasma cells do not secrete abnormal proteins.[28] An M protein cannot be detected by serum protein electrophoresis in about 25 percent of

Table 2 Criteria for Diagnosis of Multiple Myeloma

Major Criteria

1. Plasmacytomas on tissue biopsy

2. Bone marrow plasmacytosis (> 30% plasma cells)

3. Monoclonal immunoglobulin spike on serum electrophoresis—IgG>3.5 g/dl or IgA > 2.0 g/dl; κ or λ light-chain excretion > 1.0 g/day on 24-hr urine protein electrophoresis

Minor Criteria

a. Bone marrow plasmacytosis (10%–30% plasma cells)

b. Monoclonal immunoglobulin spike present but of lesser magnitude than given above

c. Lytic bone lesions

d. Normal IgM < 50 mg/dl, IgA < 100 mg/dl, or IgG < 600 mg/dl

Any of the following sets of criteria will confirm the diagnosis

Any two major criteria

Major criterion 1 plus minor criterion b, c, or d

Major criterion 2 plus minor criterion b, c, or d

Major criterion 3 plus minor criterion a or c

Minor criteria a, b, and c or a, b, and d

ditions other than myeloma, such as benign monoclonal gammopathy [*see* Benign Monoclonal Gammopathy, *below*]. The information used to diagnose myeloma has also been used to construct a staging system, allowing for better initial assessment of the patient and more accurate comparison of study groups [*see Table 3*].[30,31]

Two prognostic indicators in myeloma are serum levels of β_2-microglobulin (β_2M) and lactic dehydrogenase (LDH).[7,32,33] An elevated β_2M level indicates a large malignant cell mass, renal impairment, or both. A very high LDH level predicts an aggressive, lymphomalike course.

The diagnosis of hyperviscosity syndrome is indicated by a clinical picture of visual disturbances, somnolence, headache, irritability, and mucosal bleeding; retinopathy with hemorrhages, exudates, edema, and engorged (sausage-shaped) retinal veins may also be present, as well as an expanded blood volume and possibly congestive heart failure. Serum viscosity measurements are usually three to five times the normal value. Rarely, when the M protein can form a cryoprecipitate, Raynaud's syndrome, peripheral gangrene, and even vasculitis may be present.[21]

Unexplained high-output cardiac failure has also been observed in patients with multiple myeloma.[34]

Management

Bed rest should be avoided because it leads to increased mobilization of calcium and predisposes to the development of hypostatic pneumonia and urinary tract infection, which are major causes of death among immunocompromised multiple myeloma patients.[35] A graded exercise program should be instituted to increase muscle tone and reduce osteoporosis, and efforts should be made to avoid hospitalization. Therapy for specific types of multiple myeloma and for various complications of this disorder are discussed in detail below.

Solitary Plasmacytoma

A bone plasmacytoma is frequently discovered in a clinically treacherous location,

patients at presentation. However, most of these patients have an excessive amount of light-chain protein in their urine, which can be detected by urine protein electrophoresis or immunoelectrophoresis. When multiple myeloma is suspected, a normal serum protein electrophoresis profile does not exclude the diagnosis.

Alternative diagnostic criteria have been proposed. One authority has suggested that the criteria be the presence of at least 10 percent abnormal, immature plasma cells in the marrow, or biopsy evidence of plasmacytoma, and one of the following findings: M protein concentration greater than 3 g/dl, M protein in the urine, or osteolytic lesions.[29] An M protein spike may also occur in con-

Table 3   Clinical Myeloma Staging System

Stage I	Low myeloma cell mass ($< 0.6 \times 10^{12}$ cells/m^2)
	 All of the following criteria
	     Hb > 10 g/dl
	     Serum calcium (corrected) ≤ 12 mg/dl*
	     X-rays reveal normal bone structure or a solitary lesion
	     M component production values
	         IgG < 5 g/dl
	         IgA < 3 g/dl
	         Urine light-chain excretion < 4 g/24 hr

Stage II	Intermediate myeloma cell mass ($0.6–1.2 \times 10^{12}$ cells/m^2) Criteria fit neither stage I nor stage III

Stage III	High myeloma cell mass ($> 1.2 \times 10^{12}$ cells/m^2)
	 Any of the following criteria
	     Hb < 8.5 g/dl
	     Serum calcium (corrected) > 12 mg/dl*
	     Advanced lytic bone lesions
	     M component production values
	         IgG > 7 g/dl
	         IgA > 5 g/dl
	         Urine light-chain excretion > 12 g/24 hr

Note: staging system proposed by Durie and Salmon (see reference 23).

Stages are subclassified as A or B according to renal function: A = creatinine < 2 mg/dl or BUN < 30 mg/dl; B = creatine > 2 mg/dl or BUN > 30 mg/dl.

*Corrected calcium = calcium (mg/dl) - albumin (g/dl) + 4.0.

such as the paravertebral area, inside the vertebrae, in the chest wall, or in the hip. Indications that the plasmacytoma is a solitary lesion are the absence of an M paraprotein in the serum or urine and the absence of a plasma cell infiltrate on several marrow biopsy specimens taken from remote sites. Even a solitary plasmacytoma can produce an M protein, but in such cases, local radiation therapy causes the M protein to disappear. Some researchers believe that solitary plasmacytoma of bone is a variant of multiple myeloma with an initially indolent course.[36] Other researchers believe, however, that some cases of solitary plasmacytoma will not progress to multiple myeloma and that, with careful staging, approximately 50 percent of such patients with solitary plasmacytoma can be cured by radiation.[7] For a solitary extramedullary plasmacytoma of the upper respiratory and upper digestive tracts, local radiotherapy is the treatment of choice and may be curative.[37,38]

Myelomatosis

Radiography is still the method of choice for evaluating the extent and site of bony lesions in myeloma, especially if cost is a factor. However, computed tomography is superior for detailing vertebral involvement,[39] and magnetic resonance imaging (MRI), although costly, provides an excellent view of the vertebrae and spinal cord, dramatically revealing areas of potential cord compression.[40] The availability of CT scans and MRI has decreased the use of myelography. Radioisotopic bone scans are not sensitive in detecting myeloma, perhaps because there is very little osteoblastic reaction surrounding the destructive lesions.

Localized radiotherapy should be employed for lytic lesions that threaten the spinal cord or axial skeleton. For the management of cord compression, localized radiotherapy alone appears to be as effective as the combination of laminectomy and radiotherapy [*see Chapter 37*].[41] Decompression laminectomy is performed as an emergency procedure if the signs and symptoms of cord compression progress despite the use of radiotherapy or chemotherapy.

Clinically active myeloma usually requires systemic therapy. A simple, effective regimen that can be safely followed on an outpatient basis is one that combines the alkylating cytotoxic agent melphalan with prednisone. Melphalan, 0.25 mg/kg/day, and prednisone, 2.0 mg/kg/day, are administered orally together in three or four divided doses for four days; this four-day pulse of therapy is then repeated every four to six weeks. Prednisone decreases the synthesis and hence the urine level of the Bence Jones protein.[42] Side effects of the large prednisone dose include unpleasant mental symptoms; in addition, the patient may experience symptoms suggestive of mild adrenal insufficiency, such as mild arthralgias, the day after the drug is withdrawn. Because the white blood cell and platelet counts usually decline within 10 to 14 days after the first dose of melphalan, both of these values should be monitored carefully. The dangers of infection and bleeding must be explained to the patient.

Response begins between the first and third pulse of therapy in approximately 40 to 50 percent of patients. In several recent clinical trials, therapeutic response or remission has been defined as a 75 percent or greater reduction in the level of M protein in the serum or the disappearance of Bence Jones protein from the urine.[43,44] However, two studies have challenged the use of the serum M protein level as a marker for therapeutic efficacy or disease progression.[45,46] It appears that a decrease in the serum level of M protein does not correlate with improvement in survival. Therefore, when one is reviewing the literature, it is probably necessary to rely on traditional survival data.

Other indicators of a therapeutic response include a reduction in bone pain; an increased ability to ambulate; cessation of bone destruction; a decline in the serum levels of urea nitrogen, creatinine, and calcium; and an increase in the serum albumin level and the hemoglobin concentration.

The melphalan-prednisone regimen rarely produces healing of lytic bone lesions. The white blood cell count usually falls to about 2,500/mm³, and the platelet count generally stays in the range of 50,000 to 200,000/mm³. Increases or decreases in dosage may be necessary, depending on clinical response and blood counts. Signs and symptoms of hyperadrenocorticism or hypoadrenocorticism are not prominent.

Patients who have severe pancytopenia and a packed myelomatous marrow require prompt therapy, but the therapy must be carefully monitored because it may intensify and further prolong the pancytopenia and lead to death. A reasonable approach in such cases is to start with full doses of prednisone and one fourth the full dose of melphalan (0.06 mg/kg/day for four days). From day 9 to day 14, the patient should be hospitalized or closely followed at office or clinic visits. If the patient tolerates this pulse of therapy, one half the normal dose of melphalan can be given with the next pulse after a rest of four to six weeks, three fourths of a dose can be given with the third pulse, and finally a full dose can be given with the fourth pulse if prohibitive pancytopenia does not occur.

Several studies have suggested that the use of more aggressive, complex, and expensive chemotherapeutic programs may be justified because they can achieve an increased frequency of response and longer survival than can the standard melphalan-prednisone regimen. An Eastern Cooperative Oncology Group study investigated the M-2 protocol [*see Table 4*] and concluded that this program produced more responses than the standard regimen but did not prolong survival.[47] The Cancer and Acute Leukemia Group B reported that a triple alkylator program similar to the M-2 regi-

Table 4　Some Combination Chemotherapy Regimens Used for Multiple Myeloma

Regimen Eponym	Drugs	Dosage and Schedule	Usual Treatment Schedule
M-2	Vincristine	1.2 mg/m^2 I.V. on day 1	Cycle is repeated at 35-day intervals
	Carmustine (BCNU)	20 mg/m^2 I.V. on day 1	
	Cyclophosphamide	400 mg/m^2 I.V. on day 1	
	Melphalan	8.0 mg/m^2 p.o. on days 1–4	
	Prednisone	40 mg/m^2 p.o. on days 1–7 and 20 mg/m^2 on days 8–14 for cycles 1–3 only	
VMCP	Vincristine	1.0 mg/m^2 I.V. on day 1 (1.5 mg maximum)	Alternating cycles of VMCP and VBAP are given at three-week intervals
	Melphalan	6.0 mg/m^2 p.o. on days 1–4	
	Cyclophosphamide	125 mg/m^2 p.o. on days 1–4	
	Prednisone	60 mg/m^2 p.o. on days 1–4	
VBAP	Vincristine	1.0 mg/m^2 I.V. on day 1 (1.5 mg maximum)	
	Carmustine	30 mg/m^2 I.V. on day 1	
	Doxorubicin (Adriamycin)	30 mg/m^2 I.V. on day 1	
	Prednisone	60 mg/m^2 p.o. on days 1–4	
VAD	Vincristine	0.4 mg/day by continuous I.V. infusion on days 1–4	Cycles are repeated at 21-day intervals depending on the extent of myelosuppression
	Doxorubicin	9.0 mg/m^2/day by continuous I.V. infusion on days 1–4	
	Dexamethasone	40 mg p.o., q.d. on days 1–4, 9–12, and 17–20	

men improved survival for stage III patients [see Table 3] relative to the melphalan-prednisone regimen,[48] but these results were not confirmed by a Canadian study.[49] A Southwest Oncology Group study indicated that the use of alternating cycles of combination chemotherapy, including vincristine, doxorubicin, melphalan, cyclophosphamide, carmustine (BCNU), and prednisone, produced more responses and a longer survival than conventional chemotherapy with melphalan and prednisone.[43] A more recent study by this group found that alternating cycles of VMCP (vincristine, melphalan, cyclophosphamide, and prednisone) and VBAP (vincristine, carmustine [BiCNV], doxorubicin [Adriamycin], and prednisone)

given at three-week intervals prolonged survival relative to the standard melphalan-prednisone regimen,[43,50] but another study failed to confirm the superiority of the VMCP-VBAP regimen.[44] One review of therapeutic programs indicated that none of the more aggressive programs lead to substantial improvement in course and survival when compared with the standard melphalan-prednisone regimen.[7]

Pending a more definitive resolution of this therapeutic problem, I prefer to start treatment with the simpler, less expensive melphalan-prednisone program and switch to the more aggressive, complex programs if the patient does not respond or becomes refractory to therapy (see below).[51] The incorporation of fluoride, calcium, vitamin D, or androgenic steroids into a chemotherapy regimen does not promote the healing of bony lesions,[52] nor does the use of the immunopotentiating agent levamisole.[50] There are several innovative programs, however, that appear to improve response rate and prolong survival. One program utilizes two modifications of the M-2 protocol. The length of the first cycle is still 35 days; subsequent cycles alternate between 21 and 22 days, and interferon-alfa (5 million U/m^2 subcutaneously three times weekly) is added to the 22-day cycle.[53] The complete response rate to this regimen is higher than is generally seen, but the actual survival rate is not yet known. The addition of interferon-alfa causes severe granulocytopenia and thrombocytopenia. A second program involves allogeneic bone marrow transplantation; however, most patients with multiple myeloma are older than 50 years and have poor tolerance for graft versus host disease. A third program combines high-dose melphalan and total body irradiation with rescue using autologous bone marrow transplantation[7] or peripheral blood stem cells (blood stem cells may have fewer myeloma clonal stem cells than does bone marrow).[7,54,55] Preliminary results of this approach are encouraging.[54,55] Another approach employs interferon alfa-2b in maintenance treatment of patients who have responded to conventional induction chemotherapy. A randomized study of 101 patients who had responded to induction therapy has shown that maintenance therapy with recombinant interferon alfa-2b (3 megaunits/m^2 administered subcutaneously three times a week) prolongs response and survival.[56]

Occasionally, the diagnosis of multiple myeloma is made in a patient whose disease seems to be quiescent. Such a patient can be identified readily because the M protein spike is relatively low, the bone marrow is not heavily infiltrated with plasma cells (usually less than 15 percent), few if any lytic bone lesions are present, and the serum creatinine and hemoglobin values are usually normal.[51]

Criteria for this indolent variant, which is also called smoldering multiple myeloma, include a serum M protein level of 2 to 3 g/dl and approximately 10 percent atypical plasma cells in the bone marrow.[29] A low plasma cell labeling index provides unambiguous identification of patients with indolent disease, but such measurements can only be performed by a research laboratory.[10] Although it might appear that therapy should be successful in such cases because the malignant cell burden is low, current therapies can achieve only a 1 to 2 log (90 to 99 percent) kill of malignant plasma cells. Because chemotherapy carries a significant risk, it probably should not be employed in patients with indolent myeloma. Such patients should be followed and treated only when there is evidence of disease progression.[29,57]

Hyperviscosity

The modalities chosen to treat hyperviscosity depend on clinical urgency. If the hyperviscosity appears to be life threatening, plasmapheresis should be started promptly. Plasmapheresis is generally effective in controlling hyperviscosity when the myeloma protein is IgM because IgM is predominantly intravascular. For the same reason, aggregated or polymerized IgA or IgG3 may be effectively removed by plasmapheresis.[21]

Hypercalcemia

Usually, hypercalcemia is caused by the release of calcium from eroded bone. However, although many patients with myeloma have destructive bony lesions, only 20 percent have hypercalcemia. Hypercalcemia is commonly associated with impaired glomerular filtration, and hence, its management requires correction of renal functional abnormalities. Hypercalcemia should always be treated promptly, using the following measures in sequence as required:

1. Administration of 3 to 4 L of saline I.V. together with 20 to 40 mg of furosemide I.V.; administration of adequate intravenous flu-

ids, the most important step, is frequently sufficient to control hypercalcemia.[58]

2. Addition of 60 mg of prednisone daily (if it is not already being administered as part of a melphalan-prednisone pulse).

3. A single intravenous injection of 15 to 25 mg/kg of plicamycin (formerly termed mithramycin).

4. Subcutaneous or I.M. injection of calcitonin (4 IU/kg); the dose may have to be repeated in 12 hours.

Studies in Europe showed that several diphosphonate compounds can reduce the serum calcium level in patients with multiple myeloma.[59,60] However, these agents are not available in the United States. The related drug etidronate disodium, which is available, is ineffective.[61]

Central Nervous System Complications

In addition to cord compression, CNS complications include an unusual peripheral neuropathy associated with axonal degeneration and demyelination.[25,26] It develops in the rare, osteosclerotic form of myeloma, which occasionally is accompanied by erythremia. This unusual variant of myeloma (osteosclerosis, erythremia, and neuropathy) does not respond to the conventional therapies. One patient with peripheral neuropathy had an IgM κ monoclonal protein that was active against peripheral nerve myelin.[62] Plasmapheresis combined with chlorambucil therapy appeared to produce a beneficial effect in this case. I have attempted apheresis in several patients with multiple myeloma and peripheral neuropathy, without clinical benefit. This presentation remains a frustrating problem.

Renal Complications

Patients who present with myeloma kidney and renal failure (serum creatinine level greater than 10 mg/dl) may require lifelong hemodialysis. Systemic chemotherapy should still be administered, however, because it has occasionally produced substantial improvement in renal function in such cases.[63] It has been recommended that patients with myeloma and severe acute renal failure undergo dialysis until their response to chemotherapy can be evaluated. Improvement may occur in as many as 50 percent of cases, with 20 percent returning to normal creatinine values.[64] Long-term dialysis should probably be restricted to patients who show a good response to chemotherapy.[65]

Infections

Because patients with myeloma have functional hypogammaglobulinemia, injections of γ-globulin, including the newer preparations of intravenous immunoglobulin, have been used to prevent or treat bacterial infections. There are no controlled studies, however, establishing the effectiveness of immunoglobulin in these circumstances. Pneumococcal vaccine can be administered for prophylaxis against severe pneumococcal sepsis, but the antibody responses of patients with myeloma to this vaccine are impaired.

Problems Arising during Therapy

About 50 percent of patients benefit from melphalan-prednisone therapy. The remainder do not improve and generally undergo a rapidly progressive decline. A small number of patients who do not respond to melphalan-prednisone improve when switched to a more aggressive program such as M-2 or alternating cycles of VMCP and VBAP. Such patients may also respond to a program termed VAD, which employs vincristine, doxorubicin, and dexamethasone [*see Table 4*][66]; this program requires hospitalization. In addition to the risk of infection, complications of VAD include gastric disturbances, presumably caused by the dexamethasone component. Dexamethasone appears to be the critical ingredient that accounts for the improvement in previously unresponsive patients.[67] Because this agent is also highly toxic, a modified VAD regimen has been proposed in which the second and third dexamethasone pulses are dropped in every second course of therapy.

Several groups have reported good response rates using the VAD program in such refractory patients,[68,69] which suggests that VAD should be used as first-line therapy. However, in one study, VAD did not improve survival rates.[7]

After an initial response to pulse melphalan and prednisone therapy, patients may reach the so-called reverse gompertzian plateau, a state in which all measurable parameters have fallen to stable levels and do not improve with continued therapy; this plateau phase appears to be cytokinetically quiet.[70] Cessation of therapy at this point may be advisable because it avoids the hazards of continued drug administration and prevents the emergence of drug resistance without harming the patient. It is my practice to stop therapy when the patient has been stable for six to 12 months and to continue to monitor all parameters; therapy is resumed only when signs of disease progression appear.[51]

After several years of good response to melphalan-prednisone pulses, patients tend to follow one of three clinical courses. In one course, some patients no longer respond to the same, higher, or more closely spaced doses of melphalan-prednisone, and the pace of their disease increases. In such cases, the VAD program or alternating cycles of VMCP and VBAP could be used, depending on the extent of myelosuppression. The response to a variety of programs, including those containing glucocorticoids, is usually poor[71]; therefore, chemotherapy should be limited to prevent the development of significant myelosuppression and pancytopenia.[72]

Other patients undergo clinical deterioration even though their serum and urine levels of M protein continue to decline. In such patients, skin nodules, ascites with infiltration of the peritoneal wall, and other unusual myeloma infiltrates may appear, and pancytopenia recurs or becomes worse. Repeat marrow biopsy usually shows extreme anaplasia of the myeloma cells. This condition, which has been termed a reticulosarcomatous change, may represent a form of tumor dedifferentiation. The cell morphology may be bizarre. Response to therapy at this point in the disease is poor.

In the third group of patients, who have responded well to melphalan and prednisone for three to four years, progressive pancytopenia develops while the patients are receiving constant or even reduced doses of melphalan. Abnormal red blood cell shapes are sometimes seen on the blood smear. Bizarre megaloblastoid erythroid precursors and maturational abnormalities of the myeloid and megakaryocytic precursors are apparent on bone marrow aspiration and biopsy, which may also show residual multiple myeloma. An iron stain may show ringed sideroblasts, which are the erythroblastic or sideroblastic precursors of acute myeloid leukemia. The incidence of leukemic transformation in treated multiple myeloma is approximately 15 to 20 percent.[49] Treatment-associated myelodysplastic syndrome [*see Chapter 15*] and acute myeloblastic leukemia are difficult to treat.

Prognosis

Patients with multiple myeloma who respond to therapy can expect a median survival of approximately 40 months, much of it in good health and pain free. About two percent of patients survive for 10 years or longer after diagnosis.[73]

Other Variants of Plasma Cell Malignancy

Waldenström's Macroglobulinemia

Waldenström's macroglobulinemia is characterized by the proliferation of a malignant plasma cell clone that secretes IgM, and thus, hyperviscosity is relatively common in this condition. The marrow is infiltrated with malignant plasmacytoid lymphocytes, and the liver, spleen, and lungs are frequently involved.[21,74]

Therapy consists of aggressive plasmapheresis to remove the abnormal protein and the administration of chlorambucil. This drug is given in a dosage of 4 mg/day orally, and the dosage is titered to produce a reduction in IgM levels and in liver and spleen size without causing pancytopenia. Some patients who do not respond to chlorambucil or to melphalan-prednisone do respond to CVP (cyclophosphamide, vincristine, and prednisone) therapy administered according to the following schedule: cyclophosphamide, 200 to 300 mg/m^2/day orally on days 1 through 5; vincristine, 1.5 mg/m^2 intravenously on day 1 (maximum dose of 2 mg); and prednisone, 100 mg/m^2/day orally on days 1 through 5; the cycle is repeated every 21 to 28 days.

Red blood cell transfusions pose a real danger because they may accentuate the viscosity by increasing the hematocrit. If transfusions are required, they should be preceded by aggressive plasmapheresis to reduce the amount of abnormal protein.

Heavy-Chain Diseases

In γ heavy-chain disease, the paraprotein usually consists of a dimer of the Fc fragment of IgG and a portion of the N-terminal end of the heavy-chain sequence. Although the paraprotein appears in the serum, it is found mainly in the urine. Because patients with heavy-chain diseases do not produce excess light chains, the test for Bence Jones proteins is negative. The use of urine protein electrophoresis or immunoelectrophoresis of concentrated urine specimens to detect the γ heavy-chain fragments may be necessary to make the diagnosis. Clinical features include fever, lymphadenopathy, infections caused by hypogammaglobulinemia, and autoimmune hemolytic anemia, all in the context of a variety of lymphoproliferative disorders. Combination chemotherapy with CVP has been used.[75]

α Heavy-chain disease involves the production of polymers of the heavy chain–containing fragments of secretory IgA. This condition has been termed Mediterranean lymphoma because it often occurs in the southeastern portion of that region. The sites that are clinically involved are the areas where secretory IgA is normally localized, predominantly the gastrointestinal tract and, to a lesser extent, the respiratory tract. The intestinal lamina propria is infiltrated with plasmacytoid lymphocytes, and immunoelectrophoresis reveals a monoclonal

α heavy chain that is not associated with κ or λ light chains. Patients have diarrhea, malabsorption, and abdominal pain. Therapy with the melphalan-prednisone regimen may be beneficial in such cases.[75] Some patients may respond to treatment with antibiotics (e.g., tetracycline). The role of aggressive chemotherapy is being tested.[76]

μ Heavy-chain disease involves the overproduction of the heavy chain of IgM. Clinically, most patients appear to have chronic lymphocytic leukemia.

Amyloidosis

The term amyloidosis encompasses several disorders that are characterized by the accumulation of insoluble fibrillar proteins (i.e., amyloid) in various tissues. At least five different forms of amyloidosis have been distinguished: primary, secondary, hereditary systemic, local, and senile amyloidosis. The distinct pathophysiology of each form of amyloidosis is determined by the secondary structure of the amyloid proteins. In all forms of amyloidosis, the amyloid proteins display a β-pleated sheet conformation. This arrangement leads to the formation of linear, nonbranching twisted fibers of 7.5 to 10.0 nm in diameter. The β-pleated sheet conformation accounts for the characteristic features of amyloid deposits: insolubility in physiologic salt solutions and resistance to proteolysis and phagocytosis. The amyloid fibers stain with Congo red and show green birefringence under a polarizing microscope.[77,78] Because several different proteins can be modified to produce this unusual conformation, it has been proposed that the various forms of amyloidosis should instead be termed the β-fibrilloses.[77]

Composition of Amyloid Deposits

The amyloid deposits in each form of amyloidosis are composed of a characteristic major fibrillar protein. The clinical manifestations of the various disorders are closely correlated with the type of protein that makes up the major portion of the amyloid fibril. In addition, a P component, which is an α_1-glycoprotein with a pentagonal structure, constitutes five to 10 percent of the amyloid deposits in all forms of amyloidosis.[77,78] The amyloid P component appears in the serum and may also be a constituent of normal vascular and glomerular basement membranes.[79] Its structure is related to that of the acute-phase reactant C-reactive protein. The P component shows a considerable affinity for polyanions, such as heparin, and divalent cations, such as calcium; its binding at various sites may be calcium dependent.

Primary Amyloidosis

In primary amyloidosis, the amyloid protein fibrils consist of immunoglobulin light-chain fragments that include the variable region and part of the constant region. The molecular weight of intact light chains is 25,000, whereas that of the fragments ranges from 5,000 to 25,000. Such fibrils are also found in the forms of amyloidosis associated with multiple myeloma (10 percent of myeloma patients), with some cases of Waldenström's macroglobulinemia, and with related disorders. The proteins, called AL (amyloid light chains), are similar in structure and composition to Bence Jones proteins and are produced by a clone of malignant plasma cells. Presumably, the fragments result from partial degradation of light chains by macrophages. The ratio of κ to λ light chains for normal immunoglobulins is 2:1, but λ proteins are twice as frequent as κ proteins in AL amyloidosis. A special λ subclass termed λ_{VI} is quite frequently seen in AL proteins. This finding suggests that intact λ_{VI} light chains and fragments of the variable regions of these chains have a special propensity to form the intercellular amyloid fibrils.[80]

Deposits in the AL form of acquired systemic amyloidosis accumulate in the tongue, skeletal muscle, heart, skin, gastrointestinal tract, peripheral nerves, liver, spleen, and kidneys. Clinical abnormalities develop because the deposits replace or compress normal tissue and interfere with organ function.[81] Macroglossia caused by amyloid deposits in the tongue causes problems in swallowing and speaking. Cardiac involvement can lead to conduction disturbances and can occasionally produce manifestations resembling those of constrictive pericarditis. Because the patterns of amyloid infiltration do not adequately explain the conduction disturbances, other factors also appear to be involved.[82] Patients with cardiac amyloidosis are very sensitive to digitalis, which can apparently produce sudden death secondary to arrhythmias.[77,78] If digitalis is needed, it should be administered cautiously and the patient monitored closely.

Renal involvement with amyloid results in the nephrotic syndrome. Infiltration into blood vessel walls in the skin leads to the development of ecchymoses,[83] which, curiously, occur in the distribution of the superior vena cava more often than elsewhere. Salivary gland involvement with extension into the adjacent strap muscles produces airway obstruction and mimics angioneurotic edema. Amyloid deposition in periarticular and synovial tissues causes joint pain and limitation of motion. Sensory and motor disturbances may be caused by involvement of peripheral nerves, which are occasionally enlarged and even palpable. Autonomic nerve infiltration is responsible for impotence, gastrointestinal motility disturbances, and postural hypotension. Carpal tunnel syndrome may occur as a result of median nerve compression. Functional hyposplenism marked by the presence of Howell-Jolly bodies in red blood cells has been observed in as many as 24 percent of cases.[81]

Amyloidosis of the gastrointestinal tract may produce ileus, malabsorption, hemorrhage, and even intestinal obstruction. Hepatosplenomegaly is a common finding, but hepatic dysfunction is infrequent. Rarely, amyloid infiltration interferes with the passage of bile from the canaliculi to the bile ducts, producing a cholestatic picture.[84] Other very infrequent manifestations include pulmonary nodules and hormonal insufficiency resulting from infiltration of endocrine glands. Amyloid deposits may trap factor X, resulting in a severe hemorrhagic disorder.[85] Increased fibrinolysis is another cause of hemorrhage in patients with amyloidosis.[86] This abnormality is marked by short euglobulin lysis times and distinctly low fibrinogen values. In such cases, hemorrhage may be controlled by the administration of ε-aminocaproic acid.

Secondary Amyloidosis (Reactive Systemic Amyloidosis)

Secondary amyloidosis is an acquired systemic disorder that may develop in patients with chronic infections or inflammatory disease. Associated disorders have included empyema, osteomyelitis, tuberculosis, bronchiectasis, rheumatoid arthritis, paraplegia, Crohn's disease, leprosy, Hodgkin's disease, intravenous drug abuse, and renal cell cancer.

The fibrillar protein in secondary amyloidosis is amyloid A (AA), which has a molecular weight of 8,500. It is probably derived from the normal serum component serum amyloid A (SAA), an acute-phase reactant. The molecular weight of the circulating SAA protein is reported to range from 84,000 to 200,000; a molecule that appears to be a monomer of the SAA protein has a molecular weight of 11,000. SAA may circulate complexed to high-density lipoproteins and albumin. It is synthesized at least partly in the liver; addition of a macrophage product stimulates synthesis remarkably.[87] SAA is probably cleaved to AA on monocyte surfaces, after which the AA fibers are deposited between cells.

Not all patients with one of the aforementioned disorders develop secondary amyloidosis. Overproduction of SAA plays an important role, but the critical factor that determines whether secondary amyloidosis develops may be the pattern by which monocytes degrade SAA to AA.[78] The observation that the progression of secondary amyloidosis in rheumatoid arthritis correlates with persistently high levels of SAA and C-reactive protein suggests that these acute-phase reactants play an etiologic role in the amyloidosis.[88]

In one patient in whom a form of bone and joint amyloidosis developed as a com-

plication of chronic dialysis for renal failure, the amyloid protein was identified as β$_2$-microglobulin altered into a fibrillar configuration.[89]

Deposits in secondary, or AA, amyloidosis build up mostly in the liver, spleen, adrenals, and kidneys. The nephrotic syndrome is the most common cause of clinical manifestations.

Hereditary Systemic Amyloidosis

Amyloidosis associated with deposition of AA fibrils develops in patients with familial Mediterranean fever (FMF). The nephrotic syndrome is a serious, relatively common complication of the disease. In the Portuguese type of hereditary amyloidosis, fibrils composed of prealbumin (AF$_P$) formed into β-pleated sheets infiltrate peripheral nerves.[77,78] Lower limb neuropathy is a common finding in this form of amyloidosis.

Local Amyloidosis

Local forms of amyloidosis are limited to the skin (AD, or amyloid dermatologic), larynx, or lung. Hormonal forms arise in patients who have medullary cancer of the thyroid or diabetes; the fiber composition is designated AE (amyloid endocrine). Deposits that develop adjacent to areas of medullary cancer of the thyroid are composed of thyrocalcitonin fibers (termed AE$_T$).

Senile Amyloidosis

Occasionally, postmortem examinations of elderly individuals reveal amyloid deposits in the heart and brain. This condition, termed senile amyloidosis, is presumed to be an incidental finding, but the deposits may have caused organ dysfunction during life. The protein type is called AS (amyloid senile), and the subvariants are AS$_C$ (cardiac) and AS$_B$ (brain).[90,91]

Diagnosis

Features that may suggest amyloidosis include the nephrotic syndrome, unexplained heart disease, peripheral neuropathy, hepatosplenomegaly, purpura over the neck and chest, and carpal tunnel syndrome.

Polarized-microscopic examination of Congo red–stained tissue from an involved organ can establish the diagnosis but not the specific amyloid type. Some authors caution against liver biopsy because of the danger of hepatic rupture and hemorrhage.[78] If involved tissues are not easily accessible, a rectal biopsy, which reportedly yields the correct diagnosis in about 80 percent of cases, can be done.[77,78] In 50 percent of cases, the diagnosis is apparent on examination of skin biopsy specimens.[83] Marrow biopsy samples, when appropriately stained with Congo red, occasionally can also provide the diagnosis.

The choice of effective therapy may require identification of the specific amyloid type. In the AL variant, free light chains in serum and in concentrated urine can be detected by immunoelectrophoresis in 90 percent of cases.[92] Serum protein electrophoresis may reveal an M protein; bone marrow biopsy may show a plasmacytosis or a myelomatous or lymphoid infiltrate, but it is nondiagnostic in 60 percent of cases.[81] If the type of amyloidosis remains obscure, special research laboratories can furnish definitive identification of the specific amyloid protein by studying biopsied tissue. Of course, because a patient can have more than one form of amyloidosis, it is possible that more than one specific protein will be identified.

Management

Most authorities agree that the therapy for primary (AL) amyloidosis is generally ineffective.[78,81] However, a few patients have benefited from the melphalan-prednisone regimen used in the treatment of multiple myeloma.[93] This combination has produced objective signs of improvement, including disappearance of the M protein spike, disappearance of Bence Jones protein in the urine, reversal of the nephrotic syndrome, and shrinkage of gum, tongue, and neck infiltrates. A controlled study has determined that the melphalan-prednisone regimen is superior to colchicine for the treatment of primary systemic amyloidosis.[94] Cardiac amyloidosis seems particularly resistant to therapy.

Renal transplantation has been used effectively for treating the renal amyloidosis of FMF. In several patients, however, the transplanted kidney became involved with amyloidosis.[95] Colchicine can block SAA secretion by cultured hepatocytes.[87] Administered in a dosage of 0.5 mg three to four times daily, colchicine has been used as an anti-inflammatory agent in FMF[95,96] and seems to limit the advance of AA amyloidosis in patients with FMF.[97] A clinical trial demonstrated that colchicine reduced the frequency of renal amyloidosis in patients with FMF, in addition to decreasing the frequency and severity of febrile attacks.[98] Because prevention of renal amyloidosis was not directly correlated with the reduction in febrile episodes, it appears that the action of colchicine in preventing amyloidosis may involve a mechanism other than inhibition of the febrile attacks.

DMSO (dimethyl sulfoxide) has produced beneficial effects in animal studies of AA amyloidosis, and sporadic case reports suggest that it might be a useful adjunct to therapy.[99] The agent has not been released in the United States for treatment of amyloidosis, but it is undergoing critical testing by several groups. Severe hepatotoxicity has been reported after intravenous use of DMSO.[81,100]

Benign Monoclonal Gammopathy (Monoclonal Gammopathy of Undetermined Significance)

Benign monoclonal gammopathy is characterized by a stable level of M protein in the serum and no evidence of clinical progression. Waldenström reported that one percent of 7,000 normal subjects older than 25 years and three percent of patients older than 70 years had M protein in their serum. The incidence appears to be as high as six percent in persons older than 80 years and 14 percent in those older than 90 years when very sensitive techniques, such as immunofixation, are used.[101]

The presence of a serum M protein requires that the diagnosis of multiple myeloma be excluded. In contrast to patients with multiple myeloma, patients with benign monoclonal gammopathy show no bone destruction, minimal to moderate plasmacytosis of marrow, a serum M protein level of less than 3 g/dl, little or no Bence Jones proteinuria, minimal anemia, and a low plasma cell labeling index.[10,102] In addition, they do not exhibit azotemia or depressed levels of serum albumin, nor do they experience a progressive increase in M protein levels. A study in which 241 patients with monoclonal gammopathy were followed for more than 10 years revealed that in 19 percent of such patients, myeloma, macroglobulinemia, amyloidosis, or related disorders eventually developed.[102] Such malignant conversion was not found to correlate with the initial hemoglobin level, the presence of organomegaly, the size and type of the M protein peak, Bence Jones proteinuria, serum albumin levels, or the serum levels of normal immunoglobulins. In a long-term follow-up study of 430 cases of IgM monoclonal gammopathy, 56 percent retained the diagnosis, 26 percent had chronic lymphocytic leukemia or another lymphoproliferative disease, 17 percent had Waldenström's macroglobulinemia, and one percent had primary amyloidosis. Malignant lymphoproliferative disorders typically evolved four to nine years after the IgM spike was first detected. Patients with IgM gammopathy, as well as those with IgG and IgA gammopathy, should therefore be seen every six months for clinical examination and measurement of hemoglobin, immunoglobulin, and albumin levels.[103] Therapy is usually not required in the absence of clinical progression.

Hyperglobulinemic Purpura of Waldenström

Hyperglobulinemic purpura of Waldenström is characterized by prominent polyclonal elevation of γ-globulins in association with petechiae and purpura over the extremities, particularly the lower extremities. It is not a clearly defined condition, and associations have been reported with Sjögren's syndrome, Raynaud's phenomenon, benign thymoma, and rheumatoid dis-

eases.[104] Serum analysis reveals the presence of complexes of γ-globulin with IgG anti–γ-globulin.[21]

Cryoglobulinemia

Cryoglobulins are proteins that precipitate on exposure to cold.[105] The cryoglobulinemias have been classified into three different subgroups. In type 1 disease, the serum contains isolated monoclonal immunoglobulins of IgM, IgG, IgA, or Bence Jones composition. In type 2 disease, there are mixed cryoglobulins: a monoclonal immunoglobulin (usually of IgM but occasionally of IgG origin) with antibody activity against polyclonal IgG interacts and cryoprecipitates with the polyclonal IgG. Type 3 cryoglobulins are mixed polyclonal cryoglobulins containing one or more classes of immunoglobulins; type 3 cryoglobulins are occasionally mixed with complement and lipoproteins. Type 2 and type 3 cryoglobulinemia are probably immune complex diseases in which the complexes form cryoprecipitates.

The pathogenetic mechanisms relate to systemic immune complex deposition followed by complement activation and inflammation; platelet aggregation and consumption of clotting factors by the cryoglobulins, causing coagulation disorders; small vessel thromboses and vasculitis produced by immune complexes; and a hyperviscosity syndrome. Type 1 and type 2 cryoglobulinemia are associated with cutaneous and vasomotor symptoms. Patients with type 2 and type 3 cryoglobulinemia may have vascular purpura and Raynaud's phenomenon. Renal and neurologic problems also occur in all three kinds of disorders. Cryoglobulinemias are typically associated with underlying immunoproliferative or autoimmune disorders, but there may also be an association with hepatitis B infection.

The diagnosis is made by carefully drawing blood into a warmed syringe and removing the red cells using a warmed centrifuge. The remaining plasma in a Wintrobe tube is refrigerated at 4° C for 24 to 72 hours; it is then centrifuged and a cryocrit is determined. Most cryoglobulins have rheumatoid factor activity.[106] A specialized immunology laboratory can identify the type of cryoglobulinemia.

Treatment of the underlying disease is required for acute symptoms such as those caused by hyperviscosity syndrome or vascular obstruction. Plasmapheresis is beneficial when it is done at 37° C. Prednisone and immunosuppressive agents, such as azathioprine and cyclophosphamide, have been tried in uncontrolled studies without evident benefit.

References

1. Semin Hematol 8:239, 1976
2. J Clin Invest 74:1301, 1984
3. J Clin Invest 75:2024, 1985
4. Lancet 1:1174, 1978
5. Br J Haematol 36:545, 1977
6. Blood 64:352, 1984
7. Blood 73:865, 1989
8. Blood 74:1206, 1989
9. J Clin Invest 84:2008, 1989
10. Br J Haematol 58:689, 1984
11. Br J Haematol 51:361, 1982
12. N Engl J Med 317:526, 1987
13. J Clin Invest 82:1, 1988
14. Cancer 48:783, 1981
15. Arch Intern Med 138:727, 1978
16. Medicine (Baltimore) 55:217, 1976
17. Br Med J 292:2, 1986
18. J Clin Pathol 42:59, 1989
19. Am J Hematol 20:345, 1985
20. J Clin Oncol 4:80, 1986
21. Baillieres Clin Haematol 1:695, 1987
22. J Clin Invest 58:1155, 1976
23. Am J Ophthalmol 86:303, 1978
24. Ann Intern Med 110:275, 1989
25. Medicine (Baltimore) 59:301, 1980
26. Br J Haematol 48:383, 1981
27. Arch Intern Med 140:1150, 1980
28. Am J Med 63:1015, 1977
29. Haematologica 72:107, 1987
30. Cancer 36:842, 1975
31. Br J Haematol 42:199, 1979
32. Br J Haematol 69:47, 1988
33. Ann Intern Med 110:521, 1989
34. N Engl J Med 319:1651, 1988
35. Blood 55:602, 1980
36. J Clin Oncol 5:1811, 1987
37. Cancer 45:2893, 1980
38. Cancer 59:1475, 1987
39. Skeletal Radiol 11:258, 1984
40. Lancet 2:364, 1987
41. Ann Neurol 3:40, 1978
42. J Clin Invest 61:97, 1978
43. J Clin Oncol 1:453, 1983
44. Cancer 53:583, 1984
45. J Clin Oncol 5:1373, 1987
46. Br J Cancer 59:110, 1989
47. Proc Annu Meet Am Soc Clin Oncol 3:270, 1984
48. Blood 54:13, 1979
49. N Engl J Med 301:743, 1979
50. Blood 66(suppl 1):214a, 1985
51. N Engl J Med 310:1382, 1984
52. Blood 63:639, 1984
53. Proceedings of ASCO 8:272, 1989
54. Lancet 2:879, 1989
55. Blood 73:20, 1989
56. N Engl J Med 322:1430, 1990
57. Arch Intern Med 148:1963, 1988
58. J Clin Oncol 6:759, 1988
59. Arch Intern Med 147:1629, 1987
60. Lancet 2:1180, 1989
61. Lancet 1:1043, 1980
62. N Engl J Med 303:618, 1980
63. Ann Intern Med 90:793, 1979
64. Lancet 1:1201, 1988
65. Br Med J 287:1575, 1983
66. N Engl J Med 310:1353, 1984
67. Ann Intern Med 105:8, 1986
68. Lancet 2:882, 1989
69. Br J Haematol 71:25, 1989
70. Lancet 2:65, 1980
71. J Clin Oncol 6:889, 1988
72. J Clin Oncol 6:757, 1988
73. N Engl J Med 308:314, 1983
74. Lancet 2:311, 1985
75. Mayo Clin Proc 56:439, 1981
76. Cancer 63:1251, 1989
77. N Engl J Med 302:1283, 1333, 1980
78. Hosp Pract 15(9):70, 1980
79. Lancet 2:606, 1980
80. J Clin Invest 70:453, 1982
81. Mayo Clin Proc 58:665, 1983
82. Am J Med 62:677, 1977
83. Ann Intern Med 88:781, 1978
84. Am J Med 64:937, 1978
85. N Engl J Med 297:81, 1977
86. Arch Intern Med 143:678, 1983
87. Nature 285:498, 1980
88. Br Med J 286:1391, 1983
89. J Clin Invest 76:2425, 1985
90. Br Med J 282:846, 1981
91. Am J Med 75:618, 1983
92. Arch Intern Med 144:2145, 1984
93. Arch Intern Med 139:1144, 1979
94. Am J Med 79:708, 1985
95. Arch Intern Med 139:1135, 1979
96. Ann Intern Med 87:568, 1977
97. Br Med J 281:2, 1980
98. N Engl J Med 314:1001, 1986
99. Lancet 1:207, 1979
100. Lancet 2:1004, 1980
101. Am J Med 82:39, 1987
102. JAMA 251:1849, 1984
103. Mayo Clin Proc 62:719, 1987
104. Medicine (Baltimore) 50:125, 1971
105. Am J Med 57:775, 1974
106. Am J Med 69:287, 1980

Acknowledgments

Table 3 Modified from "A Clinical Staging System for Multiple Myeloma," by B. G. Durie and S. Salmon, in *Cancer* 36:852, 1975. Used by permission.

17 Nosocomial Bacteremia and Shock

CYRUS C. HOPKINS, M.D.

Overview

More than 40 percent of all primary nosocomial bacteremias are caused by gram-negative bacilli, and bacteremia occurs in two to four percent of other gram-negative infections.[1] Twenty-five to 40 percent of bacteremias are associated with hypotension or shock.[2] The overall mortality approaches 25 percent, but it is clearly correlated with the severity of underlying disease and of cardiovascular complications.

Gram-negative bacteremia is not synonymous with shock. In fact, shock or hypotension is usually absent. The most common presentation is fever and leukocytosis, accompanied by symptoms consistent with infection at the site of origin. The full hypotensive reaction may occur rarely when infection is focal and blood cultures are negative. Hypotension or septic shock can also occur in severe infections caused by gram-positive bacteria or, rarely, by nonbacterial pathogens.

Pathogenesis

Infusion of fluids contaminated by bacteria or endotoxins can cause bacteremia or shock. More often, bacteremia and shock arise from local invasive infection. In such cases, the infecting organisms reflect the flora of the portal of entry, especially when the portal of entry is the urinary tract. Organisms vary somewhat among hospitals and services.

The precipitating cause of hypotension and shock is not well understood. It appears that cachectin (tumor necrosis factor) plays a major role in mediating these effects; however, cachectin is not always detectable, and its level does not predict the major complications of sepsis.[3-5] Endotoxin by itself cannot be responsible: it is frequently absent, and when present, it often does not correlate with the severity of disease. The clinical picture of shock can be produced by organisms that do not make endotoxin. A complex cascade of metabolic and physiologic changes, including disseminated intravascular coagulation, activation of the kallikrein and complement systems, and immunologic overreaction, is involved in septic shock.[6,7] Endogenous opiates may play a role, but the first controlled trial of a low-dose opiate antagonist showed no benefit in the treatment of shock.[8]

Secondary sequelae can result from bacteremic seeding of other organs or anatomic sites. Enterobacteriaceae may produce focal abscesses. *P. aeruginosa* may cause severe vascular involvement, especially in immunosuppressed hosts. Massive infiltration of arterial and venous walls and hemorrhagic septic infarction may occur.

Clinical Features

Although such signs of systemic sepsis as chills, fever, and malaise are frequent, they may be relatively minor in elderly, debilitated, or immunosuppressed patients. Hypothermia may also occur.

In shock, the cardiac output may initially increase and peripheral resistance may decrease. Later, blood pools form in peripheral tissues, venous return declines, central venous pressure falls, and cardiac output decreases. Bedside observations such as those distinguishing warm shock from cold shock do not provide adequate data for diagnosis or treatment. A declining cardiac output indicates a poor prognosis but is reversible within seven to 10 days in some cases.[9]

Respiratory changes are often prominent and may be the earliest sign of gram-negative sepsis. Patients may present with hyperventilation and respiratory alkalosis alone or with striking hypoxemia, unaccompanied by pulmonary edema, pulmonary embolus, or pneumonia. Frank adult respiratory distress syndrome (ARDS), which is associated with a high mortality, may ensue. As circulatory changes become more prominent, metabolic acidosis supervenes.

Confusion, disorientation, and changes in consciousness are common. Vomiting, diarrhea, or both may be present. Dermal alterations may occur and reflect circulatory changes. *Pseudomonas* bacteremia is associated with characteristic skin lesions, including red macules or deep purple-red hemorrhagic bullous lesions that can progress to the necrotic lesions of ecthyma gangrenosum. Hemorrhagic lesions may also appear in association with disseminated intravascular coagulation.

Laboratory Findings

Leukocytosis is common and is sometimes accompanied by thrombocytopenia. Arterial blood gases reflect circulatory changes (see above), and acidosis, azotemia, or elevations in the level of enzymes such as aspartate aminotransferase (AST, formerly termed SGOT) reflect poor systemic perfusion. An elevated AST level may also reflect liver injury, and ECG changes indicative of ischemia may be found.

Other laboratory data reflect changes at the site of origin. Secretions from suspected sites, including sputum, urine, wound drainage, or needle aspirates from areas of cellulitis near a wound, should be carefully examined by Gram's stain and culture. Blood cultures are usually positive; to ensure a maximum yield, three sets should be obtained.[2] The first major diagnostic evidence is often the identification of gram-negative rods on staining of the appropriate specimen. However, this finding is not definitive. Diagnosis and treatment must often be based on clinical manifestations until a more specific bacteriologic diagnosis is available.

Differential Diagnosis

When full-blown septic shock is present, there is rarely doubt about the diagnosis. However, if fever and chills are minor or absent, the presentation may suggest other illnesses. For example, unexplained hypo-tension or oliguria requires a careful search for causes of blood loss or circulatory failure. Tachypnea or hypoxemia is more often related to pulmonary disease, pneumonia, pulmonary embolus, or congestive heart failure. In the absence of clinical confirmation of these entities, blood cultures should always be obtained.

When septic shock is present, consideration of all possible etiologic agents must guide initial therapy until blood culture and other bacteriologic results become available. A careful review of the patient's history or hospital record may reveal a potential precipitating factor, such as manipulation or insertion of a urinary catheter, aspiration, or a wound infection. If bacteriologic tests from such sites are available, they often reveal the involved organism. Such data are particularly helpful if prior antibiotic use may have selected for resistant organisms. Underlying disease must also be considered: leukopenia occurring during therapy for leukemia may be associated with bacteremia caused by *P. aeruginosa*. A physical examination that includes inspection of catheters and recent wounds helps to focus the diagnosis.

If no source of infection is defined at a specific anatomic site, such as the urinary tract, the lungs, or a surgical wound, primary bacteremia originating from a contaminated intravenous catheter or infusion set must be considered. Whenever possible, all indwelling intravenous catheters and intravenous fluid and tubing should be removed and cultured. Semiquantitative techniques of streaking catheter tips on solid media help to distinguish the low-grade contamination that occurs on catheter removal from a true positive catheter tip.[10] Although removal of an intravenous catheter is generally preferred, some patients with a central venous catheter who have bacteremia or exit site infections but neither shock nor tunnel infection may be treated with the catheter in place.[11]

Treatment

Therapy is based on appropriate culture results and should include early aggressive cardiovascular monitoring, effective antibiotics, drainage of infected areas, and prompt reaction to new problems.

For initial treatment, two drugs are often required: a cephalosporin active against staphylococci and an aminoglycoside provide a broad spectrum of coverage as well as a synergistic effect against many gram-negative bacilli. In immunocompromised hosts, a synergistic effect may be particularly important, and the risk of *Pseudomonas* infection is higher. Therefore, in these patients, an aminoglycoside should be combined with one of the newer so-called antipseudomonal penicillin derivatives or a third-generation cephalosporin, such as ceftazidime. Many infections caused by gram-negative bacilli are appropriately treated with two drugs, either for their synergistic effect[12] or to delay the development of resistance to a β-lactam drug.[13] None of the agents employed in immunocompromised patients provide optimal therapy for *Staphylococcus* infections.

The choice of specific antibiotics depends on several factors: intramural patterns of prevalence and antibiotic susceptibility, clinical clues suggesting the site or sites of infection, and diagnostic findings such as ecthyma gangrenosum or the results of surveillance cultures.

When specific bacteriologic identification becomes available, usually in the form of positive blood cultures, and the organism's sensitivities are known, the regimen should be simplified, if possible, to reduce the risk of toxicity. The quinolone drugs, such as ciprofloxacin, may provide a useful alternative therapy in some settings.[14]

Careful monitoring of clinical status and plasma antibiotic levels and the results of further blood cultures may provide valuable information concerning persistent or recurrent bacteremia. Failure to respond to antibiotics may reflect either inadequate plasma drug levels, especially when treatment failure occurs early in the course of infection, or a later superinfection caused by an organism that is resistant to the antibiotics initially used.

Aggressive hemodynamic monitoring and therapy are also required to prevent shock [*see Chapter 1*]. Rapid repletion of intravascular volume is often helpful because it can improve peripheral perfusion and alleviate the acidotic component. Vasoactive agents may be required to treat and prevent shock. Dopamine is particularly useful because it improves renal blood flow and causes less tachycardia and ventricular irritability than isoproterenol.

Although it had been thought that corticosteroids might be useful in the treatment of gram-negative sepsis and shock, two studies have shown that they are ineffective.[15,16] Glucocorticoids inhibit cachectin production experimentally but only when given before exposure to endotoxin.[3] They may be ineffective because an irreversible metabolic cascade has been initiated by the time the clinical syndrome has become evident. The use of steroids may increase mortality in patients with an elevated serum creatinine level[15] and may increase the risk of secondary infection.

Endogenous opiates may play a pathogenetic role in septic shock, but it is premature to use naloxone or other opiate antagonists for routine therapy.[8]

Other major physiologic abnormalities should be corrected. If respiratory symptoms, tachypnea, or hypoxia occur, it is often necessary to employ intubation and mechanical ventilation. The need for these measures can be accurately assessed by the use of serial arterial blood gas determinations.

The potential role of immunotherapy in treating or preventing serious systemic reactions to gram-negative bacillary sepsis remains under active investigation.[17,18] Antiserum prepared in human volunteers by immunization against the lipopolysaccharide core antigen of mutant *E. coli* may decrease the mortality caused by gram-negative bacteremia.[17] However, this approach has produced mixed results, perhaps because the immunologic reactions involved are complex.[19,20]

Prognosis

Prognosis is directly related to the severity of underlying disease and to the extent of metabolic and hemodynamic complications. Mortality from bacteremia has ranged from

16 percent in patients without an underlying fatal disease to 81 percent in patients with an underlying disease that might be expected to result in early mortality. Metastatic infection is a relatively uncommon complication of bacteremia caused by most gram-negative bacilli except for *P. aeruginosa*. However, high-grade bacteremia caused by any of the gram-negative bacilli may result in seeding and local abscess formation. Endocarditis is an uncommon complication of nosocomial bacteremia but can occur when intravenous drug abuse introduces organisms such as *Pseudomonas* or *S. marcescens* into the blood-stream.[21] The risk of endocarditis is greater if a prosthetic cardiac valve is present.

Prevention

Prevention requires prompt identification and treatment of primary infection sites. The risk of introducing endogenous normal flora or surface colonizers into deep tissue can be diminished by using rigorous aseptic techniques when handling catheters or performing other invasive procedures. The risk of cross-contamination and hazards of infected fluids can be controlled by techniques used in hospital infection control programs.

References

1. J Clin Microbiol 27:1421, 1989
2. Ann Intern Med 86:456, 1977
3. N Engl J Med 316:379, 1987
4. Science 229:869, 1985
5. JAMA 262:249, 1989
6. JAMA 250:3324, 1983
7. Lancet 1:1122, 1989
8. Lancet 1:1363, 1985
9. Ann Intern Med 100:483, 1984
10. N Engl J Med 296:1305, 1977
11. Am J Med 85:495, 1988
12. Am J Med 87:540, 1989
13. Rev Infect Dis 10:830, 1988
14. Lancet 1:819, 1986
15. N Engl J Med 317:653, 1987
16. N Engl J Med 317:659, 1987
17. N Engl J Med 307:1225, 1982
18. Lancet 1:981, 1984
19. J Infect Dis 158:312, 1988
20. J Infect Dis 159:168, 1989
21. Ann Intern Med 84:29, 1976

18 Acquired Immunodeficiency Syndrome

ROBERT H. RUBIN, M.D.

Epidemiology

Acquired immunodeficiency syndrome (AIDS) refers to the occurrence of a life-threatening opportunistic infection, Kaposi's sarcoma, or both in patients who have not received immunosuppressive drugs and who have no apparent immunosuppressing disease [*see Table 1*].[1] The syndrome is initiated by a human retrovirus termed the human immunodeficiency virus (HIV), previously known as lymphadenopathy-associated virus (LAV), AIDS-associated virus, human T cell lymphotropic virus type III (HTLV-III), and immunodeficiency-associated virus. Two forms of HIV have been identified. The prototype virus, HIV-1, is responsible for most of the cases of AIDS worldwide, particularly in the United States and Europe. A second retrovirus, termed HIV-2, has been isolated from patients with AIDS and is increasingly being reported from West Africa, where the pattern of transmission seems to be similar to that of HIV-1. In addition, HIV-2 has been demonstrated in the Americas, presumably spread as a result of contacts with infected West Africans. HIV-2 is actually more closely related to simian immunodeficiency virus (SIV), a retrovirus found in monkeys, than to HIV-1.[2-5]

Since the first reports of AIDS in 1981,[6-8] more than 200,000 cases have occurred throughout the world, and approximately two thirds of these cases have occurred in the United States. In 1989, 35,238 cases were reported in the United States, which is a 9.4 percent increase over the 1988 total. This rate of increase was lower than in previous years and is consistent with the slowing trend in AIDS incidence that has been noted since the middle of 1987, when the rapid upward trend in AIDS incidence began to moderate.

Although it is believed that this leveling off in the rate of increase in new AIDS cases is likely to continue, 52,000 to 57,000 new cases of AIDS and 37,000 to 42,000 deaths resulting from AIDS are predicted for 1990. More than one million individuals in the United States are thought to harbor asymptomatic HIV infection, and it is believed that more than 40,000 adults and 1,500 to 2,000 newborns will become newly infected with HIV each year.[9-11] Data suggest that AIDS will develop in 54 percent of those infected with HIV within 10 years and that AIDS will eventually develop in virtually all remaining HIV-infected persons who do not succumb to some other disease process first.[12,13]

The distribution of cases of AIDS and HIV infection in the United States and other countries is best described as a series of partially overlapping subepidemics. Thus, in different regions, varying rates of seropositivity are noted in groups at high risk of the disease. In the United States, surveys have found that the prevalence of HIV infection in male homosexual populations ranges from 10 to 70 percent. Rates of infection in populations of intravenous drug users have ranged from zero to 70 percent; the highest rates have been reported from New York City and northern New Jersey.[9]

Four population groups account for the vast majority of AIDS cases in the United States[9,10,14,15]: homosexual or bisexual men (71 percent of the total number of cases, eight percent of whom also have a history of intravenous drug use); heterosexual men or women who are intravenous drug users (17 percent, representing 60 percent of the cases among heterosexuals); recipients of transfusions, virtually all of whom received transfusions before the testing of blood became possible in 1985 (two percent); and hemo-

Table 1   CDC Surveillance Case Definition for AIDS

I. *HIV Status of Patient is Unknown or Inconclusive*

If laboratory tests for HIV infection were not performed or gave inconclusive results and the patient had no other cause of immunodeficiency listed in IA (see below), a definitive diagnosis of any disease listed in IB (see below) indicates AIDS.

  A. *Causes of immunodeficiency that disqualify a disease as an indication of AIDS in the absence of laboratory evidence of HIV infection*

    1. The use of high-dose or long-term systemic corticosteroid therapy or other immunosuppressive/cytotoxic therapy within three months before the onset of the indicator disease.

    2. A diagnosis of any of the following diseases within three months after diagnosis of the indicator disease: Hodgkin's disease, non-Hodgkin's lymphoma (other than primary brain lymphoma), lymphocytic leukemia, multiple myeloma, any other cancer of lymphoreticular or histiocytic tissue, or angioimmunoblastic lymphadenopathy.

    3. A genetic (congenital) immunodeficiency syndrome or an acquired immunodeficiency syndrome that is atypical of HIV infection, such as one involving hypogammaglobulinemia.

  B. *Diseases that indicate AIDS (requires definitive diagnosis)*

    1. Candidiasis of the esophagus, trachea, bronchi, or lungs.

    2. Cryptococcosis, extrapulmonary.

    3. Cryptosporidiosis with diarrhea persisting for more than one month.

    4. Cytomegalovirus disease of an organ other than the liver, spleen, or lymph nodes in a patient older than one month.

    5. Herpes simplex virus infection causing a mucocutaneous ulcer that persists longer than one month; or herpes simplex virus infection causing bronchitis, pneumonitis, or esophagitis for any duration in a patient older than one month.

    6. Kaposi's sarcoma in a patient younger than 60 years.

    7. Lymphoid interstitial pneumonia or pulmonary lymphoid hyperplasia (LIP/PLH complex) in a patient younger than 13 years.

    8. Lymphoma of the brain (primary) affecting a patient younger than 60 years.

    9. *Mycobacterium avium* complex or *M. kansasii* disease, disseminated (at a site other than or in addition to the lungs, skin, or cervical or hilar lymph nodes).

    10. *Pneumocystis carinii* pneumona.

    11. Progressive multifocal leukoencephalopathy.

    12. Toxoplasmosis of the brain in a patient older than one month.

II. *Patient Is HIV Positive*

Regardless of the presence of other causes of immunodeficiency (see IA, above), in the presence of laboratory evidence of HIV infection, any disease listed in IB (see above) or in IIA or IIB (see below) indicates a diagnosis of AIDS.

  A. *Diseases that indicate AIDS (requires definitive diagnosis)*

    1. Bacterial infections, multiple or recurrent (any combination of at least two

philiacs (one percent). Heterosexual transmission accounts for four percent of adult cases and generally occurs in individuals who have a history of heterosexual contact with someone in a high-risk category (an intravenous drug user in approximately 70 percent of cases) or with immigrants from such areas as Haiti and central Africa, where heterosexual transmission is the major route of spread. Since 1985, several trends have been noted: a decrease in the percentage of cases in non–drug-using homosexual and bisexual men (from 63 percent to 56 percent), and an increase in the percentage of cases among women (from seven percent to 11 percent) and among intravenous drug users (from 18 percent to 23 percent).[12] More than 2,000 cases of AIDS have been reported in children younger than 13 years. Seventy-five percent of these children acquired the

---

Table 1   (Continued)

within a two- to four-year period), of the following types in a patient younger than 13 years: septicemia, pneumonia, meningitis, bone or joint infection, or abscess of an internal organ or body cavity (excluding otitis media or superficial skin or mucosal abscesses) caused by *Hemophilus, Streptococcus* (including pneumococcus), or other pyogenic bacteria.

2. Coccidioidomycosis, disseminated (at a site other than or in addition to the lungs or cervical or hilar lymph nodes).

3. Histoplasmosis, disseminated (at a site other than or in addition to the lungs or cervical or hilar lymph nodes).

4. HIV encephalopathy.

5. HIV wasting syndrome.

6. Isosporiasis with diarrhea persisting for more than one month.

7. Kaposi's sarcoma at any age.

8. Lymphoma of the brain (primary) at any age.

9. *M. tuberculosis* disease, extrapulmonary (involving at least one site outside the lungs, regardless of whether there is concurrent pulmonary involvement).

10. Mycobacterial disease caused by mycobacteria other than *M. tuberculosis*, disseminated (at a site other than or in addition to the lungs, skin, or cervical or hilar lymph nodes).

11. Non-Hodgkin's lymphoma of B cell or unknown immunologic phenotype and the following histologic types: small noncleaved lymphoma (Burkitt's or non-Burkitt's) or immunoblastic sarcoma.

12. *Salmonella* (nontyphoidal) septicemia, recurrent.

B. *Diseases that indicate AIDS (presumptive diagnosis)*

1. Candidiasis of the esophagus.

2. Cytomegalovirus retinitis, with loss of vision.

3. Kaposi's sarcoma.

4. Lymphoid interstitial pneumonia or pulmonary lymphoid hyperplasia (LIP/PLH complex) in a patient younger than 13 years.

5. Mycobacterial disease (acid-fast bacilli with species not identified by culture), disseminated (involving at least one site other than or in addition to the lungs, skin, or cervical or hilar lymph nodes).

6. *P. carinii* pneumonia.

7. Toxoplasmosis of the brain in a patient older than one month.

III. *Patient Is HIV Negative*

With laboratory test results negative for HIV infection, a diagnosis of AIDS for surveillance purposes is ruled out *unless*

A. All the other causes of immunodeficiency listed in 1A (see above) are excluded; and

B. The patient has had either of the following:

1. *P. carinii* pneumonia diagnosed by a definitive method.

2. A definitive diagnosis of any of the other diseases indicative of AIDS listed in IB (see above) and a CD4$^+$ helper-inducer T cell count of less than 400/mm^3.

Note: Reference 1 provides a complete commentary and explanation of these criteria, including criteria for diagnosis.

---

disease perinatally, probably before birth, from infected mothers, virtually all of whom were intravenous drug users or had sexual contact with intravenous drug users. The remainder of children with AIDS acquired the disease from transfusions or after treatment for hemophilia.

In the United States, the incidence of AIDS is more than three times higher in blacks and Hispanics than in whites. Most white AIDS patients are either homosexual or bisexual or have acquired the disease from blood products. Most black or Hispanic AIDS patients have a history of intravenous drug use, have acquired the disease from heterosexual contact with someone at high risk for acquiring AIDS, or are children.[9-12,14-16]

A major epidemiologic concern has been the threat HIV infection poses to the use of blood and blood products. More than 95 percent of patients receiving HIV-contaminated blood become infected, and symptomatic AIDS develops in 50 percent of those infected within seven years. If the blood donor has AIDS or if AIDS develops in the donor within 29 months after giving blood, the incubation period for AIDS in the recipient is considerably shortened.[17,18] There have been documented cases of individuals with transfusion-associated infection who transmitted the virus to their spouses, presumably via heterosexual contact. Most patients with transfusion-associated AIDS received their transfusions and were diagnosed in areas where AIDS has been most commonly identified (i.e., New York City, San Francisco, Miami, and Los Angeles). Although AIDS has been transmitted via transfusions of whole blood, blood cellular components, plasma, or clotting factors that have not been heat treated (as in the factor VIII concentrates previously used to treat hemophiliacs), no other products prepared from blood, such as immunoglobulin, albumin, plasma protein factor, or hepatitis B vaccine, have been implicated. In particular, although antibody to HIV may have been found in many immunoglobulin preparations, it is now clear that immunoglobulin preparations, whether given intramuscularly or intravenously, do not transmit HIV.[19,20] However, HIV can be transmitted via an organ transplant from an infected donor.[21]

It is important to emphasize that three public health measures have done much to ensure the safety of the blood supply: screening of donated blood and plasma for antibody to HIV, which became possible in April 1985; heat treatment of clotting factor concentrates; and donor screening on the basis of history.[22] Although transmission of HIV by a unit of blood that had tested negative by current enzyme-linked immunosorbent assays (ELISAs) for HIV antibody has been documented, the likelihood that infection will be transmitted via transfusion is estimated to be one in 153,000 per unit of blood, which represents a significant decrease in risk (30 percent a year) since HIV testing of the blood supply was first introduced.[18,23] This is not to say, however, that more cases of AIDS from the transfusion of blood products will not continue to be observed. It is estimated that 70 to 80 percent of hemophiliacs in the United States are infected with HIV and that 12,000 individuals became infected from transfusions before the availability of HIV testing. Given the long period of asymptomatic infection, cases of AIDS from this pool of infected individuals will continue to occur for years to come.[14]

The epidemiology of AIDS shows parallels to that of hepatitis B. In this regard, the presence of HIV antibody, like the presence of hepatitis B surface antigen, serves as a marker of potentially transmissible infection. Both AIDS and hepatitis B are transmissible, blood-borne, infectious processes that can also be spread by intimate personal contact—that is, infection may occur in children born to infected mothers and in the sexual partners of putative cases.[9,14] In addition, asymptomatic viremia, particularly among potential blood donors, has played an important role in the transmission of both AIDS and hepatitis B.[9,14] Among homosexual men, epidemiologic factors associated with an increased risk of AIDS[24] include promiscuity; receptive anal intercourse; a history of syphilis, hepatitis C (formerly termed non-A, non-B hepatitis), or enteric parasitic infections; and the use of illicit intravenous drugs. These epidemiologic observations are accounted for by the isolation of HIV from the blood, semen, cervix, saliva, and tears of AIDS patients and other HIV antibody–positive individuals.[14,25] There is some evidence that the more compromised an individual's immune function is (i.e., the more advanced the disease), the more efficiently the virus is transmitted through intimate contact. Moreover, the presence of anogenital skin lesions or mucosal ulcerations may increase the rate of HIV acquisition and transmission.[9]

It is important to emphasize that the transmission of HIV by routes other than intimate contact, transfusion of blood products, or communal intravenous drug abuse is virtually unknown [*see Table 2*].[14] Thus, household, school, or work contacts of patients with HIV infection who are not the children or sexual partners of such patients are at minimal or no risk of infection.[14,26,27] Similarly, despite some claims to the contrary, there is compelling evidence that insect-borne HIV transmission does not occur.[28]

An extremely important issue is the risk of transmission of HIV to health care workers. Data suggest that the risk is very low but not nonexistent. One report noted that infection occurred in three of 351 health care workers who had needle-stick exposures to the blood of HIV-infected individuals.[9] There may be a somewhat greater risk associated with the inoculation of concentrated viral specimens in the research laboratory.[9,29] Of perhaps more concern is a report of three instances of HIV infection apparently following the exposure of skin lesions or mucous membranes to infected blood.[9] Other reports, however, suggest that transmission rates are very low[30-32]; one report based on combined data from the National Institutes of Health, the Centers for Disease Control, and the University of California found that of 2,200 persons who were injured while working with blood or other materials contaminated with HIV, 16 ultimately became seropositive for HIV infection.[33] In another report, surveillance of 963 health care workers exposed to HIV-infected blood or body fluids revealed a seroconversion rate of 0.42 percent. Of particular importance was the finding that two of the exposures resulting in seroconversion occurred when health care workers accidentally exposed coworkers to infected blood during resuscitation procedures.[32] This observation and reports of a slowly rising incidence of undiagnosed HIV infection among patients presenting to urban hospitals for emergency care underline the need for great care on the part of health care workers. Such care should include the implementation of universal blood and body fluid precautions [*see* Management, *below*] within the health

---

Table 2   Transmission of HIV

Known Routes of Transmission
  Inoculation of blood
    Transfusion of blood and blood
      products
    Needle sharing among intravenous
      drug users
    Needle stick, open wound, and mucous
      membrane exposure in health-care
      workers
    Injection with unsterilized needles
  Sexual
    Homosexual (male to male)
    Heterosexual (male to female and female to male)
  Perinatal
    Intrauterine
    Peripartum

Routes Investigated and Not Shown to Be Involved in Transmission
  Close personal contact
    Household
    Workplace
    School
    Health care workers without exposure
      to blood
  Insects

---

care setting to protect against transmissions of this type even though the likelihood of such an event occurring is actually quite small.[34,35]

Data suggest that the incubation period for the development of AIDS varies significantly with age of acquisition of HIV infection. Children who are infected by transfusion before five years of age have incubation periods of less than two years, whereas those who contract transfusion-associated infection after five years of age have incubation periods of approximately eight years. In homosexuals and hemophiliacs, the mean incubation period may be as long as nine to 10 years. Children with perinatally acquired infection have a high rate of disease progression in the first year of life.[9,36,37] Overall, AIDS appears to develop within three years in 15 to 38 percent of asymptomatic individuals who have antibody to HIV.[38] In at least another 25 percent, generalized lymphadenopathy, oral candidiasis, or other AIDS-related conditions will develop.

As suggested by the mean incubation period statistics, there is a continuing risk of development of various clinical effects of HIV infection for several years.[36-38]

Pathogenesis

AIDS encompasses a complex group of clinical entities that share a profound immune defect. The severe immunosuppression causes a high incidence of repeated bouts of opportunistic infection and a high incidence of Kaposi's sarcoma, a tumor that had previously been exceedingly rare in the population in which it is now occurring. Because of the underlying immunodeficiency, this tumor follows a particularly malignant course in AIDS patients. The risk of other tumors developing is also high. Tumors such as B cell lymphoproliferative disorders and Burkitt's lymphoma probably arise because of an impaired immune response to infection with various viruses (see below).

Initiation of AIDS by a Retrovirus

A major advance in understanding the etiology of AIDS occurred when two scientific groups, one headed by Luc Montagnier at the Pasteur Institute in Paris and the other led by Robert Gallo at the National Cancer Institute in Bethesda, Maryland, identified the new human retrovirus known as HIV as the cause of AIDS.[2,3,39,40] HIV is a member of the nontransforming, cytopathic lentivirus family of retroviruses that also includes the visna virus of sheep, the caprine arthritis encephalitis virus, the equine infectious anemia virus, and the feline immunodeficiency virus. These viruses cause slowly progressive, invariably fatal diseases characterized by progressive neurodegenerative disease, progressive immunodeficiency, or both.[41,42]

HIV is similar to other retroviruses in that it has a dense, cylindrical nucleoid that contains core proteins, genomic RNA, and the hallmark enzyme reverse transcriptase. It has the standard retroviral genes known as *gag, pol,* and *env. Gag* encodes a polyprotein gene product called p55, which is subsequently cleaved to form the viral core proteins p17, p24, and p15. *Pol* encodes three enzymes: reverse transcriptase, which transcribes the viral RNA genome into double-stranded DNA; integrase, which is essential for integration of the viral DNA into the host cell's chromosomal DNA; and protease, which is responsible for cleaving p55 and is a major target for the development of innovative anti-HIV therapeutic strategies.[43,44] *Env* codes for a polyprotein termed gp160, which is subsequently cleaved into the major envelope glycoprotein gp120 and a transmembrane protein called gp41; gp41 is the attachment site for the external spikes of gp120 on the surface of the HIV virion.[41,42,45,46]

In addition to the standard retroviral genes, HIV possesses at least six other genes that regulate various aspects of viral replication and pathogenicity. Two of these genes, *tat* and *rev*, are essential for the optimal transcription and translation of viral structural gene products. Both genes act in a *trans*-acting manner; that is, they produce diffusible proteins that act at a distance on various viral and cellular genes. The *tat* gene encodes a protein that amplifies HIV gene expression, whereas the *rev* gene is essential for the expression of *gag* and *env* proteins. In addition, the *tat* protein appears to inhibit the antigen-induced proliferation of lymphocytes, perhaps contributing to the immunosuppressed state of HIV-infected individuals.[47] The *nef* gene, in contrast, appears to maintain low-level or latent HIV infection; the loss of this function is associated with an up-regulation of viral production and increased cytopathicity. The *vif* gene appears to be necessary for infectivity, the *u* gene for the assembly or maturation of new virus, and the *r* gene for an as yet undelineated function.

It is important to emphasize that various factors and processes can exert effects on the HIV genes and gene products and thereby modulate HIV synthesis. These factors and processes include T cell activation, lymphokines, and *trans*-activating factors produced by other viral infections, particularly infections caused by herpes simplex virus, cytomegalovirus (CMV), and varicella-zoster virus.[41,42,45,46]

The immunopathologic effects of HIV infection are directly related to the interaction of the virus with cells that carry the CD4 surface molecule, which serves as a high-affinity cell surface receptor for the virus. Helper T cells (CD4$^+$ T cells) have the highest expression of CD4 on their surface, although the molecule is also found on certain populations of monocytes and macrophages and certain neurons and glial cells from particular areas of the brain. The immunologic abnormalities and resulting disease manifestations of HIV infection would thus be predicted to result from interference in the normal functioning of these CD4-bearing cells. Whether other cell surface structures can play a secondary role in the HIV infection of human cells remains unclear.[41,42,45,46]

The cardinal manifestation of HIV infection is the depletion of the CD4$^+$ T cell population. Virtually all of the immunologic abnormalities observed in AIDS [*see Table 3*] can be explained by the ablation of the helper functions normally carried out by these lymphocytes: activation of macrophages, induction of B cell function, induction of cytotoxic T cell function, induction of natural killer (NK) cell function, induction of suppressor cell function, secretion of growth and differentiation factors for lymphoid cells, secretion of hematopoietic colony-stimulating factors, and secretion of factors that induce non-lymphoid cell function.[41,42,45,46]

Infection of CD4$^+$ T cells by HIV is initiated by the interaction of the CD4 surface molecule with the HIV gp120 envelope glycoprotein. This interaction results in a marked depletion in the CD4$^+$ T cell population by mechanisms that are incompletely understood but that probably include at least some of the following events: recruitment of uninfected cells into a syncytium via interaction between gp120 on the surfaces of

Table 3   Immunologic Abnormalities in Patients with AIDS

Prevalence	*Specific Abnormality*
Almost always present	Lymphopenia
	Selective T cell deficiency based on a quantitative reduction within the antigenic subset designated by OKT4 or anti–Leu-3 monoclonal antibodies (helper-inducer subset)
	Decreased or absent delayed cutaneous hypersensitivity to both recall and new antigens
	Elevated serum immunoglobulins, predominantly IgG and IgA in adults and including IgM in children
	Increased spontaneous immunoglobulin secretion by individual B cells
Consistently observed	Decreased in vitro lymphocyte proliferative responses to mitogens and antigens (alloantigens and autoantigens)
	Decreased cytotoxic responses by natural killer cells; decreased cell-mediated cytotoxicity (T cell)
	Decreased ability to mount a de novo antibody response to a new antigen
	Altered monocyte function
	Elevated serum levels of immune complexes
Occasionally present	Increased levels of acid-labile interferon-alpha
	Antilymphocyte antibodies
	Suppressor factors
	Increased levels of β_2-microglobulin and thymosin-α_1

infected cells and CD4 antigen on uninfected cells; the formation of microholes in the cell membrane, resulting in increased calcium penetration of the cell and subsequent cell death; direct cellular killing by the accumulation of unintegrated viral DNA in the cell cytoplasm; infection of precursors or cells that normally secrete factors necessary for continued regeneration of the lymphoid cell pool; and the autoimmune attack of uninfected cells resulting from cross-reactivity between the HIV envelope and a portion of the major histocompatibility complex (MHC) class II antigen.[46]

The importance of the CD4-gp120 interaction in the initiation of HIV infection is further underlined by three in vitro observations that could lead to successful therapeutic interventions. First, it has been found that an excess of a soluble form of the CD4 molecule or derivatives of this peptide will block the binding of the virus to CD4[+] T cells and thus prevent both infection and the formation of syncytia.[48-53] Second, recombinant CD4 that has been conjugated to the A chain of the toxin ricin will kill HIV-infected cells.[54] Third, anti-idiotype antibodies directed against a murine monoclonal antibody (anti–Leu-3a) that inhibits binding of HIV to CD4[+] T cells have been generated, and these anti-idiotype antibodies, which resemble the CD4 epitope, have been found to neutralize the virus. The development of an AIDS vaccine that induces anti-idiotype antibodies in an infected host could represent a novel approach to management.[55]

It was previously thought that following infection with HIV, the virus exerted a direct cytolytic effect on CD4[+] T cells; however, in vitro studies of long-term cultures of cells infected with HIV have shed new light on the pathogenetic mechanisms involved. Infected cells can be maintained for up to 50 to 60 days in cell culture, provided they do not undergo immunologic stimulation, in which case HIV replication is up-regulated and cell death follows quickly. In vitro, such events can be demonstrated to occur after antigenic, allogeneic, or mitogenic stimulation.[56-58] In the individual with HIV infection,

infections caused by CMV, the hepatitis viruses, herpes simplex virus, human T cell lymphotropic virus type I (HTLV-I), and other viruses are believed to play a similar role, as is allogeneic stimulation after exposure to semen, blood, or allografts. Studies of CMV suggest that other mechanisms may also be operative. Normally, CD4[+] T cells are relatively resistant to CMV infection; however, CD4[+] T cells infected with HIV will support productive infection with CMV, ultimately resulting in cell death. Thus, HIV-infected cells appear to be more susceptible to superinfection with other pathogens.[41] Conversely, CMV infection can facilitate infection with HIV. Thus, human fibroblasts infected with CMV can be infected via the CMV-induced Fc receptor, which will bind HIV that is complexed to antibody.[59] In addition, the function of HIV-infected T cells may be impaired because HIV may cause uncoupling of the events that normally follow antigen-specific stimulation (i.e., so-called signal transduction). As many as one in 100 CD4[+] T cells may be infected in AIDS patients.[60]

A second cell population that becomes infected with HIV is the subset of monocytes and macrophages that bears the CD4 surface molecule. Once infected, these cells live much longer than infected CD4[+] T cells. These monocytes and macrophages are resistant to both the cytolytic and syncytium-forming effects that HIV has on lymphocytes, possibly because they have a lower density of CD4 molecules on their surface. In vitro, hematopoietic growth factors such as granulocyte-macrophage colony-stimulating factor (GM-CSF) and macrophage colony-stimulating factor (M-CSF) as well as interferon gamma can be shown to alter the production of HIV-1 by infected mononuclear phagocytes. It is believed that infected monocytes and macrophages serve as important reservoirs of persistent infection within the host and as vehicles for transporting HIV to the central nervous system.[41,42,45,46,61,62]

HIV infection of monocytes and macrophages also results in a number of other important effects that probably contribute to clinical disease. First, HIV infection causes a significant deficit in chemotactic function. Second, infection and subsequent dysfunction of alveolar macrophages is probably a factor in the pathogenesis of *Pneumocystis carinii* pneumonia as well as in the pediatric syndrome of lymphocytic interstitial pneumonitis, although in the latter condition, Epstein-Barr virus infection probably also plays an important role. Third, interleukin-1 (IL-1) release by infected monocytes could explain the chronic fevers that occur in many patients with AIDS. Finally, infected monocytes also release tumor necrosis factor (cachectin), which could be important in the pathogenesis of the severe weight loss observed in some individuals with AIDS.[41,42,45,46]

It has been shown that myeloid progenitor cells in the normal bone marrow that express the CD34 surface marker can be infected in vitro with HIV. If such infection occurs in vivo, these cells could be another important reservoir of HIV in the body.[63]

Many patients with AIDS have evidence of a profound dysregulation of B cell function despite the presence of normal numbers of these lymphocytes. The B cells in these patients are spontaneously hyperactive and manifest a decreased proliferative response to T cell–independent B cell mitogens. Various B cell abnormalities are observed in vivo, including polyclonal activation, hypergammaglobulinemia, circulating immune complexes, autoantibodies, and a deficient antibody (particularly IgM) response to primary immunizations that is only partially explainable by the defect in CD4$^+$ T cell function. These abnormalities have been correlated with an increased risk of bloodstream invasion by and dissemination of *Streptococcus pneumoniae* and *Hemophilus influenzae* type b, both of which are encapsulated bacteria that require antibody production for effective opsonization.[41,42,45,46,64-67] The B cell abnormalities are not the result of direct infection by HIV, as is the case with HIV-induced impairment of CD4$^+$ T cells, monocytes, and macrophages; rather, the virus itself and subunits of it are polyclonal

activators of B cells. One such subunit, a portion of the HIV gp120 envelope glycoprotein, is homologous to neuroleukin, a factor that enhances B cell growth and differentiation. In addition, the Epstein-Barr virus and CMV, both very common causes of infection in persons with AIDS, are potent polyclonal B cell activators and could contribute to the B cell abnormalities.[41,42]

HIV also has a direct pathologic effect on the central nervous system. At least 60 percent of AIDS patients have neuropsychiatric abnormalities. Monocytes and macrophages are the predominant cell types in the brain to be infected with the virus, and it is believed that these cells transport the virus to the brain and release a variety of monokines, enzymes, and chemotactic factors that result in neuronal damage and inflammation of brain tissue.[41,42,45,46,68-70] In addition, the fact that some neurons and glial cells apparently can express the CD4 molecule lends credence to the hypothesis that direct HIV infection of brain tissue itself could play a role in the pathogenesis of AIDS-related neurodegenerative syndromes.[41,42] HIV-specific, HLA-restricted cytotoxic T cells have been isolated from the cerebrospinal fluid of AIDS patients, and it has been suggested that such cells could mediate neuronal damage.[71] It has also been proposed that the homology between a portion of the HIV gp120 envelope glycoprotein and neuroleukin may block the ability of neuroleukin to stimulate neuronal growth, thereby contributing to brain dysfunction. In vitro studies suggest that this effect may be blocked by vasoactive intestinal peptide.[45,46,72] High levels of unintegrated HIV DNA have been demonstrated in the brains of patients with AIDS dementia and presumably play a role in the pathogenesis of the dementia.[73]

Genomic analysis of retrovirus isolates from patients with AIDS has revealed that different isolates of the virus possess significant genomic diversity, which may have an impact on efforts to develop an effective vaccine. When virus is repeatedly isolated from the same patient during a period of one to two years, changes are observed throughout the viral genome as a result of a high rate of mutation from the original infecting virus. Such changes may have an impact on the cellular tropisms and clinical effects of an isolate. Thus, in vitro studies show that viral isolates from T cells infect T cells more effectively than they infect macrophages; conversely, macrophage isolates are better adapted to infect macrophages than T cells. Similarly, viral isolates from brain tissue may be particularly adapted to the infection of brain-derived cells, a function that lymphocyte-derived virus accomplishes quite poorly, if at all. Some brain-derived isolates appear not to produce cytopathic effects in CD4[+] T cells but still cause persistent infection of neuronal cells.[41,74-77] In addition, it has been suggested that progression from an asymptomatic state to AIDS is associated with the isolation of increasingly cytopathic strains of virus from the same individual.[78] Single amino acid changes in the HIV envelope have been shown to change both the cell tropism of the virus and its susceptibility to attack by cytotoxic T cells.[79,80] Thus, the variability in the HIV genome may play an important role in determining both the sites and the extent of viral attack.

Despite the extreme immune perturbations caused by HIV, the infected host is able to mount an immune response to the virus after infection. Antibodies to a variety of viral proteins are easily detected and, indeed, form the basis of most diagnostic tests [*see* Clinical Features and Diagnosis, *below*]. The presence of neutralizing antibodies in the serum of individuals with both asymptomatic infection and AIDS suggests, however, that such antibodies offer little protection against the development of disease. Indeed, it has been suggested that antibody to HIV could facilitate entry of the virus into cells through the binding of antibody-virus complexes to Fc receptors.[81,82] Similarly, it has been shown that complement-fixing antibodies bound to HIV can facilitate infection by binding to complement receptors on certain cells.[83] HIV-specific cytotoxic T cells can be demonstrated in

infected individuals, and at least some cytotoxic activity is directed against the viral enzyme reverse transcriptase.[84] It can also be shown that in vitro, CD8[+] lymphocytes can suppress HIV replication.[85]

At this point, however, two major questions regarding the host immune response to HIV remain to be answered. First, can one or more of these responses be correlated with protection against the virus and lack of progression to disease? Second, can any of these responses be amplified or induced by a vaccine to confer protection? Answers to these questions are of critical importance and are being avidly sought.

Role of Secondary Viral Infection

Although retrovirus infection has now been implicated as the cause of the immune defect that leads to opportunistic infections in patients with AIDS, other viral infections that are commonly present in these patients probably contribute to clinical events in at least four ways: (1) by immune stimulation of HIV-infected CD4[+] T cells, which could result in cell death,[41,42,45,46] (2) by immune modulation, which contributes to the net state of immunosuppression,[86] (3) by the production of clinical infectious disease syndromes specific for the viruses themselves, and (4) by the role such secondary viral infections play in the pathogenesis of at least some of the malignant disorders that develop during the course of AIDS.

In regard to the last category, several malignant disorders have been linked to specific viral infections in patients with HIV infection. Epstein-Barr virus is highly associated with the development of Burkitt's lymphoma and B cell lymphoproliferative disease; herpes simplex virus type 2 infection is associated with cloacogenic carcinoma of the rectum and squamous cell carcinoma of the anus; and herpes simplex virus type 1 is associated with squamous cell carcinoma of the tongue. A two-step model has been proposed to explain these events. The first step involves the development of HIV-induced immunodeficiency, which is manifested by an increased incidence of opportunistic infection. The exaggerated or prolonged clinical response to viral infection that is observed in certain patients represents the second step, which results in tumor development.[87]

Perhaps the clearest example of virally induced malignant disease is the occurrence of Epstein-Barr virus–related B cell lymphomas in AIDS patients. The malignant cells in these lymphomas contain Epstein-Barr virus DNA and display characteristic chromosomal translocations.[88-90] In addition, there is a particularly high risk of such lymphomas developing in AIDS patients because they have abnormally high numbers of Epstein-Barr virus–infected B cells in their circulation as well as a profound defect of T cell immunity to this potentially oncogenic virus.[91] The net result is epidemic B cell lymphoproliferative disease.[88-91] Non-Hodgkin's lymphomas that may be related to other viruses also occur more frequently in these patients.[92]

Clinical Features

The clinical manifestations of AIDS can be divided into four general categories: those caused by the direct effects of HIV, those related to the opportunistic infections resulting from HIV-induced immunosuppression, those caused by Kaposi's sarcoma, and those that arise from the combined effects of HIV-induced immunosuppression and the malignancy-promoting effects of other viruses.

The direct clinical effects of the virus appear to be very broad. Prospective studies of homosexual male populations and of transplant recipients who received allografts from HIV-infected donors have revealed that in some individuals who are initially seronegative for the virus, an infectious mononucleosis–like illness associated with acute HIV infection develops three weeks to three months after exposure. The illness has been characterized by a sudden onset and a duration of up to 14 days; its prominent features include fevers, sweats, malaise, fatigability, myalgias, arthralgias, headache, sore throat, diarrhea, generalized lymphadenopathy, a macular erythematous truncal eruption, and thrombocytopenia. Serial studies in a few of these individuals revealed that seroconversion occurred three to eight weeks after the onset of symptoms; in addition, a decrease (inversion) in the ratio of circulating $CD4^+$ helper-inducer T cells to $CD8^+$ suppressor-cytotoxic T cells was noted shortly after the onset of acute illness.[21,93-95]

Much more common than this acute illness is a persistent version of the syndrome. About 10 to 30 percent of homosexual men who ultimately acquire AIDS have an otherwise unexplained persistent, generalized lymphadenopathy, sometimes associated with fever and malaise, for several months before the onset of the syndrome. Biopsy of lymph nodes in such patients typically reveals nonspecific hyperplasia. Approximately 15 to 25 percent of homosexual or bisexual men who have the generalized lymphadenopathy syndrome will have progressed to AIDS after one year. Patients with the lymphadenopathy syndrome resemble AIDS patients in terms of past sexual practices, history of other infections and drug use, increased prevalence of histocompatibility antigen HLA-DR5, and presence of antibody to HIV. Because of these considerations, the generalized lymphadenopathy syndrome is regarded by most investigators as a prodromal form of AIDS and has been termed the AIDS-related complex (ARC).[96,97]

The most important direct clinical effect of HIV infection is on the nervous system. The brain appears to serve as a privileged sanctuary for HIV replication after infected monocytes and macrophages transport the virus across the blood-brain barrier. Various neurologic syndromes are directly ascribable to HIV infection [see Table 4].[98] The most important syndrome is subacute encephalitis, also termed AIDS encephalopathy or the AIDS dementia complex, which is characterized by a progressive dementia, psychomotor retardation, focal motor abnormalities, and behavioral changes. Clinical manifestations of this disorder are found in at least two thirds of patients with AIDS, and pathologic evidence of the disorder is found in about 90 percent of patients. However, because neurologic manifestations may be associated with central ner-

Table 4   Neurologic Disorders Associated with HIV Infection

Neurologic Disorder	Prevalence (%)	Clinical Features	Histopathologic Features
Subacute encephalitis	90	Cognitive deficits, memory loss, psychomotor slowing, pyramidal tract signs, ataxia, weakness, depression, organic psychosis, incontinence, myoclonic seizures	Gliosis, myelin pallor, microglial nodules, perivascular inflammation, focal demyelination, multinucleate giant cells
Peripheral neuropathies	10–50		
Chronic distal symmetric polyneuropathy		Painful dysesthesias, numbness, paresthesias, weakness, autonomic dysfunction	Demyelination, axonal loss, mild inflammation
Chronic inflammatory demyelinating polyneuropathy		Weakness, sensory deficits, mononeuropathy multiplex, cranial nerve palsies, hyporeflexia or areflexia, cerebrospinal fluid pleocytosis	Marked inflammation, demyelination with secondary axonal loss
Vacuolar myelopathy	11–22	Gait ataxia, progressive spastic paraparesis, posterior column deficits, incontinence	Vacuolar degeneration of lateral and posterior columns
Aseptic meningitis	5–10	Headache, fever, meningeal signs, cranial nerve palsies, cerebrospinal fluid pleocytosis	—

vous system disease caused by such organisms as *Cryptococcus neoformans*, *Toxoplasma gondii*, *Treponema pallidum*, and JC virus (progressive multifocal leukoencephalopathy) as well as with B cell lymphoma, the clinician must search for these entities in the HIV-infected individual with neurologic complaints or findings.[41,98-101]

Various other abnormalities may also arise from the direct effects of the virus. An enteropathy that is characterized by malabsorption and mucosal abnormalities of the small intestine and that is not attributable to other infectious agents has been observed.[102] In addition, a gastropathy characterized by impaired gastric acid secretion has been defined in AIDS patients. The gastropathy results in an increased susceptibility to such enteric pathogens as *Salmonella* and *Campylo-*

bacter and also causes malabsorption of the antifungal drug ketoconazole.[103,104] Renal dysfunction, often accompanied by proteinuria, is increasingly being found in AIDS patients. Kidney biopsies reveal a focal and segmental glomerulosclerosis with significant abnormalities in the mesangium. In addition, reversible episodes of acute renal failure are not uncommon in these patients, and terminal episodes of acute renal insufficiency may occur.[105-107] Although dialysis can be useful in the management of potentially reversible acute renal failure in patients with AIDS, it is not effective in prolonging life in AIDS patients with chronic renal disease. Congestive cardiomyopathy apparently related to HIV infection of the myocardium has been reported.[108] Thyroid function is altered during the course of HIV infection by as yet unclear mechanisms. As disease progresses, there is a steady decline in reverse triiodothyronine (rT_3) levels and an increase in levels of thyroxine-binding globulin. Low serum triiodothyronine (T_3) levels correlate with mortality, whereas normal T_3 levels may contribute to cachexia in patients with AIDS.[109]

A number of rheumatologic phenomena are associated with HIV infection: various types of arthritis, ranging from Reiter's syndrome and psoriatic arthritis to an arthritis primarily affecting the lower extremities; myopathies, including polymyositis; vasculitis; a sicca syndrome resembling Sjögren's syndrome that is associated with the histocompatibility antigen HLA-DR5 and characterized by an infiltration by $CD8^+$ lymphocytes; and a syndrome mimicking systemic lupus erythematosus, with laboratory findings that include the presence of antinuclear and anticardiolipin antibodies.[110,111] Other unusual clinical manifestations of AIDS that are presumably autoimmune in nature include autoimmune thrombocytopenia,[112,113] thrombotic thrombocytopenic purpura,[114,115] various endocrine and metabolic disorders (e.g., hypercalcemia and adrenal insufficiency),[116] a nonspecific interstitial pneumonitis that clinically mimics *Pneumocystis* infection,[117,118] a recrudescence of atopy, and a marked increase in the incidence and severity of allergic reactions to trimethoprim-sulfamethoxazole.[96]

Far more commonly, the presenting clinical manifestations of AIDS are associated with a syndrome caused by an opportunistic infection [*see* Table 5]. The most common presentation is *P. carinii* pneumonia, the initial clinical disorder in about 50 percent of cases.[6-8,87-96] HIV-infected individuals are at particular risk for *Pneumocystis* infection if their $CD4^+$ T cell counts fall below $200/mm^3$ or if thrush or unexplained fevers develop.[119,120] *Pneumocystis* pneumonia is usually manifested in AIDS patients by the subacute development of a nonproductive cough and dyspnea over a period of days to weeks. Typically, interstitial pneumonitis is evident on the chest x-ray, and arterial blood

gas measurements reveal hypoxia and hypercapnia. However, despite negative findings on x-ray, a significant minority of AIDS patients with cough and dyspnea have *P. carinii* infection confirmed by biopsy. In such patients, a positive result on gallium scan or abnormal results on pulmonary function tests can also suggest the presence of *Pneumocystis* infection.

Two aspects differentiate *Pneumocystis* infection in AIDS patients from that in immunocompromised patients without AIDS. First, in AIDS patients, the number of organisms is so high that the diagnosis can often be made noninvasively through the examination of expectorated sputum, particularly by immunofluorescent techniques using monoclonal antibodies.[121] Second, AIDS patients may experience metastatic infection to other organs, particularly the skin.[122]

Approximately 12 percent of patients present with an opportunistic infection other than *P. carinii* pneumonia. Among the more common opportunistic infections appear to be recurrent mucosal candidiasis, disseminated cytomegalovirus infection, and severe, progressively ulcerating perianal herpes simplex virus infection. Other opportunistic infections that are unusually common, even for immunosuppressed individuals, are disseminated atypical mycobacterial infection, toxoplasmosis (particularly of the central nervous system), and severe, persistent diarrhea caused by *Cryptosporidium* or *Isospora belli* infection. Other gastrointestinal pathogens, such as *C. jejuni* and *Shigella* species, also have a higher incidence and greater severity in patients with AIDS.[6-8,87-96,123-126] In addition, AIDS patients are at particular risk for recurrent *Salmonella* bacteremia and disseminated salmonellosis.[127,128] Disseminated cat-scratch disease has been observed in AIDS patients.[129] Biliary tract disease, ranging from acalculous cholecystitis[130] to benign strictures of the biliary tract,[131] is increasingly being observed in AIDS patients. The pathogenesis of biliary tract disease is somewhat complex: HIV-induced immunodeficiency results in severe cytomegalovirus infection or cryptosporidiosis, and these secondary in-

Table 5   Infectious Complications of AIDS

Infecting Organism		*Type of Infection*
Viruses	Cytomegalovirus	Pneumonia, disseminated infection, retinitis, encephalitis
	Epstein-Barr virus	Important pathogenic factor in B cell lymphoproliferative disorders and Burkitt's lymphoma, oral hairy leukoplakia
	Herpes simplex virus	Recurrent severe localized infection
	Varicella-zoster virus	Localized or disseminated infection
	Papovavirus	Progressive multifocal leukoencephalopathy
Fungi	*Candida albicans*	Mucocutaneous infection, esophagitis, disseminated infection
	Cryptococcus neoformans	Meningitis, disseminated infection
	Histoplasma capsulatum	Disseminated infection
	Coccidioides immitis	Dissseminated infection
	Petriellidium boydii	Pneumonia
	Aspergillus	Invasive pulmonary infection with potential for dissemination
Protozoa	*Pneumocystis carinii*	Pneumonia, retinal infection
	Toxoplasma gondii	Encephalitis
	Cryptosporidium	Enteritis
	Isospora belli	Enteritis
Mycobacteria	*Mycobacterium avium-intracellulare*	Disseminated infection
	Mycobacterium tuberculosis	Disseminated infection
Bacteria	*Nocardia*	Pneumonia, disseminated infection
	Legionella	Pneumonia
	Streptococcus pneumoniae	Pneumonia, disseminated infection
	Hemophilus influenzae type B	Pneumonia, disseminated infection
	Salmonella	Gastroenteritis, disseminated infection

fections have a significant impact on the biliary tract.

Secondary infections caused by *Mycobacterium* species are particularly difficult to treat in AIDS patients. In patients from population groups with a high endemic rate of *M. tuberculosis* or *M. kansasii* disease, reactivation infections caused by these organisms predominate. In areas such as New York City and parts of Florida, where the prevalence of HIV-related tuberculosis is relatively high, there has been a significant increase in recent years in the overall number of cases of tuberculosis caused by these organisms. In population groups with a low prevalence of *M. tuberculosis* infection, *M. avium-intracellulare* infection is the rule. In all AIDS patients, extrapulmonary forms of tuberculosis, particularly those affecting the bloodstream, the central nervous system, the gastrointestinal tract, the lymphatic system, and the bone marrow, are much more common than classic pulmonary tuberculosis; disseminated tuberculosis is also common. Indeed, even when the lungs are involved, atypical presentations that cannot be distinguished from more common pulmonary infections in this setting, such as *P. carinii* pneumonia, are common.[132-136]

Syphilis has become a major problem in HIV-infected individuals. The problem is partly a result of the fact that the male homosexual population that has borne the brunt of the AIDS epidemic has long been recognized as having an especially high incidence of syphilis and other sexually transmitted diseases. Genital ulcers produced by syphilis increase the risk of transmission and acquisition of HIV. Syphilis testing is therefore recommended for patients with newly diagnosed HIV infection; similarly, those with newly diagnosed syphilis should be tested for HIV infection. In addition, syphilis presents unique clinical and diagnostic dilemmas in HIV-infected individuals. First, diagnosis may be difficult in these patients because the standard serologic tests that form the cornerstone of a syphilis diagnosis may be falsely negative as a result of the patient's immunocompromised state. Tissue biopsy and subsequent examination of the biopsy material for spirochetes with special stains is sometimes the only effective diagnostic modality. Second, patients with AIDS may not respond to what has traditionally been effective antimicrobial therapy. Such patients may progress to neurosyphilis after a very short incubation period, even though standard penicillin therapy for early syphilis has been given. The use of maintenance penicillin therapy to prevent the consequences of neurosyphilis in HIV-infected individuals is a concept that bears consideration, particularly in patients with demonstrable immunocompromise.[137-140]

AIDS patients are also at risk for conventional bacterial infections, which may be grouped into two general categories: infections caused by the encapsulated organisms *S. pneumoniae* and *H. influenzae* type b, which lead to a high rate of pneumonia and bacteremia as a result of impaired B cell function, and infection caused by organisms such as *Shigella* and *Campylobacter*, which rarely produce severe or prolonged disease in the normal host but commonly cause protracted clinical disease and bloodstream invasion in the patient with AIDS.[65-67]

Approximately 30 percent of AIDS patients have presented with Kaposi's sarcoma, and another seven percent have presented with both *Pneumocystis* pneumonia and Kaposi's sarcoma.[6-8,87,96] It has been suggested that the incidence of Kaposi's sarcoma in AIDS patients is now decreasing, although the reasons for such a decrease are unclear.[141] Patients who present with Kaposi's sarcoma alone generally have a less severe immune defect than patients who present with *Pneumocystis* or another opportunistic infection. Unlike classic Kaposi's sarcoma, which usually has a cutaneous presentation and indolent course, the form of the disease that develops in patients with AIDS is a multicentric disease process that frequently involves lymph nodes and visceral organs, particularly in the gastrointestinal tract. Kaposi's sarcoma can cause both pulmonary infiltrates and respiratory failure in patients with AIDS.

Reportedly, the HIV *tat* gene induces skin lesions resembling Kaposi's sarcoma in transgenic mice, a finding that suggests that this tumor may be a direct manifestation of HIV infection.[142] Evidence is also beginning to emerge that suggests a close relation between HIV-infected cells and this tumor. For example, retrovirus-infected CD4$^+$ T cells produce growth factors that support the growth of Kaposi's sarcoma cells.[143] These Kaposi's sarcoma cells themselves produce cytokines that induce not only their own growth but also the growth of normal human endothelial cells and fibroblasts.[144]

The previously described tumors, particularly the lymphomas, are also a common cause of clinical symptoms in patients with AIDS. In addition, a cutaneous vascular neoplasm distinct from Kaposi's sarcoma but also capable of visceral metastasis has been described in patients with AIDS. This entity has been termed epithelioid angiomatosis. Although experience with this tumor is limited, it has caused death from disseminated intravascular coagulation and laryngeal obstruction in some individuals with AIDS.[145]

A patient may have more than one opportunistic infection or malignant disorder associated with AIDS. In addition, multiple diseases may concurrently affect a single patient or even a single tissue or structure. Of growing concern is the occurrence of simultaneous infection with two retroviruses, particularly HIV-1 and HTLV-I. When such simultaneous infection occurs, the clinical course may be accelerated and the clinical manifestations may be more diverse.[5,146,147]

The Centers for Disease Control has proposed the following clinical classification system for HIV infection[93]:

1. Group I—acute HIV infection. Patients have a syndrome similar to infectious mononucleosis, with or without aseptic meningitis, associated with seroconversion for HIV antibody.

2. Group II—asymptomatic HIV infection. Patients have no manifestations or history of HIV infection (except for a possible history of an illness similar to infectious mononucleosis). Patients with previous designations of manifestations of groups III or IV should not be reclassified as group II when these problems resolve. Patients in group II may be subclassified further on the basis of such laboratory findings as the presence or absence of lymphopenia, thrombocytopenia, and decreased number of helper T cells.

3. Group III—persistent generalized lymphadenopathy. Patients have palpable lymphadenopathy (lymph node enlargement > 1 cm) at two or more extrainguinal sites persisting for more than three months in the absence of a concurrent illness or condition other than HIV infection. Again, patients may be further subclassified on the basis of laboratory findings, as previously noted. Patients with group IV findings that resolve should not be reclassified as group III.

4. Group IV—other HIV disease.
   a. Subgroup A—constitutional disease. One or more of the following are present: fever persisting for more than one month, involuntary weight loss of more than 10 percent of baseline, or diarrhea persisting for more than one month with no explanation other than HIV infection.
   b. Subgroup B—neurologic disease. One or more of the following are present: dementia, myelopathy, or peripheral neuropathy occurring with no explanation other than HIV infection.
   c. Subgroup C—secondary infectious disease. Patients have an infectious process associated with defects in cell-mediated immunity with no explanation other than HIV infection. These infectious diseases are subdivided into two categories. Category C-1 includes patients with symptomatic or invasive disease stemming from one or more of the 12 specified secondary infectious diseases listed in the CDC surveillance definition of AIDS: *P. carinii* pneumonia, chronic cryptosporidiosis, toxoplasmosis, extraintestinal strongyloidiasis, isosporiasis, candidiasis (esophageal, bronchial, or pulmonary), cryptococcosis, histoplasmosis, mycobacterial infection with *M. avium-intracellulare* or *M. kansasii,* cytomegalovirus infection, chronic mucocutaneous or disseminated herpes simplex virus infection, or progressive multifocal leukoencephalopathy. Category C-2 includes patients with symptomatic or invasive disease arising from six other specified secondary infectious diseases: oral hairy leukoplakia, multidermatomal herpes zoster, recurrent *Salmonella* bacteremia, nocardiosis, tuberculosis, or oral candidiasis (thrush).
   d. Subgroup D—secondary cancers. Patients have one or more of the following cancers associated with HIV infection and included as part of the CDC surveillance definition of AIDS: Kaposi's sarcoma, non-Hodgkin's lymphoma (small, noncleaved lymphoma or immunoblastic sarcoma), or primary lymphoma of the brain.

e. Subgroup E—other conditions in HIV infection. Patients have unclassifiable clinical findings or diseases, such as chronic lymphoid interstitial pneumonitis, that may be attributed to HIV infection or may indicate a defect in cell-mediated immunity. Also included are patients whose signs and symptoms could be attributed to HIV infection or another, coexisting disease not classified elsewhere and those patients with other clinical illnesses in which the course or management may be complicated or altered by HIV infection.

An alternative prognostic staging system has been devised based on such physiologic deficits as severe diarrhea, hypoalbuminemia, neurologic deficit, hypoxia, and hematologic dysfunction.[148] This prognostic index should be particularly useful for evaluating innovative therapies.

Laboratory Findings and Diagnosis

Three diagnostic issues need to be addressed when approaching a patient with possible HIV infection and clinical manifestations possibly stemming from such infection: the diagnosis of HIV infection, the diagnosis of AIDS itself, and the diagnosis of the array of complicating infections and malignant disorders that occur in patients with HIV infection. It is important to emphasize that the diagnosis of HIV infection does not constitute a diagnosis of AIDS. As outlined in the CDC clinical classification system [*see* Clinical Features, *above*], HIV infection causes a continuum of manifestations, and the exact classification of a patient with HIV infection is made on the basis of the clinical syndrome rather than on the basis of laboratory tests. Currently, there is no single test that can yield an unequivocal laboratory diagnosis of AIDS, including assays for anti-HIV antibody or even isolation of the virus. Nevertheless, specific laboratory tests enhance certain aspects of clinical assessment and management of AIDS.

The major advance in diagnosis has been the development of tests for measuring antibody to HIV. More than 90 percent of patients with AIDS harbor antibodies to the virus, and more than 95 percent of asymptomatic carriers of the virus are antibody positive. For practical purposes, anyone who is antibody positive should be assumed to have transmissible virus in his or her blood and bodily secretions. Thus, antibody testing is important in screening blood and organ donors [*see* Table 6].

Currently available ELISA tests, which measure antibody against HIV envelope antigens, appear to have a false positive rate of much less than one percent and a false negative rate of less than three percent. Serum samples that are positive by ELISA are rechecked with a more specific confirmatory test, usually the Western blot assay. In the Western blot assay, a lysate of HIV-1 is separated into its individual protein components by polyacrylamide gel electrophoresis. These proteins are transferred onto nitrocellulose paper and then exposed to the patient's serum. Any antibody that adheres to a protein band can be detected by an anti–human IgG antibody that in the presence of a substrate yields a color reaction. This technique permits assessment of the serum for antibodies to particular HIV antigens. Although a variety of criteria have been prepared by different groups, a positive test result generally requires the presence of antibody to two or more antigens. For example, one commercially licensed assay requires the presence of antibodies to the p24 core antigen (a product of the *gag* gene), the p31 antigen (a product of the *pol* gene), and the gp41, gp120, or gp160 envelope antigens (products of the *env* gene) for a positive result to be reported. A negative test would not have antibodies to any of these antigens. All other patterns are regarded as indeterminate. In general, strongly positive or clearly negative ELISA tests will be confirmed by Western blot assay, whereas weakly positive ELISA tests will be negative or indeterminate by Western blot testing. Studies of potential blood donors with persistently indeterminate Western blot tests have shown that these

---

Table 6 Recommendations for Screening Donated Blood and Plasma for Antibody to HIV

Initial Testing

Persons accepted as donors should be informed that their blood or plasma will be tested for HIV antibody. Persons not wishing to have their blood or plasma tested must refrain from donation. Donors should be told that they will be notified if their test is positive and that they may be placed on the collection facility's donor deferral list, as is currently practiced with other infectious diseases, and should be informed of the identities of additional deferral lists to which the positive donors may be added.

All blood plasma should be tested for HIV antibody by ELISA. Any blood or plasma that is positive on initial testing must not be transfused or manufactured into other products capable of transmitting infectious agents.

When the ELISA test is used to screen populations in whom the prevalence of HIV infections is low, the proportion of positive results that are falsely positive will be high. Therefore, the ELISA test should be repeated on all seropositive specimens before the donor is notified. If the repeat ELISA test is negative, the specimen should be tested by another technique.

Other Testing

Other tests have included immunofluorescence and radioimmunoprecipitation assays, but the most extensive experience has been with the Western blot technique, in which antibodies to HIV proteins of specific molecular weights can be detected. Based on available data, the Western blot should be considered positive for antibody to HIV if band p24 or gp41 is present (alone or in combination with other bands).

Notification of Donors

If the repeat ELISA test is positive or if other tests are positive, it is the responsibility of the collection facility to ensure that the donor is notified. The information should be given to the donor by an individual especially aware of the sensitivities involved. At present, the proportion of these seropositive donors who have been infected with HIV is not known. It is, therefore, important to emphasize to the donor that the positive result is a preliminary finding that may not represent true infection. To determine the significance of a positive test, the donor should be referred to a physician for evaluation. The information should be given to the donor in a manner to ensure confidentiality of the results and of the donor's identity.

Maintaining Confidentiality

Physicians, laboratory and nursing personnel, and others should recognize the importance of maintaining confidentiality of positive test results. Disclosure of this information for purposes other than medical or public health concerns could lead to serious consequences for the individual. Screening procedures should be designed with safeguards to protect against unauthorized disclosure. Donors should be given a clear explanation of how information about them will be handled. Facilities should consider developing contingency plans in the event that disclosure is sought through legal processes. If donor deferral lists are kept, it is necessary to maintain confidentiality of such lists. Whenever appropriate, as an additional safeguard, donor deferral lists should be general, without indication of the reason for inclusion.

---

individuals are rarely if ever infected with either HIV-1 or HIV-2.[149-152]

Typically, the conventional ELISA antibody tests become positive one to three months after infection with HIV, at approximately the same time some patients experience the acute HIV infectious mononucleosis–like syndrome. However, it has now become apparent that the typical pattern of seroconversion is not universal and that prolonged periods of viral infection (and potential transmissibility) may occur in the presence of a negative ELISA or Western blot antibody test.[153-155] In geographic areas with high rates of HIV infection, HIV has been isolated from seven to 15 percent of antibody-negative homosexual men.[154,156] Consistent with these observations is a report that HIV was isolated from the blood of 23 percent of seronegative homosexual men in Los Angeles who continued to engage in high-risk sexual behavior. Seronegativity was documented to

---

Table 6   (Continued)

Medical Evaluation

The evaluation might incude ELISA testing of a follow-up serum specimen and Western blot testing, if the specimen is positive. Persons who continue to show serologic evidence of HIV infection should be questioned about possible exposure to the virus or possible risk factors for AIDS in the individual or his or her sexual contacts and examined for signs of AIDS or related conditions, such as lymphadenopathy, oral candidiasis, Kaposi's sarcoma, and unexplained weight loss. Additional laboratory studies might include tests for other sexually transmitted diseases, tests of immune function, and where available, tests for the presence of the virus, such as viral culture. Testing for antibodies to HIV in the individual's sexual contacts may also be useful in establishing whether the test results truly represent infection.

Recommendations for the Individual

An individual judged most likely to have an HIV infection should be provided the following information and advice:

1. The long-term prognosis for an individual infected with HIV is not known. However, data available from studies conducted among homosexual men indicate that most persons will remain infected.

2. Although asymptomatic, these individuals may transmit HIV to others. Regular medical evaluation and follow-up are advised, especially for individuals who acquire signs or symptoms suggestive of AIDS.

3. Refrain from donating blood, plasma, body organs, other tissue, or sperm.

4. There is a risk of infecting others by sexual intercourse, sharing of needles, and possibly, exposure of others to saliva through oral-genital contact or intimate kissing. The efficacy of condoms in preventing infection with HIV is unproved, but the consistent use of them may reduce transmission.

5. Toothbrushes, razors, or other implements that could become contaminated with blood should not be shared.

6. Women with a seropositive test, or women whose sexual partner is seropositive, are themselves at increased risk of acquiring AIDS. If they become pregnant, their offspring are also at increased risk of acquiring AIDS.

7. After accidents resulting in bleeding, contaminated surfaces should be cleaned with household bleach freshly diluted 1:10 in water.

8. Devices that have punctured the skin, such as hypodermic and acupuncture needles, should be steam sterilized by autoclave before reuse or safely discarded. Whenever possible, disposable needles and equipment should be used.

9. When seeking medical or dental care for intercurrent illness, these persons should inform those responsible for their care of their positive antibody status so that appropriate evaluation can be undertaken and precautions taken to prevent transmission to others.

10. Testing for HIV antibody should be offered to persons who may have been infected as a result of their contact with seropositive individuals (e.g., sexual partners, persons with whom needles have been shared, or infants born to seropositive mothers).

---

persist for periods of at least 36 months in some of these individuals.[157] Similarly, immunosuppressed patients (e.g., transplant recipients) with HIV infection may have a greatly delayed antibody response.[158] In addition, reversion to antibody-negative status by asymptomatic individuals harboring HIV-1 has now been documented.[159] These observations place an increased emphasis on the need for the development and deployment of other HIV diagnostic tests, such as detection of circulating HIV antigens (p24 is the leading candidate at present), detection of HIV DNA by the polymerase chain reaction, or viral culture.[153,154,160-162]

Laboratory markers to assess the prognosis for patients with HIV infection are being actively pursued. At present, the most accurate marker for disease progression is the serial measurement of the level of circulating $CD4^+$ T cells; levels lower than $200/mm^3$ are highly associated with disease progression.[163,164] It has been shown that the level of HIV in plasma and peripheral blood mononuclear cells is much higher than originally thought and that quantitation of the level of virus in the plasma is a useful marker of the status of the disease.[161,165] Other markers that can be useful are the level of p24 antigen in the serum and the levels of serum neopterin and β_2-microglobulin; the last two markers provide a measure of the degree of immune activation.[159,160,164] Such prognostic markers will probably have an increasingly important role in the planning and management of antiviral therapy and in the institution of prophylactic measures against opportunistic infection in HIV-infected individuals.

Although testing for anti-HIV antibody is reasonable when examining a patient suspected of having AIDS, it is essential that the clinician first undertake an aggressive investigation of the particular symptom complex manifested by the patient. Thus, lung infiltrates merit induced sputum examination, bronchoalveolar lavage, or biopsy; central nervous system symptoms should prompt a CT scan, lumbar puncture, and, possibly, brain biopsy; diarrhea should be investigated by culture and examination for parasites; and mass lesions of any type warrant a biopsy. Because multiple or sequential infections as well as malignant disorders are the rule in AIDS patients, constant surveillance is essential to ensure that a patient does not have more than one complication.

Management

Management of AIDS requires a combination of approaches: preventive, therapeutic, and supportive. The need for a coordinated attack is underlined by the magnitude of this unprecedented epidemic. It has been projected that as many as 480,000 cases of AIDS, with up to 340,000 deaths, will have occurred in the United States by the end of 1993, six times the number of American combat deaths in the Vietnam War.[11] It has been estimated that the first 10,000 patients with AIDS in the United States accounted for or will account for 1.6 million days spent in the hospital (at a cost of more than $1.4 billion), 8,387 years of missed work, and $4.8 billion in lost potential earnings.[166] Already, the financial costs of caring for AIDS patients is having a major impact on both the medical and financial resources of many hospitals, particularly public teaching hospitals. Until more effective treatments become available, a major emphasis must be placed on prevention.

A high priority has been given to the development of an effective vaccine against HIV; however, formidable barriers to its development remain. Although individuals with AIDS mount some form of an immune response against HIV [*see* Pathogenesis, *above*], it is not clear what aspects of the immune response afford protection against disease and against which antigens a vaccine should be directed. Similarly, the genomic and antigenic heterogeneity of the virus and a lack of animal models of HIV infection, other than chimpanzees, for testing a candidate vaccine greatly complicate efforts at developing an effective vaccine against AIDS.[167]

Until an effective vaccine is developed, prevention must involve more traditional public health interventions. These methods include antibody testing to protect blood and organ recipients and education about the danger of sharing needles during intravenous drug use. Methadone treatment clinics appear to be particularly useful sites both for limiting the intravenous drug–associated spread of HIV infection and for providing primary care of individuals already infected with the virus.[168-170] Programs that educate the public about safer sexual practices, including the roles of promiscuity and anal intercourse in facilitating transmission of the virus, also need to be stressed. In addition, evidence suggests that the use of condoms and perhaps a spermicide containing the compound nonoxynol 9 will decrease the risk of sexual transmission of HIV.[171-173]

One of the most controversial aspects of attempts to prevent the spread of HIV infection is the role of antibody testing as a screening device for detecting subclinical infection. So far, compulsory testing for such purposes as premarital screening has been viewed as a relatively ineffective and inefficient use of resources. Far more difficult is the issue of whether to test patients in the hospital environment as a means of protecting health care workers. On the one hand, the risk of HIV transmission in the health care setting is extremely low: the rate of transmission is less than 0.5 percent after direct inoculation of infected blood through a needle-stick injury and even lower after other exposure. On the other hand, the risk is not zero, and there is controversy regarding the utility of knowing the HIV status of all patients. At present, emphasis has been placed on the application of universal precautions within the hospital environment rather than universal screening [*see Table 7*].[174-177]

Therapy for patients with AIDS can be divided into two categories: treatment aimed at the HIV infection itself and treatment aimed at the secondary infections and malignant disorders associated with HIV infection.

Zidovudine (also known as AZT) is the first drug to be licensed by the FDA for the treatment of HIV infection. This thymidine analogue acts by inhibiting the viral enzyme reverse transcriptase and terminating DNA chain synthesis. The clinical benefit of zidovudine was first demonstrated in a double-blind, placebo-controlled study in which 200 mg of the drug was administered every four hours to individuals with AIDS or severe ARC.[178,179] Although efficacy was clearly demonstrated, anemia and granulocytopenia were significant problems, and total bone marrow failure was also noted.[180] Because of these side effects, zidovudine was given in combination with the potent hematopoietic hormone GM-CSF, and results of these trials have been promising.[181] More recently, the administration of 500 mg/day of zidovudine for the treatment of AIDS or severe ARC has been shown to be at least as effective as the higher dosage and to be relatively free of major hematologic toxicity.[182] In a subsequent landmark study, the administration of zidovudine at this lower dosage was shown to provide clear benefit to asymptomatic, HIV-infected individuals with CD4[+] T cell counts lower than 500/mm^3, thus justifying the earlier initiation of zidovudine therapy.[182,183] An important feature of zidovudine is that the drug appears to cross the blood-brain barrier and improve neurologic function in patients with HIV infection of the CNS.[178,184]

Prolonged zidovudine therapy appears to confer continuing survival benefits,[185] although zidovudine-resistant HIV isolates may emerge after six months of therapy. It has been suggested that these resistant isolates may be responsible for the clinical deterioration observed in some patients after six to 18 months of a therapeutic response to zidovudine.[186,187] Despite the concerns regarding resistance, zidovudine has been shown to be effective in children with AIDS and in patients with thrombocytopenia.[188,189] Zidovudine by itself has been shown to have antiretroviral activity in AIDS patients with Kaposi's sarcoma,[190] and when zidovudine was administered with interferon alfa, both antiviral and antitumor responses were noted.[191]

The finding of zidovudine resistance underlines the need for alternative strategies for treating HIV infection. Such new strategies include agents that inhibit HIV attachment to or entry into cells, such as recombinant soluble CD4 and CD4 immunoadhesins; immunotoxins; inhibitors of reverse transcriptase activity other than zidovudine, including 2′,3′-dideoxycytidine (ddC), 2′,3′-dideoxyinosine (ddI), and foscarnet; inhibitors of other important HIV enzymes, such as HIV protease; and biologic response modifiers.[43,44,54,192-195] Phase I studies in a small number of patients with AIDS or ARC found that the administration of ddI led to decreases in the serum levels of p24 antigen, increases in the numbers of CD4[+] T cells, and clinical improvement.[196,197] Combination therapy will probably emerge as the best approach.

The chemoprophylactic efficacy of zidovudine after occupational or nosocomial exposure is being assessed. In one instance, a patient was accidentally given an intravenous injection of a small amount of blood (estimated to be 100 to 200 µl) from a patient infected with HIV-1. Zidovudine therapy was begun within 45 minutes of exposure

Table 7   Universal Precautions to Prevent Transmission of HIV

Universal Precautions

Because a medical history and physical examination cannot reliably identify all patients infected with HIV or other blood-borne pathogens, blood and body-fluid precautions should be consistently used for all patients, especially those in emergency-care settings in which the risk of blood exposure is increased and the infection status of the patient is usually not known.

1. Use appropriate barrier precautions to prevent skin and mucous membrane exposure when exposure to blood, body fluids containing blood, or other body fluids to which universal precautions apply (see below) is anticipated. Wear gloves when touching blood or body fluids, mucous membranes, or nonintact skin of all patients; when handling items or surfaces soiled with blood or body fluids; and when performing venipuncture and other vascular access procedures. Change gloves after contact with each patient; do not wash or disinfect gloves for reuse. Wear masks and protective eye wear or face shields during procedures that are likely to generate droplets of blood or other body fluids to prevent exposure of mucous membranes of the mouth, nose, and eyes. Wear gowns or aprons during procedures that are likely to generate splashes of blood or other body fluids.

2. Wash hands and other skin surfaces immediately and thoroughly following contaminations with blood, body fluids containing blood, or other body fluids to which universal precautions apply. Wash hands immediately after gloves are removed.

3. Take care to prevent injuries when using needles, scalpels, and other sharp instruments or devices; when handling sharp instruments after procedures; when cleaning used instruments; and when disposing of used needles. Do not recap used needles by hand; do not remove used needles from disposable syringes by hand; and do not bend, break, or otherwise manipulate used needles by hand. Place used disposable syringes and needles, scalpel blades, and other sharp items in puncture-resistant disposal containers, which should be located as close to the use area as is practical.

4. Although saliva has not been implicated in HIV transmission, the need for emergency mouth-to-mouth resuscitation should be minimized by making mouthpieces, resuscitation bags, or other ventilation devices available for use in areas in which the need for resuscitation is predictable.

5. Health-care workers with exudative lesions or weeping dermatitis should refrain from all direct patient care and from handling patient-care equipment until the condition resolves.

Universal precautions are intended to supplement rather than replace recommendations for routine infection control, such as hand washing and use of gloves to prevent gross microbial contamination of hands. In addition, implementation of universal precautions does not eliminate the need for other category- or disease-specific isolation precautions, such as enteric precautions for infectious diarrhea or isolation for pulmonary tuberculosis. Universal precautions are not intended to change waste management programs undertaken in accordance with state and local regulations.

Body Fluids to Which Universal Precautions Apply

Universal precautions apply to blood and other body fluids containing visible blood. Blood is the single most important source of HIV, hepatitis B virus, and other blood-borne pathogens in the occupational setting. Universal precautions also apply to tissues, semen, vaginal secretions, and the following fluids: cerebrospinal, synovial, pleural, peritoneal, pericardial, and amniotic.

Universal precautions do not apply to feces, nasal secretions, sputum, sweat, tears, urine, and vomitus unless they contain visible blood. Universal precautions also do not apply to human breast milk, although gloves may be worn by health-care workers in situations in which exposure to breast milk might be frequent. In addition, universal precautions do not apply to saliva. Gloves need not be worn when feeding patients or wiping saliva from skin, although special precautions are recommended for dentistry, in which contamination of saliva with blood is predictable. The risk of transmission of HIV, as well as hepatitis B virus, from these fluids and materials is extremely low or nonexistent.

Use of Gloves for Phlebotomy

Gloves should be effective in reducing the incidence of blood contamination of hands during phlebotomy (drawing of blood samples), but they cannot prevent penetrating injuries caused by needles or other sharp instruments. In universal precautions, all blood is assumed to be potentially infectious for blood-

Table 7   (Continued)

borne pathogens. Some institutions have relaxed recommendations for the use of gloves for phlebotomy by skilled health-care workers in settings in which the prevalence of blood-borne pathogens is known to be very low (e.g., volunteer blood-donation centers). Institutions that judge that routine use of gloves for all phlebotomies is not necessary should periodically reevaluate their policy. Gloves should always be available for those who wish to use them for phlebotomy. In addition, the following general guidelines apply:

1. Use gloves for performing phlebotomy if cuts, scratches, or other breaks in the skin are present.

2. Use gloves in situations in which contamination with blood may occur—for example, when performing phlebotomy on an uncooperative patient.

3. Use gloves for performing finger or heel sticks on infants and children.

4. Use gloves when training persons to do phlebotomies.

Precautions for Laboratories

Blood and other body fluids from all patients should be considered infective. To supplement the universal precautions listed above, the following precautions are recommended for workers in clinical laboratories:

1. Put all specimens of blood and body fluids in a well-constructed container with a secure lid to prevent leakage during transport. Take care when collecting each specimen to avoid contaminating the outside of the container or the laboratory form accompanying the specimen.

2. Wear gloves when processing blood and body-fluid specimens (e.g., when removing tops from vacuum tubes). Wear masks and protective eye wear if it is anticipated that mucous membranes will come in contact with blood or body fluids. Change gloves and wash hands after completion of specimen processing.

3. For routine procedures, such as histologic and pathologic studies or microbiologic culturing, a biologic safety cabinet is not necessary. However, use a biologic safety cabinet (class I or II) when procedures are conducted that have a high potential for generating droplets, such as blending, sonicating, and vigorous mixing.

4. Use a mechanical pipetting device for manipulating all liquids in the laboratory. Do not pipette by mouth.

5. Limit use of needles and syringes to situations in which there is no alternative.

6. Decontaminate laboratory work surfaces with an appropriate chemical germicide after a spill of blood or other body fluids and after work is completed.

7. Decontaminate materials contaminated during laboratory tests before reprocessing them. Place contaminated materials for disposal in bags and discard in accordance with institutional policies for disposal of infective waste.

8. Decontaminate and clean scientific equipment that has been contaminated by blood or body fluids if repair in the laboratory or transport to the manufacturer is necessary.

9. Wash hands after completing laboratory work and remove protective clothing before leaving the laboratory.

Implementation of universal precautions eliminates the need for warning labels on specimens because blood and body fluids from all patients should be considered infective.

---

but failed to prevent viremia and the subsequent development of HIV-1 antibodies.[198]

Coincident with the reports of the emergence of zidovudine-resistant HIV isolates during zidovudine therapy are reports of the isolation of ganciclovir-resistant cytomegalovirus infection,[199] acyclovir-resistant herpes simplex virus infection,[200-202] and acyclovir-resistant varicella-zoster virus infection.[203] These antiviral-resistant isolates all occurred under similar circumstances: progressive or disseminated infection in a highly immunocompromised patient who required prolonged or recurrent therapy for a high infection burden. More such instances are likely to occur in AIDS patients, emphasizing the need for new therapeutic strategies not only for HIV infection but also for the infections that occur as complications of HIV disease.

Another therapeutic consideration is the treatment and prevention of the secondary infections that account for most of the morbidity and mortality in AIDS patients. With-

Table 8   Recommendations for Routine Immunization
of HIV-Infected Children

Vaccine	*Asymptomatic HIV Infection*	*Symptomatic HIV Infection*
Diphtheria toxoid–tetanus toxoid–pertussis vaccine	Yes	Yes
Oral polio vaccine	No	No
Inactivated polio vaccine	Yes	Yes
Live measles-mumps-rubella combined vaccine	Yes	Yes
Hemophilus influenzae type B conjugate vaccine	Yes	Yes
Pneumococcal vaccine	No	Yes
Influenza vaccine	No	Yes

These recommendations, although devised specifically for children, apply to adolescents
and adults with HIV infection as well.

out detailing the specific therapy for each condition, it is important to emphasize two key points that underline such therapies: prompt diagnosis and early therapy are essential, and prolonged or indefinite therapy is usually required.

A special effort is warranted to prevent *P. carinii* pneumonia because prevention of this one opportunistic infection will significantly extend the survival of patients with AIDS. In those patients who can tolerate it, trimethoprim-sulfamethoxazole, given in a dosage of one double-strength tablet (160 mg of trimethoprim and 800 mg of sulfamethoxazole) twice a day, provides effective prophylaxis against *Pneumocystis* pneumonia.[204] Data are still incomplete, but similar benefits may be provided by other regimens, including trimethoprim plus dapsone, intermittent intravenous or aerosolized pentamidine, and the combination drug pyrimethamine-sulfadoxine (Fansidar), an agent that has been associated with severe toxic reactions. The approval by the FDA of aerosolized pentamidine (300 mg administered once every four weeks) for prophylaxis is a major advance because this agent appears to provide effective prophylaxis with less severe side effects than trimethoprim-sulfamethoxazole or other regimens. Some kind of prophylaxis against *Pneumocystis* is indicated in HIV-infected individuals with CD4+ T cell counts lower than $200/mm^3$ and in those with full-blown AIDS.[119,120,205-207]

A remaining issue of prevention that merits attention is the appropriateness of routine immunization in individuals with HIV infection. There have been reports of disseminated mycobacterial infection after bacillus Calmette-Guérin (BCG) inoculation[208] and disseminated vaccinia after smallpox immunization[209] in HIV-infected individuals. Despite such reports, judicious use of most vaccines is still recommended [*see Table 8*].[210] It is important to note that the serologic response to most vaccines is greatest in HIV-infected individuals with the least degree of clinical compromise but that the response may be impaired even in asymptomatic individuals.[211-213]

Finally, the effective clinical management of AIDS patients requires attention to the social, ethical, psychological, and public health issues raised by the epidemic. The economic, personal, and social costs of HIV infection are immense and continue to grow. The many issues that must be addressed include competent and humane care for patients, widespread educational efforts to dispel fears and misconceptions about AIDS and to prevent further spread of infection, protection of patient confidentiality, ethical dilemmas related to life-sustaining treatments, and counseling and support of patients. The

Table 9   Summary Policy Statement on AIDS

1. The American College of Physicians and the Infectious Diseases Society of America believe that physicians, other health-care professionals, and hospitals are obligated to provide competent and humane care to all patients, including patients with AIDS and AIDS-related conditions as well as HIV-infected patients with unrelated medical problems. The denial of appropriate care to patients for any reason is unethical.

2. Physicians and other health-care professionals are urged to become fully aware of potential risks and problems encountered in caring for HIV-positive patients and patients with AIDS and to take appropriate steps to minimize them. Such problems include the risks of HIV transmission, economic problems, and personal psychologic stresses.

3. Elected leaders, employers, community service organizations, welfare agencies, public housing authorities, prison officials, and school officials are urged to become fully informed and educate others about HIV infection and, particularly, to understand the limited mechanisms by which the virus can be transmitted. Dissemination of such knowledge should serve to guide public policy development, to alleviate discrimination against those who become infected with the virus, and to limit the further spread of infection.

4. Testing for HIV antibody should be used only when it will benefit the patient or contacts to whom the virus may have been transmitted or for protection of the public health.

5. Counseling and educational efforts, rather than policies promoting physical restriction or quarantine, are appropriate methods for controlling the spread of HIV infection.

6. The confidentiality of patients infected with HIV should be protected to the greatest extent possible, consistent with the duty to protect others and to protect the public health.

7. Physicians should incorporate into their practices standard procedures for taking complete sexual histories of their patients and should assume responsibility for candid communication with and education of persons known to be at risk for HIV infection. The need to modify sexual practices to prevent transmission of infection should be stressed. In addition, physicians are urged to take a major part in educating the public to eliminate misconceptions about AIDS.

8. The American College of Physicians and the Infectious Diseases Society of America encourage continued research into the causes, prevention, and treatment of AIDS and AIDS-related conditions. In addition to biomedical aspects, research into psycho-social and economic issues related to AIDS should be increased. Studies of the effectiveness of various types of educational interventions on behavior modification are critically important.

Health and Public Policy Committee of the American College of Physicians and the Infectious Disease Society of America have proposed recommendations in an attempt to clarify and work toward solving many of these problems [*see Table 9*].[175]

References

1. MMWR 36(suppl 1):1S, 1987
2. Science 220:868, 1983
3. Science 224:497, 1984
4. N Engl J Med 316:1180, 1987
5. N Engl J Med 320:953, 1989
6. N Engl J Med 305:1425, 1981
7. N Engl J Med 305:1439, 1981
8. N Engl J Med 305:1431, 1981
9. Science 239:610, 1988
10. MMWR 39:81, 1990
11. MMWR 39:110, 1990
12. MMWR 38:561, 1989
13. Science 240:1333, 1988
14. N Engl J Med 317:1125, 1987
15. Science 242:916, 1988
16. N Engl J Med 321:874, 1989
17. N Engl J Med 321:947, 1989
18. N Engl J Med 321:966, 1989
19. N Engl J Med 321:1148, 1989
20. Ann Intern Med 105:536, 1986
21. Transplantation 44:1, 1987
22. N Engl J Med 321: 917, 1989
23. N Engl J Med 321:941, 1989
24. JAMA 256:2222, 1986
25. Ann Intern Med 106:380, 1987
26. N Engl J Med 314:344, 1986
27. N Engl J Med 314:380, 1986
28. J Infect Dis 160:970, 1989
29. Science 239:68, 1988
30. Ann Intern Med 104:644, 1986
31. Ann Intern Med 105:730, 1986
32. N Engl J Med 319:1118, 1988
33. Science 241:161, 1988
34. Ann Intern Med 110:653, 1989
35. JAMA 262:516, 1989
36. Nature 328:719, 1987
37. Nature 338:251, 1989
38. Science 231:992, 1986
39. Science 224:500, 1984
40. N Engl J Med 311:1292, 1984
41. N Engl J Med 317:278, 1987
42. Science 239:617, 1988
43. Nature 343:90, 1990
44. Science 247:454, 1990
45. JAMA 261:2997, 1989

46. Adv Immunol 47:377, 1989
47. Science 246:1606, 1989
48. Nature 331:76, 1988
49. Nature 331:78, 1988
50. Nature 331:82, 1988
51. Nature 331:84, 1988
52. Science 238:1704, 1987
53. Science 241:712, 1988
54. Science 242:1166, 1988
55. Lancet 2:1047, 1987
56. J Immunol 138:1719, 1987
57. Science 239:1299, 1988
58. Science 241:573, 1988
59. Nature 343:659, 1990
60. Science 245:305, 1989
61. Science 233:215, 1986
62. Science 241:1673, 1988
63. Science 242:919, 1988
64. Science 233:1084, 1986
65. Ann Intern Med 103:738, 1985
66. Ann Intern Med 104:38, 1986
67. Ann Intern Med 104:511, 1986
68. Science 233:1089, 1986
69. JAMA 256:2365, 1986
70. JAMA 256:2390, 1986
71. Nature 335:639, 1988
72. Science 237:1047, 1987
73. Nature 343:85, 1990
74. Science 236:819, 1987
75. Lancet 2:234, 1987
76. Nature 334:440, 1988
77. Science 241:357, 1988
78. Science 240:80, 1988
79. Nature 340:571, 1989
80. Science 246:118, 1989
81. Science 242:580, 1988
82. Science 244:1357, 1989
83. Nature 340:431, 1989
84. Science 240:64, 1988
85. Science 234:1563, 1986
86. N Engl J Med 308:307, 1983
87. Ann Intern Med 99:208, 1983
88. Lancet 2:631, 1982
89. Am J Med 78:141, 1985
90. Blood 63:818, 1984
91. N Engl J Med 314:874, 1986
92. JAMA 261:719, 1989
93. MMWR 35:334, 1986
94. Lancet 1:537, 1985
95. Ann Intern Med 103:880, 1985
96. Ann Intern Med 102:800, 1985
97. Lancet 1:301, 1985
98. Ann Intern Med 107:383, 1987
99. Medicine (Baltimore) 66:407, 1987
100. JAMA 261:2396, 1989
101. Ann Intern Med 111:400, 1989
102. Ann Intern Med 111:15, 1989
103. Ann Intern Med 109:471, 1988
104. Ann Intern Med 109:502, 1988
105. N Engl J Med 316:1062, 1987
106. Am J Med 87:389, 1989
107. Ann Intern Med 112:35, 1990
108. Ann Intern Med 107:691, 1987
109. Ann Intern Med 110:970, 1989
110. Ann Intern Med 111:158, 1989
111. Ann Intern Med 112:3, 1990
112. Ann Intern Med 104:47, 1986
113. Ann Intern Med 109:190, 1988
114. Ann Intern Med 109:194, 1988
115. Ann Intern Med 109:209, 1988
116. Arch Intern Med 149:330, 1989
117. Ann Intern Med 107:7, 1987
118. Ann Intern Med 109:874, 1988
119. Ann Intern Med 111:223, 1989
120. N Engl J Med 322:161, 1990
121. N Engl J Med 318:589, 1988
122. Ann Intern Med 106:396, 1987
123. Ann Intern Med 108:585, 1988
124. J Infect Dis 157:863, 1988
125. J Infect Dis 157:1, 1988
126. Ann Intern Med 108:328, 1988
127. J Infect Dis 156:998, 1987
128. Ann Intern Med 110:1027, 1989
129. Ann Intern Med 109:449, 1988
130. Ann Intern Med 104:53, 1986
131. Ann Intern Med 105:207, 1986
132. Ann Intern Med 105:184, 1986
133. Ann Intern Med 105:710, 1986
134. N Engl J Med 320:545, 1989
135. MMWR 38:236, 1989
136. J Infect Dis 159:96, 1989
137. N Engl J Med 316:1569, 1987
138. N Engl J Med 316:1587, 1987
139. N Engl J Med 316:1600, 1987
140. J Infect Dis 160:530, 1989
141. J Infect Dis 159:569, 1989
142. Nature 335:606, 1988
143. Science 242:426, 1988
144. Science 243:223, 1989
145. Lancet 2:654, 1987
146. N Engl J Med 320:992, 1989
147. N Engl J Med 320:1005, 1989
148. N Engl J Med 320:1388, 1989
149. N Engl J Med 319:961, 1988
150. Ann Intern Med 110:617, 1989
151. MMWR 38(suppl S-7):1, 1989
152. N Engl J Med 322:217, 1990
153. N Engl J Med 317:1114, 1987
154. Lancet 2:589, 1987
155. Ann Intern Med 111:961, 1989
156. Ann Intern Med 104:194, 1986
157. N Engl J Med 320:1458, 1989
158. Transplant Int 1:36, 1988
159. Ann Intern Med 108:785, 1988
160. JAMA 262:64, 1989
161. N Engl J Med 321:1621, 1989
162. J Infect Dis 161:436, 1990
163. Ann Intern Med 110:963, 1989
164. N Engl J Med 322:166, 1990
165. N Engl J Med 321:1626, 1989
166. JAMA 255:209, 1986
167. Ann Intern Med 110:373, 1989
168. Ann Intern Med 111:761, 1989
169. JAMA 262:1664, 1989
170. Ann Intern Med 110:833, 1989
171. N Engl J Med 316:1339, 1987
172. JAMA 259:1851, 1988
173. JAMA 259:2428, 1988
174. MMWR 37:377, 1988
175. Ann Intern Med 108:460, 1988
176. JAMA 259:1819, 1988
177. JAMA 259:1861, 1988
178. N Engl J Med 317:185, 1987
179. N Engl J Med 317:192, 1987
180. Ann Intern Med 107:502, 1987
181. N Engl J Med 317:593, 1987
182. N Engl J Med 322:941, 1990
183. N Engl J Med 322:1000, 1990
184. N Engl J Med 319:1573, 1988
185. JAMA 262:2405, 1989
186. Science 243:1731, 1989
187. Science 246:1155, 1989
188. N Engl J Med 319:889, 1988
189. Ann Intern Med 109:718, 1988
190. Ann Intern Med 111:41, 1989
191. Ann Intern Med 111:280, 1989
192. Rev Infect Dis 11(suppl 7):S1648, 1989
193. Ann Intern Med 112:241, 1990
194. J Infect Dis 159:837, 1989
195. Science 245:412, 1989
196. N Engl J Med 322:1333, 1990
197. N Engl J Med 322:1340, 1990
198. N Engl J Med 322:1375, 1990
199. N Engl J Med 320:289, 1989
200. N Engl J Med 320:293, 1989
201. N Engl J Med 320:297, 1989
202. Ann Intern Med 110:710, 1989
203. Ann Intern Med 112:187, 1990
204. JAMA 259:1185, 1988
205. Ann Intern Med 105:45, 1986
206. Clin Res 35:468A, 1987
207. MMWR 38(suppl 5):1, 1989
208. MMWR 34:227, 1986
209. N Engl J Med 316:673, 1987
210. MMWR 37:181, 1988
211. Ann Intern Med 109:383, 1988
212. Ann Intern Med 109:101, 1988
213. Ann Intern Med 109:92, 1988

Acknowledgments

Table 2 Modified from "Transmission of the Human Immunodeficiency Virus," by G. H. Friedland and R. S. Klein, in *The New England Journal of Medicine* 317:1125, 1987. Used by permission.

Table 4 Modified from "Neurologic Manifestations of Infection with Human Immunodeficiency Virus: Clinical Features and Pathogenesis," by D. H. Gabuzda and M. S. Hirsch, in *Annals of Internal Medicine* 107:383, 1987. Used by permission.

Table 9 Modified from "The Acquired Immunodeficiency Syndrome (AIDS) and Infection with the Human Immunodeficiency Virus (HIV)," a policy statement by the Health and Public Policy Committee, American College of Physicians, and the Infectious Diseases Society of America, in *Annals of Internal Medicine* 108:460, 1988. Used by permission.

19 Chemotherapy for Microbial Diseases

HARVEY B. SIMON, M.D.
MORTON N. SWARTZ, M.D.

Selection of Antimicrobial Drugs and Treatment Guidelines

The essential feature of effective chemotherapeutic agents is selective toxicity, that is, the ability to inhibit microorganisms at concentrations that are tolerated by the host. The most successful antimicrobial agents are those whose targets are anatomic structures or biosynthetic functions unique to microorganisms. Penicillins, cephalosporins, and vancomycin act by interfering with synthesis of the mucopeptide layer of the bacterial cell wall, a structure absent in host cells. Polymyxins act by altering the permeability of the bacterial cell membrane, allowing cell contents to leak out. Aminoglycoside antibiotics and the tetracyclines appear to exert their chemotherapeutic effects on the 30S subunit of the bacterial ribosome, inhibiting protein synthesis at the translational level. Chloramphenicol, erythromycin, and lincomycin also block bacterial protein synthesis at the translational level, by interfering with the function of the 50S subunit of the bacterial ribosome. Rifampin selectively inhibits the bacterial DNA–dependent RNA polymerase but does not affect this enzyme in the host cell. The sulfonamides inhibit microbial synthesis of folic acid both by competing with their structural analogue, aminobenzoic acid, for transport into the bacterial cell and by subsequently inhibiting the enzymatic incorporation of aminobenzoic acid into a precursor of folic acid. The quinolones impair bacterial DNA synthesis by inhibiting DNA gyrase, the enzyme responsible for maintaining the helical structure of DNA.

The choice of appropriate chemotherapy for an infection is based on several considerations:

1. Identification of the infecting organism.
2. Knowledge of the antimicrobial susceptibility pattern of the microorganism.
3. Relative merits of the use of bactericidal drugs as opposed to bacteriostatic drugs.
4. Definition of the site of infection. A bactericidal drug is required in the treatment of endocarditis but not in the treatment of a urinary tract infection. Central nervous system infections must be treated with agents that can cross the blood-brain barrier to achieve therapeutic concentrations in the cerebrospinal fluid. In the management of a localized abscess, surgical drainage is frequently more important than the use of antimicrobial drugs.
5. Host factors. Patients who have neutropenia or other impairments of host defense mechanisms generally need combinations of bactericidal drugs at dosages that achieve high serum levels. Drug allergies and underlying illnesses, especially renal or hepatic dysfunction, often influence antimicrobial selection.
6. Indications for combinations of antibiotics.
7. Clinical pharmacology (e.g., dosage, routes of administration, adverse reactions, drug interactions, and serum levels).
8. Appropriate duration of therapy (extensive data on which to base decisions are often lacking, but some empirical guidelines are available for certain types of infection).
9. Public health considerations in a closed community (e.g., a hospital). The widespread use of certain antibiotics may select out a highly resistant flora that poses a threat of nosocomial infection. In some hospitals, the administration of one or two recently released antimicrobial agents is limited to very specific indications.

10. Cost. The price of antimicrobial agents varies widely, and new drugs are often much more expensive than older agents. If the efficacy and toxicity of two or more agents are equal, the least expensive one should be selected.

Identification of the Infecting Organism

Prompt identification of the causative organism is essential to the appropriate selection of antimicrobial drugs and successful management of clinical infections. Gram's stain of infected body fluids can provide early clues to the etiologic agent and aid in selection of initial therapy before culture results are available. Occasionally, in overwhelming pneumococcal or staphylococcal bacteremias, the density of organisms is so great as to allow their detection on smears of the buffy coat by using Wright-Giemsa or Gram's stain. Other relatively simple laboratory procedures, such as immunodiagnostic tests and the quellung reaction (capsular swelling), may provide further identification of organisms detected by Gram's stain. For example, in a young patient with clinical meningitis who has received partial antibiotic therapy and whose CSF sediment shows only one or two pleomorphic gram-negative bacilli, the latex agglutination test can demonstrate *Hemophilus influenzae* type b capsular polysaccharide and rapidly provide evidence for the etiologic diagnosis. Similarly, the observation of gram-positive cocci in pairs and short chains in the CSF of an elderly man with acute meningitis and a history of chronic prostatic obstruction can be promptly and more precisely evaluated by the latex agglutination test or the use of the quellung reaction. The findings revealed by a Gram's stain of a smear could be consistent with either pneumococcal or enterococcal meningitis, both of which require consideration in view of the patient's history. If a latex agglutination test demonstrates the presence of pneumococcal capsular polysaccharide or if a quellung reaction is produced by the addition of pooled pneumococcal antiserum, the organism is *Streptococcus pneumoniae*; otherwise, the etiologic agent may be an enterococcus, and initial treatment should include gentamicin along with ampicillin.

If examination of involved body fluids or abscess contents by Gram's stain cannot be done or does not suggest the etiologic diagnosis in a seriously ill patient, initial decisions regarding chemotherapy are based on the clinical features and the usual bacteriology of the illness, pending results of appropriate cultures. For example, in a patient with a brain abscess, initial therapy with penicillin and either metronidazole or chloramphenicol is begun before surgery and before exact definition of the infecting bacterium has been made. The therapy for brain abscess is directed at the organisms commonly implicated in this infection: streptococci and various anaerobes, including Bacteroidaceae and Enterobacteriaceae.

Culture results must be interpreted with full recognition of the indigenous flora on various mucosal surfaces and on the skin. *H. influenzae* and *Staphylococcus aureus* are often carried in the upper respiratory tract of adults; their isolation on culture may merely reflect a clinically silent carriage and not a pathogenetic role in an ongoing pharyngitis. The isolation of *S. pneumoniae* from the throat during the respiratory virus season may also reflect a clinically silent carriage. The presence of anaerobic species in cultures of expectorated sputum or of a periodontal abscess (obtained by intraoral drainage) is meaningless because such specimens are invariably contaminated by oral secretions that normally include a number of anaerobic organisms.

Cultural identification of the infecting organism can offer a clue to the pattern of antimicrobial susceptibilities that may be anticipated [*see Table 1*]. On the basis of such information, changes in antimicrobial therapy may be considered. When examining a pure culture of a single type of organism (e.g., in a blood culture), a bacteriology laboratory can at times provide antimicrobial susceptibility data even earlier than it can identify the isolate.

Bacterial Susceptibility to Antimicrobial Agents

Determination of the in vitro susceptibility of bacteria isolated from sites of infection is usually necessary in seriously ill patients because of the inconstancy of antimicrobial susceptibility among species. This variability is found even among strains of the same species, particularly among gram-negative bacilli [*see Table 1*]. In a few instances, susceptibility of certain species (for example, *Neisseria meningitidis* or group A streptococci) to the drug of choice (in this case, penicillin G) has been so clear-cut and uniform that routine in vitro testing has not been necessary.

In vitro susceptibility data provide a necessary, but not sufficient, basis for the definitive selection of chemotherapeutic agents. Additional information about the clinical re-

Table 1   Representative Antimicrobial Susceptibilities of Clinical Isolates at the Massachusetts General Hospital

Organism	Strains Susceptible to Various Antimicrobials (%)							
	Pen	*Meth*	*Eryth*	*Cef*	*Tetra*	*Chlor*	*Clind*	*Vanco*
Staphylococcus aureus	12	89	76	89	94	99	82	100
S. epidermidis	22	51	51	53	79	94	58	100
Pneumococci	100	—*	98	—*	100	100	—*	100

Organism	*Cef*	*Tetra*	*Amp*	*Gent*	*Tobra*	*Amik*	*Tic*	*Trim-Sulf*	*Cefotax*	*Amox-Clav*	*Imi*	*Cipro*
Escherichia coli	96	78	74	99	99	99	75	92	99	84	100	99
Klebsiella pneumoniae	89	80	0	95	92	99	5	92	99	89	100	99
Proteus mirabilis	100	1	92	96	96	99	93	91	100	95	86	99
Providencia rettgeri	20	0	33	95	100	100	91	81	100	25	100	100
Pseudomonas aeruginosa	—*	—*	—*	93	98	98	93	—*	—*	—*	96	97
Enterobacter cloacae	7	82	0	95	96	99	80	94	88	5	100	99
Acinetobacter calcoaceticus (Herellea)	0	78	0	88	92	93	96	92	0	84	99	97
Serratia marcescens	0	4	0	97	96	99	87	99	99	2	98	98

*Isolate has not been tested; all untested isolates are expected to be resistant.

Note: this listing represents the results of standard disk susceptibility tests performed on clinical isolates (from both hospitalized and ambulatory patients) and reported routinely at the Massachusetts General Hospital in 1991. Drugs selected for testing often represent a class of antibiotics (e.g., methicillin for the penicillinase-resistant penicillins such as oxacillin and nafcillin; cephalothin for the first-generation cephalosporins such as cefazolin and cephradine). The listing does not routinely include the susceptibilities of all isolates to certain selected antimicrobials. Thus, for example, although many strains of *A. calcoaceticus* appear to be resistant to the drugs for which susceptibility is regularly determined, some of these very resistant strains are susceptible in vitro to minocycline. Amik—amikacin Amox-Clav—amoxicillin–clavulanic acid Amp—ampicillin Cef—cefazolin Cefotax—cefotaxime Chlor—chloramphenicol Cipro—ciprofloxacin Clind—clindamycin Eryth—erythromycin Gent—gentamicin Imi—imipenem Meth—methicillin Pen—penicillin Tetra—tetracycline Tic—ticarcillin Tobra—tobramycin Trim-Sulf—trimethoprim-sulfamethoxazole Vanco—vancomycin

sponse of certain types of infection to specific therapeutic agents must be considered. For example, although essentially 100 percent of *Salmonella* isolates are susceptible in vitro to gentamicin, chloramphenicol, ampicillin, and third-generation cephalosporins, gentamicin is not effective in systemic salmonellosis. Similarly, although essentially 100 percent of viridans streptococci show in vitro susceptibility to chloramphenicol, poor clinical results eliminate this drug as an alternative to penicillin for subacute bacterial endocarditis. Susceptibility data may not accurately predict the therapeutic outcome for infections caused by other organisms, such as *S. epidermidis*, enterococci (especially when enterococci infect the bloodstream or deep tissue), and *Enterobacter* species, which rapidly develop penicillin and cephalosporin resistance because of inducible β-lactamase enzymes.

Most laboratories test antimicrobial susceptibility using the disk diffusion method. When necessary, organisms can be tested by tube dilution techniques to determine the minimal inhibitory concentration (MIC) and the minimal bactericidal concentration (MBC) of various antibiotics.

Antimicrobial Susceptibility Patterns

The pattern of antimicrobial susceptibility of various bacterial species has changed during the past several decades because of the selection pressures applied by intense antibiotic usage and because of the widespread occurrence among the Enterobacteriaceae and *Pseudomonas* species of transmissible resistance determinants, called R factors.[1,2] For instance, R factor–mediated resistance to penicillin (from β-lactamase production) has appeared in clinical isolates of *H. influenzae* type b and *N. gonorrhoeae*.[3,4] About 20 percent of clinical isolates of *H. influenzae* are now ampicillin resistant.

Changes in antibiotic susceptibility extend beyond the gram-negative bacilli. When penicillin G was introduced in the mid-1940s, less than 10 percent of *S. aureus* strains isolated from patients or carriers were penicillin resistant. By the early 1960s, most *S. aureus* strains isolated from hospitalized patients in the United States were resistant to penicillin G. At that time, however, most strains isolated from patients in the community were still susceptible to penicillin. In 1978, more than 80 percent of strains of *S. aureus*, regardless of the source, were resistant to penicillin G because of penicillinase production [*see Table 1*]. The advent of the penicillinase-resistant semisynthetic penicillins provided potent antibiotics for use in infections caused by penicillin-resistant *S. aureus*. In a few years, however, methicillin-resistant *S. aureus* strains (also resistant to the other penicillinase-resistant penicillins and to the cephalosporins) began to appear.[5] Vancomycin is the drug of choice for these strains, which are a cause of increasing concern, although they are currently responsible for only a small minority of *S. aureus* infections.

From the time of the introduction of penicillin until 1977, clinical isolates of *S. pneumoniae* had remained susceptible to penicillin, and this antibiotic had been the treatment of choice without concern for resistance. However, a mild decrease has been noted in the level of susceptibility to penicillin of *S. pneumoniae* isolated in the United States and abroad.[6] Nevertheless, the levels of penicillin achieved in current therapeutic programs are sufficient to provide adequate therapy. Much more disturbing was the appearance, in 1977, in several pediatric hospitals in South Africa, of strains of *S. pneumoniae* highly resistant to penicillin G (and often to such usual alternatives as the cephalosporins, erythromycin, chloramphenicol, and tetracycline). These strains can produce highly invasive infections, such as pneumonia, empyema, and meningitis.[7] Resistant pneumococcal strains were also found in asymptomatic carriers in the same hospitals. The only antibiotics to which some of the multiply resistant strains proved susceptible were rifampin, vancomycin, and fusidic acid (an antimicrobial agent employed in Europe but not approved for use in the United States). No evidence links such resistance to R factors or to β-lactamase production. Although such resistance is not currently a problem in the United States, it could pose future difficulties in the management of pneumococcal infections. Previously, antimicrobial susceptibility testing was not performed routinely, because pneumococcal strains were uniformly sensitive to penicillin. Penicillin susceptibility can no longer be assumed, and in vitro testing of pneumococcal isolates (certainly, CSF or blood isolates) is reasonable.

It is helpful to keep track of the changing antimicrobial susceptibilities of common bacterial species in a hospital [*see Table 1*]. This information can assist in the initial selection of chemotherapeutic agents for treating infections caused by specific pathogens, particularly gram-negative bacilli. Because the susceptibilities of bacteria vary from hospital to hospital (usually reflecting patterns of antibiotic usage), the data from one institution may not be directly applicable to another.

Relative Superiority of Bactericidal to Bacteriostatic Agents

Antimicrobials can be classified on the basis of their in vitro action as either bactericidal or bacteriostatic drugs [*see Table 2*]. For bactericidal drugs, the minimal bactericidal, or lethal, concentration is close to or identical to the minimal inhibitory concentration. For bacteriostatic drugs, little if any killing occurs at the MIC; only bacteriostasis occurs, which is reversed on removal of the chemotherapeutic agent. This distinction is blurred in vivo because bacteria whose multiplication has been arrested by bacteriostatic drugs are killed by cellular and humoral defenses of the host. In certain clinical situations, there appears to be both a rationale and evidence to support the use of bactericidal drugs over bacteriostatic drugs. Thus, in bacterial endocarditis, in which there is little leukocytic penetration into infected vegetations, bactericidal drugs produce superior results, even though bacteriostatic agents are inhibitory in vitro. Similarly, in serious infections in patients

Table 2   Bactericidal and Bacteriostatic Drugs

Bactericidal Agents	Bacteriostatic Agents
Aminoglycosides*	Chloramphenicol
Aztreonam	Clindamycin
Bacitracin	Erythromycin
Cephalosporins	Sulfonamides
Imipenem	Tetracyclines
Penicillins	Trimethoprim
Polymyxins†	
Quinolones‡	
Vancomycin	

*Include streptomycin, neomycin, kanamycin, gentamicin, tobramycin, amikacin, and netilmicin.

†Include polymyxin B and colistimethate.

‡Include norfloxacin, ciprofloxacin, ofloxacin, and lomefloxacin.

who have granulocytopenia, bactericidal drugs appear to produce a better outcome than bacteriostatic drugs. In other situations, such as urinary tract infections caused by susceptible *Escherichia coli* strains, bacteriostatic drugs (e.g., the sulfonamides or the tetracyclines) appear to be as effective as bactericidal drugs (e.g., ampicillin, cephalosporins, or aminoglycosides).

Definition of the Site of Infection

Knowledge of the site of infection affords two kinds of assistance in antibiotic selection and usage. It provides clues to the infecting organism; for instance, in children who have primary meningitis, the three principal considerations are *H. influenzae, S. pneumoniae,* and *N. meningitidis.* It also suggests guidelines for proper administration to ensure therapeutic concentrations at the site of infection. Transport across the blood-brain barrier varies considerably among antibiotics. Penicillin is effective in the treatment of meningitis caused by *S. pneumoniae* or other susceptible organisms only when it is administered in a dose high enough to achieve therapeutic levels in the CSF without producing toxicity. In the doses usually used to treat systemic infections, penicillin does not sufficiently penetrate the blood-brain barrier. Active inflammation, however, significantly enhances transport of penicillin or ampicillin into the CSF. Reduction of the initially high doses of these antibiotics as soon as the patient shows clinical improvement is inappropriate because the CSF levels of these drugs may be reduced before the infecting organism has been completely eradicated. Aminoglycosides and polymyxins also cross the blood-brain barrier poorly; however, unlike penicillin, they cannot be rendered more effective by administration of larger doses, because beyond a certain level, toxicity becomes a limiting factor. Clindamycin and other cephalosporins do not penetrate even inflamed meninges well enough to provide therapeutic levels in the CSF and thus should not be used in the treatment of bacterial meningitis. For effective treatment of meningitis caused by most gram-negative bacilli, the third-generation cephalosporins are emerging as the agents of choice.

Penetration by antibiotics of all serous surfaces is not uniform. Most antibiotics employed parenterally in the treatment of septic arthritis enter inflamed joints in adequate concentrations, and intra-articular injections are rarely necessary.

The efficacy of antibiotic therapy depends on drug delivery to the infection site as well as on the attainment of therapeutic blood levels. Necrotic lesions such as sequestrums in bone or large abscesses hinder penetration of antimicrobial agents and prevent eradication of the infection unless drainage, debridement, or both are combined with vigorous chemotherapy. Infection in or around a foreign body or prosthesis is almost always resistant to antibiotic therapy unless these materials are removed or replaced.

In the absence of obstruction, infections in the biliary tree, urinary tract, and respiratory tract usually respond to antimicrobial therapy; in the presence of obstruction, such infections become refractory to chemotherapy until the obstruction is eliminated or the infection is otherwise drained. In addition to the mechanical factors favoring extension of infection under these circumstances, antibiotic penetration into obstructed areas such as the biliary tree is often markedly reduced.

Anatomic considerations may determine the appropriate duration of therapy in certain situations. Although viridans and similar streptococci are exquisitely sensitive to penicillin and can be readily eradicated from many sites of infection, their presence in the vegetations of endocarditis requires many weeks of therapy. In the urinary tract, the distinction between renal and bladder sites of infection also appears to be of importance in determining the response to abbreviated courses of antimicrobial therapy.[8]

At the cellular level, the anatomic site of infection also determines the response to antimicrobial therapy with certain drugs. Tetracycline, which readily penetrates cells, is an effective chemotherapeutic agent in infections such as rickettsioses and brucellosis, which are predominantly intracellular. Similarly, courses of therapy with isoniazid and rifampin are successful in the treatment of tuberculosis.

The Use of Antibiotics in Combination

The simultaneous use of multiple antibiotics in a shotgun fashion should be avoided because of the problems of drug toxicity and sensitizations, microbial superinfections, and antagonisms between certain agents. Most bacterial infections can be treated satisfactorily with a single antimicrobial agent. There are a limited number of situations, however, in which the simultaneous administration of more than one chemotherapeutic agent is warranted[9,10]: (1) synergism between two antimicrobials against a specific infecting agent, (2) prevention of emergence of resistance to one or both drugs, (3) treatment of polymicrobial infections for which one antibiotic is not sufficient, and (4) initial treatment of life-threatening infections before isolation of the etiologic agent.

Antibiotic Antagonism and Synergism

The use of a combination of two antimicrobial drugs may result in two kinds of additive effect: antagonism (i.e., the combined antimicrobial drug effect is less than the sum of the effects of the individual drugs) or synergism (the combined antimicrobial drug effect is greater than the sum of the effects of the individual drugs). Antagonism is commonly observed in vitro when an inhibitory concentration of a bacteriostatic drug [*see Table 2*] interacts with a minimal bactericidal concentration of a penicillin or another inhibitor of cell wall synthesis or an aminoglycoside. Antagonism is usually not observed when high concentrations of either the bactericidal drugs or the bacteriostatic drugs are studied in vitro. In general, antagonism is manifested in vitro by a reduction of the number of viable bacteria to the level produced by the bacteriostatic drug alone. This interaction may not prevent successful therapy in the presence of an adequate level of antibody and an adequate number of leukocytes, but in immunosuppressed or granulocytopenic hosts, it can contribute to therapeutic failure.

The mechanism of antibiotic antagonism varies with the specific pair of antibiotics involved. Bacteriostatic drugs such as tetracycline probably exert an antagonistic effect by inhibiting the bacterial multiplication needed to permit the bactericidal action of penicillin and other drugs that interfere with cell wall synthesis. Chloramphenicol can antagonize the bactericidal action of gentamicin in vitro either by blocking the small amount of protein synthesis needed for the bactericidal effect of an aminoglycoside or by binding to the ribosome, which blocks aminoglycoside uptake elsewhere on the ribosome complex.

In experimental infections (e.g., pneumococcal meningitis), antagonism can be observed when a bacteriostatic drug (e.g., chloramphenicol) and a bactericidal drug (e.g., penicillin) are administered simultaneously. This antagonism, however, is not observed when the bactericidal drug is administered and acts first or when multiple doses of both drugs are given.[11] Similarly, in experimental *Proteus mirabilis* meningitis, chloramphenicol can interfere with the bac-

tericidal action of gentamicin.[12] Such antagonism, however, is not important when the effects of the bacteriostatic drug (in the presence of normal host defenses) are sufficient to cure the infection. Because of very specific timing and relation of doses, antimicrobial antagonism is not commonly observed clinically. The most convincing evidence for clinically important antagonism is the combined use of two specific antibiotics, chlortetracycline and penicillin, for the treatment of meningitis resulting from a specific infection by *S. pneumoniae*.[13] Very few other clinical examples of antimicrobial antagonism have been documented.

Conversely, several different mechanisms of antimicrobial synergism are known.

Enhancement by one drug of the entry of a second drug into microbial cells The synergistic action of penicillin and an aminoglycoside has been most extensively studied with enterococci, both in vitro and in vivo.[14] Penicillin alone inhibits growth of enterococci but is not bactericidal. Aminoglycosides alone cannot enter enterococci because of a permeability barrier. Penicillin-induced changes in the enterococcus cell wall, however, enable the aminoglycosides to enter and kill the bacteria unless the enterococcal strain has an R factor–mediated resistance to the aminoglycoside.[15] In some hospitals, about 50 percent of enterococcal isolates are resistant to high levels of streptomycin (< 2,000 µg/ml); these strains are not susceptible to penicillin-streptomycin synergism.[16] Many strains of enterococci are similarly resistant to kanamycin and amikacin and thus are immune to the synergism of combined therapy with penicillin. Gentamicin and either penicillin or ampicillin has been the combination of choice for synergistic treatment of serious enterococcal infections, but isolates with high levels of resistance to penicillin[17] and gentamicin[18] have recently been identified. Synergism between vancomycin and an aminoglycoside against enterococci has also been shown,[19] but cephalosporins do

Table 3   In Vivo Drug Interactions Involving Antimicrobials

Antimicrobial Agent	Interacting Drug	Adverse Effect	Proposed Mechanism
Acyclovir	Probenecid	Increased acyclovir toxicity	Decreased renal excretion
Amantadine	Anticholinergics	Hallucinations, nightmares, confusion	?
	Thiazides	Possible increased amantadine toxicity	Decreased renal excretion
	Triamterene	Possible increased amantadine toxicity	Decreased renal excretion
Aminoglycosides	Amphotericin B	Increased nephrotoxicity	Synergism
	Ascorbic acid	Decreased antibacterial effect in urinary tract	Urinary acidification
	Bumetanide	Increased ototoxicity	Additive actions
	Carbenicillin, ticarcillin	Decreased aminoglycoside effect	Inactivation of aminoglycosides by the penicillin at high concentrations
	Cephalosporins	Increased nephrotoxicity	?
	Cisplatin	Increased nephrotoxicity	?
	Curarelike drugs	Increased neuromuscular blockade	Additive actions
	Digoxin	Probable decreased digoxin effect with neomycin or gentamicin	Decreased absorption
	Ethacrynic acid	Increased ototoxicity	Additive actions
	Furosemide	Increased nephrotoxicity, increased ototoxicity	Additive actions
	Magnesium sulfate	Possible increased neuromuscular blockade	Additive actions
	Methotrexate	Possible increased methotrexate toxicity with kanamycin	?
		Decreased methotrexate effect with oral aminoglycosides	Decreased absorption
	Polymyxins	Increased nephrotoxicity, neuromuscular blockade	Additive actions
Aminosalicylic acid	Probenecid	Increased aminosalicylic acid toxicity	Decreased renal excretion
	Rifampin	Decreased rifampin effect	Decreased absorption
Amphotericin B	Aminoglycosides	Increased nephrotoxicity	Synergism
	Digitalis glycosides	Increased digitalis toxicity	Hypokalemia
	Miconazole	Decreased anticandidal effect	?
	Neuromuscular blocking agents	Increased neuromuscular blockade	Hypokalemia

Antimicrobial Agent	Interacting Drug	Adverse Effect	Proposed Mechanism
Azole anti-fungals (ketocon-azole, fluconazole)	Antacids	Decreased azole levels	Decreased absorption
	Carbamazepine	Altered effects of azole, carbamazepine, or both	Altered metabolism
	Cimetidine, ranitidine	Decreased azole levels	Decreased absorption
	Cyclosporine	Possible increased renal toxicity	Possible increased cyclo-sporine absorption
	Isoniazid	Decreased azole levels	?
	Phenytoin	Altered effects of azole, phenytoin, or both	Altered metabolism
	Rifampin	Decreased azole and rifampin levels	?
	Terfenadine	Ventricular arrhythmias (with ketoconazole)	Decreased terfenadine metabolism
Cephalosporins	Alcohol	Disulfiramlike effect with cefamandole, cefoperazone, and moxalactam	Probable inhibition of inter-mediary metabolism of alcohol
	Aminoglycosides	Increased nephrotoxicity	?
	Oral anticoagulants	Possible increased anticoag-ulant effect with moxalactam	?
	Aspirin, heparin	Possible increased bleeding risk with moxalactam	Additive actions
	Ethacrynic acid	Increased nephrotoxicity	?
	Furosemide	Increased nephrotoxicity	?
	Penicillins	Possible increased cefotaxime toxicity with azlocillin in azotemic patients	Decreased excretion
Chloramphenicol	Acetaminophen	Possible increased chloram-phenicol toxicity	Decreased metabolism
	Oral antico-agulants	Increased anticoagulant effect	Inhibition of microsomal enzymes
	Barbiturates	Increased barbiturate effect	Decreased metabolism
		Decreased chloramphenicol effect	Increased metabolism
	Cimetidine	Possible aplastic anemia (single case report)	?
	Etomidate	Prolonged anesthesia	Decreased metabolism
	Oral hypogly-cemic agents	Increased sulfonylurea-induced hypoglycemia	?
	Phenytoin	Possible increased chloramphenicol toxicity	?
		Increased phenytoin toxicity	Decreased metabolism
Clindamycin	Neuromuscular blocking agents	Increased neuromuscular blockade	Additive actions

Table 3   (continued)

Antimicrobial Agent	Interacting Drug	Adverse Effect	Proposed Mechanism
Cycloserine	Alcohol	Increased alcohol effect or seizures	?
	Isoniazid	CNS toxicity	?
Erythromycin	Oral anti-coagulants	Increased anticoagulant effect	Possible decreased metabolism
	Carbamazepine	Increased carbamazepine toxicity	Decreased metabolism
	Corticosteroids	Increased methylprednisolone effect and possible toxicity	Decreased excretion
	Digoxin	Increased digoxin effect	Increased absorption
	Disopyramide[266]	Possible increased disopyramide levels and possible increased cardiac arrhythmias	Possible decreased metabolism
	Theophyllines	Increased theophylline effect and possible toxicity	Decreased metabolism
	Terfenadine	Ventricular arrhythmias	Possible decreased terfenadine metabolism
Griseofulvin	Oral anticoagulants	Decreased anticoagulant effect	?
	Oral contraceptives	Decreased contraceptive effect	Increased metabolism
	Cyclosporine	Increased cyclosporine levels and toxicity	Possible decreased metabolism
Isoniazid	Alcohol	Possible decreased isoniazid effect in some chronic alcohol abusers	Increased metabolism
		Increased incidence of hepatitis	?
	Aluminum antacids	Decreased isoniazid effect	Inhibition of isoniazid absorption
	Oral anticoagulants	Possible increased anticoagulant effect	Decreased metabolism
	Benzodiazepines	Increased triazolam effect	Decreased metabolism
	Carbamazepine	Increased isoniazid and carbamazepine toxicity	Altered metabolism
	Cycloserine	CNS toxicity	?
	Diazepam	Possible increased I.V. diazepam effect	Decreased metabolism
	Disulfiram	Psychotic episodes, ataxia	Altered dopamine metabolism
	Ketoconazole	Decreased ketoconazole levels	?
	Phenytoin	Increased phenytoin toxicity	Decreased metabolism
	Rifampin	Possible increased hepatotoxicity	Possible increased toxic metabolites

Antimicrobial Agent	Interacting Drug	Adverse Effect	Proposed Mechanism
Lincomycin	Kaolin-pectin	Decreased lincomycin effect	Decreased lincomycin absorption
	Neuromuscular blocking agents	Increased neuromuscular blockade	Additive actions
Methenamine mandelate or methenamine hippurate	Acetazolamide, thiazides, sodium bicarbonate	Decreased antibacterial effect	Urinary alkalinization
Metronidazole	Alcohol	Nausea, cramps, headache, flushing	Possible inhibition of intermediary metabolism of alcohol
	Oral anticoagulants	Increased anticoagulant effect	Inhibition of microsomal enzymes
	Cimetidine	Possible increased metronidazole toxicity	Decreased metabolism
	Disulfiram	Organic brain syndrome	?
	Phenobarbital	Decreased metronidazole effect	Probable increased metabolism
Miconazole	Amphotericin B	Decreased anticandidal effect	?
	Oral anticoagulants	Increased anticoagulant effect	?
	Hypoglycemic agents (sulfonylureas)	Severe hypoglycemia	?
	Phenytoin	Increased phenytoin toxicity	Decreased metabolism
Nalidixic acid	Oral anticoagulants	Increased anticoagulant effect	Displacement of warfarin from albumin binding site
Penicillins	Beta-adrenergic blockers	Possible decreased atenolol effect with ampicillin	Decreased absorption
	Allopurinol	Increased incidence of rashes with ampicillin	?
	Aminoglycosides	Decreased aminoglycoside effect with carbenicillin or ticarcillin at high concentrations	Aminoglycoside inactivation
	Oral anticoagulants	Decreased anticoagulant effect with nafcillin	Increased metabolism
	Cephalosporins	Possible increased cefotaxime toxicity with azlocillin in azotemic patients	Decreased excretion
	Oral contraceptives	Decreased contraceptive effect with ampicillin	Decreased enterohepatic circulation of estrogen
	Lithium	Hypernatremia with ticarcillin	Large sodium load and decreased renal excretion
	Methotrexate	Possible increased methotrexate toxicity	Decreased excretion

Table 3 *(continued)*

Antimicrobial Agent	*Interacting Drug*	*Adverse Effect*	*Proposed Mechanism*
Polymyxins	Aminoglycosides	Increased nephrotoxicity, increased neuromuscular blockade	Additive actions
	Neuromuscular blocking agents	Increased neuromuscular blockade	Additive actions
Pyrimethamine	Antacids (kaolin-pectin)	Possible decreased pyrimethamine effect	Decreased absorption
Quinolones (norfloxacin, ciprofloxacin, ofloxacin, and lomefloxacin)	Nonsteroidal anti-inflammatory agents	Possible increased CNS toxicity	Possible effects on receptor sites
	Metronidazole	Possible increased CNS toxicity	?
	Probenecid	Increased quinolone levels	Decreased renal excretion
	Theophyllines	Increased theophylline levels (except with lomefloxacin)	Probable alteration of hepatic metabolism
	Warfarin	Possible increased anticoagulant effect	Possible alteration of hepatic metabolism
	Antacids	Decreased quinolone levels	Decreased absorption
	Sucralfate	Possible decreased quinolone levels	Possible decreased absorption
Rifampin	Aminosalicylic acid	Decreased rifampin effect	Decreased absorption
	Antacids	Possible decreased rifampin levels	Possible decreased gastric emptying
	Oral anticoagulants	Decreased anticoagulant effect	Induction of microsomal enzymes
	Barbiturates	Decreased barbiturate effect	Increased metabolism
	Beta-adrenergic blockers	Decreased beta blockade	Increased metabolism
		Possible increased beta blockade with metoprolol	Decreased metabolism
	Oral contraceptives	Decreased contraceptive effect	Increased estrogen metabolism
	Corticosteroids	Decreased corticosteroid effect	Induction of microsomal enzymes
	Cyclosporine	Decreased cyclosporine effect	Increased metabolism
	Dapsone	Decreased dapsone levels	Increased metabolism
	Diazepam	Possible decreased effect of I.V. diazepam	Increased metabolism
	Digoxin, digitoxin	Decreased digitalis effect	Increased metabolism
	Diltiazem	Decreased diltiazem effect	Increased metabolism
	Disopyramide	Decreased disopyramide effect	Probable increased metabolism
	Fluconazole	Possible decreased fluconazole levels	?

Antimicrobial Agent	Interacting Drug	Adverse Effect	Proposed Mechanism
Rifampin (*continued*)	Haloperidol	Possible decreased haloperidol levels	Possible increased metabolism
	Oral hypoglycemic agents	Decreased hypoglycemic effect	Induction of microsomal enzymes
	Isoniazid	Possible increased hepatotoxicity	Possible increased toxic metabolites
	Ketoconazole	Decreased ketoconazole and rifampin levels	?
	Mexiletine	Decreased antiarrhythmic effect	Increased metabolism
	Narcotics	Narcotic withdrawal symptoms	Induction of microsomal enzymes
	Phenytoin	Decreased phenytoin effect	Increased metabolism
	Quinidine	Decreased quinidine effect	Increased metabolism
	Theophylline	Decreased theophylline effect	Increased metabolism
	Tocainide	Decreased tocainide levels	Increased metabolism
	Verapamil	Decreased verapamil effect	Increased metabolism
Spectinomycin	Lithium	Increased lithium toxicity	Decreased renal excretion
Sulfonamides	Oral anticoagulants	Increased anticoagulant effect	Displacement from binding sites, decreased metabolism
	Digoxin	Possible decreased digoxin effect with sulfasalazine	Decreased absorption
	Oral hypoglycemic agents	Increased sulfonylurea-induced hypoglycemia	?
	Methotrexate	Possible increased methotrexate toxicity	Displacement from binding sites, decreased renal clearance
	Phenytoin	Increased phenytoin effect (except possibly with sulfisoxazole)	Decreased metabolism
	Monoamine oxidase inhibitors	Possible increased phenelzine toxicity	Decreased metabolism
	Pyrimethamine	Increased hypersensitivity reaction, including fatalities, with sulfadoxine	?
	Thiopental sodium	Increased thiopental sodium effect	Decreased albumin binding
Tetracyclines	Antacids	Decreased tetracycline effect	Decreased tetracycline absorption
	Oral anticoagulants	Increased anticoagulant effect	?
	Barbiturates	Decreased doxycycline effect	Induction of microsomal enzymes
	Bismuth subsalicylate	Decreased tetracycline effect	Decreased absorption

Table 3　(continued)

Antimicrobial Agent	Interacting Drug	Adverse Effect	Proposed Mechanism
Tetracyclines (*continued*)	Carbamazepine	Decreased doxycycline effect	Induction of microsomal enzymes
	Oral contraceptives	Decreased contraceptive effect	Possible decreased enterohepatic circulation of estrogen
	Digoxin	Increased digoxin effect	Increased absorption
	Oral iron salts	Decreased tetracycline and iron effects	Decreased absorption of tetracycline and iron
	Lithium	Increased lithium toxicity	Decreased renal excretion
	Phenytoin	Decreased doxycycline effect	Induction of microsomal enzymes
	Zinc sulfate	Decreased tetracycline effect	Decreased absorption
Thiabendazole	Theophyllines	Increased theophylline toxicity	Decreased metabolism
Trimethoprim	Amiloride, thiazides	Hyponatremia	Additive actions
	Oral anticoagulants	Increased anticoagulant effect	Decreased metabolism
	Cyclosporine	Increased nephrotoxicity	Synergism
	Mercaptopurine	Decreased antileukemic effect	?
	Digoxin	Possible increased digoxin effect	Decreased renal excretion
	Procainamide	Increased procainamide levels	Decreased renal excretion
Trimethoprim-sulfamethoxazole	Oral anticoagulants	Increased anticoagulant effect	Decreased metabolism
Vidarabine	Allopurinol	Increased vidarabine toxicity	Decreased metabolism
	Theophyllines	Increased theophylline effect	Decreased metabolism

not show synergistic activity with aminoglycosides in the treatment of enterococcal infections. Other examples of in vitro penicillin-aminoglycoside synergism include the combination of penicillin and streptomycin against viridans streptococci and *Listeria*, nafcillin and gentamicin against *S. aureus*, and carbenicillin and gentamicin against gentamicin-susceptible (but not gentamicin-resistant) *Pseudomonas aeruginosa*. In these instances, there is no clinical evidence of superiority of combined therapy over penicillin alone, whereas clinical evidence of superiority does exist for enterococcal endocarditis.

Synergism between a cephalosporin and an aminoglycoside occurs with some strains of *Klebsiella* and may provide a rationale for combined therapy in serious *Klebsiella* infections, such as pneumonia and bacteremia. In vitro synergism between flucytosine and amphotericin B can be shown against certain strains of *Cryptococcus* and *Candida*.[20] When this combination is administered to treat *Cryptococcus* meningitis, the toxic side effects of amphotericin B are reduced, without compromising therapeutic efficacy, by a decrease in dosage.

Inhibition by one drug of a microbial enzyme that inactivates a second drug Organisms that produce β-lactamase (penicillinase) are highly resistant to penicillin. However, if β-lactamase is exposed to a substrate that has a high binding affinity but is not hydrolyzable, the enzyme may be so tightly bound that it is unavailable for destruction of a readily cleavable penicillin. In this way, a penicillinase-susceptible penicillin may be protected from enzymatic hydrolysis and is allowed to exert its antibacterial effect. Clavulanic acid and sulbactam, which are very potent inhibitors of microbial β-lactamases, can maintain the efficacy of otherwise hydrolyzable penicillins against *S. aureus* and various resistant gram-negative bacilli.[21]

Inhibition of successive steps in a metabolic sequence Sulfonamides act as competitive inhibitors of aminobenzoic acid, which many bacteria require as a precursor in the biosynthesis of folic acid. The conversion of folic acid to its coenzyme form, which is involved in purine synthesis, requires enzymatic reduction of dihydrofolate to tetrahydrofolate, a step that is inhibited by trimethoprim. Thus, the combination of a sulfonamide and trimethoprim blocks two sequential steps in purine and nucleic acid synthesis, resulting in more effective suppression of microbial growth than can be achieved by either drug alone. This combination has been effective in the treatment of urinary tract infections caused by enteric gram-negative bacilli, typhoid fever caused by chloramphenicol-resistant bacteria, and pneumonia caused by *Pneumocystis* organisms.

Prevention of Emergence of Drug-Resistant Mutants

In a few chronic infections in which large numbers of organisms are present, continued use of a single drug is likely to select out resistant mutants. This development can be prevented by the simultaneous administration of a second drug that acts at a different locus in the microbial cell and is able to suppress or kill any mutants resistant to the first drug. The best example of this approach is the administration of isoniazid and rifampin for the treatment of pulmonary tuberculosis.

Treatment of Mixed Infections

Some polymicrobial infections, such as community-acquired aspirational lung abscess, can be treated satisfactorily with a single drug (in this case, penicillin) because of the composition of the normal upper respiratory tract flora. In contrast, other polymicrobial infections (e.g., intra-abdominal abscesses and peritonitis) result from a mixed bowel flora (e.g., enteric gram-negative bacilli, *Bacteroides* species, gram-positive cocci, and clostridia), which have a wide spectrum of antimicrobial susceptibilities. Therapy with ampicillin-sulbactam and gentamicin or with other combinations is employed—not only for synergistic action against a bacterial species but also for coverage of the many organisms involved.

Initial Treatment of Life-Threatening Infections

In critically ill patients with severe infections, such as bacterial meningitis of unknown etiology, brain abscess, or presumed bacteremia in an immunosuppressed patient, several antimicrobial agents are initially employed together to adequately treat the most likely etiologic agents while awaiting the results of cultures. Often, two or occasionally three antimicrobials are employed together under these circumstances. In the treatment of a brain abscess before surgery and definitive bacteriologic diagnosis, penicillin combined with either metronidazole or chloramphenicol is employed to cover the array of organisms implicated in this infection (i.e., streptococci, *Bacteroides* and other anaerobes, and Enterobacteriaceae). Treatment of unknown sepsis in neutropenic patients receiving antineoplastic chemotherapy generally involves combinations of drugs aimed at *P.*

aeruginosa and other causes of severe infections in this setting.[22] Such combinations include ticarcillin, piperacillin, or mezlocillin and either gentamicin, tobramycin, or amikacin; an aminoglycoside and either cefazolin or ceftazidime; and imipenem-cilastatin and an aminoglycoside. The choice of an aminoglycoside for initial empirical therapy depends on local epidemiological considerations and on whether one of those agents—gentamicin, tobramycin, or amikacin—has been employed previously.

Clinical Pharmacology of Antimicrobials

Dosage

The required dosage of an antimicrobial agent can vary considerably, depending on the susceptibility of the causative organism, the location of the infection, the route of administration, the blood levels achieved, the route of elimination, and the therapeutic-toxic ratio of the drug. In general, drug dosages are aimed at achieving serum levels that exceed the MIC for the infecting organism by severalfold. In the treatment of subacute bacterial endocarditis, serum levels that are at least eight times higher than the bactericidal concentration are sought. However, the serum level is not the only determinant of a drug's antimicrobial effect. Serum levels of bacteriostatic drugs are often close to the MICs for susceptible organisms, but they are adequate because the drugs work in combination with normal host defenses. In the treatment of the usual types of urinary tract infection uncomplicated by obstruction or bacteremia, the level of drug in the urine is the important determinant. Therapy is successful even in the absence of blood levels exceeding the MIC for the infecting organism because of the predominantly renal route of excretion of the drugs employed for such infections. With the penicillins, a very wide dosage range is possible because of the extremely low toxicity of this family of compounds. A daily oral dosage of one million units of penicillin G is employed for group A streptococcal pharyngitis, but 24 million units I.V. daily is given for men-ingitis caused by the same organism. In the presence of renal insufficiency, however, the high levels of penicillin achieved may cause neurotoxicity or side effects secondary to hyperkalemia (penicillin is usually given as the potassium salt). In contrast, the usual dosage of the aminoglycoside gentamicin in a patient with normal renal function has a much narrower therapeutic range of 3 to 5 mg/kg/day.

Absorption and Route of Administration

Many antibiotics are absorbed sufficiently well by the oral route to provide effective blood levels, but their absorption from the intestinal tract is impeded by food and some medications (e.g., antacids). These drugs should therefore be administered at least one hour before or several hours after meals. Dicloxacillin, doxycycline, and some other antibiotics are almost completely absorbed from the gastrointestinal tract and produce similar peak serum levels after oral or intravenous administration.[23] Other antibiotics, such as ampicillin, are less well absorbed and produce significantly lower blood levels when given via the enteral route than when administered intravenously. Certain antibiotics are essentially nonabsorbable and are used primarily for their effects on bowel flora. Such agents include oral vancomycin, which is used in the treatment of antibiotic-induced pseudomembranous enterocolitis, and oral neomycin, which is used in the treatment of hepatic precoma and in preoperative bowel preparation.

Many intravenously administered antibiotics, such as erythromycin, tetracycline, and cephalothin, cannot be given intramuscularly in clinically effective dosages because of local pain or necrosis at the injection site. Chloramphenicol sodium succinate is ineffective when administered intramuscularly. Metabolic factors may influence the dosage of the parenteral antibiotic required; for example, dosages should be increased in diabetic adults because serum levels of penicillin G attained after I.M. injection are lower than in nondiabetic adults.

The intravenous route of administration should be utilized in the treatment of such life-threatening infections as septic shock, meningitis, and endocarditis to ensure delivery of high concentrations of the drug to the sites of infection. To prevent incompatibilities between one another, antimicrobial agents should not be administered simultaneously through the same intravenous line. Gentamicin, for example, may lose activity when mixed with carbenicillin. Mixing of chloramphenicol sodium succinate and erythromycin lactobionate or erythromycin gluceptate results in precipitation of the drugs.

The stability of antibiotics may vary with the diluent employed in intravenous administration. Ampicillin at room temperature is stable for up to eight hours at concentrations of 30 mg/ml in 0.9 percent NaCl solution, but it is stable for less than four hours at concentrations of up to 2 mg/ml in five percent dextrose solution.

Serum Levels and Protein Binding

The relative merits of intermittent versus continuous intravenous infusion have been debated for years. Intermittent intravenous infusion of antibiotics is commonly the preferred method because it produces greater peak levels in the blood.[24] Data on the penetration of antibiotics into fibrin clots in vivo support this contention. Intermittent infusion is commonly employed in the treatment of bacterial meningitis, bacterial endocarditis, and other infections.

Antimicrobial blood levels can be determined in the laboratory. They can confirm that therapeutic levels are being achieved and can also provide guidance in avoiding excessive levels of potentially toxic drugs. The latter is most important in the regulation of the dosage of aminoglycosides and vancomycin, particularly in the presence of renal insufficiency. A variety of radio-enzymatic, immunologic, and chromatographic assays are available to measure antibiotic concentrations in blood and body fluids; older microbiological assays are still used for some antimicrobials.

The binding of antimicrobial agents to serum proteins is reversible and varies considerably from drug to drug. Among the penicillins, it may be 20 percent (ampicillin), 40 percent (methicillin), 60 percent (penicillin G), or 90 percent (oxacillin and nafcillin). Although binding of chemotherapeutic agents to serum protein inhibits their antimicrobial activity in vitro, antibiotics that are highly protein bound (e.g., oxacillin and nafcillin) are nonetheless effective in vivo. Because the percent binding reflects an equilibrium reaction, passage of free drug into the tissues is accompanied by further release of the drug from its protein-bound state, maintaining a serum level of free drug characteristic of that antimicrobial agent. The significance of protein binding of antibiotics is still uncertain; there is no clear correlation between the degree of protein binding and in vivo activity.

Excretion and Inactivation

Most antimicrobial agents that are in common use (e.g., penicillins, cephalosporins, aminoglycosides, vancomycin, polymyxins, and tetracyclines) are excreted as active drugs primarily by the kidneys. However, three tetracyclines—chlortetracycline, minocycline, and doxycycline—are excreted principally in the bile and feces. Nafcillin is also excreted predominantly in bile. Only a small percentage of administered chloramphenicol and rifampin is excreted unchanged in the urine; the major portion of these drugs is removed by the liver. Neither urinary nor biliary excretion accounts for the disappearance from the circulation of significant amounts of erythromycin, lincomycin, clindamycin, or amphotericin B; the mechanisms of inactivation of these antibiotics remain unknown.

Renal elimination of antimicrobial agents occurs by tubular secretion, by glomerular filtration, or by a combination of the two. Tubular secretion is important in the excretion of the penicillins and cephalosporins; gentamicin and other aminoglycosides are eliminated mainly by glomerular filtration. The extent of tubular secretion plays an important role in determining the serum half-life and blood levels achieved with the different penicillins. Penicillin G is the form of these drugs most rapidly excreted by the tubules. Ampicillin is less readily excreted by the tubules; after a comparable intravenous dose, ampicillin attains about twice the peak blood level that penicillin G does, and the serum half-life of ampicillin is also twice as long. Probenecid blocks tubular secretion of most penicillin and cephalosporin derivatives and increases the blood levels of these agents. This effect is greatest with those penicillin and cephalosporin derivatives for which tubular secretion is most marked (e.g., penicillin G and cephalothin, rather than ampicillin and cefazolin).

The excretion of an antibiotic by the renal route is an important consideration in determining dosage in a patient with renal insufficiency. Guidelines for dosage adjustment in patients who have severe renal failure and are undergoing hemodialysis or peritoneal dialysis are listed elsewhere [*see Chapter 32*]. Nomograms and calculations for dosage of aminoglycosides in patients with renal failure will be considered later [*see* Specific Antimicrobial Drugs, Aminoglycoside Antibiotics, *below*]. If the infecting organism is susceptible, certain antibiotics whose major route of excretion is extrarenal (e.g., nafcillin) may be used to advantage.

The level of antibacterial activity in the urine is mainly determined by the degree of renal clearance of the particular drug. The activity of a given amount of an antimicrobial agent, however, may be altered by the ambient pH. Certain drugs are more active at an acid pH, which can be achieved by the addition of acidifying agents such as ascorbic acid. These drugs include methenamine mandelate, methenamine hippurate, tetracycline, and nitrofurantoin. Antibiotics such as aminoglycosides and erythromycin are more active at an alkaline pH, attainable by oral administration of sodium bicarbonate.

Some antibiotics are inactivated by the liver. The clearest example is chloramphenicol, which is converted to its inactive form, the monoglucuronide, and subsequently excreted in this form by the kidney. Fatal chloramphenicol toxicity, called the gray syndrome, is manifested by vasomotor collapse and cyanosis; the syndrome may develop in neonates, particularly premature infants. It is caused by exposure to excessive dosages, defined as greater than 25 mg/kg/day. The mechanisms that produce this toxicity are considered to be (1) failure of inactivation of the drug stemming from immaturity of the hepatic glucuronyl transferase system in the first few weeks of life and (2) inadequate renal excretion of the unconjugated drug. For these two reasons, considerable caution is required in the administration of chloramphenicol to premature infants and to full-term infants younger than two weeks. Fortunately, the third-generation cephalosporins have largely replaced chloramphenicol in the treatment of serious infections in infants; if chloramphenicol is required in this setting, determination of blood levels is helpful in guiding therapy. In adults with hepatic dysfunction, chloramphenicol metabolism is not markedly altered, and dosage alteration is not required unless hematotoxicity is observed.

Adverse Drug Interactions

The simultaneous use of several drugs can result in interactions that alter anticipated responses to one or more of the pharmacological agents administered. Such interactions may involve several antimicrobial agents or an antimicrobial agent and one or more drugs of an unrelated class [*see* Table 3].[25-27] The consequences of such interactions may be an unexpected reaction or an increase or a decrease in the usual response to one of the drugs. Several mechanisms may account for observed drug interactions: (1) accelerated metabolism of one agent produced by the induction of microsomal enzymes by administration of a second agent, (2) decreased metabolism of one drug produced by inhibition of microsomal enzymes by another drug, (3) decreased absorption of one drug produced by the presence of a second drug in the gastrointestinal tract, (4) increased circulating levels of one drug in its active form produced by its displacement from plasma proteins or secondary tissue receptor sites, (5) interference by one drug with transport to or uptake at target sites of a second drug, and (6) decreased renal excretion of one drug produced by the administration of a second drug. Some interactions occur only with high doses of the involved drugs; others may be conditioned by genetic differences in drug metabolism. Because of the many adverse drug interactions that may occur, as few drugs as possible should be administered concurrently. If interacting drugs must be prescribed together, dose adjustments will probably be required.

In addition to the in vivo drug interactions previously described [*see Table 3*], in vitro incompatibilities may occur on mixing several drugs or on adding certain drugs to specific diluents (see above).

Adverse Reactions to Antimicrobial Agents

There are three general types of adverse reactions to antimicrobial agents: hypersensitivity responses that are not directly dose related; direct drug toxicity, usually dose related and manifest in a single or, occasionally, in several target organs; and microbial superinfection.[28]

Hypersensitivity Responses

The more severe allergic reactions tend to occur after parenteral administration of a drug, but they can certainly also appear after oral ingestion. A history of allergy should be taken before initiating antimicrobial therapy in any patient. Incidences of atopy or other allergic manifestations should be noted, and particular attention should be given to previous drug allergies. More information is available regarding allergy to the penicillins than to other agents, but skin eruptions, drug fever, and even anaphylaxis may be produced by many drugs other than penicillin. Furthermore, sulfonamides, streptomycin, isoniazid, stibophen, chloroquine, penicillin, and rifampin have all been implicated at some time in the immunothrombocytopenias that can develop during antimicrobial therapy. Cholestatic jaundice from use of erythromycin estolate is probably a manifestation of drug hypersensitivity. Respiratory reactions of fever, eosinophilia, cough, dyspnea, and pleural effusions that occur in some patients receiving nitrofurantoin reflect pulmonary hypersensitivity to the drug. Cephalosporins have rarely been reported to cause an interstitial pneumonitis resulting from a hypersensitivity reaction.[29]

Allergic reactions to penicillin develop in one to 10 percent of patients receiving the drug.[30] Fatal anaphylactic reactions are much less frequent; only one death was reported among approximately 95,000 patients who received penicillin in venereal disease clinics.[31] Immunologic reactions to penicillin may take a variety of forms, such as anaphylaxis, urticaria, Coombs'-positive hemolytic anemia, serum sickness, and morbilliform eruptions. Methicillin and, less commonly, other penicillins can result in interstitial nephritis. A patient who has had an allergic reaction to a penicillin is at increased risk for a hypersensitivity reaction on subsequent administration of another penicillin, such as ampicillin or oxacillin. In most clinical situations, however, effective alternative drugs are available, and therefore, allergic patients should not be put at risk.

In many instances, cephalosporins are employed in place of a penicillin when the infecting organism is susceptible. This substitution, however, carries its own risks. A patient who is allergic to one allergenic drug is more likely to be allergic to other sensitizing drugs, and cephalosporins, like penicillins, are potent immunogens. Furthermore, cephalosporins and penicillins have cross-reacting major antigenic determinants. Although the clinical significance of such reactions is still debated, there have been a few reports of anaphylaxis on initial exposure to cephalosporins in patients allergic to penicillin.[32] For this reason, many physicians do not employ a cephalosporin as an alternative to a penicillin in a patient who has had a clear-cut allergic response to penicillin, particularly if the reaction was immediate anaphylaxis or accelerated urticaria with associated wheezing or pharyngeal edema. Of the newer β-lactam antibiotics, carbapenems (e.g., imipenem) have the potential for cross-immunogenicity with penicillins and cephalosporins, but monobactams (e.g., aztreonam) do not.

Skin-sensitizing IgE antibodies, which can attach to the surface of tissue mast cells, appear to mediate penicillin anaphylaxis. These antibodies to penicillin are specific for either the major haptenic determinant (benzylpenicilloyl) or the minor haptenic determinants (e.g., benzylpenicillin and benzylpenicilloate). Skin testing to reveal the presence of such skin-sensitizing antibodies may be helpful in evaluating a patient with an uncertain history of penicillin allergy. Testing with both the major and the minor haptenic determinants is necessary for complete evaluation.[33] At present, only the benzylpenicilloyl-polylysine skin-test antigen is commercially available; the minor determinant mixture is used only as a research reagent. Facilities and equipment necessary for treatment of anaphylaxis should always be on hand when skin testing is performed. Patients with positive skin tests have a 41 to 67 percent chance of exhibiting significant penicillin allergy if they are rechallenged with the drug. The risk to patients with negative skin tests is only one to four percent, and no life-threatening reactions have been reported.[34]

In the rare instance of penicillin allergy in which cephalosporins or other drugs cannot serve as first-line substitutes for treatment of life-threatening infections, desensitization to penicillin can be attempted. Successful desensitization is thought to be achieved by one of two processes: (1) blocking IgG antibodies successfully competing with IgE for the antigen or (2) successive doses of penicillin depleting the available quantity of IgE. Desensitization is carried out with the equipment and medications for the treatment of anaphylaxis at bedside: laryngoscope, oxygen, endotracheal tube, epinephrine 1:1,000, and sodium bicarbonate solution; an intravenous infusion should be running. Penicillin

doses are administered in graded increases on the forearm at a site low enough that a tourniquet can be applied proximally should a reaction occur.[35] The initial dose of one unit is applied by scratch test. If there is no wheal-and-flare reaction within 15 minutes, two units of penicillin are injected intradermally. If no local or systemic reaction occurs after another 15 minutes, five units of penicillin are injected intradermally. If no reactions occur, successive doses that approximately double each prior dose are injected intradermally at 15-minute intervals. When the amount injected becomes large, it is administered subcutaneously. When a dose of 100,000 units has been injected without reaction, penicillin can be given intravenously. If an immediate local or systemic reaction occurs, it can be controlled. Use of an alternative drug is then advisable. Oral desensitization regimens are also available.[34] Neither corticosteroids nor antihistamines will prevent anaphylaxis in an individual who is highly sensitive to penicillin.

Morbilliform or urticarial rashes that occur during a course of penicillin therapy indicate only a very slight risk of anaphylactoid reactions. If morbilliform or urticarial rashes develop and penicillin administration must be continued, these eruptions may often be controlled by the use of antihistamines or, if necessary, corticosteroids. Of the various penicillins, ampicillin produces the highest frequency of skin rashes (five to 10 percent); in patients with infectious mononucleosis, the incidence is increased to 50 to 80 percent.

Direct Drug Toxicity

The kidney The principal antibiotics directly toxic to the kidney are aminoglycosides, polymyxins, and amphotericin B. Azotemia and renal tubular damage are induced by all of these drugs. Outdated and polymerized tetracycline has produced proximal renal tubular damage and Fanconi's syndrome. Demethylchlortetracycline can produce nephrogenic diabetes insipidus; this effect of the drug has been used in treatment of water retention in patients with inappropriate secretion of antidiuretic hormone. Azotemia from preexisting renal failure can be aggravated by tetracyclines through their antianabolic effects; blood urea levels are elevated without corresponding increases in the level of creatinine. Renal effects of high-dose carbenicillin treatment can produce hypokalemic alkalosis, especially in patients with preexisting renal or cardiac disease. Rifampin can cause renal failure if it is given intermittently.

Patients with preexisting renal insufficiency are at increased risk for many toxic reactions to antimicrobials, including nephrotoxicity, coagulopathies and other hematologic toxicities, seizures, ototoxicity, and other neurotoxicities.[36]

The hematopoietic system Chloramphenicol produces two kinds of bone marrow suppression. One form is relatively common, dose related, and reversible on discontinuance of the drug; this suppression is caused by chloramphenicol inhibition of mitochondrial protein synthesis.[37] The bone marrow suppression usually appears after several weeks of treatment and is manifested by a rise in serum iron, an increased percent saturation of iron-binding globulin, and a drop in the level of hemoglobin. Cytoplasmic vacuolization develops in white cell and red cell precursors in the marrow. This hematologic picture is most evident in those patients who have extensive liver disease and a reduced capacity to conjugate chloramphenicol.

A grave and rarer form of bone marrow depression produced by chloramphenicol is an irreversible fatal aplastic anemia. It occurs in one in 20,000 to 40,000 courses of therapy, and its occurrence is not directly dose related. Leukopenia or granulocytopenia may precede pancytopenia. This reaction principally occurs after prolonged courses of therapy, particularly in individuals who have been previously exposed to the drug. It may appear weeks or months after chloramphenicol has been administered. The occurrence of this form of drug reaction in identical twins suggests a possible genetic predisposition.[38]

Because of the risk of bone marrow depression, a complete blood count and differential should be performed three times weekly in all patients receiving chloramphenicol.

Chloramphenicol, sulfonamides, nitrofurantoin, and primaquine can cause hemolytic anemia in patients who have deficiencies of erythrocyte glucose-6-phosphate dehydrogenase (G6PD). Hemolytic anemia, thrombocytopenia, and leukopenia that involve an immune mechanism can be caused by penicillins, cephalosporins, and rifampin, but these reactions are uncommon. Tetracycline is an uncommon cause of hemolytic anemia.[39] Trimethoprim-sulfamethoxazole and macrolides have been statistically associated with agranulocytosis.[40]

Amphotericin B commonly produces a reversible normocytic normochromic anemia, probably secondary to injury to the red cell membrane. Trimethoprim can produce anemia, leukopenia, and thrombocytopenia from folate deficiency; the effect is reversible by folinic acid. Flucytosine (5-FC) causes bone marrow suppression (leukopenia or pancytopenia) when its excretion is reduced by renal failure. The conversion by intestinal flora of 5-FC to fluorouracil (5-FU) and accumulation of the latter may be responsible for the marrow toxicity.

Neutropenia can occur during therapy with penicillins or cephalosporins.[41] Although neutropenia is usually an isolated abnormality, it is accompanied in some patients by thrombocytopenia, eosinophilia, rash, or fever. Neutropenia develops in fewer than 0.1 percent of patients receiving brief courses of β-lactam antibiotics, but the risk to patients receiving prolonged high-dose therapy has been estimated at five to 15 percent. Bone marrow aspirates reveal that maturation arrest occurs early in granulocyte differentiation; in vitro studies demonstrate that β-lactam antibiotics suppress granulopoiesis by a direct mechanism that is dose related. Neutropenia may be severe, but it is self-limited; recovery occurs one to seven days after the antibiotic is withdrawn.

Penicillins inhibit platelet aggregation by adenosine diphosphate, which may account for the postoperative bleeding that occurs in some patients receiving these antibiotics. Because carbenicillin is administered in high doses, it is the agent most often responsible for such bleeding; other penicillins may have a similar effect if given in very high doses.

Various cephalosporin antibiotics may produce coagulopathies by prolonging the prothrombin time; the methylthiotetrazole side chain present in such cephalosporins as cefotetan, cefamandole, and moxalactam appears to be responsible.

The nervous system Antibiotics may produce a wide range of toxic effects on the central and peripheral nervous systems.[42] Ototoxicity can be produced by all of the aminoglycoside antibiotics. Streptomycin and gentamicin more commonly affect the vestibular portion of the eighth cranial nerve, but hearing loss can also occur with these drugs. With neomycin, kanamycin, amikacin, and tobramycin, hearing loss is a more frequent side effect than vestibular changes. Loss of hearing has reportedly been produced by absorption of an aminoglycoside solution employed to irrigate a wound in a patient with normal renal function. The risks of ototoxicity and nephrotoxicity from aminoglycosides are greatest in the elderly, in patients with preexisting renal damage, in those with blood levels in the toxic range, in those receiving prolonged therapy, and in patients receiving sequential courses of therapy with one or more aminoglycoside antibiotics.

Although aminoglycosides are the most common causes of antibiotic-induced ototoxicity, other drugs can cause these reactions. Minocycline has occasionally been reported to produce significant vestibular reactions. Vertigo and dizziness were prominent side effects among a group of patients in the United States who were receiving this drug as meningococcal prophylaxis.[43] In extensive studies in other countries, however, vestibular reactions to minocycline have been infrequent.[44] Erythromycin is an uncommon cause of sensorineural hearing loss.[45] Vancomycin can cause auditory neurotoxicity; patients who are older than 65 years, have azotemia, or have high vancomycin blood levels are at the greatest risk.

Several other uncommon forms of neurotoxicity are associated with the aminoglycosides. Circumoral paresthesias may occasionally occur shortly after injections of streptomycin, but they usually do not require discontinuance of the drug. A more serious side effect that may follow either intraperitoneal or intravenous administration of an aminoglycoside is neuromuscular blockade accompanied by respiratory arrest, similar to that produced by tubocurarine. This side effect is usually dose related and is most frequently observed during anesthesia; it may be reversed by the administration of neostigmine and calcium gluconate. Colistimethate and polymyxin B can also produce transient paresthesias and, occasionally, neuromuscular blockade. This neuromuscular blockade, unlike that produced by the aminoglycosides, is resistant to neostigmine but may respond to calcium gluconate. Both lincomycin and clindamycin have weak neuromuscular blocking effects but may potentiate tubocurarine.

Penicillin G can produce seizures after intrathecal injections of more than 30,000 to 40,000 units (and after one third of this dose if the drug is administered intraventricularly). Intravenous administration of massive doses of penicillin (more than 40 million units daily in an adult) may produce neurotoxicity characterized by premonitory myoclonic jerking of the face and extremities, followed by focal and generalized seizures. These seizures are most likely to occur in patients with renal insufficiency or in those who receive the drug during cardiopulmonary bypass, when the permeability of the blood-brain barrier is increased and higher levels of penicillin in the cerebrospinal fluid are achieved. The neurotoxicity observed with penicillin G can be induced by other penicillins and cephalosporins in the presence of renal insufficiency. Another β-lactam, imipenem, may also produce seizures, especially when administered in very high doses or when given to azotemic patients or to patients with underlying epilepsy.

Peripheral neuropathy can occur as a complication of therapy with nitrofurantoin, particularly when renal failure is present. The neuropathy that occurs with isoniazid can be prevented by the daily administration of 100 mg of pyridoxine. A toxic encephalopathy may be associated with high doses of isoniazid. Cycloserine, a drug occasionally used to treat tuberculosis, can produce dysarthria, toxic encephalopathy, and seizures; 100 mg of pyridoxine daily may prevent the seizures.

Tetracycline may rarely produce reversible benign intracranial hypertension with headache and papilledema in infants, children, and even adults. Nalidixic acid may also produce intracranial hypertension and seizures in children. Metronidazole can infrequently cause ataxia, encephalopathy, seizures, or peripheral neuropathies.

Optic neuritis, usually manifested by decreased visual acuity and decreased perception of the color green, may occur as a side effect of ethambutol. This side effect is uncommon with a daily dosage of 15 mg/kg, and when it occurs, it is usually reversible by withdrawal of the medication. Optic neuritis is a rare side effect of isoniazid administration. A rare, untoward effect of prolonged chloramphenicol administration in children is an optic neuritis that may cause permanent blindness.

The liver The principal antimicrobials that produce adverse effects on the liver are those used in the treatment of tuberculosis: isoniazid, rifampin, aminosalicylic acid (PAS), and pyrazinamide. Isoniazid produces mild hepatic injury, as judged by elevation of serum aspartate aminotransferase (AST) levels, in 10 to 20 percent of patients receiving the drug.[46] Most patients who show biochemical evidence of liver injury recover from this side effect during the course of therapy with isoniazid, and overt hepatitis does not develop. In a small number of patients, clinical hepatitis does develop; chills, fever, and deterioration of

hepatic function shortly after rechallenge with the drug suggest a hypersensitivity mechanism. It has been suggested, however, that most cases of isoniazid hepatitis are caused by the hydrolysis of acetylisoniazid (the initial isoniazid metabolite in humans) releasing free acetylhydrazine, which is subsequently converted to a potent hepatotoxic acylating agent.[47] Persons who acetylate isoniazid rapidly, such as some Asians, appear to be more susceptible to isoniazid hepatitis than individuals who acetylate the drug slowly.[47] The incidence of isoniazid toxicity increases with age and is of particular concern in patients older than 50 years. Most instances of hepatotoxicity occur within two months after initiating therapy, but this side effect may be delayed for as long as 11 months. Routine monitoring of serum aminotransferase levels to detect hepatic injury is not recommended, because moderate transient elevations of AST occur in many patients receiving the drug.[48] Patients should be monitored for evidence of possible toxicity, such as fever, anorexia, nausea, vomiting, and abdominal pain. If such symptoms occur, liver function tests should be performed promptly and the medication stopped.

Rifampin may cause a transient mild hyperbilirubinemia but may also infrequently produce significant hepatic injury, usually within three weeks after the start of treatment. Liver injury is more frequent in patients with alcoholism or preexisting liver disease or in patients concurrently receiving another hepatotoxic drug, such as isoniazid. Hepatic damage may occur rarely as part of a hypersensitivity reaction to PAS. The other elements of the reaction are malaise, fever, pruritus and rash, and eosinophilia.

Liver injury caused by the tetracyclines may occur in patients receiving 2 g or more daily, usually by the intravenous route. The histologic changes amount to an extensive fatty metamorphosis. Hepatotoxicity is most likely to occur in pregnant women receiving high doses of intravenous tetracycline in the treatment of pyelonephritis.[49] The fatty changes in the liver from pregnancy and some decreased renal function secondary to the kidney infection may predispose to hepatotoxicity.

Patients receiving high-dose intravenous oxacillin therapy may experience reversible anicteric hepatitis, presumably a hypersensitivity reaction.

Nitrofurantoin may cause chronic active hepatitis in some patients.[50]

The gastrointestinal tract Gastrointestinal reactions to antibiotics result from either direct irritation by the drug, usually dose related, or bacterial overgrowth. From a therapeutic viewpoint, it is essential to distinguish between the diarrheas caused by these two mechanisms. Irritative gastrointestinal side effects are usually produced when antibiotics are administered orally rather than parenterally. The predominant site of irritation varies from drug to drug. Erythromycin more commonly produces gastric irritation with epigastric distress and nausea. The tetracyclines may produce diarrhea as well as upper gastrointestinal symptoms. The oral administration of neomycin in a daily dosage greater than 3 g can produce diarrhea and intestinal malabsorption with prominent steatorrhea.

Some qualitative and quantitative changes in the intestinal flora occur after antibiotic administration; they may contribute to flatulence and other lower gastrointestinal symptoms that are quite common when broad-spectrum antibiotics are administered orally. Extreme overgrowth of a single bacterial species can result in serious superinfection. Typical examples are staphylococcal enterocolitis and pseudomembranous enterocolitis. Staphylococcal enterocolitis is an uncommon infection of the intestinal mucosa that follows suppression of the normal bowel flora by antimicrobial therapy. The drugs most often involved are tetracycline, chloramphenicol, and neomycin. Examination of the feces by a Gram's stain of a smear and culture usually discloses a predominance of *S. aureus*. Treatment involves fluid replacement, omission of the antimicrobials being used, and antibi-

otic therapy against *S. aureus*. In many patients, oral vancomycin, 0.5 g every six hours for three to five days, is adequate therapy.[51] In patients with severe disease, bacteremia and systemic infection occasionally occur; therefore, parenteral therapy with a penicillinase-resistant penicillin, such as nafcillin, 6 g I.V. daily, is warranted.

Several agents, including ampicillin, cephalosporins, and other antimicrobials, have been associated with antibiotic-induced enterocolitis; clindamycin, however, has most frequently been associated with this disease. Diarrhea has been reported in 21 percent of patients and pseudomembranous enterocolitis in 10 percent of patients who take clindamycin[52]; other studies, however, indicate a much lower incidence of these side effects.[53] Antibiotic-induced pseudomembranous enterocolitis is caused by overgrowth of toxin-producing *Clostridium difficile*.[54] Oral administration of vancomycin or metronidazole has been effective for antibiotic-induced pseudomembranous enterocolitis. Oral administration of bacitracin may be useful in the occasional patient who fails to respond to metronidazole or vancomycin.[55] Cholestyramine binds the clostridial toxin and may also be therapeutically beneficial.

Microbial Superinfection

Continued antimicrobial therapy eliminates susceptible organisms from the normal flora of the skin, oral and genitourinary mucosa, and gastrointestinal tract and selects instead an altered flora consisting of drug-resistant organisms. Such resistant organisms can occasionally establish a superinfection at the site of the original infection, which was caused by a susceptible bacterial species. For example, pneumonia caused by resistant gram-negative bacilli (e.g., *P. aeruginosa*) has occasionally followed intense antibiotic treatment of an initial pneumonia caused by a more susceptible organism. The effects of antibiotic administration on the respiratory tract flora of tracheotomized patients have long been known.[56] However, even in the absence of antimicrobial drugs, there is evidence that upper respiratory tract flora shift predominantly toward gram-negative bacilli in hospitalized patients who are severely ill.[57]

Elimination of normal flora can also produce disease caused by overgrowth of resistant microorganisms at sites remote from those of the initial infection for which antimicrobials were prescribed. Antibiotic-associated pseudomembranous enterocolitis and oral or vaginal candidiasis after the use of broad-spectrum antibiotics exemplify this type of clinical disease.

Duration of Antimicrobial Therapy

Adequate data for establishing the optimal duration of antimicrobial therapy are generally not available. Some guidelines have been based on microbiological evidence; for example, a 10-day regimen of penicillin therapy for acute streptococcal pharyngitis is required to eradicate *S. pyogenes* and to prevent the subsequent development of acute rheumatic fever. In urinary tract infections, the appropriate duration of therapy depends on the specific location of the process: a single dose of an appropriate antimicrobial may eradicate bladder infections in women, but much longer courses of therapy are required for infections of the kidney or prostate.[8] In other instances, empirical evidence is all that underlies such programs as four weeks of penicillin for treatment of subacute bacterial endocarditis caused by viridans streptococci or four to six weeks of a penicillinase-resistant penicillin for acute *S. aureus* osteomyelitis. In most acute infections, treatment lasting three to five days after the patient is afebrile is adequate if clinical signs of active infection have abated. For bacteremia, longer periods of chemotherapy are warranted, depending on the nature of the infecting organism.

Antimicrobial Resistance in Hospitals

The extensive use of antimicrobial agents in a hospital environment strongly favors the selection of resistant microbial species, particularly bacterial strains harboring transmissible resistance plasmids.[58] Outbreaks of nosocomial infections from highly resistant strains of *Serratia, Klebsiella, Acinetobacter, Enterobacter,* and *S. aureus* have become important problems. With extensive overuse at a particular hospital, a new effective antibiotic may lose its efficacy in that institution. The situation then becomes a matter of public health policy in the institution. In some hospitals, one or more of the newer antimicrobial agents are kept on reserve, for use only in patients in whom susceptibility testing indicates that the agent is the only effective or least toxic one for combating the specific infecting organism. Thus, one or several of the newer β-lactams are not in general hospital use except in life-threatening situations or for treating infections caused by more resistant organisms. Monitoring antibiotic susceptibility patterns is essential because a significant decrease in the percentage of bacterial strains susceptible to the conventional drug would warrant wider use of the newer drug, especially in initial therapy for serious infections.

Antibiotics in Pregnancy

The administration of antimicrobial agents during pregnancy and in the postpartum period poses several problems.[59,60] Foremost is the question of safety, both for the mother and for the fetus or neonate. Although most antibiotics cross the placenta and enter maternal milk, the concentrations to which the fetus or neonate is exposed vary widely, depending on the extent of protein binding, lipid solubility, ionization, and other factors. Because the immature liver may lack the enzymes required to metabolize certain drugs, fetal pharmacokinetics and toxicities are often very different from those in older children and adults. In addition to direct drug toxicities, teratogenicity is a major concern when any drug is administered during pregnancy. Finally, the dosage schedules may have to be altered when administering those drugs that appear to be safe to use during pregnancy; increases in maternal blood volume, glomerular filtration rate, and hepatic metabolic activity often reduce the maternal serum levels of antimicrobials by 10 to 50 percent, especially late in pregnancy and in the early postpartum period. In some women, delayed gastric emptying may reduce the absorption of antibiotics that have been administered orally during pregnancy.

Even though 25 to 40 percent of women receive antibiotics during pregnancy, data regarding their safety and efficacy in this setting are often scarce. Some general recommendations have been proposed for the administration of antimicrobials during pregnancy, but they are intended as a guide only [see Table 4]; in all cases, therapy must be individualized, and both the indications for antibiotics and the possible risks to mother and fetus must be considered.

Antibiotics in the Elderly

Physiologic changes that occur with age have the potential for altering the pharmacokinetics of antimicrobial agents. For example, decreased gastric acidity and intestinal motility could impair drug absorption, increased body fat and decreased serum albumin levels could alter drug distribution, and decreased hepatic blood flow and enzymatic action could delay drug metabolism. Although these factors have not consistently affected antibiotic levels in the elderly, the decrease in glomerular filtration rate that occurs with age can lead to the accumulation of drugs excreted by the kidney.[61] In the case of the penicillins and cephalosporins, the high therapeutic index obviates the need for major changes in dosage schedules in elderly patients who have normal serum creatinine levels. However, in the case of aminoglycosides and vancomycin, decreased dosage schedules are often required; ideally, drug levels should be measured, and renal function should be monitored when these agents are given. The dosage of amantadine should also be reduced in elderly patients.

Outpatient Intravenous Antibiotic Therapy

Prolonged intravenous antibiotic therapy is required for a variety of infections; for example, four- to six-week regimens are standard for the treatment of osteomyelitis and endocarditis. In many cases, however, patients are clinically stable during the last weeks of treatment but remain hospitalized solely because they require parenteral antibiotics. It is now possible to discharge such patients and to administer parenteral antibiotics on an outpatient basis.[62] Supervision by special teams of physicians, nurses, and pharmacists is required; antibiotics can be administered either in the hospital outpatient department or at home if competent family members are available. New antibiotics with long half-lives can be used in simplified regimens, leading to substantial economic benefits, enhanced patient comfort, and good therapeutic results with few complications.

Specific Antimicrobial Drugs

The considerations presented thus far provide the basis for selection of antimicrobials of choice for various infections and of suitable alternatives for patients unable to tolerate the primary drug [see Table 5].[63,64] The agents and the chemotherapy for specific diseases will be discussed (see below).

Penicillins

The penicillins are bactericidal antibiotics that impair synthesis of the bacterial cell wall constituent peptidoglycan by binding to penicillin-binding proteins in the cell wall. The penicillin-binding proteins are located on the inner surface of the cell membrane. They are enzymes that are responsible for linking individual elements of the bacterial cell wall together. At least seven penicillin-binding proteins have been identified; penicillins and other β-lactam antibiotics have different affinities for various penicillin-binding proteins.[40]

The penicillins may be classified into subgroups on the basis of their structure, β-lactamase susceptibility, and spectrum of action [see Figure 1]. Dosages of these agents vary according to the type and severity of infection [see Table 6]. The side effects of penicillin are generally shared by all its de-

Table 4 Antibiotics in Pregnancy

Drug	Major Toxic Potential		Pharmacology	
	Maternal	*Fetal*	*Maternal Serum Levels*	*Excreted in Mother's Milk*
Considered Safe				
Cephalosporins	Allergies	None known	Decreased	Trace
Erythromycin base	Allergies, GI intolerance	None known	Decreased	Yes
Penicillins	Allergies	None known	Decreased	Trace
Spectinomycin	?	None known	?	?
Use with Caution				
Aminoglycosides	Ototoxicity and nephrotoxicity	Ototoxicity	Decreased	Yes
Clindamycin	Allergies, colitis	None known	Unchanged	Trace
Ethambutol	Optic neuritis	Probably safe	?	?
Isoniazid	Allergies, hepatotoxicity	Neuropathy, seizures	Unchanged	Yes
Rifampin	Hypersensitivity, hepatotoxicity	Probably safe	Unchanged	Yes
Sulfonamides (contraindicated at term)	Allergies, crystalluria	Kernicterus (at term), hemolysis (G6PD deficiency)	Unchanged	Yes
Avoid if Possible				
Metronidazole	Hypersensitivity, alcohol intolerance, neuropathy	None known (teratogenic in animals)	Probably unchanged	Yes
Contraindicated				
Chloramphenicol	Blood dyscrasias	Gray syndrome	Unchanged	Yes
Erythromycin estolate	Hepatotoxicity	None known	Decreased	Yes
Nalidixic acid	GI intolerance	Increased intracranial pressure	?	?
Norfloxacin, ciprofloxacin, ofloxacin, lomefloxacin	GI intolerance	Arthropathies in immature animals	?	?
Nitrofurantoin	Allergies, neuropathy, GI intolerance	Hemolysis (G6PD deficiency)	Decreased	Trace
Tetracyclines	Hepatotoxicity, renal failure	Tooth discoloration and dysplasia, impaired bone growth	Probably unchanged	Yes
Trimethoprim	Hypersensitivity	Teratogenicity	Unchanged	Yes

Table 5 Antimicrobial Drugs of Choice for Various Infections in Adults

	Causative Organism	Drug of Choice	Alternative Drugs
Gram-Positive Cocci	*Staphylococcus aureus*		
	Methicillin-resistant (uncommon)[1]	Vancomycin,[2] with or without rifampin, gentamicin, or both	Trimethoprim-sulfamethoxazole,[2] with or without rifampin[2]; ciprofloxacin[2]; minocycline[3]
	Non–penicillinase-producing (uncommon)	Penicillin G[4]	A cephalosporin,[5] clindamycin, vancomycin,[6] imipenem, a fluoroquinolone[7]
	Penicillinase-producing (common)	Penicillinase-resistant penicillin[8]	A cephalosporin,[5] clindamycin, vancomycin,[6] imipenem,[9] ticarcillin–clavulanic acid, ampicillin-sulbactam, amoxicillin–clavulanic acid, ciprofloxacin[7]
	S. epidermidis[10]	Vancomycin,[6] with or without rifampin[2] or gentamicin	A cephalosporin, a penicillinase-resistant penicillin, imipenem,[9] a fluoroquinolone[7]
	Anaerobic streptococcus (*Peptostreptococcus*)	Penicillin G[4]	Clindamycin, a cephalosporin,[5] vancomycin[6]
	Streptococcus bovis	Penicillin G[4,11]	A cephalosporin,[5] vancomycin[6]
	Enterococcus		
	Endocarditis or other serious infection	Penicillin or ampicillin, plus gentamicin[12] or amikacin	Vancomycin,[6] with gentamicin
	Uncomplicated urinary tract infection	Ampicillin (or amoxicillin) or penicillin G	A fluoroquinolone,[7] trimethoprim-sulfamethoxazole or nitrofurantoin[13]
	Groups A, G, and C streptococci	Penicillin G[4,14] or penicillin V	A cephalosporin,[5] vancomycin,[6] an erythromycin,[15] clindamycin, clarithromycin, azithromycin
	Group B streptococcus	Penicillin G[4,14] or ampicillin	A cephalosporin,[5] vancomycin,[6] an erythromycin
	S. pneumoniae (pneumococcus)	Penicillin G[4,14] or penicillin V	An erythromycin,[14,15] a cephalosporin,[5] chloramphenicol,[6,14] vancomycin[6,14]
	Viridans streptococcus	Penicillin G,[4,11] with or without gentamicin	A cephalosporin,[5] vancomycin[6]
Gram-Positive Bacilli	*Bacillus anthracis*	Penicillin G	Tetracycline, an erythromycin[2]
	Clostridium difficile	Vancomycin[16] or metronidazole[16]	Bacitracin
	C. perfringens	Penicillin G	Chloramphenicol,[6] clindamycin, metronidazole, a tetracycline[3]
	C. tetani	Penicillin G	A tetracycline[3]
	Corynebacterium diphtheriae	An erythromycin	Penicillin G
	Corynebacterium, JK strain	Vancomycin	
	Listeria monocytogenes	Ampicillin, with or without gentamicin	Penicillin G, with gentamicin; trimethoprim-sulfamethoxazole
	Propionibacterium	Penicillin G	Clindamycin, an erythromycin

Note: all superscript numbers refer to footnotes that follow table.

	Causative Organism	Drug of Choice	Alternative Drugs
Gram-Negative Cocci	*Moraxella* (formerly *Branhamella*) *catarrhalis*	Trimethoprim-sulfamethoxazole	Amoxicillin–clavulanic acid, an erythromycin, a tetracycline, cefuroxime, third-generation cephalosporins, clarithromycin, azithromycin
	Neisseria gonorrhoeae[17]	Ceftriaxone[5]	Penicillin G or amoxicillin or ampicillin (plus probenecid when given p.o. or I.M.), spectinomycin,[18] cefoxitin,[5] cefixime, trimethoprim-sulfamethoxazole, chloramphenicol,[6] ciprofloxacin,[7] ofloxacin
	N. meningitidis Carrier state	Rifampin	Minocycline, ciprofloxacin
	Meningitis, bacteremia	Penicillin G	Chloramphenicol,[6] cefuroxime,[5] a third-generation cephalosporin,[5] trimethoprim-sulfamethoxazole

Enteric Gram-Negative Bacilli	*Bacteroides*
	  GI tract strains
	    (*B. fragilis*)
		Metronidazole	Clindamycin, cefoxitin or cefotetan; chloramphenicol[19]; ticarcillin, mezlocillin, or piperacillin; imipenem[9]; ticarcillin–clavulanic acid; ampicillin-sulbactam, ceftizoxime, cefmetazole

	Respiratory tract strains	Penicillin G	Clindamycin, cefoxitin,[5] cefotetan,[5] metronidazole, chloramphenicol[6]
	Campylobacter jejuni	A fluoroquinolone,[7] an erythromycin	A tetracycline,[3] gentamicin[6]
	Citrobacter	Gentamicin, a third-generation cephalosporin[5]	A fluoroquinolone,[7] imipenem,[9] tobramycin, chloramphenicol,[6] amikacin
	Enterobacter	Imipenem[9]	A third-generation cephalosporin[5]; for serious infections, use with ciprofloxacin or gentamicin; gentamicin, tobramycin, amikacin, a fluoroquinolone,[7] a carboxypenicillin or acylaminopenicillin,[20] aztreonam,[21] trimethoprim-sulfamethoxazole, chloramphenicol[6]
	Escherichia coli[22]	Ampicillin, a cephalosporin,[5] a fluoroquinolone,[7] trimethoprim-sulfamethoxazole[24]	Gentamicin,[23] tobramycin, amikacin, imipenem,[9] aztreonam,[21] chloramphenicol[6]
	Klebsiella[22]	A cephalosporin[5]	Gentamicin,[23] tobramycin, amikacin, chloramphenicol,[6] trimethoprim-sulfamethoxazole,[24] a carboxypenicillin or acylaminopenicillin,[20] amoxicillin–clavulanic acid, ampicillin-sulbactam, ticarcillin–clavulanic acid, imipenem,[9] aztreonam,[21] a fluoroquinolone[7]

Note: all superscript numbers refer to footnotes that follow table.

	Causative Organism	Drug of Choice	Alternative Drugs
Enteric Gram-Negative Bacilli (continued)	Proteus mirabilis [22]	Ampicillin	Gentamicin or tobramycin, a cephalosporin, chloramphenicol,[6] a carboxypenicillin or acylaminopenicillin,[20] imipenem,[9] trimethoprim-sulfamethoxazole, aztreonam,[21] a fluoroquinolone[7]
	non-mirabilis,[22] including P. vulgaris, Morganella morganii, and Providencia rettgeri	A second- or third-generation cephalosporin[5]	Gentamicin, tobramycin, amikacin, a carboxypenicillin or acylaminopenicillin,[20] chloramphenicol,[6] imipenem,[9] aztreonam,[21] ampicillin-sulbactam, ticarcillin–clavulanic acid, amoxicillin–clavulanic acid, a fluoroquinolone[7]
	Providencia stuartii	A second- or third-generation cephalosporin	An aminoglycoside, trimethoprim-sulfamethoxazole,[24] imipenem,[9] aztreonam,[21] a carboxypenicillin or acylaminopenicillin,[20] a fluoroquinolone[7]
	Salmonella typhi	Ceftriaxone (ciprofloxacin[7] for the carrier state)	Chloramphenicol or ampicillin,[25] trimethoprim-sulfamethoxazole, a fluoroquinolone[7]
	Other Salmonella species	Ceftriaxone or cefotaxime	Ampicillin or amoxicillin, a fluoroquinolone,[7] trimethoprim-sulfamethoxazole, a third-generation cephalosporin, chloramphenicol[6]
	Serratia	A third-generation cephalosporin	Gentamicin or amikacin, a carboxypenicillin or acylamino-penicillin,[20] chloramphenicol,[6] imipenem,[9] aztreonam, a fluoroquinolone[7]
	Shigella	A fluoroquinolone[7]	Trimethoprim-sulfamethoxazole, ampicillin, ceftriaxone
Other Gram-Negative Bacilli	Acinetobacter (Herellea)	Imipenem[9]	Tobramycin, gentamicin, amikacin, doxycycline, minocycline, a carboxypenicillin or acylamino-penicillin,[20] trimethoprim-sulfamethoxazole
	Aeromonas hydrophilia	Trimethoprim-sulfamethoxazole[2]	A fluoroquinolone,[7] gentamicin, tobramycin, imipenem,[9] a tetracycline
	Brucella	A tetracycline, with gentamicin	Chloramphenicol,[6] with or without streptomycin; trimethoprim-sulfamethoxazole[2]; rifampin[2] with a tetracycline

Note: all superscript numbers refer to footnotes that follow table.

<table>
<tr><td rowspan="20">Other Gram-Negative Bacilli (continued)</td></tr>
</table>

Causative Organism	*Drug of Choice*	*Alternative Drugs*
Eikenella corrodens	Ampicillin	An erythromycin, a tetracycline,[3] amoxicillin–clavulanic acid, ampicillin-sulbactam, ceftriaxone
Francisella tularensis (*tularemia*)	Streptomycin or gentamicin	A tetracycline,[3] chloramphenicol[6]
Fusobacterium	Penicillin	Clindamycin, metronidazole, chloramphenicol[6]
Gardnerella (formerly *Hemophilus*) *vaginalis*	Metronidazole[2]	Ampicillin[2]
Hemophilus influenzae		
Bronchitis, otitis media	Trimethoprim-sulfamethoxazole	Ampicillin or amoxicillin; a tetracycline[3]; a sulfonamide, with or without erythromycin; amoxicillin–clavulanic acid; cefuroxime axetil, ceftizoxime, clarithromycin, azithromycin
Meningitis, epiglottitis, life-threatening infections	Cefuroxime[5] or a third-generation cephalosporin	Chloramphenicol plus ampicillin initially[26]; a tetracycline[3]
Legionella pneumophila (Legionnaires' disease)	Erythromycin	Rifampin,[27] trimethoprim-sulfamethoxazole,[2] clarithromycin, a fluoroquinolone,[7] azithromycin
L. micdadei	Erythromycin	Rifampin,[2] trimethoprim-sulfamethoxazole[2]
Pasteurella multocida	Penicillin G	A tetracycline,[3] a cephalosporin,[5] amoxicillin–clavulanic acid, ampicillin-sulbactam
Calymmatobacterium granulomatis (granuloma inguinale)	A tetracycline[3]	Streptomycin, trimethoprim-sulfamethoxazole, an erythromycin
H. ducreyi (chancroid)	Ceftriaxone or an erythromycin	Ciprofloxacin[7]
Pseudomonas aeruginosa Urinary tract infections	A fluoroquinolone,[7] a carboxypenicillin or acylaminopenicillin[20]	Gentamicin or tobramycin; amikacin; ceftazidime,[5] with or without gentamicin or tobramycin; imipenem[9]; aztreonam[21]
Other infections	Gentamicin or tobramycin, with or without a carboxypenicillin or acylaminopenicillin[20]; ceftazidime, imipenem[9]; aztreonam,[21] alone or with gentamicin or tobramycin	Amikacin, with or without a carboxypenicillin or acylaminopenicillin[20]; ciprofloxacin[7]
P. cepacia	Trimethoprim-sulfamethoxazole	Chloramphenicol,[6] ceftazidime,[2] imipenem[2,9]
Streptobacillus moniliformis (rat-bite fever)	Penicillin G	A tetracycline,[3] streptomycin
Vibrio cholerae	A tetracycline[3]	Trimethoprim-sulfamethoxazole, a fluoroquinolone[7]
V. vulnificus	A tetracycline[3]	Cefotaxime
Agents of Vincent's stomatitis (trench mouth)	Penicillin G	A tetracycline,[3] an erythromycin
Yersinia enterocolitica	Trimethoprim-sulfamethoxazole[2]	Ciprofloxacin,[7] gentamicin,[2] tobramycin,[2] amikacin,[2] tetracycline,[3] cefotaxime[2,5]
Y. pestis (plague)	Streptomycin	A tetracycline,[3] chloramphenicol,[6] gentamicin[2]

Note: all superscript numbers refer to footnotes that follow table.

	Causative Organism	Drug of Choice	Alternative Drugs
Other Gram-Negative Bacilli (continued)	Mycobacterium avium-intracellulare	Multiple-drug regimens[28]	
	M. fortuitum	Amikacin,[2] doxycycline,[2] or both	Rifampin,[2] an erythromycin,[2] cefoxitin, a sulfonamide
	M. kansasii	Isoniazid with rifampin, with or without ethambutol	Streptomycin
	M. leprae	Dapsone[6] with rifampin, with or without clofazimine	Minocycline,[3] ofloxacin[7]
	M. marinum (balnei)[29]	Minocycline	Trimethoprim-sulfamethoxazole, rifampin, ethambutol, clarithromycin
	M. tuberculosis[30]	Isoniazid with rifampin, with or without pyrazinamide	Ethambutol, streptomycin, pyrazinamide
Acid-Fast Bacilli	Actinomyces israelii	Penicillin G	A tetracycline[3]
	Nocardia	Trimethoprim-sulfamethoxazole	Minocycline, sulfisoxazole, imipenem,[9] amikacin,[2] cycloserine
Fungi	Aspergillus	Amphotericin B[6]	No dependable alternative
	Blastomyces dermatitidis	Amphotericin B[6]	Ketoconazole, fluconazole[2]
	Candida	Amphotericin B[6,31] or fluconazole	Ketoconazole, flucytosine,[32] nystatin (oral or topical), miconazole (topical),[33] clotrimazole (topical)
	Coccidioides immitis	Amphotericin B[6]	Fluconazole, ketoconazole, miconazole[33]
	Cryptococcus neoformans	Amphotericin B,[6] with or without flucytosine[34]	Fluconazole, ketoconazole, flucytosine,[32] miconazole[33]
	Histoplasma capsulatum	Amphotericin B	Ketoconazole
	Phycomycetes (e.g., Mucor)	Amphotericin B	No dependable alternative
	Sporothrix schenckii (sporotrichosis)	Saturated solution of potassium iodide[35]	Amphotericin B,[6] ketoconazole
Chlamydia	Chlamydia psittaci (psittacosis)	A tetracycline[3]	Chloramphenicol[6]
	C. trachomatis		
	Inclusion conjunctivitis	An erythromycin (oral or I.V.)	A sulfonamide (topical plus oral)
	Lymphogranuloma venereum	A tetracycline[3] or an erythromycin	
	Pneumonia	An erythromycin	A sulfonamide
	Trachoma	A tetracycline[3] (topical plus oral)	A sulfonamide (topical plus oral)
	Urethritis or pelvic inflammatory disease	A tetracycline[3] or an erythromycin	Azithromycin, ofloxacin, sulfisoxazole
	C. pneumoniae	An erythromycin or clarithromycin; a tetracycline	
Myco-plasma	Mycoplasma pneumoniae	An erythromycin[36] or a tetracycline[3]	Clarithromycin
	Ureaplasma urealyticum	An erythromycin	A tetracycline[3]; clarithromycin

Note: all superscript numbers refer to footnotes that follow table.

	Causative Organism	Drug of Choice	Alternative Drugs
Rickettsia	Various rickettsial organisms Rocky Mountain spotted fever, epidemic and endemic (murine) typhus, rickettsial pox, Q fever, scrub typhus	A tetracycline[3]	Chloramphenicol,[6] a fluoroquinolone[7]
Spirochetes	*Borrelia burgdorferi* (Lyme disease)	A tetracycline,[3] amoxicillin or ceftriaxone	Penicillin, an erythromycin, clarithromycin, azithromycin
	B. recurrentis (relapsing fever)	A tetracycline[3]	Penicillin G
	Leptospira	Penicillin G	A tetracycline,[3] an erythromycin
	Treponema pallidum	Penicillin G	A tetracycline,[3] an erythromycin, ceftriaxone
Misc. Organisms	*Afipia felis* (cat-scratch disease)	Ciprofloxacin[7]	Trimethoprim-sulfamethoxazole, gentamicin
	Rochalimaea henselae (bacillary angiomatosis)	An erythromycin	A tetracycline
Viruses	Herpes simplex Disseminated	Acyclovir	Vidarabine, foscarnet[2]
	Encephalitis	Acyclovir	Vidarabine
	Genital	Acyclovir	Vidarabine, foscarnet[2]
	Keratitis	Trifluridine (topical)	Idoxuridine (topical), vidarabine (topical)
	Neonatal	Acyclovir	Vidarabine
	Human immunodeficiency virus (HIV)[37]	Zidovudine (AZT)	Dideoxyinosine
	Cytomegalovirus	Ganciclovir	Foscarnet[2]
	Influenza A	Amantadine	No dependable alternative
	Respiratory syncytial virus	Ribavirin	None
	Varicella-zoster	Acyclovir	Vidarabine

1. Occasional strains of *S. aureus* and many strains of *S. epidermidis* are resistant to penicillinase-resistant penicillins; these strains are also resistant to cephalosporins.

2. Not approved for this indication by the FDA.

3. Tetracycline hydrochloride is preferred for most uses. Doxycycline is the safest of the tetracyclines for use in treatment of extrarenal infections in patients with renal insufficiency. Tetracyclines should generally be avoided in pregnant women and in children younger than eight years.

4. Crystalline penicillin G is administered parenterally in serious infections. For less severe infections caused by pneumococci, group A streptococci, gonococci, or *T. pallidum*, procaine penicillin is administered I.M. once or twice daily. For mild infections caused by streptococci and pneumococci, oral penicillin V is preferable to oral penicillin G. Benzathine penicillin G is given I.M. (once monthly for the prophylaxis of rheumatic fever; a single injection for the treatment of group A streptococcal pharyngitis) when patient compliance for oral medication is questionable and, for treatment of syphilis, in one to three doses at weekly intervals, depending on the stage of disease.

5. Cephalosporins are sometimes used as alternatives to penicillin in patients in whom penicillin allergy is suspected but not in patients with serious hypersensitivity (especially immediate anaphylactic or accelerated urticarial reactions). Patients who have had allergic reactions to penicillin may have hypersensitivity reactions to cephalosporins. Only third-generation cephalosporins are effective in the treatment of bacterial meningitis.

6. In view of the occurrence of adverse reactions, this drug should be used only for serious infections and when other less toxic drugs are ineffective.

7. Not recommended for children.

8. For severe infections, I.V. nafcillin or oxacillin should be used. For mild infections (e.g., those involving skin and soft tissue), oral cloxacillin, dicloxacillin, or oxacillin may be employed. One to two percent of strains of *S. aureus* are resistant to penicillinase-resistant penicillins (and usually

to cephalosporins as well) but are susceptible to vancomycin. High doses of penicillin G, ampicillin, amoxicillin, carbenicillin, or ticarcillin do not overcome the clinical resistance of penicillinase-producing staphylococci to these drugs.

9. Imipenem is a β-lactam antibiotic that should be used with caution in patients who are allergic to penicillins and cephalosporins.

10. In vitro sensitivity testing with cephalosporins or penicillins may be misleading because of heteroresistance and because these antibiotics may be bacteriostatic only. For serious infections, such as endocarditis, vancomycin is preferred (see text for details).

11. The combination of penicillin G with streptomycin for the first two weeks of treatment of endocarditis caused by viridans streptococci is preferred by some.

12. Various aminoglycosides (streptomycin, kanamycin, and gentamicin) have been used in synergistic combination with penicillin or vancomycin. Because of the appearance of enterococcal strains resistant to the synergistic action with streptomycin (but not gentamicin), gentamicin is preferred for use in the combination.

13. Contraindicated in pregnancy or in the presence of renal insufficiency.

14. In patients with major allergy to penicillin, erythromycin is the alternative for respiratory tract infections; and chloramphenicol is the preferred alternative for meningitis. Occasional strains of pneumococci have high-level resistance to penicillin and to most other antibiotics except vancomycin.

15. Occasional strains of pneumococci and group A streptococci are erythromycin resistant.

16. Antibiotics may be administered orally for antibiotic-associated pseudomembranous enterocolitis. Vancomycin has been the drug of choice, but metronidazole appears to be as effective and is much less expensive.

17. Large doses of penicillin G or ampicillin (or amoxicillin) may be required because some strains are relatively resistant to these drugs. Penicillinase-producing gonococci, which are much more resistant to penicillin, have now appeared in the United States; spectinomycin is the treatment of choice for patients known to be infected with such strains.

18. Rare strains of gonococci are resistant to spectinomycin; cefoxitin, cefuroxime, cefotaxime, or trimethoprim-sulfamethoxazole should be used to treat these strains.

19. When CNS infection is present, metronidazole or chloramphenicol should be used.

20. The carboxypenicillins are carbenicillin and ticarcillin; the acylaminopenicillins are mezlocillin, azlocillin, and piperacillin. When one of these drugs is used for a severe infection, an aminoglycoside is often recommended as well.

21. Aztreonam is a β-lactam antibiotic; although cross-sensitivity has not been a problem, it should be used with caution in patients who are allergic to penicillins, cephalosporins, or imipenem.

22. An oral sulfonamide such as sulfisoxazole is often the initial therapy for an acute uncomplicated urinary tract infection, before the results of culture and susceptibility testing have been obtained. Alternatives include oral ampicillin or amoxicillin. Should the causative agent be a *Klebsiella* organism, an oral cephalosporin can be used; should it be a non-*mirabilis Proteus* organism, then carbenicillin indanyl can be employed.

23. In severely ill patients, an aminoglycoside is combined with a cephalosporin.

24. Principally in treatment of uncomplicated urinary tract infections.

25. Ampicillin or amoxicillin may be effective in milder cases.

26. Some encapsulated *H. influenzae* (type b) strains and some unencapsulated strains are resistant to ampicillin, and rare strains are resistant to chloramphenicol. Chloramphenicol plus ampicillin (or chloramphenicol alone) should be used for initial treatment of meningitis or epiglottitis in children until the organism is identified and its susceptibility is determined. In adults who have meningitis of unknown etiology and an indeterminate Gram's stain of a smear and in whom *H. influenzae* is a suspected pathogen, chloramphenicol is added to ampicillin (or penicillin G) for the first 24 hours until the results of culture become available. Ampicillin is preferred for treatment when the infecting strain of *H. influenzae* is known to be susceptible.

27. Not a use approved by the FDA. Evidence for possible efficacy comes thus far only from in vitro susceptibility testing and from treatment of infections produced in experimental animals. In both situations, *L. pneumophila* is highly susceptibile to rifampin.

28. Most strains are highly drug resistant. Agents such as clarithromycin or azithromycin, rifampin or rifabutin, clofazimine, ethambutol, ciprofloxacin, and amikacin are generally employed in multidrug regimens.

29. Most infections are self-limited without therapy.

30. A variety of combination treatment regimens are available.

31. I.V. amphotericin B is the drug of choice for systemic candidal infections. If in vitro synergism can be demonstrated with flucytosine, the combination may be indicated in therapy. For GI infections or oral thrush, oral nystatin may be adequate. Topical nystatin, miconazole, or clotrimazole is useful for skin or vaginal infections.

32. Some strains of *Candida* may be resistant to flucytosine, or resistance may develop during treatment. Bone marrow depression may be produced by flucytosine administration in the presence of renal insufficiency.

33. I.V. miconazole appears to have promise in treatment of coccidioidomycosis, particularly when amphotericin B has failed or cannot be tolerated. Its role in treatment of cryptococcal meningitis in patients who cannot tolerate amphotericin B is under study.

34. Combined therapy for cryptococcal meningitis with amphotericin B and flucytosine may provide more rapid sterilization of CSF. Combined therapy appears to decrease amphotericin B toxicity by allowing some reduction in dose without loss in therapeutic effect.

35. For treatment of lymphocutaneous form only.

36. Erythromycin and tetracycline have been equally effective in the treatment of mycoplasmal pneumonia. Because of the initial clinical similarity between mycoplasmal pneumonia and some cases of Legionnaires' disease and because erythromycin is effective in both diseases, it is the drug of choice in patients presumed to have mycoplasmal pneumonia.

37. Guidelines for the treatment of HIV infections are evolving rapidly.

rivatives [*see Table 7*]; however, methicillin is more likely to produce interstitial nephritis, broad-spectrum penicillins such as ampicillin are more likely to cause pseudomembranous colitis, and penicillins with α-carboxyl substitutions such as carbenicillin and ticarcillin are more likely to impair platelet function.[65] Patients who are known to be allergic to one penicillin compound are likely to be allergic to other such compounds as well. Thus, the patient's history is most important in excluding possible penicillin allergies; skin testing can be useful as well.[66,67] In patients allergic to penicillin, desensitization procedures can be used if alternative antimicrobials cannot be employed (see below).[68]

Penicillin G and Penicillin V

Penicillin G, which was the first antibiotic to be used for systemic infections, still remains the drug of choice for a variety of infections. Resistance to penicillin among group A streptococci, meningococci, and *Treponema pallidum* has not been observed, and penicillin G is highly effective in the treatment of subacute bacterial endocarditis caused by susceptible bacteria. Oral penicillin G continues to be effective against streptococcal pharyngitis. Penicillin V (phenoxymethyl penicillin) has the same spectrum of activity as penicillin G but is more stable than penicillin G in the acid pH of the stomach and is thus better absorbed from the gastrointestinal tract; however, penicillin V is the more expensive of the two. Blood levels of penicillin V are more predictable and, on the average, are two to five times higher than those achieved by an identical dose of penicillin G. Although all forms of penicillin introduced since the release of penicillin G are prescribed by weight, penicillin G is still commonly prescribed for parenteral administration by unitage. For interconversion, 1 mg of penicillin G is equivalent to approximately 1,600 units.

An intramuscular injection of penicillin G procaine is almost painless; because the drug is slowly absorbed, injections are required only every 12 to 24 hours for treatment of highly susceptible infections. Meningitis and endocarditis pose special problems of penetration across the blood-brain barrier and into vegetations, respectively. Thus, when these conditions are caused by susceptible organisms, high doses of aqueous penicillin G are administered intravenously at intervals of two to four hours. In patients with renal dysfunction, such high doses, particularly when administered rapidly, may produce neurotoxicity and enhance hyperkalemia (10 million units of penicillin G contain 16 mEq of K^+). In most instances, the hyperkalemia accompanying renal failure can be treated readily, and the use of penicillin G presents no problem. If necessary, a sodium salt of penicillin G or a sodium salt of a similar penicillin, such as ampicillin or carbenicillin, can be substituted for the aqueous penicillin G.

Penicillinase-Resistant Penicillins

Methicillin, oxacillin, nafcillin, cloxacillin, and dicloxacillin are the five penicillinase-resistant penicillins available in the United States. Methicillin was the first of these agents to be used clinically. Its introduction had an enormous impact in the early 1960s, when infections from penicillin-resistant *S. aureus* had reached epidemic proportions. Parenteral methicillin has largely been superseded by oxacillin and nafcillin. These two penicillins are as effective as methicillin against penicillinase-producing *S. aureus*. They are more active than methicillin, but less active than penicillin G or ampicillin, against pneumococci, various streptococci, and penicillinase-negative staphylococci. Thus, they may have some advantage in the treatment of mixed infections involving *S. aureus* and other gram-positive cocci. An allergic interstitial nephritis, methicillin nephritis (hematuria with proteinuria, rash, fever, and renal insufficiency), appears to be more frequent after the administration of methicillin but also occurs when the other penicillins or cephalosporins are given.[69,70] Hemorrhagic cystitis has also occurred as a complication of methicillin therapy.[71] More than 80 per-

Table 6   Antimicrobial Drug Dosages for Treatment of Bacterial and Fungal Infections in Adults with Normal Renal Function

| | | | Mild Infections* | | | |
| | | | Oral | | Intramuscular | |
Class of Drug	Specific Agent	Trade Names	Daily Dose	Interval	Daily Dose	Interval
Penicillinase-susceptible penicillins	Penicillin G	Pentids, Crystifor, Pfizerpen, etc.	0.8–3.2 million units	6 hr	1.2 million units	8 hr
	Penicillin G benzathine	Bicillin	—	—	1.2–2.4 million units	See fn. 1
	Penicillin G procaine	Crysticillin, Duracillin, etc.	—	—	0.6–4.8 million units	6–24 hr
	Penicillin V	Pen-Vee K, V-Cillin K, etc.	0.8–3.2 million units (0.5–2.0 g)	6 hr	—	—
Penicillinase-susceptible penicillins with activity against gram-negative bacilli	Amoxicillin	Amoxil, Larotid, etc.	750–1,500 mg	8 hr	—	—
	Ampicillin	Omnipen, Polycillin, etc.	1–4 g	6 hr	1–2 g	6 hr
	Azlocillin	Azlin	—	—	—	—
	Carbenicillin	Pyopen, Geopen	—	—	See fn. 2	See fn. 2
	Carbenicillin indanyl sodium	Geocillin	—	—	—	—
	Mezlocillin	Mezlin	—	—	—	—
	Piperacillin	Pipracil	—	—	See fn. 4	See fn. 4
	Ticarcillin	Ticar	—	—	See fn. 5	See fn. 5
Penicillinase-resistant penicillins	Cloxacillin	Tegopen	1–3 g	6 hr	—	—
	Dicloxacillin	Dynapen, Pathocil	1–2 g	6 hr	—	—
	Methicillin	Celbenin, Staphcillin	—	—	4 g	6 hr
	Nafcillin	Nafcil, Unipen	2–4 g[6]	6 hr	2–3 g	4–6 hr
	Oxacillin	Bactocill, Prostaphlin	2–4 g	6 hr	1–2 g	6 hr
Penicillin with β-lactamase inhibitors	Amoxicillin–clavulanic acid	Augmentin	750–1,500 mg (amoxicillin)	8 hr	—	—
	Ampicillin–sulbactam	Unasyn	—	—	1 g (ampicillin)	6 hr
	Ticarcillin–clavulanic acid	Timentin	—	—	—	—

Note: all superscript numbers refer to footnotes after table.

Uncomplicated Urinary Tract Infections		Major and Systemic Infections[†]			
Oral		Intramuscular		Intravenous	
Daily Dose	Interval	Daily Dose	Interval	Daily Dose	Interval
—	—	—	—	4–24 million units	2–4 hr
—	—	—	—	—	—
—	—	—	—	—	—
—	—	—	—	—	—
750–1,500 mg	8 hr	—	—	—	—
2–4 g	6 hr	—	—	4–12 g	2–4 hr
—	—	—	—	12–18 g	4 hr
—	—	—	—	12–18 g	4 hr
4–8 tablets[3]	6 hr	—	—	—	—
—	—	—	—	12–18 g	4 hr
—	—	See fn. 4	See fn. 4	12–18 g	4 hr
—	—	—	—	16–24 g	3–6 hr
—	—	—	—	—	—
—	—	—	—	—	—
—	—	—	—	6–12 g	4–6 hr
—	—	—	—	4–12 g	4–6 hr
—	—	—	—	4–12 g	4–6 hr
750 mg (amoxicillin)	8 hr	—	—	—	—
—	—	1–2 g (ampicillin)	6 hr	1–2 g (ampicillin)	6 hr
—	—	—	—	12–18 g (ticardillin)	4–6 hr

*Infections of the upper respiratory tract, soft tissues, etc.

†Osteomyelitis, peritonitis, bacteremia, endocarditis, etc.

Table 6 (continued)

Class of Drug	Specific Agent	Trade Names	Mild Infections*			
			Oral		Intramuscular	
			Daily Dose	Interval	Daily Dose	Interval
Cephalo-sporins	Cefaclor	Ceclor	750 mg–1.5 g	8 hr	—	—
	Cefadroxil	Duricef	500 mg–2 g	12–24 hr	—	—
	Cefamandole	Mandol	—	—	2–4 g	6 hr
	Cefazolin	Ancef, Kefzol	—	—	750 mg–1.5 g	8 hr
	Cefixime	Suprax	400 mg	24 hr	—	—
	Cefmetazole	Zefazone	—	—	—	—
	Cefonicid	Monocid	—	—	See fn. 8, 9	See fn. 8, 9
	Cefoperazone	Cefobid	—	—	See fn. 8, 9	See fn. 8, 9
	Ceforanide	Precef	—	—	See fn. 8, 9	See fn. 8, 9
	Cefotaxime	Claforan	—	—	See fn. 8, 9	See fn. 8, 9
	Cefotetan	Cefotan	—	—	See fn. 8, 9	See fn. 8, 9
	Cefoxitin	Mefoxin	—	—	2–4 g	6 hr
	Cefprozil	Cefzil	500 mg–1 g	12–24 hr	—	—
	Ceftazidime	Fortaz, Tazidime	—	—	See fn. 8, 9	See fn. 8, 9
	Ceftizoxime	Cefizox	—	—	See fn. 8, 9	See fn. 8, 9
	Ceftriaxone	Rocephin	—	—	See fn. 8, 9	See fn. 8, 9
	Cefuroxime	Zinacef, Ceftin (p.o.)	250–500 mg	12 hr	See fn. 8, 9	See fn. 8, 9
	Cephalexin	Keflex	1–4 g	6 hr	—	—
	Cephalothin	Keflin	—	—	2–3 g	6 hr
	Cephapirin	Cefadyl	—	—	2–3 g	6 hr
	Cephradine	Anspor, Velosef	1–4 g	6 hr	2 g	6 hr
	Moxalactam	Moxam	—	—	See fn. 8, 9	See fn. 8, 9
Carbapenems	Imipenem-cilastatin	Primaxin	—	—	—	—
Monobactams	Aztreonam	Azactam	—	—	1–2 g	8–12 hr
Aminogly-cosides	Amikacin	Amikin	—	—	—	—
	Gentamicin	Garamycin	—	—	3–5 mg/kg[12]	8 hr
	Kanamycin	Kantrex	—	—	—	—
	Neomycin	—	See fn. 16	See fn. 16	—	—
	Netilmicin	Netromycin	—	—	4–6 mg/kg[12,13]	8 hr
	Streptomycin	—	—	—	1–2 g	12 hr
	Tobramycin	Nebcin	—	—	3–5 mg/kg[12]	8 hr

Note: all superscript numbers refer to footnotes after table.

| Uncomplicated Urinary Tract Infections | | Major and Systemic Infections[†] | | | |
| Oral | | Intramuscular | | Intravenous | |
Daily Dose	Interval	Daily Dose	Interval	Daily Dose	Interval
750 mg–1.5 g	8 hr	—	—	—	—
500 mg–2 g	12–24 hr	—	—	—	—
—	—	—	—	4–12 g	2–4 hr
See fn. 7	See fn. 7	2–3g	6–8 hr	2–6 g	6–8 hr
400 mg	24 hr	—	—	—	—
—	—	—	—	4–8 g	6–12 hr
—	—	—	—	0.5–2.0 g	12–24 hr
—	—	—	—	2–12 g	6–8 hr
—	—	—	—	1–2 g	12 hr
—	—	—	—	2–12 g	4–6 hr
—	—	—	—	2–6 g	12 hr
—	—	—	—	4–12 g	4 hr
—	—	—	—	—	—
—	—	—	—	2–6 g	8–12 hr
—	—	—	—	2–6 g	8–12 hr
—	—	—	—	1–4 g	12–24 hr
—	—	—	—	3–6 g	6 hr
1–4 g	6 hr	—	—	—	—
—	—	—	—	4–12 g	2–4 hr
—	—	—	—	4–12 g	2–4 hr
2 g	6 hr	—	—	3–8 g	4–6 hr
—	—	—	—	2–12 g	8 hr
—	—	—	—	1–4 g	6–8 hr
—	—	—	—	3–8 g	6–8 hr
—	—	15 mg/kg[10]	8–12 hr	15 mg/kg[11]	8 hr
—	—	3–5 mg/kg	8 hr	3–5 mg/kg[13]	8 hr
—	—	15 mg/kg[14]	8–12 hr	15 mg/kg[15]	8 hr
—	—	—	—	—	—
—	—	4–6 mg/kg	8 hr	4–6 mg/kg[17]	8 hr
—	—	1–2 g	12 hr	—	—
—	—	3–5 mg/kg	8 hr	3–5 mg/kg[17]	8 hr

*Infections of the upper respiratory tract, soft tissues, etc.

†Osteomyelitis, peritonitis, bacteremia, endocarditis, etc.

Table 6   (continued)

Class of Drug	Specific Agent	Trade Names	Mild Infections*			
			Oral		Intramuscular	
			Daily Dose	Interval	Daily Dose	Interval
Tetracyclines	Demeclo-cycline	Declomycin	600 mg	6 hr	—	—
	Doxycycline	Vibramycin, etc.	100–200 mg[18]	12 hr	—	—
	Minocycline	Minocin	200 mg[20]	12 hr	—	—
	Oxytetra-cycline	Terramycin	1–2 g	6 hr	See fn. 22	See fn. 22
	Tetracycline	Achromycin, Panmycin, Sumycin, Tetracyn, etc.	1–2 g	6 hr	See fn. 22	See fn. 22
Macrolides	Erythromycin	E-Mycin, Erythrocin, Ilotycin	1–2 g	6 hr	See fn. 22	See fn. 22
	Erythromycin estolate[24]	Ilosone	1–2 g	6 hr	—	—
	Clarithro-mycin	Biaxin	500 mg–1 g	12 hr	—	—
	Azithromycin	Zithromax	500 mg day 1 250 mg days 2–5	24 hr	—	—
Lincomycins	Clindamycin	Cleocin	600 mg–1.8 g	6 hr	600 mg–1.2 g	6–8 hr
	Lincomycin[25]	Lincocin	1.5–2.0 g	6–8 hr	600 mg–1.2 g	8–12 hr
Polymyxins	Colistimethate	Coly-Mycin	—	—	—	—
	Polymyxin B	Aerosporin, etc.	—	—	—	—
Sulfonamides	Sulfadiazine	—	2–4 g[27]	6 hr	—	—
	Sulfisoxazole	Gantrisin	2–6 g[27]	6 hr	—	—
	Trimethoprim-sulfameth-oxazole	Bactrim, Septra	4 tablets[28]	12 hr	—	—
Miscellaneous antibacterial agents	Chloram-phenicol	Chloromycetin	1.5–3.0 g	6 hr	See fn. 29	See fn. 29
	Metronidazole	Flagyl	250 mg	8 hr	—	—
	Spectinomycin	Trobicin	—	—	2 g[31]	Single injection
	Trimethoprim	Proloprim, Trimpex	200 mg	12 hr	—	—
	Vancomycin	Vancocin	2 g[32]	6 hr	—	—

Note: all superscript numbers refer to footnotes after table.

Uncomplicated Urinary Tract Infections		Major and Systemic Infections[†]			
Oral		Intramuscular		Intravenous	
Daily Dose	Interval	Daily Dose	Interval	Daily Dose	Interval
600 mg	6 hr	—	—	—	—
100–200 mg[18]	12 hr	—	—	100–200 mg[19]	12 hr
200 mg[20]	12 hr	—	—	200 mg[21]	12 hr
1–2 g	6 hr	—	—	—	—
1–2 g	6 hr	See fn. 22	See fn. 22	750 mg–1 g[23]	6–12 hr
—	—	See fn. 22	See fn. 22	2–4 g	6 hr
—	—	—	—	—	—
—	—	—	—	—	—
—	—	—	—	—	—
—	—	1.2–2.4 g	6–8 hr	1.8–3.0 g	6–8 hr
—	—	1.2–1.8 g	8 hr	1.8–3.0 g	8 hr
—	—	2.5–5.0 mg/kg[26]	6 hr	2.5–5.0 mg/kg	6 hr
—	—	1.5–2.5 mg/kg	6–8 hr	1.5–2.5 mg/kg	6–8 hr
2–4 g[27]	6 hr	—	—	—	—
2–6 g[27]	6 hr	—	—	100 mg/kg[27]	4–6 hr
4 tablets[28]	12 hr	—	—	8–12 mg/kg[28] (trimethoprim)	6 hr[28]
1.5–2.0 g[30]	6 hr	See fn. 29	See fn. 29	2–4 g	6 hr
—	—	—	—	30 mg/kg	6 hr
—	—	—	—	—	—
200 mg	12 hr	—	—	—	—
—	—	—	—	1–2 g	6–12 hr

*Infections of the upper respiratory tract, soft tissues, etc.

†Osteomyelitis, peritonitis, bacteremia, endocarditis, etc.

Table 6   (continued)

Class of Drug	Specific Agent	Trade Names	Mild Infections*			
			Oral		Intramuscular	
			Daily Dose	Interval	Daily Dose	Interval
Urinary tract disinfectants	Methenamine mandelate	Mandelamine	—	—	—	—
	Methenamine hippurate	Hiprex	—	—	—	—
	Nitrofurantoin	Furadantin, Macrodantin	—	—	—	—
Antifungal drugs	Amphotericin B	Fungizone	—	—	—	—
	Fluconazole[34]	Diflucan	100–200 mg	24 hr	—	—
	Flucytosine	Ancobon	50–150 mg/kg[34]	6 hr	—	—
	Ketoconazole	Nizoral	200 mg[35]	24 hr	—	—
	Miconazole	Monistat	—	—	—	—
	Nystatin	Mycostatin	1.5–3.0 million units[38]	8 hr	—	—
Quinolones	Ofloxacin	Floxin	400–800 mg	12 hr	—	—
	Lomefloxacin	Maxaquin	400 mg	24 hr	—	—
	Nalidixic acid	NegGram	—	—	—	—
	Norfloxacin	Noroxin	—	—	—	—
	Ciprofloxacin[39]	Cipro	500 mg	12 hr	—	—

Note: all superscript numbers refer to footnotes after table.

1. Benzathine penicillin G is used primarily in three circumstances: (1) treatment of streptococcal pharyngitis in cases in which patient compliance is questionable (a single dose of 1.2 million U I.M.); (2) prophylaxis for rheumatic fever recurrences (1.2–2.4 million U I.M. once monthly); (3) treatment of syphilis: for primary, secondary, or early (less than one year) latent syphilis, a single dose of 2.4 million U I.M.; for late syphilis (late latent, cardiovascular, neurosyphilis, etc.), 2.4 million U I.M. weekly for three doses has been recommended, but many physicians now treat neurosyphilis with high-dose I.V. penicillin.

2. Parenteral carbenicillin is usually used in the treatment of serious infections caused by susceptible *Pseudomonas*, *Enterobacter*, and non-*mirabilis Proteus* strains and is given in maximal dosage (30–40 g daily I.V.). It is often used in synergistic combination with gentamicin or tobramycin for I.V. treatment of *Pseudomonas* infections. Occasionally, it is given in smaller dosages (1–2 g I.M. or I.V. q 6 hr) to treat an uncomplicated urinary tract infection caused by the same organisms.

3. Each tablet of carbenicillin indanyl sodium is equivalent to 382 mg of carbenicillin (usual dosage is one to two tablets p.o., q.i.d.).

4. Piperacillin is most often used in the treatment of serious infections caused by susceptible *Pseudomonas*, *Klebsiella*, *Enterobacter*, and non-*mirabilis Proteus* strains; the agent is given in maximal dosage (12–18 g daily I.V.). It is commonly used in synergistic combination with tobramycin or gentamicin for treatment of *Pseudomonas* infections. Occasionally, it is given in smaller dosages (1.0–1.5 g I.M. or I.V. q 6 hr) to treat an uncomplicated urinary tract infection caused by the same organisms.

5. Ticarcillin, piperacillin, mezlocillin, and azlocillin are usually used in the treatment of serious infections caused by susceptible *Pseudomonas*, *Enterobacter*, and non-*mirabilis Proteus* strains and are given in maximal dosage (12–24 g daily I.V.). One of these agents is commonly used in synergistic

| Uncomplicated Urinary Tract Infections | | Major and Systemic Infections [†] | | | |
| Oral | | Intramuscular | | Intravenous | |
Daily Dose	Interval	Daily Dose	Interval	Daily Dose	Interval
4 g	6 hr	—	—	—	—
2 g	12 hr	—	—	—	—
200–400 mg	6 hr	—	—	Not recommended	—
—	—	—	—	$0.25–1.0$ mg/kg[33]	24 hr
—	—	—	—	200 mg[34]	24 hr
—	—	—	—	—	—
—	—	See fn. 35	See fn. 35	See fn. 35	See fn. 35
—	—	—	—	600 mg–3.6 g[37]	8 hr
—	—	—	—	—	—
12 hr	—	—	—	800 mg	12 hr
400 mg	24 hr	—	—	—	—
2–4 g	6 hr	—	—	—	—
800 mg	12 hr	—	—	—	—
250–500 mg	12 hr	—	—	400 mg	12 hr

*Infections of the upper respiratory tract, soft tissues, etc.

†Osteomyelitis, peritonitis, bacteremia, endocarditis, etc.

combination with tobramycin or gentamicin for treatment of Pseudomonas infections. Occasionally, they are given in small dosages (1 g I.M. or I.V. q 6 hr) to treat an uncomplicated urinary tract infection caused by the same organisms.

6. Nafcillin is not reliably absorbed by the oral route.

7. Cefazolin may be used to treat acute uncomplicated urinary tract infections caused by susceptible gram-negative bacilli (*Escherichia coli, Proteus mirabilis,* and *Klebsiella*). It is administered I.M. in a dosage of 2 g daily (given as aliquots q 8 hr).

8. Although the second- and third-generation cephalosporins can be used for milder infections at the lower end of their recommended dosage range, these potent but expensive agents should generally be reserved for serious infections or for the treatment of resistant organisms when the alternative is a more toxic antimicrobial drug.

9. The I.M. route is acceptable for milder illnesses, but the I.V. route is recommended for serious infections, including bacteremias and meningitis. The I.M. dosage range is the same as that for the I.V. dosage.

10. Dosage must be reduced in the presence of renal insufficiency. The daily parenteral dose should not exceed 15 mg/kg, and the total daily amount administered should not exceed 1.5 g, regardless of the patient's weight.

11. The I.V. dose should be infused over a period of 30–60 min q 8 hr.

12. For urinary tract infections caused by resistant organisms.

13. Dosage must be reduced in the presence of renal insufficiency. The I.V. dose should be administered over a period of 30–60 min q 8 hr. In patients with meningitis caused by susceptible gram-negative bacilli, intrathecal gentamicin (5 mg for adults, 1–2 mg for infants) is often administered once daily along with parenteral gentamicin until CSF cultures are negative.

14. Dosage must be reduced in the presence of renal insufficiency. The daily parenteral dose should not exceed

15 mg/kg (daily dose should not exceed 1.5 g, regardless of weight); the total quantity administered in a therapeutic course should not exceed 15 g.

15. The I.V. route should be employed only when I.M. administration is not possible. The I.V. should be administered over a period of at least 60 min q 8 hr.

16. There are no clinical indications for the parenteral administration of neomycin in view of its marked toxicity and the availability of safer alternative drugs. The drug is given p.o. or by nasogastric tube (4–6 g daily in four divided doses) to reduce the number of ammonia-forming bacteria in the intestine in the short-term treatment of acute hepatic coma. It is also given in a total daily dose of 2–3 g in long-term therapy for chronic hepatic encephalopathy or episodic hepatic coma. Nephrotoxicity and ototoxicity have followed prolonged high-dose therapy in hepatic coma, particularly in patients with some renal impairment.

Neomycin is also used along with vigorous mechanical cleansing of the large bowel as preoperative prophylaxis for bowel surgery. In this situation, it is administered for one to three days preoperatively (40 mg/kg p.o. daily in six divided doses).

17. Dosage must be reduced in the presence of renal insufficiency. The intravenous dose should be administered over a period of 30–60 min q 8 hr.

18. Usually administered as 100 mg p.o. q 12 hr on the first day of treatment, followed by 50 mg q 12 hr. For more difficult infections, the dosage may be continued at 100 mg q 12 hr.

19. Usually administered as 100 mg I.V. q 12 hr on the first day of treatment. Thereafter, it may be given as 50–100 mg q 12 hr I.V. Each I.V. dose should be given over a period of one to four hours.

20. Usually administered initially as 200 mg p.o., followed by 100 mg q 12 hr.

21. Usually given initially as 200 mg I.V., followed by 100 mg q 12 hr. Maximal dose in any 24-hour period is 400 mg.

22. I.M. administration is generally unsatisfactory because of poor absorption and local irritation.

23. In special circumstances, it may be given in higher doses but not in excess of 500 mg q 6 hr.

24. Cholestatic hepatitis may develop as a hypersensitivity response to erythromycin estolate but not to the other erythromycin preparations. For this reason, erythromycin base or erythromycin stearate is preferable.

25. Clindamycin has supplanted lincomycin in clinical usage.

26. Dosage usually is 2.5–3.5 mg/kg daily parenterally. Occasionally, the dosage required is as high as 5 mg/kg daily; at this level, paresthesias and more serious neurotoxicity and nephrotoxicity may be manifest in some patients.

27. A loading dose of half the daily dosage is given initially. In severe infections, the dosage of sulfonamide is adjusted to provide a blood level of 10–15 mg/dl. Sulfonamides must be used with caution in patients with renal insufficiency. Sulfisoxazole is the preferred sulfonamide.

28. Each tablet contains 80 mg trimethoprim and 400 mg sulfamethoxazole. Double-strength tablets are also available (usual dosage is one tablet q 12 hr). Pediatric suspensions contain 40 mg trimethoprim and 200 mg sulfamethoxazole per 5 ml. Trimethoprim-sulfamethoxazole has also been used in the treatment of typhoid fever in the same dosage as recommended for urinary tract infections. It has been used in a dosage of four to eight standard tablets daily in the treatment of brucellosis. For pneumonia caused by *Pneumocystis carinii*, the dosage is 20 mg/kg trimethoprim and 100 mg/kg sulfamethoxazole per 24 hr (equally divided doses q 6 hr). The I.V. dosage of trimethoprim-sulfamethoxazole ranges from 8 mg/kg trimethoprim and 40 mg/kg sulfamethoxazole per 24 hr to 20 mg/kg trimethoprim and 100 mg/kg sulfamethoxazole per 24 hr. The lower dosage range is used in the treatment of urinary tract infections that require parenteral antimicrobial therapy and in the treatment of shigellosis; the larger dosage is employed in the treatment of *P. carinii* pneumonia.

29. Chloramphenicol sodium succinate, the parenteral preparation, should only be used I.V. It is ineffective when administered I.M.

30. Chloramphenicol should not be used in the treatment of a urinary tract infection that could be managed with another safer, effective antimicrobial.

31. The only approved indication for the use of spectinomycin is in the treatment of anogenital and urethral gonorrhea in a penicillin-allergic patient or when the infecting organism is highly penicillin resistant. In geographic areas where antibiotic-resistant gonococci are prevalent, treatment with 4 g of spectinomycin (2 g in each gluteal region) may be indicated.

32. Vancomycin is not absorbed through the GI tract. Its use orally is for treatment of staphylococcal enterocolitis or antibiotic-associated enterocolitis.

33. The dry powder is reconstituted by addition of Sterile Water for Injection, USP, *without a bacteriostatic agent*. The solution is then added to a bottle of 5% Dextrose Injection, USP. The pH of the dextrose solution should first be checked to verify that it is above 4.2. If it is not, a buffer solution (as described in package insert) should be added. Amphotericin B solutions should be administered promptly after preparation and should be protected from light during administration. It is given once a day over 6 hr. (Later in the course of administration, double the daily dose is sometimes given on an alternate-day schedule.) Dosage is 1 mg on the first day and then increased in 5 mg increments each day until maintenance dosage is reached. The daily dose is determined by the susceptibility of the organism and the occurrence of toxic side effects. In some instances (e.g., cryptococcal meningitis), combination therapy with flucytosine p.o. may allow employment of smaller daily doses (0.3–0.4 mg/kg) of amphotericin B. In fungal meningitis, intrathecal administration may be necessary (0.1 mg initially, increased gradually to 0.5 mg q 48–72 hr), depending on the evaluation of the patient's condition.

34. Fluconazole is very useful for the treatment of oropharyngeal, esophageal, and disseminated infections caused by candida and for control of cryptococcus, especially chronic suppression of cryptococcal meningitis in patients with AIDS. To initiate therapy, a loading dose of twice the usual daily dose should be used. A daily dose of 400 mg can be used for cryptococcal meningitis, depending on the patient's response to therapy. The dose should be reduced in patients who have renal insufficiency.

35. Used in the treatment of urinary tract infections and visceral infections caused by *Candida*. Also used in cryptococcal infections in which amphotericin B is not toler-

ated. Resistance to flucytosine may develop during treatment of candidal and cryptococcal infections. Sometimes used in combination with amphotericin B to treat systemic fungal infections.

36. Ketoconazole is indicated in the treatment of patients with susceptible fungal infections that have failed to respond to amphotericin B or in the treatment of patients unable to tolerate the toxic effects of amphotericin B. In either role, it is generally preferred over therapy with miconazole when the patient can take oral medications. It is also the drug of choice in the long-term treatment of chronic mucocutaneous candidiasis. It has been useful in the treatment of oroesophageal candidiasis and candiduria. It has also been useful in the treatment of histoplasmosis, coccidioidomycosis, chromomycosis, and paracoccidioidomycosis. In view of its poor penetration of the CSF, it should not be used in the treatment of coccidioidal or cryptococcal meningitis. Ketoconazole requires gastric acidity for dissolution and absorption. Antacids and cimetidine, if needed, should be given at least 2 hr after a dose of ketoconazole. The most frequent side effects have been nausea and vomiting. Several cases of liver injury of varying severity, possibly the result of idiosyncratic reactions, have occurred during ketoconazole therapy. Liver function tests, therefore, should be evaluated before and periodically during treatment, especially in patients who are on prolonged therapy or who have preexisting hepatic disease. Ketoconazole, in daily dosages of 200–1,800 mg p.o., is used in major and systemic fungal infections for which the mycotic agent is susceptible and amphotericin B cannot be employed.

37. Miconazole is available for parenteral therapy for systemic mycoses. Experience is relatively limited, and it should probably be reserved for patients who cannot tolerate or who do not respond to amphotericin B and flucytosine. Miconazole is metabolized by extrarenal mechanisms, and patients with fungal bladder infections require supplementary bladder irrigation with the drug. Side effects of miconazole include phlebitis, fever, rash, nausea and vomiting, anemia, thrombocytopenia, and transient hyperlipidemia caused by the diluent used.

38. Not absorbed from the GI tract. Use only in treatment of intestinal tract colonization by *Candida* species and not for any systemic mycotic infection. Nystatin suspension (400,000–600,000 units q.i.d.) is used as a mouthwash in treatment of oral thrush. The suspension can also be swallowed for use in the treatment of candidal esophagitis.

39. Ciprofloxacin has been used with success in a variety of serious systemic infections, including pneumonias and osteomyelitis. The use of oral antibiotics in seriously ill patients must be weighed against the much greater experience with parenteral therapy; in particular, oral therapy may not be effective in those patients who have adynamic ileus and therefore may not reliably absorb drugs from the gastrointestinal tract.

cent of an intravenous dose of nafcillin is excreted in the bile, which may be an advantage when high-dose therapy is necessary in a patient with impaired renal function.

Oxacillin and nafcillin can be administered orally as well as parenterally. Cloxacillin and dicloxacillin are available only as oral preparations. Oxacillin and its two chlorinated derivatives are preferred to nafcillin for oral administration because of variability in gastrointestinal absorption of nafcillin. Cloxacillin and dicloxacillin (1 to 2 g daily) are often preferred to oxacillin for the oral treatment of mild staphylococcal infections because they produce blood levels two and four times higher, respectively. All three drugs, however, have been used successfully as primary treatments of soft tissue infections or as extensions of previous intravenous therapy.

Penicillinase-Susceptible Broad-Spectrum Penicillins (Second-Generation Penicillins)

Ampicillin has a broader range of activity than penicillin G. Its spectrum encompasses not only pneumococci, meningococci, gonococci, and various streptococci but also a number of gram-negative bacilli, such as *H. influenzae, Salmonella* species, *Shigella* species, *E. coli*, and *P. mirabilis*. Like penicillin G, ampicillin is readily cleaved by β-lactamase and is useless in the treatment of infections caused by *S. aureus* or other organisms elaborating this enzyme. Plasmids conferring ampicillin resistance have now appeared in *S. typhi, H. influenzae*, and *N. gonorrhoeae*, organisms previously uniformly susceptible to this drug.[2-4] As use of ampicillin has become more frequent, increasing resistance has appeared among strains of *E. coli* and nontyphoidal *Salmonella* strains.

Oral ampicillin produces a lower peak plasma level than penicillin V. Oral daily doses of more than 2 to 3 g of ampicillin are frequently accompanied by diarrhea and are thus ineffective; serious infections require intravenous therapy.

Amoxicillin is chemically identical to ampicillin except for an -OH substituent instead of an -H on the side chain. Its spectrum of

Table 7   Adverse Effects of Penicillins

Frequency	*Adverse Effects*
Frequent	Rashes (more common with ampicillin), allergic reactions (rarely anaphylactic), diarrhea (most common with oral ampicillin)
Occasional	Hemolytic anemia (with high parenteral doses), drug fever
Rare	Myoclonic jerking and seizures (with high parenteral doses, especially in patients with renal insufficiency); interstitial nephritis; hemorrhagic cystitis (with methicillin); hyperkalemia with possible arrhythmias (with large doses of rapidly administered penicillin G); granulocytopenia; bleeding from platelet dysfunction (with high-dose I.V. therapy) or prolonged prothrombin time, or both; hepatitis (with semisynthetic penicillins such as oxacillin or with amoxicillin–clavulanic acid); sodium overload or hypokalemic alkalosis, or both (with high doses of carbenicillin); pseudomembranous colitis (with ampicillin)

activity is identical to that of ampicillin, but it is more efficiently absorbed from the gastrointestinal tract than ampicillin, and effective concentrations are present in the circulation for twice as long.[72] Amoxicillin is thus administered every eight hours. In a few situations, the prolonged blood level and the rarer occurrence of diarrhea may allow more effective oral therapy than can be achieved with ampicillin. Single-dose amoxicillin can be used to treat uncomplicated acute lower urinary tract infections in women.[8,73]

Bacampicillin is hydrolyzed in vivo to ampicillin and therefore has an identical spectrum of action. The serum level of orally administered bacampicillin is about twice that of ampicillin, but bacampicillin has no advantages over amoxicillin and is more expensive. Cyclacillin is also similar to ampicillin and amoxicillin, but it is more expensive than these agents.

Extended-Spectrum Carboxypenicillins (Third-Generation Penicillins)

The change from an amino to a carboxyl substituent on the side chain converts ampicillin to carbenicillin [*see Figure 1*]. Carbenicillin is active against most ampicillin-susceptible organisms, but it is much less active than ampicillin when compared by weight. The advantage of carbenicillin, however, is its extended spectrum of activity against gram-negative bacilli, including *P. aer-uginosa*, *Proteus* species other than *P. mirabilis*, and some strains of *Enterobacter*, as well as against *E. coli* and other bacilli that are susceptible to ampicillin. Carbenicillin is also active against anaerobes, including 50 percent of *Bacteroides fragilis* strains. More than 70 percent of *Pseudomonas* isolates are susceptible to 100 µg/ml of carbenicillin, a blood level readily achieved or exceeded without clinical toxicity with a daily dose of 24 to 36 g, administered intravenously. Half the dose may suffice in the treatment of more susceptible gram-negative bacilli. Urine levels of 2,000 to 4,000 µg/ml are obtained with intramuscular administration of 2 g of carbenicillin; 1 to 2 g given parenterally at six-hour intervals can be used to treat urinary tract infections caused by *Pseudomonas* and other susceptible organisms. Carbenicillin itself is not absorbed from the gastrointestinal tract. The indanyl carbenicillin ester is acid stable and suitable for oral administration in treatment of urinary tract infections caused by susceptible gram-negative bacilli, including *Pseudomonas* [*see Table 6*], but blood levels are too low for use in infections at other sites.

Resistant strains of *Pseudomonas* and other gram-negative bacilli can appear rapidly during treatment with carbenicillin, especially in infections that communicate with the outside environment, such as pulmonary infections, burn-surface infections, and

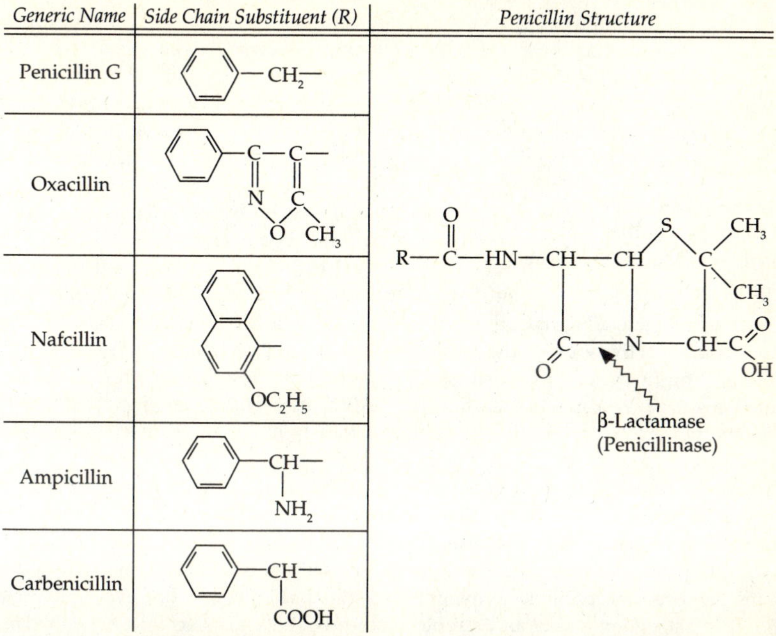

Generic Name	Side Chain Substituent (R)	Penicillin Structure
Penicillin G	phenyl—CH_2—	
Oxacillin	isoxazole structure (phenyl—C—C— with N, O, CH_3)	
Nafcillin	naphthalene with OC_2H_5	
Ampicillin	phenyl—CH— with NH_2	
Carbenicillin	phenyl—CH— with COOH	

The penicillin structure at right:

$$R—\overset{\displaystyle O}{\overset{\|}{C}}—HN—CH—CH \quad \overset{S}{\diagup} \quad \overset{CH_3}{\underset{CH_3}{C}}$$

with β-Lactamase (Penicillinase) site of action indicated at the $C—N$ bond.

β-Lactamase
(Penicillinase)

Figure 1 *Various semisynthetic penicillins have been produced by modifying the structure of the side chain (R) attached to the penicillin nucleus (right). In this way, penicillins have been developed that lack some of the drawbacks of penicillin G, such as poor gastrointestinal absorption, limited spectrum of antibacterial activity, and inactivation by penicillinase-producing microorganisms; for example, oxacillin and nafcillin are resistant to inactivation by penicillinase. This bacterial enzyme (also termed β-lactamase) cleaves the β-lactam ring of penicillin to form an inactive product; the site of action of penicillinase is shown at right.*

osteomyelitis with draining sinuses. Because they delay the emergence of such resistance and because they act synergistically in vitro against some strains of *P. aeruginosa*, carbenicillin and gentamicin (or tobramycin) are often used in concert to treat serious infections caused by this organism. Gentamicin (or tobramycin) and carbenicillin must not be mixed in the same infusion, because this combination results in rapid inactivation of the aminoglycoside. In patients with severe renal failure who are receiving these drugs concomitantly, the serum half-life of gentamicin may be reduced. The sodium load given with 30 to 40 g of carbenicillin is considerable because more than 10 percent of carbenicillin is sodium (about 5 mEq/g); sodium content may be an important consideration in patients with borderline congestive heart failure. The adverse effects of carbenicillin are similar to those of the other penicillins. In addition, patients who are receiving full doses of carbenicillin may experience hemorrhagic manifestations related to platelet dysfunction or hypokalemic alkalosis. Both toxicity reactions are associated with high blood levels of the drug and are more common in patients with renal dysfunction.

Ticarcillin is another semisynthetic penicillin, with virtually the same spectrum of microbiological activity, pharmacological properties, and side effects as carbenicillin. It is about twice as active per gram against *P. aeruginosa* as carbenicillin. Because it is used in a dosage about half that of carbenicillin (16 to 24 g/day), ticarcillin differs little from carbenicillin in clinical use except that it delivers a lower sodium load.

Extended-Spectrum Acylaminopenicillins (Fourth-Generation Penicillins)

The acylaminopenicillins (mezlocillin, piperacillin, and azlocillin) have the broadest spectrum of activity of all the penicillins.[74,75] Although these three drugs are grouped together as a new generation of penicillins, they are in fact very similar to the somewhat older carboxypenicillins, carbenicillin and ticarcillin. Like the carboxypenicillins, the acylaminopenicillins are ampicillin derivatives. All five drugs in the two groups are active against most organisms that are susceptible to ampicillin, including most pneumococci and streptococci, *N. meningitidis*, most *E. coli* and *P. mirabilis* strains, and non–penicillinase-producing strains of *H. influenzae* and *N. gonorrhoeae*; however, none of these drugs is superior to ampicillin or penicillin in treating infections caused by these organisms. All five drugs are ineffective against penicillinase-producing strains of *S. aureus*.

All five extended-spectrum penicillins differ from ampicillin in their increased effectiveness against many anaerobes, including about 50 percent of *B. fragilis* strains. However, the major role of these drugs depends on their spectrum of activity against resistant gram-negative bacilli, which is somewhat broader for the acylaminopenicillins than it is for the carboxypenicillins. Mezlocillin, azlocillin, and piperacillin are active against most isolates of *Klebsiella* and many strains of *Serratia*, whereas carbenicillin and ticarcillin are inactive against most of these organisms. Some *E. coli* strains are resistant to carbenicillin and ticarcillin, and many of these strains are susceptible to the acylaminopenicillins. Piperacillin has the greatest activity of any of the penicillins against *P. aeruginosa*, and

azlocillin is nearly as active; however, mezlocillin is somewhat less active against this organism, and its effectiveness is comparable to that of ticarcillin and carbenicillin.

Despite these in vitro differences, clinical studies have not demonstrated that the acylaminopenicillins are superior to the carboxypenicillins in treating organisms susceptible to both groups. The newer cephalosporins, however, appear to be preferable for treating infections caused by resistant *Klebsiella* and *Serratia* strains. The emergence of resistance is a concern with the acylaminopenicillins; like the carboxypenicillins, these newer drugs should generally be used with an aminoglycoside to treat seriously ill patients, especially those with neutropenia.

The serum levels, tissue distribution, half-life, and recommended dosage ranges of piperacillin, mezlocillin, and azlocillin are similar to those of ticarcillin. Unlike carbenicillin and ticarcillin, however, piperacillin, mezlocillin, and azlocillin are excreted in the bile and the urine and do not accumulate in patients with renal failure. The acylaminopenicillins have a lower sodium content than that of the carboxypenicillins. The toxicities of the acylaminopenicillins and the carboxypenicillins appear to be identical except that mezlocillin seems less likely to impair platelet function than the other members of the two groups[65,76]; this property may be a particular asset in the treatment of thrombocytopenic patients. As many as 50 percent of patients who receive high doses of an acylaminopenicillin for prolonged periods develop an adverse reaction severe enough to warrant a change in therapy; the major adverse reactions include rash, drug fever, eosinophilia, leukopenia, thrombocytopenia, and abnormal liver function tests.[77]

Penicillin–β-Lactamase Inhibitor Combinations

The major mechanism of resistance to the penicillins is bacterial production of β-lactamase enzymes that hydrolyze the β-lactam ring, rendering the molecule inactive. Clavulanic acid and sulbactam are β-lactam compounds that have little intrinsic antibacterial activity. Both, however, bind irreversibly to the β-lactamases that are produced by many bacteria, thus inactivating these enzymes and rendering the organisms sensitive to β-lactamase–susceptible penicillins.[78]

Clavulanic acid is available with amoxicillin in an oral formulation.[79] Sulbactam is available with ampicillin in a parenteral formulation.[80] In addition to showing activity against ampicillin-susceptible organisms, the combinations are also active against various ampicillin-resistant organisms, including *Moraxella catarrhalis*, β-lactamase–producing strains of *H. influenzae*, *E. coli*, *K. pneumoniae*, some *Proteus* species, and *S. aureus* (except methicillin-resistant strains). The combinations are also active against gonococci, enterococci, and many anaerobes, including *B. fragilis*. However, *P. aeruginosa* is resistant, as are many strains of *Serratia* and *Enterobacter*.

The clavulanic acid–amoxicillin therapy has been used successfully to treat such conditions as upper and lower respiratory tract infections, urinary tract infections, and human and animal bites. The recommended dosage for the clavulanic acid–amoxicillin combination is similar to that for amoxicillin alone. The combination may cause a higher incidence of gastrointestinal side effects than amoxicillin alone. It is not clear whether clavulanic acid–amoxicillin is clinically superior to older antimicrobials, which may be less expensive.

The ampicillin-sulbactam combination has been used successfully to treat gynecologic and intra-abdominal infections as well as infections of the upper and lower respiratory tract, urinary tract, skin and soft tissues, and bones and joints. The fixed-dose combination contains 1 g of sulbactam for each 2 g of ampicillin. The usual adult dosage for I.V. treatment of serious infection is 1 to 2 g of the ampicillin component every six hours.

Clavulanic acid is available in combination with ticarcillin for intravenous administration. The combination is active against ticarcillin-susceptible organisms and against various ticarcillin-resistant organisms, such as *S. aureus* (except methicillin-resistant strains), and some resistant gram-negative bacilli, including various *Klebsiella*, *Serratia*, *Proteus*, and *Pseudomonas* species. Clavulanic acid–ticarcillin has been successful in the treatment of pulmonary, urinary tract, bone and soft tissue, and bloodstream infections.[81] The toxicities and recommended dosages are similar to those of ticarcillin alone.

Amdinocillin

Amdinocillin, a novel semisynthetic penicillin known outside the United States as mecillinam, is more active than ampicillin against many species of enteric gram-negative bacilli, including *E. coli*, *Salmonella*, *Shigella*, *Citrobacter*, *Campylobacter*, *K. pneumoniae*, *E. cloacae*, and *P. mirabilis*.[82,83] However, amdinocillin is not active against *H. influenzae*, gonococci, anaerobes, *Pseudomonas*, indole-positive *Proteus* species, or gram-positive organisms. Amdinocillin, administered intravenously either alone or in combination with other β-lactam antibiotics, has been effective in the treatment of various infections caused by susceptible organisms. However, older penicillins or cephalosporins are also effective in these situations, and the clinical role of amdinocillin appears to be quite limited.

Cephalosporins

The cephalosporins and closely related cephamycins (e.g., cefoxitin and cefotetan) and oxa-β-lactams (e.g., moxalactam) are a large and rapidly expanding group of β-lactam antibiotics. Like the penicillins, which they resemble structurally, the cephalosporins are bactericidal antibiotics that inhibit bacterial cell wall synthesis and have a low intrinsic toxicity. The adverse effects of the cephalosporins are mainly local pain (with intramuscular use), renal impairment, and allergic reactions. Pseudomembranous colitis has also been reported [*see Table 8*]. Because the cephalosporins share immunologic cross-reactivity, patients who are allergic to one cephalosporin are likely to be allergic to others; there is also a possibility of cross-reactivity in penicillin-allergic patients. Like the newer penicillins, the newer cephalosporins have an extraordinarily broad spectrum of antimicrobial activity but are very expensive.

The cephalosporins are grouped into generations on the basis of their antibacterial spectrum [*see Table 9*]; in general, activity against gram-positive cocci diminishes from the first to the third generation, whereas the spectrum of activity against gram-negative organisms increases. Agents in each group exhibit pharmacological differences that are related to differences in serum levels and half-lives, and thus, recommended doses vary substantially. The third-generation cephalosporins also display good cerebrospinal fluid activity; none of the first-generation drugs and only one second-generation agent (cefuroxime) are effective in meningitis.

First-Generation Cephalosporins

The antibacterial spectrum of the first-generation cephalosporins includes most gram-positive bacteria (*S. aureus*, pneumococci, all streptococci except enterococci, *Actinomyces*, and most gram-positive anaerobes). The cephalosporins are resistant to the penicillinase of *S. aureus* and thus are active against penicillin-resistant *S. aureus* strains; however, they are ineffective against methicillin-resistant *S. aureus* strains. Clinical efficacy against *S. epidermidis* and against penicillin-resistant pneumococci and *Listeria* species is poor. Although the first-generation cephalosporins are active against many strains of *E. coli*, *K. pneumoniae*, and *P. mirabilis*, they are ineffective against many other gram-negative species because these organisms produce chromosomally determined, membrane-bound β-lactamases. These β-lactamases are active against many of the earlier (first- and second-generation) cephalosporins.

Cephalothin was introduced in 1962 and remains the prototype of first-generation cephalosporins. Like most other cephalosporins, cephalothin is excreted largely unaltered and primarily by the renal route.[84] Dosage must be reduced in the presence of renal failure [*see Chapter 32*]. Probenecid blocks tubular secretion of cephalothin and most other cephalosporins, prolonging and enhancing the blood levels achieved. Because the first-generation cephalosporins show poor penetration into the cerebrospinal fluid, they should not be used to treat bacterial meningitis. However, all cephalosporins do cross the placenta readily [*see Table 4*]. These drugs also penetrate readily into the pericardium and the joints.

Two other first-generation cephalosporins, cephapirin and cephradine, are almost identical to cephalothin in their antibacterial spectrum, pharmacology, and toxicity; a possible determinant in choosing among members of this group of very similar antibiotics may be differences in cost.

Table 8 Adverse Effects of Cephalosporins

Frequency	Adverse Effects
Frequent	Thrombophlebitis with I.V. use, pain on I.M. injection, minor GI symptoms (particularly diarrhea)
Occasional	Allergic reactions, including morbilliform and urticarial rashes, serum sickness, and anaphylaxis; drug fever and eosinophilia; reversible neutropenia and thrombocytopenia; pseudomembranous colitis; hemorrhagic diathesis (prolonged prothrombin time, primarily from moxalactam)
Rare	Hemolytic anemia with direct Coombs'-positive reaction, transient rise in SGOT and alkaline phosphatase, interstitial pneumonitis, interstitial nephritis, disulfiramlike reaction with alcohol ingestion, gallstones (reported after use of ceftriaxone)

Table 9 Properties of Cephalosporin Antibiotics

	Specific Agent	Trade Names	Comment*
First Generation	Oral		
	Cefadroxil	Duricef, Ultracef	Longer half-life
	Cephalexin	Keflex	Most experience with this agent
	Cephradine	Anspor, Velosef	Properties are similar to those of cephalexin
	Parenteral		
	Cefazolin	Ancef, Kefzol	Longer half-life; well tolerated when given I.M.
	Cephalothin	Keflin, Seffin	Painful when given I.M.
	Cephapirin	Cefadyl	Properties are similar to those of cephalothin
	Cephradine	Anspor, Velosef	Properties are similar to those of cephalothin
Second Generation	Oral		
	Cefaclor	Ceclor	Moderately active against *Hemophilus influenzae*
	Cefuroxime axetil	Ceftin	Active against *H. influenzae*
	Cefprozil	Cefzil	Active against *H. influenzae*
	Parenteral		
	Cefamandole	Mandol	Active against *H. influenzae*; may cause bleeding
	Cefmetazole	Zefazone	Spectrum and half-life similar to cefoxitin; may cause bleeding
	Cefonicid	Monocid	Spectrum similar to that of cefamandole
	Ceforanide	Precef	Spectrum similar to that of cefamandole
	Cefotetan	Cefotan	Spectrum similar to that of cefoxitin; longer half-life than cefoxitin; may cause bleeding
	Cefoxitin	Mefoxin	Active against *Bacteroides fragilis*, *Serratia*, *Neisseria gonorrhoeae*
	Cefuroxime	Zinacef, Kefurox	Active against *H. influenzae*; only second-generation drug approved for meningitis (selected pathogens)
Third Generation	Oral		
	Cefixime	Suprax	More active against gram-negative bacilli, gonococci, *Moraxella catarrhalis*, and *H. influenzae* than other oral cephalosporins but much less active against *Staphylococcus aureus*
	Parenteral		
	Cefoperazone	Cefobid	Increased activity against *Pseudomonas aeruginosa* but less against Enterobacteriaceae; may cause bleeding
	Cefotaxime	Claforan	More active against gram-positive cocci
	Ceftazidime	Fortaz, Tazidime, Tazicef	More active against *Pseudomonas*
	Ceftizoxime	Cefizox	Properties are similar to those of cefotaxime
	Ceftriaxone	Rocephin	Longer half-life; less active against *Pseudomonas*, *B. fragilis*
	Moxalactam	Moxam	More active against anaerobes; less active against gram-positive cocci; may cause bleeding

Note: detailed information about the various cephalosporins is covered in the text.

*Agents are being compared with other members of the same generation of cephalosporins.

Cefazolin has essentially the same antibacterial spectrum as cephalothin and is employed in treating similar infections.[85] Cefazolin has two major advantages over other first-generation cephalosporins: relative lack of pain on intramuscular administration and higher blood levels because of its somewhat slower renal elimination. The adult dosage for moderate infections is 0.5 to 1.0 g every eight hours, administered intramuscularly or intravenously; for severe infections, daily dosages of up to 6 g, but usually no more than 4 g, are given intravenously.

Oral first-generation cephalosporins are used to treat urinary tract infections caused by susceptible gram-negative bacilli when less expensive agents cannot be given. They are also used to treat infections of the respiratory tract or skin and soft tissues in patients with a mild penicillin allergy.

Three oral cephalosporins—cephalexin, cephradine, and cefadroxil—are classified as first-generation drugs because of their spectrum of activity. The usual oral dosage for cephalexin and cephradine is 250 to 500 mg every six hours. Larger doses may be given orally, but it is generally preferable to switch to a parenteral cephalosporin if larger doses are needed. Cefadroxil has a much longer half-life than the other two agents, and hence, it may be given in a dosage of 500 mg to 1 g every 12 to 24 hours.[86] Cefadroxil's greater convenience is offset by its higher cost.

Second-Generation Cephalosporins

Cefoxitin and cefamandole, the first parenteral cephalosporins with extended activity against gram-negative bacteria (termed second-generation agents), were introduced into clinical use in 1978, and within two years, they accounted for nearly 60 percent of antibiotic sales in the United States.[87] Since then, five additional parenteral agents (cefotetan, cefmetazole, cefonicid, ceforanide, and cefuroxime) and three oral agents (cefaclor, cefprozil, and cefuroxime axetil) with similar properties have been introduced and have been classified as second-generation cephalosporins.

Cefoxitin, a cephamycin, is active against most organisms that are susceptible to first-generation cephalosporins, but it is somewhat less active against gram-positive cocci. Because it is resistant to the β-lactamase produced by various gram-negative bacilli, cefoxitin is active against many cephalothin-resistant strains of *E. coli*, *Klebsiella*, *Serratia*, and *Proteus*. Cefoxitin is active against gonococci, including penicillinase-producing strains, but not against *H. influenzae* or most strains of *Enterobacter*. The major advantage of cefoxitin, however, is its enhanced activity against gram-positive and gram-negative anaerobes, including most strains of *B. fragilis*; as a result, cefoxitin is valuable for the management of abdominal and pelvic infections in which these organisms play a role. Cefoxitin is ineffective in the treatment of meningitis. Its dosage range and toxicity are similar to those of cephalothin.

Cefotetan, a cephamycin introduced in 1986, has a spectrum of action that is very similar to that of cefoxitin.[88] It is as active as cefoxitin against *B. fragilis* but is less active against other strains in the *B. fragilis* group. Unlike cefoxitin, cefotetan is active against *H. influenzae*; both drugs are active against gonococci and many enteric gram-negative bacilli, but neither is effective against *Enterobacter*, *Pseudomonas*, *Acinetobacter*, or enterococci. Because cefotetan has a longer half-life (4.5 hours) than cefoxitin, it can be administered in a dosage of 1 to 3 g every 12 hours. Another advantage to cefotetan is that it is significantly less expensive than cefoxitin. Cefotetan has proved effective and safe in a variety of clinical settings, including gynecologic infections[89] and surgical prophylaxis.[90] Because it has a methylthiotetrazole side chain, bleeding[91] and disulfiramlike reactions associated with concurrent alcohol ingestion are a concern, but in the limited clinical experience with this drug, such reactions have not been a problem. Further experience will be needed to determine if cefotetan is as safe and effective as cefoxitin. Cefmetazole, a newer cephamycin, exhibits good activity against *B. fragilis* and other anaerobes; like cefotetan, it has a methylthiotetrazole side chain.

Cefamandole is pharmacologically very similar to cefoxitin, but it has a somewhat different spectrum of activity; cefamandole is ineffective against *B. fragilis*, many gonococci, and some *Serratia* strains, but it is more active against *Enterobacter* and *H. influenzae* strains than cefoxitin. Its major advantage is its activity against *H. influenzae*, including ampicillin-resistant strains. However, the third-generation cephalosporins have greater activity against *H. influenzae*. Cefamandole is ineffective in meningitis. Its dosage range and toxicity are similar to those of cephalothin, but its methylthiotetrazole side chain poses a risk of bleeding and disulfiramlike reactions with concurrent use of alcohol.

Cefonicid has a spectrum of activity very similar to that of cefamandole, but it is less active against gram-positive cocci and more active against *H. influenzae*.[92] The half-life of cefonicid (4.5 hours) is much longer than that of cefamandole, probably as a result of increased protein binding. Hence, cefonicid can be administered intravenously in a dosage of 1 to 2 g every 24 hours.

Ceforanide is less active than cefamandole against *S. aureus* and *H. influenzae*, but the spectrum of activity of these two cephalosporins is otherwise similar.[93] The half-life of ceforanide (three hours) is greater than that of cefamandole but less than that of cefonicid. At present, this drug appears to have no advantages over the older cephalosporins.

Cefuroxime is more active than cefamandole against *H. influenzae* and is the only second-generation cephalosporin to be approved for use in meningitis.[94] It is as effective as ampicillin plus chloramphenicol in childhood meningitis that is caused by *H. influenzae*, pneumococci, and meningococci.[95] These potential advantages, however, are shared by the third-generation cephalosporins, which are active against a broader range of gram-negative bacilli than cefuroxime. The toxicities of cefuroxime appear to be similar to those of the other cephalosporins.

Unlike cefuroxime, cefuroxime axetil, an ester with increased lipid solubility, is well absorbed from the GI tract.[96] The antibacterial spectrum of the oral preparation is similar to that of the parent compound. A newer oral cephalosporin, cefprozil, has a similar spectrum of action. Both have been effective in treating infections of the upper and lower respiratory tract, urinary tract, and skin and soft tissues. Another oral drug, cefaclor, may be classified as a second-generation cephalosporin because of enhanced activity against *H. influenzae*. In all other respects, however, cefaclor resembles the three first-generation oral cephalosporins. Cefuroxime axetil and cefaclor may be more effective than the other oral cephalosporins in the treatment of otitis media or bronchitis caused by *H. influenzae*,[86,97] but ampicillin, amoxicillin, and trimethoprim-sulfamethoxazole are less expensive alternatives; clavulanic acid–amoxicillin is similar in cost and is also active against β-lactamase–producing *H. influenzae* and staphylococci. The usual adult dosage of cefuroxime axetil is 250 to 500 mg every 12 hours; of cefprozil, 500 mg every 12 to 24 hours; and of cefaclor, 250 to 500 mg every eight hours.

Third-Generation Cephalosporins

The third-generation cephalosporins differ from other cephalosporins in some important respects. Their enhanced ability to resist hydrolysis by the β-lactamase of many gram-negative bacilli gives them an expanded antibacterial spectrum.[98] Pharmacologically, these drugs also have an important advantage: unlike older cephalosporins, they achieve therapeutic levels in the cerebrospinal fluid and can be used to treat meningitis. Unfortunately, these advantages come at the disadvantage of increased cost.

The third-generation agents are less active than the older cephalosporins against gram-positive cocci; like the earlier cephalosporins, they are inactive against enterococci, methicillin-resistant *S. aureus*, and *Listeria*. However, they have enhanced potency against many gram-negative bacilli, including *E. coli*, *Klebsiella*, *Proteus* (indole-positive and indole-negative species), *Serratia*, and *Citrobacter* organisms. They are also very active against penicillinase-producing and non–penicillinase-producing strains of *H. influenzae* and gonococci. The third-generation cephalosporins are active against most *Salmonella* species and have been clinically effective in the treatment of typhoid fever and other *Salmonella* infections.[99] Although most *Enterobacter* species are initially sensitive to third-generation cephalosporins, they rapidly develop resistance because of inducible cephalosporinases; hence, it may be prudent to avoid using a cephalosporin as the sole therapy for these organisms.[100] Although these drugs do exhibit activity against *B. fragilis* and other anaerobes, cefoxitin and cefotetan, which are second-generation cephalosporins, are more active. Ceftazidime is the third-generation cephalosporin with the greatest activity against *P. aeruginosa*; cefoperazone also demonstrates activity, but the other third-generation cephalosporins have been disappointing. Other nosocomial gram-negative pathogens that are resistant to these drugs include *Acinetobacter* and strains of *Pseudomonas* other than *P. aeruginosa*.

The third-generation cephalosporins seem to have the same relatively low toxicities as the older cephalosporins, but moxalactam appears more likely to prolong the prothrombin time than any of the other cephalosporins.

Cefotaxime, released in 1981, was the first member of the group to become available in the United States. Cefotaxime has been effective in a broad range of infections,[101] including meningitis caused by gram-negative bacilli other than *Pseudomonas*.[102] Although the third-generation cephalosporins have been used chiefly for gram-negative infections, cefotaxime has been effective in the treatment of pneumococcal meningitis[103] and of pneumonias and bacteremias caused by pneumococci and methicillin-sensitive *S. aureus*.[104] Cefotaxime compares favorably with nafcillin plus tobramycin for serious bacterial infections

in nonneutropenic patients.[105] The pharmacological properties of cefotaxime resemble those of cephalothin; 1 to 2 g may be administered every four to six hours.

Ceftizoxime structurally resembles cefotaxime,[106] and their antibacterial spectrums are very similar. Cefotaxime, however, is metabolized by the liver and excreted by the kidneys, whereas ceftizoxime depends solely on renal elimination. As a result, it has a longer half-life and can be administered in a dosage of 1 to 4 g every eight hours.

Moxalactam, which was introduced in 1981, was the first totally synthetic β-lactam antibiotic. Of the third-generation cephalosporins, moxalactam has the greatest activity against anaerobes, but it is less active than cefotaxime and ceftizoxime against gram-positive cocci.[107] Moxalactam has been effective in the treatment of a broad range of infections, including abdominal and pelvic infections and meningitis.[108] Moxalactam has the greatest propensity of any cephalosporin to produce bleeding resulting from prolongation of the prothrombin time; this effect can be prevented or reversed by vitamin K administration and is probably related to moxalactam's methylthiotetrazole side chain. Because of its potential for causing bleeding, moxalactam has been supplanted by newer cephalosporins.

Ceftriaxone has the longest half-life of any third-generation cephalosporin.[109] Its antibacterial spectrum is similar to that of cefotaxime; it is highly active against enteric gram-negative bacilli, *Neisseria*, *Salmonella*,[110] and *Hemophilus* species but is less active against *B. fragilis* and *P. aeruginosa*. Ceftriaxone is effective in meningitis caused by susceptible pathogens, including *H. influenzae*, pneumococci, and meningococci; as little as seven days of intravenous therapy has been effective in childhood meningitis.[111] Ceftriaxone appears to be superior to cefuroxime for the treatment of bacterial meningitis in children.[112] The recommended dosage for systemic infections in adults is 2 to 4 g/day, administered every 12 to 24 hours. A single intramuscular dose of 125 to

250 mg is very effective in gonococcal urethritis, cervicitis, pharyngitis, and proctitis.[113] Ceftriaxone is now the treatment of choice for gonorrhea in regions in which the prevalence of penicillinase-producing gonococci is one percent or higher; its efficacy in the treatment of incubating syphilis has not yet been established.[114] Ceftriaxone is considered the drug of choice for Lyme disease that involves the central nervous system. A case of ceftriaxone-induced cholelithiasis has been reported.[115]

Cefoperazone is less active against many enteric gram-negative bacilli than the other third-generation cephalosporins. Its major asset has been its activity against *P. aeruginosa*, but ceftazidime has appreciably greater antipseudomonal activity. The recommended dosage is 2 to 4 g/day, administered every 12 hours.

Ceftazidime, the newest third-generation cephalosporin, has been effective in a broad range of infections, including meningitis.[116] The feature that distinguishes ceftazidime is its enhanced activity against *P. aeruginosa*, which exceeds that of all other cephalosporins, including cefoperazone; it is also the only cephalosporin that is active against *P. cepacia*.[117] Its spectrum of activity is otherwise typical of third-generation cephalosporins; many strains of *B. fragilis* are resistant. Ceftazidime may act synergistically with aminoglycosides against *P. aeruginosa*; more experience is needed to determine how this combination compares with piperacillin-tobramycin or similar combinations. A prospective study of non-neutropenic patients showed that ceftazidime alone compared favorably with the combination of tobramycin and ticarcillin.[118] Ceftazidime-aminoglycoside therapy has been effective in neutropenic cancer patients with gram-negative bacteremia[119]; monotherapy with ceftazidime may be as effective.[120] The recommended dosage of ceftazidime is 1 to 2 g every eight to 12 hours.

Because of its broad activity against gram-negative organisms, cefixime is the first oral cephalosporin to be classified as a third-generation agent.[121] It is as active as other cephalosporins against pneumococci and group A streptococci but is much less active against *S. aureus*. It is more active than other oral cephalosporins against *E. coli*, *Klebsiella*, *P. mirabilis*, and *Serratia* but is not active against anaerobes, *Pseudomonas*, and *Enterobacter*. Cefixime is very active against *H. influenzae*, *N. gonorrhoeae*, and *M. catarrhalis*. It can be administered in a single daily dose; the usual adult dose is 400 mg. Like other oral cephalosporins, cefixime is expensive. Its spectrum of action and single daily dose make it attractive for upper respiratory tract infections, but less expensive alternatives are available. Cefixime shows great promise as a single-dose oral agent for the treatment of uncomplicated gonorrhea.[122]

Choosing a Cephalosporin

The clinician who is confronted with 17 parenteral and seven oral cephalosporins may understandably find such an array of drugs confusing. Although the choice of an antimicrobial agent for any one patient must be individualized, a few general guidelines may be helpful.[123]

To help avoid confusion, most hospital pharmacies should stock only selected cephalosporins so that the clinical staff can become familiar with the relative merits of these agents. Microbiology laboratories should perform routine bacterial susceptibility testing only with representative cephalosporins from each generation. The decision as to which agents to stock and test should be based on considerations of the antibacterial spectrum, pharmacological properties, and cost of these drugs.

In general, the least expensive cephalosporin that will be effective should be prescribed. Similarly, to minimize toxicity (including superinfection) and cost, the lowest effective dose should be used. Finally, when choosing an antibiotic, the cephalosporins should be compared with other antibiotics, including β-lactams and aminoglycosides, in terms of effectiveness, toxicity, and cost.

The selection of a cephalosporin depends on the clinical setting.

Surgical prophylaxis Cephalosporins are widely used perioperatively to prevent infection. For surgical prophylaxis, the newer cephalosporins provide no advantages over the much less expensive first-generation cephalosporins.[124] A possible exception is colorectal and abdominal operations, for which the prominence of anaerobes makes cefoxitin, cefotetan, or cefmetazole a rational choice; however, even in such cases, bowel preparation with oral antibiotics may provide a less costly alternative.

In general, adequate surgical prophylaxis can be achieved with regimens ranging from a single dose to 48 hours of cephalosporin administration.

Meningitis The third-generation cephalosporins have emerged as the agents of choice for gram-negative bacillary meningitis caused by susceptible organisms. *P. aeruginosa* meningitis has been an exception, but ceftazidime, alone or combined with an aminoglycoside, has proved useful in this difficult situation.[116] Penicillin remains the drug of choice for pneumococcal and meningococcal meningitis; ampicillin is the drug of choice for meningitis caused by non–penicillinase-producing strains of *H. influenzae*. In penicillin-allergic patients who can tolerate cephalosporins, a third-generation cephalosporin may be preferable to chloramphenicol in the treatment of meningitis caused by one of these pathogens. None of the cephalosporins should be used for *Listeria* or enterococcal meningitis. First- and second-generation cephalosporins (except cefuroxime) should never be used as therapy for meningitis.

Gram-negative pneumonia Excellent results have been obtained in the treatment of gram-negative pneumonia with the newer cephalosporins. Because aminoglycosides are likely to be less active in the acid pH of infected lungs, the newer cephalosporins may be preferred for the treatment of nosocomial pneumonias other than those caused by either Acinetobacter, which is cephalosporin resistant, or Enterobacter, which rapidly develops resistance.

Other infections Ceftriaxone is the drug of choice for Lyme disease involving the CNS and for gonorrhea in regions where the prevalence of penicillinase-producing strains of *N. gonorrhea* is one percent or higher. Although cephalosporins have been effective in treating many other infections, they are not clearly identifiable as the drug of choice in any of these infections. For example, penicillin remains the preferred drug for pneumococcal infection, and nafcillin or oxacillin is the drug of choice for infections caused by susceptible *S. aureus* strains, although a first-generation cephalosporin is an excellent alternative in patients who cannot tolerate these drugs. Cephalosporins are ineffective against methicillin-resistant *S. aureus* strains, most *S. epidermidis* infections, and enterococcal infections. Although cefoxitin and cefotetan have been very useful for the treatment of anaerobic infections, penicillin or clindamycin appears to be preferable for the treatment of aspiration pneumonia. Antimicrobial combinations that contain clindamycin, metronidazole, clavulanic acid–ticarcillin, ampicillin- sulbactam, or chloramphenicol are reasonable alternatives to cefoxitin for treating abdominal and pelvic infections. Finally, for cases of suspected sepsis and for infection in immunologically impaired hosts, the effectiveness of a cephalosporin, with or without an aminoglycoside, must be compared with the effectiveness of various penicillin-aminoglycoside combinations.

Other β-Lactam Antibiotics

Carbapenems

Introduced in 1985, imipenem is the first member of the carbapenem group of antibiotics to become available for clinical use in the United States.[125,126] Like other β-lactam antibiotics, imipenem is bactericidal and acts by inhibiting bacterial cell wall synthesis. Three properties account for the extraordinarily broad antibacterial spectrum of imipenem: there is no permeability barrier excluding the drug from bacteria; it has a high affinity for the penicillin-binding protein 2 (PBP-2), which is a crucial component of cell wall structure; and it is extremely resistant to hydrolysis by β-lactamases.

Imipenem is extensively degraded in the renal tubule, which results in low urinary levels of the drug. This drawback can be prevented by using cilastatin, an inhibitor of the brush-border enzyme dehydropeptidase-1. Cilastatin also appears to prevent the tubular damage that is occasionally observed in experimental animals given imipenem alone in high doses. For clinical use, imipenem is administered simultaneously with cilastatin in equal doses; the drugs have similar pharmacokinetic properties and are marketed together in a combination formulation known as Primaxin.

Imipenem has the broadest antibacterial spectrum of any β-lactam antibiotic. It is active against most gram-positive bacteria, both aerobes and anaerobes. Exceptions include some enterococci; many *Enterococcus faecalis* strains are sensitive, but most *E. faecium* strains are resistant. Some diphtheroids are resistant. Although most *S. aureus* strains are very sensitive to imipenem, the susceptibility of methicillin-resistant *S. aureus* and *S. epidermidis* strains is highly variable. Methicillin-resistant *S. aureus*, *E. faecalis*, and *Listeria* also exhibit imipenem tolerance: the drug is bacteriostatic at low concentrations but bactericidal only at concentrations at least 32-fold higher. Finally, some strains of *C. difficile* are resistant.

Imipenem is also extraordinarily active against gram-negative bacteria. Virtually all Enterobacteriaceae are sensitive. *Hemophilus* and *Neisseria* species are also susceptible to imipenem but at somewhat higher concentrations than those needed for third-generation cephalosporins. *Acinetobacter*, which is resistant to most other β-lactam antibiotics, is imipenem sensitive, as are *Serratia, Salmonella, Citrobacter, Yersinia,* and *Brucella* species. Gram-negative anaerobes, including *B. fragilis*, are susceptible to imipenem. *P. aeruginosa* is also susceptible to imipenem, but some resistant strains have emerged during therapy. Other *Pseudomonas* species such as *P. maltophilia* and *P. cepacia* are resistant, as are *Flavobacterium* species.

When administered with cilastatin, imipenem is widely distributed in body fluids; CSF penetration is variable,[127] and therefore, imipenem should not be used in the treatment of meningitis. The drugs are excreted by glomerular filtration; the dosage should be reduced in patients with renal failure, but supplementary doses are required in patients who are undergoing hemodialysis. The safety of imipenem-cilastatin seems comparable to that of other β-lactam antibiotics. Because the structure of the carbapenems resembles that of the penicillins and cephalosporins, there is a potential for cross-reactivity in patients allergic to other β-lactam antibiotics. Clinical experience in this situation is scant, but it appears prudent to avoid imipenem in patients with anaphylactic sensitivity to β-lactam drugs and to use it with caution in patients with milder allergies to penicillins or cephalosporins. Nausea and vomiting, local pain at injection sites, and hypersensitivity are the most common reactions. Seizures, although unusual, are a potential concern. They have been observed in 0.9 percent of patients receiving the drug; risk factors for seizures include excessive dosages of the drug, preexisting CNS lesions, epilepsy, and renal insufficiency.[128] Transient elevations of liver function tests and leukopenia can occur in patients who are given imipenem-cilastatin. Antibiotic-associated pseudomembranous colitis has occurred, necessitating the cessation of therapy in some patients. In one study, resistant organisms have emerged in nine percent of patients who were treated for *P. aeruginosa* infections. Such resistance is probably caused by impaired penetration of the drug into *P. aeruginosa*, which is related to alterations in the outer membrane proteins of this organism.[129] Because of this problem, imipenem should not be used alone to treat serious *P. aeruginosa* infections. Synergism can be demonstrated in vitro between imipenem and either ciprofloxacin or amikacin against some strains of *Pseudomonas*[130]; double β-lactam therapy with imipenem and either ceftazidime or aztreonam can also be considered, but experience with all of these combinations is still limited. Superinfection otherwise seems uncommon.

Imipenem-cilastatin has been used successfully in patients with pneumonia, intra-abdominal infections, urinary tract infections, endocarditis, bacteremia, osteomyelitis, and cellulitis. Imipenem-cilastatin has also been effective in treating infections in neutropenic cancer patients,[131] and in this setting, it appears to be as effective as double therapy with piperacillin and cefoperazone or ceftazidime.[132] The broad spectrum and apparent low toxicity of imipenem-cilastatin are impressive, but it should be used with restraint and selectivity.

Monobactams

The monobactams are monocyclic β-lactam antibiotics that lack the thiazolidine ring found in penicillins and the dihydrothiazine ring found in cephalosporins. Licensed in the United States in 1987, aztreonam was the first monobactam to become available for clinical use.[133] The antibacterial activity of aztreonam depends on its ability to penetrate the outer membrane of gram-negative bacilli, on its high affinity for penicillin-binding protein 3 (PBP-3), and on its resistance to hydrolysis by the β-lactamases of gram-negative bacilli.[134]

The antibacterial activity of aztreonam is restricted to aerobic or facultatively aerobic gram-negative bacteria. Most strains of *H. influenzae*, gonococci, and meningococci are susceptible to aztreonam, as are most enteric gram-negative bacilli, including *E. coli*, *Klebsiella*, *Proteus*, and *Enterobacter*. Most strains of *P. aeruginosa* are also susceptible, but somewhat higher concentrations of aztreonam are required to kill this bacteria. *Acinetobacter* (also known as *Herellea*), *P. maltophilia*, and *P. cepacia* are generally resistant to aztreonam, as are all gram-positive bacteria and anaerobes.

Aztreonam is not absorbed from the GI tract, but excellent blood levels are achieved after intramuscular or intravenous administration. The drug is widely distributed in body tissues and fluids, including the CSF.[135] The serum half-life of aztreonam is about 90

minutes; glomerular filtration is the major means by which the drug is eliminated.

Aztreonam is well tolerated. Its toxicities resemble those of other β-lactam antibiotics, including occasional instances of local reactions at the site of injection, rash, diarrhea, nausea, and vomiting.[136] Neither nephrotoxicity nor bleeding disorders have been reported. Aztreonam does not cross-react with serum antibodies of penicillin- and cephalosporin-allergic patients,[137] and the drug has been well tolerated in penicillin-allergic patients.[138,139] Because experience in this setting is limited, the drug should be used with caution. Although superinfections were reported in only two to six percent of 2,734 patients who received aztreonam,[136] much smaller studies have reported superinfections in as many as 30 percent, with enterococci predominating.[140-142]

Aztreonam has been used successfully in the treatment of a wide variety of infections caused by gram-negative bacteria,[143] including pneumonias, skin and soft tissue infections, bone and joint infections, urinary tract infections, and bacteremias. Aztreonam has been effective and safe when combined either with vancomycin in the treatment of febrile episodes in neutropenic cancer patients[144] or with clindamycin or metronidazole in the treatment of pulmonary or abdominal infections. Although aztreonam achieves therapeutic concentrations in the CSF, experience in the treatment of meningitis has been very limited.

The recommended dosages for aztreonam range from 500 mg every 12 hours for urinary tract infections to 1 to 2 g every eight to 12 hours for systemic infections; it would seem reasonable to select dosage schedules in the higher ranges when the pathogen is *P. aeruginosa*. Maximum dosages of 2 g every six hours may be given for life-threatening infections. The dosage of aztreonam must be reduced in azotemic patients; the drug is efficiently removed by hemodialysis but not by peritoneal dialysis.

Because aztreonam combines the activity of the aminoglycosides with the low toxicity of the β-lactams, it may eventually replace aminoglycosides in many gram-negative infections. A potential disadvantage to aztreonam is the risk of enterococcal superinfections. Aztreonam is significantly more expensive than gentamicin. Synergy can be demonstrated between aztreonam and aminoglycosides for some gram-negative bacilli.[145] More clinical experience will be needed to determine the circumstances in which aztreonam should be a substitute for or a supplement to aminoglycosides.

Allergic Reactions to β-lactam Antibiotics

Hypersensitivity is the most common adverse reaction to β-lactam antibiotics. Most often, it is a delayed reaction characterized by maculopapular eruptions, fever, or both; eosinophilia may also be present. Much less common, but much more serious, is immediate hypersensitivity that is mediated by IgE; manifestations may include early-onset urticaria, laryngeal edema, or anaphylaxis. Immune complexes can produce serum sickness in some patients. Antibodies to β-lactam antibiotics can also cause hemolytic anemia.

Many patients with vague histories of penicillin allergies are not truly hypersensitive. A careful history is the best way to establish true drug allergy. A recollection of rash, urticaria, arthralgias, wheezing, or anaphylaxis confirms the diagnosis of hypersensitivity, whereas treatment failure, diarrhea, vaginitis or other superinfections, or vague symptoms do not. Skin tests have a limited role in predicting true penicillin allergy, but they can help exclude IgE-mediated (anaphylactic) hypersensitivity. To document severe allergy, both benzyl penicilloylpolylysine (a major-determinant antigen) and the so-called minor-determinant antigens should be injected[146]; unfortunately, only the former is available commercially. A wheal-and-flare reaction signifies IgE-mediated allergies; negative reactions to both major and minor determinants make anaphylaxis unlikely, but small test doses of penicillin may be administered for additional safety. Patients with penicillin allergy,

whether documented by history or by skin testing, should receive other antibiotics for infections; in rare cases in which there is no acceptable alternative to a penicillin, desensitization can be attempted.[146]

Patients who are allergic to one penicillin should be considered allergic to all penicillins; this generalization may not be true for some children in whom a rash has developed after taking ampicillin or amoxicillin, particularly in the setting of infectious mononucleosis. Patients who are allergic to penicillin have a three to seven percent likelihood of having an allergic reaction to a cephalosporin antibiotic[146]; cephalosporins are best avoided in patients who have IgE-mediated (anaphylactic) hypersensitivity to penicillin. Although there is much less experience with carbapenems (e.g., imipenem), the same guidelines apply for the use of these drugs in patients who are allergic to other β-lactams. However, monobactams (e.g., aztreonam) have not provoked cross-reacting hypersensitivity reactions. There are no reliable skin tests for cephalosporin, carbapenem, or monobactam allergies.

Aminoglycoside Antibiotics

Streptomycin Streptomycin was the first parenterally administered antibiotic that was active against many species of gram-negative bacilli and *Mycobacterium tuberculosis*. Although extensively employed 25 to 30 years ago, its current use is limited because of the rapid emergence of highly resistant organisms, the widespread occurrence among Enterobacteriaceae of R factor–mediated transmissible streptomycin resistance, the relatively frequent occurrence of vestibular damage during prolonged treatment, the availability of less toxic broad-spectrum antibiotics, and the development of aminoglycosides with wider ranges of activity and greater potency. Use of streptomycin is restricted principally to three situations: the initial treatment of serious tuberculous infections in which adequate therapy with isoniazid, rifampin, ethambutol, and pyrazinamide cannot be employed because of adverse effects or because of resistance of the infecting strain; the treatment of enterococcal and other infections in which synergism between a penicillin and an aminoglycoside is desired; and the treatment of a few uncommon infections, such as bubonic plague and tularemia, for which streptomycin is the drug of choice.

Kanamycin Kanamycin has a broader spectrum of activity than streptomycin against gram-negative bacilli other than *Pseudomonas*; it also has some activity against *S. aureus* but not against streptococci and pneumococci. However, with the availability of penicillinase-resistant penicillins and cephalosporins, there is no indication for kanamycin or its successors, such as gentamicin, as the primary drug in the treatment of staphylococcal infections. R factor–mediated resistance to kanamycin occurs among the Enterobacteriaceae; as with other antibiotics, widespread use of the drug in a hospital selects for a population of resistant organisms and can result in nosocomial infections.[147]

Kanamycin is given intramuscularly or occasionally intravenously in a daily dosage of 15 mg/kg, with a maximum dosage of 1.5 g/day. A course of therapy ordinarily does not exceed a total of 15 g in patients with normal renal function. Kanamycin—and the other ototoxic and nephrotoxic aminoglycosides—should be given only in a hospital where the clinical and laboratory data on adverse effects can be closely monitored. Kanamycin is excreted primarily by the kidney. In the presence of renal insufficiency, the dosage of all aminoglycoside antibiotics must be decreased because of the narrow margin between therapeutic and toxic levels. Kanamycin has been largely replaced in clinical use by gentamicin and other aminoglycosides that are less ototoxic and that have a wider range of antibacterial activity.

Gentamicin Gentamicin is active against *P. aeruginosa* as well as the gram-negative bacilli susceptible to kanamycin.[148] Gentamicin penetrates pleural, ascitic, and synovial fluids in the presence of inflammation. It diffuses poorly into certain other body fluids, such as CSF, respiratory tract secretions, and the aqueous humor. Intrathecal administration of gentamicin is recommended for treatment of some types of gram-negative bacillary meningitis in adults.[149,150] In the treatment of endophthalmitis, subconjunctival injection is necessary to achieve therapeutic levels in the aqueous humor.

Gentamicin is excreted almost totally by glomerular filtration. Peak serum concentrations are reached 30 to 60 minutes after an intramuscular injection. The daily dosage of gentamicin for a patient with normal renal function is 3 to 5 mg/kg, divided into equal aliquots administered at eight-hour intervals. With a dosage of 1.5 mg/kg every eight hours, a peak serum gentamicin level of 5 to 7 µg/ml is expected. Peak levels may be lower than anticipated in febrile patients, in patients with an expanded extracellular volume, in patients with major burns, and in patients receiving high-dose carbenicillin or ticarcillin. Gentamicin can reach a toxic serum concentration in patients who receive dosages higher than those recommended, particularly if there is some underlying renal impairment.

Patients receiving gentamicin or any aminoglycoside should be checked frequently for vestibular or auditory dysfunction because hearing loss has been documented in up to 47 percent of patients receiving aminoglycosides. A shortened five-frequency monitoring protocol can detect early, high-frequency ototoxicity in 82 percent of affected ears.[151] If impairment occurs, the drug should be stopped. To prevent toxicity, serum creatinine levels, creatinine clearance, and urine volume should be closely monitored. Many hospitals can provide serum levels of gentamicin. Therapeutic peak serum levels are important determinants of a clinical response to aminoglycosides.[152] Monitoring serum levels is also the best way to avoid potentially toxic peak levels of the drug (> 8 to 9 µg/ml) in patients who exhibit decreased renal function.

If serum levels cannot be determined, gentamicin dosage can be adjusted on the basis of serum creatinine level. (The serum half-life of gentamicin, in hours, is equal to four times the serum creatinine level; a dose of 1.0 to 1.5 mg/kg given every second half-life maintains an effective serum level of the drug.[153]) The adjustment can be made either by giving a constant dose at extended intervals or by varying the dose at constant eight-hour intervals. In the former case, the serum creatinine level is multiplied by a constant factor of eight to give the interval between injections of a usual maintenance dose. Thus, for a patient with a serum creatinine level of 3.0 mg/dl, the gentamicin dosage would be 1.5 mg/kg at intervals of 24 hours (instead of the usual eight hours). The second method of adjusting the dosage involves dividing the maintenance dose by the serum creatinine level and giving this altered dose every eight hours. A serum creatinine level of 3.0 mg/dl would require a gentamicin dosage of 0.5 mg/kg at eight-hour intervals, that is, 1.5 mg/kg divided by 3.0.

Tobramycin Tobramycin is very similar to gentamicin in pharmacology. The dosage is the same as for gentamicin, and similar adjustments must be made in patients with renal impairment. Tobramycin resembles gentamicin in its spectrum of activity against most aerobic gram-negative bacilli, but it is somewhat more active against *P. aeruginosa*. In particular, tobramycin may be active against strains of *P. aeruginosa* that are resistant to gentamicin. Like gentamicin, tobramycin can act synergistically with carbenicillin against *P. aeruginosa*. The combination of penicillin and tobramycin has been found to be less effective than the combination of penicillin and gentamicin against some enterococcal strains, especially *S. faecium*.[154]

Tobramycin and gentamicin appear to have similar ototoxic potential; although some studies suggest that tobramycin may be somewhat less nephrotoxic than gentamicin,[155,156] other studies have noted similar nephrotoxicity for the two drugs.[157] Tobramycin is significantly more expensive than

gentamicin and appears to offer few advantages, except against *P. aeruginosa* or gentamicin-resistant gram-negative bacilli.

Amikacin Amikacin is a semisynthetic derivative of kanamycin. It is a poor substrate for the bacterial enzymes that inactivate aminoglycoside antibiotics; whereas gentamicin is affected by six of these enzymes and tobramycin by five, amikacin is inactivated by only one of them.[158] Indeed, amikacin resistance has not increased significantly even in hospitals that have used the drug routinely.[159]

Amikacin's spectrum of activity, like that of gentamicin, is broad. Amikacin is active against *S. aureus* in vitro, but clinical effectiveness against this organism has not been demonstrated. Amikacin is effective in vitro and in vivo against *P. aeruginosa* and against many gentamicin- and tobramycin-resistant Enterobacteriaceae (particularly *Serratia*, *Proteus* species other than *mirabilis*, and *Providencia* strains).[160] It should not be used to treat infections caused by streptococci or pneumococci. Also, it should not be used in combination with penicillin to treat enterococci, because it can antagonize the bactericidal effects of penicillin against some strains of *E. faecalis*.[161]

The pharmacological properties of amikacin are essentially identical to those of kanamycin. The recommended dosage in adults with normal renal function is 15 mg/kg/day, administered intramuscularly in equally divided doses every eight to 12 hours. A prolonged peak serum level greater than 30 μg/ml should be avoided. Amikacin can be administered intravenously when indicated—for example, in a patient with thrombocytopenia or shock. Divided doses are infused over 60 minutes every eight to 12 hours. In patients with impaired renal function, the dosage must be reduced and should be based on determination of serum levels. When serum level determinations are not available, it is appropriate to follow the same guidelines for dose adjustment that are recommended for gentamicin (see above). With amikacin, however, a constant factor of nine is used in administering normal dosage at prolonged intervals. Thus, if the serum creatinine level were 3 mg/dl, the maintenance dose normally used on a 12-hour schedule—7.5 mg/kg—would be administered every 27 hours.

The principal use of amikacin is in the treatment of infections caused by gentamicin- or tobramycin-resistant gram-negative bacilli. It is also used in the initial treatment of presumed gram-negative bacillary bacteremia in compromised hosts when a gentamicin-resistant organism is suspected because of antibiotic susceptibility patterns at a specific institution.

The major adverse effects of amikacin are the same as those of the other aminoglycosides: ototoxicity and nephrotoxicity [*see Table 10*]. These side effects can usually be avoided by proper monitoring and by limiting treatment to two weeks or less. Gentamicin and amikacin appear to have the same incidence of ototoxicity and nephrotoxicity.[162]

Netilmicin Netilmicin, a semisynthetic aminoglycoside, is pharmacologically similar to gentamicin. The antibacterial spectrum of the drugs is also similar, except netilmicin is less active against *P. aeruginosa*. Compared with amikacin, netilmicin appears to be more nephrotoxic and less efficacious; the two drugs have similar ototoxic potentials.[163] It is generally used only for organisms resistant to other aminoglycosides. The recommended dosage of 1 to 2 mg/kg every eight hours must be reduced in patients with impaired renal function.

The changing role of aminoglycosides The aminoglycosides are extremely active antibiotics that have proved clinically effective against many serious infections caused by gram-negative bacilli, and as patents have expired, these agents have become inexpensive. These assets, however, must be weighed against the potential of aminoglycosides to produce renal and otovestibular toxicity. New efforts to improve the toxic-to-therapeutic ratio of aminoglycosides include once-daily dose schedules[164]

Table 10   Adverse Effects of Aminoglycosides

Frequency	Adverse Effects
Occasional	Renal damage, rash (maculopapular), nausea and vomiting, ototoxicity (both auditory and vestibular to varying degrees—kanamycin effects more likely to be auditory; streptomycin and gentamicin effects more likely to be vestibular)
Rare	Neuromuscular blockade and apnea (to be considered particularly in patients receiving succinylcholine or other blocking agents and in patients with myasthenia gravis)

and reevaluations of the recommended therapeutic ranges.[165] To determine the future role of aminoglycosides, the cost-effectiveness of aminoglycosides needs to be compared directly with that of the new β-lactams and the fluoroquinolones.

Tetracyclines

Tetracyclines were originally widely employed because of their broad spectrum of activity against both gram-positive and gram-negative bacteria. They are used less extensively now because of the availability of the more effective bactericidal penicillins, cephalosporins, and fluoroquinolones. The emergence of resistance among gram-negative bacilli, group A streptococci, and pneumococci and the frequency of superinfection have also tended to decrease indications for their use.

Tetracyclines are the drugs of choice in the treatment of Rocky Mountain spotted fever and other rickettsioses. They are useful in the treatment of mycoplasmal pneumonia and such chlamydial diseases as psittacosis, trachoma, and lymphogranuloma venereum. They are used in the treatment of urinary tract infections caused by susceptible organisms and are effective in the treatment of nongonococcal urethritis. Other indications for their use include brucellosis, plague, cholera, granuloma inguinale, and Lyme disease; they may also be used in the treatment of syphilis and gonococcal pelvic inflammatory disease in patients allergic to penicillin. Tetracyclines are used as adjuvant therapy in the treatment of severe cystic acne.

There are numerous tetracycline compounds, but it is advisable to become familiar with one standard preparation (e.g., tetracycline) and one long-acting preparation (e.g., doxycycline) for use in practice. Tetracycline is administered either orally, 0.25 to 0.50 g four times daily, or intravenously in seriously ill patients, 1.0 g daily in divided doses every six to 12 hours. Concomitant ingestion of milk and antacids impairs tetracycline absorption. Therapeutic doses cannot be administered satisfactorily by the intramuscular route. Tetracycline is excreted in the urine and feces; it accumulates in patients with renal insufficiency and can cause hepatic toxicity, which can also occur when a daily dose of more than 1 g is administered intravenously. The tetracyclines should not be given to children who are younger than nine years or to pregnant women, because permanent discoloration of teeth may result.

The serum half-life of orally administered long-acting tetracyclines such as minocycline and doxycycline is 11 to 22 hours; administration is needed only every 12 to 24 hours to sustain therapeutic levels. The usual oral dose of minocycline for adults is 200 mg initially, followed by 100 mg every 12 hours; for doxycycline, the usual oral dose is 200 mg initially, followed by 50 to 100 mg every 12 hours. One distinct advantage of doxycycline over other tetracyclines is that the serum half-life remains close to normal values in patients whose renal function is severely impaired. Therefore, if a tetracycline must be administered in the presence of renal insufficiency, doxycycline would appear to be the preparation of choice; in rare instances, however, renal function may deteriorate further in those

azotemic patients who are receiving doxycycline.[166]

Both minocycline and doxycycline are available in intravenous preparations, which are given in a daily dose of 100 to 200 mg when the oral route cannot be employed. The spectrum of antibacterial activity of the long-acting tetracyclines is generally the same as that for the standard tetracyclines. Doxycycline has been found useful in the prophylaxis of traveler's diarrhea in Kenya.[167] Minocycline has been used as an alternative to sulfonamides for nocardial infections and for chemoprophylaxis in asymptomatic nasopharyngeal carriers of *N. meningitidis*. It should not be used for meningococcal infections. Side effects are almost identical for all of the tetracyclines, except for minocycline, which is occasionally associated with vestibular toxicity [*see Table 11*]. The long-acting tetracyclines are more costly than standard tetracycline.

Macrolides

The macrolides are composed of 14, 15, or 16 carbon atoms joined together in a complex, central, circular molecule that is linked to various side chains. A 14-member macrolide, erythromycin, has been available since 1952; at least 10 other macrolides are marketed in several countries, but in the United States, erythromycin was the only macrolide available until clarithromycin was approved in 1991 and azithromycin in 1992. Several newer macrolides are undergoing clinical trials.

Erythromycin

Erythromycin,[168] the oldest and most widely used macrolide, has a spectrum of activity that includes most gram-positive bacteria: *S. pneumoniae, S. aureus, Corynebacterium diphtheriae*, and diphtheroids. In the United States, most streptococci remain susceptible to erythromycin, but in Finland, erythromycin-resistant group A streptococci have been emerging since 1988.[169] In the United States, the extensive use of erythromycin in hospitals has led to the selection and predominance of *S. aureus* strains that

Table 11   Adverse Effects of Tetracyclines

Frequency	Adverse Effects
Frequent	GI irritation (nausea, vomiting, diarrhea); inhibition of bone growth and discoloration and deformity of teeth in children younger than 8 yr and in newborns, when administered after the first trimester of pregnancy; mucocutaneous candidiasis
Occasional	Intestinal malabsorption; staphylococcal enterocolitis; pseudomembranous enterocolitis; photosensitivity (fever, sunburn reactions), most frequent with demeclocycline; negative nitrogen balance and increased azotemia with preexisting renal insufficiency (rarely with doxycycline); liver injury when large I.V. doses (> 1 g/day) are administered, especially when given to pregnant patients or to those with renal disease; prolongation of prothrombin time with extended use; vestibular reactions with minocycline; tooth discoloration in young adults with minocycline[267]
Rare	Allergic reactions; fixed drug eruptions; increased intracranial pressure (pseudotumor cerebri) in infants and extremely rarely in adults; Fanconi's syndrome after ingestion of outdated tetracycline; diabetes insipidus–like symptoms with demeclocycline

are highly resistant to this drug. Erythromycin remains active against *Mycoplasma pneumoniae, Chlamydia trachomatis*, and some gram-negative bacilli, including *Legionella pneumophila, Campylobacter, Flavobacterium,* and *H. pertussis. Neisseria* and *T. pallidum* are also susceptible to erythromycin, as are occasional strains of atypical mycobacteria.

Erythromycin is excreted to a large extent in the bile and only to a minor degree in the urine. The dosage need not be altered in the presence of renal insufficiency. Erythromycin penetrates pleural and peritoneal fluids. In the presence of meningeal inflammation associated with pneumococcal meningitis, sufficient concentrations can be achieved in the CSF with large intravenous dosages (4 g/day), but this treatment is not the preferred one [*see Chapter 35*]. Because erythromycin crosses the placenta, it is used to treat syphilis in pregnant women allergic to penicillin.

Erythromycin is the drug of choice for treating *Legionella* infections and is excellent for treating *Mycoplasma* infections; hence, it is the preferred treatment for patients with so-called atypical pneumonia who are not producing sputum. Erythromycin is also effective for *Campylobacter* gastroenteritis, for the treatment of diphtheria and chlamydial infections, and for chemoprophylaxis in per-

tussis carriers. In patients who cannot tolerate penicillins and cephalosporins, erythromycin is an effective alternative for the treatment of streptococcal pharyngitis, bronchitis, and pneumonia; infections of skin and soft tissue; and syphilis. Other uses of erythromycin include granuloma inguinale and chancroid (administered with a sulfonamide), prophylaxis for elective bowel surgery (administered with neomycin), and acne (administered topically or orally).

Erythromycin is administered orally in a dosage of 0.25 to 0.50 g four times daily. Therapeutic blood levels can be achieved with any of the oral erythromycin preparations.[170] Gastrointestinal intolerance is the most common side effect; enteric-coated preparations are available, but a comparative trial failed to confirm the clinical impression that it produces fewer gastrointestinal side effects.[171] Because of the occasional occurrence of cholestatic hepatitis after administration of the estolate form, however, erythromycin base or stearate is preferred for adults [*see Table 12*]. Intravenous preparations of erythromycin (lactobionate or glucceptate salts, 1 to 4 g daily) are used in the treatment of severe infections, but prolonged therapy is difficult because of the frequent occurrence of thrombophlebitis at infusion sites. As many as 16 percent of patients receiving erythromycin intravenously in dosages of 4 g/day develop tinnitus or hearing loss that resolves when the drug is discontinued.[172] Up to 37 percent of patients receiving erythromycin intravenously experience nausea, sometimes with vomiting, that is severe enough to interrupt therapy; pretreatment with 0.1 mg of intravenous glycopyrrolate followed by a one-hour infusion of erythromycin significantly reduces the gastrointestinal toxicity of intravenous erythromycin.[173] A case of hepatic failure induced by intravenous erythromycin lactobionate has been reported.[174] Therapeutic levels of the drug are not achieved with intramuscular doses that patients can tolerate.

Clarithromycin

Clarithromycin, which is a semisynthetic 14-member macrolide, was approved for clinical use in the United States in 1991.[175,176] The drug is acid stable and well absorbed from the gastrointestinal tract; meals do not significantly affect its bioavailability. Like erythromycin, clarithromycin achieves wide tissue penetration; because of its longer half-life, however, clarithromycin may be administered twice a day rather than four times a day.[177] Clarithromycin appears to produce fewer gastrointestinal side effects than erythromycin, but clinical experience with the new antibiotic is still limited.

Clarithromycin is highly active against those organisms that are sensitive to erythromycin; these include streptococci, pneumococci, staphylococci, *Legionella*, *Campylobacter*, *Mycoplasma*, and *Chlamydia pneumoniae*. Clarithromycin also exhibits excellent activity against *M. catarrhalis* and *H. influenzae*,[177-180] which therefore makes it an attractive agent for the treatment of respiratory tract infections. Although there is only limited clinical experience, clarithromycin has been used successfully for the treatment of sinusitis, pharyngitis, bronchitis, and pneumonia caused by susceptible organisms.[181-183] Clarithromycin has also been used successfully in a small number of patients who have Legionnaires'

Table 12 Adverse Effects of Macrolides

Frequency	Adverse Effects
Occasional	GI irritation (particularly epigastric distress), stomatitis, cholestatic hepatitis in adults treated with erythromycin estolate, reversible ototoxicity occurring after I.V. administration of 4 g of erythromycin a day
Rare	Allergic reactions with fever and rash (sometimes resembling Stevens-Johnson syndrome), pseudomembranous colitis, potentiation of warfarin effect, pancreatitis

disease.[184] Because it displays in vitro activity against several other pathogens, the drug is being studied for the monotherapy of *Helicobacter pylori* gastric infections as well as for the treatment of Lyme disease and of *Mycobacterium avium-intracellulare* and *Toxoplasma gondii* infections in patients who have acquired immunodeficiency syndrome (AIDS). The usual adult dosage is 250 to 500 mg administered orally twice a day.

At present, the Food and Drug Administration has approved clarithromycin for the treatment of only those infections of the skin, the soft tissues, and the upper and lower respiratory tract that are caused by susceptible pathogens. In order to determine the best use of this promising drug, additional experience will be necessary. Clarithromycin is substantially more expensive than erythromycin.

Azithromycin

Azithromycin, a 15-member macrolide that was approved in 1992 for clinical use in the United States, is active against the same broad range of organisms that clarithromycin inhibits. Azithromycin is also active against *C. trachomatis*, *H. ducreyi*, and some anerobes.[185]

Like the other macrolides, azithromycin is acid stable and well absorbed from the GI tract. Unlike clarithromycin, however, its bioavailability is decreased by food; thus, azithromycin should be taken one hour before or two hours after meals. Azithromycin clears rapidly from serum and moves promptly into interstitial and intracellular tissue compartments.[186] Tissue levels are extraordinarily prolonged, with an average terminal half-life of 68 hours. Therefore, tissue levels of azithromycin can be expected to remain in the therapeutic range from four to seven days after a five-day treatment course. These unique pharmacokinetics support the current program of administering azithromycin once daily for five days. Like clarithromycin, azithromycin appears to be well tolerated and to have fewer gastrointestinal side effects than erythromycin.

Although clinical experience with azithromycin is limited, it has been effective in the treatment of streptococcal pharyngitis,[187] sinusitis,[188] bronchitis and pneumonia,[189] and skin and soft tissue infections.[190] In addition to these indications, which the Food and Drug Administration has approved, azithromycin has been used successfully as a single-dose therapy for urethritis and cervicitis caused by *C. trachomatis*[191]; if the FDA approves these uses, azithromycin would provide a significant advantage because no approved single-dose regimens now exist for these infections. The greatest promise for azithromycin, however, may lie in the treatment of difficult-to-treat chronic infections, such as *M. avium-intracellulare* and *T. gondii* in patients with AIDS.

The usual dosage of azithromycin is 500 mg on day 1 and 250 mg on days 2 through 5. Azithromycin is substantially more expensive than erythromycin.

Lincomycin and Clindamycin

Clindamycin generally has replaced the parent compound lincomycin in clinical usage because clindamycin has greater antibacterial activity against anaerobes, higher blood levels, and a somewhat lower frequency of gastrointestinal side effects than lincomycin.[192] Clindamycin is active against the following pathogens: *S. aureus, S. pneumoniae*, group A and other streptococci (except enterococci), *Bacteroides* (including *B. fragilis*) and *Fusobacterium* species, anaerobic streptococci and peptococci, and *C. perfringens* and *C. tetani* (but not other clostridial strains).

Only about 10 percent of administered clindamycin is excreted in active form in the urine; the remainder is changed into inactive metabolites. In patients with marked renal insufficiency, the half-life of clindamycin is only slightly prolonged, and little change in dosage is necessary. In patients with severe liver disease, however, dosage should be determined with care; serum levels are helpful. Because clindamycin does not penetrate readily into the central nervous system, even when there is marked meningeal inflammation, it should not be used to treat meningitis.

Because severe pseudomembranous colitis can be a complication of clindamycin therapy, the drug should be used only for infections that cannot be treated satisfactorily by other agents. It is indicated in the treatment of serious infections caused by susceptible anaerobes, particularly those originating in the gastrointestinal and female genital tracts. Clindamycin has also been very effective in the treatment of aspiration pneumonia and lung abscess. This agent should not be used in the treatment of pharyngitis; in penicillin-allergic patients who have streptococcal pharyngitis, erythromycin is the preferred alternative. Clindamycin should be used only topically for acne therapy. Clindamycin has also been used to treat protozoan infections, such as toxoplasmosis and babesiosis.

Clindamycin is administered orally in an average adult daily dose of 600 to 1,200 mg; in more severe infections, 1,800 mg daily may be used. The daily intramuscular dose is 1.2 to 2.4 g, and the daily intravenous dose is 1.8 to 3.0 g. Clindamycin should be avoided, or used with considerable caution, in patients with a history of bowel disease, particularly colitis [*see Table 13*]. If significant diarrhea occurs, the antibiotic should be discontinued. Diarrhea and colitis are more likely to occur with the oral form of the drug but can develop with parenteral administration as well.

Chloramphenicol

Although chloramphenicol remains a valuable broad-spectrum antibiotic,[193] its use has decreased as the availability of less toxic alternatives has increased. Because of the rare occurrence of aplastic anemia [*see Adverse Reactions to Antimicrobial Agents, above*], clinical use of chloramphenicol should be limited to serious infections, for which alternative antibiotics may be less effective: typhoid fever; nontyphoidal salmonelloses caused by ampicillin-resistant strains; meningitis caused by ampicillin-resistant strains of *H. influenzae*; meningitis caused by *H. influenzae*, *N. meningitidis*, or *S. pneumoniae* in patients who are allergic to penicillin and cephalosporins; and infections caused by *B. fragilis*. Even for these traditional uses, however, chloramphenicol must be evaluated in comparison to other antibiotics. For example, the newer cephalosporins and fluoroquinolones should be considered for salmonellosis; second- and third-generation cephalosporins should be considered for ampicillin-resistant strains of *H. influenzae*; and cefoxitin, cefotetan, clindamycin, or metronidazole could be used to treat infections caused by *B. fragilis*.

Chloramphenicol is usually given orally or intravenously; although intramuscular administration had been considered unreliable in adults, this route does produce therapeutic serum levels in children.[194] The average oral dosage is 30 to 50 mg/kg daily. In children with severe infection, the intravenous dose may be as high as 100 mg/kg initially; in adults with severe infection, the intravenous dose is 2 to 4 g. Chloramphenicol diffuses rapidly into most tissues, cerebrospinal fluid, ascitic fluid, and aqueous humor. The drug is lipid soluble and achieves levels in the brain up to nine times higher than in the serum. Chloramphenicol

Table 13 Adverse Effects of Clindamycin

Frequency	Adverse Effects
Frequent	Diarrhea; hypersensitivity reactions (maculopapular rashes)
Occasional	Pseudomembranous colitis, nausea and vomiting
Rare	Reversible neutropenia

is inactivated in the liver by conjugation with glucuronic acid; blood levels may increase in patients with marked cirrhosis and jaundice.

In view of the risk of aplastic anemia [*see Table 14*], the following guidelines should be employed in the use of chloramphenicol:

1. Use only in the treatment of infections for which it is clearly indicated.
2. Avoid repeated courses.
3. Check blood counts two to three times weekly.
4. Observe the patient closely for evidence of sore throat (granulocytopenia) or other new infections.

Although additional data are needed, chloramphenicol administered parenterally

Table 14 Adverse Effects of Chloramphenicol

Frequency	Adverse Effects
Occasional	Reversible anemia or leukopenia (dose-related toxic effect on bone marrow); gray syndrome in neonates; nausea, vomiting, diarrhea; glossitis; oropharyngeal candidiasis
Rare	Aplastic anemia, rashes, drug fever, enterocolitis, neurotoxic reactions (with prolonged use: confusion, headache, peripheral neuritis, or optic neuritis)

seems to be associated only very rarely with aplasia of the bone marrow.[193]

Vancomycin

Vancomycin is a bactericidal glycopeptide that impairs cell wall synthesis of gram-positive bacteria; its narrow spectrum of action includes staphylococci, streptococci, pneumococci, enterococci, clostridia, *Corynebacterium* species, and some other gram-positive bacteria.[195,196] It is bacteriostatic but not bactericidal against some strains of enterococci, *S. epidermidis*, and corynebacteria.

Vancomycin is poorly absorbed when administered orally. The oral route is employed only for the treatment of staphylococcal enterocolitis and antibiotic-associated pseudomembranous enterocolitis; a dosage of 125 to 250 mg every six hours is recommended for this purpose. Vancomycin is administered intravenously, 0.5 g every six hours or 1.0 g every 12 hours, in the treatment of severe staphylococcal infections or viridans streptococcal or enterococcal endocarditis in patients highly allergic to penicillin. To avoid hypotension and histaminelike reactions, the drug should always be infused slowly over a period of one hour. Pretreatment with antihistamines can help avert the so-called red man syndrome;[197] in rare cases, desensitization may be necessary.[198] Concomitant administration of an aminoglycoside is often necessary when vancomycin is used in the treatment of enterococcal endocarditis. It is also the drug of choice in the treatment of infections caused by methicillin-resistant *S. aureus*. Vancomycin can be very useful in therapy for prosthetic valve endocarditis caused by *S. epidermidis*; in this setting, the agent is frequently administered in combination with either gentamicin or rifampin. Vancomycin is also used for prophylaxis against endocarditis in penicillin-allergic patients who have valvular heart disease and are undergoing dental procedures.

Vancomycin does not penetrate normal meninges but does enter the CSF when the meninges are inflamed; however, experience with vancomycin in the treatment of meningitis is very limited. Most of the drug is known to be eliminated through the kidneys. In the presence of renal failure, the drug accumulates in the circulation, and the dose must be reduced.[199] The serum half-life (six hours) in normal adults is prolonged to nine days in anuric patients. Determination of serum levels is an important guide to dosage when the drug must be administered in the presence of impaired renal function; peak serum levels of 20 to 30 μg/ml are considered ideal, as are trough levels of 10 μg/ml or less. Because of its side effects, vancomycin should be avoided, if possible, in patients who have a history of hearing loss or renal insufficiency [*see Table 15*]. Particular attention to ototoxicity and nephrotoxicity is required when vancomycin is administered with an aminoglycoside.

Polymyxin B and Colistimethate

The antibacterial spectrum of polymyxin B and colistimethate (polymyxin E) covers most of the common aerobic gram-negative bacilli. Until they were superseded by the newer and more effective aminoglycosides and carbenicillin, the polymyxins were employed principally to treat infections caused by *P. aeruginosa*. However, because the polymyxins do not readily enter body tissue and fluid compartments (e.g., the respiratory tract, CSF) and because they have toxic side effects, these drugs are now rarely used systemically. Polymyxin B is used topically in eye or ear drops.

Spectinomycin

Although spectinomycin is active in vitro against a variety of gram-negative bacteria, it is less effective than many other drugs. Its one clinical use is for the treatment of gonorrhea. It is used in the treatment of urethral and anogenital gonorrhea in patients allergic to penicillins and cephalosporins. Spectinomycin is not effective in the treatment of gonococcal pharyngitis but can be used as an alternative drug for pelvic inflammatory disease or the arthritis-dermatitis-bacteremia syndrome. The dose of spectinomycin that is used in treating acute gonococcal urethritis, cervicitis, and procti-

Table 15 Adverse Effects of Vancomycin

Frequency	Adverse Effects
Occasional	Thrombophlebitis; chills and fever; ototoxicity (principally hearing loss with large doses or prolonged therapy, especially in patients with impaired renal function and in the elderly); nausea; nephrotoxicity (usually mild and reversible); urticaria and other rashes; hypotension, which may be accompanied by paresthesias, pruritus, and upper body rash (after rapid I.V. administration)
Rare	Neutropenia; thrombocytopenia

tis is a single intramuscular injection of 2 g; for the arthritis-dermatitis syndrome, the dosage is 2 g given intramuscularly twice a day for three days. Side effects have been minor: pain at the injection site, chills and fever, urticaria, and dizziness.

Sulfonamides

Although the sulfonamides no longer play a major clinical role, they are still useful antimicrobials. Because of their efficacy and low cost, individual sulfonamides are used principally to treat uncomplicated urinary tract infections caused by *E. coli*. Sulfonamides are also useful for nocardial infections. The emergence of ampicillin-resistant *H. influenzae* has brought about a return to sulfonamides (in combination with erythromycin or trimethoprim) for treating otitis media in children.

The short-acting sulfonamides consist of sulfisoxazole, sulfadiazine, and trisulfapyrimidines. The last is a mixture of sulfonamides (sulfadiazine, sulfamerazine, and sulfamethazine) designed to minimize renal damage resulting from sulfonamide crystalluria [*see* Table 16]. Its use has been superseded by more soluble sulfonamides, such as sulfisoxazole. Generally, sulfisoxazole has also replaced the less soluble sulfadiazine and can be considered the sulfonamide for systemic use. After oral or intravenous administration, sulfisoxazole is rapidly and almost totally excreted in its free and acetylated forms in the urine. Both forms are much more soluble at normal urine pH than are free and acetylated sulfadiazine. The oral dosage of sulfisoxazole for adults is a loading dose of 2 to 4 g, followed by 0.5 to 1.0 g every four to six hours. The intravenous daily dosage is 100 mg/kg in equally divided doses every six hours. In patients with serious infections (e.g., nocardiosis), the sulfonamide blood level should be checked [*see* Table 6] to ensure proper therapy. The rapid excretion of sulfisoxazole may require that larger intravenous doses be given at shorter intervals. Because of the high solubility of the drug, crystalluria and hematuria occur only rarely; still, a good fluid intake should be maintained.

The intermediate-acting sulfonamide in use is sulfamethoxazole, which is excreted more slowly than sulfisoxazole and requires

Table 16 Adverse Effects of Sulfonamides

Frequency	Adverse Effects
Frequent	Hypersensitivity reactions (rashes, Stevens-Johnson syndrome, photosensitivity, drug fever, serum sickness–type response), nausea and vomiting
Occasional	Crystalluria (with sulfadiazine and sulfonamides of similar solubility; risk is minimal with sulfisoxazole), hemolytic anemia, agranulocytosis (usually reversible), kernicterus in the newborn if administered to mother at term and during nursing period
Rare	Hepatitis (from toxic or hypersensitivity reaction), aplastic anemia, renal tubular necrosis, necrotizing angiitis, possible activation of SLE, pancreatitis, aseptic meningitis

less frequent administration. Unfortunately, crystalluria is more frequent with this drug than with sulfisoxazole. For mild infections in adults, sulfamethoxazole is given as a loading dose of 2 g orally, followed by 1 g every 12 hours.

Topical sulfonamides are still used in a few situations. Sulfacetamide eye drops are sometimes employed to treat superficial ocular infections. Topical silver-sulfadiazine cream is administered to burn surfaces to suppress bacterial growth and prevent subsequent invasive infection. Both the silver ion and the sulfadiazine components of the compound probably contribute to the antibacterial activity.

Trimethoprim

The single-drug preparation of trimethoprim was not released until 1980, even though the fixed-dose combination of trimethoprim-sulfamethoxazole (see below) has been available in the United States since 1973.[200] Trimethoprim is a pyrimidine analogue that, like the sulfonamides, acts to block bacterial folic acid synthesis. Trimethoprim is well absorbed from the gastrointestinal tract and is widely distributed in tissues (including the prostate); most of the drug is excreted unchanged in the urine. Its antibacterial spectrum encompasses many aerobic gramnegative bacilli; it does not have activity against *P. aeruginosa*. Trimethoprim is well tolerated; side effects include skin rash (less common than with sulfonamides) and megaloblastic marrow changes (uncommon). The agent is teratogenic in rats and therefore should not be given to pregnant women.

Trimethoprim is approved only for the initial treatment of uncomplicated urinary tract infections; the oral dosage is 100 mg twice daily. Resistance has not been a major problem thus far, but it may be a concern if the drug is used on a large scale or for prolonged periods, especially in a hospital setting; for example, the emergence of high-level trimethoprim resistance in *E. coli* isolates from the stools of persons receiving trimethoprim (or trimethoprim-sul-

famethoxazole) was observed during a two-week diarrhea-prevention study in Mexico.[201] If trimethoprim resistance were to become widespread, the usefulness of trimethoprim-sulfamethoxazole, a very valuable antimicrobial, would be impaired. Hence, it may be prudent to reserve trimethoprim for situations in which other agents, such as sulfonamides, ampicillin, amoxicillin, or tetracycline, are not effective.

Trimethoprim-Sulfamethoxazole

Use of the trimethoprim-sulfamethoxazole combination extended the list of clinical situations in which sulfonamides appear to be of value: uncomplicated urinary tract infections caused by organisms other than *E. coli* (i.e., *Klebsiella*, *Enterobacter*, and *Proteus* species), prevention of recurrent bacteriuria and urinary tract infections, prostatitis, acute otitis media, sinusitis or bronchitis caused by susceptible strains of *H. influenzae* and *S. pneumoniae*, systemic infections caused by chloramphenicol- and ampicillin-resistant *Salmonella* strains, and shigellosis.[202] Trimethoprim-sulfamethoxazole can be used to prevent or treat traveler's diarrhea.[203] High-dose oral trimethoprim-sulfamethoxazole may be used to treat uncomplicated gonorrhea, but other regimens are more effective. Trimethoprim-sulfamethoxazole may be useful in the treatment of infections caused by gram-negative bacilli resistant to other antimicrobials; it may be administered intravenously to treat serious infections,[204] including meningitis,[205] when other drugs are not effective. It is the treatment of choice for *Pneumocystis carinii* pneumonia and nocardiosis.

The trimethoprim-sulfamethoxazole synergistic combination is currently available in oral or intravenous preparations in a 1:5 ratio (80 mg trimethoprim and 400 mg sulfamethoxazole, or 160 mg trimethoprim and 800 mg sulfamethoxazole). Sulfamethoxazole was selected as the sulfonamide in the compound because its half-life (10 hours) is close to that of trimethoprim. Both drugs are excreted primarily by the kidneys. The dosage of trimethoprim-sulfamethoxazole for treatment of urinary tract infection in an adult is two single-strength tablets (or one double-strength tablet) every 12 hours; a similar dosage is effective for the treatment of otitis. For serious systemic infections, the intravenous dosage is 8 to 10 mg/kg (based on the trimethoprim component) in two to four equal doses every six to 12 hours. For *Pneumocystis* pneumonia, the dosage is 20 mg/kg (based on the trimethoprim component) in equally divided doses every six hours. Reduction in dosage is necessary if renal function is impaired.

Adverse reactions to trimethoprim-sulfamethoxazole are similar to those that are caused by sulfonamides alone; megaloblastic anemia is rare. Patients with AIDS, however, have a very high incidence of adverse reactions to this drug combination.[206]

Metronidazole

Metronidazole was first approved in 1959 for use as an antiparasitic agent against *Trichomonas vaginalis*; the drug later proved to be effective against the parasitic organisms *Entamoeba histolytica* and *Giardia lamblia*. In 1981, the FDA approved an intravenous preparation of metronidazole for the treatment of serious infections caused by anaerobic bacteria.[207] Orally administered metronidazole is excellent for treating pseudomembranous colitis caused by *C. difficile*. Metronidazole is also useful as part of preoperative prophylactic regimens for elective colorectal surgery. The drug is being studied for use in the treatment of nonspecific vaginitis, which is associated with *Gardnerella vaginalis*.

Metronidazole appears to act by disrupting bacterial DNA and inhibiting nucleic acid synthesis.[208] The drug is bactericidal against almost all anaerobic gram-negative bacilli, including *B. fragilis*, and against most *Clostridium* species. Although true anaerobic streptococci are generally susceptible to it, microaerophilic streptococci as well as *Actinomyces* and *Propionibacterium* species are often resistant.[209] Metronidazole has cured a variety of infections caused by anaerobes: central nervous system infections,

bone and joint infections, abdominal and pelvic sepsis, and endocarditis. Failures have been reported in the treatment of pleuropulmonary infections.

Side effects of metronidazole include dry mouth (associated with a metallic taste) and nausea. Concurrent use of alcohol may cause a reaction similar to that produced when alcohol is drunk after disulfiram ingestion. Neurologic symptoms, including peripheral neuropathy and encephalopathic reactions, and neutropenia are uncommon. Pancreatitis has been reported.[210] Metronidazole is mutagenic for bacteria and carcinogenic for rats and mice.[211] Carcinogenicity in humans has not been demonstrated but remains a concern.

When metronidazole is administered orally, it is well absorbed and is widely distributed in body tissues, including those of the CNS. For serious anaerobic infections, the drug is administered intravenously; a loading dose of 15 mg/kg is given, followed by 7.5 mg/kg every six hours until the patient is well enough to take an oral dosage of 7.5 mg/kg every six hours. The dosage need not be reduced in azotemic patients, but it should be reduced in patients with hepatic insufficiency.

Because of its bactericidal action and excellent tissue penetration, intravenous metronidazole may be the treatment of choice for *B. fragilis* endocarditis and *B. fragilis* CNS infections, both of which are uncommon. Metronidazole is also excellent for anaerobic infections of the abdomen and pelvis, but alternative drugs are available.

Quinolones

The quinolones are an important, rapidly expanding group of antimicrobial agents. The first quinolone to be used clinically was nalidixic acid, which was introduced in the United States in 1963. Poor serum levels limited the use of nalidixic acid to urinary tract infections, and the rapid development of bacterial resistance relegated it to a minor role; cinoxacin, a closely related synthetic organic acid, did not represent a significant improvement. However, the addition of a fluorine group and a piperazine substituent has greatly improved the antibacterial spectrum of the quinolones; the addition of a methyl group on the piperazine ring appears to further enhance the bioavailability of these compounds.[212] Norfloxacin was the first and ciprofloxacin was the second of the newer quinolones to be released for clinical use in the United States; they have now been joined by ofloxacin and lomefloxacin. A fifth compound, temafloxacin, was approved in 1992 for clinical use in the United States but was rapidly withdrawn because toxicities were reported. Many other fluoroquinolones are being studied actively.

The quinolones are bactericidal compounds that act by inhibiting DNA gyrase, the bacterial enzyme that is responsible for maintaining the supertwisted helical structure of DNA. The quinolones rapidly kill bacteria, probably by impairing DNA synthesis and possibly by mechanisms involving cleaving of bacterial chromosomal DNA. Bacterial resistance to the quinolones depends on a change in their DNA gyrase; in the case of nalidixic acid, this single-step mutation occurs with a frequency of 10^{-7}, but resistance to the newer fluoroquinolones occurs much less frequently (about 10^{-11}). Bacterial strains that are resistant to one fluoroquinolone tend to be cross-resistant to related compounds; however, because resistance is mediated by chromosomes rather than by plasmids, transfer of quinolone resistance has not been recognized.

The fluoroquinolones are broad-spectrum antimicrobials. Most enteric gram-negative bacilli, including *E. coli*, *Proteus*, *Klebsiella*, and *Enterobacter*, are highly susceptible; common gastrointestinal pathogens, such as *Salmonella*, *Shigella*, and *Campylobacter* species, are also very sensitive. Other gram-negative organisms that are killed by low concentrations of the fluoroquinolones include *N. gonorrhoeae* and *N. meningitidis*, *H. influenzae*, *Pasteurella multocida*, *M. catarrhalis*, and *Y. enterocolitica*. Organisms that are somewhat less susceptible include *P. aeruginosa*, *Acinetobacter* (also known as *Herellea*), *Serratia*, and staphylo-

cocci (*S. aureus* and *S. epidermidis*) and streptococci (including pneumococci and enterococci); many pneumococci and other streptococci are resistant to lomefloxacin. Even fastidious intracellular pathogens can be inhibited by certain quinolones; *Chlamydia*, *Mycoplasma*, *Listeria*, *Legionella*, and *M. tuberculosis* are in this category. The activity of the fluoroquinolones against anaerobic bacteria is variable and generally unimpressive; *C. difficile* is resistant. Aerobic bacteria that are resistant include *P. cepacia* and *P. maltophilia*.

The fluoroquinolones are rapidly absorbed from the gastrointestinal tract.[213] Penetration into body fluids and tissues is generally excellent; therapeutic concentrations are readily achieved in blister fluid, bile, urine, saliva and sputum, bone, and muscle. Excellent concentrations of these drugs are achieved in the prostate, and stool levels are extraordinarily high. The fluoroquinolones appear to penetrate the CSF in the presence of meningeal inflammation.

Although serum protein binding is modest, the fluoroquinolones have long serum half-lives that range from three to four hours for norfloxacin and ciprofloxacin to five hours for ofloxacin and eight hours for lomefloxacin. The major route of elimination of these drugs is renal, including glomerular filtration and tubular secretion. The dosage of the quinolones should be reduced in the presence of moderately severe renal failure. Although experience is limited, the fluoroquinolones appear to be very well tolerated, with mild gastrointestinal side effects (nausea, vomiting, or anorexia) and CNS side effects (light-headedness, dizziness, somnolence, or insomnia) occurring in fewer than 10 percent of treated patients. Crystalluria has been reported after the use of very large doses, and cartilage toxicity has been noted in some animal studies.[213] Because quinolones have caused arthropathy in young animals, these drugs should be avoided in children and in women who are pregnant or nursing.

The fluoroquinolones have been useful clinically in a variety of infections. Most data on the efficacy of these drugs have been obtained from studies of genitourinary and gastrointestinal infections, but respiratory tract, soft tissue, and bone infections have also responded to these agents.

Except for temafloxacin, which is no longer available, toxicities associated with the quinolones have been minimal [*see Table 17*]. Clearly, additional experience will be needed to define the indications for these promising antimicrobial agents.

Norfloxacin

The spectrum of action and the pharmacological properties of norfloxacin are typical of the fluoroquinolones.[214] Excellent results have been achieved with norfloxacin in the treatment of urinary tract infections, with cure rates of about 95 percent. In one study, for example, norfloxacin was as effective as trimethoprim-sulfamethoxazole, and there were fewer adverse reactions.[215] A single 800 mg dose of norfloxacin is effective for uncomplicated *E. coli* cystitis in women, but three days of therapy with 400 mg twice daily is needed to achieve comparable cure rates for cystitis caused by *S. saprophyticus*.[216] Although many less expensive antimicrobials can be used for uncomplicated urinary tract infections, norfloxacin is especially useful for urinary tract infections caused by resistant organisms such as *P. aeruginosa* and enterococci.

Although norfloxacin is currently approved by the FDA for urinary tract infections only, it has been found to be useful in the treatment of gonorrhea. Because of its excellent penetration, it should also be effective for prostatitis. Norfloxacin has been successful in treating enteric infections caused by *Shigella* and enterotoxigenic *E. coli*; it has also been successful in treating acute *Salmonella* gastroenteritis and in eradicating the chronic typhoid carrier state.[217] In addition, norfloxacin is effective in preventing traveler's diarrhea. The drug appears to help prevent gram-negative infections in patients with granulocytopenia.[218,219] Superinfection with resistant gram-negative organisms is not common, possibly because

Table 17   Adverse Effects of Quinolones

Frequency	Adverse Effects
Occasional	Gastrointestinal: nausea and vomiting, anorexia, diarrhea
	Central nervous system: restlessness, tremor, headache, lethargy, light-headedness or dizziness
	Rash
	Mucosal candidiasis
	Arthropathy (observed in studies of young animals)
Rare	Crystalluria, hematuria, abnormal renal function, allergic interstitial cystitis
	Pseudomembranous colitis
	Abnormal liver function tests
	Eosinophilia, neutropenia
	Possible seizures and anaphylactoid reactions
	Possible eosinophilic meningitis
	Possible delirium

norfloxacin dramatically reduces the aerobic bowel flora but leaves anaerobes intact, thus preserving colonization resistance. However, gram-positive bacteremias continue to be a problem in patients with granulocytopenia.[220] Moreover, in a randomized, multicenter trial, ciprofloxacin appeared to be more effective than norfloxacin in preventing infections in neutropenic patients with hematologic malignancies.[221]

The usual dosage of norfloxacin is 400 mg twice daily. Because food can delay oral absorption, norfloxacin should be administered either one hour before or two hours after eating; concurrent use of antacids should be avoided. A high fluid intake may help prevent crystalluria. The dosage should be reduced to 400 mg once daily in patients who have creatinine clearances below 30 ml/min.

Norfloxacin is not recommended for use in children or in women who are either pregnant or nursing.

Ciprofloxacin

The antibacterial spectrum of ciprofloxacin is nearly identical to that of norfloxacin. Like norfloxacin, ciprofloxacin[222-224] has been highly successful in the treatment of urinary and genital tract infections, including prostatitis, and gastrointestinal infections; both drugs are being studied for infection prophylaxis in neutropenic patients, with encouraging preliminary results.[221,225] Like other fluoroquinolones, ciprofloxacin has been used successfully to treat both acute salmonellosis and the typhoid carrier state;[226,227] it was ineffective, however, in an outbreak of gastroenteritis caused by *Salmonella java*.[228] The major advantages of ciprofloxacin are its greatly enhanced serum concentration and its availability in an intravenous preparation. Because of high blood levels and good tissue penetration, ciprofloxacin has been successful in treating a wide variety of systemic infections, including upper and lower respiratory tract infections, skin and soft tissue infections, and bone and joint infections. Success has been reported in certain infections that are often difficult to treat, such as *Pseudomonas* pulmonary infections in patients with cystic fibrosis,[229] the meningococcal carrier state,[230] and lower-extremity infections in patients with vascular insufficiency.[231] Most strains of *M. tuberculosis* and about one third of *M. avium-intracellulare* strains are susceptible to ciprofloxacin, which is being used experimentally for certain mycobacterial infections. Also experimental are the use of oral ciprofloxacin to treat acute and chronic osteomyelitis[232,233] and the long-term use of ciprofloxacin to suppress selected incurable chronic infections.[234] Ciprofloxacin has been less successful in treating some staphylococcal infections.[223,235] The methicillin-resistant *S. aureus* carrier state has not responded to ciprofloxacin alone, but preliminary studies using ciprofloxacin and rifampin have been promising.[236]

The usual oral dosage of ciprofloxacin is 250 mg twice daily for uncomplicated urinary tract infections; for more serious infections, the dosage should be increased to 500 or 750 mg every 12 hours. Antacids impair absorption of oral ciprofloxacin, which is best administered one hour before or two hours after meals. The usual intravenous dosage is 400 mg every 12 hours, infused over 60 minutes; blood levels after the 400 mg intravenous dosage are similar to the levels achieved by an oral dose of 500 mg, which is considerably less expensive.[237] The dosage should be decreased in patients with moderate or severe renal insufficiency. Ciprofloxacin is not recommended for children or for women who are pregnant or nursing. An ophthalmic preparation is also available.

Adverse reactions to ciprofloxacin are uncommon and resemble those of other fluoroquinolones. Because of its low toxicity, very broad spectrum, and good tissue penetration, ciprofloxacin shows great promise in many systemic infections. However, as the use of this agent has increased, ciprofloxacin-resistant strains of *S. aureus* and gram-negative bacilli[238] have begun to emerge. Furthermore, the advantages of ciprofloxacin should be carefully weighed against the known benefits of more established antibiotics, many of which are less expensive.

Ofloxacin

Ofloxacin is a tricyclic fluoroquinolone that bears many similarities to ciprofloxacin. The two agents share a similar wide spectrum of antimicrobial activity; ciprofloxacin, however, appears more active against *P. aeruginosa*,[239] whereas ofloxacin is more active against chlamydiae.[240] Ofloxacin is well absorbed from the gastrointestinal tract; peak serum levels are achieved within two hours; and its half-life is about five hours. Ofloxacin is widely distributed in body tissues and fluids, but data on CSF penetration are sparse. Because ofloxacin is excreted in the urine, its dosage should be reduced in patients with moderate to severe renal dysfunction. The side effects of ofloxacin appear similar to those of the other fluoroquinolones.

Ofloxacin has been used successfully to treat infections of the urinary tract, lower respiratory tract, and skin and soft tissues.[241] It has also been effective for prostatitis and for genital tract infections caused by *Chlamydia trachomatis* and *N. gonorrhoeae*.[242] Ofloxacin is more effective than trimethoprim-sulfamethoxazole for the prevention of infection in patients with chemotherapy-induced neutropenia,[243] and three days of ofloxacin therapy is effective for traveler's diarrhea.[244] The usual oral dosage for adults with normal renal function is 200 mg every 12 hours for urinary tract infections, 300 mg every 12 hours for prostatitis and genital tract infections, and 400 mg every 12 hours for infections of the skin and soft tissue and lower respiratory tract. A single dose of 400 mg is approved for the treatment of uncomplicated gonorrhea.

Ofloxacin may be administered intravenously in the same dosages; because serum levels are no higher after intravenous administration than after oral administration, intravenous ofloxacin should be reserved for patients who cannot absorb or tolerate the oral form.

Lomefloxacin

Lomefloxacin is a difluoroquinolone that is similar to the other fluoroquinolones in most important aspects.[245] Potential advantages of lomefloxacin include its longer half-life, which permits once-daily administration,[246] and its lack of influence on xanthine pharmacokinetics.[247] A disadvantage of lomefloxacin is its decreased activity against pneumococci and other streptococci, *Mycoplasma*, and *Chlamydia*.[248] The FDA approved lomefloxacin in 1992 for the treatment of urinary tract infections and of bronchitis caused by *M. catarrhalis* and *H. influenzae*. The usual dosage is 400 mg once daily; like the other fluoroquinolones, its dosage should be reduced in patients with renal dysfunction, and it should not be administered to patients who are pregnant or younger than 18 years.

Other Quinolones

Although experience is still limited, amifloxacin, enoxacin, and pefloxacin all appear to be effective new fluoroquinolones; clinical trials with these agents are in progress.

Nitrofurantoin

Nitrofurantoin is readily absorbed from the gastrointestinal tract and rapidly excreted. Antibacterial levels are not attained in the blood; therapeutic utility results from the high urinary concentrations achieved. This drug should be employed only in the treatment of uncomplicated, mild urinary tract infections. The spectrum of antibacterial activity includes *E. coli*, enterococci, and some strains of *Klebsiella* and *Enterobacter*. *Proteus* and *Pseudomonas* species are usually resistant. R factor–mediated resistance to nitrofurantoin has not been observed. Nitrofurantoin is administered orally in a dosage of 50 to 100 mg four times daily. It should not be administered when there is significant impairment of renal function. Nitrofurantoin can produce a variety of adverse effects [*see Table 18*].[249,250] Nausea and vomiting are common side effects, but their incidence may be decreased by using the macrocrystalline formulation and by taking the drug with food.

Antimicrobial Chemoprophylaxis

The term antimicrobial chemoprophylaxis refers to the use of antibiotics for preventing infection either before or very shortly after introduction of pathogenic organisms—for example, after the occurrence of a compound fracture but before the appearance of clinical infection. Chemoprophylaxis is most effective when a specific drug is selected for its activity against a particular organism. When prophylaxis is aimed at preventing all possible organisms from initiating infection, it is likely to be unsuccessful because it merely selects out the most drug-resistant organism as the cause of any infection that follows. Thus, prophylaxis is ineffective in the prevention of complicating bacterial or mycotic infections in patients with viral respiratory tract infections, in comatose patients or patients with congestive heart failure, and in patients requiring prolonged use of indwell-

Table 18   Adverse Effects of Nitrofurantoin

Frequency	*Adverse Effects*
Frequent	GI irritation (principally gastritis; less commonly diarrhea)
Occasional	Pulmonary hypersensitivity reactions (acute with chills, fever, dyspnea, pulmonary infiltrate, pleural effusion, and eosinophilia; chronic subacute process with dyspnea and diffuse fibrosis in patients on long-term therapy), rashes, drug fever, hemolytic anemia (associated with red blood cell G6PD deficiency), peripheral neuropathy
Rare	Cholestatic jaundice, chronic active hepatitis, parotitis

ing urinary catheters. Most current uses of chemoprophylaxis fall into three general categories: prevention of infection after exposure to a specific pathogen, prevention of specific types of infection in highly susceptible individuals, and prevention of postoperative infectious complications. In many instances, prophylactic use of antimicrobials is widely practiced, but convincing data validating the efficacy of this approach are not available.[251]

Prevention of Infection after Exposure to a Specific Pathogen

Group A streptococcal disease Patients with a history of rheumatic fever or signs of rheumatic heart disease are given penicillin to prevent reactivation of the rheumatic process that might follow any reinfection with group A streptococci.[252] Penicillin prophylaxis is also indicated to protect normal individuals from sequelae during a streptococcal epidemic in a closed group. Benzathine penicillin G, 1.2 million units given intramuscularly every three to four weeks, is the most reliable prophylaxis. Oral penicillin V, 250 mg twice daily, is also used. Such prophylaxis should be continued for at least five years after an episode of rheumatic fever. An oral sulfonamide, 1 g/day, is an alternative in a penicillin-allergic patient.

Pneumococcal infections Because young children with sickle cell anemia are extremely vulnerable to pneumococcal infections, penicillin prophylaxis has become part of standard medical care in this group of patients.[253]

Meningococcal infections Rifampin, four doses of 600 mg orally every 12 hours, is the preferred prophylaxis for meningococcal infections. Prophylaxis is indicated only for close contacts of a patient with meningococcal disease.[254]

H. influenzae infections Rifampin can eliminate the *H. influenzae* nasopharyngeal carrier state and can be used to reduce the risk of infection in close contacts of patients who have severe *H. influenzae* infections. A dosage of 20 mg/kg once daily (not to exceed 600 mg) for four days has been recommended.[255]

Gonococcal infections Individuals with a recent known exposure to gonorrhea should receive the same treatment used for the established disease [*see Table 5*]. Silver nitrate (one percent) ophthalmic solution is still recommended for the prevention of gonococcal ophthalmia in newborns.

Syphilis Epidemiological treatment of recent contacts of persons with suspected or proven syphilis employs the same program used in the treatment of primary syphilis: benzathine penicillin G, 2.4 million units given intramuscularly once only.

Tuberculosis Prophylactic isoniazid should be considered for tuberculin converters and certain tuberculin reactors.

Bacterial diarrheal diseases caused by enterotoxigenic *E. coli* and *Shigella* Prevention of traveler's diarrhea caused by enterotoxigenic *E. coli* is best effected by adherence to the principles of food sanitation. Antimicrobial prophylaxis with doxycycline, 100 mg/day orally, has been successful in preventing traveler's diarrhea.[167] Its therapeutic efficacy appears to stem from its transport across the small bowel mucosa into the intestinal lumen and from the current susceptibility of most enterotoxigenic *E. coli* strains. Doxycycline should not be routinely or extensively used to forestall the emergence of antibiotic resistance; rather, its use should be individualized. The combination of trimethoprim and sulfamethoxazole or trimethoprim alone can also be used to prevent (or treat) traveler's diarrhea.[203] Because of the increasing prevalence of sulfonamide-tetracycline resistance and ampicillin resistance among *Shigella* organisms, these drugs are not of much value in the prophylaxis of shigellosis in endemic areas. The combination of trimethoprim and sulfamethoxazole can be used for this purpose, but it should be individualized as well. Widespread use of this combination will inevitably select for resistant strains; trimethoprim-sulfamethoxazole should be kept available for its special role in the treatment of infections caused by strains of *Salmonella* and *Shigella* that are resistant to chloramphenicol and ampicillin.

Plague pneumonia Contacts, including medical personnel, of patients with plague pneumonia are at risk for this highly lethal form of the disease. They should receive tetracycline, 0.5 g orally daily, beginning within one day after exposure and continuing for five days.

Prophylaxis for Individuals with Increased Susceptibility to Particular Infections

Bacterial endocarditis with valvular heart disease or prosthetic heart valves Patients who have abnormal cardiac valves are at risk for bacterial endocarditis. Antibiotic prophylaxis for these patients is described elsewhere [*see Chapter 20*].

Recurrent urinary tract infection Prolonged antimicrobial prophylaxis may be used successfully in certain women who experience frequent recurrence of urinary tract infections.[256,257] Methenamine mandelate (1 g orally four times daily), trimethoprim-sulfamethoxazole (one-half to one single-strength tablet daily), trimethoprim (100 mg daily), or nitrofurantoin (100 mg at bedtime) may be sufficient to reduce markedly the incidence of symptomatic recurrences. Recurrent cystitis after sexual intercourse is a problem in some women. A single dose of an antimicrobial—for example, a double-strength tablet of trimethoprim-sulfamethoxazole, 250 mg of cephalexin, 100 mg of nitrofurantoin, or 1,000 mg of nalidixic acid—after sexual intercourse can be highly effective in preventing infection in the bladder.[257]

Chronic obstructive pulmonary disease A viral respiratory tract infection may predispose the patient to bacterial infections with an exacerbation of symptoms of chronic bronchitis. *H. influenzae* and *S. pneumoniae* are often isolated from the sputum at such times. Prophylaxis with tetracycline (500 mg twice daily), ampicillin (250 mg three times daily), or the combination of trimethoprim and sulfamethoxazole (two tablets twice daily), given at the first sign of a viral upper respiratory tract infection and continued for 10 to 14 days, may reduce the frequency of such bacterial infections and decrease morbidity; however, it probably cannot prevent progressive episodes of the underlying disease in these patients. Occasionally, acute exacerbations are so frequent that they may warrant continuous antimicrobial prophylaxis during the winter season.

Infections in patients with severe granulocytopenia Various measures have been employed in attempts to decrease the incidence and severity of infections in patients undergoing therapy for neoplasms or leukemia, in whom granulocytopenia develops (neutrophil count < 1,000/mm^3). These measures have included intense hygiene, protective isolation, and antimicrobial prophylaxis. Prophylaxis has taken three forms. The first approach is the use of oral nonabsorbable antimicrobials (e.g., gentamicin with vancomycin and nystatin or neomycin with polymyxin and nystatin) during the period of neutropenia.[258,259] The second approach is prophylactic trimethoprim-sulfamethoxazole therapy, with or without nystatin,[260,261] during episodes of granulocytopenia. Despite earlier reports of success, these regimens have proved only moderately beneficial at best and are not recommended for routine use.[262] Norfloxacin and ciprofloxacin are now being studied for prophylaxis against infections in patients who have granulocytopenia[218,219,263]; ciprofloxacin appears superior for this purpose.[221] The third method consists of empirical systemic antimicrobial therapy for a new febrile episode. Combinations of an aminoglycoside with a cephalosporin or antipseudomonal penicillin, or both, are commonly employed because of the frequency of bacteremias caused by gram-negative bacilli.

Antimicrobial Prophylaxis for Surgical Procedures

The use of antimicrobial prophylaxis in surgery involves a risk-to-benefit appraisal that varies depending on the nature of the operative procedure. To help prevent wound infections in patients undergoing elective surgery, antibiotics should be administered within two hours of the incision.[264] If prophylactic antibiotics are to be effective, administration should be timed so that therapeutic levels are attained at surgery but selection of bacteria resistant to the drugs is avoided. Antibiotics should usually be stopped 24 hours after the procedure.

The indications for prophylaxis with different operations have been reviewed, but in many instances, the available data are insuf-

ficient.[250,265] For clean elective surgical procedures—such as mastectomy and thyroidectomy—in which no tissue (other than the skin) carrying an indigenous flora is penetrated, the risks of routine antibiotic prophylaxis outweigh the possible benefits. When cardiovascular prostheses are emplaced, vancomycin is administered intravenously beginning two hours before surgery and continuing for three to five days. First-generation cephalosporins (e.g., cefazolin or cephapirin) may be used for prophylaxis, and similar regimens may be employed for major vascular surgery. Because of the grave consequences of infection in a prosthetic joint, vancomycin or a first-generation cephalosporin is used prophylactically when a total hip replacement is performed. In the repair of open fractures, which are commonly contaminated, prophylactic treatment with a cephalosporin for seven days is warranted. Controlled clinical studies have indicated that the administration of oral antibiotics (enteric-coated erythromycin plus neomycin, or tetracycline plus neomycin) just before colonic surgery significantly reduces the incidence of infectious complications. The erythromycin-neomycin combination, 1 g of each administered orally at 1:00 P.M., 2:00 P.M., and 11:00 P.M. on the day before surgery, strikingly reduced the number of aerobic and anaerobic organisms remaining in the colon at the time of surgery. The emergence of tetracycline resistance among intestinal *Bacteroides* organisms may limit the future utility of the tetracycline plus neomycin combination.

When patients cannot be prepared for surgery using oral antibiotics, parenteral cefoxitin, cefotetan, or cefmetazole prophylaxis may be useful in certain circumstances—for example, for patients undergoing colorectal surgery or repair of a ruptured viscus.

Cefazolin prophylaxis is recommended for patients undergoing pelvic surgery or high-risk gastric or biliary operations.

References

1. J Infect Dis 119:89, 1969
2. Infectious Multiple Drug Resistance. Pion Limited, London, 1975
3. Pediatrics 58:388, 1976
4. J Infect Dis 137:170, 1978
5. Ann Intern Med 67:81, 1967
6. N Engl J Med 284:175, 1971
7. MMWR 26:285, 1977
8. N Engl J Med 298:413, 1978
9. Pediatr Clin North Am 30:121, 1983
10. Medicine (Baltimore) 57:179, 1978
11. J Lab Clin Med 70:408, 1967
12. J Infect Dis 137:251, 1978
13. Arch Intern Med 88:489, 1951
14. J Clin Invest 50:2580, 1971
15. J Clin Invest 61:1645, 1978
16. Antimicrob Agents Chemother 10:335, 1971
17. Ann Intern Med 110:515, 1989
18. Arch Intern Med 149:1397, 1989
19. Am J Med Sci 259:346, 1970
20. Antimicrob Agents Chemother 8:117, 1975
21. Antimicrob Agents Chemother 11:852, 1977
22. J Infect Dis 161:381, 1990
23. Major Problems in Internal Medicine, Vol. VIII. WB Saunders Co, Philadelphia, 1976, p 68
24. J Infect Dis 129:73, 1974
25. The Medical Letter Handbook of Adverse Drug Interactions. The Medical Letter, Inc, New Rochelle, New York, 1985
26. Clin Infect Dis 14:165, 1992
27. Clin Infect Dis 14:272, 1992
28. Surg Clin North Am 60:65, 1980
29. Chest 86:138, 1984
30. Bull WHO 38:159, 1968
31. JAMA 223:499, 1973
32. JAMA 206:130, 1968
33. JAMA 196:679, 1966
34. N Engl J Med 312:1229, 1985
35. Ann Intern Med 67:235, 1967
36. Rev Infect Dis 12:236, 1990
37. Arch Intern Med 126:272, 1970
38. N Engl J Med 281:7, 1969
39. N Engl J Med 312:840, 1985
40. Arch Intern Med 149:1036, 1989
41. J Infect Dis 152:90, 1985
42. Ann Intern Med 101:92, 1984
43. MMWR 24:9, 1975
44. J Infect Dis 137:238, 1978
45. Arch Otolaryngol 110:258, 1984
46. Ann Intern Med 84:181, 1976
47. Clin Pharmacol Ther 18:70, 1975
48. MMWR 23:97, 1974
49. N Engl J Med 269:999, 1963
50. Ann Intern Med 92:14, 1980
51. Ann Intern Med 65:1, 1966
52. Ann Intern Med 81:429, 1974
53. J Infect Dis 135(suppl):S99, 1977
54. J Infect Dis 136:701, 1977
55. N Engl J Med 301:414, 1979
56. N Engl J Med 257:861, 1957
57. N Engl J Med 281:1137, 1969
58. Microbiology—1974. American Society for Microbiology, Washington, DC, 1975, p 179
59. Rev Infect Dis 7:287, 1985
60. Med Lett Drugs Ther 29:61, 1987
61. Rev Infect Dis 9:250, 1987
62. JAMA 248:336, 1982
63. Med Lett Drugs Ther 28:33, 1986
64. Med Lett Drugs Ther 28:41, 1986
65. Ann Intern Med 105:924, 1986
66. Arch Intern Med 152:1025, 1992
67. Arch Intern Med 152:930, 1992
68. Journal of Critical Illness 7:791, 1992
69. N Engl J Med 279:1245, 1968
70. Am J Med 65:756, 1978
71. Antimicrob Agents Chemother 12:438, 1977
72. Ann Intern Med 90:356, 1979
73. JAMA 244:561, 1980
74. Ann Intern Med 97:755, 1982
75. Rev Infect Dis 6:13, 1984
76. J Infect Dis 155:1242, 1987
77. Rev Infect Dis 13:68, 1991
78. Rev Infect Dis 13(suppl 9):S723, 1991
79. Med Lett Drugs Ther 26:99, 1984
80. Med Lett Drugs Ther 29:79, 1987
81. Med Lett Drugs Ther 27:69, 1985
82. Ann Intern Med 101:389, 1984
83. Med Lett Drugs Ther 27:30, 1985
84. N Engl J Med 294:24, 1976
85. Ann Intern Med 89:650, 1978
86. Med Lett Drugs Ther 21:85, 1979
87. Ann Intern Med 103:70, 1985
88. Med Lett Drugs Ther 28:70, 1986
89. Am J Obstet Gynecol 154:946, 1986
90. Am J Obstet Gynecol 154:960, 1986
91. Ann Intern Med 105:924, 1986
92. Med Lett Drugs Ther 26:71, 1984
93. Med Lett Drugs Ther 26:91, 1984
94. Med Lett Drugs Ther 26:15, 1984
95. J Pediatr 109:123, 1986
96. Med Lett Drugs Ther 30:57, 1988
97. Arch Intern Med 148:343, 1988
98. Annu Rev Med 32:559, 1981
99. Rev Infect Dis 9:719, 1987
100. Ann Intern Med 115:585, 1991
101. Med Lett Drugs Ther 23:61, 1981
102. Am J Med 80:398, 1986
103. Infection 13(suppl 1):S73, 1985
104. Infection 13(suppl 1):S28, 1985
105. Ann Intern Med 101:469, 1984
106. Med Lett Drugs Ther 25:109, 1983
107. Med Lett Drugs Ther 24:13, 1982
108. Am J Med 71:693, 1981
109. Am J Med 77(4C):1, 1984
110. Antimicrob Agents Chemother 28:540, 1985
111. JAMA 253:3559, 1985
112. N Engl J Med 322:141, 1990
113. Sex Transm Dis 13(suppl):199, 1986
114. Rev Infect Dis 11:299, 1989
115. Ann Intern Med 115:712, 1991
116. Rev Infect Dis 7:604, 1985
117. Med Lett Drugs Ther 27:85, 1985
118. Antimicrob Agents Chemother 28:33, 1985
119. N Engl J Med 317:1692, 1987
120. J Infect Dis 164:907, 1991
121. Med Lett Drugs Ther 31:73, 1989
122. N Engl J Med 325:1337, 1991
123. Med Lett Drugs Ther 32:107, 1990
124. JAMA 252:3277, 1984
125. Ann Intern Med 103:552, 1985
126. Med Lett Drugs Ther 28:29, 1986
127. J Antimicrob Chemother 16:751, 1985
128. J Antimicrob Chemother 27:405, 1991
129. J Infect Dis 154:289, 1986
130. Antimicrob Agents Chemother 31:632, 1987
131. Arch Intern Med 152:283, 1992
132. Ann Intern Med 115:849, 1991
133. Med Lett Drugs Ther 29:45, 1987
134. Rev Infect Dis 7(suppl 4):S594, 1985
135. Antimicrob Agents Chemother 29:281, 1986
136. Rev Infect Dis 7(suppl 4):S648, 1985
137. Rev Infect Dis 7(suppl 4):S613, 1985
138. J Allergy Clin Immunol 83:735, 1989

139. Am J Med 88(suppl 3C):12S, 1990
140. Antimicrob Agents Chemother 29:359, 1986
141. J Antimicrob Chemother 17:661, 1986
142. Lancet 1:1315, 1984
143. Am J Med 88(suppl 3C):2S, 1990
144. Am J Med 81:243, 1986
145. Rev Infect Dis 6(suppl 3):S678, 1984
146. Ann Intern Med 107:204, 1987
147. Ann Intern Med 71:1, 1969
148. Ann Intern Med 89:528, 1978
149. Yale J Biol Med 50:31, 1977
150. Ann Intern Med 77:295, 1972
151. J Infect Dis 165:1026, 1992
152. J Infect Dis 155:93, 1987
153. Ann Intern Med 74:192, 1971
154. Antimicrob Agents Chemother 3:526, 1973
155. N Engl J Med 302:1106, 1980
156. JAMA 244:1808, 1980
157. Mayo Clin Proc 56:556, 1981
158. J Infect Dis 134(suppl):S249, 1976
159. Am J Med 79(suppl 1A):1, 1985
160. Ann Intern Med 95:328, 1981
161. Antimicrob Agents Chemother 28:78, 1985
162. N Engl J Med 296:349, 1977
163. Am J Med 86:809, 1989
164. Antimicrob Agents Chemother 35:399, 1991
165. Clin Infect Dis 14:320, 1992
166. Arch Intern Med 138:793, 1978
167. N Engl J Med 298:758, 1978
168. Mayo Clin Proc 60:189, 1985
169. N Engl J Med 326:292, 1992
170. Med Lett Drugs Ther 27:1, 1985
171. J Fam Pract 31:265, 1990
172. Am J Med 92:61, 1992
173. Am J Med 92:249, 1992
174. Arch Intern Med 150:215, 1990
175. Med Lett Drugs Ther 34:45, 1992
176. Ann Intern Med 116:517, 1992
177. J Antimicrob Chemother 27(suppl A):1, 1991
178. J Antimicrob Chemother 27(suppl A):11, 1991
179. J Antimicrob Chemother 27(suppl A):43, 1991
180. J Antimicrob Chemother 27(suppl A):47, 1991
181. J Antimicrob Chemother 27(suppl A):67, 1991
182. J Antimicrob Chemother 27(suppl A):83, 1991
183. J Antimicrob Chemother 27(suppl A):109, 1991
184. Chest 100:1503, 1991
185. Am J Med 91(suppl 3A):3A-12S, 1991
186. Am J Med 91(suppl 3A):3A-5S, 1991
187. Am J Med 91(suppl 3A):3A-23S, 1991
188. Am J Med 91(suppl 3A):3A-27S, 1991
189. Am J Med 91(suppl 3A):3A-31S, 1991
190. Am J Med 91(suppl 3A):3A-36S, 1991
191. Am J Med 91(suppl 3A):3A-19S, 1991
192. Rev Infect Dis 4:1133, 1982
193. Rev Infect Dis 3:479, 1981
194. N Engl J Med 313:410, 1985
195. Antimicrob Agents Chemother 35:605, 1991
196. Med Lett Drugs Ther 28:121, 1986
197. J Infect Dis 164:1180, 1991
198. Arch Intern Med 150:2197, 1990
199. Ann Intern Med 94:343, 1981
200. Med Lett Drugs Ther 22:69, 1980
201. N Engl J Med 306:130, 1982
202. N Engl J Med 303:426, 1980
203. N Engl J Med 307:841, 1982
204. Rev Infect Dis 4:332, 1982
205. Ann Intern Med 100:881, 1984
206. Ann Intern Med 100:495, 1984
207. Med Lett Drugs Ther 23:13, 1981
208. N Engl J Med 303:1212, 1980
209. Ann Intern Med 93:585, 1980
210. Rev Infect Dis 13:1213, 1990
211. Mayo Clin Proc 63:147, 1988
212. Antimicrob Agents Chemother 28:581, 1985
213. Antimicrob Agents Chemother 28:716, 1985
214. Med Lett Drugs Ther 29:25, 1987
215. J Infect Dis 155:170, 1987
216. Arch Intern Med 152:1233, 1992
217. J Infect Dis 157:1221, 1988
218. Am J Med 80:884, 1986
219. Ann Intern Med 106:1, 1987
220. Am J Med 84:847, 1988
221. Ann Intern Med 115:7, 1991
222. Med Lett Drugs Ther 30:11, 1988
223. Rev Infect Dis 10:505, 1988
224. Rev Infect Dis 10:528, 1988
225. Ann Intern Med 106:7, 1987
226. J Infect Dis 157:1235, 1988
227. Rev Infect Dis 12:873, 1990
228. Ann Intern Med 114:195, 1991
229. Lancet 1:235, 1987
230. J Infect Dis 156:211, 1987
231. Am J Med 86:801, 1989
232. Ann Intern Med 114:986, 1991
233. J Bone Joint Surg 72-A:104, 1990
234. Am J Med 84:786, 1988
235. J Antimicrob Chemother 20:595, 1987
236. Antimicrob Agents Chemother 33:181, 1989
237. Med Lett Drugs Ther 33:75, 1991
238. Antimicrob Agents Chemother 35:256, 1991
239. Med Lett Drugs Ther 33:71, 1991
240. Clin Infect Dis 14:526, 1992
241. Clin Infect Dis 14:539, 1992
242. Am J Obstet Gynecol 164:1380, 1991
243. Antimicrob Agents Chemother 34:215, 1990
244. Antimicrob Agents Chemother 36:87, 1992
245. Met Lett Drugs Ther 34:58, 1992
246. Am J Med 92(suppl 4A):4A-26S, 1992
247. Am J Med 92(suppl 4A):4A-22S, 1992
248. Am J Med 92(suppl 4A):4A-58S, 1992
249. Am J Med 69:733, 1980
250. Ann Intern Med 92:62, 1980
251. Rev Infect Dis 2:1, 1980
252. Circulation 55:1, 1977
253. J Pediatr 118:736, 1991
254. JAMA 236:1053, 1976
255. JAMA 251:2381, 1984
256. N Engl J Med 291:597, 1974
257. JAMA 231:934, 1975
258. N Engl J Med 288:477, 1973
259. Lancet 2:837, 1977
260. Am J Med 66:248, 1979
261. N Engl J Med 304:1057, 1981
262. J Infect Dis 150:372, 1984
263. Ann Intern Med 106:7, 1987
264. N Engl J Med 326:281, 1992
265. Med Lett Drugs Ther 34:5, 1992
266. Am J Med 86:465, 1989
267. JAMA 254:2930, 1985

Acknowledgments

Figure 1 Janet Betries.

Table 4 Modified from a table in "Pharmacokinetics and Safety of Antimicrobial Agents during Pregnancy," by A.W. Chow and P.J. Jewesson, in *Reviews of Infectious Diseases* 7:287, 1985. © 1985 The University of Chicago Press. Used by permission.

Table 5 Modified from "The Choice of Antimicrobial Drugs," in *The Medical Letter on Drugs and Therapeutics* 32:41, 1990. Courtesy of The Medical Letter, Inc., New Rochelle, New York. Used by permission.

20 Infective Endocarditis

ADOLF W. KARCHMER, M.D.
MORTON N. SWARTZ, M.D.

Etiology and Epidemiology

Infective endocarditis is a microbial infection implanted on a heart valve or on the mural endocardium. Analogous infections called infective endaortitis and infective endarteritis occur on the endothelial surface of the aorta and large arteries. Although most such infections are caused by bacteria, the general term infective endocarditis is appropriate because endocarditis may also be caused by fungi, rickettsias, or chlamydiae.

Based on its clinical course, endocarditis has been classified as either subacute (duration of more than six weeks) or acute. Subacute endocarditis is commonly caused by relatively avirulent organisms, such as viridans streptococci, and develops on congenital or rheumatic endocardial lesions, whereas the acute form is caused by more aggressive pathogens that can establish infection in the absence of any gross underlying endocardial abnormality. From a clinical perspective, two other forms of endocarditis have been distinguished because they are unique and warrant individual consideration: prosthetic valve endocarditis and endocarditis associated with narcotic abuse. These two entities may present in either a subacute or an acute form.

Almost all species of bacteria have been implicated in cases of bacterial endocarditis (BE). The bacteriology of native valve endocarditis has changed strikingly since the advent of antimicrobial therapy. Before 1960, viridans streptococcus was the etiologic agent in 60 to 70 percent of all cases of BE, *Streptococcus pneumoniae* was responsible for eight to 12 percent of cases, and *Neisseria gonorrhoeae* was the agent in four to 10 percent of cases.[1,2] Since the 1970s, viridans and all other streptococci exclusive of enterococci have accounted for about 40 percent of cases and *S. pneumoniae* for one to five percent,

whereas *N. gonorrhoeae* endocarditis is rarely encountered.[2] Group A streptococci only rarely cause infective endocarditis. In contrast, staphylococci have become more frequent causes of endocarditis in the past three decades, particularly in hospitalized patients and drug addicts. In a compilation from several series published in the 1960s and 1970s, *Staphylococcus aureus* was the etiologic agent in 20 percent of cases and *S. epidermidis* in seven percent.[1-3] In some large urban centers, the incidence of *S. aureus* endocarditis is even higher. The enterococci currently account for 10 percent of cases of endocarditis.

The increased frequency of endocarditis from gram-negative bacilli can be attributed particularly to cases in drug addicts caused by *Pseudomonas aeruginosa*, *P. cepacia*, and *Serratia marcescens*.[4-6] Improvement in the laboratory techniques for isolating fastidious species such as *Hemophilus aphrophilus* and *Actinobacillus actinomycetemcomitans* has also contributed to a growing number of reports of gram-negative endocarditis. In addition, these fastidious species have emerged as important causes of prosthetic valve endocarditis.

The bacteriology of endocarditis associated with intravenous drug abuse tends to show a regional variability, probably related to contamination of narcotics or the shared use of injection equipment. For example, for a period, *Serratia* and *Candida* were prominent causes of addict-associated endocarditis in San Francisco, whereas elsewhere they were uncommon.[6]

Fungal endocarditis occurs in addicts; in patients who receive intravenous fluids, antibiotics, or hyperalimentation mixtures for prolonged periods; and in patients who have undergone open heart surgery. The fungal species involved differ from setting to setting. For example, *C. albicans* endocarditis occurs most frequently in patients who have received intravenous alimentation or undergone cardiac surgery, whereas *C. parapsilosis* and other nonalbicans candidal species are isolated most commonly from addicts with fungal endocarditis. *Aspergillus* endocarditis typically occurs in patients who have recently undergone cardiovascular surgery.[7]

About 10 percent of cases of endocarditis are reported as culture negative, but it is likely that this figure is exaggerated. Diagnostic and scientific advances will probably reduce the reported incidence of culture-negative endocarditis to five percent or less. Among these advances are better techniques for isolating bacterial species with relatively fastidious growth requirements, including anaerobes, capnophilic bacteria, and pyridoxal-requiring streptococci. Contributing to the trend toward more accurate reporting is the fact that nonbacterial causes of infective endocarditis have been recognized, including *Aspergillus*, *Histoplasma*, and other fungi that are difficult to isolate; rickettsias such as *Coxiella burnetii*; and chlamydiae such as *Chlamydia psittaci*. Better diagnosis of atrial myxoma, nonbacterial thrombotic endocarditis, and certain other conditions mimicking endocarditis has also helped to increase the accuracy of reporting.

Subacute Bacterial Endocarditis

The clinical course of endocarditis may provide a clue to the nature of the infecting organism as well as to prognosis. Subacute bacterial endocarditis (SBE), which has a duration of more than six weeks, may be caused by a variety of relatively avirulent bacteria. Commonly, the causative bacteria are members of the indigenous flora. These agents lack sufficient invasiveness to initiate infection on normal heart valves or endocardium but can establish a focus on deformed heart valves or at sites of congenital cardiac lesions. The most common agents are streptococcal species, including viridans streptococci, enterococci, nonhemolytic streptococci, β-hemolytic streptococci (other than group A streptococci), microaerophilic streptococci, and anaerobic streptococci. These organisms belong to

the normal flora and are found in the oral cavity and in the gastrointestinal and genitourinary tracts. Viridans streptococci are not a single species of bacteria but a loose grouping of strains sharing two properties: the capacity to produce an alpha reaction on blood agar and the lack of heat resistance and other properties associated with enterococci. Viridans streptococci are normally found in the gingival sulci, and they can transiently enter the bloodstream during dental manipulations.

The streptococci that cause endocarditis can be accurately categorized using Lancefield serogrouping. About 40 percent belong to group D, about 10 percent belong to group H (*S. sanguis*), and about 15 percent belong to other serogroups (including B, C, G, and K). About five percent are anaerobic streptococci, and the remaining 30 to 35 percent are nongroupable streptococci.

The enterococci, primarily *Enterococcus faecalis* and *E. faecium*, and the nonenterococcal group D streptococcus *S. bovis* are important causes of endocarditis. The enterococci, formerly classified as streptococcal species, bear a Lancefield group D surface antigen, as does *S. bovis*. The enterococci are relatively resistant to penicillin and require a combination of penicillin and an aminoglycoside for optimal treatment, whereas *S. bovis* is as susceptible as ordinary viridans streptococci to penicillin.[8] The portal of entry for *S. bovis* causing endocarditis or bacteremia is often a malignant or premalignant colonic lesion.[9] Enterococci are commonly found in the lower gastrointestinal tract, in the female genitourinary tract, and about the perineum; enterococci are also a cause of urinary tract infection in females and in males with prostatic obstruction. Bacteremia that arises at these sites, particularly after instrumentation, may be the source for endocarditis. Enterococcal endocarditis usually follows a subacute course, but at times, the picture may more closely resemble the acute disease, with accelerated local valve destruction and metastatic foci of infection.

Various other bacterial species produce SBE but much less frequently than streptococcal species. These species include fastidious small gram-negative bacilli such as *H. aphrophilus, A. actinomycetemcomitans, H. influenzae, H. parainfluenzae,* and *Cardiobacterium hominis,* all of which require special culture methods for isolation. If such culture methods are not employed, the diagnosis of culture-negative, or abacteremic, endocarditis may be made erroneously.[10-12] Occasionally, *S. epidermidis* is the etiologic agent of SBE. Most cases of *S. aureus* endocarditis are acute, but *S. aureus* may rarely cause SBE. Diphtheroid endocarditis is a rare disease, and in most cases, it is associated with prosthetic heart valves.[13] SBE may also be caused by *Erysipelothrix insidiosa,* the agent of erysipeloid. Very rare nonbacterial types of infective endocarditis produce a clinical picture of SBE. Q fever endocarditis, which is caused by *C. burnetii* and occurs in the setting of preexisting valvular disease, is one of the most indolent forms of infective endocarditis. The interval from original infection with *C. burnetii* to clinical signs of endocarditis often extends beyond a year.[14] Infective endocarditis from *C. psittaci* has occurred in several patients.[15]

Acute Bacterial Endocarditis

Acute bacterial endocarditis (ABE) is commonly caused by organisms that are more invasive than the agents of subacute bacterial endocarditis. The agents of acute bacterial endocarditis can attack normal heart valves and mural endocardium and establish suppurative foci at sites of embolic deposition. Such agents include *S. aureus,* the most frequent cause of ABE; *S. pneumoniae;* group A *Streptococcus; N. gonorrhoeae; Salmonella;* other members of the Enterobacteriaceae[16]; and *P. aeruginosa. Salmonella* organisms have also been implicated as a cause of infective endaortitis; they produce a continuous bacteremia in the absence of a cardiac murmur or apparent intracardiac focus.[17] Endocarditis from enteric gram-negative bacilli is distinctly uncommon and occurs less frequently than *Pseudomonas* endocarditis, which is seen mainly in intravenous drug abusers.

Pathogenesis

Subacute Bacterial Endocarditis

Previous damage to a heart valve, such as that in mitral insufficiency, or an abnormal hemodynamic situation produced by a congenital abnormality, such as a ventricular septal defect, appears to predispose to the development of SBE. Such defects give rise to a Venturi effect when blood is driven from a high-pressure area through an orifice into a low-pressure sink. This low-pressure sink appears to be the site of bacterial deposition. Platelets adhere to the abnormal valve or adjacent endocardium, and a fibrin clot forms in the area of the low-pressure sink.[18] During transient bacteremia, organisms adhere to the valve or mural endocardium or to the overlying fibrin-platelet aggregate. This sequence of events has been simulated in the rabbit model of endocarditis. First, a polyethylene catheter is placed in the heart to induce a sterile endocardial platelet-fibrin vegetation, and this vegetation is then infected with an intravenous injection of bacteria.[19] Large colonies of bacteria grow within the fibrin mesh, which appears to present an effective physical barrier against polymorphonuclear leukocytes.

Among the streptococci that most frequently cause SBE are four species: *S. mutans* and *S. mitior* (viridans streptococci), *S. sanguis* (group H), and *S. bovis* (group D). These organisms commonly produce extracellular dextrans, which may contribute to the pathogenesis of streptococcal endocarditis by helping the bacteria to stick to the heart valves.[20] In contrast, other streptococcal species that are not dextran producers cause endocarditis much less frequently. Those species frequently involved in endocarditis, such as enterococci, viridans streptococci, and *S. aureus,* show greater adherence to aortic valves in vitro than those species that rarely cause endocarditis, such as *Escherichia coli* and *Klebsiella pneumoniae.*[21]

SBE most commonly involves the left side of the heart and particularly affects insufficient valves. The mitral valve is more frequently involved than the aortic valve. A regurgitant jet stream through an incompetent aortic valve typically produces lesions on the ventricular aspect of the aortic valve and on the aortic leaflet of the mitral valve. Right-sided endocarditis, which involves the tricuspid valve more commonly than the pulmonary valve, is usually caused by pyogenic organisms and occurs most often in intravenous drug abusers. Aortic valves distorted by syphilis or calcareous aortic stenosis may also be susceptible to infection. Various congenital malformations predispose to endocarditis, including ventricular septal defect, bicuspid aortic valve, aortic stenosis, pulmonary stenosis, tetralogy of Fallot, complex cyanotic congenital heart disease, systemic to pulmonary artery shunts, patent ductus arteriosus, and coarctation of the aorta. An uncomplicated ostium secundum–type atrial septal defect is only rarely the site of endocarditis. Hypertrophic cardiomyopathy may predispose to endocarditis either on the aortic valve or on the anterior mitral valve leaflet. In two studies of endocarditis occurring after 1974, mitral valve prolapse, usually accompanied by mitral insufficiency, was the predisposing valvular abnormality in about 25 percent of cases.[22,23] Endocarditis can become engrafted on prosthetic heart valves of all types at the time of their placement or later during a transient bacteremia.

Acute Bacterial Endocarditis

ABE may develop on an entirely normal heart, or it may be engrafted on underlying acquired or congenital cardiac lesions. History or examination often reveals an antecedent pyogenic infection such as pneumococcal pneumonia or meningitis, staphylococcal abscesses, or furunculosis. Alternatively, predisposing factors such as intravenous drug abuse or nosocomial bacteremia secondary to intravenous alimentation may be uncovered.

Clinical Presentations

Subacute Bacterial Endocarditis

The symptoms of SBE usually begin insidiously, are nonspecific, and may persist for months. Feverishness, sweats, weakness, myalgias, arthralgias, malaise, and fatigability are prominent. Fewer than five percent of patients are afebrile, and such patients often have azotemia, which may quench the fever. Anorexia is almost universal; indeed, its absence should raise serious doubts about a diagnosis of SBE, unless it is very early in the course of the disease. Chilly sensations are not uncommon, but frank rigors are unusual. Occasionally, a patient with left-sided SBE has a nonproductive cough of sufficient prominence to suggest that the lung is the primary disease site. The mechanism of the cough is not clear, because it occurs in patients without pulmonary congestion, pneumonitis, a dilated pulmonary artery, or evidence of associated right-sided endocarditis. Whether small bronchial artery embolization is a factor is not known. The cough clears in one to two weeks after therapy is initiated.

An apparent portal of entry for the infection, such as recent dental extraction or scaling, cystoscopy, rectal surgery, or tonsillectomy, is suggested by the patient's history or is found on examination in about two thirds of patients with BE. The route of infection is identified more often in ABE than in SBE.[3]

Occasionally, the onset of SBE can be sharply defined. Indeed, because of greater awareness of this disease, the diagnosis is now made earlier than in the past; consequently, many of the classic features of SBE, such as clubbing and Osler's nodes, are not observed. Fever and nonspecific symptoms in the presence of a predisposing cardiac lesion may be the only manifestations in some patients with SBE. A variety of organs are commonly involved in endocarditis and may be the source of the patient's presenting symptoms. Thus, the diagnosis may be obscure either because only nonspecific symptoms are present or because symptoms arise primarily from an organ other than the heart. For example, if there are signs of meningitis, cerebral emboli, or glomerulonephritis, the physician's attention may be focused on the central nervous system or kidneys as the primary site of the illness.

Cutaneous Manifestations

Anemia is commonly present and produces pallor. Petechiae occur in the conjunctivas, in the oropharynx, and on the skin; they are particularly common on the extremities and may be present in large numbers on the lower extremities in particular. Petechiae may continue to appear for some weeks during successful antibiotic treatment, and under these circumstances, they do not indicate uncontrolled infection. Linear subungual splinter hemorrhages in the middle of the nail bed are a feature of SBE; those in the distal part of the nail bed are induced by trauma. Osler's nodes are tender, purplish, subcutaneous nodules that develop in the pulp of the fingers and disappear within several days. They occur in about five percent of patients with endocarditis. In acute endocarditis, Osler's nodes can be the result of microemboli; aspiration of the lesions may reveal the causative organism—for example, *S. aureus*. In SBE, it is still not clear whether the lesions are embolic in nature or are manifestations of an immunologically mediated small-vessel vasculitis.[24] Small, slightly nodular, nonpainful, erythematous or hemorrhagic areas on the palms or soles, called Janeway lesions, may occur in SBE or more commonly in ABE.

Musculoskeletal Features

Myalgias, arthralgias, arthritis, or low back pain occurs in 40 to 50 percent of patients with endocarditis, and in about half of these patients, such symptoms represent either initial or prominent manifestations of the disease.[25] Arthritis may be either monoarticular or polyarticular. Frank joint effusions occur, but such effusions are less common than the finding of painful, red, warm, tender joints. Septic arthritis may occur in ABE, but it is not a feature of SBE. Several findings suggest that immunologic processes may be involved in the genesis of articular symptoms: rheumatoid factor is present in 25 to 50 percent of patients with endocarditis of more than six weeks' duration, antinuclear antibody is found in some patients with infective endocarditis, and circulating immune complexes occur in more than 90 percent of patients with the disease.[26] As a result of earlier diagnosis and effective treatment, clubbing of the fingers is now seen in only 15 percent of patients who have SBE. Low back pain is a feature in about 10 percent of patients with endocarditis. It can be prominent enough to lead to a diagnosis of herniated intervertebral disk. During ABE, metastatic vertebral osteomyelitis associated with disk space infection occasionally is the cause of the back pain. All the musculoskeletal manifestations of SBE tend to disappear within the first one to two weeks of antimicrobial therapy.

Eye Findings

Petechial and flame-shaped hemorrhages occur in the retina of patients with endocarditis. Cotton-wool exudates, originally called cytoid bodies, develop in the fundus. Roth's spots are oval or boat-shaped white areas in the retina that are surrounded by a zone of hemorrhage[27]; small numbers of such lesions appear in about five percent of patients with bacterial endocarditis. Roth's spots are not pathognomonic of endocarditis and may be observed in patients with such disorders as severe anemia or collagen vascular diseases.

Endophthalmitis is an occasional complication of endocarditis caused by invasive organisms such as *S. pneumoniae*, enterococcus, or group B, C, or G streptococci. Unless endophthalmitis is promptly diagnosed and treated, it can result in blindness.

Splenomegaly

The spleen is palpably enlarged in about one third of patients with endocarditis; this finding is more common in SBE than in ABE. Rarely, a splenic abscess may be the cause of fever that persists after the endocarditis has been controlled by antibiotic therapy.

Renal Manifestations

Microscopic hematuria is observed in about 50 percent of patients with bacterial endocarditis. Four types of renal lesions occur.

Renal infarcts secondary to embolization Flank pain and hematuria are the clinical features of renal infarcts caused by embolization, and renal failure is uncommon.

Diffuse membranoproliferative glomerulonephritis The deposition of IgG, IgM, and complement in a granular or nodular, lumpy-bumpy fashion in the glomerular basement membrane indicates that the diffuse membranoproliferative glomerulonephritis associated with bacterial endocarditis is an immune complex nephritis.[28] Serum complement levels are reduced. Streptococcal bacterial antigen has been identified by indirect immunofluorescent techniques in glomerular deposits in the diffuse membranoproliferative glomerulonephritis of SBE.[29] The frequent occurrence of circulating immune complexes and rheumatoid factor in SBE supports the view that the renal lesion is an immune deposit disease. Diffuse membranoproliferative glomerulonephritis during endocarditis may cause severe renal failure, which generally improves after treatment of the infection.[18,29]

Focal embolic glomerulonephritis It was originally thought that focal glomerular lesions in so-called embolic glomerulonephritis resulted from small bacterial emboli that destroyed segments of glomerular loops. This condition is now considered an additional form of immune complex disease and is occasionally associated with renal failure.

Renal abscesses Renal abscesses occur in cases of ABE caused by a pyogen such as *S. aureus.* The renal infection develops either from septic embolization or from localization of organisms that are being spread by the continuous bacteremia characteristic of endocarditis. Such an abscess may cause continuing fever in ABE even after the valvular infection has been controlled by antibiotic therapy.

Thromboembolic Phenomena

Significant embolic episodes occur in about one third of patients with endocarditis. A cerebral embolus (see below) producing neurologic signs, including hemiparesis, monoplegia, and aphasia in an elderly person, may be diagnosed as a stroke unless careful attention is paid to the presence of low-grade fever, anemia, heart murmur, and a history of antecedent illness. Sudden monocular blindness may be produced by emboli in the central retinal artery. Mesenteric emboli may produce acute abdominal pain, ileus, and melena. Emboli in the spleen, with or without abscess formation, produce left upper quadrant abdominal pain with radiation to the left shoulder; pleuritic chest pain and a splenic friction rub may be present, and a small pleural effusion may develop. Peripheral emboli may produce pain in the digits or gangrene of the extremities. Emboli that occlude large arteries suggest fungal endocarditis, marantic endocarditis, left atrial myxoma, or, occasionally, *S. aureus* endocarditis. Septic infarction is not a feature of SBE because of the bland nature of the infecting organisms, but it is a feature of ABE, in which the etiologic agents are usually highly invasive and capable of abscess formation.

Pulmonary emboli occur in right-sided endocarditis and frequently cause pulmonary infarcts and pneumonia. Invasive organisms such as *S. aureus* and *P. aeruginosa* produce septic emboli that may be associated with lung abscess, empyema, and pyopneumothorax. The prominence of the pulmonary manifestations may misdirect attention initially to the lung as the primary site of infection and lead to an incorrect diagnosis of pneumonia. Coronary emboli, which can be sterile in SBE and sterile or septic in ABE, are found in as many as 50 percent of autopsied patients.[18] Coronary emboli are seldom suspected based on clinical findings, but occasionally, they result in frank myocardial infarction.

Mycotic Aneurysms

Peripheral mycotic aneurysms in SBE may result from embolic occlusion of the vasa vasorum or from deposition of immune complexes in the arterial wall.[18] In

ABE, an aneurysm may result from direct bacterial invasion of the arterial wall. In SBE, an aneurysm can develop during the active stage of infection but may not become evident for months after the valvular infection has been eradicated; at this point, the aneurysm is sterile.

Aneurysms may form in any artery. Palpation of brachial, external iliac, and popliteal arteries and auscultation for abdominal bruits should be a routine part of both the initial examination of patients suspected of having endocarditis and the final examination at completion of antibiotic therapy. The clinical features include pain, a pulsatile mass, evidence of pressure on adjacent structures, or the sudden development of an expanding hematoma or signs of major blood loss. Surgical excision to prevent rupture is usually indicated for accessible aneurysms of significant size.

Neurologic Manifestations

Neurologic complications develop in 30 to 40 percent of patients with endocarditis. Cerebral embolism is the most frequent complication, occurring in about 15 percent of patients.[30] Emboli most commonly obstruct the middle cerebral artery or one of its branches, producing a contralateral hemiparesis and hemisensory deficit. Bacteria are rarely found in the occluded vessel or surrounding tissue. Cerebral embolism may be the initial manifestation of endocarditis. It may also appear during the course of treatment, and in such cases, it does not necessarily indicate failure of the therapeutic program. Cerebral emboli are most common in patients with mitral valve infection and in patients with ABE.[30] In addition to patients who have emboli to major cerebral arteries, there are a smaller number of patients who have multiple microscopic embolic infarcts. Such microinfarcts are manifested by an altered level of consciousness, seizures, fluctuating focal neurologic signs, or a combination of these symptoms.

Cerebral mycotic aneurysms occur in two to 10 percent of patients with BE. They may become clinically apparent as a sudden cerebral or subarachnoid hemorrhage or as an embolic stroke followed by an intracerebral hemorrhage. A persistent focal headache may signal the presence of an aneurysm before rupture.[31] Aneurysms occur more frequently in ABE than in SBE. Treatment of a mycotic aneurysm that has been defined by angiography depends on its location, the presence or absence of hemorrhage, and the clinical course. Healing of mycotic aneurysms during the treatment of endocarditis has been demonstrated by angiography.[32] A leaking aneurysm, however, should be removed surgically, provided it is accessible.

Macroscopic brain abscess is very uncommon in BE. In ABE, usually in cases caused by *S. aureus*, septic emboli may give rise to multiple small abscesses, but surgery is not indicated because of their small size, their multiplicity, and their response to antimicrobial therapy.

Seizures, which are usually triggered by emboli, and toxic encephalopathy are other cerebral complications of endocarditis. A cerebrospinal fluid pleocytosis is observed in some patients. Some patients have meningitis with a purulent CSF profile; the infecting agent is usually a pyogenic organism and not a viridans streptococcus. Other patients have nuchal rigidity and an aseptic CSF profile, both of which result from embolic cerebral infarction without bacterial meningitis.

Cardiac Findings

The cardiac features in SBE are those of the underlying valvular or congenital lesion. Murmurs are present in more than 90 percent of patients with SBE, but at least one third of patients with ABE have no murmur. The murmur may be minor in intensity and may be characterized mistakenly as functional or innocent, particularly in elderly patients who have some degree of calcareous aortic disease. Changing murmurs are not common in SBE, but they can occur in ABE, in which they represent a major diagnostic finding. Mild changes in the intensity of a murmur, particularly a systolic murmur, are associated with the development of anemia, high fever, or tachycardia and are often of little significance. The appearance of a new aortic diastolic murmur suggests dilatation of the aortic anulus or eversion or fenestration of an aortic leaflet. The sudden onset of a loud mitral pansystolic murmur with a midsystolic peak suggests rupture of a chorda tendinea.

Acute Bacterial Endocarditis

The onset of ABE is usually abrupt, and rigors are common. Temperatures reach 39.4° to 40.6° C (102.9° to 105.1° F) and are often remittent in patients with ABE, and the illness is rapidly progressive. Cutaneous manifestations, particularly petechiae, may be prominent, especially when *S. aureus* is the agent. Occasionally, the clinical features in a patient with acute *S. aureus* endocarditis mimic those of acute meningococcemia on several counts: grossly similar skin lesions, including petechiae, purpura, and focal gangrene; similar hematologic changes, including disseminated intravascular coagulation; and the common neurologic findings of nuchal rigidity and CSF pleocytosis.[33] A Gram's stain of the CSF, however, does not reveal organisms in patients whose meningeal signs and pleocytosis are caused by embolic cerebral infarction or microabscesses rather than by staphylococcal meningitis.

Careful examination of the skin lesions may provide the correct diagnosis and prevent institution of inappropriate antibiotic therapy during the first 24 hours. Pustular petechiae or purulent purpura should strongly suggest *S. aureus* bacteremia, particularly that associated with endocarditis, rather than meningococcemia. A Gram's stain and culture of the aspirate from a skin lesion are imperative because they can promptly reveal the etiologic agent.

Embolic manifestations, especially in the central nervous system and kidneys, are common in ABE. Metastatic infections in the bones, kidneys, brain, and lungs may arise from either septic embolization or the sustained bacteremia. Osler's nodes occur but less often than in SBE. Janeway lesions occur on the palms and soles of five to 10 percent of patients who have *S. aureus* endocarditis.

Acute bacterial endocarditis may be present even if the patient does not have a cardiac murmur. The sudden appearance—within days of the onset of illness—of a new murmur, particularly a murmur characteristic of valvular insufficiency, strongly suggests valve destruction and confirms the diagnosis of ABE. Valve damage can lead to severe congestive heart failure and necessitates prompt valve replacement.

Endocarditis Associated with Drug Abuse

The annual incidence of endocarditis among intravenous drug abusers is estimated at between 0.2 and two percent. At the time of their initial attack of endocarditis, 70 to 80 percent of drug addicts have no history or findings of preexisting valvular heart disease. It has been suggested that repeated intravenous injections of particulate foreign material predispose to the development of endocarditis by initiating microscopic endocardial injury and platelet thrombi, on which circulating organisms become engrafted. This hypothesis seems more applicable to right-sided endocarditis than to left-sided endocarditis. Indeed, in drug addicts, the tricuspid valve is the site of infection more frequently (55 percent) than the aortic valve (35 percent) or mitral valve (30 percent).[34] These findings contrast markedly with the rarity of right-sided involvement in cases of infective endocarditis that are not associated with drug abuse.[2] Frequent transient bacteremias combined with valvular damage that resulted from the prior endocarditis give rise to the development of multiple episodes of endocarditis among intravenous drug abusers.

The data from 11 reported series of addict-associated endocarditis indicate that *S. aureus* is responsible for approximately 50 percent of cases [*see Table 1*].[33] Although polymicrobial endocarditis, such as simultaneous infection by *P. aeruginosa* and *S. aureus*, is extremely rare among nonaddicts with native valve endocarditis, it accounts for five percent of cases of endocarditis in addicts. Certain organisms have a predilection for particular valves in cases of addict-associated endocarditis: enterococci and other streptococcal species predominantly involve the mitral and aortic valves, *S. aureus* infects the tricuspid valve in 80 percent of cases, and *Candida* organisms predominantly affect the valves of the left side of the heart. *Pseudomonas* organisms are associated with biventricular and multiple valve infection in addicts.[35]

Regional differences have been noted in the bacteriology of addict-associated endocarditis, but the reasons for this variation are not clear. *Serratia* endocarditis cases were clustered in San Francisco in the 1970s,[6] and *P. aeruginosa* was an important cause of endocarditis in Detroit and Chicago in the 1980s.[35,36] Methicillin-resistant *S. aureus* organisms were responsible for almost half of the cases of addict-associated staphylococcal endocarditis in Detroit in the mid-1980s. Endocarditis caused by these methicillin-resistant *S. aureus* organisms is associated with self-administration of nonprescribed antibiotics and is now being encountered widely in the United States. In both Chicago and Detroit, the *P. aeruginosa* strains that cause endocarditis have belonged predominantly to the serotype O-11, and infection with this organism has been significantly correlated with abuse of pentazocine and tripelennamine (T's and blues).[35]

Although the manifestations of endocarditis in addicts are generally similar to those in nonaddicts, there are noteworthy differences caused by variations in the frequency of tricuspid involvement and the nature of the infecting organisms in the two groups. Fever (often accompanied by chills), malaise, cough, and pleuritic chest pain are the most common presenting complaints in right-sided endocarditis of addicts. Septic pulmonary emboli occur in about 75 percent of cases, particularly those with *S. aureus* infection, and cause sputum production, hemoptysis, and initial radiologic findings that may suggest pneumonia. Cavitation of embolic pulmonary lesions is common. Significant cardiac murmurs are heard in most patients at some time during their illness,

Table 1   Etiology of Addict-Associated Endocarditis

Causative Organism	Cases (%)
Staphylococcus aureus	54
Streptococci (other than enterococci)	10
Enterococci	11
Gram-negative bacilli (e.g., *Pseudomonas, Serratia,* and *Enterobacter* species)	6
Fungi (primarily *Candida* species)	6
Polymicrobial	5
Culture negative	6
Miscellaneous	2

Note: see reference 33.

but the murmurs may not be detected on initial examination. The auscultatory sign of tricuspid involvement—a short ejection systolic murmur that is louder on inspiration—may be difficult to detect. Frank tricuspid insufficiency is manifested by large V waves in the neck veins and a pulsating liver.

Because *S. aureus* and other pyogenic bacteria are the predominant causes of infective endocarditis in addicts, metastatic infections are common. Peripheral emboli are observed frequently, and neurologic manifestations are common. Large peripheral emboli that occlude major vessels have been observed not only in fungal endocarditis but also as a complication of mural endocarditis of the left atrium caused by *P. aeruginosa*.[4]

Blood cultures generally reveal the causative organism in addict-associated endocarditis, even when the involvement is exclusively on the right side.

Prosthetic Valve Endocarditis

Infection involving mechanical prosthetic valves and porcine bioprosthetic valves accounts for a significant percentage of the cases of endocarditis. The cumulative incidence of prosthetic valve endocarditis (PVE) is estimated at three percent at one year after valve implantation and at four to 5.5 percent at four years after surgery.[37,38] A prosthetic valve remains at risk for infection throughout the life of the patient. The overall risk of infection is similar for mechanical and bioprosthetic valves and for aortic and mitral valve prostheses.[38]

Prosthetic valve endocarditis is conveniently subdivided into two categories: early prosthetic valve endocarditis (EPVE), which becomes clinically manifest within 60 days after valve replacement, and late prosthetic valve endocarditis (LPVE), which is manifested clinically more than 60 days after valve replacement. EPVE is usually a consequence of intraoperative contamination, particularly from the extracorporeal bypass unit, or the result of a septic complication of surgery, such as sternotomy wound infection, pneumonia, urinary tract infection, or infection about intravenous catheters. In contrast, the predisposing factors in LPVE are usually dental procedures, genitourinary tract manipulations, or other incidental septic events identical to those producing the transient bacteremias that are incriminated in the genesis of conventional SBE.[39] Patients with coagulase-negative staphylococcal (usually *S. epidermidis*) PVE that develops between the second and 12th months after surgery were probably infected perioperatively but have a delayed onset of symptoms.[38] An indolent form of nosocomially acquired PVE caused by *Legionella pneumophila* or *L. dumoffii* has also occurred months after prosthetic valve placement.[40]

In cases of EPVE that occurred before 1975, the principal agents were staphylococci, *Candida*, gram-negative bacilli (Enterobacteriaceae and *Pseudomonas* species), and diphtheroids (also referred to as *Corynebacterium* species).[41] This spectrum reflected the hypothesized pathogenic circumstances. In contrast, the bacteriology of LPVE resembled that of conventional endocarditis. Before 1975, streptococci, including the enterococci, accounted for about 36 percent of cases of LPVE, whereas they were found in only about 10 percent of cases of EPVE [see Table 2].

Since 1975, *S. aureus*, fungi, and gram-negative bacilli have been implicated less frequently as causes of EPVE; the predominant organism isolated from cases with an onset during the initial two months and throughout the first year after surgery has been the coagulase-negative staphylococcus. Although coagulase-negative staphylococci are still significant causes of PVE that has an onset a year or more after surgery, 64 percent of such cases are caused by *S. aureus*, streptococci (including enterococci), and fastidious gram-negative coccobacilli (organisms frequently associated with native valve endocarditis) [*see Table 2*].[38] Coagulase-negative staphylococci, which rarely cause native valve endocarditis, are responsible for 25 to 45 percent of cases of PVE and therefore cannot be dismissed as contaminants when they are isolated from a patient with a prosthetic valve.

Infection of prosthetic valves is often associated with valvular dysfunction and pathological changes that cannot be corrected by antibiotic therapy alone. In native valve endocarditis, the infection is commonly restricted to the valve leaflet, but infection engrafted on prosthetic valves often invades perivalvular tissues.[42] Necrosis of the anulus because of invasive infection causes partial dehiscence of the prosthesis and hemodynamically significant valvular regurgitation. Deeper invasion leads to myocardial abscess. Infection of porcine and mechanical prosthetic valves is associated with invasion and destructive changes, particularly when valves at the aortic position are infected and when onset occurs during the first postoperative year.[38,43] Occasionally, vegetations may partially obstruct the valve orifice or restrict valve movement, causing functional stenosis. Such changes are more likely to occur when a mitral, rather than an aortic, prosthesis is infected.[42] When infection is restricted to the leaflets of a porcine bioprosthetic valve, abnormalities such as leaflet fenestration or destruction, the development of obstructing vegetations, or the delayed onset of leaflet stiffness may cause clinically significant valvular dysfunction.

The clinical features of EPVE differ from those of LPVE.[39,44] Although EPVE may be

Table 2   Etiology of Prosthetic Valve Endocarditis

Causative Organism	Onset after Surgery (Cases before 1975)		Onset after Surgery (Cases 1975–1982)		
	< 2 months	≥ 2 months	< 2 months	2–12 months	>12 months
Coagulase-negative staphylococci	41	36	22	19	10
Gram-negative bacilli	30	19[*]	2	1	1
Diphtheroids	12	6	4	0	1
Fungi	18	9	2	2	1
Staphylococcus aureus	30	22	2	3	5
Streptococci (other than enterococci)	9	41	0	1	12
Pneumococci	2	0	0	0	0
Enterococci	6	14	0	2	4
Fastidious gram-negative coccobacilli	—	—	0	1	7
Polymicrobial	—	—	3	2	1
Culture negative	3	7	3	3	2
Total cases	151	154	38	34	44

Note: based on data from references 38 and 41.

*Includes fastidious gram-negative coccobacilli.

initially obscured by coexisting postoperative infectious complications, the disease is generally rapidly progressive. Fever, a prosthetic regurgitant murmur, and prosthetic valve dysfunction with resulting congestive heart failure strongly suggest the diagnosis. Valve dysfunction may be manifested by a new or changing murmur related to valve incompetence or by a muffling of the opening or closing of the prosthesis. The latter is a consequence of vegetations that restrict valve motion.

Unexplained fever during the postoperative period may be the only initial manifestation of EPVE. Frequent blood cultures are the only means of making the diagnosis. Some febrile patients who manifest no signs of endocarditis after valve replacement experience a transient gram-negative bacillus bacteremia from an extracardiac source, but EPVE does not develop. In other patients, however, the bacteremia is sustained even after the extracardiac focus of infection has been eradicated, and endocarditis is undoubtedly present. Such patients should be considered to have EPVE and should be treated accordingly. Patients who have sustained gram-negative bacillus bacteremia with no identifiable extracardiac source should also be considered to have EPVE, regardless of whether a new regurgitant murmur or other signs of endocarditis are present.[44]

Petechiae occur in about half of patients with EPVE, but Roth's spots, Osler's nodes, Janeway lesions, and other peripheral signs of endocarditis are observed less frequently than in LPVE or native valve endocarditis. Conjunctival petechiae are common findings for several days immediately after surgery in patients who have been on cardiopulmonary bypass, and their presence at that time does not indicate EPVE. Emboli are common in EPVE. Emboli that occlude large peripheral arteries suggest fungal endocarditis. This diagnosis, particularly in cases of *Aspergillus* endocarditis, must be based on histologic examination or culture of the clot recovered at embolectomy because blood cultures seldom reveal the organism.

The clinical features of LPVE are quite similar to those of native valve endocarditis. The onset is often gradual and marked by fever, malaise, fatigue, and anorexia. The course is typically indolent and more slowly progressive than that of EPVE. However, patients with LPVE from an invasive organism such as *S. aureus* or group A *Streptococcus* have an acute illness with a rapidly progressive course. Splenomegaly, petechiae, Roth's spots, Janeway lesions, and Osler's nodes occur as frequently in LPVE as in native valve endocarditis.

Special Diagnostic and Therapeutic Considerations

The diagnosis of PVE is based on clinical findings and the demonstration of a continuous bacteremia. Cultures are negative in two to five percent of cases. Negative cultures are usually caused by prior antibiotic therapy or the presence of an infecting organism that is difficult or slow to isolate, such as *Aspergillus* and other fungi. PVE caused by *Candida* organisms, diphtheroids, or fastidious gram-negative coccobacilli (*Actinobacillus*, *Cardiobacterium*, and *Hemophilus* species) is usually associated with positive blood cultures. Because these organisms grow slowly, however, their isolation may require prolonged incubation of cultures (i.e., 14 to 21 days). Routine blood cultures from patients with PVE caused by *Legionella* species are also negative. However, *Legionella* species can be recovered from the blood of infected patients using specialized techniques. For example, these organisms can generally be isolated if either an aliquot from an aerobic blood culture flask that has been incubated for 24 hours or a pellet from a lysis-centrifugation culture tube is cultured on buffered charcoal–yeast extract agar. The diagnosis can also be made by culturing the endocarditic vegetation on this special agar. Finally, the diagnosis is suggested by high titers of antibody to *L. pneumophila* in the serum of patients who have clinical signs of PVE but negative blood cultures and who would not otherwise be expected to have antibody to this organism.[40]

Prosthetic valve dysfunction, identified by auscultatory findings or noninvasive tests, strongly supports a suspected diagnosis of PVE. New ECG changes indicative of conduction disturbances suggest extension of a ring abscess into the septum, with involvement of the conduction system. Although large vegetations on prosthetic valves can occasionally be imaged by M mode or transthoracic two-dimensional echocardiography, these studies have limited usefulness because the prosthesis itself produces echoes that obscure the vegetations. Indirect evidence of prosthetic valve dysfunction, such as fluttering of the anterior mitral valve leaflet or mitral valve preclosure indicative of aortic regurgitation, may be demonstrable. Doppler echocardiography, which allows noninvasive assessment of blood flow and pressure across valves, may be extremely useful in the serial evaluation of the function of infected prosthetic valves. As compared with transthoracic echocardiography, transesophageal two-dimensional and Doppler echocardiography more effectively assess the prosthetic valve and perivalvular tissue, especially when a mitral valve prosthesis is present. Among 22 patients with PVE, the transesophageal technique identified definite or probable vegetations in 86 percent of patients, compared with a 36 percent identification rate using transthoracic echocardiography.[45] Acoustic shadowing produced by mitral prosthetic valves is less of a limitation for transesophageal Doppler evaluation of mitral valve function than for transthoracic Doppler assessment. Consequently, transesophageal echocardiography is the procedure of choice for investigating suspected mitral PVE.[46]

The same general principles that govern antimicrobial therapy for BE [*see* Treatment, *below*] are employed in the treatment of PVE. Occasionally, PVE is treated for longer periods than native valve BE caused by similar organisms. Follow-up therapy with orally administered antibiotics for several months is not recommended routinely. Occasionally, a patient who experiences a relapse of PVE and who cannot or will not undergo a second or third valve replacement will have to be managed by another course of parenteral antimicrobial treatment followed by months to years of suppressive therapy with oral antibiotics. The patients most likely to be cured by antibiotic therapy are those who have LPVE from highly sensitive organisms such as streptococcal species or fastidious gram-negative coccobacilli and no evidence of valve dysfunction or invasive infection.

Early aggressive surgical treatment is an essential element of therapy in selected patients with PVE. Surgery is necessary for those patients who have invasive perivalvular infection, prosthesis dysfunction causing congestive heart failure, or PVE caused by an antibiotic-resistant organism. Surgical intervention is indicated in 45 percent of patients with PVE [*see* Treatment, Surgical Intervention, *below*]. When surgery is required, the optimal results are obtained when the operation is performed early rather than as a last heroic effort.[47,48]

The use of antithrombotic therapy in the management of PVE was evaluated by a national conference sponsored by the American College of Chest Physicians and the National Heart, Lung and Blood Institute that issued its recommendations in 1986 [see Treatment, Antithrombotic Therapy, *below*].[49]

Diagnosis

Laboratory Findings

The leukocyte count in subacute bacterial endocarditis is usually normal, whereas a leukocytosis is commonly present in acute bacterial endocarditis. Normocytic normochromic anemia is often present in subacute bacterial endocarditis.

The erythrocyte sedimentation rate is elevated in almost all patients with endocarditis except those with congestive heart failure. Immunoglobulin abnormalities are frequent in infective endocarditis. Rheumatoid factor is found in 50 percent of patients with endocarditis of more than six weeks' duration; it disappears after successful treatment. Circulating immune complexes have been demonstrated in more than 90 percent of patients with infective endocarditis.[26] Hyperglobulinemia is common when the illness is prolonged. Occasionally, there have been reports of patients with IgG or IgM M components in their serum.[50] Serum complement levels are low in some patients, particularly when endocarditis is complicated by immune complex glomerulonephritis.

Renal abnormalities are common, and most patients have proteinuria and microscopic hematuria. Elevated levels of creatinine accompany the development of extensive immune deposit glomerulonephritis. The occasional occurrence of drug-induced interstitial nephritis during treatment with a penicillin must be distinguished from the complicating nephropathy associated with infective endocarditis.

In most patients with SBE, all blood cultures taken before initiation of antibiotic therapy are positive, reflecting the sustained bacteremia associated with an infected endothelial surface. Four to six sets of cultures taken before the start of therapy are adequate for demonstrating the bacteremia. Cultures should be taken in both aerobic and anaerobic media and should be incubated in five to 10 percent carbon dioxide; this procedure allows isolation of anaerobic organisms, particularly peptostreptococci, and strains whose growth is enhanced in the presence of added carbon dioxide, such as capnophilic streptococci, *H. aphrophilus*, and *A. actinomycetemcomitans*. Isolation of the etiologic agent on blood culture may be delayed or prevented by prior antimicrobial therapy (up to 10 days previously) even if the drug and dose employed represent inadequate treatment of the disease. Blood cultures may also be negative in cases of right-sided endocarditis caused by relatively noninvasive organisms. At present, however, most cases of right-sided endocarditis occur among intravenous drug abusers and are caused by pyogenic bacteria, such as

S. aureus and *P. aeruginosa*, which are readily isolated from the blood. Because venous blood cultures demonstrate the bacteremia as readily as arterial blood cultures, the latter are unnecessary. Bone marrow cultures usually do not provide more information than can be obtained from blood cultures.

Several additional factors can thwart isolation of the infecting agent from blood and lead to a diagnosis of apparent culture-negative infective endocarditis: the fastidious growth requirements of *Hemophilus*, *Legionella*, and *Brucella* species, diphtheroids, strict anaerobes, and other bacteria; the particular properties of certain fungal organisms such as *H. capsulatum* and *Aspergillus* that make them difficult to isolate; and the nonbacterial and nonmycotic nature of etiologic agents such as *C. burnetii* and *C. psittaci*. Endocarditis caused by *Legionella*, *C. psittaci*, and *C. burnetii* can be diagnosed by serologic tests.

Differential Diagnosis

The differential diagnosis of infective endocarditis is straightforward in the patient who manifests the full panoply of fever, heart murmurs, petechiae, anemia, microscopic hematuria, and splenomegaly; however, the physician must be alert to atypical cases in which the most prominent clinical findings are in organs other than the heart. Such cases include cerebrovascular accident (embolic stroke) in an elderly patient whose low-grade fever is attributed to the stroke; meningitis (CSF pleocytosis and stiff neck), as a result of either true meningeal infection or bland embolic infarction in silent areas of the brain; unexplained renal insufficiency from immune complex glomerulonephritis; musculoskeletal disease that suggests such diagnoses as polymyalgia rheumatica, vertebral osteomyelitis, and disk space infection; apparent pneumonia that is actually septic pulmonary infarcts accompanying acute right-sided *S. aureus* endocarditis; and fever of undetermined origin in which the peripheral stigmata of endocarditis may be minimal and a heart murmur is misinterpreted as functional.

> ### *Table 3*   Clinical Mimics of Infective Endocarditis
>
> Acute rheumatic fever with carditis
>
> Nonbacterial thrombotic (marantic) endocarditis
>
> Collagen vascular diseases (SLE with cardiac involvement; systemic vasculitis)
>
> Atrial myxoma
>
> Organizing left atrial thrombus
>
> Certain neoplastic diseases (hypernephroma, carcinoid)
>
> Postpericardiotomy and postperfusion (cytomegalovirus infection) syndromes in patients who have recently undergone valve replacement

The diagnosis of infective endocarditis must be considered in any patient with a heart murmur and fever. In contrast to younger patients, elderly patients (i.e., those older than 60 years) with endocarditis are less likely to report fever and are more likely to present with confusion as a prominent symptom and to have acquired the infection nosocomially. The manifestations of endocarditis in the elderly may be so muted that the diagnosis is not suspected. In fact, in more than 60 percent of elderly patients who are subsequently determined to have endocarditis, the initial diagnosis was incorrect.[51]

A variety of noninfectious illnesses can mimic infective endocarditis [*see Table 3*]. Acute rheumatic fever sometimes resembles ABE because it can cause fever, cardiac murmurs, and congestive failure, but acute rheumatic fever can be distinguished on clinical grounds and by blood cultures, anti–streptolysin O antibody titer, and response to salicylates. Rarely, recurrence of acute rheumatic fever may coincide with BE. Marantic endocarditis is usually associated with underlying neoplasm or wasting disease but occasionally complicates acute illness. Marantic endocarditis may resemble infective endocarditis because it also can give rise to multiple embolic episodes. The presence of fever, anemia, and renal involvement in polyarteritis nodosa may suggest a diagnosis of subacute bacterial endocarditis, and the findings on biopsy of a lesion of a large artery may even resemble those of a mycotic aneurysm.

A cardiac myxoma, usually in the left atrium, may mimic infective endocarditis in both clinical and laboratory features. Such manifestations of endocarditis as low-grade fever, weight loss, arthralgias, cutaneous lesions (petechiae, Osler's nodes, Janeway lesions), clubbing of the fingers, emboli to major arteries, and the auscultatory findings of mitral stenosis and regurgitation can also occur in patients with a cardiac myxoma.[52] Cardiac myxoma syndrome may further parallel infective endocarditis by giving rise to cerebral aneurysms at the sites of myxomatous emboli. Increased sedimentation rate, anemia, and hyperglobulinemia are seen in both diseases. Negative blood cultures, changes of murmurs with position, the presence of large-vessel emboli, and absence of splenomegaly are more suggestive of an atrial myxoma than of endocarditis. Echocardiography and angiocardiography can help establish the diagnosis.

Other neoplasms may mimic infective endocarditis by induction of marantic endocarditis or by their hemodynamic effects. For example, a richly vascular hypernephroma may be associated with cardiomegaly, a flow murmur, anemia, and fever. The renal mass may be mistaken for the spleen. Carcinoid tumors occasionally mimic endocarditis when they produce endocardial and valvular fibrosis that leads to tricuspid insufficiency and pulmonary stenosis.

Fever that develops in a patient after valve replacement surgery raises the question of prosthetic valve endocarditis, and blood cultures are essential for diagnosis. Cytomegalovirus infection acquired on exposure to blood during bypass pump perfusion or through postoperative transfusions may mimic endocarditis because it can produce fever and splenomegaly. However, in patients infected with cytomegalovirus, prosthesis function is normal, liver function abnormalities are often present, and atypical lymphocytes appear in the blood. This diagnosis is confirmed by recovering cytomega-

lovirus in viral cultures of peripheral blood white cells (buffy coat).

Cardiac Complications of Endocarditis

Congestive heart failure is the most frequent cardiac complication of infective endocarditis. Aortic valve infection causes more serious hemodynamic consequences than mitral valve infection [*see Table 4*], probably because of the effect of the high aortic diastolic pressure on the weakened or fenestrated valve. A mycotic aneurysm of a sinus of Valsalva or an aortic ring abscess may rupture through the membranous septum into the right atrium or ventricle. Such rupture causes a sudden rise in the jugular venous pressure and a to-and-fro murmur and thrill along the left sternal border; the lungs remain relatively clear. The murmur produced by rupture into the right atrium is heard closer to the right sternal border. Valvular damage and subsequent dysfunction, as well as intracardiac fistula formation, can be accurately defined by use of two-dimensional and Doppler echocardiography from a transthoracic or transesophageal approach.

Conduction abnormalities are complications of BE that are important to recognize because they may signal the extension of valvular infection to the septum and its major conduction tissues. In one group of 142 adults with BE,[53] first-, second-, or third-degree AV block occurred in 14 percent of patients. The aortic valve was involved in 90 percent of the patients with heart block. In patients with complete heart block who were examined at autopsy or at surgery, the infection was found to have extended to the AV node or bundle of His and to adjacent structures, resulting in cardioaortic fistulas. The proximity of the right cusp and the noncoronary cusp of the aortic valve to the conduction system accounts for the development of complicating conduction abnormalities. Similarly, extension of infection from the mitral anulus, which is close to the bundle of His and to the AV node, may also produce conduction defects, but such extension occurs less frequently than from the aortic

Table 4　Intracardiac Complications of Infective Endocarditis

Aortic Valve

Anatomic changes producing valvular dysfunction and cardiac decompensation

- Fenestration of valve cusp
- Eversion (occurring even after bacteriologic cure) or disintegration of cusps or commissural detachment by microbial vegetations
- Mycotic aneurysm of sinus of Valsalva
    - Extension through the membranous septum, producing a right-sided vegetation and right-sided endocarditis
    - Rupture through the membranous portion of the septum, producing a left-to-right shunt (left ventricular to right atrial; less commonly, a ventricular septal defect)
- Valve obstruction by vegetation (fungal endocarditis)
- Valve ring abscess
    - With extension to aortic-mitral intervalvular fibrosa with secondary formation of a mycotic aneurysm of the left ventricle
    - Extension into epicardium, producing pericarditis
    - Extension into the area of the AV node or bundle, producing a variety of conduction defects (first-degree, second-degree, or complete heart block)

Mitral Valve

Anatomic changes producing valvular dysfunction and cardiac decompensation

- Perforation of leaflet
- Mycotic aneurysm of leaflet
- Disruption or disintegration of leaflet
- Valve obstruction by vegetation (fungal endocarditis)
- Rupture of chordae tendineae, producing a flail leaflet
- Burrowing abscess of valve anulus
    - Rarely, extension into area of AV node or bundle, producing conduction defects
- Papillary muscle rupture (rare occurrence; either the result of a myocardial infarct on which endocarditis has been engrafted or the result of an infarct secondary to a coronary embolus complicating endocarditis)

Coronary Arteries

Myocardial dysfunction caused by coronary emboli with myocardial infarction or a mycotic aneurysm of a coronary artery

Myocardium

Myocardial dysfunction caused by myocardial abscesses

Pericardium

Pericarditis from direct spread of infection by a pyogenic organism into the pericardium; hemorrhagic fibrinous pericarditis from extension of aortic ring infection to the epicardium

valve. The development of PR interval prolongation or the appearance of a new left bundle branch block or of a new right bundle branch block with left anterior hemiblock suggests that the infection has spread from the aortic valve into the ventricular septum. In the absence of digitalis toxicity or a recent inferior myocardial infarction, the development of nonparoxysmal junctional tachycardia, a Wenckebach block, or complete heart block with a narrow QRS complex serves as a clue to the spread of infection from the mitral anulus into the AV node and proximal bundle of His.[54] The development of new and persistent conduction abnormalities, particularly in patients with infected aortic valves, usually indicates the presence of a deep-seated abscess and the need for debridement and valve replacement.[55] Conduction abnormalities are an indication for pacing. Another rhythm disturbance that may be seen in infective endocarditis is ventricular premature beats, which in the absence of electrolyte abnormalities or digitalis toxicity are caused by myocarditis, myocardial abscesses, or small coronary emboli.

Abscess of the aortic valve ring may be suggested by the recent onset of aortic regurgitation, by the presence of a high degree of AV block, and by the development of pericarditis[56]; most abscesses are caused by highly invasive organisms such as *S. aureus*. Pericarditis, manifested by pericardial rub or effusion, may occur in the course of active infective endocarditis and is most commonly caused by extension of a valve ring abscess into the epicardium. This pericarditis is more often hemorrhagic and fibrinous rather than purulent. Occasionally, pericarditis in the course of infective endocarditis is the result of transmural myocardial infarction secondary to coronary emboli. Rarely, pericarditis may be produced by extension of a myocardial abscess into the epicardium.

Treatment

Two major modalities are used to treat endocarditis: (1) antibiotic therapy and (2) surgical debridement of infected perivalvular tissue and replacement of the infected valve. Effective treatment of BE requires definition of the etiologic agent and its antimicrobial susceptibility. Therefore, when BE is suspected in a patient with indolent disease, antibiotic therapy may be delayed briefly pending the results of blood cultures. In cases in which the recent administration of antibiotics has rendered the initial cultures negative, this delay may be particularly important because it provides an opportunity to obtain additional blood cultures after the effects of the antibiotics have dissipated. If the infection is fulminant or if there is valvular dysfunction that may require urgent surgical intervention, empirical antibiotic therapy must be initiated promptly after blood cultures have been obtained (see below). Bactericidal antibiotics are used parenterally in high doses for four to six weeks. The clinical response must be evaluated, and the suitability of the serum level of bactericidal activity is usually measured by in vitro testing against the infecting organism.

Selection of Antimicrobial Agents

Streptococci other than enterococci are quite susceptible to penicillin G. Enterococci are usually susceptible to the synergistic combination of penicillin or ampicillin and an aminoglycoside antibiotic, such as streptomycin or gentamicin [*see Table 5*]. The choice of aminoglycoside to be used with penicillin or ampicillin against the enterococcus depends on the characteristics of the organisms isolated in a given locality. In many hospitals, up to 40 percent of enterococcal isolates are resistant to streptomycin in a concentration of 2,000 µg/ml. These highly resistant strains are not killed when streptomycin is used as the aminoglycoside in combination therapy.[57] Only rare enterococcal strains, however, are highly resistant to gentamicin. Therefore, in cases of enterococcal endocarditis, therapy with penicillin and gentamicin is preferred unless it can be demonstrated that the infecting strain is not highly resistant to streptomycin. When the enterococcal strain is not highly resistant to streptomycin, the combination of penicillin and streptomycin is effective. Tobramycin should not be used interchangeably with gentamicin. Penicillin and tobramycin are not synergistic against *E. faecium*, a species that accounts for five to 15 percent of enterococcal isolates from specimens. In highly penicillin-allergic patients with enterococcal endocarditis, the combination of vancomycin and gentamicin, which is synergistic against most enterococci, is preferred. Ceph-

Table 5 Antimicrobial Therapy for Bacterial Endocarditis in Adults

Infectious Agent	Drug	Dosage and Route of Administration	Duration of Therapy† (wk)
Penicillin-susceptible viridans and other nonenterococcal streptococi (MIC < 0.2 µg/ml)	*Preferred Regimen*		
	Penicillin G	12–16 million units I.V. daily (in divided doses q 4 hr)	4
	or		
	Penicillin G plus streptomycin‡	12–16 million units I.V. daily (in divided doses q 4 hr)	4
		7.5 mg/kg (not to exceed 500 mg) I.M. q 12 hr	2
	or		
	Penicillin G plus streptomycin‡	Doses same as in previous regimen	2
	*Alternative Regimen**		
	Vancomycin	2 g I.V. daily (in divided doses q 6 hr)	4
Relatively penicillin-resistant streptococci			
	Preferred Regimen		
MIC 0.2–0.5 µg/ml	Penicillin G plus streptomycin‡§	20–30 million units I.V. daily (in divided doses q 4 hr)	4
		7.5 mg/kg (not to exceed 500 mg) I.M. q 12 hr	2
MIC > 0.5 µg/ml	Penicillin G plus streptomycin	Doses same as in previous regimen	4
	*Alternative Regimen**		
	Vancomycin§	2 g I.V. daily (in divided doses q 6 hr)	4
Enterococci	*Preferred Regimen*		
	Penicillin G plus	20–30 million units I.V. daily (in divided doses q 4 hr)	4–6
	gentamicin	3 mg/kg I.M. or I.V. daily (in divided doses q 8 hr)	4–6
	or		
	Ampicillin plus	8–12 g I.V. daily (in divided doses q 4 hr)	4–6
	gentamicin	3 mg/kg I.M. or I.V. daily (in divided doses q 8 hr)	4–6
	*Alternative Regimen**		
	Vancomycin plus	2 g I.V. daily (in divided doses q 6 hr)	4–6
	gentamicin	3–5 mg/kg I.M. or I.V. daily (in divided doses q 8 hr)	4–6

Infectious Agent	Drug	Dosage and Route of Administration	Duration of Therapy† (wk)
Staphylococcus aureus (methicillin susceptible)	*Preferred Regimen* Nafcillin or oxacillin *Alternative Regimen*[*] Cephalothin or Vancomycin	12 g I.V. daily (in divided doses q 4 hr) 12 g I.V. daily (in divided doses q 4 hr) 2 g I.V. daily (in divided doses q 6 hr)	4–6 4–6 4–6
S. aureus (methicillin resistant)	Vancomycin	2 g I.V. daily (in divided doses q 6 hr)	4–6

[*] Alternative drug is for use in patients with a history of penicillin hypersensitivity.

† Treatment programs are longer for prosthetic valve endocarditis (6–8 wk).

‡ Gentamicin, 1 mg/kg I.M. or I.V. q 8 hr., can be used instead of streptomycin.

§ Some investigators recommend omission of streptomycin if the MIC is > 0.2 but < 0.5 µg/ml; the role of streptomycin in combination with vancomycin has not been fully established.

alothin and other cephalosporins should not be used for enterococcal endocarditis.

Enterococci that are highly resistant to streptomycin, gentamicin, and all other aminoglycosides are becoming more frequent. These strains are not killed by combinations of penicillin, ampicillin, or vancomycin with an aminoglycoside. Optimal treatment of endocarditis caused by these strains has not been established. Continuous I.V. infusion of ampicillin in high doses along with excision of the infected valve has been suggested when the clinical response is suboptimal or when relapse occurs.[58]

Most viridans streptococci and non-enterococcal streptococci are highly susceptible to penicillin G. Two highly effective regimens have been widely used to treat endocarditis caused by viridans streptococci and other types of penicillin-sensitive streptococci (i.e., minimum inhibitory concentration [MIC] of penicillin < 0.2 µg/ml). One regimen employs parenteral penicillin alone in high doses for four weeks,[59,60] and the second regimen adds streptomycin during the initial two weeks of the four-week course.[60,61] The latter regimen utilizes the in vitro synergism achieved against most strains of nonenterococcal streptococci by the combination of penicillin and strepto-

mycin. A third approach employs only two weeks of parenteral penicillin plus streptomycin, instead of four weeks of parenteral therapy. Although the relapse rate in early studies using a similar two-week regimen was unacceptable,[62] a subsequent study showed that this regimen is an effective and economical treatment for selected patients with endocarditis caused by penicillin-sensitive streptococci.[63] Gentamicin (1 mg/kg I.M. or I.V. every eight hours in patients with normal renal function) can be used in lieu of streptomycin in these regimens. The short-duration treatment should be considered for only those cases of native valve endocarditis with the most favorable prognoses: those without complicating hypotension, renal failure, thrombocytopenia, mycotic aneurysms, or congestive heart failure caused by valve dysfunction. The streptococci should not be pyridoxal dependent or thiol dependent and should be highly susceptible to penicillin. Prosthetic valve endocarditis should not be treated with the two-week regimen. S. bovis is highly penicillin sensitive, and the endocarditis it causes can be treated with regimens recommended for other penicillin-sensitive streptococci.[60]

Occasionally, strains of viridans streptococci and S. bovis that cause endocarditis are highly resistant to streptomycin (i.e., resistant to 1,000 µg/ml). Combination therapy with streptomycin and penicillin is not synergistic against these strains. These strains, however, have not become highly resistant to gentamicin, and the combination of gentamicin and penicillin does act synergistically to kill them.[64,65] When combination therapy is being used to treat endocarditis caused by nonenterococcal streptococci, the streptococcus should be screened for high-level resistance to streptomycin. Such screening is particularly important when short-duration therapy is planned. Alternatively, if screening is not feasible, gentamicin could be substituted for streptomycin in regimens that require an aminoglycoside.

Rarely, endocarditis caused by relatively penicillin-resistant (MIC $\geq$ 0.2 µg/ml) viridans or other nonenterococcal streptococci occurs, usually in the setting of prolonged prophylactic use of oral penicillin.[66] These infections are treated with an increased dosage of penicillin G, 20 to 30 million units I.V. daily, combined with an aminoglycoside. If the strain is even more resistant to penicillin (MIC > 0.5 µg/ml), the infection is treated with the same regimen that is employed for enterococcal endocarditis (see above).[60,66] Nutritionally dependent streptococci, such as those dependent on pyridoxal, are often relatively penicillin resistant.[67] Endocarditis caused by such organisms should be treated with intravenous penicillin and an aminoglycoside for four weeks.[68] Pneumococcal endocarditis and group A streptococcal endocarditis are treated with intravenous penicillin G in a dosage of 20 million units daily for four weeks. A penicillinase-resistant penicillin should be the initial agent used to treat S. aureus endocarditis, unless the presence of methicillin-resistant S. aureus strains is suspected. In the latter case, vancomycin should be used until the susceptibility of the actual strain has been clarified. Penicillin G (20 to 30 million units daily) is substituted only if the particular isolate has been shown to be penicillin susceptible by tube dilution testing and if it has been demonstrated not to produce penicillinase. The addition of gentamicin, 3 to 5 mg/kg daily in divided doses every eight hours, to a penicillinase-resistant penicillin may be indicated in a seriously ill patient because the antibiotics display synergism in vitro against methicillin-sensitive S. aureus strains. In limited retrospective and prospective studies of methicillin-sensitive S. aureus endocarditis in drug addicts, combination therapy with a penicillinase-resistant penicillin and gentamicin has not proved significantly better than therapy with a penicillinase-resistant penicillin alone.[69,70] Studies comparing the use of the two regimens for S. aureus endocarditis in nonaddicts produced similar findings.[70,71] Despite these findings, the role of combination therapy for S. aureus endocarditis remains controversial. If combination therapy is to be used initially, gentamicin should be restricted to the first three to five days because a two-week course of gentamicin in nonaddicts was found to be associated with nephrotoxicity.[70] Some clinicians prefer to initiate treatment with a penicillinase-resistant penicillin and to add gentamicin to the regimen if a patient has not demonstrated a satisfactory clinical response after five days of therapy.

S. epidermidis endocarditis, which is usually engrafted on a prosthetic valve, may persistently frustrate antibiotic management. More than 80 percent of the staphylococcal strains causing PVE within one year after valve implantation are resistant to all β-lactam antibiotics, including cephalosporins.[38,72] Only when the onset of this form of PVE occurs more than a year after surgery does the frequency of β-lactam resistance in the coagulase-negative staphylococci fall below 30 percent.[38,72] Moreover, the β-lactam resistance is often not detected by routine disk and tube dilution susceptibility testing. Most of these coagulase-negative staphylococci are sensitive to vancomycin, gentamicin, and rifampin, although plasmid-mediated resistance to gentamicin has been noted frequently in some hospitals. For PVE caused by β-lactam–resistant organisms that are susceptible to rifampin and gentamicin, the most effective treatment is vancomycin

(2 g daily I.V. in divided doses every six hours) in combination with rifampin (300 mg every eight hours orally) and gentamicin (1 mg/kg every eight hours I.M. or I.V.). Although treatment is administered for six weeks, the gentamicin is usually deleted from the regimen after the initial two weeks.[73] Gentamicin should not be used if the infecting strain is resistant to this agent. If another aminoglycoside is effective against the strain, it could be substituted for gentamicin, but clinical data to support this practice are not available. Rigorous susceptibility testing is required,[72] but the coagulase-negative staphylococci that cause native valve endocarditis are usually sensitive to β-lactam antibiotics unless the infection has been acquired nosocomially. Endocarditis caused by these sensitive staphylococci can be treated with the regimens that are employed to treat *S. aureus* endocarditis.[74]

Because only a limited number of cases have been studied, the treatment of endocarditis caused by the fastidious gram-negative coccobacilli (*H. influenzae, H. aprhophilus, H. parainfluenzae, A. actinomycetemcomitans,* and *C. hominis*) is not clearly established. Currently recommended therapy is ampicillin, 12 g daily intravenously, or ampicillin plus streptomycin.[75] The occurrence of ampicillin resistance in strains of *H. influenzae* makes in vitro susceptibility testing mandatory for any isolates of *Hemophilus*. Patients who have a nonanaphylactic type of ampicillin allergy or endocarditis caused by an ampicillin-resistant strain of *Hemophilus* species can be treated with a third-generation cephalosporin in high doses.

The diagnosis of diphtheroid, or *Corynebacterium,* endocarditis, which is usually engrafted on a prosthetic valve, is difficult because the organisms are fastidious, requiring five to 15 days for growth, and because they often are found as contaminants in blood cultures. Many diphtheroid isolates from patients with endocarditis are resistant to penicillin and to other β-lactam antibiotics. The combination of penicillin and gentamicin in vitro acts synergistically to kill those diphtheroids that are suscepti-

ble to gentamicin (MIC ≤ 4 μg/ml). Synergism is not achieved against strains that are resistant to gentamicin. For PVE caused by gentamicin-sensitive strains, therapy with intravenous penicillin G (20 million units daily) and gentamicin (1.3 mg/kg I.M. or I.V. every eight hours) is recommended. Vancomycin, which is bactericidal against diphtheroids, is recommended as the initial treatment of diphtheroid PVE pending results of antibiotic susceptibility tests, and it is the drug of choice if the infecting strain is resistant to gentamicin.[76]

Endocarditis caused by gram-negative bacilli should be treated with one of the potent β-lactam antibiotics, such as a third-generation cephalosporin, with or without an aminoglycoside. The particular antimicrobial regimen that should be used is determined by susceptibility testing and by published experience for the specific gram-negative bacillus involved. Effective treatment of endocarditis caused by *P. aeruginosa* requires the synergistic combination of ticarcillin, 3 g I.V. every four hours, and tobramycin, 2.7 mg/kg I.M. or I.V. every eight hours (8 mg/kg daily), for at least six weeks.[77] Because pseudomonal endocarditis is often destructive and is associated with perivalvular abscess, aggressive early surgical intervention is recommended.[36,77]

The response of fungal endocarditis to therapy is most discouraging. More than 80 percent of patients with fungal endocarditis die of their infection.[7] Prompt valve debridement and valve replacement along with antifungal chemotherapy are indicated for treatment of native or prosthetic valve endocarditis caused by fungi.[7,78] Several considerations support this approach: the limitations of antifungal chemotherapy, the tendency for bulky vegetations to form and to fragment into major arterial emboli, and the propensity of fungal organisms to invade local tissue. Amphotericin B is the drug of choice for treatment of systemic fungal infection. In treating endocarditis, the daily dosage of amphotericin B is raised during a period of two to three days to 1 mg/kg intravenously. Synergism in vitro between flucytosine and amphotericin B has been reported against some strains of *Candida*, and the combined use of these two agents in this life-threatening situation seems warranted. In patients who have normal renal function, the dosage of flucytosine is 150 mg/kg daily, administered orally in divided doses every six hours. The drug should not be given in the presence of renal failure, because it can induce severe bone marrow depression.

Culture-Negative Endocarditis

When blood cultures are negative or culture results are not available, the selection of empirical therapy requires careful consideration of the clinical clues and factors predisposing to endocarditis that might suggest the identity of the causative organism. In the absence of information suggesting a probable cause for native valve SBE, treatment with ampicillin and gentamicin as for enterococcal endocarditis is advised. If the course is fulminant or *S. aureus* is an etiologic consideration, combined therapy with nafcillin and gentamicin is recommended. Because blood cultures rarely remain negative in patients with fulminant endocarditis, such empirical therapy can usually be revised later based on the culture results.

The spectrum of microorganisms causing PVE differs from that implicated in native valve endocarditis, and culture-negative PVE should be treated with a combination of vancomycin, gentamicin, and ampicillin, each administered in maximum dosages. The ampicillin is directed against the fastidious gram-negative coccobacilli, which are important causes of LPVE and difficult to isolate from blood cultures. When embarking on therapy for culture-negative endocarditis, it is important to consider the possibility that the endocarditis is caused by a nonbacterial organism or that one of the conditions that mimic this disease is present [*see Table 3*].

Monitoring Clinical Response and Serum Bactericidal Activity

A decrease in fever is usually evident within one week of instituting appropriate antibiotic therapy; some patients become afebrile 24 to 48 hours after the start of therapy. Petechiae and embolic phenomena may occur for several weeks after initiation of recommended treatment; such findings do not necessarily indicate that therapy is ineffective, particularly if other signs indicate the patient is getting better. Blood cultures should be taken on several occasions after antibiotic therapy is initiated if the patient does not become afebrile within a few days. To establish that biologically effective concentrations of antibiotics are being achieved by a given therapeutic program, serum bactericidal activity is often determined. In this test, dilutions of serum are tested for bactericidal activity against the organism previously isolated from the patient's blood. It is desirable to have bactericidal activity at a serum dilution of 1 : 8 or greater when the antibiotic concentration in blood is at its nadir. To achieve this level of bactericidal activity, the antibiotic dose can be increased within the limits of toxicity; alternatively, a second drug may be added to the regimen. The test only serves to indicate whether antibiotic activity in blood is satisfactory and does not ensure that the patient will survive the infection. Bactericidal activity at a serum dilution of 1 : 8 or greater can usually be achieved against highly susceptible organisms but may not be obtainable against relatively resistant bacteria. Although it may not be possible to achieve the desired level of serum bactericidal activity at the nadir for serum antibiotic concentrations in patients with *S. aureus* endocarditis, such patients may nevertheless be cured by antibiotic therapy. An increase in the dosage to enhance bactericidal activity against *S. aureus* may increase the risk of antibiotic toxicity and is not recommended routinely if the clinical course has been satisfactory.[79]

Antithrombotic Therapy

A decision regarding the use of antithrombotic therapy in patients with native or prosthetic valve endocarditis should be individualized. It should be based on whether the patient has cardiac or extracardiac disease that would warrant use of such therapy in the absence of endocarditis. A national conference sponsored by the American College of Chest Physicians and the National Heart, Lung and Blood Institute issued recommendations for the use of antithrombotic therapy in such cases[49]:

Infective endocarditis Antithrombotic therapy to prevent systemic emboli is not indicated in patients with normal sinus rhythm who have uncomplicated infective endocarditis involving a native or bioprosthetic valve.

In patients with prosthetic valves who have cardiac disease that requires long-term warfarin therapy, such therapy should be continued during endocarditis unless there are specific contraindications. Warfarin therapy, however, carries a significant risk of intracranial hemorrhage; thus, the prothrombin time should be maintained at 1.5 times the control value using rabbit-brain thromboplastin (INR=3.0).

The indications for anticoagulant therapy are uncertain when systemic embolism occurs during the course of infective endocarditis involving a native or bioprosthetic heart valve. The therapeutic decision should consider comorbid factors, including atrial fibrillation, evidence of left atrial thrombus, evidence and size of valvular vegetations, and the distribution and severity of embolism. Two other factors should also be considered when making this decision: there is an increased risk of hemorrhage in these patients, and there is a lack of evidence that antithrombotic therapy will prevent embolization of vegetations.

Surgical Intervention

Operative intervention to debride infected perivalvular tissue or to replace or reconstruct a dysfunctioning valve has a major role in the management of complicated infective endocarditis that involves either a native or a prosthetic valve.[36,43,47,48,80-84] Several observations have prompted the increased use of surgery in the treatment of active endocarditis: (1) the mortality of patients undergoing valve surgery during active endocarditis is not greater than that of patients treated medically,[80-84] (2) the risk that residual endocarditis from the initial infecting organism will develop on the newly implanted prosthesis is low,[43,82,84,85] and (3) some intracardiac complications of endocarditis that cannot be remedied by antibiotic therapy can be corrected surgically. Long-term survival rates for patients who undergo valve replacement during active endocarditis are satisfactory.[82,83,85]

The indications for surgical treatment of active native and prosthetic valve endocarditis have been developed through a retrospective analysis of therapy. Moderate to severe congestive heart failure resulting from valve dysfunction is the most widely accepted indication for valve replacement and accounts for 90 percent of the decisions to operate.[48,80-82,85] Bulky vegetations that obstruct the valve orifice may also produce congestive heart failure and are an equally compelling indication for surgery. Surgical intervention should also be considered when there is clinical evidence of perivalvular invasion and abscess formation and when infection remains uncontrolled despite maximal antimicrobial therapy. Fever, other than drug-induced fever, that persists despite antimicrobial therapy is often an indication of perivalvular invasion.[86] Perivalvular abscess or invasion is also strongly suggested by new-onset and persistent electrocardiographic conduction disturbances, especially in the setting of aortic valve infection.[55] Perivalvular invasion or intracardiac fistula formation requiring surgical intervention may be detected by two-dimensional and Doppler echocardiography.[46] Fungal endocarditis is treated surgically because it responds poorly to medical therapy.[7,78] Similarly, PVE that occurs within a year after valve implantation and is caused by coagulase-negative staphylococci is frequently complicated and usually requires surgery for cure.[72,84] Because left-sided native valve endocarditis and PVE caused by *S. aureus* are frequently invasive, early surgery should be considered for patients with these infections who do not show prompt and sustained improvement during antibiotic therapy.[48,85] Endocarditis caused by *P. aeruginosa* or other gram-negative bacilli that has not responded after seven to 10 days of maximal antibiotic therapy should be treated surgically.[36] Although patients with native valve endocarditis who relapse after appropriate antibiotic therapy can often be cured by repeat courses of antibiotics, patients with PVE who relapse respond better if treated surgically.[84]

The occurrence of an arterial embolus, particularly to the cerebrum, is another factor to be considered when making the decision to operate. Occasionally, systemic embolization itself is an indication for surgery, especially if echocardiography confirms the presence of a persistent vegetation after the embolic event. Although it has been suggested that echocardiographic confirmation of a vegetation is an indication for surgery, this recommendation remains controversial.[87] Surgery may be beneficial if the vegetations are unusually large and mobile or if they are accompanied by echocardiographically imaged evidence of complicated endocarditis, such as valvular dysfunction or an anulus abscess.[45,46] Occasionally, a single clinical or microbiological finding constitutes an absolute indication for surgery, but more often, the decision to operate is based on a consideration of multiple clinical and microbiological observations.[83]

Among patients with endocarditis, the operative mortality is proportional to the degree of preoperative hemodynamic impairment. If surgery is indicated, it should be performed promptly. Prolonged antibiotic therapy before surgery has not been associated with a more favorable operative outcome.[74,85] In fact, delaying surgery to administer additional antibiotic therapy in the presence of uncontrolled infection or deteriorating hemodynamic status may result in a less favorable outcome.[88]

Although implantation of a prosthetic valve in a drug addict may occasionally be lifesaving, this approach is hazardous: endocarditis is likely to recur if intravenous drug abuse continues, and it is more difficult to eradicate an infection involving a prosthetic valve than it is to cure native valve endocarditis. To avoid the complication of recurrent endocarditis in a patient with a prosthetic valve, tricuspid or pulmonary valvulectomy (without valve replacement) has been employed in the treatment of antibiotic-resistant right-sided endocarditis that occurs in addicts.[36,77,89] However, in addicts with isolated right-sided endocarditis, valvulectomy or prosthetic valve implantation should be postponed and antibiotic therapy continued for a prolonged period despite persistent fever and pulmonary emboli in an effort to achieve a medical cure and thus avoid cardiac surgery. In addicts with *S. aureus* tricuspid valve endocarditis, the detection, by two-dimensional echocardiography, of tricuspid valve vegetations exceeding 1 cm in diameter is not an indication for surgery. In most intravenous drug addicts, *S. aureus* tricuspid valve endocarditis can be cured medically. Occasionally, however, cardiac surgery is beneficial in patients with fever that persists after three weeks of therapy or patients with evidence of right ventricular failure.[90]

Prophylaxis

Transitory bacteremia may be caused by a variety of manipulations or surgical procedures, and in an individual with structural heart disease, such bacteremia may initiate bacterial endocarditis. Certain procedures are associated with a high risk of bacteremia: dental extraction (60 to 90 percent), periodontal surgery (35 to 85 percent), tonsillectomy (30 to 40 percent), and transurethral prostatic resection (10 to 60 percent).[91]

The indications for antibiotic prophylaxis for endocarditis are based on two criteria: an increased risk of endocarditis developing on specific cardiac lesions [*see Table 6*] and the likelihood that selected manipulative procedures give rise to bacteremia with organisms that commonly cause endocarditis [*see Table 7*]. Viridans-type streptococci are responsible for most cases of endocarditis originating in the oral cavity; enterococci are responsible

---

Table 6   Anatomic Lesions, Devices, and Conditions for Which Antibiotic Prophylaxis Is Recommended

Most congenital heart disease (e.g., ventricular septal defect, tetralogy of Fallot, complex cyanotic congenital heart disease, aortic or pulmonary stenosis, patent ductus arteriosus, systemic-to-pulmonary artery shunts, coarctation of the aorta)*

Rheumatic or other acquired valvular heart disease

Hypertrophic cardiomyopathy

Mitral valve prolapse with mitral insufficiency (the incidence of endocarditis appears to be low)†

Prosthetic heart valves of all types

Previous episode of endocarditis (even in the absence of overt heart disease)

---

*Prophylaxis is not recommended for the following congenital heart lesions: isolated ostium secundum atrial septal defect; ostium secundum atrial septal defect that was closed without a patch at least 6 mo earlier; or patent ductus arteriosus that was ligated and divided at least 6 mo earlier.

†Individuals who have mitral valve prolapse associated with thickening of the valve leaflets, redundancy of the valve leaflets, or both, particularly men who are 45 yr of age or older, may be at increased risk for bacterial endocarditis.

---

for those episodes arising in the genitourinary tract. A statement presenting the rationale and indications for prophylaxis and the specific recommendations for antibiotic use has been prepared by a committee of the American Heart Association [*see Tables 8 and 9*][92]; other organizations have developed similar guidelines for prophylaxis.[93,94] Although amoxicillin, ampicillin, and penicillin show comparable in vitro efficacy against viridans-type streptococci, amoxicillin has replaced penicillin V as the recommended agent for oral prophylaxis because it is better absorbed from the gastrointestinal tract and provides higher and more sustained serum antibiotic concentrations. Erythromycin stearate, erythromycin ethylsuccinate, and clindamycin are specifically recommended for use in patients who are allergic to penicillin because these agents are reliably absorbed and their use results in sustained serum concentrations. Tetracyclines and sulfonamides are not recommended for endocarditis prophylaxis.

Table 7   Procedures for Which Antibiotic Prophylaxis Is Recommended

Dental procedures likely to produce gingival bleeding (including routine professional cleaning)

Surgery of the upper respiratory tract (e.g., tonsillectomy, adenoidectomy)

Surgical procedures that involve intestinal or respiratory tract mucosa, including esophageal dilation and sclerotherapy

Bronchoscopy with a rigid bronchoscope

Surgery or instrumentation of the genitourinary tract, especially in the presence of local infection

Obstetric infections (e.g., septic abortions or peripartum infection) and surgery through or on the vagina

Surgery involving infected tissues*

---

*Prophylaxis should be directed against the likely bacterial pathogen or pathogens, particularly against suspected *Staphylococcus aureus*.

Table 8   Prophylactic Antibiotics Recommended for Adults Undergoing Upper Respiratory Tract or Dental Procedures

Type of Regimen	Drug Dosages
Standard regimens	Amoxicillin, 3 g p.o. 1 hr before the procedure; then 1.5 g 6 hr after the initial dose[*] *or* Erythromycin ethylsuccinate, 800 mg p.o., or erythromycin stearate, 1 g p.o., 2 hr before the procedure; then half the dose 6 hr after the initial dose *or* Clindamycin, 300 mg p.o. 1 hr before the procedure; then 150 mg 6 hr after the initial dose
Standard regimens for patients unable to tolerate oral medications	Ampicillin, 2 g I.V. or I.M. 30 min before the procedure; then 6 hr after the initial dose, ampicillin, 1 g I.V. or I.M., or amoxicillin, 1.5 g p.o. *or* Clindamycin, 300 mg I.V. 30 min before the procedure; then 150 mg I.V. or p.o. 6 hr after the initial dose
Special regimens for patients considered at high risk[†]	Ampicillin, 2 g I.V. or I.M., plus gentamicin, 1.5 mg/kg (not to exceed 80 mg) I.V. or I.M., 30 min before the procedure; then amoxicillin, 1.5 g p.o. 6 hr after the initial dose, or repeat the parenteral regimen 8 hr after the initial dose[‡] *or* Vancomycin, 1 g I.V., infused over 1 hr starting 1 hr before the procedure; no repeat dose is necessary

[*]In patients who have been taking oral penicillin for rheumatic fever prophylaxis or other conditions, viridans streptococci that are relatively resistant to penicillin may have emerged in the oral cavity. In such patients, a standard regimen of erythromycin or clindamycin or a special regimen is suggested.

[†]Individuals who have prosthetic heart valves, a history of endocarditis, or surgically constructed systemic-pulmonary shunts or conduits are at high risk for endocarditis; see text for comments regarding prophylaxis for these patients.

[‡]Repeat doses of gentamicin may require modification if renal function is significantly impaired.

The dose of penicillin used to prevent recurrences of acute rheumatic fever is insufficient to prevent bacterial endocarditis. However, patients taking oral penicillin for this reason or other reasons may harbor relatively penicillin-resistant strains of bacteria in their oral cavity. Prophylaxis with erythromycin, clindamycin, or a special regimen is suggested when relatively penicillin-resistant streptococci are anticipated.

Patients who have prosthetic heart valves, surgically constructed systemic-pulmonary shunts or conduits, or a history of endocarditis are at high risk for endocarditis and experience high mortality and morbidity as a result of endocarditis. Accordingly, more intensive prophylaxis, often with parenteral regimens, has been recommended. Although parenteral regimens may be desirable for these patients, logistic and financial considerations have been major obstacles to providing this form of prophylaxis. A committee of the American Heart Association has recommended the use of the standard oral regimens for these high-risk patients. Nevertheless, a special parenteral regimen has been provided for high-risk patients in cases in which practitioners consider more intensive parenteral prophylaxis desirable [*see Table 8*].

Prophylaxis is not recommended for the following procedures because they are not considered to be risks for subsequent endocarditis: dental procedures that are not likely to cause gingival bleeding, simple adjustment of orthodontic appliances, injections of intraoral anesthetics (except intraligamentary injections), shedding of primary teeth, endotracheal intubation, bronchoscopy with a flexible bronchoscope, and tympanostomy tube insertion. Similarly, the occurrence of endocarditis after certain procedures involving the gastrointestinal tract or the genitourinary tract is rare enough that antibiotic prophylaxis is not required in most patients with underlying heart disease. Such low-risk procedures include uncomplicated vaginal delivery or cesarean section, upper gastrointestinal tract endoscopy without biopsy, percutaneous liver biopsy, proctosigmoidoscopy without biopsy, brief (so-called in-and-out) bladder catheterization in patients whose urine is sterile, barium enema, pelvic examination, dilatation and curettage of the uterus, and uncomplicated insertion or removal of intrauterine devices. However, when patients are at high risk for endocarditis, physicians may administer prophylactic antibiotics in conjunction with these low-risk procedures.

Although various procedures [see Table 7] are associated with transient bacteremia and subsequent endocarditis, most cases of endocarditis are not related to defined events. It is likely that these infections arise from bacteremias associated with ordinary activities (e.g., vigorous chewing in patients with gingival disease, use of oral irrigating jets,[91] or minor unrecognized infections). Maintaining optimal dental health is essential if the risk of endocarditis is to be minimized among patients with vulnerable cardiac lesions. Dental evaluations, including extractions and other necessary work, should be performed under appropriate antibiotic prophylaxis several weeks before the insertion of prosthetic heart valves. In addition, the following efforts to minimize the occurrence of bacteremia in patients at risk for endocarditis should be undertaken: prompt treatment of all infections, use of fiberoptic flexible instruments rather than rigid instruments for endoscopy, establishment of a sterile urine before urinary tract instrumentation, and use of sequential peripheral sites for intravenous access rather than long-duration centrally placed polyethylene catheters.

Prognosis

Overall survival for patients with infective endocarditis is about 75 percent. The rate depends in large measure on the promptness of initiation of therapy and the

Table 9 Prophylactic Antibiotics Recommended for Adults Undergoing Gastrointestinal or Genitourinary Tract Surgery or Instrumentation

Type of Regimen	Drug Dosages
Standard regimen	Ampicillin, 2 g I.M. or I.V., plus gentamicin, 1.5 mg/kg (not to exceed 80 mg) I.M. or I.V., 30 min before the procedure; then amoxicillin, 1.5 g p.o. 6 hr after the initial dose, or repeat the parenteral regimen 8 hr after the initial dose*
Regimen for penicillin-allergic patients	Vancomycin, 1 g I.V. infused slowly over 1 hr starting 1 hr before the procedure, plus gentamicin, 1.5 mg/kg (not to exceed 80 mg) 1 hr before the procedure; the regimen may be repeated 8 hr later*
Regimen for minor or low-risk procedures	Amoxicillin, 3 g p.o. 1 hr before the procedure; then 1.5 g p.o. 6 hr after the initial dose

*Repeat doses of gentamicin or vancomycin may require modification if renal function is significantly impaired. For procedures in which mucosal healing will be delayed, more than two doses may be beneficial, whereas for brief outpatient procedures, a single dose may be sufficient.

nature of the infecting organism. It approaches 90 percent when the infecting organism is a viridans-type streptococcus or *S. bovis* but is about 50 percent in endocarditis from *S. aureus* among nonaddicts. Cardiac failure is a grave prognostic sign and is the most common cause of death; other causes of death include major emboli and rupture of mycotic aneurysms. The short-term outlook is relatively good for intravenous drug addicts with right-sided endocarditis. Endocarditis from fungi or gram-negative bacilli, such as Enterobacteriaceae or *Pseudomonas* species, is extremely difficult to cure despite optimal antimicrobial therapy and aggressive surgical intervention. Overall survival in patients with prosthetic valve endocarditis approaches 70 percent.

References

1. Am J Med 51:83, 1971
2. N Engl J Med 274:199, 259, 323, 388, 1966
3. Medicine (Baltimore) 56:287, 1977
4. Medicine (Baltimore) 52:173, 1973
5. Am J Med 59:29, 1975
6. Ann Intern Med 84:29, 1976
7. Medicine (Baltimore) 54:331, 1975
8. Am J Med 57:239, 1974
9. J Clin Microbiol 27:305, 1989
10. Am J Cardiol 35:72, 1975
11. Medicine (Baltimore) 56:115, 1977
12. Am J Clin Pathol 63:131, 1975
13. Johns Hopkins Med J 139:61, 1976
14. Am J Med 72:396, 1982
15. Lancet 2:844, 1971
16. Am J Med Sci 273:203, 1977
17. Ann Surg 171:219, 1970
18. N Engl J Med 291:832, 1122, 1974
19. Br J Exp Pathol 53:44, 1972
20. American Heart Association Monograph No 52, 1977, p 9
21. J Clin Invest 56:1364, 1975
22. Am J Med 82:681, 1987
23. J Crit Illness 2:18, 1987
24. Ann Intern Med 85:471, 1976
25. Ann Intern Med 87:754, 1977
26. N Engl J Med 295:1500, 1976
27. Infective Endocarditis, University Park Press, Baltimore, 1976, p 55
28. Medicine (Baltimore) 51:1, 1972
29. Arch Intern Med 136:334, 1976
30. Medicine (Baltimore) 57:329, 1978
31. Current Clinical Topics in Infectious Diseases, Vol 2, McGraw-Hill Book Co, New York, 1981, p 151
32. Neurology (Minneap) 24:1103, 1974
33. Arch Intern Med 137:844, 1977
34. Endocarditis, Churchill Livingstone, New York, 1984, p 183
35. Rev Infect Dis 8:374, 1986
36. Circulation 66(suppl I):135, 1982
37. Circulation 69:223, 1984
38. Circulation 72:31, 1985
39. Circulation 48:365, 1973
40. N Engl J Med 318:530, 1988
41. American Heart Association Monograph No 52, 1977, p 58
42. Am J Cardiol 38:281, 1976
43. Ann Thorac Surg 35:87, 1983
44. Infections of Prosthetic Heart Valves and Vascular Grafts, University Park Press, Baltimore, 1977, p 61
45. J Am Coll Cardiol 14:631, 1989
46. J Am Coll Cardiol 15:1234, 1990
47. J Thorac Cardiovasc Surg 73:416, 1977
48. Endocarditis, Churchill Livingstone, New York, 1984, p 163
49. Chest 89(suppl):36S, 1986
50. JAMA 223:156, 1973
51. Am J Med 83:626, 1987
52. Ann Thorac Surg 5:255, 1968
53. Circulation 46:939, 1972
54. JAMA 235:1603, 1976
55. Am J Cardiol 58:1213, 1986
56. Circulation 54:140, 1976
57. Antimicrob Agents Chemother 12:401, 1977
58. Eur J Clin Microbiol Infect Dis 7:525, 1988
59. JAMA 241:1801, 1979
60. Circulation 63:730A, 1981
61. Ann Intern Med 81:178, 1974
62. Trans Am Clin Climatol Assoc 83:95, 1972
63. JAMA 245:360, 1981
64. J Infect Dis 155:954, 1987
65. J Infect Dis 155:948, 1987
66. N Engl J Med 300:296, 1979
67. Rev Infect Dis 1:955, 1979
68. Rev Infect Dis 9:908, 1987
69. Ann Intern Med 90:789, 1979
70. Ann Intern Med 97:496, 1982
71. Am J Med Sci 273:133, 1977
72. Ann Intern Med 98:447, 1983
73. 24th Interscience Conference on Antimicrobial Agents and Chemotherapy, American Society of Microbiology, Washington, DC, October 1984
74. Am J Med 83:619, 1987
75. Medicine (Baltimore) 58:145, 1979
76. Am J Med 69:838, 1980
77. Rev Infect Dis 5:314, 1983
78. Infections of Prosthetic Heart Valves and Vascular Grafts, University Park Press, Baltimore, 1977, p 163
79. Am J Med 81:43, 1986
80. Prog Cardiovasc Dis 22:145, 1979
81. Ann Intern Med 96:650, 1982
82. Current Clinical Topics in Infectious Diseases, Vol 1, McGraw-Hill Book Co, New York, 1980, p 124
83. Endocarditis, Churchill Livingstone, New York, 1984, p 201
84. J Thorac Cardiovasc Surg 92:776, 1986
85. Ann Thorac Surg 40:429, 1985
86. Lancet 1:1341, 1986
87. Am Heart J 112:1291, 1986
88. J Thorac Cardiovasc Surg 73:23, 1977
89. Am J Cardiol 35:481, 1975
90. Chest 93:247, 1988
91. Medicine (Baltimore) 56:61, 1977
92. JAMA 264:2919, 1990
93. Lancet 335:88, 1990
94. Med Lett Drugs Ther 31:112, 1989

Acknowledgments

Text on page 583 adapted from "Antithrombotic Therapy in Valvular Heart Disease," by H. J. Levine, S. G. Pauker, and E. W. Salzman. A national conference sponsored by the American College of Chest Physicians and the National Heart, Lung and Blood Institute. Reprinted from Chest 89(suppl):36S, 1986. Used by permission.

21 Sexually Transmitted Diseases

ADOLF W. KARCHMER, M.D.

Of the many diverse diseases that are transmitted sexually, the ones that will be discussed in this subsection are gonorrhea, chancroid, granuloma inguinale, nongonococcal urethritis, acute pelvic inflammatory disease, vaginitis, anorectal disease, and selected infections in homosexual men. Sexually transmitted diseases discussed elsewhere include syphilis, lymphogranuloma venereum, herpes simplex virus infection, and the acquired immunodeficiency syndrome (AIDS) [*see Chapter 18*].

Infections Due to *Neisseria gonorrhoeae*

N. gonorrhoeae is the causative agent of gonorrhea; humans are the only known reservoir for this organism. The gonococcus usually invades the transitional and columnar epithelial surfaces of the genitourinary tract and its appendages; however, gonococcal infection may be acquired through invasion of other mucosal sites, such as the conjunctiva, pharynx, and anal canal. Nonmucosal sites are infected by hematogenous dissemination.

Causative Agent

Gonococci are fastidious and fragile; in smears of clinical specimens, the gonococci typically appear as intracellular, gram-negative, kidney bean–shaped diplococci paired with their flattened surfaces in apposition. Gonococci grow most readily on chocolate agar in an atmosphere enriched by five to 10 percent carbon dioxide. Only the two *Neisseria* species pathogenic for humans, *N. gonorrhoeae* and *N. meningitidis*, can grow on Thayer-Martin or transgrow selective medium. Although all *Neisseria* species yield a positive oxidase test, the gonococcus can be differentiated from the meningococcus by its ability to metabolize glucose but not maltose, sucrose, or lactose.

The surface of the gonococcus is complex and greatly contributes to the pathogenicity of the organism.[1,2] Hairlike structures called fimbriae, or pili, which project from the surface of the gonococcus, facilitate attachment of the organism to nonciliated human epithelial cells and shield it from phagocytosis by polymorphonuclear leukocytes and macrophages. In addition, proteins I and II and the lipopolysaccharide of the gonococcal outer membrane play important roles in pathogenesis. Protein II also mediates attachment of gonococci to human epithelial cells. Once the organisms adhere to endothelial cells, protein I migrates from the gonococcal membrane to the cytoplasmic membrane of human cells, an event that may prompt an endocytic process in which viable organisms are transported across the epithelium. After attachment of gonococci to epithelial cells, lipopolysaccharide, a potent endotoxin, causes decreased ciliary activity as well as sloughing of ciliated cells. Gonococci also release IgA proteases, which inactivate secretory IgA antibodies. Specific types of protein I are associated with the resistance of gonococci to the bactericidal activity of normal serum, a property that plays a role in dissemination of gonococci beyond the genitourinary tract. Lipopolysaccharide stimulates the inflammatory process that characterizes clinical gonorrhea.

Gonococci isolated in the United States have gradually become less susceptible to penicillin G, ampicillin, and tetracycline. These changes initially resulted from chromosomal mutations that decreased the permeability of the organisms to these agents.[3] In contrast to the gradual evolution of penicillin resistance, gonococci that were highly resistant to penicillins, by virtue of plasmid-mediated penicillinase production, were isolated in 1975. Until 1979, the frequency of infection caused by penicillinase-producing

N. gonorrhoeae (PPNG) had increased slowly in the United States; many of these infections were traced to Southeast Asia. Thereafter, PPNG became endemic in many areas of the United States, and in 1986, 1.8 percent (16,608) of all cases of gonorrhea reported to the Centers for Disease Control were caused by PPNG.[4] Gonococci with high-level resistance to penicillin that was chromosomally mediated (so-called chromosomally mediated resistant *N. gonorrhoeae*, or CMRNG) were noted in an outbreak in North Carolina in 1983.[5] By late 1984, CMRNG that were also highly resistant to tetracycline had been identified in 23 states.[6] Since then, plasmid-mediated high-level resistance to tetracycline has been noted in gonococci from many areas.[7] These gonococci are termed tetracycline-resistant *N. gonorrhoeae*, or TRNG. Spectinomycin-resistant gonococci, which were a frequent cause of gonorrhea in American military personnel in South Korea, have been isolated only sporadically in the United States. Although resistance to spectinomycin is caused by a specific chromosomal mutation, the organisms recovered in the United States have been resistant to penicillins, tetracycline, and cefoxitin. This finding suggests that spectinomycin resistance arose in gonococci that already possessed chromosomal resistance to other antibiotics.[8] The increasing frequency of infections in the United States resulting from antibiotic-resistant gonococci has prompted prospective surveillance of antimicrobial resistance in *N. gonorrhoeae*[9] as well as changes in the recommended therapy for gonorrhea (see below).[10]

Epidemiology

In the United States, gonorrhea has reached pandemic proportions. It is particularly prevalent in low socioeconomic urban settings but is found in every social milieu. It is found in all age groups, although 90 percent of cases occur among teenagers and young adults.

Both men and women who have asymptomatic gonorrhea actively spread gonorrhea. Extensive bacteriologic screening of women in various clinical settings has disclosed a vast reservoir of asymptomatic gonococcal infection. Most men with urethral gonococcal infection seek therapy when symptoms develop, but some men are infected for extended periods and experience either mild symptoms or none at all. Urethral cultures of asymptomatic male contacts of women with symptomatic gonorrhea revealed that 40 percent of the men were infected.[11] Gonococci were recovered from the urethra of 2.2 percent of sexually active male military personnel who had minimal symptoms or none at all.[11] Therapy for gonorrhea, regardless of the patient's sex, requires identification and treatment of asymptomatically infected sexual contacts to prevent reinfection and further spread.

Clinical Features

The clinical features of gonorrhea depend on the site of inoculation, the age and sex of the patient, the duration of infection, and the local or systemic extension of disease.

Gonorrhea in Men

Gonorrhea in heterosexual men typically presents as urethritis with a spontaneous purulent urethral exudate and dysuria. The urethritis is preceded by an incubation period that averages three to four days but may extend to 14 days or more. Pharyngeal infection is uncommon. Before the use of antibiotic therapy, gonorrhea resulted in epididymitis, prostatitis, and infection of the paraurethral glands and adjacent soft tissues; these complications are now very rare. Untreated gonococcal urethritis may result in urethral stricture. Nongonococcal urethritis (NGU) is the major entity to be distinguished from gonococcal urethritis in men. Among homosexual men, gonococcal infection may involve not only the urethra but also the anal canal (30 to 55 percent)[12] and the pharynx (20 percent).[13]

Gonorrhea in Women

The clinical picture of gonococccal infection in women is extremely diverse. The sites from which the organisms are most commonly isolated, in decreasing frequency, are the endocervical canal, urethra, anal canal, and pharynx.[14] In a study of gonococcal infection detected in all patient-care areas of the Boston City Hospital,[15] female patients with asymptomatic anogenital infection accounted for 19 percent of those infected.

The frequent presence of multiple sexually transmitted pathogens in the genital tract of women who have gonorrhea makes the assignment of symptoms to a specific agent difficult. Given this caveat, it may be stated that gonococcal infection in women is often associated with vaginal discharge, lower abdominal discomfort, and abnormal uterine bleeding. Anal canal infection, which causes symptoms of proctitis similar to those seen in homosexual males, may result from autoinoculation by infected vaginal secretions or from penis-anus contact with or without rectal intercourse. Pharyngeal infection occurs in women who practice fellatio. It may cause acute exudative pharyngitis but is often asymptomatic.[13]

Gonorrhea in women may also present as urethritis or trigonitis with dysuria, urgency, frequency, pyuria, and occasionally, hematuria. In the absence of bacteriuria, these symptoms are termed the acute urethral syndrome and, in a sexually active woman, should prompt an evaluation for infection by *N. gonorrhoeae* and *Chlamydia trachomatis*. Milking of the urethra via the vagina may yield an exudate containing gonococci, which are visible on Gram's stain. In the Boston City Hospital review of gonorrhea in women, 37 percent of patients had infectious complications, including acute pelvic inflammatory disease, abscess of Bartholin's glands, conjunctivitis, and disseminated infection. Acute pelvic inflammatory disease accounted for almost all of the complications.[15]

Women who have undergone hysterectomy remain vulnerable to infection by *N. gonorrhoeae*. In one study, the frequency of gonorrhea in women who had had a hysterectomy approximated that noted in a matched control group. In these patients, gonococci are most likely to be isolated from the urethra but may be recovered from the vagina or the anal canal.[16]

Gonococcal Infection in Infants and Children

Gonococcal infection in infancy results from contamination of the neonate during birth or from accidental contamination by an infected adult at a later date. Maternal gonococcal infection at parturition may cause gonococcal ophthalmia neonatorum, despite silver nitrate prophylaxis of the eyes, or it may produce primary infection of the child's anogenital, oropharyngeal, or umbilical area.[17] Infection at these sites may lead to disseminated gonococcal infection in the neonate.[18] To reduce the morbidity caused by neonatal gonorrhea, as well as by salpingitis, chorioamnionitis, and disseminated infection, infected pregnant women should be identified and treated.

Infection in prepubertal children is usually the result of precocious sexual activity or molestation. Except for gonococcal vulvovaginitis, which occurs only in prepubertal girls, gonococcal infection in prepubertal children resembles that in adults.[19] The anal canal and pharynx are often infected but rarely symptomatic. These areas and the genital areas should be routinely cultured when gonococcal disease is suspected in prepubertal children.

Disseminated Gonococcal Disease

Disseminated gonococcal disease, often called the arthritis-dermatitis syndrome, develops when the bloodstream is invaded; organisms may invade from any of the primary sites of infection, whether the site is symptomatic or asymptomatic. The syndrome is more common in women; the risk is greatest during menstruation and in the second and third trimesters of pregnancy. Disseminated gonococcal infection is currently the most common cause of infectious arthritis in young adults. It is characterized by a febrile, variably toxic, bacteremic initial phase, during which skin lesions, polyarticular arthralgias, and tenosynovitis are noted.[20] Joint effusions are rare, and synovial fluid, if obtained at this stage, contains fewer than 20,000 leukocytes/mm^3 and is usually sterile. The sparse, predominantly acral skin lesions are 5 to 15 mm in diameter and erythematous; they are often tender papules with a pustular, hemorrhagic, or necrotic center. Gonococci are rarely recovered by culturing scrapings from skin lesions; the yield can be increased by culturing skin from a punch biopsy. In 55 percent of cases, the organism can be identified by specific direct fluorescent antibody staining of biopsies from the pustular skin lesions.[21] During the first two to three days of the arthritis-dermatitis syndrome, 50 percent of patients have positive blood cultures.

The later stage, seen a week or more after onset, is characterized by spontaneous clearance of bacteremia, resolution of skin lesions, and the emergence of a monoarticular or oligoarticular arthritis with purulent synovial fluid. Although blood cultures at this stage are usually sterile, the synovial fluid yields gonococci in at least 50 percent of cases. More than 90 percent of patients with disseminated infection have some joint or periarticular symptoms. In about 20 percent of patients, the disease does not conform to the sequential pattern but combines various aspects of both stages or is initially manifested as purulent arthritis, with the bacteremic stage absent.

Disseminated gonococcal disease merits consideration in all sexually active persons who have acute arthritis or polyarthralgias and skin rash. The differential diagnosis is extensive. A combination of skin and joint symptoms mimicking disseminated gonococcal disease is occasionally seen in serum sickness, acute hepatitis B, erythema multiforme, sarcoidosis with erythema nodosum, cutaneous vasculitis such as Schönlein-Henoch purpura, and septicemia caused by a variety of organisms, especially *Staphylococcus aureus* or *Pseudomonas aeruginosa*. Chronic meningococcemia, although usually accompanied by a petechial eruption, may be associated with skin lesions indistinguishable from those of gonococcemia. If only urethritis and arthritis are noted, Reiter's syndrome may be confused with disseminated disease.[22] Gonococcemia rather than Reiter's syndrome is suggested if fever and arthritis respond within 72 hours after taking antibiotics.

Endocarditis or meningitis develops infrequently as a consequence of gonococcemia. New valvular murmurs, arterial emboli, splenomegaly, or continued positive blood cultures after the fifth day of gonococcemic symptoms suggest endocarditis. The presence of arthralgias or arthritis at the outset of a gram-negative diplococcal meningitis favors gonococcus as the causative agent (joint symptoms are relatively rare during the acute phase of meningococcal meningitis). Thus, joint symptoms accompanying a gram-negative diplococcal meningitis are an indication for culture of all potential portals of entry for gonococci.

Diagnosis

Cultures should be obtained from sexually active persons whenever the diagnosis of *N. gonorrhoeae* infection is suspected. Because asymptomatic infection is prevalent and screening cultures are inexpensive and sensitive, the strategy of obtaining endocervical cultures from selected sexually active women during routine gynecologic care and treating those with positive results will not only decrease morbidity but also reduce medical costs.[23] A cost benefit can be anticipated when the prevalence of gonorrhea exceeds 1.5 percent. This prevalence can be expected among women who report contact with a person who has a sexually transmitted infection, recent multiple sexual partners, a history of gonorrhea or syphilis, or intercourse at 16 years of age or younger.

Definitive diagnosis is contingent on recovery of gonococci from the patient. Gram's-stained smears of exudates from the urethra or from the freshly cleansed cervix are helpful. A tentative diagnosis can be made when typical gram-negative diplococci are seen within three or more polymorphonuclear leukocytes. The specificity and sensitivity of these findings in smears of urethral exudates from men exceed 90 percent.[24] The specificity of Gram's-stained smears of cervical exudates exceeds 90 percent; the sensitivity is only 65 percent.[25] Gram's-stained smears of synovial and cerebrospinal fluids may reveal *Neisseria* organisms, but these smears cannot provide a tentative etiologic diagnosis, because meningococci frequently infect these fluids.

The use of selective culture media, such as Thayer-Martin or transgrow, has greatly enhanced recovery of *N. gonorrhoeae* from the endocervix, urethra, rectum, and pharynx; therefore, specimens from these sites should always be placed on a selective medium when a mixed bacterial flora is present. The culture medium, warmed to room temperature, should be immediately and heavily inoculated, and the culture should be promptly placed in the CO_2-supplemented air of a candle jar. Transgrow medium is available in a small vial that has been supplemented with CO_2. This system is ideal for office practice. Cultures should be placed in an incubator no later than the end of the day on which they are obtained. Typical gonococcal colonies on these media are confirmed by Gram's stain, oxidase reaction, and sugar metabolism or by specific fluorescent antibody techniques. It is important to confirm isolates specifically as *N. gonorrhoeae*, especially when they are taken from sites where *N. meningitidis* may also be found. Synovial and CSF specimens should not be cultured on selective media that will suppress non-*Neisseria* pathogens. When both gonococci and other pathogens are sought or when competing bacterial flora is not expected, samples should be grown on routine media and chocolate agar.

All infected and potentially infected sites should be cultured, whether or not local symptoms are present. Endocervical cultures are positive on a single examination in 80 to 95 percent of infected women.[14,26] The yield may be higher in cultures taken during or immediately before menstruation. A simultaneously obtained rectal culture will identify an additional five percent of infected women despite negative cervical cul-

tures.[26] If fellatio is practiced, pharyngeal cultures should also be obtained. Cultures of the female urethra are indicated if there is clinical urethritis or if the uterus has been removed. Urethral cultures should be taken in all men; rectal and pharyngeal cultures should be taken in homosexual males.

The diagnosis of disseminated gonococcal infection can be established by isolating *N. gonorrhoeae* from blood or synovial fluid, although in a patient with a typical clinical presentation this diagnosis is often based on isolation of gonococci from the urogenital tract, pharynx, or rectum or from the patient's sexual partner. If resolution of systemic symptoms does not occur promptly (within 48 to 72 hours) when antimicrobial therapy is given, infection by antibiotic-resistant gonococci or an incorrect diagnosis should be suspected.

Appropriately obtained specimens are essential. To obtain a specimen from a male who has no urethral exudate, a calcium alginate–tipped urethrogenital swab (Calgiswab) should be inserted 2 to 4 cm into the anterior urethra. To obtain an endocervical culture, the cervix is cleansed with sterile cotton, and then, a sterile cotton-tipped swab is inserted 2 cm into the endocervical canal and rotated. Rectal cultures are obtained by inserting a sterile cotton-tipped swab 2 to 3 cm into the anal canal. A fecal-contaminated swab should be discarded and another specimen obtained.

Treatment

Although gonococci have gradually developed increased resistance to penicillin, ampicillin, amoxicillin, and tetracycline, these agents remained major elements of recommended treatment for gonococcal infections in the United States until the mid-1980s. At that time, gonococci that were highly resistant in vitro to penicillins and tetracycline (PPNG, CMRNG, TRNG) were found to be relatively prevalent and widely distributed in the United States. Unacceptably high failure rates have occurred with ampicillin, amoxicillin, and tetracycline when these agents have been used to treat infections caused by such highly resistant gonococci. Consequently, ceftriaxone and spectinomycin, to which PPNG, CMRNG, and TRNG remain susceptible, have become the agents recommended for treatment of gonococcal infections in the United States [*see Table 1*].[10,27] In areas where highly resistant gonococci, particularly PPNG, constitute less than one percent of all isolates, the previously recommended aqueous procaine penicillin G, amoxicillin, and ampicillin regimens remain effective [*see Table 1*].[2,10,28] Physicians, however, are unlikely to know the susceptibility pattern of gonococci in a given area. Therefore, ceftriaxone, 250 mg I.M., which is the only single-dose regimen effective for uncomplicated anogenital or pharyngeal gonorrhea caused by susceptible strains or by the highly resistant PPNG, CMRNG, and TRNG, has become the treatment of choice.[10,27,28] This single-dose regimen and the higher-dose, multiple-day regimens recommended for disseminated infection are also effective against incubating syphilis.[29]

Patients who are allergic to penicillin and cephalosporins are generally treated with spectinomycin [*see Table 1*]. Spectinomycin in the recommended doses provides effective therapy for urethral, genital, anorectal, and disseminated gonococcal infection in men and women, including in women who are pregnant. However, it does not eradicate pharyngeal infection, nor is it effective against incubating syphilis. Gonococci resistant to spectinomycin have rarely been encountered in the United States; these organisms usually have epidemiologic links to Southeast Asia or Korea.[8] Patients who do not respond to spectinomycin therapy should be treated with ceftriaxone, and the gonococcus should be tested for spectinomycin resistance.

In areas with a low prevalence of penicillin-resistant gonococci (less than one percent of all isolates), single-dose intramuscular procaine penicillin G remains effective for genital, anorectal, and pharyngeal gonorrhea in men and women. It is also effective against incubating syphilis. Its use is limited by pain at the injection site and by potential allergic and procaine-related side effects, which include hallucinations, seizures, fear of impending death, and violent behavior. These symptoms are related to inadvertent intravenous administration of procaine penicillin; they begin immediately after injection and subside in minutes.[30] Single-dose oral ampicillin or amoxicillin is effective treatment, in men and women, for anogenital infections caused by penicillin-susceptible gonococci; however, these regimens do not eradicate gonococci from the pharynx and may not be effective against incubating syphilis. If single-dose ampicillin or amoxicillin is supplemented by the respective agent (500 mg p.o., q.i.d., for three days), pharyngeal infections will be eradicated.[31]

Gonococcal isolates that cause disseminated disease are more susceptible to penicillin, erythromycin, and tetracycline than isolates that do not cause disseminated infection.[32] This observation resulted in treatment of the arthritis-dermatitis syndrome with a shorter course and a lower dose of intravenous penicillin than had been initially thought to be necessary.[33] Although these regimens remain effective for disseminated disease caused by penicillin-susceptible gonococci, disseminated gonorrhea caused by PPNG and CMRNG have been reported.[34,35] It seems prudent, therefore, to initiate therapy with ceftriaxone when penicillin-resistant gonococci are relatively prevalent. If disseminated infection fails to respond to penicillin within 48 to 72 hours, infections caused by resistant organisms must be considered and penicillin therapy must be changed to ceftriaxone or spectinomycin therapy.

Initial outpatient therapy with oral antibiotics for disseminated gonococcal infection is generally not advocated. Hospitalization and treatment with a parenteral antibiotic is preferable until the patient shows definite improvement. Purulent arthritis requires, in addition to these antibiotic regimens, supportive treatment as described for septic arthritis. Open drainage is not required, but repeated joint aspirations

Table 1   Recommended Treatment of Gonococcal Infection

Type of Infection	Therapeutic Regimens (Do not use less than recommended dosages)	Comments
Uncomplicated anogenital infection	Ceftriaxone, 250 mg I.M., in a single dose plus doxycycline, 100 mg p.o., b.i.d., or tetracycline, 500 mg p.o., q.i.d., for seven days to treat presumed coinfection by *Chlamydia trachomatis** *or* Spectinomycin, 2 g I.M., in a single dose plus doxycycline or tetracycline as noted above*	If penicillin-resistant gonococci constitute < 1% of isolates: (1) amoxicillin (3 g p.o.) or ampicillin (3.5 g p.o.) as a single dose plus probenecid (1 g p.o.), or (2) aqueous procaine penicillin G (4.8 million units I.M.) divided between two sites plus probenecid (1 g p.o.) Erythromycin stearate or erythromycin base, 500 mg p.o., q.i.d., for seven days, or erythromycin ethylsuccinate, 800 mg p.o., q.i.d., for seven days, can be used for *C. trachomatis* if tetracyclines are contraindicated or not tolerated Ceftriaxone is probably effective for incubating syphilis
Pharyngeal infection	Ceftriaxone, 250 mg I.M., in a single dose *or* Trimethoprim-sulfamethoxazole (80 mg/400 mg), nine tables p.o. in a single daily dose for five days†	Single-dose amoxicillin, ampicillin, and spectinomycin are ineffective against pharyngeal infection
Uncomplicated anogenital infection during pregnancy	Ceftriaxone, 250 mg I.M., in a single dose *or* Spectinomycin, 2 g I.M., in a single dose†	Trimethoprim-sulfamethoxazole is contraindicated during pregnancy Tetracycline should not be given; erythromycin in doses noted above can be used for coinfecting *C. trachomatis*
Disseminated infection (arthritis-dermatitis syndrome)	Ceftriaxone, 1 g I.V. or I.M. daily for seven days, or cefotaxime, 500 mg I.V. q 6 hr for seven days *or* Spectinomycin, 2 g I.M. q 12 hr for seven days†	In areas where penicillin-resistant gonococci constitute < 1% of isolates, aqueous crystalline penicillin G, 2.5 million units I.V. q 6 hr for at least three days, followed by ampicillin or amoxicillin, 500 mg p.o., q.i.d., for at least four more days, can be used Treat for presumed coinfection with *C. trachomatis* Longer courses and higher doses of ceftriaxone, cefotaxime, or penicillin are required if meningitis, osteomyelitis, or endocarditis is present
Conjunctivitis	Ceftriaxone, 1 g I.V. or I.M. daily for five days, or cefotaxime, 500 mg I.V. q 6 hr for five days plus irrigation of the eye with saline or buffered ophthalmic solution	Aqueous crystalline penicillin G, 2.5 million units I.V. q 6 hr for five days, can be used if infection is caused by penicillin-susceptible gonococci Topical antibiotic therapy alone is inadequate Wound precautions should be instituted for 24 hr to decrease the risk of contagion

Table 1   (continued)

Type of Infection	Therapeutic Regimens (Do not use less than recommended dosages)	Comments
Acute epididymitis	Ceftriaxone, 250 mg I.M., in a single dose *or* Spectinomycin, 2 g I.M., in a single dose†	Treat for presumed coinfection by *C. trachomatis* with doxycycline or tetracycline in doses noted above for anogenital infection; continue treatment for 10 days For epididymitis in homosexual men, use trimethoprim-sulfamethoxazole, an aminoglycoside, or a broad-spectrum cephalosporin unless *C. trachomatis* or gonococci are detected
Neonatal ophthalmitis	Cefotaxime, 25 mg/kg q 8 hr for seven days *or* Ceftriaxone, 125 mg I.M., in a single dose When infection is caused by penicillin-susceptible gonococci, aqueous crystalline penicillin G, 100,000 U/kg/day in four doses for seven days, can be used	Eye irrigations as noted for adult conjunctivitis Patients should be isolated during the initial 24 hr of therapy because of the risk of contagion; parents of patients should also be treated *C. trachomatis* infection should be considered if the response to treatment is unsatisfactory
Neonatal colonization (from an infected mother)	Ceftriaxone, 125 mg I.M., in a single dose	All infants born to mothers with gonorrhea should be treated; prophylaxis for neonatal ophthalmia should be given; evidence of illness necessitates additional treatment
Neonatal disseminated infection	Cefotaxime, 25–50 mg/kg I.V. q 8 hr for 10 to 14 days; for meningitis, cefotazime, 50 mg/kg I.V. q 8 hr for 10 to 14 days	If infection is caused by penicillin-susceptible gonococci, aqueous crystalline penicillin G I.V. can be used; the penicillin dose for an infant younger than one week is 100,000 U/kg/day in two divided doses; penicillin dose for an infant one to four weeks of age is 250,000–300,000 U/kg/day in four divided doses; therapy should be given for at least 10 days
Childhood vulvovaginitis, urethritis, proctitis, pharyngitis‡	Ceftriaxone, 125 mg I.M., in a single dose *or* Spectinomycin, 40 mg/kg I.M., divided between two sites† In areas where penicillin-resistant gonococci are not prevalent (< 1% of isolates): (1) aqueous procaine pencillin G, 100,000 U/kg I.M., divided between two sites and given at one visit, plus probenecid, 25 mg/kg, before the injection, or (2) amoxicillin, 50 mg/kg p.o., plus probenecid, 25 mg/kg, simultaneously	Topical or systemic estrogens are not beneficial in vulvovaginitis The preferred agents for pharyngitis are ceftriaxone and penicillin; as in adults, single-dose amoxicillin and spectinomycin are relatively ineffective against pharyngeal infections

Type of Infection	Therapeutic Regimens (Do not use less than recommended dosages)	Comments
Childhood disseminated infection, ophthalmitis, peritonitis‡	Ceftriaxone, 50 mg/kg (maximum 2 g) I.V. q.i.d. for seven days *or* Cefotaxime, 50 mg/kg/day I.V. in divided doses q 8 hr for seven days In areas where penicillin-resistant gonococci are not prevalent: aqueous penicillin G, 150,000 U/kg/day I.V. in four divided doses for seven days For meningitis: ceftriaxone, 100 mg/kg (maximum, 2 g) I.V. q.i.d., or cefotaxime, 200 mg/kg/day I.V. in divided doses q 6 hr for at least 10 days	Spectinomycin, 40 mg/kg I.M., divided between two sites and given daily for seven days; spectinomycin is not advised for ophthalmitis† Therapy for ophthalmitis includes eye irrigations as noted for adult conjunctivitis

*Doxycycline and tetracycline are contraindicated in pregnancy; staining of the teeth and enamel dysplasia may occur if it is given to children younger than eight years. Tetracycline should be given on an empty stomach, one hour before or two hours after eating.
†Can be used in patients who are allergic to penicillin and cephalosporins but is ineffective against incubating syphilis.
‡Children more than 100 lb (45 kg) should be considered adults for purposes of dose calculations.

may be beneficial. Intra-articular antibiotic injections are not indicated.

Gonococcal meningitis and endocarditis demand prolonged antibiotic treatment and supportive therapy. Antibiotic therapy should be initiated with 2 g of intravenous ceftriaxone daily. If the isolate is subsequently demonstrated to be susceptible to penicillin, treatment may be completed with 20 million units of intravenous penicillin G daily. Patients with endocarditis who have a history of immediate-type hypersensitivity to penicillin (e.g., urticaria and respiratory distress) will require desensitization before ceftriaxone or penicillin therapy is initiated. In lieu of desensitization, patients with meningitis who have this severe form of penicillin allergy may be treated with 4 to 6 g of intravenous chloramphenicol daily for at least 10 days.

The quinolone antibiotics are highly active in vitro against *N. gonorrhoeae*, including strains that are susceptible to penicillins, penicillinase-producing strains, and strains that have chromosomally mediated resistance to penicillins. Oral norfloxacin, given in two 600 mg doses separated by four hours, was as effective as spectinomycin in eradicating urethral infection caused by penicillin-resistant gonococci.[36] Additionally, oral norfloxacin, 800 mg in a single dose, cured uncomplicated urethral infection in men and anogenital infection in women.[37] Oral ciprofloxacin, 250 mg in a single dose, was as effective as the single-dose ampicillin-probenecid regimen in the treatment of men with uncomplicated urethral infection caused by β-lactamase–negative gonococci.[38] Although the quinolone antibiotics provide effective therapy for uncomplicated gonorrhea, they do not eradicate coinfecting *C. trachomatis*.

Fifteen to 30 percent of heterosexual men with gonococcal urethritis are simultaneously infected with *C. trachomatis*. In 25 to 50 percent of women with gonorrhea, there is a simultaneous *C. trachomatis* cervical infection. Only five to 10 percent of homosexual men with gonorrhea have urethral or rectal coinfection with *C. trachomatis*. Ceftriaxone, spectinomycin, penicillin, ampicillin, and amoxicillin are ineffective against *C. trachomatis*. Given the frequency of coinfection with *N. gonorrhoeae* and *C. trachomatis* and the morbidity of untreated *Chlamydia* infection, tetracycline or doxycycline is recommended as supplemental therapy for patients with gonorrhea. Erythromycin can be used as supplemental therapy when tetracycline is contraindicated (e.g., during pregnancy or in young children) or when it is not tolerated. Supplemental treatment will prevent postgonococcal urethritis in men and mucopurulent cervicitis and chlamydial pelvic inflammatory disease in women. Because of the prevalence of gonococci resistant to tetracyclines, these agents are no longer recommended as primary therapy for gonorrhea.

All patients treated for gonorrhea, including persons treated a second time because of failure of initial therapy, should be evaluated five to 14 days later. Cultures should be obtained from previously infected areas; rectal cultures should always be obtained from females and homosexual males. Gonococcal isolates from patients in whom treatment has failed should be tested for antibiotic resistance. Patients with infection caused by antibiotic-resistant gonococci must be reported to local public health authorities. Their contacts must be identified and treated.

When a patient is treated for gonorrhea, evidence of syphilis should be sought on physical examination and by serologic testing. In patients who exhibit no evidence of syphilis and who receive the recommended ceftriaxone or aqueous procaine penicillin G regimen, a follow-up evaluation is unnecessary; the ceftriaxone and penicillin G regimens eradicate incubating *Treponema pallidum*.[29,39] Patients treated for gonorrhea with ampicillin, amoxicillin, or spectinomycin, however, require follow-up serologic tests at six weeks and at three months after therapy. If infectious syphilis is discovered or if a serologic test is positive, therapy dictated by the stage of syphilis should be administered in addition to the therapy for gonorrhea. The possibility of coinfection with human immunodeficiency virus (HIV) should be considered, particularly in homosexual men; more vigorous therapy for syphilis is required when HIV is present.[40,41]

Other Sexually Transmitted Diseases

Infection in Homosexual Men

Homosexual men are at increased risk for pharyngeal and anorectal infection with the classic sexually transmitted pathogens and for enteric infection with pathogens transmitted through the fecal-oral route. Promiscuity, direct oral-anal contact, fellatio, and anal intercourse are contributing factors. Simultaneous infection with multiple pathogens is common and must always be considered. HIV infection should also always be considered.

Anorectal gonorrhea is common in homosexual men, and 20 percent of patients are asymptomatic. The 80 percent of infected patients who are symptomatic frequently complain of pruritus ani, pain on defecation, mucopurulent discharge, and constipation. Sigmoidoscopic abnormalities are usually limited to the anal canal and rectum, where an inflamed, edematous, friable, and sometimes ulcerated mucosa may be seen. These findings, however, are not specific for gonococcal infection. Twenty percent of patients with proved anorectal infection show normal findings on anoscopy. Mucopus for Gram's-stained smear and culture may be obtained under direct vision via the anoscope. Although such smears may suggest gonorrhea, they are not diagnostic. Cultures of mucopus planted on Thayer-Martin or transgrow medium should be used for the diagnosis.

Although uncommon, anogenital infection caused by *N. meningitidis* has been increasing in frequency among homosexual males. Meningococci have been isolated from the anal canal in two percent of this group.[42] Meningococci infecting the urogenital tract and anal canal cause a spectrum of illness similar to that produced by gonococci and should be treated with the regimen recommended for the analogous gonococcal infection [*see Table 1*].

After gonococci, herpes simplex virus is most frequently isolated from the rectum of homosexual men with symptomatic anorectal disease. Patients with primary anorectal herpes simplex virus infection experience marked local pain, tenesmus, constipation, and mucopurulent rectal discharge. Fever, chills, sacral paresthesias, and acute urinary retention are common. Perianal and rectal vesicular lesions or ulcerations may be absent. Ulceration and extensive inflammation of the bowel mucosa are confined to the distal 20 cm, particularly the distal 10 cm, of the rectosigmoid colon. Diagnosis is established by culture of the virus or demonstration of seroconversion.[43]

Severe acute ulcerative proctitis with granulomatous inflammation histologically resembling Crohn's disease has been associated with *Chlamydia* of the lymphogranuloma venereum (LGV) immunotypes. In contrast, *C. trachomatis* organisms that do not have LGV immunotypes have been isolated from asymptomatic men who practice anal-receptive intercourse. Infection with non-LGV *Chlamydia* is associated with polymorphonuclear leukocytes in the rectal mucopus, mild mucosal abnormalities noted at sigmoidoscopy, and mild nongranulomatous inflammation of the rectal mucosa. Isolation of *Chlamydia* from the rectal mucosa or demonstration of seroconversion in paired serum samples establishes the diagnosis. Tetracycline, 500 mg four times daily for two to three weeks, is suggested.[44]

The diagnosis of anorectal *T. pallidum* infection may be difficult. Symptoms are mild, and a local chancre may be missed. The diagnosis is based on anoscopy with dark-field examination of perianal lesions and on serologic findings.

In homosexual men, acute epididymitis is likely to be caused by coliform bacteria or *Hemophilus* species and is associated with fever and prominent symptoms.[45] In contrast, acute epididymitis in sexually active heterosexual men younger than 35 years usually occurs in conjunction with urethritis and is caused by *N. gonorrhoeae* and *C. trachomatis*. Epididymitis in homosexual men is often associated with urethritis and bacteriuria, and organisms are visible on Gram's stain of the urine and recoverable on urine culture; how-

ever, underlying obstructive genitourinary pathology is not present. Trimethoprim-sulfamethoxazole, an aminoglycoside, or a broad-spectrum cephalosporin might be appropriate treatment of epididymitis in homosexual men, pending the results of diagnostic tests (i.e., urethral studies to detect gonococci and *C. trachomatis* and urine cultures).

Homosexual men are at increased risk of infection with enteric bacterial pathogens and parasites. Among these are *Shigella*, *Salmonella*, *Campylobacter jejuni*, *Entamoeba histolytica*, and *Giardia lamblia*. These men are also at increased risk for hepatitis A, hepatitis B, and cytomegalovirus infection.

Acute Pelvic Inflammatory Disease

Except in cases involving recent abortion, parturition, or pelvic surgical procedure, acute pelvic inflammatory disease (PID) arises when microorganisms migrate from the vagina and endocervix to the endometrium, fallopian tubes, and adjacent structures. Persistent salpingitis causes luminal scarring and blocks the fimbriated ends, which may cause tubal abscess. Infertility caused by fallopian tube damage, the major residual morbidity linked to acute PID, increases with the severity and number of infections. PID is also associated with an increased risk of ectopic pregnancy and a high frequency of lower abdominal pain.

Formerly, acute PID was considered almost exclusively gonococcal in etiology. It is now recognized that many microorganisms, including aerobic and anaerobic bacteria found in fecal and cervicovaginal flora (especially *Bacteroides* species and anaerobic gram-positive cocci), are implicated in at least half of the cases. The recovery of *N. gonorrhoeae*, alone or with other organisms, from the pelvic peritoneum of women with acute PID has been associated with the presence of gonococci in the endocervical canal.[25] These observations suggest that the endocervical gonococci play a causative role in acute PID. Cultures from the cul-de-sac and peritoneal cavity, however, generally yield gonococci less frequently than do cultures from the endocervix. It has been postulated that an initial gonococcal infection damages the salpinx and thus plays a preparatory role in the development of acute or recurrent PID caused by cervicovaginal commensals. The isolation of gonococci from the endocervix of patients with acute PID certainly neither guarantees that salpingitis is caused by *N. gonorrhoeae* nor excludes a role for other microorganisms. In practice, however, gonococci isolated from the endocervix of women with acute PID are considered to be primary pathogens or to play a preparatory role in the infection. The recovery of bacteria other than gonococci from the endocervix does not indicate the participation of these organisms as pathogens in the upper genital tract.

Endocervical cultures yield *N. gonorrhoeae* in 40 to 60 percent of women with PID.[25,46] Recovery of gonococci is more likely when the onset of symptoms occurs during menstruation, the patient lacks a history of PID, there is an endocervical exudate with gram-negative diplococci resembling gonococci within three or more leukocytes, or the patient's sexual partner has gonorrhea.[25,47]

C. trachomatis is another primary cause of salpingitis. It has been isolated from the fallopian tubes of 30 percent of women with acute salpingitis in Scandinavia, and it appears to cause a milder but more protracted illness than that associated with *N. gonorrhoeae*.[48,49] *C. trachomatis* is an important cause of acute PID in nonhospitalized women in North America. Serologic data suggest chlamydial involvement in as many as 50 percent of acute PID episodes.[50,51] Like gonococci, *C. trachomatis* plays a preparatory role for acute PID caused by cervicovaginal commensals and a significant etiologic role in tubal infertility.

Although their causative role in acute PID is less certain, *Mycoplasma hominis* and *Ureaplasma urealyticum* have been isolated from the fallopian tubes of four and eight percent of patients with PID, respectively, which suggests that these pathogens do play a causative role in some cases.[52]

The factors associated with an increased risk of acute PID include intercourse at a young age, multiple sexual partners, and a sexual partner or partners with untreated urethritis.[51] The method of contraception may also alter the risk of acute PID and may influence which pathogens cause infection. Intrauterine contraceptive devices (IUDs) increase the risk of nongonococcal acute PID, especially during the initial months after insertion and with prolonged use. IUDs have been associated specifically with rare cases of acute PID caused by *Actinomyces* species.[53] Oral contraceptives have been reported to decrease the risk of acute PID; however, careful analysis suggests that the decreased risk may be related only to gonococcal PID and that the risk of acute PID from *C. trachomatis* may be enhanced by use of oral contraceptives.[51,54] Barrier or mechanical methods of contraception (i.e., condoms, diaphragms, and spermicidal agents) reduce the risk of PID, compared with other methods or with no form of contraception.[51]

The clinical features of acute PID vary in severity and lack diagnostic specificity. Symptoms of acute PID begin most often during or immediately after menstruation. Lower abdominal pain and tenderness, adnexal tenderness on pelvic examination, and pain on movement of the cervix are found in 90 percent of patients. Less common symptoms are increased vaginal discharge (55 percent), fever or chills (40 percent), and irregular vaginal bleeding (35 percent). Anorexia, nausea, and vomiting with marked pelvic peritonitis occur in 25 percent of cases. A leukocytosis and an elevated erythrocyte sedimentation rate are common but not always present. The uterus is tender but not enlarged. Swelling of the adnexa or a true adnexal mass is noted in 50 percent of patients. Occasionally, infection spreads along the paracolic gutters to the upper abdomen. This upper abdominal infection can produce two syndromes: (1) upper quadrant abdominal pain with or without pain referred to the corresponding shoulder and (2) perihepatitis with mild liver function test abnormalities (Fitz-Hugh–Curtis syndrome). Recognition of acute PID and prompt response to antibiotics help distinguish gonococcal perihepatitis from cholecystitis. Perihepatitis has accompanied both gonococcal and chlamydial salpingitis.[50]

It is difficult to diagnose acute PID. In a large series, the clinical diagnosis of acute salpingitis was confirmed at laparoscopy in only 65 percent of patients.[55] Other lower abdominal or pelvic processes, such as appendicitis, hemorrhagic corpus luteum, pelvic endometriosis, ectopic pregnancy, mesenteric adenitis, and ovarian tumors, were found in 12 percent of patients and were indistinguishable clinically from acute PID. In the remaining 23 percent, laparoscopic findings were normal. In this study, although no single symptom or noninvasive laboratory test finding was diagnostic of acute PID, the likelihood of a negative laparoscopy diminished as the number of symptoms and signs increased. The full constellation of findings occurred in only 20 percent of patients with acute PID; even so, acute PID was indistinguishable from other pelvic diseases. Other reports of laparoscopic findings in women with clinically diagnosed acute PID also reveal the poor correlation between the visualized pathology and the clinical impression.[51] It has been suggested that the clinical diagnosis of acute PID be reserved for women with direct lower abdominal tenderness (with or without rebound tenderness), cervical motion tenderness, adnexal tenderness, and at least one of the following signs: Gram's stain of an endocervical smear that contains intracellular gram-negative diplococci, elevated temperature, leukocytosis, purulent material on culdocentesis, or a pelvic inflammatory complex (abscess) revealed by sonogram or bimanual examination.[56] Confirmation of the diagnosis is suggested by a response to antibiotics. When the patient's symptoms do not fit the above criteria, when the distinction between acute PID and other pelvic diseases is uncertain, or when the disease is unusually severe, a definitive diagnosis should be established by laparoscopy or laparotomy.

Hospitalization for the treatment of acute PID is recommended when (1) the diagnosis is uncertain or a surgical emergency must be excluded, (2) a pelvic abscess is suspected, (3) the patient is an adolescent, (4) an IUD is in place, (5) there is severe illness, (6) the patient is pregnant, (7) vomiting or patient unreliability precludes adherence to an oral regimen, (8) outpatient therapy fails, (9) there is generalized peritonitis, or (10) clinical reevaluation in 48 to 72 hours cannot be arranged.

Because gonococcal and nongonococcal acute PID are clinically indistinguishable and direct culture from the site of infection is often infeasible or inappropriate, initial antibiotic therapy should cover the broad range of potential pathogens most likely to be present on the basis of epidemiologic and clinical data [*see Table 2*]. Whether acute PID is gonococcal or nongonococcal, patients usually show improvement within 48 to 72 hours and are usually asymptomatic within five days after treatment is started; 80 percent of effectively treated patients have a normal pelvic examination by the seventh day of therapy.

The ambulatory patient with mild PID may be treated with single-dose antigonococcal therapy followed by the tetracycline or doxycycline regimen [*see Table 1*]. If antigonococcal therapy is selected with appropriate consideration for the frequency of PPNG and CMRNG in the area, this combination will provide activity against *N. gonorrhoeae, C. trachomatis, and M. hominis.*

This recommendation is based on the observation that mild, uncomplicated PID is most likely the result of either gonococci or *Chlamydia,* or both, and that unacceptably high failure rates are associated with therapy that does not eradicate both of these organisms.[51]

The acutely ill hospitalized patient requires parenterally administered, broad-spectrum antimicrobial coverage [*see Table 2*]. The antibacterial spectrum of cefoxitin includes, in addition to gonococci, many gram-negative bacilli and many anaerobic bacteria, including *B. fragilis.* Cefoxitin is well tolerated and can be given in conjunction with doxycycline or tetracycline, either of which will treat *Chlamydia, Mycoplasma,*

Table 2   Treatment of Acute Pelvic Inflammatory Disease

	Regimen	Comment
Outpatient	Cefoxitin, 2 g I.M., and probenecid, 1 g p.o., each in a single dose plus either doxycycline, 100 mg p.o., b.i.d., for 10 to 14 days, or tetracycline, 500 mg p.o., q.i.d., for 10 to 14 days[*] *or* Ceftriaxone, 250 mg I.M., in a single dose plus doxycycline or tetracycline as noted above[*]	In areas where penicillin-resistant gonococci are not prevalent ($< 1\%$ of all gonococci), the single-dose procaine penicillin G regimen or the ampicillin or amoxicillin regimen for anogenital gonorrhea [*see Table 1*] can be used instead of cefoxitin or ceftriaxone Spectinomycin, 2 g I.M. in a single dose, is used instead of cephalosporins in allergic patients Sexual contacts should be treated with the regimen used for anogenital gonorrhea [*see Table 1*]
Hospitalized patient	Cefoxitin, 2 g I.V. q 6 hr, plus tetracycline, 1.5–2.0 g/day (maximum dose) I.V. in divided doses q 6 hr, or doxycycline, 100 mg I.V. q 12 hr. Continue I.V. therapy until patient shows definite improvement; then, complete a minimum of 10 to 14 days of therapy with doxycycline, 100 mg p.o., b.i.d.	If the patient is unusually ill or if initial therapy is ineffective: 1. Confirm the diagnosis 2. Reassess the etiology of the infection with culdocentesis or laparoscopic specimens 3. Revise antibiotic therapy based on bacteriologic data; if none are available, consider parenteral clindamycin plus an aminoglycoside or imipenem-cilastatin

[*]Both tetracycline and doxycycline are contraindicated in pregnancy and generally are not recommended for use in azotemic patients; either drug should be given on an empty stomach, one hour before or two hours after eating.

and *U. urealyticum* infections and will enhance antibiotic activity against cervicovaginal commensal bacteria. These antibiotics are continued intravenously for at least four days and for 48 hours after fever resolves. Thereafter, a 10- to 14-day antibiotic course can be completed with the administration of doxycycline.

The more severe and difficult to treat episodes of PID, especially those that are recurrent, are usually caused by multiple cervicovaginal commensals. Ideally, in this setting, antibiotic therapy is based on specific bacteriologic data obtained at laparoscopy or culdocentesis. If specific data are not available, empirical therapy with either clindamycin (900 mg I.V. every eight hours) and gentamicin (1.5 mg/kg I.V. every eight hours, which should be adjusted for patients with renal dysfunction) or with imipenem-cilastatin (500 mg I.V. every six hours) will provide broad coverage against facultative gram-negative rods and anaerobic bacteria. Neither regimen is effective treatment for *C. trachomatis*; hence, follow-up therapy with a tetracycline should be administered. Clindamycin and gentamicin are not optimal therapy for *N. gonorrhoeae*; therefore, if previous therapy for gonococci has not been given, ceftriaxone should be given with the initial doses of these drugs. Antibiotic therapy for these difficult episodes of PID should be carefully designed with consideration of the pathogens that are likely to have played a preparatory role, including gonococci and *Chlamydia*. The potential toxicities of the antimicrobials selected should also be considered.

Bed rest and abstinence from sexual intercourse are recommended during treatment for PID. IUDs should be removed after initiating antibiotic therapy, and an alternate method of contraception should be provided. Sexual partners, even if asymptomatic, must be evaluated for gonococcal and chlamydial infections and appropriately treated.

Patients with acute PID should be reexamined on the third day of therapy to assess the response to treatment. Failure of initial therapy is indicated by persistent fever after four days of treatment, fever with a rising white blood cell count, worsening abdominal pain, or the appearance of an adnexal mass during therapy.[51] Failure to respond requires reevaluation of the initial diagnosis with laparoscopy, sonography, or computed tomography to search for a tubo-ovarian abscess or other lower abdominal or pelvic disorder. It should be noted that more than 50 percent of tubo-ovarian abscesses will respond to intensive antibiotic therapy; however, careful follow-up is required to ensure progressive improvement. Tubo-ovarian abscesses that do not respond to antibiotics require surgical treatment.[57] Patients with acute PID should also be reexamined a week after completion of therapy to evaluate final response to therapy and to reculture for *N. gonorrhoeae*.

Nongonococcal Urethritis and Cervicitis

Nongonococcal urethritis (NGU) and nongonococcal cervicitis are more prevalent than gonococcal infections of the urethra and endocervix. *C. trachomatis* causes about 50 percent of cases of NGU[58] and cervical infections.[59] *U. urealyticum* has been associated with a *Chlamydia*-negative NGU syndrome.

There are clinical and epidemiologic differences between gonococcal urethritis and NGU, but they are insufficient for making a definitive diagnosis.[24,58] Males with NGU are more likely than males with gonococcal urethritis to be white, less sexually active, and either employed or in school. Patients with gonococcal urethritis complain of dysuria and a spontaneous purulent urethral discharge of recent onset (most often, less than four days) more frequently than patients with NGU. In patients with NGU, the symptoms of urethritis last longer (in most, more than four days), and the urethral discharge is scanty, nonspontaneous, and mucoid. Minimally symptomatic or asymptomatic *C. trachomatis* urethral infection is not uncommon in sexually active males.

The diagnosis of NGU is made when *N. gonorrhoeae* is absent and any of the following three features is found: (1) urethral discharge, (2) 15 or more polymorphonuclear leukocytes (PMNs) per high-power microscopic field in the sediment from the first 10 to 15 ml of voided urine, or (3) an average of four or more PMNs in five high-power fields of a Gram's-stained urethral exudate or swab specimen.[58] An increased number of PMNs in the urethral exudate is central to this diagnosis. Dysuria in the absence of these diagnostic criteria should not be equated with NGU. Culture of the urethral discharge for *N. gonorrhoeae* is required to differentiate definitively between gonococcal and nongonococcal urethritis. In 85 percent of males with urethritis, a tentative classification of infection can be made by examination of Gram's-stained smears of the discharge for the presence or absence of gram-negative intracellular diplococci with the typical appearance of gonococci.[24] Cultures are required for classification of the remaining 15 percent who have equivocal smears.

Postgonococcal urethritis (PGU), an NGU syndrome in men that emerges after treatment of gonorrhea with penicillins, cephalosporins, or spectinomycin, is primarily caused by *C. trachomatis*, although other agents may play a causative role. PGU develops when men who have simultaneous gonococcal and nongonococcal urethral infections are treated with an antibiotic that eradicates only the gonococci.[60,61] PGU may present as a continued symptomatic urethritis after eradication of gonococcal infection or, more commonly, as a recrudescence of urethritis without evidence of gonorrhea two to three weeks after treatment of gonorrhea. Gonococcal urethritis caused by treatment failure or reinfection must be distinguished from PGU.

The frequency of coinfection with gonococci and *C. trachomatis* in heterosexual men and, to a lesser extent, in homosexual men has resulted in the recommendation that all patients with gonorrhea be treated with a regimen directed against both *N. gonorrhoeae* and the organisms that commonly cause NGU, *C. trachomatis* and *U. urealyticum*. This practice will eliminate most cases of PGU and reduce the transmission of *Chlamydia*.

C. trachomatis infection of the genitourinary tract in women causes 30 to 50 percent of the cases of mucopurulent cervicitis[50] and an acute urethral syndrome (dysuria and frequency when the urine contains fewer than 10^5 bacteria/ml).[62] Mucopurulent cervicitis, which may be asymptomatic, is characterized by a mucopurulent endocervical exudate, local edema, and ectopic columnar epithelium on the exocervix. Herpes simplex virus or gonococcus may cause cervical infection and should be considered in the differential diagnosis.

Many women with the acute urethral syndrome and pyuria (urine sediment with 10 PMNs per high-power microscopic field) have *C. trachomatis* infection or bacteriuria. The urine from these women, however, is marked by fewer than 105 organisms/ml.[62] Another study suggests that the diagnostic criterion for lower urinary tract coliform infection in women with acute dysuria and frequency should be 102 coliform organisms per milliliter of midstream clean-catch urine.63 In patients who had bacteriuria, abrupt onset of symptoms and microscopic or gross hematuria were typical findings. In those with chlamydial infection, association with a new sexual partner during the previous month was characteristic.

In patients with the acute urethral syndrome and pyuria[64] or with mucopurulent cervicitis, tetracycline effectively eliminates symptoms.[65] The regimen used for NGU (see below) is recommended. The agent does not alleviate symptoms in women who have the acute urethral syndrome but do not have pyuria.

C. trachomatis urethritis and cervicitis can be effectively treated with sulfisoxazole, tetracycline, or erythromycin. Most *Ureaplasma* organisms are susceptible to tetracycline, erythromycin, and aminoglycosides but not to sulfisoxazole. Because the techniques used to distinguish chlamydial infections from *Ureaplasma* infections are generally unavailable, an antimicrobial effective against both organisms is employed in the treatment of NGU or mucopurulent cervicitis.[50] Tetracycline (500 mg p.o., q.i.d., for seven days) is recommended and is the least expensive regimen. Treatment with doxycycline (100 mg p.o., b.i.d., for at least seven days) is also effective. Erythromycin base or stearate (500 mg p.o., q.i.d., for seven days) and erythromycin ethyl succinate (800 mg p.o., q.i.d., for seven days) are suitable alternatives and are preferred for pregnant women.[50]

Symptomatic or asymptomatic infection with *C. trachomatis* is frequently found in the sexual partner of an individual with chlamydial infection. Therapy for NGU or mucopurulent cervicitis should therefore be extended simultaneously to the partner to prevent reinfection. Even when both partners are appropriately treated, NGU relapse is common. Recurrence is most common in patients from whom neither *Chlamydia* nor *Ureaplasma* organisms were initially isolated and is usually not associated with an identifiable etiologic agent. A second treatment with the same regimen for a longer period or with an alternate regimen is recommended. Symptomatic NGU that persists during tetracycline therapy may be caused by tetracycline-resistant *U. urealyticum* and warrants treatment with erythromycin, to which this organism is susceptible.[66] Rarely, *Trichomonas vaginalis* has been the cause of persistent nongonococcal urethritis.[67]

Infection with *C. trachomatis* has become the most prevalent sexually transmitted disease. This organism is a major cause of morbidity and has led to an increase in health-care costs, particularly in sexually active women but also in men and infants; it is an important cause of neonatal ophthalmitis and pneumonia in infants. Considerations of morbidity, cost of treatment, and the public health suggest that cervical and urethral smears should be used to screen sexually active individuals who on presentation would not otherwise require antichlamydial therapy.[50] Screening should be considered for those attending sexually transmitted disease and family planning clinics, sexually active persons younger than 30 years (especially adolescents), and persons with multiple sexual partners. Among sexually active persons, considerations of the morbidity and frequency of infection suggest that the priorities for screening should be women, then heterosexual men, and lastly, homosexual men. Previously, *C. trachomatis* infections were considered more prevalent in lower socioeconomic urban settings. However, the prevalence of *Chlamydia* infections in sexually active suburban adolescents and college students has increased, and screening of this population is recommended.[68] The prevalence of *C. trachomatis* infection in neonates suggests that pregnant women should be screened if they are younger than 20 years, are unmarried, are married and have multiple sexual partners, or have a history of another sexually transmitted disease. Studies indicate that in neonates, topical ocular prophylaxis with silver nitrate drops, tetracycline ointment, or erythromycin ointment is only partially effective in preventing chlamydial ophthalmitis and does not prevent chlamydial pneumonitis.[69,70]

Vaginitis

Vaginitis is characterized by an abnormal vaginal discharge and is a manifestation of local infection with *T. vaginalis*, *Candida* species (primarily *C. albicans*), or *Gardnerella vaginalis* (formerly *H. vaginalis* or *Corynebacterium vaginale*). *N. gonorrhoeae* does not usually infect the vagina in women, but true gonococcal vulvovaginitis may be seen in prepubertal girls.

Vaginitis caused by sexually transmitted *T. vaginalis* is as common as gonorrhea in sexually active women. Although many women with *T. vaginalis* demonstrable in vaginal secretions are asymptomatic, most women with heavy infection complain of labial pruritus or vaginal discharge, or both.

Dyspareunia is often noted, and dysuria from labial irritation occurs frequently. Symptoms often coincide with or immediately follow menstruation. A copious, yellow-green, foul-smelling, frothy vaginal discharge is a classic symptom. Usually, however, vaginal secretions are less characteristic. The vagina and cervix may appear granular, and punctate mucosal hemorrhages are occasionally seen. *T. vaginalis* can be cultured from the vagina and paraurethral glands in 98 percent of infected patients, from the urethra in 82 percent, and from the endocervix in 13 percent. In 65 percent of women with trichomonal infection, *T. vaginalis* can be seen on a Papanicolaou smear.

Candidal vaginitis usually results from an overgrowth of endogenous *Candida* rather than from venereal infection. *Candida* organisms in small quantities are recovered from the vaginal secretions of 25 to 50 percent of asymptomatic women. Increased colonization and symptomatic vaginitis are associated with diabetes, hypoparathyroidism, altered host defenses, corticosteroid therapy, broad-spectrum antibiotic therapy, oral contraceptive medications, and pregnancy. Pruritus and discharge are the major symptoms of candidal vaginitis. Dyspareunia occurs occasionally. Erythema of the vulva and vulvovaginal thrush may be seen. A typical candidal intertriginous eruption with small satellite pustules may involve the perineal skin. The onset of candidal vaginitis usually precedes the menstrual period and is associated with a thick, white, curdlike discharge.

A third form of vaginitis, nonspecific vaginitis, is seen in the absence of gonorrhea, trichomoniasis, candidiasis, and genital herpesvirus infection. It is characterized by a scanty, nonirritating, malodorous discharge. Pruritus is mild, and dyspareunia is exceptionally rare. *G. vaginalis* has been associated with nonspecific vaginitis; however, the significance of this association is controversial. In one study, *G. vaginalis* was recovered from vaginal cultures as frequently in women without abnormal discharge as in women with abnormal discharge.[71] Furthermore, inoculating large numbers of these bacteria into the vagina of normal women initiates vaginitis at a low frequency. Some observations imply that nonspecific vaginitis is a synergistic infection that requires the presence of both *G. vaginalis* and anaerobic bacteria.[72,73] Supporting this idea is the finding that increased concentrations of *Bacteroides* species and *Peptococcus* species and their organic acid metabolites can be demonstrated in the vaginal secretions of female patients with nonspecific vaginitis.[66]

Identifying the Disease Agent

Determination of the causative agent of vaginitis is based on microscopic examination of the vaginal discharge. A saline wet mount of the vaginal secretions should be promptly examined for motile, ovoid flagellated trichomonads, which indicate trichomoniasis. Use of a douche within 24 hours before examination reduces the frequency with which trichomonads are seen. In nonspecific vaginitis, the saline wet mount contains a small number of leukocytes and large epithelial cells stippled with bacteria that obscure the cell borders (clue cells). A potassium hydroxide wet mount aids recognition of the yeast and pseudohyphal forms of *Candida*. *T. vaginalis* can be seen on Giemsa-stained smears of vaginal secretions. *Candida* and *G. vaginalis* can be seen on Gram's stains.

The pH of vaginal secretions from women with candidal vaginitis is lower than 4.5; the pH of secretions from women with nonspecific vaginitis or *T. vaginalis* infection is usually at least 5.5. When the discharge from patients with nonspecific vaginitis is mixed with potassium hydroxide in the preparation of a wet mount, a fishy, aminelike odor is generated.[72] The odor may be considered an additional clue to nonspecific vaginitis, although it is occasionally noted in trichomoniasis; the odor is not found in candidal vaginitis. Multiple pathogens coexist in some patients. Studies designed to exclude gonorrhea are always indicated for sexually active patients who present with vaginitis.

Treatment

Metronidazole is the drug of choice for trichomonal vaginitis. Because of its simplicity, the recommended regimen is a single 2 g oral dose.[74] However, multiple-dose metronidazole (250 mg p.o., t.i.d., for 10 days) is slightly more effective than the single-dose regimen. Each regimen is associated with an 80 to 95 percent cure rate.[74] Patients in whom treatment fails usually respond to a second course of therapy. *T. vaginalis* resistant to metronidazole has been observed, however, and may be responsible for some failures of metronidazole therapy. The male sexual partner, regardless of symptoms, should be simultaneously treated to prevent reinfection of the woman. A single 2 g oral dose of metronidazole is used. Women with asymptomatic *T. vaginalis* infection should be treated as noted. Metronidazole has been associated with a reaction similar to that of disulfiram (Antabuse) when alcoholic beverages are drunk during therapy. Metronidazole should not be taken during pregnancy. Although experience is limited, clotrimazole is considered acceptable during pregnancy. This agent may provide symptomatic relief; it cures 50 percent of trichomonal infections. Clotrimazole, in a 100 mg dose, is administered intravaginally at bedtime for seven days.

Candida vaginitis is treated topically with nystatin, miconazole, or clotrimazole; the last two agents are more effective than nystatin. Boric acid powder, 600 mg in a gelatin capsule administered intravaginally at bedtime for two weeks, is also effective in providing symptomatic relief and eradicating yeast. Boric acid is inexpensive, and adverse reactions are rare.[74] Treatment failures or relapses are common. They are usually associated with abbreviated courses of therapy or failure to eliminate a precipitating factor, such as corticosteroid or antibiotic therapy. Rarely, the male sexual partner has a *Candida* balanitis, which should be treated topically with an anti-*Candida* agent.

Asymptomatic male sexual partners do not need treatment.

Nonspecific vaginitis is treated with metronidazole (500 mg p.o., b.i.d., for seven days).[71] Ampicillin (500 mg p.o., q.i.d., for seven days) has been used but is less effective. The efficacy of metronidazole may be the result of its action against the anaerobic bacteria noted in vaginal secretions of these women. The benefits produced by metronidazole in treatment of this mild infection must be weighed against the drug's potential toxicity. Although nonspecific vaginitis may be sexually transmissible, the benefits of routinely treating the male sexual partners have not been established. Simultaneous treatment of the male sexual partner with ampicillin may be indicated in a patient with recurrent nonspecific vaginitis.

Chancroid

Chancroid, an acute venereal infection caused by *H. ducreyi*, is manifested by a ragged exudative ulcer usually involving the external genitalia. *H. ducreyi* is a small, pleomorphic gram-negative rod that is difficult to recover from infected patients; it requires special culture media on which to grow.[75] Although the distribution of chancroid is worldwide, it is more common in tropical and subtropical areas and has been associated with poor standards of hygiene. The infection is more common in men than in women.

The initial lesion of chancroid, a small papule at the inoculation site, is usually seen after a two- to five-day incubation period. This papule rapidly undergoes a sequence of vesiculation, pustulation, and finally, ulceration. The ulcer enlarges rapidly, forming an irregular, purulent, exudative, painful lesion with ragged, undermined edges. In contrast to the characteristic syphilitic chancre, these lesions are not infiltrated—hence the name chancroid, or soft chancre. Multiple lesions may develop as a result of autoinoculation. In men, lesions involve the prepuce, coronal sulcus, and frenulum, whereas in women, the labia, clitoris, fourchette, vestibule, and

perianal region are most commonly involved. Within one to two weeks, inguinal adenopathy, usually unilateral, develops in about 50 percent of untreated patients. The involved node is initially firm and tender. Progressive infection results in further enlargement and tenderness of the node (bubo), and subsequently, a fluctuant unilocular mass is formed. The overlying skin may become thin and erythematous, and the node may drain spontaneously, causing a large irregular inguinal crater. Systemic manifestations of chancroid are minimal except for a moderate fever and malaise, which may accompany the bubo. Occasionally, the initial ulcer is secondarily infected by fusobacteria, spirochetes, and *Bacteroides,* and it becomes phagedenic. Such ulcers enlarge rapidly, destroy tissue, and cause a foul-smelling discharge. To avoid mutilating tissue loss, they must be promptly recognized and treated.

Chancroid is suggested by the presence of painful exudative genital ulcers. Diagnosis requires isolation of *H. ducreyi* from the ulcer or inguinal bubo. To obtain material, debris should first be cleaned away by abrading the ulcer with gauze soaked in normal saline. Then, with a cotton-tipped swab, material for culture can be obtained and planted on a special selective medium. Pus aspirated from a bubo may reliably reveal the organism on Gram's stain and provide more optimal material for culture than a specimen from the ulcer. Often, the diagnosis is presumptive, based on history, clinical findings, and absence of other pathogens. Before treatment, dark-field examinations for *T. pallidum* and a Giemsa-stained smear for the Donovan bodies associated with granuloma inguinale are required. By microscopic examinations of scrapings from the ulcers and by the clinical features of the illness, chancroid can be distinguished from other genital ulcers of venereal origin [*see Table 3*]. The extragenital features of Behçet's and Reiter's syndromes and erythema multiforme (Stevens-Johnson syndrome) allow these two illnesses to be distinguished from chancroid.

Table 3   Clinical Features of Genital Ulcers

Disease	Nature of Genital Ulcer	Incubation Period (Range)	Painful	Extent of Inguinal Adenopathy	Laboratory Studies	Other Considerations
Chancroid	Irregular; purulent; undermined edges; not indurated; multiple ulcers	2–12 days	Yes	Present in 50%; usually unilocular; if fluctuant, very painful; may form crater	Small gram-negative rods; parallel ("school of fish") alignment	—
Granuloma inguinale	Extensive, progressive indolent granulation-like tissue; rolled edges	1–12 weeks	Mildly	Pseudobuboes; inguinal subcutaneous granuloma after 1 to 2 months	Donovan bodies in macrophages	—
Syphilis	Indurated, relatively clean base; heals spontaneously	2 weeks or longer	No	Firm, rubbery nodes; not tender	Dark field reveals spirochete (*Treponema pallidum*)	Serologic test positive in the late stage of the ulcer; condyloma latum of the vulva and anal region during secondary disease
Lympho-granuloma venereum (LGV)	Usually not observed; small and shallow; rapid spontaneous healing	5–21 days	No	More common in males than in females; nodes in matted clusters; unilateral or, often, bilateral multiloculated fluctuance; painful groove sign; sinus tracts common	LGV serology positive; Frei test positive 40 days after primary lesion	—

Table 3 *(continued)*

Disease	Nature of Genital Ulcer	Incubation Period (Range)	Painful	Extent of Inguinal Adenopathy	Laboratory Studies	Other Considerations
Herpes simplex virus type 2 infection	Multiple, small, grouped vesicles coalesce and form shallow ulcers; can have extensive vulvovaginitis	2–7 days	Yes	Tender bilateral adenopathy	Tzanck preparation with multi-nucleate giant cells	Recurs in same area; primary infection associated with fever and malaise
Trauma	Purulent; foul smell; secondarily infected	Days	Mildly	Reactive nodes common	Bacteria of mixed morphology on Gram's stain	History of human bite

The efficacy of antibiotic therapy for chancroid correlates with the in vitro susceptibility of *H. ducreyi* to the respective antibiotic. Therapy, therefore, should be selected from among agents to which essentially all isolates, regardless of country of origin, are susceptible. These agents include erythromycin, trimethoprim-sulfamethoxazole, clindamycin, rifampin, gentamicin, tobramycin, amikacin, cefoxitin, and cefotaxime.[76] Currently, recommended treatment is oral erythromycin, 500 mg four times daily, or one double-strength tablet of trimethoprim-sulfamethoxazole (160 mg/800 mg) twice daily.[77] Therapy should continue for a minimum of 10 days or until the ulcer and adenopathy have resolved. Tetracycline and sulfonamides have been considered as alternatives but may be less effective.[76] Chancroid has also been treated successfully with kanamycin,[78] streptomycin, or cephalothin.[79] The combination of clavulanic acid, a β-lactamase inhibitor, and ampicillin is effective in treatment of chancroid caused by β-lactamase–producing strains of *H. ducreyi*.[80] Sexual partners of a patient with chancroid should be treated with an effective antibiotic for at least 10 days. Local relief can be obtained with soaks of cool saline or Burow's solution (five percent aluminum acetate solution) applied three times daily. A fluctuant chancroid bubo should not be incised, but decompression and relief of pain can be accomplished by aspiration through the uninvolved skin above the lesion. In addition to routine therapy, patients with secondarily infected phagedenic chancroid should be treated with penicillin G, 10 million U/day I.V., and with clindamycin, 1.8 g/day I.V. Syphilis should be excluded by initial and follow-up serologic tests.

Granuloma Inguinale

Granuloma inguinale, a slowly progressive ulcerative granulomatous infection involving the genitalia, is thought to be caused by *Calymmatobacterium granulomatis* (formerly *Donovania granulomatis*). It is a dark-staining, encapsulated, intracellular rod-shaped inclusion in macrophages, the so-called Donovan body.[81] This organism, an encapsulated gram-negative bacterium, is difficult to recover from the lesions. *C. granulomatis* can be seen in Wright's-stained or Giemsa-stained scrapings or crush preparations of tissue from the infected granulomatous lesions.

The disease, spread by sexual contact, does not seem highly contagious. Of the fewer than 100 patients seen yearly in the United States, the majority are men. Highly promiscuous male homosexuals are seen frequently among those with the disease.

The initial lesion, a painless papule at the site of inoculation, appears after an incubation period of one to 12 weeks. The papule ulcerates, resulting in a beefy-red granular lesion with rolled, raised, sharply defined borders. Other painless exuberant lesions form, coalesce, and spread locally on the penis, scrotum, vulva, vagina, or rectum. Extension of the granulomatous reaction subcutaneously into the inguinal area gives rise to pseudobuboes, which may be confused with local adenopathy. Progressive infection can be very mutilating and in late stages is associated with genital lymphedema.[82] If secondary fusospirochetal infection occurs, the ulcerated lesions become foul smelling, painful, and even more destructive.

The diagnosis is suggested by the clinical presentation and is confirmed by the demonstration of Donovan bodies in the tissues on crush preparations or in fixed-tissue sections. Special fixation techniques and stains facilitate the finding of Donovan bodies in tissue sections.[81,82] Other ulcerating diseases of the genitalia and perianal area must be excluded [*see Table 3*]. The promiscuity associated with granuloma inguinale frequently results in simultaneous infection with other sexually transmitted pathogens. A coincidental syphilitic chancre or condyloma latum must be excluded by dark-field examination and serologic test for syphilis.

Tetracycline (500 mg p.o., q.i.d.) is the treatment of choice. Therapy is continued until Donovan bodies are no longer seen and the skin lesions heal. With effective antibiotic therapy, healing occurs within several weeks, but continued therapy for three to four weeks may be required. Alternative antibiotic regimens have included streptomycin, erythromycin, and chloramphenicol. Recently, gentamicin (40 mg I.M. b.i.d. for two weeks) has been advocated for recalcitrant infection.[83] The continued presence of skin lesions in the absence of Donovan bodies requires that malignant disorders be excluded. Late follow-up examinations should assess both relapse and the malignant degeneration of previously infected tissues. Surgery is occasionally required to resect pseudobuboes that persist despite effective antibiotic therapy; it may also be required to correct cicatricial complications of healing granuloma inguinale.

References

1. N Engl J Med 312:1683, 1985
2. Ann Intern Med 102:229, 1985
3. J Bacteriol 124:740, 1975
4. MMWR 36:107, 1987
5. N Engl J Med 313:607, 1985
6. J Infect Dis 153:340, 1986
7. J Infect Dis 155:819, 1987
8. J Infect Dis 156:1002, 1987
9. MMWR 36:585, 1987
10. Ann Intern Med 110:5, 1989
11. N Engl J Med 290:117, 1974
12. Ann Intern Med 86:340, 1977
13. N Engl J Med 288:181, 1973
14. Adv Intern Med 19:259, 1974
15. Lancet 1:1182, 1977
16. Br J Vener Dis 55:434, 1979
17. Am J Obstet Gynecol 108:595, 1970
18. Pediatrics 53:436, 1974
19. JAMA 236:1359, 1976
20. Ann Intern Med 74:979, 1971
21. J Infect Dis 129:583, 1974
22. Arch Intern Med 137:858, 1977
23. Am J Med 86:297, 1989
24. Ann Intern Med 82:7, 1975
25. N Engl J Med 293:166, 1975
26. J Infect Dis 125:499, 1972
27. Med Lett Drugs Ther 30:5, 1988
28. MMWR 36(suppl 5):1S, 1987
29. J Infect Dis 158:881, 1988
30. Sex Transm Dis 5:4, 1978
31. Ann Intern Med 104:655, 1986
32. N Engl J Med 288:1221, 1973
33. Ann Intern Med 84:661, 1976
34. MMWR 36:161, 1987
35. Ann Intern Med 104:365, 1986
36. N Engl J Med 311:137, 1984
37. Antimicrob Agents Chemother 30:514, 1986
38. Antimicrob Agents Chemother 30:267, 1986
39. JAMA 218:711, 1971
40. Ann Intern Med 109:855, 1988
41. Ann Intern Med 109:849, 1988
42. JAMA 244:2060, 1980
43. N Engl J Med 308:868, 1983
44. N Engl J Med 305:195, 1981
45. J Infect Dis 155:1341, 1987
46. Sex Transm Dis 4:105, 1977
47. Clin Obstet Gynecol 18:35, 1975
48. N Engl J Med 296:1377, 1977
49. Genitourin Med 61:179, 1985
50. MMWR 34(suppl 3):53S, 1985
51. Rev Infect Dis 8:86, 1986
52. Br J Vener Dis 46:179, 1970
53. Obstet Gynecol 48:341, 1976
54. JAMA 253:2246, 1985
55. Obstet Gynecol 105:1088, 1969
56. Am J Obstet Gynecol 61:113, 1983
57. Am J Obstet Gynecol 151:1098, 1985
58. Sex Transm Dis 5:27, 1978
59. N Engl J Med 311:1, 1984
60. N Engl J Med 292:1199, 1975
61. Br J Vener Dis 48:437, 1972
62. N Engl J Med 303:409, 1980
63. N Engl J Med 307:463, 1982
64. N Engl J Med 304:956, 1981
65. Ann Intern Med 97:216, 1982
66. Ann Intern Med 94:192, 1981
67. Sex Transm Dis 7:135, 1980
68. J Pediatr 111:617, 1987
69. N Engl J Med 320:769, 1989
70. N Engl J Med 320:802, 1989
71. J Infect Dis 136:740, 1977
72. N Engl J Med 298:1429, 1978
73. N Engl J Med 303:601, 1980
74. Sex Transm Dis 8(suppl):316, 1981
75. Rev Infect Dis 2:867, 1980
76. Rev Infect Dis 4(suppl):S848, 1982
77. 1982. MMWR 31(suppl 2), 1982
78. J Urol 107:807, 1972
79. Med J Aust 1:808, 1975
80. Lancet 2:509, 1982
81. JAMA 211:632, 1970
82. Arch Dermatol 111:1464, 1975
83. Clin Obstet Gynecol 18:73, 1975

Acknowledgment

Tables 1, 2 Based in part on "Treatment of Sexually Transmitted Diseases," in *Medical Letter on Drugs and Therapeutics* 30:5, 1988; and "Antibiotic-Resistant Strains of Neisseria gonorrhoeae: Policy Guidelines for Detection, Management, and Control," in *Morbidity and Mortality Weekly Report* 36(suppl 5):IS, 1987.

22 Fever of Undetermined Origin

MORTON N. SWARTZ, M.D.

Fever occurs in about one third of all hospitalized patients; in most cases, diagnostic studies reveal the cause of fever, but in 12 to 18 percent of patients, the cause of fever cannot be determined.[1,2] In the vast majority of these patients, however, the fever is short lived.

Prolonged fever of undetermined origin (FUO) presents one of the most challenging and perplexing problems in clinical medicine. Such fevers may persist for weeks or months in the absence of characteristic clinical findings or clues. Ultimately, most such obscure fevers prove to be caused by common diseases presenting in an atypical fashion rather than by rare and exotic illnesses.

Petersdorf and Beeson in their classic monograph[3] specified three criteria to define FUO:

1. Duration: at least three weeks. This requirement eliminates from consideration febrile illnesses of obvious cause, most short-lived fevers of indeterminate or viral origin, and pyrexias of postoperative patients, in whom fevers of one or two weeks' duration may stem from sequential processes.

2. Magnitude: a temperature that exceeds 38.3° C (101.0° F) on at least several occasions. This criterion eliminates from consideration those individuals (most commonly young females) with habitual hyperthermia, in whom the body temperature normally ranges from 37.3° to 38.0° C (99.1° to 100.4°F). If such individuals are not clinically ill, their elevated body temperature should not cause too much concern.[4]

3. Obscure nature: perplexing enough to defy diagnosis after one week of routine study.

Etiologic Classification

It is helpful to approach the problem of obscure fever in a particular patient by reviewing the established causes and their relative frequencies. These diagnostic considerations can then be viewed in the light of evidence from the patient's history, clinical findings, and initial laboratory data. Further specific studies are then obtained, with the aim of confirming or eliminating the more likely diagnoses. Although geographic factors are relevant, the leading causes of FUO are reasonably uniform throughout the United States. The relative frequencies of the etiologic categories responsible for FUO seemed quite stable from the 1950s[3] to the 1970s[5]; however, a subtle change was noted in a more recent study,[6] with neoplasms replacing infections as the leading cause of FUO [see Table 1]. In addition, despite the increasing sophistication of diagnostic studies, the percentage of patients with FUO who remain undiagnosed may be increasing.

Infections

Infections always merit initial consideration because of their frequency and specific therapeutic implications.

Systemic infections The two major systemic infections to consider in the evaluation of FUO are tuberculosis (usually disseminated but sometimes confined predominantly to the liver and spleen) and infective endocarditis [see Table 2]. Most FUO cases caused by miliary tuberculosis arise in elderly patients in whom dissemination has followed breakdown of quiescent foci.[7] Often, in cases caused by miliary tuberculosis, the intermediate-strength (five tuberculin units) purified protein derivative skin test is negative, and miliary pulmonary lesions are not present on the chest x-ray.[8]

Table 1   Causes of Fever of Undetermined Origin

Cause	Study		
	New Haven, 1961[3] (% of 100 Patients)	Boston, 1973[5] (% of 128 Patients)	Seattle, 1982[6] (% of 105 Patients)
Infections	36	35	30
Neoplasms	19	23	31
Collagen vascular diseases	13	16	9
Other specific causes	25	18	18
Undiagnosed	7	8	12

Anemia and leukopenia caused by bone marrow involvement or, less often, by hypersplenism may be evident. A leukemoid reaction (usually myelocytic and, rarely, lymphocytic) may indicate bone marrow involvement and provide a valuable clue to diagnosis[9]; bone marrow biopsy is a very helpful diagnostic test in patients in whom miliary tuberculosis is suspected. An isolated elevation of the serum alkaline phosphatase level may indicate miliary involvement of the liver by tuberculosis, other infection, or neoplasm. The histologic findings on liver biopsy often suggest the diagnosis, and a portion of the specimen should always be cultured for the presence of tubercle bacilli.

Infective endocarditis, usually subacute, is also an important diagnostic consideration. Most patients with subacute bacterial endocarditis have a heart murmur. In about five percent of cases, however, particularly in the elderly, the murmur may be absent or may be considered functional. If the murmur is disregarded, the febrile illness without localizing features is often attributed to influenza, a urinary tract infection, or some other plausible cause. Blood cultures would be expected to provide the diagnosis in a patient with subacute bacterial endocarditis, particularly because only five percent of patients with endocarditis have negative blood cultures.[10] The leading cause of negative blood cultures in patients with endocarditis is the administration of antibiotics[10-13]; such drugs may also inhibit bacterial growth sufficiently to cause cultures taken some days after cessation of the antibiotics to remain negative. It is therefore very important that multiple blood cultures be obtained, including some as long as five to 10 days after antibiotics have been withdrawn. Other causes of culture-negative endocarditis that should be considered in patients with FUO include infection with fastidious bacteria, chlamydial infection, and Q fever.

Careful scrutiny for the peripheral stigmas of endocarditis, such as petechiae, subungual splinter hemorrhages, Osler nodes, Janeway lesions, Roth's spots in the fundi, splenomegaly, peripheral emboli, and microscopic hematuria, is essential in the evaluation of any patient with FUO. Rheumatoid factor is present in the serum of 50 percent of patients with subacute bacterial endocarditis and may provide a valuable diagnostic clue. Circulating immune complexes also may be present. Echocardiography may reveal valvular vegetations in patients with endocarditis. Left atrial myxomas mimic culture-negative endocarditis but may be detected with echocardiography.

Other systemic infections, including bacteremias that occur in the absence of any obvious primary site of involvement, only rarely cause FUO [*see Table* 2]. Viral infections are usually self-limited and do not produce fevers that last longer than three weeks. An important exception to this generalization is cytomegalovirus (CMV) infection.

CMV infection may occasionally present as FUO (often with some mononucleosislike features) in otherwise well individuals. More frequently, CMV infection develops in patients who have received multiple blood transfusions or who have undergone organ transplantation. CMV disease, either alone or accompanied by other systemic infections or by allograft rejection, is the cause of 50 percent of all febrile episodes in renal transplant recipients; it underlies 70 percent of those episodes that last longer than three weeks.[14] CMV infection is a major diagnostic consideration in a renal transplant patient with prolonged obscure fever unaccompanied by localized findings, particularly when the fever occurs between two and 20 weeks after transplantation.

Localized infections The more common types of localized infection that present as FUO include hepatic abscess, subphrenic abscess, and subhepatic and pericholecystic abscess [*see Table* 2]. Sites of previous surgery may harbor an abscess in a patient with FUO[15]; the surgery may have been performed as long ago as 12 months before the onset of fever. An unvarying gastric air bubble may suggest a subdiaphragmatic abscess.

Liver abscesses are often occult[16]; the physician should look for a history that includes biliary tract disease symptomatology, recent blunt abdominal trauma, or travel, which might suggest the diagnosis of amebiasis. Hepatomegaly may be absent initially. The serum alkaline phosphatase level is usually elevated even when the abscess is solitary. Serologic tests for amebiasis are positive in patients with amebic liver abscess. Elevation of the diaphragm, particularly when accompanied by overlying pulmonary atelectasis or a pleural effusion, should raise suspicion of a subphrenic ab-

---

Table 2   **Infections Causing Fever of Undetermined Origin**

Systemic Infections

Tuberculosis (miliary)

Infective endocarditis (primarily bacterial endocarditis but also endocarditis with a fungal, Q fever, or chlamydial etiology)

Bacteremia from an inapparent primary focus

   Chronic meningococcemia

   Brucellosis

   Listeriosis, vibriosis, leptospirosis, relapsing fever (caused by *Borrelia recurrentis*), rat-bite fever (caused by either *Streptobacillus moniliformis* or *Spirillum minus*)

Miscellaneous

   Psittacosis, toxoplasmosis (disseminated acquired form), Q fever, disseminated deep mycotic infections (e.g., histoplasmosis, blastomycosis, cryptococcosis), cytomegalovirus infection

Localized Infections and Abscesses

Hepatic infections

   Liver abscess

   Cholangitis

Intraperitoneal infections

   Upper abdomen: empyema of gallbladder, pericholecystic and subhepatic abscesses, right or left subphrenic abscesses, lesser sac abscess

   Lower abdomen: periappendiceal and peridiverticular abscesses

Other intra-abdominal abscesses

   Tubo-ovarian abscess, pelvic inflammatory disease, pelvic abscess

   Retroperitoneal abscess, pancreatic abscess

Urinary tract infectons

   Perinephric abscess

   Renal carbuncle

   Pyelonephritis with ureteral obstruction and pyonephrosis

   Prostatic abscess

---

scess. Ultrasonography and computed tomography are valuable in identifying such collections; gallium scans are less useful.

Localized infection in the urinary tract is an important consideration in a patient with

FUO. Perinephric abscess and renal carbuncle are difficult to diagnose, even with intravenous pyelography. Ultrasonography, CT, or renal angiography may be necessary to establish the diagnosis.

Many other localized infections occasionally present as FUO; occult dental infections[17] are one such example and illustrate the need for thoroughness in the evaluation of patients with obscure fevers.

Neoplasms

Lymphoma, particularly Hodgkin's disease, is the most common neoplastic cause of obscure fever. Lymphoma may be difficult to diagnose when the principal site of involvement is the retroperitoneal nodes, but abdominal CT scans greatly facilitate this diagnosis. Because the rapid DNA turnover in lymphoma could produce an increase in the serum uric acid level, an isolated, unexplained elevation of this level may also suggest the diagnosis. Although so-called Pel-Ebstein recurrent fevers suggest Hodgkin's disease, they are observed in only a minority of patients with this disorder.

The development of fever in a patient who has myeloma or chronic lymphocytic leukemia is usually caused by superimposed infection and not by the neoplastic process. In some patients, however, the febrile course appears to be caused by the leukemia itself. Occasionally, a patient with the preleukemia syndrome will present with fever and atypical blood and bone marrow changes, suggesting myeloid metaplasia or a leukemoid response. Only after some months can the hematologic picture be established as leukemia.

Fever associated with hypernephroma may be mild or marked. Occasionally, such tumors are extremely vascular and produce changes characteristic of a high-output state (e.g., cardiomegaly and flow murmurs). A renal vascular bruit in the upper quadrants may provide a diagnostic clue. Recrudescence of fever months or years after removal of a hypernephroma may indicate local recurrence or distant metastases. Up to 10 percent of patients with colorectal carcinoma present with fever[18]; either extension of the tumor through the bowel wall, producing a paracolonic abscess, or necrosis and abscess formation in a polypoid intraluminal lesion may be the underlying mechanism.

Widespread metastatic cancer may be responsible for continuing fever; hepatic involvement is not necessary for fever to occur.[19] Occasionally, a neuroblastoma involving bone or soft tissues or a pheochromocytoma may have a febrile course.

Fevers caused by malignant disease often respond to therapy with nonsteroidal anti-inflammatory drugs; fevers caused by infections are less likely to respond completely to these agents.[20]

Collagen Vascular Disease

A variety of connective tissue disorders and vasculitides may produce prolonged fevers before the development of articular or other characteristic manifestations. In the elderly, polymyalgia rheumatica and the closely related disorder giant cell arteritis (temporal arteritis) are the most common connective tissue disorders presenting as FUO. Malaise, weight loss, muscle weakness, mild arthralgias without overt arthritis, and a markedly elevated sedimentation rate (usually < 100 mm/hr) are usual features. Jaw claudication, visual symptoms, and a tender or thickened temporal artery suggest the diagnosis of giant cell arteritis. Up to 15 percent of cases of giant cell arteritis present as FUO, and in some patients, the vasculitis itself remains occult.[21] Similarly, virtually all patients with adult-onset Still's disease are febrile,[22] and systemic symptoms such as fever and weakness may antedate by weeks or months the evolution of the more characteristic clinical manifestations of rheumatoid arthritis in patients with the adult type of juvenile rheumatoid arthritis[23]; the occurrence of an evanescent salmon-colored maculopapular rash, particularly on the trunk, may point toward the diagnosis. In other patients, involvement of the paranasal sinuses and mastoid or the rapid excavation of a pulmonary lesion suggests

Wegener's granulomatosis. Many other connective tissue diseases, ranging from classic vasculitides such as systemic lupus erythematosus to uncommon disorders such as relapsing polychondritis,[24] can also present as FUO.

Less Common Etiologic Categories

Granulomatous diseases Other than those granulomatous diseases caused by known infectious agents, granulomatous diseases that may be responsible for FUO include sarcoidosis, granulomatous hepatitis of unknown etiology, and starch peritonitis. The presence of noncaseating granulomas in lymph nodes or the liver is characteristic but not pathognomonic of sarcoidosis. There are about 40 diseases that may be associated with hepatic granulomas.[25] Treatable infectious granulomatous diseases (e.g., tuberculosis, brucellosis, and histoplasmosis) must be ruled out by cultures, skin tests, serologic tests, and special stains of biopsied tissues. Rarely, despite extensive investigation and therapeutic trials with antituberculous drugs, an etiologic diagnosis cannot be made in patients with noncaseating hepatic granulomas who have a febrile illness of many months' duration. Whether such cases of granulomatous hepatitis of unknown origin represent a single entity or merely the hepatic response to a variety of agents is not clear. Beneficial results have been achieved in such cases by giving corticosteroids after exclusion of the other specific granulomatous diseases.[25]

Prolonged fever is uncommon in sarcoidosis, but when it does occur, prominent hilar adenopathy, ocular involvement, erythema nodosum, and hepatic granulomas are usually also present. Biopsy of involved lymph nodes, muscle, or liver usually shows noncaseating granulomas. Such lesions are not specific for sarcoidosis, but the histologic diagnosis is reinforced if a zone of dense collagenized connective tissue surrounds the granulomas.

Starch peritonitis represents a febrile granulomatous response to starch introduced on surgical gloves. The nature of the process may not be appreciated for weeks; the initial supposition is that a doughy abdominal mass and fever are caused by a postoperative abscess.

Inflammatory bowel disease Bowel symptoms are prominent in almost all patients with idiopathic ulcerative colitis, granulomatous colitis, or regional enteritis, and the diagnosis is obvious in such febrile patients. In an occasional patient, however, bowel symptoms may not be marked or may be of such long duration that they have become accepted as the norm. In this setting, FUO may be the presenting complaint in a patient with inflammatory bowel disease. The evaluation of any patient with an obscure fever must include detailed questioning regarding bowel function as well as an examination of the stool for mucus and occult blood.

Alcoholic hepatitis and cirrhosis Fever is observed occasionally in chronic liver disease. Attention should first be directed to possible complicating infections, such as enterogenous bacteremias, salmonellosis, or tuberculosis, or to an unrelated process. Active hepatocellular necrosis may occur in the course of alcoholic hepatitis and may account for low-grade fever. Occasionally, a patient shows a higher temperature than one might expect on the basis of the SGOT level. In such a situation, other causes of fever should be pursued, but often, alcoholic hepatitis ultimately proves to be the cause.

Pulmonary emboli Rarely, a patient may have multiple small pulmonary emboli but not exhibit any significant changes in arterial blood gases or on the chest film and will present primarily with a problem of unexplained fever. The fever may exceed 39.0° C (102.2° F), but high-grade fevers caused by pulmonary emboli rarely persist longer than one week.[26] The thrombi may be in symptomless calf veins or, more often, in pelvic veins in patients who have recently undergone pelvic surgery or in postpartum patients. Pelvic thrombophlebitis itself may be a source of protracted fever, even in the absence of pulmonary emboli.

Drug fever Drug fever frequently occurs in the absence of other manifestations of hypersensitivity, such as rash and eosinophilia.[27] Antimicrobial agents (e.g., β-lactams, sulfonamides, nitrofurantoin, or isoniazid), antihypertensives (e.g., hydralazine or methyldopa), anticonvulsants (e.g., phenytoin), and allopurinol are among the most common offenders,[28] but many other drugs have been implicated in isolated cases. In most instances, the diagnosis of drug fever is considered within the first several weeks of onset of FUO, and any recently administered drugs are discontinued. Several drugs, however, such as phenytoin, methyldopa, and isoniazid, may not produce drug fever until weeks or months after their initial use. Drugs such as these may be overlooked just because they have been administered for some time without producing side effects.

Intramuscular injections of analgesics can produce FUO, which may or may not be accompanied by the presence of a sterile abscess or other gross evidence of tissue injury.[29]

Factitious fever Rarely, a patient may simulate illness by deliberately producing false elevations in temperature. Factitious fever is one of the most challenging etiologic categories of FUO.[30] The patients are usually female and are often paramedical personnel. The underlying problem may be malingering or a more complicated emotional disorder. Discordance between the marked temperature elevations and the pulse rate, distortion of the usual diurnal temperature curve, and absence of diaphoresis when the fever abates suggest the diagnosis. Some patients generate a factitious fever by applying friction to the tip of the thermometer within the mouth or anal canal; others enter the hospital with their own thermometers, which are then preheated and given to the attendant at the appropriate time. Comparison of the serial number of the thermometer that is given with that of the one reclaimed from the patient may substantiate suspicion. Measurement of simultaneous rectal and urinary temperatures may distinguish between true and factitious fevers.

Miscellaneous causes The diagnosis of familial Mediterranean fever is suggested by ethnic background, episodic occurrence of fever in association with abdominal pain or other signs of polyserositis, and well-being between attacks. Maintenance therapy with colchicine may succeed in preventing attacks.

Whipple's disease is a multisystem infection caused by unidentified bacilli; it may present as a prolonged febrile illness with weight loss, arthralgias, and weakness.[31] Malabsorption is usually present but may not be a prominent feature in some patients. Anergy during the active phase of the disease and the finding of noncaseating granulomas in lymph nodes may erroneously suggest a diagnosis of sarcoidosis. Periodic acid–Schiff (PAS) stains of biopsy material may reveal characteristic PAS-positive macrophages; electron microscopy may reveal bacilliform bodies even when PAS stains are negative.[32]

Rarely, endocrinologic abnormalities, such as subacute thyroiditis,[33] or metabolic disorders, such as hypertriglyceridemia, hypercholesterolemia, or glycosphingolipid storage disease (Fabry's disease), present as FUO.[34]

Unusual infections such as visceral leishmaniasis (kala-azar) or trypanosomiasis, acquired in endemic areas abroad, are responsible for a few cases of persisting FUO seen in the United States.[34,35]

Central nervous system lesions are decidedly uncommon causes of FUO, except in very obtunded patients with extensive brain damage. However, a small number of conscious patients with primary disorders of thermoregulation and recurring episodes of unexplained fever have been reported.[36] These patients cannot maintain body temperature in the cold; thus, they respond to a reduction in environmental temperature as if they were poikilotherms.

Patterns of Fever

Although different types of fever have been described, neither the degree of elevation of the temperature[37] nor the pattern of fever[38] generally permits discrimination among the causes of FUO. Many patterns are altered by the use of antipyretics. A sustained fever is one in which the temperature is consistently elevated and the usual diurnal variation is absent; this pattern is seen in untreated typhoid fever and in some cases of miliary tuberculosis. The use of salicylates, however, can convert such fevers to a remittent pattern with two or more daily peaks. An intermittent fever is one in which the daily fluctuations are wide but the morning temperatures are usually normal. Such a pattern is commonly observed with abscesses and other pyogenic infections. Pel-Ebstein fever, occasionally observed in patients with Hodgkin's disease, may be sufficiently distinctive in its periodicity (five to 10 days of fever alternating with similar periods of afebrility) to suggest the diagnosis. The characteristic periodicities of relapsing fever, malaria, and familial Mediterranean fever will suggest the diagnosis of these entities.

Diagnostic Studies

Detailed review of the history is essential, particularly regarding travel, animal exposure, occupational risks, and other epidemiologic factors; previous trauma or surgery; or features relevant to each of the diagnoses outlined (see above). When physical findings are being evaluated, particular attention should be paid to structures that may be inapparent sources of obscure fever, such as the cardiovascular system, abdominal viscera, and genitourinary tract. Lymph nodes should be examined in the usual distribution but also in the epitrochlear areas and along the medial aspect of the upper arm. Search of the skin, nail beds, and mucous membranes for petechiae and vasculitic lesions may provide important clues to the diagnosis of endocarditis or of colla-

gen vascular diseases. Funduscopic examination may reveal choroidal tubercles or signs of vasculitis or endocarditis. Rectal examination is particularly important in the elderly or obtunded patient, in whom a perirectal or prostatic abscess may be overlooked. The testes should be carefully palpated for tumor or for evidence of epididymitis, which may indicate tuberculosis, brucellosis, or collagen vascular disease.

Common Laboratory Studies

Blood cultures Blood cultures should include aerobic (five to 10 percent CO_2 tension) and anaerobic cultures that have been incubated for at least two weeks. Newer blood culture techniques, including the use of antibiotic removal devices, may be helpful in some patients.

Serologic tests Serologic tests employed in cases of FUO include *Brucella* agglutination, *Salmonella* agglutination (usually not very helpful), antistreptolysin-O (ASO) titer if acute rheumatic fever is suspected, Venereal Disease Research Laboratories (VDRL) test for syphilis, serologic tests for less common infections (e.g., psittacosis, toxoplasmosis, and cytomegalovirus), test for rheumatoid factor, antinuclear antibody test, and the test for the lupus erythematosus (LE) cell. A serum specimen obtained during an acute-phase host response can be frozen for subsequent comparison with a late or convalescent-phase specimen to look for rising titers to specific pathogens.

Sedimentation rate A sedimentation rate greater than 100 mm/hr suggests vasculitis but does not differentiate between this disorder and neoplasms, tuberculosis, or pyogenic infections.[39]

Serum enzymes and chemistries The results of liver function tests may indicate primary involvement (e.g., caused by hepatitis or a liver abscess) or secondary infiltration (e.g., miliary tuberculosis) of the liver.

Measurement of the serum alkaline phosphatase level is particularly helpful in the diagnosis of secondary hepatic infiltration.

Skin tests Skin testing may aid in diagnosis if positive results are obtained (e.g., a positive tuberculin test would suggest tuberculosis) or if anergy, a characteristic finding in sarcoidosis, Whipple's disease, and Hodgkin's disease, is demonstrated.

Spinal fluid examination Examination of the spinal fluid is usually unrewarding unless the patient has CNS signs or symptoms, such as headache or stiff neck.

Radiologic Studies

Various radiologic studies in addition to chest films may assist in making the diagnosis:

1. Ultrasonography and CT scans have become very valuable for detecting intra-abdominal and pelvic abscesses and retroperitoneal adenopathy. The use of CT scans has decreased the number of biopsies of normal tissues in patients studied for FUO.[40] The use of magnetic resonance imaging (MRI) in patients with FUO is under investigation.

2. Radionuclide bone scans are considerably more sensitive than bone x-rays in the detection of osseous metastases or foci of osteomyelitis. Liver-spleen scans can help define hepatic metastases. Gallium scans are occasionally useful in detecting occult abscesses, but this technique has not generally been helpful in patients with FUO[41]; scans utilizing indium-111–labeled leukocytes are being investigated.[42]

3. Intravenous pyelograms may indicate intrarenal or perirenal abscesses or renal tumors. Some parenchymal lesions can be demonstrated only with the use of a renal angiogram.

4. Upper and lower gastrointestinal tract x-rays may indicate regional enteritis, ulcerative colitis, or large-bowel neoplasms.

5. Lymphangiograms may be helpful in suggesting retroperitoneal lymphoma; however, significant morbidity is associated with this procedure in some patients. Definitive histologic diagnosis of lymphoma will still require laparotomy.

6. Bone x-rays generally are not helpful in the absence of skeletal symptoms.

7. Other radiographic examinations, such as cholangiograms, aortograms, and celiac angiograms, may also be useful; these studies, however, should only be performed on the basis of clinical clues that suggest specific diagnoses.

Biopsies

All biopsied material should be cultured for bacteria, mycobacteria, and fungi and examined histologically. Biopsies that may help determine the diagnosis in patients with FUO include the following:

1. Percutaneous liver biopsy. Neoplastic or granulomatous diseases can generally be detected more easily by percutaneous liver biopsy than by bone marrow biopsy, particularly if hepatomegaly or abnormalities of hepatic function, or both, are present.

2. Bone marrow biopsy. This technique may also be used to detect granulomatous diseases or metastatic tumor; it may be rewarding in patients in whom hematologic abnormalities are evident.

3. Lymph node biopsy. Enlarged, matted, or unusually situated nodes are the most favorable for biopsy. Because of the frequent occurrence of chronic inflammation in inguinal lymph nodes, biopsy of these nodes is unsatisfactory.

4. Skin and muscle biopsy. Biopsy of skin and muscle may prove useful in diagnosing collagen vascular disease (e.g., polyarteritis or dermatomyositis); biopsy may also be useful in sarcoidosis.

5. Temporal artery biopsy. Biopsy of the temporal artery may be the only way to establish the diagnosis of giant cell arteritis in an elderly patient who has FUO, an

elevated sedimentation rate, and some thickening of the temporal artery.

Therapeutic Trials

Therapeutic trials have generally proved more misleading than helpful when applied to the patient with prolonged FUO. Coincidental temporary defervescence can suggest a specific therapeutic response, thus delaying measures that might provide the correct diagnosis. Occasionally, a therapeutic trial may be reasonable when directed at a specific diagnosis. Thus, a one- to two-week trial of penicillin and an aminoglycoside might be employed when endocarditis is a realistic possibility; aspirin might be tried in patients who may have adult-type juvenile rheumatoid arthritis; and isoniazid and rifampin might be tried in cases in which miliary tuberculosis is definitely a possibility. Patients with disseminated tuberculosis presenting as FUO often show a clinical response within two weeks after appropriate chemotherapy.

Exploratory Laparotomy

On occasion, laparotomy has been advocated and employed successfully to provide the diagnosis of FUO.[43,44] Newer noninvasive radiologic techniques, especially when combined with percutaneous needle biopsies (see above), have generally supplanted laparotomy for the diagnosis of FUO. Early abdominal exploration in the absence of clinical or laboratory clues pointing to the abdomen is usually unrewarding. Laparotomy should be reserved for those patients in whom the clinical and laboratory findings point to an intra-abdominal or retroperitoneal source for the fever, particularly when the fever has followed a prolonged and debilitating course.

Undiagnosed FUO

In a few patients with FUO, no helpful clues are found during hospitalization and the disease process is not very prolonged, is not progressive, and is not associated with marked weight loss; in these patients, the wisest course may be to pause temporarily. Readmission to the hospital and reevaluation of the patient some weeks later may provide the diagnosis.

Five to 10 percent of patients with FUO seem to recover in the absence of a diagnosis of the specific fever source; therefore, fevers that abate after several months do not necessarily recur and do not always indicate a serious underlying process such as neoplasm or collagen vascular disease.

References

1. J Gen Intern Med 3:119, 1988
2. Am J Med 82:580, 1987
3. Medicine (Baltimore) 40:1, 1961
4. Rev Infect Dis 7:692, 1985
5. N Engl J Med 289:1407, 1973
6. Medicine (Baltimore) 61:269, 1982
7. Medicine (Baltimore) 59:352, 1980
8. Br Med J 2:273, 1969
9. Arch Intern Med 125:691, 1970
10. Ann Intern Med 94:505, 1981
11. Am J Med 66:43, 1979
12. Aust NZ J Med 14:223, 1984
13. Arch Intern Med 144:2083, 1984
14. Am J Med 71:345, 1981
15. Am J Surg 125:70, 1973
16. Am J Med 57:601, 1974
17. Am J Med 66:463, 1979
18. Isr J Med Sci 21:421, 1985
19. Cancer 55:2830, 1985
20. Am J Med 76:597, 1984
21. Arthritis Rheum 24:1414, 1981
22. Arthritis Rheum 30:186, 1987
23. Medicine (Baltimore) 52:431, 1973
24. Ann Intern Med 104:74, 1986
25. Medicine (Baltimore) 52:1, 1973
26. Am J Med 67:232, 1979
27. Ann Intern Med 106:728, 1987
28. Rev Infect Dis 4:69, 1982
29. Rev Infect Dis 8:68, 1986
30. Ann Intern Med 90:230, 1979
31. N Engl J Med 300:920, 1979
32. Am J Med 83:165, 1987
33. Am J Med 66:257, 1979
34. Annu Rev Med 26:277, 1975
35. Mayo Clin Proc 55:455, 1980
36. Am J Med 36:956, 1964
37. JAMA 236:2419, 1976
38. Arch Intern Med 139:1225, 1979
39. Arch Intern Med 146:1581, 1986
40. J Infect Dis 156:408, 1987
41. Ann Intern Med 79:403, 1973
42. Scand J Infect Dis 19:339, 1987
43. JAMA 169:1306, 1959
44. Johns Hopkins Med J 125:159, 1969

23 Intoxication by Centrally Acting Agents

EDWARD RUBENSTEIN, M.D.

Drug Overdose

Drug overdose is a leading cause of unconsciousness in patients brought to emergency rooms. Most instances represent suicidal acts, but in some cases, especially those involving the consumption of large volumes of alcohol, suicidal intention may not be clear. Manifestations and therapy are virtually the same for overdoses of short-acting barbiturates, benzodiazepines, glutethimide, meprobamate, and ethchlorvynol. Other agents produce unique problems requiring specific therapy.

Evaluation and Initial Treatment

Clinical assessment and initial treatment should proceed simultaneously [*see Figure 1*]. The head should be tilted backward, the jaw moved forward, and the mouth opened. The oropharynx must be cleared of food, secretions, loose dentures, or other obstructions; if the patient is or is becoming obtunded, an oropharyngeal airway must be inserted and the upper air passages suctioned. The patient must be positioned on his or her side; the prone or supine position increases the hazard of aspiration. If severe respiratory depression is present, a cuffed endotracheal tube must be passed and controlled mechanical ventilation begun. A nasal tube should be used if there is a risk of seizures. (Manual ventilation with a self-inflating bag and mask should be used by personnel inexperienced with intubation. The definitive procedure can be carried out later.)

Next, the pulse rate and arterial blood pressure should be determined, the jugular venous pressure and blood volume estimated, the lungs examined for pulmonary vascular congestion and aspiration, and the size and the reactivity of the pupils recorded. If hemodynamic failure with shock is present, I.V. saline should be started and a central venous pressure (CVP) catheter inserted. The choice and flow rate of I.V. solutions depend on the ingested agents and the patient's status.

Systematic assessment of CNS depression is important. A widely used classification system is the following:

Group 0: asleep but arousable; responds to painful stimuli; sits up in bed.

Group I: comatose but withdraws from painful stimuli; reflexes intact; circulation normal.

Group II: comatose; does not withdraw from painful stimuli; most or all reflexes intact; normal circulation and ventilation.

Group III: most or all reflexes absent; normal circulation and ventilation.

Group IV: circulatory and ventilatory failure, often accompanied by cyanosis and shock.

Another useful classification scheme is the Glasgow Coma Scale [*see Chapter 25*].

CNS status should be recorded on a flowchart, together with serial measurements of body temperature, pulse rate, respiratory rate, and arterial blood pressure. CVP, hourly urine volume and pH, arterial blood gases, serum electrolyte levels, complete blood counts, liver function tests, serum creatinine levels, serum myocardial enzyme levels, and blood drug levels may be needed.

Physical examination should focus on evidence of trauma, especially of the head and neck, previous venipunctures and needle tracks (at sites such as the saphenous vein, popliteal fossa, dorsal vein of the penis, sublingual veins, and neck veins),

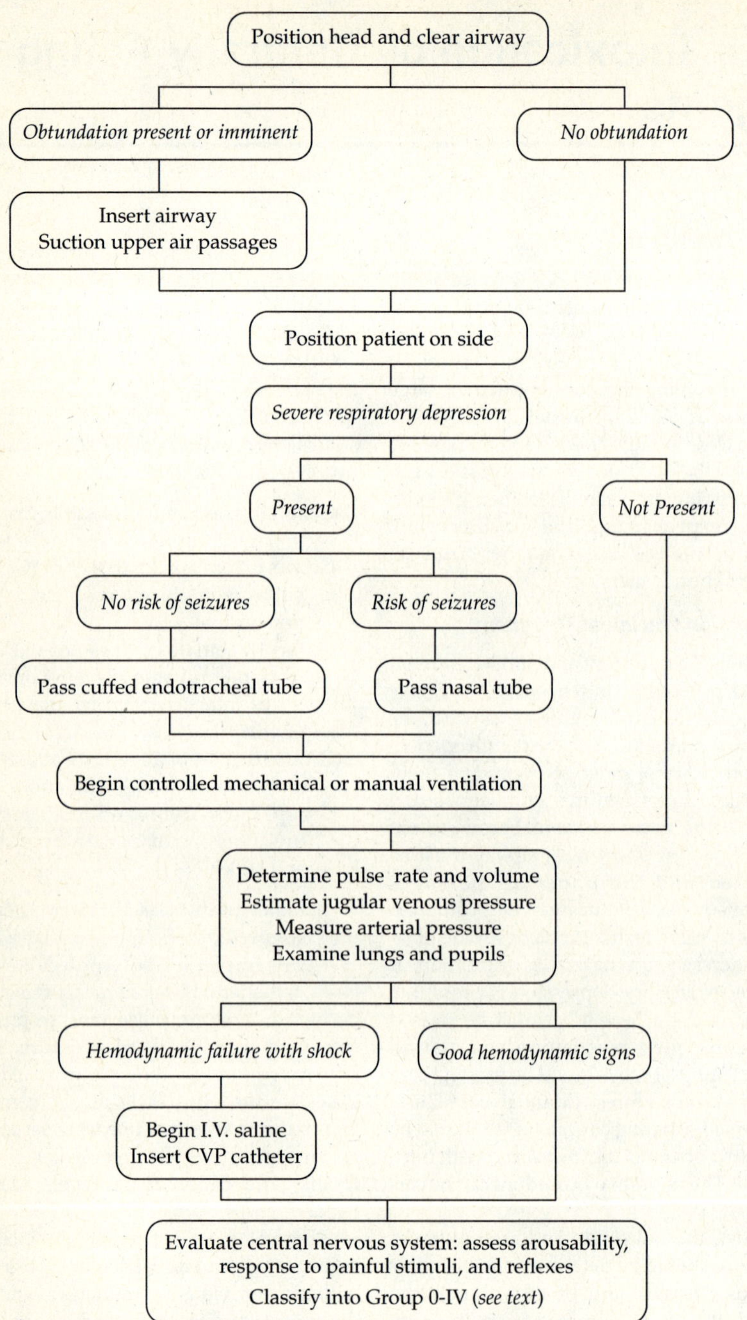

Figure 1 *Flowchart presents the clinical evaluation and initial treatment of patients with central nervous system intoxication from drug overdose.*

scars on the wrist, peristaltic activity, and signs of preexisting cardiovascular, hepatic, or renal disease. Erythematous and bullous skin lesions, especially at sites of pressure or agitation-related trauma, are characteristic of drug-induced coma.

It is important to determine the agents used (the contents of the patient's wallet or purse may provide useful clues), the doses taken, and the time of ingestion. Around-the-clock toxicology services can be invaluable in managing some high-risk patients and in identifying unknown intoxicants; whether general toxicology screening should be done routinely in instances of drug overdose is controversial.[1]

Supportive Therapy

Supportive and conservative measures ensure survival of most (probably more than 90 percent) of the patients who reach the emergency room. The key objectives are to maintain a clear airway, with adequate ventilation, and to support the circulation.

Support of Respiratory Function

It is essential to keep the upper air passages open and to watch for alveolar hypoventilation, as indicated by a rising arterial Pco_2 and a falling Po_2. If respiratory failure develops, assisted or controlled mechanical ventilation should be provided via a cuffed endotracheal tube. Adjustments of tidal volume and oxygen concentration are guided by arterial blood gas measurements [*see Chapter 38*]. Most patients require intubation for only two or three days. Rarely, longer periods of intubation and tracheostomy are required.

Pulmonary infection Lower respiratory tract infection is a major cause of morbidity, especially in patients who require intubation. Infection is probably related to the absence or inadequacy of gag and cough reflexes, which may have caused previous aspiration. Early signs are fever, leukocytosis, and purulent secretions. Chest x-rays may disclose pneumonic infiltrates and, in advanced cases, necrotizing pneumonia and abscesses.

Therapy for complicating airway or lung infections hinges on promptly identifying the invading organisms and on selecting appropriate antimicrobials. Percutaneous transtracheal aspiration (with immediate processing of specimens taken by aspiration without saline lavage) is recommended. Anaerobic organisms are the only pathogens in almost half the cases. Gram-positive cocci and gram-negative rods are also found, and mixed infections are common. Penicillin is effective for most anaerobic infections. Prednisone, 60 mg/day for two days, has been used for aspiration pneumonitis caused by gastric acid, but its effectiveness remains unproved. A bronchoscopy should be done to remove foreign material from the air passages.

Circulatory Support

Most patients require only enough I.V. fluid to maintain normal hydration and normal urine flow. Hemodynamic failure may occur and can rapidly evolve into shock. Decreased effective blood volume caused by hypovolemia or by expansion of the capacity of the vascular bed, or both, is common. Venous return is reduced, and cardiac output falls. Impaired myocardial function may also play a role in shock in severely intoxicated patients, especially if there is preexisting heart disease. Loss of peripheral arteriolar tone has been implicated, but its importance in drug-intoxication shock remains unclear. There is indirect evidence that drugs, hypotension, hypoxia, and hypothermia cause endothelial damage and increased capillary permeability. Such transcapillary leakage leads to interstitial fluid collections, pulmonary edema, and further hypovolemia.

Therapy for shock is best guided by monitoring the CVP. If the initial CVP is not elevated, 10 percent dextrose in normal saline can be infused at a rate of 20 ml/min while the CVP is monitored. If the CVP increases by more than 5 cm H_2O above the initial level, the infusion should be discontinued. If the CVP does not exceed the control value by more than 2 cm H_2O at the end of 10 minutes or if it declines, an additional 200 ml of fluid should be administered. This method, which challenges the heart, can be used cautiously during the first several hours to correct arterial hypotension. Elderly patients and patients with heart disease require special care because dangerous fluid overload can occur.

Vasoactive drugs, especially dopamine, have been used in initial treatment. Very small doses are given to increase arterial systolic pressure modestly to between 90 and 100 mm Hg. Fluid repletion should then correct the hemodynamic abnormality.

Congestive heart failure is usually heralded by an initially elevated CVP or a CVP that quickly increases to 20 cm H_2O or more before the first liter of I.V. fluid has been administered. It usually responds to I.V. dopamine. In some cases, digitalization is required.

Cardiac arrhythmias are likely to occur in the presence of severe hypoxemia, severe acid-base disorders, or severe hypovolemia. The alkaline overshoot that is caused by ventilator-induced sudden lowering of Pco_2 after several days of alveolar hypoventilation is particularly apt to cause cardiac arrhythmias. Anticholinergic drugs may also precipitate these arrhythmias.

Preventing Absorption

Stomach evacuation is most effective if done within a few hours of the time of ingestion and can be useful even after long intervals if the ingestants, such as narcotics, anticholinergics, and aspirin, delay gastric emptying. Stomach evacuation is not used if the patient has taken corrosive agents such as strong acids or strong bases (in such cases, lavage may be safely performed within a half hour of ingestion), convulsants, or petroleum distillates. The trachea should be intubated before the stomach is emptied if the gag or cough reflex is depressed.

If the patient is awake, it is simplest and safest to induce vomiting by the prompt administration of 15 to 20 ml of syrup of ipecac along with large volumes of water.[2] This procedure can be repeated in 15 to 30

minutes. In infants nine to 12 months of age, the usual dose is 10 ml; ipecac is not recommended for infants younger than nine months. The fluid extract of ipecac should not be used; it is 14 times stronger than ipecac syrup, and it is toxic.

If vomiting fails to occur, gastric lavage is appropriate. The patient should be placed on his or her left side, with the head hanging beneath the edge of the table and with the foot of the table elevated. A tube about 1 cm in diameter and of adequate length should be marked to indicate the distance between the epigastrium and the nostril, lubricated with a water-miscible jelly, and gently advanced into the stomach (most patients tolerate the nasal route better than the oral). Coughing and rapid breathing indicate that the larynx has been entered; peristaltic sounds from the epigastrium when air is injected will confirm the intragastric position. Tap water can be used for lavage, and the volume administered but not recovered should be recorded. Small washings (50 to 100 ml) are used for each lavage to avoid propelling the gastric contents into the small intestine. Each aliquot of returned washings should be saved for laboratory analysis. In cases of massive overdose, the tube can be left in place and repeated washings executed hourly.

Aspiration pneumonia, gastritis, and bleeding are potential hazards of gastric lavage. *In obtunded patients, neither lavage nor induced emesis should be attempted without the prior insertion of a cuffed endotracheal tube.* If marked drowsiness occurs after ipecac has been given, the trachea should be intubated before emesis begins.

Activated charcoal effectively adsorbs many agents. It usually is prepared as a slurry of 50 g wetted with 400 ml of distilled water and is given in doses of about 5 ml/kg. When given by lavage, it can be removed and the dose repeated. Multiple doses given during a period of several days appear to enhance clearance of phenobarbital, carbamazepine,[3] amitriptyline, and aspirin. In some patients, this regimen has apparently reduced the duration of coma; in others, however, there has been no clinical benefit.[4-6] It has been proposed that repeated doses exert their effect by blocking the reabsorption of biliary metabolites or by binding drug that has back-diffused into the gut.[5] Charcoal is relatively ineffective for the removal of alkali, boric acid, cyanide, DDT, electrolytes, elemental metals (e.g., boron, iron, lithium), ferrous sulfate, malathion, methanol, n-methyl carbamate, mineral acids, tolbutamide, and water-insoluble compounds.[7,8] It should not be used concurrently with antidotes such as ipecac and acetylcysteine.

The binding of drugs to charcoal is not irreversible. For example, 15 to 20 percent of aspirin is subsequently released by activated charcoal, leading to a delay in the time course of its absorption.[9] The clinical significance of charcoal desorption remains to be defined. Complications of charcoal therapy include fatal pulmonary aspiration of charcoal and the formation of a charcoal bezoar, which was reported in an instance of amitriptyline overdose.[10,11] Black stools can be expected after charcoal therapy.

Although it is difficult to document the benefits of cathartics in cases of drug overdose, these agents are recommended by many experts as a means of decreasing intestinal transit time and diminishing the absorption of the ingestant. A dose of 150 to 300 ml of a magnesium citrate solution (1.745 g/oz) is given by mouth to adults; half of this amount is usually prescribed for children six to 12 years of age. A 1 : 4 dilution of Fleet Phospho-Soda can be used in doses of 15 to 60 ml. Sorbitol, which is available as a mixture with ipecac, can be given instead of a saline laxative. Cathartics may be hazardous if dehydration, hypovolemia, hypotension, renal failure, or fluid and electrolyte disorders are present.

Other Supportive Measures

Patients with deep depression of the central nervous system will have to be turned from side to side about every two hours to avoid the development of bedsores. Passive leg exercises and properly fitted elastic stockings may reduce the risk of venous thrombosis. Alternating air mattresses and topical creams may help prevent pressure-induced skin damage. If the corneal reflex is absent, five percent boric acid ophthalmic ointment should be applied to the eyelids four times a day or viscous methylcellulose eyedrops instilled. Atonic eyelids should be taped closed.

An indwelling bladder catheter is necessary if prolonged unconsciousness is anticipated.

Aggressive Therapy

Forced diuresis induced by rapid infusion of fluids, by the use of mannitol, or by potent diuretics such as furosemide and ethacrynic acid has been advocated to hasten renal excretion of ingested drugs in seriously intoxicated patients but is rarely necessary, and because of significant risks, it remains controversial. Making decisions on the basis of amounts of ingested agents or blood drug levels is difficult because these factors do not always correlate with the clinical course.[12] However, in patients who are not addicted and in whom there is no other cause of CNS depression, the serum level of short-acting barbiturates apparently correlates well with the severity of intoxication.[13]

Hemodialysis may be necessary in seriously intoxicated patients with severe kidney failure if the excretion route is renal and the drug dialyzable. Because dialysis often fails to eliminate many drugs, hemoperfusion through a column containing Amberlite XAD-4 has been tried.[14] It may remove impressive amounts of barbiturates, glutethimide, ethchlorvynol, tricyclic antidepressants, chloral hydrate, and digitoxin.[14-16] The potentially serious complications (anemia, sometimes requiring transfusions; thrombocytopenia; and hypocalcemia) indicate that the method should be used only in the most dire instances of poisoning.

Psychiatric Evaluation

A high percentage of patients suffering from drug overdose or intoxication are would-be suicides. These patients are apt to try again and often do succeed in killing themselves. The risk is high for all such patients, including those whose attempts appear to have been hysteric or psychopathic gestures or the result of alcoholism. The danger of eventual suicide, however, is highest in individuals who have made serious attempts. In one study in which 88 patients who were initially hospitalized for a drug overdose were followed for an average period of 10 months, five percent died of a subsequent overdose, and 42 percent were readmitted for a nonfatal overdose or psychiatric illness.[17] Psychiatric evaluation is strongly advised for all patients who have taken an overdose.

Problems Related to Specific Drugs and Poisons

Phenobarbital

Biologic membranes are generally impermeable to ionized compounds. Shifting the equilibrium to favor formation of the ionized form of a drug will tend to prevent its penetration into cells such as the neurons of the brain or its reabsorption by cells such as those that line renal tubules. Because alkalinization of the urine strongly favors the dissociation of phenobarbital (but not of other barbiturates), sodium bicarbonate should be given intravenously to block tubular reabsorption; alkalinization markedly increases urinary excretion of this long-acting sedative. Repeated doses of activated charcoal probably enhance drug clearance.

Salicylates

At pH 7.4, virtually all salicylic acid is in the ionized, nonpenetrating form and remains in the blood. A fall in blood pH from 7.4 to 7.2 doubles the proportion of nonionized salicylic acid and causes salicylate to enter the tissues, including the brain.

The severity of intoxication correlates roughly with salicylate blood levels. In general, serum levels exceeding 85 mg/dl indicate dangerous poisoning. It is worth determining the interval since ingestion because serum levels decline with time, but

precision is often impossible. In any case, blood drug levels may be misleading—a declining serum level may reflect undesirable cellular penetration caused by acidemia unless the decline results from increased urinary loss. Because of these considerations, the arterial pH and gases should be determined frequently.

Salicylate intoxication, occasionally from therapeutic use rather than suicidal intent, increases CO_2 production, enhances sensitivity of the respiratory center, and causes hyperventilation. This sequence is protective in that respiratory alkalosis favors the extracellular distribution of the drug. Renal compensation leads to alkalinization of tubular urine and causes increased excretion of salicylate.

In severe poisoning, metabolic acidosis may supervene. Respiratory acidosis may occur if other drugs with CNS-depressant properties are ingested along with the salicylates. Combined ingestions are common in suicide attempts.[18]

Significant cation losses, especially of potassium, may occur. The severity of the potassium deficit may be difficult to estimate because potassium shifts into or out of body cells with changing arterial pH. Alkalemia shifts the ion from extracellular to intracellular fluid, lowering the serum level; acidemia moves the ion from intracellular to extracellular fluid, raising the serum level. Thus, potassium repletion should be guided by frequent measurements of serum electrolyte levels and arterial pH.

The initial phase of respiratory alkalosis rarely requires specific treatment. Metabolic acidosis associated with ingestion of large amounts of salicylates, however, can be dangerous. For this reason and because of the problems related to potassium imbalance, the arterial blood pH and gases should be determined frequently, and sodium bicarbonate should be administered at a rate sufficient to correct acidemia. The dose can be roughly estimated by means of the following formula:

$$\text{mEq bicarbonate} = 0.3 \times \text{kg body weight} \times \text{mEq/l bicarbonate deficit}$$

The goal is to bring the arterial blood pH to 7.4; the infusion rate must be adjusted on the basis of frequent monitoring of the arterial blood pH and gases.

Other intervention may be needed in very severe poisoning, especially if metabolic acidosis or renal failure supervenes. Repeated doses of activated charcoal have been reported to result in rapid reduction of plasma salicylate levels after aspirin overdose.[19] Alkaline diuresis should be considered if the plasma salicylate level exceeds 75 mg/dl (or 50 mg/dl in the presence of metabolic acidosis).[20] Bicarbonate can be used to enhance renal excretion of salicylate, which dramatically increases when urine pH exceeds 7.0.[21] The amount required varies widely, but 225 mEq given during a three-hour period to adults is usually effective and is unlikely to cause problems, provided that the arterial pH and gases and serum electrolytes are monitored.[21] Hemodialysis (or hemoperfusion) should be considered if the plasma salicylate level exceeds 90 mg/dl (or 75 mg/dl in the presence of renal failure).[20]

If CNS depression and alveolar hypoventilation develop, mechanical ventilation through a cuffed endotracheal tube may be lifesaving. Because salicylic acid may interfere with brain glucose metabolism, glucose should be included in the intravenous solutions.

Noncardiogenic pulmonary edema may develop during the first 24 hours of treatment, even if plasma salicylate levels are declining.[22] The mechanism appears to be increased pulmonary vascular permeability. The role of volume loading with colloids remains unclear.

Polycyclic Antidepressants

It is not surprising that the polycyclic antidepressants are a leading cause of serious drug overdose, given the fact that they are widely prescribed to depressed patients, the group most likely to attempt suicide.[23] Ingestion of excessive amounts may result in fatal cardiovascular and CNS dysfunction.

Most of these drugs are tricyclic, having a central three-ring structure. Amoxapine, a congener, induces less cardiotoxicity than the tricyclics when taken in overdose, but fatal cardiotoxicity has been reported after the ingestion of two grams of amoxapine.[24] Amoxapine poisoning has caused serious CNS effects, including intractable seizures that have resulted in hyperthermia, coagulopathy, and rhabdomyolysis.[25,26] Overdoses of maprotiline, a tetracyclic compound with toxicity similar to that of the tricyclics, have caused the dangerous *torsade de pointes* form of ventricular tachycardia.[27] Trazodone is chemically dissimilar from the polycyclic drugs and appears to be significantly less cardiotoxic when taken in excessive doses.[28]

The mechanism of action of the polycyclic drugs is controversial. They inhibit reuptake of norepinephrine and serotonin; however, the time course of their antidepressant effects suggests that they modify the sensitivity of perisynaptic receptors as well as inhibit neurotransmitter reuptake. They also exert potent anticholinergic effects and inhibit H_1 and H_2 histamine receptors. The drugs are readily absorbed when taken orally and are inactivated principally by the liver. Almost all of the drug is bound by protein in the plasma, and less than five percent is eliminated by the kidneys [*see Chapter 32*]. Dissociation of the protein-bound form is favored at lowered pH. Thus, acidemia, such as that associated with intractable seizures, increases the proportion of free compound and intensifies toxicity, whereas alkalemia increases protein binding and lowers the concentration of free drug in the plasma. This pH dependence provides a therapeutic opportunity in cases of serious overdose, which may respond favorably to induced alkalosis.

Symptoms of overdose usually appear within a few hours of ingestion. The initial manifestations are the result of anticholinergic effects and consist of dry mouth, blurred vision, and impaired micturition. Fever, pupillary dilatation, and hypoperistalsis, which may prolong the period of absorption, are often present. Rapid progression to more serious problems may occur. Evidence of major toxicity is usually apparent within two hours of hospital admission; in lethal cases, the mean time between hospital arrival and death is about six hours.[29] CNS impairment can lead to restlessness, agitation, confusion, hallucinations, seizures, coma, and respiratory depression. Other manifestations include severe clonus and extrapyramidal and cerebellar signs.

Cardiovascular toxicity may be an early manifestation and can be rapidly fatal. Most ECG changes appear within the first 24 hours.[30] Conduction disorders are common, and the QRS duration in ECG limb leads has been found to correlate closely with the severity of the poisoning. A QRS duration of 0.10 sec or greater indicates serious intoxication.[31] Other ECG findings include ST and T wave abnormalities, prolongation of the PR and QT intervals, and bundle branch block. Conduction defects may persist for as long as one week after ingestion. Ventricular tachycardia and ventricular fibrillation can occur suddenly. Hypotension, resulting from myocardial depression as well as vasodilatation, is often associated with arrhythmias and pulmonary edema.[32]

Because the drug plasma levels are not precisely correlated with the seriousness of the overdose, in most instances the QRS duration rather than drug plasma concentrations should be used to monitor the patient.[23]

Standard supportive measures should be instituted, including the administration of charcoal and a cathartic. Repeated doses of charcoal have been reported to hasten the elimination of amitriptyline.[33] Ipecac should not be given because of the risk of aspiration should obtundation or seizures rapidly ensue.

Seizures should be suppressed initially with diazepam. Because diazepam has a brief duration of action (about 20 minutes), phenytoin has been employed for sustained antiseizure effect. The I.V. solution should contain 1,000 mg of phenytoin sodium in 130 ml of saline and should be infused at a rate of 40 to 50 mg/min or less.[34,35] A total loading dose of 10 to 15 mg/kg usually achieves therapeutic blood levels of phenytoin (10 to

20 µg/ml).[35] Maintenance doses of about 100 mg may be required every six to eight hours; plasma phenytoin levels should be used to adjust the dose.

Ventricular arrhythmias and severe conduction disorders have responded to alkalemia induced by the administration of bicarbonate or by the use of mechanical hyperventilation.[36] The optimal pH is not known, but keeping the pH above 7.45 has been recommended.[18] Lidocaine can be used to gain rapid control of arrhythmias. Intravenous phenytoin may correct conduction defects as well as suppress arrhythmias [*see Chapter 2*].[23,34]

The efficacy and risks of beta blockers and of bretylium tosylate are ill defined.[23]

Temporary pacemaking may be needed in instances of Mobitz II heart block or complete heart block. Atropine is ineffective in this setting; isoproterenol may be helpful while pacemaking is being established [*see Chapter 3*].

Hypotension should be treated by alkalinization and volume expansion. If hypotension persists, alpha-adrenergic agents such as norepinephrine or phenylephrine may be beneficial.[23]

The cholinesterase inhibitor physostigmine salicylate (1 to 3 mg I.V. infused slowly) has been used to control CNS manifestations.[37] However, this agent has fallen into disfavor because the cardiovascular complications of polycyclic drug overdose are not related to anticholinergic effects and because bradyarrhythmias, including asystole, have been associated with its use.[38]

Ethyl Alcohol

The clinical expressions of acute ethyl alcohol (ethanol) intoxication depend on the amount consumed, the rate and duration of consumption, the rates of absorption and of hepatic oxidation, inherent or acquired CNS tolerance, and the presence of coexisting disease.[39]

The degree of CNS and respiratory depression is critical. A blood level of 5 mg/ml is lethal in about half of cases. The maintenance of adequate ventilation, as indicated by arterial blood gases, is paramount. Mechanical ventilation may be necessary. Intravenous naloxone, given in doses of 0.4 mg, can arouse intoxicated patients.[40] Its mechanism of action is uncertain.

Acutely intoxicated patients are often belligerent and difficult to examine but should be scrutinized for injury, especially of the head and neck. Hypoglycemia may be profound if heavy alcohol consumption accompanies food deprivation. Alcohol withdrawal reactions require prompt management. Alcoholic ketoacidosis is covered under Metabolism [*see Chapter 30*].

Methyl Alcohol

Methyl alcohol (methanol), widely used in industry and currently being evaluated as an energy source, is sometimes consumed as a substitute for liquor. Unlike ethyl alcohol, it produces only mild initial inebriation, but after a period that may last as long as 24 hours, signs of toxicity occur. The distinguishing clinical feature is visual impairment, ranging from blurring to blindness. The eye grounds may show retinal edema and hyperemia of the optic disk, and CT brain scans may reveal areas of infarction.[41,42] Hyperamylasemia may occur, but this finding should not be equated with the presence of pancreatitis, because plasma salivary amylase activity may be increased after methanol poisoning.[43] Headache, nausea, vomiting, severe abdominal pain (suggesting a surgical crisis or ureteral colic), and CNS depression are common. Severe metabolic acidosis develops as the compound degrades to formaldehyde, formic acid, and other acids. These substances are probably also responsible for the toxic effects on the retina, the optic nerve, and the brain. Death is common.

Hemodialysis has been strikingly effective in removing the agent and preventing visual and cerebral damage.[44] Prompt hemodialysis via percutaneous vessel cannulation should be considered when the amount of methanol ingested exceeds the minimal lethal dose (30 ml), when blood levels exceed 50 mg/dl, or when there is acidosis or evidence of visual or cerebral dysfunction.[45] Peritoneal dialysis is only one eighth as effective as hemodialysis.[46]

Other treatment should be instituted immediately, using sodium bicarbonate to control the acidosis and ethyl alcohol to retard the rate of generation of methanol's degradation products. Ethyl alcohol has a far higher affinity for the enzyme system shared by these two alcohols; ethanol, given early and continued for several days, may prevent dangerous accumulations of formaldehyde and formic acid. A loading dose of oral ethanol, 0.6 g/kg body weight, or about four 1 oz shots of 80-proof liquor for a 70 kg person, should be given whenever the oral route is appropriate. The maintenance dose of ethanol needed to sustain blood levels of 100 g/dl is about 100 mg ethanol/kg body weight/hr (for a 70 kg person, this is equivalent to about half an ounce of 80-proof liquor). In comatose patients, intravenous therapy can be used. A loading dose of about 500 ml of 10 percent ethanol may be given during a one-hour period.[47,48] The excess free water, however, may induce hyponatremia. During dialysis, the maintenance dose of ethanol should be increased to about 250 mg/kg/hr; 95 percent ethanol is added to the dialysate (to attain a dialysate level of 100 mg/ml.[41] Ethanol must be administered cautiously to patients with CNS, hepatic, or myocardial damage. Experimental data indicate that immediate administration of folinic acid may prevent the accumulation of formate.[46]

Ethylene Glycol

Ethylene glycol, used in many commercial products, is most widely available as antifreeze. Its warm, sweet, pleasant taste accounts for many accidental ingestions, especially when it is stored in beverage bottles. It has been drunk as a substitute for ethanol and in suicide attempts. Intoxications have occurred as a consequence of the inadvertent cross-connection of heating systems containing antifreeze and potable water supplies.[49] As little as 2 oz may be lethal.

The parent compound seems relatively nontoxic, but its metabolites, including aldehydes and organic acids, especially oxalate, are highly cytotoxic. Glycolic and lactic acids are important causes of severe metabolic acidosis in this form of poisoning.[50]

Initially, patients exhibit signs of inebriation without an alcoholic breath. Progressive CNS depression develops, followed by cardiac, respiratory, and renal failure. Clues to the diagnosis are (1) metabolic acidosis with anion gap, (2) calcium oxalate crystals in the urine, and (3) hypocalcemia—sometimes with tetany—from oxalate chelation of calcium.

Therapy can be lifesaving. Prompt hemodialysis removes ethylene glycol, glycolic acid, oxalate, and aldehydes. Correction of acidosis with sodium bicarbonate, restoration of plasma calcium levels by injections of calcium gluconate, and repletion of thiamine and pyridoxine reserves (which may be exhausted by the metabolic degradation of ethylene glycol) are all useful. Ethanol is a competitive inhibitor of the degradation of ethylene glycol; ethanol infusion (see above) has been advocated. Complete CNS recovery is possible if cardiac, respiratory, and renal support is successful.

The rapid inhibition of alcohol dehydrogenase by 4-methylpyrazole (4-MP) has prompted the use of this agent in the treatment of ethylene glycol poisoning. The oral administration of 4-MP has resulted in rapid urinary excretion of ethylene glycol; if further studies confirm its efficacy and safety, 4-MP could become a specific antidote for ethylene glycol poisoning in patients who have intact renal function.[51]

Heroin and Other Opioids

Opioid overdose produces pinpoint pupils, respiratory depression, and sensorial impairment. The acute syndrome and its management are essentially the same for morphine, heroin, methadone, codeine, pentazocine, propoxyphene, and related compounds. Heroin overdose is especially common, and heroin-related deaths have reached epidemic proportions in urban centers.

The initial crisis is severe respiratory depression and even apnea. (Most patients with fatal heroin overdose probably die before reaching medical facilities.) In a dire emergency, the patient should be ventilated with a manual, self-inflating resuscitative bag into which 100 percent oxygen is delivered. An endotracheal tube attached to a mechanical ventilator set for controlled ventilation should then be inserted. Next, I.V. naloxone should be given in a dosage of 0.8 mg (range, 0.4 to 2.0 mg) repeated every two to three minutes until respiratory rate increases or sensorial level improves. (For children, the usual initial dose is 0.01 mg/kg; if this dose does not produce sufficient clinical improvement, a subsequent dose of 0.1 mg/kg may be given.) In adults, failure to respond to a total dose of 10 mg suggests that the disorder is not opiate related or that other drugs have also been taken. The plasma half-life of naloxone is one hour, and the peak effect may last only 10 minutes. Intravenous infusions at dose rates of up to 5 mg/hr may be required, and treatment for several days may be needed for overdoses caused by long-acting agents such as methadone.[52] In addicts, naloxone may produce an acute withdrawal reaction within minutes; it usually subsides after one to two hours.

Pulmonary edema is common and is associated with a high mortality. Hypoxia, hypotension, neurogenic mechanisms, and drug-related endothelial damage have been implicated. Management is the same as that employed in the adult respiratory distress syndrome, and standard support measures for CNS drug overdose are appropriate.

Heroin use is associated with hepatitis, hypoglycemia, endocarditis, arrhythmias, pulmonary emboli (including septic and foreign-body emboli), pulmonary artery mycotic aneurysms, gas gangrene, tetanus (especially in females), tuberculosis, and malaria.[53] Heroin-associated nephropathy has become an important cause of end-stage renal failure in urban populations, especially among black males. The initial presentation is asymptomatic proteinuria or the nephrotic syndrome. The nephropathy is unresponsive to therapy and usually progresses rapidly to renal failure.[54] There is a positive association between heroin-related deaths and the average amount of quinine in illicit packages. A 10-second intravenous injection can deliver a quinine dose that is up to 182 times the therapeutic maximum.

Placental transfer of heroin has caused high drug levels in fetal tissue and has likely led to fetal death.[55]

Propoxyphene overdose usually occurs in persons who have a chronic physical or psychologic illness. Polypharmacy and the additive effects of alcohol are often important factors.[56] Toxic manifestations of propoxyphene overdose are progressive sensorial impairment, seizures, respiratory depression, shock, and pulmonary edema. Respiratory and lactic acidosis may be severe, especially if salicylates have been ingested concomitantly. Death may occur within one hour of ingestion.

Treatment should begin with the restoration of ventilation and the administration of naloxone. Other standard supportive measures should then be instituted.

Intravenously Injected Marijuana

Sporadic instances of toxic disorders from intravenous administration of marijuana have been reported.[57] The syndrome starts within an hour after injection and comprises nausea, vomiting, generalized pains, shaking chills, fever, tachycardia, and diarrhea. Other features include initial leukopenia followed by leukocytosis, thrombocytopenia without evidence of disseminated intravascular coagulation, and probably rhabdomyolysis. Profound hypotension and renal insufficiency ensue; both are reversible. Vasoactive amines may correct the hypotension, which is relatively refractory; mannitol infusion may prevent renal failure. Complete recovery has been reported.

Phencyclidine

Phencyclidine, also known as PCP or angel dust, is a common cause of poisoning.[58] The drug is available in tablet, capsule, or powder form and is ingested, smoked (often with tobacco or marijuana), sniffed, or injected intravenously.

Phencyclidine can produce acute psychoses, dyskinesia, seizures, laryngospasm, and respiratory distress. Nystagmus, ataxia, contracted pupils, and hyperreflexia are common. Opisthotonos, decerebrate rigidity, and rhabdomyolysis and myoglobinuria (attributed to severe dystonia) have been seen.[59] Severe hypertension sometimes occurs, and hypertensive crises may ensue. Large doses of phencyclidine result in stupor or coma, mimicking head injury.[60] Intracranial hemorrhage and hyperthermia-associated submassive liver necrosis have occurred.[61,62]

Because chromatographic assay of blood, urine, or gastric contents may not be readily available, treatment is often based on a clinical impression. Mild intoxication is usually treated by confinement in an environment in which visual and aural stimuli are minimized. A calm atmosphere and a reassuring manner on the part of the staff are helpful.

More severe cases may require specific therapy. Because phencyclidine is a weak base that is readily ionized in mildly acidic solutions, it is subject to ion trapping in the urine and the gastric lumen (i.e., the ionized form of the drug is trapped outside of the circulation because it cannot traverse membranes). Urine drug levels have been reported to be increased 200-fold by lowering the urine pH below 5.0. Acidification is achieved with ammonium chloride; 2.75 mEq/kg is dissolved in 60 ml of saline and administered via a gastric tube, which is then clamped for one hour. The dose is repeated at six-hour intervals until the urine pH is below 5.0. Usually, two doses are required. Both oral (6 g/day for four days) and intravenous (2 g/20 min) ascorbic acid have been advocated for acidification, but these regimens do not appear to lower plasma or urine pH.[63] Urine acidification could be undesirable in patients who have ingested salicylates or phenobarbital. After urine pH is lowered, furosemide-induced diuresis greatly enhances renal excretion.

In dire emergencies, such as profound coma or intractable seizures, ammonium chloride can be given intravenously in a dose of 2.75 mEq/kg as a one to two percent solution in saline. During ammonium chloride therapy, arterial blood gases, blood ammonia and electrolyte levels, and renal function should be closely monitored.

Phencyclidine is secreted into the gastric lumen, where it can be trapped and removed by gastric lavage and continuous suctioning. A saline laxative should be instilled after the initial gastric aspiration. Continuous gastric suction may be needed for several days after consciousness returns. Seizures are usually treated with diazepam; hypertensive crises require diazoxide.

Chronic brain dysfunction may persist after repetitive use. Memory gaps, dysphasia, impaired impulse control, and belligerence are among the long-lasting, perhaps permanent, effects.

Methaqualone

Prescribed under the trade names Quaalude and Sopor as a sedative-hypnotic, methaqualone is widely used by adolescents and young adults. Most methaqualone-related deaths occur in white males (average age, 25 years). The blood level is usually about 2.3 mg/dl, six times the therapeutic level. Although some fatalities result from accidental or suicidal overdose, the majority are caused by vehicular accidents.[64] Intoxication with methaqualone impairs judgment, coordination, impulse control, and the ability to cope with the unexpected. Its effects are additive to those of other psychotropic agents, including alcohol. Overdose produces vomiting, hepatic and renal damage, generalized and pulmonary edema, restlessness, hypertonia, tonic seizures, stupor, coma, and respiratory depression. Management includes general support measures and control of seizures.

Acetaminophen

Often, the victim selects acetaminophen, a readily available household analgesic, on a sudden suicidal impulse. Overdose does not produce rapid loss of consciousness, as does an overdose of salicylates or central nervous system depressants. Patients feel quite well at first, but nausea, vomiting, abdominal pain, and diarrhea rapidly develop. Many suffer hepatic damage, indicated by prolongation of the prothrombin time and elevation of the serum enzyme and bilirubin levels within 24 to 48 hours after ingestion. Renal failure is less frequent and is usually mild, although severe tubular necrosis may ensue. In some patients, centrilobular hepatic necrosis proceeds to fulminant hepatic failure, but the vast majority recover fully; many fatal cases in the United States are caused by the coingestion of propoxyphene.[65] However, ingestion of as little as 25 g of acetaminophen may be fatal.

Therapy involves emptying the gastrointestinal tract with ipecac or by means of lavage with a large-bore tube. If drug blood levels exceed 250 µg/ml four hours after ingestion, the overdose is probably severe. Because hepatotoxicity is caused by a glutathione-depleting metabolite of acetaminophen, the sulfhydryl donor acetylcysteine is an effective antidote.[66] Acetylcysteine is given orally as a five percent solution diluted with three volumes of a soft drink. The initial loading dose is 140 mg/kg; thereafter, 70 mg/kg is given every four hours for an additional 17 doses. If the patient is unable to swallow, the solution is administered by gastric or enteral tube. Treatment is most effective when it is begun within eight hours of ingestion but can still be beneficial if it is delayed for as long as 24 hours. In one series of 2,540 poisonings, there were no deaths among persons who received the antidote within 16 hours.[66]

Intravenous acetylcysteine (300 mg/kg, given during a 20-hour period) has been used in Europe and Canada. The 72-hour oral treatment appears to be as effective as the 20-hour intravenous regimen.[66]

In Great Britain, oral methionine is used. Ten 250 mg tablets are given immediately, followed by 10 tablets every four hours, for a total of 40 tablets (10 g).[67]

Severe, sometimes fatal, hepatic injury has occurred in alcoholics who have taken only moderate doses of acetaminophen.[68-70] Exceedingly high aminotransferase values characterize the hepatitis.

Cocaine

The dangerous effects of cocaine were well known early in the 20th century, but when the drug came into widespread use in the 1970s and 1980s, a common misconception about its safety prevailed. Nonusers and skeptics were dismissed as uninformed and "square." Deaths associated with cocaine use have become common, and it is estimated that 30 million Americans have tried cocaine and that five million use it regularly.[71,72]

Cocaine, an alkaloid derived from the leaves of the *Erythroxylon coca* plant, is available in various forms.[73] The usual preparation is a hydrochloride salt that is sold as a powder (often in diluted form) and inhaled or snorted. Local vasoconstriction and relatively poor absorption prevent rapid increases in plasma levels when the drug is used in this form. Euphoric effects last up to an hour and a half. Cocaine hydrochloride has a high melting point (approximately 195° C) and decomposes on heating and thus cannot be smoked.

Free-base cocaine, also known as rock or crack, is formulated by alkalinizing the hydrochloride salt with ammonia or baking soda and precipitating the alkaloid cocaine. Free-base cocaine has a melting point of 95° to 100° C and therefore can be smoked in a tobacco cigarette or a glass water pipe. It is readily absorbed in the lungs. Plasma drug levels rapidly surge, inducing almost immediate euphoria, which usually lasts only about 20 minutes and is abruptly followed by a profoundly dysphoric state, a sequence that may initiate cycles of repetitive use. Free-base cocaine became widely available during the mid-1980s, and a large number of sudden deaths have been attributed to its use.[74] It must be stressed, however, that intranasal use of cocaine is also highly dangerous and has caused sudden cardiac deaths.[75]

Central effects of cocaine appear to result from excessive dopaminergic neurotransmission in the reward pathways; presynaptic reuptake of dopamine is blocked.[73] Circulatory effects probably result from blocked reuptake of norepinephrine at adrenergic synapses.[75] In addition, cocaine produces small-vessel vasoconstriction.

Cocaine is powerfully addictive. Rats given free access to intravenous heroin or intravenous cocaine are three times more likely to die of drug-associated causes if they use cocaine than if they use heroin.[76]

Acute cocaine toxicity results in apprehension, headache, dizziness, syncope, blurred vision, and dysphoric states (e.g., depression, paranoid ideation, confusion, and suicidal, aggressive, and assaultive behavior). Focal neurologic signs and symptoms may appear.[77] Benzodiazepines may suppress some of these effects; haloperidol has been used to control paranoia.[73,77,78] Seizures, sometimes associated with fatal intoxication, are usually treated with diazepam. Coma, respiratory depression, and apnea may rapidly follow cocaine use, especially I.V. use, and can be associated with sudden death.

Cardiovascular toxicity appears to be common and has been observed after intake of nonmassive doses of the drug in its intranasal, intravenous, or free-base form.[75] Fatalities have occurred in persons without preexisting cardiovascular disease and in the absence of seizures.[75] Adverse effects have included sinus tachycardia, ventricular premature beats, ventricular tachycardia, ventricular fibrillation, and asystole.[73,75] Numerous instances of acute myocardial infarction have been documented in young individuals (mean age, 32 years).[73,75,79] Myocardial infarction has also occurred in persons with preexisting angina. The mechanism of myocardial infarction is not clear; however, it is believed to involve acute thrombosis, vasospasm, and sudden increases in myocardial oxygen requirements related to increased workload caused by sudden hypertension and tachycardia. In addition, cardiomyopathy has been found in some individuals who have abused cocaine.[75] Rupture of the ascending aorta has also been reported.[80]

Propranolol and amitriptyline have been used to treat life-threatening arrhythmias.[73] Calcium antagonists have been effective in treating cardiovascular toxicity in rats.[81] Artificial pacemaking may be required for conduction disorders.

Intravenous use of cocaine appears to be associated with an especially high risk of endocarditis when compared with other intravenous drugs of abuse.[82]

Severe hypertension and vasospasm may be responsible for the cerebrovascular accidents that have occurred in young persons shortly after using cocaine. Subarachnoid hemorrhage, cerebral vasculitis, and cerebral infarction have been reported.[73,83]

Spontaneous pneumomediastinum, pulmonary edema, and decreased diffusing capacity are among the severe lower respiratory tract complications. Damage to the upper respiratory tract includes anosmia, atrophy of the nasal mucous membranes, and ulceration and perforation of the nasal septum.

Other complications that can occur include bowel ischemia and gangrene (presumably from intense local vasoconstriction), hyperthermia, skin and muscle infarction, rhabdomyolysis, acute renal failure, liver dysfunction, and disseminated intravascular coagulation.[72,84,85]

Cocaine use during pregnancy can cause a number of problems. Onset of labor with abruptio placentae has immediately followed I.V. use. Studies in ewes indicate that cocaine reduces uterine blood flow and impairs maternal-fetal oxygen delivery.[86] The rate of spontaneous abortion is high, and exposed infants are at increased risk of congenital malformation and perinatal mortality.[73] Infants whose mothers used cocaine during pregnancy show significant depression of interactive behavior and impaired responses to environmental stimuli. It is not known whether these effects are permanent.[87]

Deaths have occurred among so-called body packers, smugglers who conceal cocaine by swallowing drug-filled balloons, condoms, or plastic bags. Such containers, which have also been carried in the rectum or vagina, are made of semipermeable material and can release their contents without rupturing, thus causing seizures and fatal intoxication. Although laparotomy and surgical removal have both been advocated, the packets can be passed uneventfully with conservative management.[88]

A hot line, 1-800-COCAINE, can provide additional information and serve as a referral source for patients.

Petroleum Products and Solvents

The advent of fuel shortages during 1979 precipitated a rash of petroleum ingestions associated with gasoline siphoning. In most cases, only small volumes (5 to 10 ml) are swallowed, and treatment is not required.[89] Ingestion of larger amounts, however, leads to gastrointestinal symptoms (burning mouth, nausea, vomiting, eructation), respiratory tract irritation (hoarseness, cough, dyspnea, burning in the chest), and CNS dysfunction (headache, vertigo, convulsions, coma, death). Ingestion of petroleum products such as turpentine, kerosene, mineral seal oil, lighter fluid, and furniture polish, usually by young children, produce similar syndromes.

The principal hazard is aspiration during spontaneous vomiting or during induced gastric emptying. Hydrocarbon pneumonia has been attributed in large part to alteration of the physical properties of surfactant, which results in atelectasis, edema, and airway closure. Bronchiolar and alveolar necrosis, interstitial pneumonia, and chronic scarring with fibrosis and bronchiectasis all may occur. Permanent sequelae are probably more likely in adults than in young children.[90]

The key management decision relates to emptying the stomach. Because of the hazard of inducing aspiration, most patients should be treated conservatively.[91] When a large volume has been swallowed (about 1 ml/kg—it can be difficult to ascertain the amount ingested) or other toxic agents have been ingested, gastric emptying with syrup of ipecac may be indicated. If central nervous system depression is present, a cuffed endotracheal tube should be inserted before gastric lavage is begun.

Gasoline sniffing can cause sudden fatal arrhythmias.[92] Habitual solvent abuse can cause cardiomyopathy[93] and lead poisoning; chelation therapy is appropriate in the latter.[94,95]

The sudden deaths of several adolescents have been attributed to arrhythmias triggered by the sniffing of typewriter correction fluid, which contains the solvents 1,1,1-trichloroethane and trichloroethylene.[96]

Strychnine

Once widely prescribed as a tonic in various medicinal forms of nux vomica, strychnine was an important cause of accidental poisoning in children and of suicide and homicide in adults. Used now as a garden and agricultural bait poison to control rodents and other ground animals, strychnine rarely causes poisoning in humans.

When it is ingested, strychnine is rapidly absorbed from the gastrointestinal tract, poorly bound by plasma proteins, and promptly cleared from the blood. It is principally metabolized in the liver; about 20 percent is excreted unchanged in the urine. Strychnine blocks inhibitory neurons in the central nervous system, principally in the spinal cord, brainstem, and thalamus. The result is extreme neuronal hyperexcitability, tetanic spasms, and convulsions. The mean lethal oral dose for adults is probably between 100 and 120 mg, although death has resulted from far smaller doses and individuals have survived ingestion of much larger amounts.

Symptoms appear rapidly, usually within 10 to 30 minutes.[97] In some, the first symptoms are agitation and apprehension, followed by pain and stiffness in the facial, nuchal, and paravertebral musculature. In others, convulsions appear without warning, beginning with clonic movement. These symptoms are followed by extreme tonic spasm and then by opisthotonos, trismus, and risus sardonicus. Tetanic spasm of the respiratory muscles causes apnea and cyanosis. In typical cases, there is a series of as many as 10 convulsions, which are interrupted by periods of muscle relaxation and profound exhaustion lasting about 10 minutes. The victims remain alert during the seizures and experience extreme pain and apprehension. Most patients survive the series of seizures, which may last as long as six hours. Death results from apnea during a protracted seizure; in instances of massive overdose, apnea may occur within minutes of ingestion, presumably because of exhaustion of medullary neurons. In one incident, eight persons sniffed strychnine in the belief that it was cocaine. The person who inhaled the largest amount experienced convulsions within minutes and died nine hours later.[98] Severe intoxication has also occurred after the snorting of cocaine that had been cut with strychnine.[99]

The principal complications of strychnine poisoning are rhabdomyolysis with myoglobinuria, lactic acidosis, and fractures, including those caused by compression of the spine. The differential diagnosis includes epilepsy, tetanus, rabies, bacterial meningitis, and hysteria.

Because of the rapid gastrointestinal absorption and plasma clearance of strychnine, toxicologic studies are often done on urine rather than on gastric contents or on blood. Lactic acidosis may cause a sharp increase in the blood lactate level, an anion gap, and a low arterial pH. Rhabdomyolysis results in myoglobinuria and in striking plasma elevations of creatine kinase and other muscle enzymes. Transient hypernatremia has been attributed to seizure-induced intracellular hyperosmolarity, which causes inflow of water from the extracellular space.[97]

Seizure control is usually achieved with diazepam (5 to 10 mg I.V. repeated as needed). Occasionally, general anesthesia, curariform drugs (succinylcholine, 60 to 80 mg I.V.), and mechanical ventilation are required.

Gastric lavage and charcoal administration may be helpful if given early; however, the rapid absorption of strychnine may defeat these measures. Furthermore, the hazards of aspiration and of inducing seizures necessitate prior convulsion control and intubation.

Because sudden sensory stimulation may evoke a violent motor response, treatment should proceed in a darkened, quiet, reassuring setting. General supportive care should be given, including oxygen, fluids, glucose, and electrolytes. Severe metabolic acidosis can be corrected with I.V. bicarbonate. Peritoneal dialysis and hemodialysis are not useful. If the patient survives the initial seizures (usually lasting six hours), recovery without sequelae can be expected.

Other Toxic Agents

There are thousands of toxic agents that can cause significant poisoning; consequently, a detailed description of the manifestations and management of all, or even most, such poisonings is not feasible within the constraints of this subsection. For a discussion of the diagnosis and management of other poisonings, the reader is referred to the *Handbook of Poisoning: Diagnosis and Treatment*, by Dreisbach and Robertson.[100]

References

1. Arch Intern Med 148:437, 1988
2. JACEP 5:22, 1976
3. Lancet 1:1027, 1987
4. N Engl J Med 307:642, 1982
5. JAMA 247:2400, 1982
6. JAMA 251:3104, 1984
7. West J Med 145:493, 1986
8. Arch Intern Med 145:43, 1985
9. Arch Intern Med 147:1390, 1987
10. Br Med J 297:459, 1988
11. Dig Dis Sci 33:106, 1988
12. JAMA 248:83, 1982
13. JAMA 248:55, 1982
14. Arch Intern Med 136:263, 1976
15. Ann Intern Med 91:549, 1979
16. Acta Med Scand 207:455, 1980
17. JAMA 251:1983, 1984
18. Arch Intern Med 138:1481, 1978
19. Br Med J 291:1472, 1985
20. Br Med J 289:366, 1984
21. Br Med J 285:1383, 1982
22. Am J Med 66:1046, 1979
23. JAMA 257:521, 1987
24. Ann Emerg Med 17:274, 1988
25. JAMA 248:1092, 1982
26. JAMA 250:1069, 1983
27. Am J Cardiol 51:904, 1983
28. Ann Emerg Med 12:221, 1983
29. Ann Emerg Med 14:1, 1985
30. JAMA 254:1772, 1985
31. N Engl J Med 313:474, 1985
32. Am J Emerg Med 6:439, 1988
33. J Clin Psychopharmacol 4:336, 1984
34. Ann Emerg Med 10:82, 1981
35. JAMA 249:762, 1983
36. West J Med 134:60, 1981
37. JAMA 235:1474, 1976
38. Ann Emerg Med 9:588, 1980
39. N Engl J Med 294:757, 1976
40. Ann Intern Med 96:464, 1982
41. Ann Neurol 8:161, 1980
42. Medicine (Baltimore) 60:373, 1981
43. Arch Intern Med 146:193, 1986
44. Arch Intern Med 134:293, 1974
45. Am J Med 64:749, 1978
46. Lancet 1:910, 1983
47. N Engl J Med 304:976, 1981
48. N Engl J Med 304:977, 1981
49. MMWR 36:611, 1987
50. Ann Intern Med 105:16, 1986
51. N Engl J Med 319:97, 1988
52. Br Med J 289:990, 1984
53. Am J Med 76:1124, 1984
54. JAMA 250:2935, 1983
55. Clin Toxicol 18:911, 1981
56. J Forensic Sci 26:739, 1981
57. Arch Intern Med 136:337, 1976
58. Ann Emerg Med 10:243, 1981
59. Ann Emerg Med 10:290, 1981
60. JAMA 243:2323, 1980
61. JAMA 248:585, 1982
62. Am J Med 77:167, 1984
63. Arch Intern Med 141:211, 1981
64. JAMA 249:621, 1983
65. Arch Intern Med 141:401, 1981
66. N Engl J Med 319:1557, 1988
67. Br Med J 289:907, 1984
68. Arch Intern Med 145:2019, 1985
69. Ann Intern Med 104:399, 1986
70. JAMA 255:2636, 1986
71. Natl Inst Drug Abuse Res Monogr Ser 61:35, 1985
72. DHHS Publication No (ADM) 80-976. National Institute of Drug Abuse, Rockville, Maryland, 1980
73. N Engl J Med 315:1495, 1986
74. JAMA 256:711, 1986
75. N Engl J Med 315:1438, 1986
76. JAMA 254:81, 1985
77. Am J Med 83:841, 1987
78. Med Lett Drugs Ther 28:69, 1986
79. Ann Intern Med 107:13, 1987
80. Am J Cardiol 57:496, 1986
81. N Engl J Med 313:519, 1985
82. Ann Intern Med 106:833, 1987
83. JAMA 258:2104, 1987
84. Ann Intern Med 108:564, 1988
85. N Engl J Med 319:673, 1988
86. JAMA 257:957, 1987
87. N Engl J Med 313:666, 1985
88. Ann Intern Med 100:73, 1984
89. N Engl J Med 298:1037, 1978
90. Clin Pediatr (Phila) 16:57, 1977
91. Pediatrics 60:554, 1977
92. N Engl J Med 299:203, 1978
93. Br Med J 294:739, 1987
94. Can Med Assoc J 127:1195, 1982
95. Am J Med 79:740, 1985
96. JAMA 253:1604, 1985
97. Can Med Assoc J 124:1268, 1981
98. Br Med J 285:478, 1982
99. Am J Med 74:507, 1983
100. Handbook of Poisoning: Diagnosis and Treatment, 12th ed. Lange Medical Publications, Los Altos, California, 1987

24 Food Poisoning

EDWARD RUBENSTEIN, M.D.

Botulism

Botulism is caused by a neurotoxin produced by the bacillus *Clostridium botulinum*. The toxin blocks release of acetylcholine at peripheral nerve endings. Death may be rapid. Victims have died as a result of tasting only very small amounts of toxin-containing food. Although the toxin is extremely potent, improved respiratory care has helped reduce mortality from 60 percent to 20 percent. A trivalent antitoxin is available; it probably modifies the disease when given promptly.[1]

Ingestion of improperly home-processed vegetables, fruits, meats (e.g., ham, bacon, and sausage), and seafood (e.g., mussels) is the cause of most cases.[2] Commercially canned foods are rarely implicated. Fresh foods grown in the ground, which can be contaminated with the ubiquitous spores of *C. botulinum*, can also produce food-borne botulism.

Danger arises when cooked foods remain at room temperature for more than 16 hours. The spores can withstand boiling temperatures for several hours; after cooling to room temperature, they can germinate and begin to produce toxin. Botulism has resulted from the consumption of commercial pot pies, a commercial preparation of chopped garlic in soybean oil, potato salad, sauteed onions, restaurant-bottled mushrooms, turkey loaves, stews, and baked potatoes that were heated and then left at room temperature.[3-6] Three separate incidents of botulism have been attributed to the ingestion of uneviscerated, salted, air-dried whitefish, known as ribyetz or kapchunka, an ethnic food favored by Russian immigrants.[7] The toxin, unlike the spores, is heat labile and can be inactivated by boiling for 10 minutes or by heating at 80° C for 30 minutes. Thus, cooked foods should be eaten promptly or refrigerated promptly and then reheated thoroughly before they are eaten.

There are seven types of *C. botulinum*. Types A, B, E, and F are the principal causes of botulism. The organism is anaerobic and gram positive. Although botulism appears throughout the United States, it is far more common in the West, especially in Alaska, California, Colorado, Oregon, and Washington. In Alaska, cases have been linked to raw fish aged in plastic bags, seal meat stored in oil, and smoked salmon wrapped in seal skins.[8] Most cases of botulism are caused by types A and B toxins. Fish products, however, tend to contain type E toxin. One outbreak caused by type F toxin was traced to home-prepared venison jerky.

Between 1943 and 1983, 27 cases of wound botulism were reported to the Centers for Disease Control.[9] The wounds, usually located on an extremity, often involved compound fractures and other major trauma; however, even a puncture wound of the foot has been associated with wound botulism.[10] Instances of botulism have been reported in chronic parenteral and intranasal drug abusers.[11] *C. botulinum* organisms in infected wounds, which may appear to be inconsequential, and in paranasal sinusitis have been implicated as sources of the toxin.[9,12] Wound botulism is usually caused by type A, type B, or both types of toxin. Its clinical features resemble those of the food-borne syndrome.

Clinical Manifestations

Prospective and retrospective studies provide a systematic account of this rare illness.[13-15]

Symptoms may appear within six hours, or they may be delayed as long as eight days. The usual incubation period is 18 to 36 hours. The earlier the onset of symptoms, the more severe the poisoning. The first vic-

Table 1   Symptoms Associated with Type A and Type B Food-Borne Botulism

	Incidence (%)*
Neurologic symptoms	
Dysphagia	96
Dry mouth	93
Diplopia	91
Dysarthria	84
Upper extremity weakness	73
Lower extremity weakness	69
Blurred vision	65
Dyspnea	60
Paresthesia	14
Gastrointestinal symptoms	
Constipation	73
Nausea	64
Vomiting	59
Abdominal cramps	42
Diarrhea	19
Miscellaneous symptoms	
Fatigue	77
Sore throat	54
Dizziness	51

*Values indicate the percentage of patients with either Type A or Type B botulism who have symptoms.

tims in an outbreak are usually the sickest; subsequent victims are usually the easiest to diagnose. Typically, only one or two persons become ill.

The victims are alert and afebrile. The most common neurologic symptoms are dry mouth, diplopia, difficulty in focusing on a near point, dysphagia, and dysarthria. About two thirds report nausea, vomiting, abdominal cramps, or diarrhea before or shortly after the onset of neurologic dysfunction [see Table 1]. Sore throat and dizziness may also appear.

Related findings are descending weakness or paralysis of the extremities and of ventilation [see Table 2]. Constipation and difficulty in urinating may also develop. Pupillary abnormalities and ptosis appear in about one half of patients; nystagmus

and ataxia affect about one fifth. Motor deficits are symmetric in about 80 percent. Although sensory abnormalities do not occur, some patients complain of paresthesias. The differential diagnosis of botulism includes the Guillain-Barré syndrome, the Eaton-Lambert syndrome, basilar artery stroke, chemical intoxication, tick paralysis, trichinosis, diphtheria, pharyngitis, acute abdomen, and various neuropsychiatric syndromes.

Laboratory Assessment

Routine laboratory tests are not helpful. The cerebrospinal fluid is usually normal, although infrequently the protein level may be raised to 50 to 60 mg/dl.

Electromyographic findings are nonspecific: (1) diminished muscle action potential after a single supramaximal stimulus and (2) augmentation after repetitive stimuli.[15] The

Table 2   Physical Findings Associated with Type A and Type B Food-Borne Botulism

	Incidence (%)*
Upper extremity weakness	75
Ptosis	73
Lower extremity weakness	69
Hypoactive gag reflex	65
Extraocular muscle weakness	65
Facial nerve dysfunction	63
Tongue weakness	58
Pupils fixed or dilated	44
Nystagmus	22
Ataxia	17
Initial mental status	
Alert	90
Lethargic	4
Obtunded	6
Deep tendon reflexes	
Normal	54
Hypoactive or absent	40
Hyperactive	6

*Values indicate the percentage of patients with either Type A or Type B botulism who have physical findings.

edrophonium chloride test is positive in most patients.

Demonstration that the patient's serum is toxic to mice confirms the diagnosis. Antigen specificity is established by neutralization tests conducted in mice injected with botulinum antitoxins.

Specimens suspected of containing botulinum toxin can be tested in a similar manner. Because of the extreme potency of the poison, such material should be handled with maximum caution. Foods should be kept in their original containers, refrigerated (preferably not frozen), shipped by the fastest means, and tested immediately for the presence of toxin.

Course

Older patients seem to be affected more adversely than younger patients. Type A botulism appears to mandate ventilatory support and prolonged hospitalization more often than does type B disease. In one group of 55 patients, 10 died.[14] Of the 21 cases reported during 1979 and 1980 to the CDC, there were three fatalities.[16]

Deaths have been attributed to the failure to recognize the need for mechanical ventilation, to ventilator malfunction, to ventilator misuse, and to intercurrent pulmonary and systemic infection.

Management

Because botulism is usually food-borne, cases tend to cluster. All persons at risk should be carefully observed. Vomiting can be induced with syrup of ipecac [*see Chapter 23*]; cathartics help remove the toxin.

Administration of antiserum to asymptomatic persons who may have been exposed must be carefully weighed against the hazard of anaphylactic reaction to this horse serum. Once the diagnosis is established, antitoxin is indicated. The earlier antitoxin is given, the more likely it is to be effective; however, apparent benefit has been noted even when antitoxin is given several weeks after the onset of symptoms. Botulism antitoxin is available from the CDC quarantine stations located throughout the United States. To obtain the antitoxin, physicians should call the Centers for Disease Control and Prevention at (404) 639-3311, Monday through Friday, and (404) 639-2888, weekdays after 4:30 P.M. and weekends.[17]

Initially, trivalent (ABE) antitoxin should be given. Type-specific antitoxin can be administered after the identity of the toxin has been determined. Antitoxin efficacy has not been proved in controlled studies.[13]

Of paramount importance is the maintenance of ventilation. Serial measurements of vital capacity are needed to detect respiratory failure, which can develop insidiously. A vital capacity of less than 30 percent suggests that the need for intubation and for mechanical ventilation may be imminent [*see Chapter 38*].

Because of the possibility that ingested *C. botulinum* might release toxin from germinating spores, penicillin has been advocated in food-borne cases. The efficacy of this therapy has not been established. Wound botulism should be treated by drainage of the lesion and by administration of penicillin along with antitoxin.

Infant Botulism

Botulism in infants has been diagnosed frequently since it was first recognized in 1976[16,18,19]; it is probably responsible for some cases of sudden infant death.

Although infant botulism has been reported in 18 states and probably appears worldwide, most cases occur in California, where spores are present in the soil and on many vegetables. Because honey has been implicated in at least one third of cases, honey should not be fed to infants younger than one year.[20]

The disease in infants is thought to be caused not by ingestion of toxin but by colonization of the intestine by *C. botulinum*, with later absorption of the toxin. Presumably, some infants are predisposed to such infection.

The syndrome is characterized by the onset of constipation between one and 38 weeks of age.[16,21] Thereafter, cranial neuropathy (which causes impaired sucking, swallowing, and crying) and generalized muscle weakness appear. The infants are often described as floppy. A characteristic pattern of brief, small, abundant motor-unit action potentials on electromyography has been noted.[21,22] Hypoventilation and apnea may occur, occasionally resulting in sudden death.

The presence of *C. botulinum* organisms or toxin in the feces confirms the diagnosis. Treatment is directed at maintaining nutrition and ventilatory function.

A clinical trial is under way in California to assess the effectiveness of immune globulin for infant botulism, which should be administered as early in the course of the illness as possible. Physicians seeking to enter infants in this trial should call the following 24-hour telephone number: (510) 540-2646.[23]

Seafood Poisoning

Since 1970, there has been an increase in the number of reports of poisoning caused by the ingestion of vertebrate fish or shellfish. The complicated taxonomy of species and exotic poisons has been reviewed.[24] The discussion here presents the common toxins.

Vertebrate Fish Poisoning

Ciguatera

Ciguatera, an acute poisoning characterized by gastrointestinal and neurologic symptoms, is the most frequently reported food-borne disease associated with seafood consumption in the United States.[25] During the 1970s, 94 outbreaks (418 cases) were recorded by the CDC. The incidence is undoubtedly far higher.[26] Most of these cases were diagnosed in southeastern Florida and in Hawaii; in Florida, the disease is most commonly encountered in the spring and summer. Ciguatera also frequently occurs inland because the toxin is heat stabile and can be found in both frozen and fresh fish.

Poisoning is caused by ciguatoxin, which is probably produced by dinoflagellates and blue-green algae that are eaten by small herbivorous fish. These fish are consumed by larger fish, which concentrate the toxin in their tissues.

Ciguatoxin is unaffected by heating, freezing, or storage and can persist for weeks. It does not alter the taste, color, or odor of contaminated tissue. The chemical structure of the ciguatoxin molecule is unknown.

Large, bottom-dwelling fish (barracuda, red snapper, amberjack, and grouper), usually caught near ocean reefs between latitudes 35° N and 35° S, are the main vectors for ciguatera poisoning. Because barracuda are so often contaminated, Miami has banned their sale. Restaurant-associated cases in Vermont have been linked to consumption of barracuda sent from Florida.[27]

An outbreak in the U.S. Virgin Islands involving 33 patients provides detailed clinical data depicting the course of the illness.[28] The illness usually develops within one to six hours but may appear within a few minutes or be delayed as long as 30 hours after ingestion. It typically begins with nausea, vomiting, abdominal cramps, and diarrhea.[24,26] Myalgias, weakness, diaphoresis, and chills may also be reported. Complaints of neurologic symptoms make the diagnosis apparent. Foremost are itching and various dysesthesias involving the mouth, the perioral region, and the extremities. Hot and cold sensations are often reversed; patients frequently perceive cold beverages to be hot and carbonated in the mouth. Another disagreeable symptom is the illusion of looseness of the teeth. Burning paresthesias of the extremities, especially of the feet, are common. Other symptoms include arthralgias, pruritus, blurred vision, photophobia, transient blindness, and cranial nerve palsies. In very severe cases, which are rare, bradycardia, hypotension, and respiratory paralysis may occur. The usual duration of illness is about eight days. Deaths caused by ciguatera seem extremely rare in the United States; in the Pacific islands, only three deaths were reported among some 3,000 cases surveyed.[29]

Emesis should be induced with syrup of ipecac [*see Chapter 23*], with care being taken to avoid aspiration. Cathartics should be used to empty the intestinal tract, unless vomiting and diarrhea have already begun. Intravenous mannitol (20 percent solution), given in a dose of 1 g/kg over a period of 30 minutes, has been reported to reverse neurologic manifestations, including coma, within 10 minutes and to alleviate gastrointestinal symptoms thereafter. The mechanism of mannitol's action is unknown.[30] If the benefits of mannitol are corroborated, life-supporting interventions, such as mechanical ventilation, should not be needed. Other agents that may relieve symptoms include tocainide and amitriptyline; the effectiveness of these two drugs and of mannitol has not been established.[31,32]

A radioimmunoassay is being developed; screening with this test may prove to be effective in the prevention of outbreaks in endemic areas.

Scombroid Poisoning

Improper handling and processing of fish, especially inadequate cooling, are probably responsible for the accumulation of toxins that results in the syndrome of scombroid poisoning, probably the most common form of seafood poisoning worldwide.[24,33] Storage at room temperature for only three to four hours may be sufficient to allow the scombrotoxin to reach levels that cause symptoms.[34] It is believed that normal enteric marine microflora degrade histidine, which is present in high concentrations in the dark meat of a variety of fish. Histidine is decarboxylated to the putative toxin histamine, which is found in very high concentrations in the urine of victims.[33] This association has led to the conclusion that histamine is the toxin responsible for the syndrome. Other putative toxins include putrescine and cadaverine, but their roles have not been established.

Both scombroid and nonscombroid fish have been implicated. The Scombroidea are large, bony fish with oily flesh and include albacore, tuna, bonito, mackerel, and skip-jack. Nonscombroid fish that have been associated with scombroid-type poisoning include mahimahi, bluefish, Japanese saury, amberjack, and marlin.[33,35]

The toxins are not destroyed by freezing or smoking and can be present in canned fish. Outbreaks have been attributed to consumption of canned tuna; fresh tuna eaten in South Carolina; mahimahi eaten in Hawaii, California, Colorado, Illinois, Michigan, Minnesota, and Washington; Pacific amberjack served in restaurants in Alabama and Tennessee; bluefish served in an inn in New Hampshire; and marlin served in Tennessee.[33,35-38] Contaminated fish may have a metallic, peppery taste.[33]

Symptoms appear within minutes to a few hours and resemble a histamine reaction: flushing, conjunctival suffusion, headache, dizziness, oropharyngeal burning or blistering, nausea, vomiting, abdominal cramps, diarrhea, pruritus, and urticaria. In cases of severe scombroid poisoning, bronchospasm may develop. Patients and their physicians may mistakenly conclude that the histaminelike syndrome is caused by an allergy to fish. The symptoms usually subside spontaneously after about four hours; in rare instances, symptoms may continue for several days.

If vomiting and diarrhea have not already occurred, syrup of ipecac and cathartics may be useful. Antihistamines, including H_2-receptor blocking agents, and bronchodilators are effective.[33,39] Fatalities have not been reported.

Shellfish Poisoning

Outbreaks of alarming and sometimes dangerous illness have been caused by the ingestion of mussels, clams, oysters, cockles, scallops, and shellfish broth that have been contaminated by neurotoxin-producing dinoflagellates.[40] These planktonic flagellates are abundant in latitudes above 30° N and below 30° S, but cases have been recorded from warmer regions, including the tropics. In the Northern Hemisphere, most outbreaks occur between May and October, when large numbers of these dinoflagellates bloom, causing a red discoloration of the sea. Toxic conditions may prevail, however, in the absence of this so-called red tide, and not all red tides are contaminated. Saxitoxin, one of the alkaloid neurotoxins responsible for the poisoning, is heat stabile and is therefore unaffected by cooking or steaming; the toxin can be concentrated in broth.

Symptoms usually begin one-half hour to two hours after ingestion. Paresthesias involve the head and the extremities, frequently accompanied by nausea, vomiting, and diarrhea. Low back pain may be a prominent complaint. In severe cases, ataxia and muscle paralysis develop and lead to dysphonia, dysphagia, and ventilatory impairment. Neurologic symptoms usually abate within six to 24 hours, but death caused by respiratory paralysis may occur within the first 12 hours. The prognosis is favorable for those who survive beyond 12 to 18 hours.

The GI tract should be emptied of unabsorbed toxin (taking care to avoid aspiration), and measures to support the cardiovascular and respiratory systems should be instituted. A mechanical ventilator may be needed. There is no specific antidote.

Other shellfish-associated toxins produce milder syndromes characterized by paresthesias, nausea, vomiting, diarrhea, and ataxia.

One dinoflagellate appears to aerosolize its toxin. Surf bathers who inhale contaminated sea spray may acquire an upper respiratory syndrome of brief duration, with conjunctival irritation, copious rhinorrhea, and dry cough. This self-limited illness does not require therapy.

Other Shellfish-Related Diseases

Other enteric diseases that can be acquired by eating contaminated shellfish are those caused by hepatitis A virus, *Salmonella typhi*, enterotoxigenic and invasive *Escherichia coli*, *Vibrio parahaemolyticus*, *V. vulnificus*, *V. cholerae*, and Norwalk virus.[41] Outbreaks may be related to surface runoff and sewage overflow after rainstorms.

Widespread outbreaks of gastroenteritis in the United States have been attributed to the consumption of raw clams and oysters.[42] A Norwalk-like virus has been implicated in an oyster-related epidemic in London, England.[43] The attack rate was high (79 percent), and in many cases, gastroenteritis was caused by the ingestion of only a single oyster.

Hepatitis A virus Although the exact temperature and heating time required to inactivate hepatitis A virus in shellfish are unknown, cooking lessens the risk of live virus ingestion. Obviously, eating raw shellfish taken from contaminated waters is hazardous. Steaming clams until their shells are open, a process that usually takes less than one minute, is inadequate for inactivating the virus. Outbreaks of hepatitis A that have been linked to steamed clams have confirmed this finding.[44]

Vibrio organisms *V. parahaemolyticus* is an important worldwide cause of food poisoning and is probably the leading cause of gastroenteritis in Japan. In the United States, it has been reported from the Atlantic seacoast and the Gulf of Mexico to the Pacific Northwest, as well as in Hawaii.[45,46]

Implicated foods, which usually have been cooked, include crab, shrimp, lobster, and oysters. Poor refrigeration and improper food handling or preparation have prompted outbreaks.

The incubation period of *V. parahaemolyticus* is usually about half a day but ranges from four to 96 hours. Complaints include abdominal cramps, diarrhea, nausea, and vomiting. Stools are very rarely bloody. The disorder usually runs its course in about three days. Prognosis is excellent; very few deaths have been reported among thousands of cases. Antimicrobial therapy is not indicated. Intravenous fluid replacement may be needed if fluid loss is severe.

Other important causes of shellfish poisoning include *V. vulnificus* and non-O group 1 *V. cholerae*.

Mushroom Poisoning

Enthusiasm for organic foods and experimentation with natural hallucinogens have probably contributed to the increased incidence of serious and fatal mushroom poisoning during the past 20 to 30 years in the United States.[47] Because species identification in the field can be exceedingly difficult even for expert mycologists and because a large number of toxic varieties grow abundantly, foraging for mushrooms is a hazardous venture. There is no way that the mushroom gatherer can be absolutely certain of the safety of his or her collection.[48] Cases of poisoning tend to occur in the fall, when the mushrooms, which are the reproductive part of the fungus, can be easily harvested.

Toxicology and Pathophysiology

Susceptibility to mushroom toxins appears to vary strikingly. Severity may also depend on the season, on the maturity of the mushrooms, and probably on the number of mushrooms eaten.

Cytotoxins

Of the many cytotoxins produced by mushrooms, the most important is the potent amatoxin found in some mushrooms belonging to the genera *Amanita* and *Galerina*. Amatoxin is a cyclic octapeptide. When ingested, this toxin inhibits RNA polymerase II in the victim's cells, thus interfering with protein synthesis. This process results in damage to membranes of cell walls, of organelles, and of nuclei. Lethal hepatic and renal tubule destruction may occur after the ingestion of only a single mushroom cap containing amatoxin. Phalloidin, a cyclic heptapeptide that accompanies amatoxin and may interfere with actin polymerization, is probably responsible for the initial gastrointestinal symptoms.

Neurotoxins

Mushroom neurotoxins are less dangerous than mushroom cytotoxins.[49] The neurotoxins include a complex group of substances that produce unique syndromes. Muscarinic toxins evoke the manifestations of parasympathetic stimulation. Other neurotoxins cause anticholinergic and halluci-

nogenic disturbances. One neurotoxin, possibly monomethylhydrazine, is thought to cause a disulfiramlike reaction (flushing, palpitation, tachycardia, and hyperventilation) but only when the patient consumes alcohol after eating the mushrooms.

Clinical Features

Amatoxin Poisoning

Symptoms of amatoxin poisoning appear from six to 24 hours after ingestion. Often, the victim has subsequently eaten several meals and has forgotten about the wild mushrooms. The initial symptom is abdominal pain, followed by severe vomiting, diarrhea, and fever. Dehydration, hypovolemia, and electrolyte loss may ensue; hematuria and blood-streaked diarrhea may also occur. After a day or two, the gastrointestinal symptoms abate and the patient's condition appears to improve. At this stage, serum levels of aspartate aminotransferase (AST, formerly termed SGOT), alanine aminotransferase (ALT, formerly termed SGPT), and lactic dehydrogenase (LDH) begin to rise.

By the third or fourth day, hepatic and renal failure become evident. Jaundice, hypoglycemia, oliguria, bleeding, delirium, and coma supervene. The overall mortality in a series of 205 cases of amatoxin poisoning in Europe from 1971 to 1980 was 22.4 percent. Mortality was 16.5 percent for patients older than 10 years and 51.3 percent for those younger than 10 years.[50]

Confirmation of the presence of amatoxin and phalloidin can be obtained by thin-layer chromatographic analysis of samples of wild mushrooms or of vomitus, gastrointestinal aspirates, or stool specimens.[47]

Treatment Toxins should be eliminated from the GI tract as soon as possible by nasogastric lavage and subsequent administration of activated charcoal [*see Chapter 23*].[47,51] Ipecac has also been used for this purpose.

There have been no reported controlled trials of the various treatments suggested for mushroom poisoning; their efficacy is therefore in doubt. Penicillin (300,000 to 1,000,000 U/kg/day) and silibinin (20 to 50 mg/kg/day) have been reported to be effective against amatoxin poisoning.[47] These agents can be given concurrently. Their modes of action are unclear.

Although thioctic acid has been widely used in Europe for a number of years and is available in the United States as an experimental agent,[52,53] there have been no controlled studies validating its efficacy. The exact dosage in cases of amatoxin poisoning is unknown, but one protocol calls for I.V. administration of thioctic acid in a solution of glucose and water for two days (25 mg four times on the first day and, depending on clinical status, up to 75 mg four times on the second day). In another regimen, thioctic acid is given in dosages of 50 to 150 mg every six hours.[54] Therapy should be guided by frequent measurements of AST, ALT, LDH, creatinine, and blood glucose levels in conjunction with blood counts, assessment of the clotting mechanism, and urinalyses. Treatment can be continued for two weeks. Thioctic acid is relatively nontoxic; hypoglycemia has been the principal side effect.

Because of the high mortality associated with fulminant hepatic failure and coma from mushroom poisoning, liver transplantation has been employed in several patients.[48] Hemodialysis has been used to treat acute renal failure, but this procedure does not remove the toxin, which is rapidly fixed in tissues.

Neurotoxin Poisoning

Most neurotoxins produce symptoms within minutes or a few hours after ingestion. The muscarinic group causes parasympathomimetic phenomena, including lacrimation, salivation, nausea, vomiting, abdominal pain, bronchospasm, headache, miosis, blurred vision, bradycardia, hypotension, and shock. The prognosis is usually good. Atropine is thought by some to be an effective antidote.

Another group of neurotoxins, the isoxazole derivatives, produce anticholiner-

gic manifestations and moderate states of confusion. Atropine is contraindicated.

Other Syndromes

Gastrointestinal disorders, alcohol-dependent disulfiramlike reactions, and confusional states are among the syndromes that have been attributed to various other mushroom toxins.

Rapid onset of symptoms and the presence of neurologic manifestations are associated with the milder disorders of mushroom poisoning. However, caution is necessary when formulating the prognosis based on these manifestations because the victim may have ingested some of the lethal amatoxin-containing species in addition to a variety of mildly toxic mushrooms.

The Chinese-Restaurant Syndrome

Diners at Chinese restaurants often experience a group of symptoms that have come to be known as the Chinese-restaurant syndrome.[55-57] A prospective, uncontrolled study demonstrated that monosodium glutamate (MSG) probably causes this evanescent ailment.[57] During the trial, symptoms of varying severity appeared in 55 of 56 normal test subjects who ingested 3 g or less of MSG. Severity was greatest in those who consumed MSG on an empty stomach. This result may explain why wonton soup is frequently identified as the offending food.

The syndrome, which begins within 15 to 25 minutes after ingestion, rarely persists for more than two hours. Burning sensations usually begin in the chest and spread to the neck, shoulders, forearms, abdomen, and, rarely, the thighs. Lacrimation and diaphoresis often follow. A sense of tightness and pressure in the face and behind the eyes is experienced by some diners. Others report precordial or substernal pressure, which can radiate to the axillae or neck. Less common are headache, syncope,[56] palpitations, and ventricular tachycardia.[58]

Although the syndrome is usually harmless, some individuals appear to be highly susceptible.[59] The manifestations of the syndrome should be described to persons who have cardiac disease.[60]

The Japanese-Restaurant Syndrome

Vasomotor near-collapse with pallor, diaphoresis, staggering, and confusion have followed the ingestion in a single swallow of an entire serving of wasabi, a horseradish mixture that accompanies sushi. Lovers of Japanese food have been advised to "watch the wasabi."[61]

Delayed Neurologic Syndromes

Toxic-oil Syndrome

In mid-1981, about 20,000 people in Spain were suddenly stricken with an unusual illness. Manifestations of the disorder, which came to be known as the toxic-oil syndrome, occurred in three phases. During the first week, symptoms included dry cough, dyspnea, pleuritic chest pain, headache, fever, and generalized lymphadenopathy. Bilateral pulmonary infiltrates appeared on chest x-ray. The middle phase, which extended from the second week through the eighth week, was characterized by gastrointestinal symptoms (nausea, vomiting, diarrhea, and abdominal pain), abnormal liver function tests (prothrombin time and serum enzyme and total bilirubin levels), and hematologic abnormalities (marked eosinophilia, leukocytosis, mild anemia, and splenomegaly). During the late phase, which began about two months after the initial onset of symptoms, striking neuromuscular abnormalities (paresthesias, dysesthesias, muscle cramps, myalgias, and motor deficits) appeared in about one fourth of the patients. Elevated aldolase levels were also found in these patients. Weakness began distally and spread proximally. Atrophy of major muscle groups and contractures of the jaw and extremities ensued. Severe weight loss and alopecia occurred in some patients. In about 1.5 percent of the cases, respiratory failure led to fatal infections that were associated with the use of mechanical ventilation.

Autoimmune abnormalities followed the illness in some patients, especially in those with neuromuscular manifestations. Sclerodermalike skin changes, pulmonary hypertension, Raynaud's phenomenon, the sicca syndrome, and dysphagia were associated with elevated levels of both antinuclear antibodies and IgE. Evidence of vasculitis was found in microscopic sections.

One-year follow-up studies indicated that of those patients who were initially hospitalized, 3.2 percent continued to manifest severe myopathy and neuropathy and 39.4 percent continued to have mild myalgias; 52.9 percent of patients had no residual abnormalities.[62] High-dose glucocorticoid therapy is thought to have been beneficial when administered during the acute phase.[62]

Toxic-oil syndrome has been attributed to the ingestion of industrial denatured rapeseed oil that had been inadequately processed and sold for use as cooking oil.[63] The specific chemical substance responsible for the syndrome has not been identified. Rapeseed oil has been used as a food oil in parts of Asia and is used in industry worldwide as a lubricant and in the manufacture of synthetic rubber, margarine, soaps, oils, and fabrics.[64]

Eosinophilia-Myalgia Syndrome

During 1989, an apparently new illness appeared in the United States, characterized by eosinophilia ($< 1,000$ cells/mm^3), generalized, severe myalgias, and other manifestations.[65,66] The syndrome appeared in the absence of infectious or neoplastic processes, and epidemiological studies established an association with the use of products containing L-tryptophan. The outbreak was subsequently linked to a tryptophan dimer impurity, in which a methine bridge spans the two tryptophan molecules between the indole nitrogens [*see Figure 1*].[67] Whether the double tryptophan molecule is a by-product of the gene-splicing technique used in the manufacturing process or is the result of an unrelated fermentation reaction is currently unclear. The discovery of this contaminant suggests a novel mechanism that may be relevant to

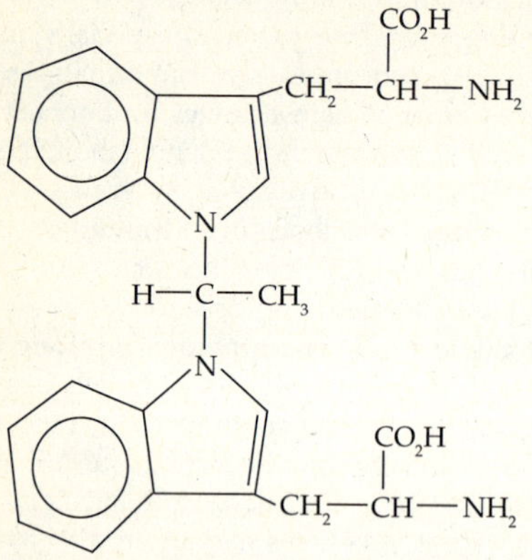

Figure 1 *The contaminant suspected of causing the eosinophilia-myalgia syndrome consists of a dimer of tryptophan residues linked by a methine bridge to the indole nitrogens. The compound is referred to as di-L-tryptophan aminal of acetaldehyde (DTAA).*

other autoimmune disorders: misincorporation of an altered amino acid into proteins may disturb their function and alter their structure, so that they are recognized as nonself antigens.

There have been a number of case and series reports as well as a summary from the CDC describing the clinical features of 1,531 cases of eosinophilia-myalgia syndrome (including 27 deaths) that had occurred nationwide as of July 10, 1990.[68-72] Patients' ages ranged from four to 85 years (median age, 48 years; mean age, 49 years), and 84 percent of the cases occurred in females. By definition, all patients had myalgia and eosinophilia greater than or equal to 1.0×10^9 cells/L. The most common signs and symptoms were arthralgia, rash, peripheral edema, and cough or dyspnea [*see Table 3*]. The most common laboratory abnormalities were leukocytosis, an elevated aldolase level, and abnormal liver function tests.

Biopsy specimens of muscle and fascia show eosinophilic infiltrates, nonspecific inflammation, vasculitis, and atrophy, although some specimens are normal.

Deaths have been attributed to bulbar paresis and aspiration pneumonia. MRI revealed changes consistent with cerebral vasculitis in one obtunded patient.

Treatment consists of discontinuation of L-tryptophan and provision of supportive care, especially for patients with ventilatory impairment. Prednisone therapy reportedly reduces eosinophilia and may diminish myalgia in some patients. The role of plasmapheresis in patients with progressive polymyopathies needs to be evaluated.

Table 3   Clinical Findings Associated with the Eosinophilia-Myalgia Syndrome

Clinical Findings	Frequency (%)
Signs and Symptons	
Myalgia	100
Arthralgia	73
Rash	60
Peripheral edema	59
Cough or dyspnea	59
Fever	36
Sclerodermalike skin changes	32
Periorbital edema	28
Alopecia	28
Neuropathy	27
Hepatomegaly	5
Splenomegaly	1
Laboratory Values	
Eosinophilia ($\geq 10^9$ cells/L)	100
Leukocytosis	85
Elevated aldolase level	46
Elevated liver function tests*	43
Elevated erythrocyte sedimentation rate	37
Elevated IgE level	17
Pulmonary infiltrate	17
Pleural effusion	12
Elevated creatine kinase level	10

Statistics are based on 1,075 patients.

*Liver function tests: bilirubin, alanine transaminase, aspartate transaminase, alkaline phosphatase, and γ-glutamyltransferase.

Attention has been called to the similarity between this symptom complex and the late manifestations of the toxic-oil syndrome (see above).

Triorthocresyl Phosphate Poisoning

The outbreak of toxic-oil syndrome is reminiscent of an epidemic of neurologic disease with delayed onset that afflicted as many as 50,000 people in the United States in 1930 and 1931. Jamaica ginger, a medicinal alcohol extract of the ginger root used as a tonic, was widely consumed as a tipple during the early years of the 20th century. After prohibition in 1920, only a highly concentrated and very irritating fluid extract form of the substance could be legally shipped to the United States.[73] Poisoning was caused by the consumption of illicit batches of Jamaica ginger that had been adulterated with triorthocresyl phosphate (TOCP).[73,74] Neurologic symptoms, preceded by abdominal pain, nausea, vomiting, and protracted diarrhea, appeared one to two weeks after ingestion of TOCP. Muscle cramps and burning dysesthesias and paresthesias were followed by rapidly progressing weakness, first in the feet and legs and then in the hands and arms. Atrophy of distal muscles and a gait characterized by footdrop and scissors spasticity typified what became known as Jake paralysis, or Jake leg. Recovery occurred in mild cases, but permanent neurologic damage was the usual outcome. The principal pathologic finding was hyperplastic fibrosis of small arteries and capillaries in the spinal cord and peripheral nerves.[75]

Outbreaks of TOCP poisoning caused by adulteration of olive oil[76,77] and mustard oil[78] and by accidental contamination of dry flour[79,80] have been reported in widely separated parts of the world. TOCP is used as a solvent and plasticizer in nitrocellulose spray paints, in jet engine lubricants, and in cooling fluids for machine guns.[80] Its presence in aircraft hydraulic fluids has led to other outbreaks. The decommissioning of an air base in Morocco in 1959 resulted in the local sale of hydraulic fluid, which was subsequently added to cooking oil as a diluent; 10,000 cases of paralysis followed.[73,76,77] Poisoning also occurred in 1970 and 1971 in Vietnam after helicopter hydraulic fluid was added to cooking oil sold on the black market.[81] The most recent outbreak, in Sri Lanka during 1977 and 1978, was caused by contamination of gingili oil, an extract of sesame seeds used by Tamil girls in puberty ritual ceremonies and by Moslem women after childbirth.[82]

Polychlorinated Biphenyls Poisoning

Outbreaks of illness related to the ingestion of cooking oils contaminated with polychlorinated biphenyls (PCBs) and polychlorinated dibenzofurans (PCDFs) occurred in Japan in 1968[83] and in Taiwan in 1979.[84] Follow-up studies have revealed unexpected consequences to the offspring of individuals exposed to these agents. PCBs pass through the placenta, cause congenital poisoning, and remain in human tissues for long intervals. The half-lives of the related dioxins are about seven years.[83]

Offspring of female patients exposed to PCBs and PCDFs during the outbreak in Taiwan have been studied to determine the effect of exposure via the placenta or possibly through breast-feeding. Data on 117 children have been compared with data on control subjects from families who lived in the same neighborhoods.[84] The affected children displayed a number of long-lasting effects from in utero exposure to PCBs and PCDFs. Poisoning resulted in lower birth weight and natal teeth. Hyperpigmentation, conjunctivitis, and nail abnormalities were also present at birth. Subsequently, the children had a high rate of bronchitis, 10 percent displayed psychomotor delay, and seven percent had speech problems. Exposed children scored lower than control subjects on developmental and cognitive tests. These findings appear to be consistent with a generalized disorder of ectodermal tissue.

In humans, developmental abnormalities caused by transplacental exposure to PCBs are consistent with those seen in monkeys. This syndrome is among the few documented disorders that have resulted from transplacental exposure to pollutants.

References

1. Handbook for Epidemiologists, Clinicians, and Laboratory Workers. Centers for Disease Control, Atlanta, 1974
2. Ann Intern Med 108:363, 1988
3. Arch Intern Med 148:578, 1988
4. JAMA 253:1275, 1985
5. MMWR 34:156, 1985
6. MMWR 36:103, 1987
7. MMWR 36:812, 1987
8. JAMA 235:35, 1976
9. MMWR 31:87, 1982
10. N Engl J Med 289:1005, 1973
11. Ann Intern Med 109:984, 1988
12. Ann Intern Med 102:616, 1985
13. JAMA 241:475, 1979
14. Ann Intern Med 95:442, 1981
15. Neurology 21:43, 1971
16. MMWR 30:121, 1981
17. MMWR 35:490, 1986
18. N Engl J Med 295:770, 1976
19. MMWR 27:17, 1978
20. MMWR 27:249, 1978
21. JAMA 237:1946, 1977
22. Neurology (Minneap) 25:173, 1975
23. West J Med 156:197, 1992
24. N Engl J Med 295:1117, 1976
25. JAMA 244:273, 1980
26. JAMA 244:254, 1980
27. MMWR 35:263, 1986
28. Arch Intern Med 142:1090, 1982
29. Am J Trop Med Hyg 28:1067, 1979
30. JAMA 259:2740, 1988
31. Am J Med 84:1087, 1988
32. N Engl J Med 315:65, 1986
33. N Engl J Med 324:716, 1991
34. Am J Public Health 77:1335, 1987
35. JAMA 258:3409, 1987
36. MMWR 29:167, 1980
37. MMWR 35:264, 1986
38. MMWR 38:140, 1989
39. Ann Emerg Med 12:104, 1983
40. MMWR 40:157, 1991
41. MMWR 31:449, 1982
42. N Engl J Med 314:678, 1986
43. Br Med J 287:1532, 1983
44. JAMA 237:1980, 1977
45. Appl Environ Microbiol 35:1226, 1978
46. Am J Epidemiol 109:171, 1979
47. Am J Med 86:187, 1989
48. Sci Am 232(March):90, 1975
49. Ann Intern Med 90:332, 1979
50. JAMA 253:3252, 1985
51. MMWR 31:287, 1982
52. West J Med 137:282, 1982
53. JAMA 251:1057, 1984
54. JAMA 253:3252, 1985
55. N Engl J Med 278:796, 1968
56. N Engl J Med 278:1122, 1968
57. Science 163:826, 1969
58. South Med J 70:879, 1977
59. Fed Proc 35(September):2205, 1976
60. N Engl J Med 294:225, 1976
61. JAMA 259:218, 1988
62. Arch Intern Med 144:254, 1984
63. N Engl J Med 309:1408, 1983
64. The Merck Index: An Encyclopedia of Chemicals and Drugs, 10th ed. Windholz M, Budavari S, Blumetti RF, et al, Eds. Merck & Co, Inc, Rahway, New Jersey, 1983, p 1172
65. MMWR 38:785, 1989
66. MMWR 38:842, 1989
67. MMWR 39:789, 1990
68. West J Med 153:269, 1990
69. Medicine (Baltimore) 69:187, 1990
70. Arch Intern Med 150:2178, 1990
71. Arch Intern Med 150:2175, 1990
72. JAMA 264:1698, 1990
73. JAMA 248:1864, 1982
74. Ann Intern Med 85:804, 1976
75. Brain 65:34, 1942
76. Lancet 2:1019, 1959
77. Can Med Assoc J 85:1249, 1961
78. J Neurol Neurosurg Psychiatry 25:234, 1962
79. Trans R Soc Trop Med Hyg 59:98, 1965
80. Med J Aust 1:506, 1969
81. Ann Intern Med 86:665, 1977
82. J Neurol Neurosurg Psychiatry 44:775, 1981
83. JAMA 259:1661, 1988
84. Science 241:334, 1988

Acknowledgment

Tables 1, 2 Modified from "Clinical Features of Types A and B Food-Borne Botulism," by J. M. Hughes, J. R. Blumenthal, M. H. Merson, et al, in *Annals of Internal Medicine* 95:442, 1981. Used by permission.

25 Water-Related Accidents

ANDREW B. NEWMAN, M.D.

The growing interest in water sports as a recreational activity has led to a corresponding increase in the number of water-related accidents and deaths. Physicians can reduce the number of mishaps by advising patients about water safety and about their fitness to participate in such activities as swimming, skin or scuba diving, riding waterslides, and soaking in hot tubs. In addition, medical problems occurring during or after participation in water sports must be recognized and treated.

Drowning and Near-Drowning

Approximately 7,000 people drown each year in the United States, making drowning the third leading cause of accidental death.[1,2] The victims may be recreational swimmers, water-skiers, sailors, or some of the one million recreational, military, and commercial divers who use a self-contained underwater breathing apparatus (scuba).

Many of these deaths can be prevented by water safety training, improvement of swimming ability, and awareness of potential dangers. Swimming alone should be discouraged, and all boaters and wind surfers should wear personal flotation devices.[3-5] The highest drowning rate is for children younger than one year (6.2 per 100,000 population). The drowning rate for children in the United States is higher than it is in other countries and appears to be rising.[6] In many states, drowning is the leading cause of death for children younger than five years.[7] An increasing number of infants and young children drown in outdoor hot tubs[8,9] and bathtubs, but most drownings occur in residential pools.[5,8-10] Plastic five-gallon buckets in particular have become a hazard for toddlers, who look inside such containers, fall in, and drown.[10,11] Children with seizure disorders are particularly at risk.[12]

Alcohol use is associated with 50 percent of drownings among teenagers and adults, and mortality is especially high among males 15 to 24 years of age. The overall drowning rate for blacks is approximately twice that for whites. The incidence of drowning is four times higher for males than for females. The probability that a drowning will occur in an unfenced pool may be two to five times higher than that in a fenced pool.[13]

Drowning frequently occurs either in areas that have not been designated for swimming and therefore are not supervised by lifeguards trained in cardiopulmonary resuscitation (CPR) or in natural bodies of water that are often far from emergency medical services. Lakes and oceans present environmental hazards such as cold water, currents, and storms. Potential accidents include falling from or being struck by recreational watercraft. Occasionally, experienced swimmers drown on attempting to swim long distances underwater.[14]

Most drowning victims experience a sense of panic and then initiate an exhausting struggle to keep their head above the water or to reach safety. Frantic breathing that leads to hyperventilation occurs while the victim's head is above water; breath-holding begins with submersion. After a variable period, the victim swallows water, vomits, and coughs violently. Finally, involuntary gasping causes the air passages and lungs to become flooded. The subsequent unconsciousness and convulsive movements are followed by death.

Pathophysiology

Profound hypoxemia is the most important abnormality in victims of drowning or near-drowning.[1,15] Laryngospasm occurs initially and appears to be the sole cause of death in about 10 percent of cases. So-called dry lungs are found during autopsy in such cases. Aspiration of fluid into alveoli intensifies hypoxemia because blood is shunted through perfused but nonventilated regions. Fresh water lowers the surface tension of surfactant, causing atelectasis; salt water floods the alveoli. In most instances, resultant increases in arterial carbon dioxide tension are transient. Severe acidosis occurs in the majority of survivors and usually is metabolic, reflecting the intense hypoxemia. Some patients experience combined metabolic and respiratory acidosis. Pulmonary abnormalities include shunting, airway obstruction, and decreased compliance.

Changes in the volume and composition of blood depend on the amount and tonicity of the fluid aspirated: freshwater drowning leads to hypervolemia, whereas aspiration of salt water results in hypovolemia. These changes may be associated with changes in electrolyte concentration. Electrolyte shifts are rarely prominent, but an exception has been noted among victims of near-drowning in the Dead Sea, a lake between Israel and Jordan that contains high concentrations of various solutes. Pronounced elevations of serum calcium and magnesium have been observed in such cases. Such marked electrolyte abnormalities may not be present on initial examination, however, presumably because the increased serum concentration of these ions is caused mainly by their absorption from swallowed, rather than aspirated, water and because absorption from the gastrointestinal tract occurs more slowly than absorption from the lungs.[16,17] These patients may have marked electrocardiographic abnormalities, including P wave changes, prolonged QRS complexes, inverted T waves, prominent U waves, and lethal ventricular tachyarrhythmias.[18]

Hypoxemia and acid-base and electrolyte disorders may lead to cardiac arrhythmias and conduction defects. Ventricular fibrillation is probably an important cause of death after freshwater submersion. In a rabbit model, the heart displays myocyte hypercontraction and hypereosinophilia

after near-drowning.[19] Cerebral hypoxia can lead to edema and cortical necrosis, causing varying degrees of permanent brain damage in some patients but no permanent injury in others. Hypothermia may also be an important consideration (see below), especially in persons who have been immersed in cold water.[20]

Treatment of Near-Drowning

The following recommendations for the treatment of victims of near-drowning or hypothermia are excerpts from the Standards and Guidelines for Cardiopulmonary Resuscitation (CPR) and Emergency Cardiac Care (ECC) that were published in the *Journal of the American Medical Association* [*see Chapter 8*] and from the *Textbook of Advanced Cardiac Life Support*.[21,22]

The most important consequences of prolonged underwater submersion without ventilation are hypoxic acidosis and pulmonary edema. Pulmonary edema occurs in up to 75 percent of near-drowning cases. There are four emergency elements in the management of a near-drowning victim.

Rescue from the water When attempting to rescue a near-drowning victim, the rescuer should get to the victim as quickly as possible, preferably with some conveyance (e.g., boat, raft, surfboard, or flotation device). The rescuer must always be aware of personal safety in attempting a rescue and should exercise caution to minimize the danger.

Rescue breathing Initial treatment of the near-drowning victim consists of rescue breathing using the mouth-to-mouth or mouth-to-nose technique [*see Chapter 8*]. Rescue breathing should be started as soon as possible, even before the victim is moved out of the water, into a boat, or onto a surfboard, provided it can be accomplished without undue risk to the rescuer. Once on land (typically, on a beach), the victim must be moved above the wave line and positioned with the head down (usually, toward the water).

Appliances, such as a snorkel in the use of the mouth-to-snorkel technique, may permit specially trained rescuers to perform rescue breathing in deep water; however, rescue breathing should not be delayed for lack of such equipment if it can otherwise be provided safely. Untrained rescuers should not attempt the use of such adjuncts.

If neck injury is suspected, however, the victim's neck should be supported in a neutral position (without flexion or extension), and the victim should be floated supine on a horizontal back support before being removed from the water. If the victim must be turned, the head, neck, chest, and body should be aligned, supported, and turned as a unit to the horizontal supine position. If artificial respiration is required, maximal head tilt should not be used. Rescue breathing should be provided with the head maintained in a neutral position; that is, jaw thrust without head tilt, or chin lift without head tilt, should be used.

Foreign matter in the airway The need for clearing the lower airway of aspirated water has not been proved, although there are anecdotal reports of clinical response to a subdiaphragmatic abdominal thrust.[23] At most, only a modest amount of water is aspirated by the majority of both freshwater and saltwater drowning victims, and fresh water is rapidly absorbed from the lungs into the circulation.[24] Furthermore, 10 to 12 percent of victims do not aspirate at all because of laryngospasm or breath-holding.[24,25] An attempt to remove water from the breathing passages by any means other than suction may be unnecessary and dangerous because it could eject gastric contents and cause aspiration.[25] Most near-drowning victims have swallowed a tremendous amount of water during the struggling phase and are very likely to vomit during CPR.

Controlled studies of the Heimlich maneuver in animals have shown that in the absence of particulate matter blocking the airway, the maneuver does not improve survival. The only time it definitely should be used is when the rescuer suspects that foreign matter is obstructing the airway or if the victim does not respond appropriately to mouth-to-mouth ventilation. Then, if necessary, CPR should be reinstituted after the Heimlich maneuver has been applied.[26-28] The Heimlich maneuver is performed on the near-drowning victim as described in the treatment of foreign-body airway obstruction (unconscious supine) [*see Chapter 8*], except that in cases of near-drowning, the victim's head should be turned sideways.

Chest compressions External chest compressions should not be attempted in the water unless the rescuer has had special training in techniques of in-water CPR, because the chest is not compressed effectively unless the victim is maintained in the horizontal position and the back is supported. It is usually not possible to keep the victim's body horizontal and still keep the victim's head above water and in position for rescue breathing.

On removal from the water, the victim must be assessed immediately for adequacy of circulation. The pulse may be difficult to appreciate in a near-drowning victim because of peripheral vasoconstriction and a low cardiac output. If a pulse cannot be felt, CPR should be started at once.

Definitive advanced life-support care Every submersion victim, even one who requires only minimal resuscitation and regains consciousness at the scene, should be transferred immediately to an advanced life-support medical facility for follow-up care because a number of patients who initially appear well experience delayed respiratory distress within four hours after the event. It is imperative that life-support measures be continued en route to the medical facility and that oxygen be administered in the transport vehicle if it is available.

Successful resuscitation with full neurologic recovery has occurred in near-drowning victims who had suffered prolonged submersion in cold water.[29-31] An absolute time limit beyond which resuscitation is not indicated has not been established. Because it is often difficult for rescuers to discern how long the victim has been submerged, attempts at resuscitation should be initiated by rescuers at the scene unless there is obvious physical evidence of death (e.g., putrefaction). The victim should receive continued CPR while being transported to an advanced life-support treatment facility, where a physician can decide whether to continue resuscitation. Aggressive continued attempts at resuscitation on hospital arrival should be encouraged. Once the victim is in the hospital, the physician should manage the following common complications: acidosis, arrhythmias, bronchospasm, pulmonary edema or adult respiratory distress syndrome (ARDS), gastric distention, cerebral edema, and hypothermia (see below). The patient should also be evaluated for underlying heart disease because this condition is a potential cause of drowning. Standard treatment measures should be employed.

Complications

Ingestion of small quantities of polluted water or the use of wet mouthpieces that were previously in contaminated water can lead to gastrointestinal illness.[32] Infections, including *Vibrio cholerae*– and *V. parahaemolyticus*–induced diarrhea and sepsis or wound infections from *V. parahaemolyticus* and *V. vulnificus*, have occurred after exposure to pathogens in the water.[33] The risk of infection is greater with exposure to warm, polluted, or murky water and increases if such water enters the mouth or is swallowed. Wound infections, sepsis, respiratory tract infections, and ear infections have also occurred after activity in nonpolluted water.[34]

Francisella philomiragia (formerly termed *Yersinia philomiragia*) may cause febrile illness after an instance of near-drowning.[35] Brain abscess caused by the fungus *Pseudallescheria boydii* has occurred as long as six months after a submersion event and is treated with high dosages of miconazole (80 to 90 mg/kg/day) for a prolonged period.[36,37]

Prognosis

A prognosis for near-drowning victims may be difficult to formulate, but current data justify guarded optimism. In a study of 83 adults (mean age, 31 years) admitted to the hospital for drowning or near-drowning, all of those with respiratory arrest and 33 percent with cardiopulmonary arrest survived resuscitation and were discharged. Predictors of survival included young age, immersion for less than 10 minutes, absence of evidence of aspiration, and a core body temperature less than 35° C (95° F) at the time of admission.[38] In a study of 40 victims who were admitted to a metropolitan hospital, those who arrived with a beating heart were apparently neurologically intact on discharge.[39] A study of 135 children younger than 20 years found that submersion duration was a major predictor of outcome. The incidence of death was 10 percent for those submerged zero to five minutes, 56 percent for those submerged six to nine minutes, 88 percent for those submerged 10 to 25 minutes, and 100 percent for those submerged longer than 25 minutes. Patients who received more than 25 minutes of CPR either suffered severe neurologic impairment or died.[40]

In a study of 101 pediatric victims of drowning and near-drowning, investigators rated 94 patients according to the Glasgow coma scale [*see Chapter 34*] on status at the time of admission.[41] A score of less than 5 identified a high-risk group in which 80 percent died or experienced permanent neurologic sequelae. A score of 6 or higher defined a low-risk group in which no deaths or apparent neurologic sequelae ensued.

Generally, a clinical picture that includes one or more of the following portends severe neurologic impairment or mortality[42-44]: fixed and dilated pupils (while the patient is in the emergency room), arterial pH less than 7.1, coma, or the need for in-hospital resuscitation or ventilatory support.[38-40] These indicators have not been absolutely reliable; patients have recovered completely despite such ominous signs.[38,45] Thus, prognostic criteria must be regarded with caution when the possibility of resuscitation is being considered. One study has shown that the blood glucose level at admission may be another prognostic indicator: patients with levels higher than approximately 400 mg/dl were more likely to die or enter a persistent vegetative state than patients with a lower blood glucose level.[46]

Recovery can occur in seemingly hopeless cases of near-drowning accompanied by circulatory arrest when victims undergo extreme and rapid chilling in low-temperature water. Young children especially exhibit this capacity to survive prolonged submersion in cold water,[47,48] but full recovery is also possible for adults.[49] The outlook is worse for victims who have been submersed in warm water.

Treatment of Hypothermia

Immersion in water in almost all cases will cause a net total body heat loss. Even warm water (the water in most swimming pools is kept at about 27° C, and the temperature of tropical ocean water is similar or higher) is significantly below core body temperature. Water, a good heat conductor, conducts heat 32 times better than air. Therefore, immersed individuals experience rapid heat loss through the skin. Skin temperatures approach water temperature within the first five minutes of immersion in both lean and overweight swimmers.[50] Swimmers are frequently unaware of this insidious heat loss until they begin to show physiologic signs of cooling, such as shivering, goose bumps, or blue lips.[51] A study of 12 monitored subjects who were immersed in 10° C water indicated that the subjects were unaware of the onset of hypothermia.[52]

Severe accidental hypothermia (below 30° C, or 86° F) is associated with marked depression in cerebral blood flow and cerebral oxygen requirement, reduced cardiac output, and decreased arterial pressure. Victims can appear to be lifeless as a result of marked depression of brain function. Peripheral pulses may be difficult to detect because of bradycardia and vasoconstric-

tion.[53] J waves are noted on the ECG in more than 80 percent of hypothermic patients. These waves increase in size with decreasing core temperature. Arrhythmias, ventricular fibrillation, and a combined metabolic and respiratory acidosis appear when the core temperature falls below 28° C (82.4° F). Alcohol consumption significantly increases the risk of water-related accidents, and it worsens hypothermia by producing peripheral vasodilatation.[22] Victims should be screened for coagulopathies because this complication can occur after hypothermia.[54]

Basic life support If the victim is not breathing, rescue breathing should be started. Immediate chest compression is indicated in the suspected hypothermia victim in the field who is pulseless and unmonitored. Up to one minute may be necessary to establish pulselessness in such circumstances.[55] The victim should continue to receive CPR while being transported as quickly as possible to an advanced life-support treatment facility. The individual should be insulated to prevent further core heat loss. Although prehospital rewarming by application of external warm objects (e.g., hot-water bottles or warm packs)[56,57] has been a longtime standard of care, a study of eight individuals cooled to clinical hypothermia in ice water and then warmed suggests that external or inhaled heat does little to prevent a subsequent drop in the core temperature and does not significantly change the rate of rewarming.[58,59]

Advanced life support Physical manipulations, including endotracheal or nasogastric intubation and temporary pacemaker or pulmonary artery flow–directed catheter insertion, may precipitate ventricular fibrillation in the hypothermic victim who has not yet gone into cardiac arrest.[60] However, when specifically and urgently indicated, such procedures should not be withheld. For example, in an unconscious hypothermic patient with inadequate ventilation, endotracheal intubation should be performed to provide effective ventilation and prevent aspiration. In such cases, prior ventilation with 100 percent oxygen may lessen the likelihood of precipitating ventricular fibrillation. Rewarming should continue after the victim has reached the hospital by use of a combination of heated blankets, heat packs, warm gastric lavage, and warm-water immersion.[61] Core rewarming is recommended for victims who are severely hypothermic to reduce the likelihood of rewarming shock (see below).

Nonessential medications should generally be avoided because the pharmacological activity of drugs and drug metabolism are reduced in patients with hypothermia.[62] Even vital medications should be used with caution, because accumulation to toxic levels can readily occur.

Management of cardiac arrest caused by hypothermia is different from the management of normothermic cardiac arrest. Defibrillation is often unsuccessful at body temperatures less than 30° C (86° F). At what temperature defibrillation should first be attempted and how often it should subsequently be tried have not been established. There are conflicting reports about the efficacy of bretylium tosylate in this setting.[63] Treatment should be directed at rapid core rewarming using warm-water immersion, warmed intravenous fluids, peritoneal dialysis, thoracotomy, and irrigation of the heart with warm fluids or extracorporeal blood warming with partial bypass.[64-66] Continuous closed thoracic cavity lavage has been successful in several studies and may provide an effective alternative to cardiopulmonary bypass.[67,68] Extracorporeal venovenous rewarming has proved effective in extremely hypothermic patients who are not in cardiac arrest.[69]

Some clinicians believe that patients who appear to be lifeless after prolonged exposure to cold temperatures should not be considered dead until their core body temperature is nearly normal and they are still unresponsive to cardiopulmonary resuscitation.[30] However, a person who experiences arrest while normothermic in a cold environment will quickly begin to cool. If the arrest was not witnessed, rescuers and hospital personnel will not know if the arrest was caused by hypothermia or if hypothermia is a sequel to the arrest. For this reason, physicians should use clinical judgment to decide when resuscitative efforts should cease in a hypothermic arrest case.

Scuba-Diving Accidents

Medical problems related to scuba diving have been radically changed by the advent of frequent air travel. Because of the relatively large number of people who fly to and from diving vacations, physicians need to be able to recognize the symptoms of the bends, which can occur during the flight home. Other diving injuries, such as sinus and ear trauma, might also become evident after the diver's return. Regardless of where they are practicing medicine, physicians should understand the conditions that would disqualify a person from diving.[70,71]

Several medical conditions should disqualify people from scuba diving; other conditions may be relative contraindications that should be evaluated by an expert in undersea medicine before a person is allowed to participate in the sport.[71,72] Most conditions that disqualify persons from diving are illnesses that predispose them to problems from gas expansion or from the formation of gas bubbles in closed body spaces [*see Table 1*]. Diver qualification and safety have been reviewed in great detail.[73-76] A comprehensive table on fitness for diving is available from the Diving Accident Network (DAN) at Duke University Medical Center.[77] Prospective divers should be able to obtain medical evaluation forms for diver eligibility from the major certifying organizations and from diving schools. A new extensive diving medical examination is available from the South Pacific Underwater Medicine Society (SPUMS).[78]

In addition to being at significant risk of drowning, scuba divers are also exposed to the risks of air embolism, decompression sickness, otorhinologic barotrauma, and cold-induced pulmonary edema.[79-82] These

Table 1   Contraindications to Diving

Contraindication	*Rationale*
Asthma, significant chronic obstructive pulmonary disorder, or emphysema	Risk of pneumothorax and air embolism; alveolar gas overexpansion may occur behind mucus-plugged or spastic airways
History of pneumothorax, pulmonary blebs, or cystic lesions	Risk of recurrence under water; subsequent development of tension pneumothorax, mediastinal shift, and cardiac arrest during diving
Seizure disorders	Risk of death, drowning, or aspiration during active seizure activity; increased pressure and depth may lower seizure threshold
Migraine headache	If symptoms include vomiting, death may result under water; if symptoms such as loss of sensation or function, vertigo, or diplopia are present, the patient may appear to have decompression sickness
History of cerebrovascular accident	Poor perfusion to certain partially damaged areas may increase the risk of CNS decompression sickness
Structural cardiac diseases, unrepaired atrial or ventricular septal defects, or patent foramen ovale	Gas bubbles forming on ascent may cross from right to left in the heart and cause cerebral air embolism
Angina, significant cardiac arrhythmias, S/P myocardial infarction, or congestive heart failure	Stress response to cold and physical exertion while swimming against currents or waves makes large demands on cardiac reserve and may precipitate angina or infarction under water
Chronic otitis media or otitis externa	Changes in pressure without the ability to clear ears may cause rupture of the round or oval window with severe vertigo and permanent hearing loss or may lead to a perforated tympanic membrane with hearing loss
Ruptured tympanic membrane or history of otosclerotic surgery	Risk of otitis developing from marine pathogens; inability to clear ears
Ménière's disease	Worsening of vertigo under pressure
Pregnancy	Possible danger to fetus, but this is still under study
Insulin-dependent diabetes	Risk of hypoglycemia in response to high-level exercise in a cold environment; inability to increase sugar level safely under water
Hemophilia or other bleeding disorders	Bleeding may occur in the sinuses or ears with barotrauma or in the lungs after overpressurization; cuts or bruises from coral may bleed profusely

medical emergencies require rapid recognition and treatment. The speed with which therapy is started is critically important. If recompression therapy is begun within 30 minutes after the onset of symptoms, improvement can be expected in 80 percent of

Table 2 Gas Parameters at Various Altitudes

Altitude (ft)	Barometric Pressure		Partial Pressure of Inspired O_2 (mm Hg)	Partial Pressure of Inspired N_2 (mm Hg)	Gas Volume (% of volume at sea level)	Bubble Diameter (% of diameter at sea level)
	(mm Hg)	(ATM)				
Commercial aircraft, 8,000 ft (maximum cabin pressure)	564	0.74	118	444	135	107.8
Denver, 5,280 ft	631	0.83	133	498	120	104.6
Small plane, 4,000 ft	656	0.86	138	516	116	103.7
Sea level	760	1	160	600	100	100
Depth						
33 ft	1,520	2	320	1,200	50	79.3
66 ft	2,280	3	480	1,800	33	69.3
99 ft	3,040	4	640	2,400	25	63

patients; if it is delayed for six hours, only 50 percent will respond.[83-86] DAN sponsors a 24-hour hot line for diving accidents (919-684-8111) and also has a number for general information about scuba diving (919-684-2948). In addition, a monthly publication by DAN, entitled *Alert Diver*, reviews medical information and current statistics about diving medicine as well as current therapies.[87]

Acute Hazards of Diving

Physical Properties of Gases and Liquids

To understand the problems that are likely to occur with air embolism or decompression sickness, several principles of the physics of gases and liquids must be understood. The atmospheric pressure at sea level, termed one atmosphere (14.7 psi, or 760 mm Hg), represents the total weight of the 18,000 ft of atmospheric gases above. As one descends underwater, pressure increases further with depth because of the combined weight of the air and the water. For each additional 33 ft in depth, the ambient pressure increases one absolute atmosphere.

The relation between the volume and the pressure of a gas is described by Boyle's law: as the pressure exerted on a gas increases, the volume of the gas decreases in inverse proportion according to the formula $P_1V_1 = P_2V_2$, where P_1 and V_1 are the initial pressure and volume and P_2 and V_2 are the final pressure and volume. Therefore, as depth and ambient gas pressure increase, any initial volume of gas, such as that in a lung or in a middle ear, will decrease. Conversely, the volume of gas in a lung that is full of air inhaled from a scuba tank in 33 ft of water doubles by the time the diver reaches the surface. The relation between atmospheric pressure, oxygen tension (P_{O_2}), nitrogen tension (P_{N_2}), and gas volume or bubble size varies according to altitude and depth [see Table 2].

The amount of gas that can be dissolved in solution is directly proportional to the pressure on the solution (stated as Henry's law). A familiar example of this phenomenon is seen on opening a champagne bottle in which there are no visible bubbles; when the cork is popped, the bubbles appear. These bubbles represent supersaturated carbon dioxide coming out of solution. A similar scenario occurs in divers with decompression sickness.

Air Embolism

Many scuba-related drownings seem to result from loss of consciousness secondary to air embolism. Emboli usually appear in the cerebral circulation (cerebral arterial gas embolism, or CAGE) because the ascent is made with the head up. In an ascent in which the diver rises gradually and exhales air at a normal rate, no significant pressure gradient builds up across the alveolar walls. However, if the diver ascends suddenly without exhaling, perhaps because of panic over a mechanical failure or other hazard or because of laryngospasm resulting from aspiration, alveoli may rupture. Localized areas of alveolar overdistention and rupture may also occur if air is trapped behind mucus plugs in the bronchi or because of airway spasm. Air then leaks from the alveolar sacs, causing pneumothorax, pneumopericardium, pneumomediastinum, or subcutaneous emphysema. If a communication develops between alveoli and the pulmonary vasculature, life-threatening emboli occur as the diver takes a breath, forcing air from the airway and alveoli into the pulmonary veins and then through the left side of the heart into the systemic arterial circulation.[88]

Clinical manifestations CAGE symptoms appear within two minutes after an embolism develops. Neurologic symptoms predominate.[89] Collapse or sudden unconsciousness immediately upon surfacing is the most marked presentation, but symptoms may include vague mood or personality changes, impaired sensorium, seizures, weakness, paresthesias, and paralysis of the limbs.[90] Complex neurologic disorders result from multiple emboli. Other symptoms relate to pneumothorax, pneumopericardium, and subcutaneous emphysema. Such manifestations as hemodynamic failure and shock may mark severe cases of air embolism. In addition, air embolism may frequently occur in combination with other forms of decompression sickness or the bends.

Decompression Sickness

With increasing depth, the nitrogen tension increases and nitrogen is driven into tissues. Because nitrogen is far more soluble in lipid than in water, it becomes most concentrated in such highly vascular, lipid-rich tissues as the central nervous system, the bone marrow, and, to a lesser extent, certain fat depots. Nitrogen's solubility increases as tissue temperature falls.

Estimates of the amount of time required for nitrogen to accumulate in tissue have been used to construct the United States Navy decompression tables. These tables specify the so-called no-decompression times for all diving depths, that is, the length of time a diver can remain at a particular depth without having to stop on the way to the surface to allow for decompression.[91,92]

If a diver ascends too rapidly from a dive that has exceeded the no-decompression time limit, tissues may become supersaturated with nitrogen. Nitrogen bubbles may form in these tissues faster than the gas can be transported to and excreted by the lungs. The bubbles may be generated both in the extravascular tissues and the intravascular fluids. Nitrogen bubbles may block blood flow, alter blood rheology, and produce endothelial changes. The results are intravascular coagulation, secondary clotting and hemorrhage, and complement activation.[93,94] A number of mathematical models for bubble growth have been proposed,[95] but knowledge of the exact mechanisms of initiation of decompression sickness is still incomplete. Silent bubble formation occurs even in divers who adhere to no-decompression time limits. In a study of 110 dives monitored with Doppler bubble detectors, venous gas emboli were seen in all dives, regardless of the dive profile (i.e., depth of dive, length of time, and rate of change in depth).[96]

Clinical manifestations Symptoms usually appear within one hour after surfacing but may be delayed up to 36 hours. The characteristics of the various syndromes depend on the location of either bubble formation or vascular occlusion.

Symptoms are divided into type 1 and type 2. Type 1 symptoms include joint pain, or the bends, and skin symptoms. The bends are characterized by deep aching and throbbing musculoskeletal pain, reflecting decompression sickness in major limb joints, periarticular tissues, and bones. Bubbles in the skin cause mottling, so-called migrating geographic rashes, pruritus, and paresthesias.

Type 2 symptoms include more serious manifestations, such as neurologic dysfunction. CNS involvement, most often affecting the spinal cord in cases of decompression sickness, is a major complication. Such signs as sensorial impairment, mood or cognitive changes, focal deficits, and seizures reveal the location of neurologic lesions. Nitrogen emboli that develop in the microcirculation of the lungs result in the syndrome known as chokes, which is characterized by substernal pain, cough, dyspnea, cyanosis, and, in severe cases, decreased cardiac output and shock. In some cases of repeated pressure exposure, aseptic bone necrosis may ultimately develop in the large joints.

A study of decompression sickness in Spain revealed that of 276 dysbaric diving accidents, 70 (25 percent) were type 1 cases, 149 (54 percent) were type 2 cases, and 39 (14 percent) were cases of acute air embolism.[97] In a similar study of 570 cases conducted by DAN, 127 (22 percent) were type 1 cases, 340 (60 percent) were type 2 cases, and 97 (17 percent) were cases of acute gas embolism.[98] In both studies, divers typically waited 15 to 18 hours before seeking treatment. A study of 100 divers with decompression sickness or cerebral arterial gas embolism in Australia found the most common symptoms to be pain (72 percent), lethargy (68 percent), headache (60 percent), and altered sensation (42 percent). Many of these cases occurred in divers with risk factors for the bends, including multiple dives (55 percent), rapid ascent (17 percent), previous episodes of decompression sickness (12 percent), alcohol consumption (6 percent), or subsequent as-

cent to high altitude (5 percent). At least 25 percent of the divers with decompression sickness had exceeded the time allowed by the dive tables without proper decompression stops.[99]

Echocardiography that is enhanced by the intravenous injection of saline can be used to examine patients who have decompression sickness. This technique produces microscopic bubbles that provide contrast and allow visualization of shunts in the heart. A study of 30 divers who had decompression sickness revealed that 37 percent had a right-to-left shunt through a patent foramen ovale.[100] A follow-up study of divers who had decompression sickness revealed that 66 percent of those who experienced neurologic symptoms within 30 minutes after surfacing had shunts, compared with 24 percent of healthy divers.[101] The results of these studies raise the question of whether commercial or serious amateur divers should be screened with this echocardiographic technique if they anticipate making dives that carry a high risk of decompression sickness.

Management

If air embolism is suspected, the patient should be placed on the left side. Studies suggest that the Trendelenburg position (head down, body elevated) should be avoided.[102-104] The airway should be kept open; 100 percent oxygen should be given at high flow rates; and dehydration and intravascular fluid depletion, which are common after extended immersion and cold exposure,[105-107] should be corrected with volume replacement, vasoactive drugs, or both. Seizures can be controlled with anticonvulsive agents. The results of a study on dogs in which inhalation of 100 percent oxygen more than halved the time that nitrogen bubbles remained in the pulmonary vasculature[108] suggest that the administration of 100 percent oxygen at the scene of an air embolism accident may be beneficial until recompression therapy can be started.

As soon as possible, the patient should be transferred to a hyperbaric facility, where recompression therapy, guided by standard tables,[91,93] should be rapidly instituted. Time is important, but hyperbaric therapy may still reverse neurologic injury even if delayed for as long as nine hours.[83] If air transportation is needed, the aircraft cabin should be maximally pressurized or the aircraft should be flown at altitudes near sea level. Bubbles further increase in size with ascent from sea level [*see Table 2*], and this situation may worsen existing symptoms or produce new problems.[87]

Advice about hyperbaric therapy can be obtained 24 hours a day by contacting DAN (919-684-8111); the Navy Experimental Diving Unit, United States Navy, Panama City, Florida (904-234-4351); or the Hyperbaric Medicine Division, Armstrong Laboratories, Brooks Air Force Base, San Antonio, Texas (512-536-3281 on weekdays and 512-536-3278 at night and on weekends).

According to Navy guidelines, divers should abstain from diving for seven days after successful treatment of type 1 symptoms and four weeks after successful treatment of type 2 symptoms.[91]

Precautions and Diver Training

According to the Centers for Disease Control, most underwater diving deaths have been attributed to the diver's inexperience, carelessness, or both. Other factors, such as strong currents or rough water, compound this risk. Failure of equipment has also played a role in diving accidents.[109]

Many of the dive-training organizations, such as the National Association of Underwater Instructors (NAUI) and the Professional Association of Diving Instructors (PADI), sponsor advanced training courses in dive conditions that involve certain hazards and therefore require special training and diving gear. These courses include cave diving, ice diving, and advanced open water certification. Anyone considering diving under these conditions should be strongly advised to seek this specialized training.

Dive computers have become more common among sport divers. These instruments typically allow longer bottom times than conventional decompression tables for repetitive dives; they may therefore underestimate the length of time needed for decompression, especially in repetitive-dive situations. Dive computers should only be used by divers who have a good working knowledge of the decompression tables. When used properly, these devices appear to be safe.[85,110-113]

Physicians should present a number of safety guidelines to divers to help prevent decompression sickness:

1. Prevent dehydration by replacing fluid and abstaining from alcohol and caffeine before and after the dive. In one study, 50 percent of injured divers had consumed alcohol the day of the dive or the night before.[111]
2. Make the deepest part of your dive first. Ascend slowly, and measure your ascent speed. Make a safety stop for a few minutes at 15 ft.[114,115]
3. Rest adequately before the dive, and keep warm during the dive by wearing dry or wet suits in cold-water areas or Lycra skins in warmer waters. Allow at least a one-hour interval at the surface between dives.
4. Undergo adequate in-water conditioning before the dive (i.e., a swimming program).
5. Avoid remaining underwater for longer than recommended by decompression tables or dive computers, and carefully plan repetitive or multiday dives. A diver who uses a computer should first read the owner's manual and should also be able to refer to Navy decompression tables in case the computer fails.[116]
6. Avoid restricting movement after the dive, such as sitting in one position for a long time on a dive boat or in a plane after the dive, which decreases regional blood flow and nitrogen removal.[117]

Over the past two years, there has been interest among sport divers in the use of gas mixtures other than compressed air that can extend the amount of time they can spend underwater without decompression or that can shorten decompression times. These gas mixtures, called nitrox (32 percent oxygen and 68 percent nitrogen) and EAN (enriched air nitrox), contain more oxygen and less nitrogen than ordinary air, which is composed of 21 percent oxygen and 78 percent nitrogen.

Nitrox has been used for years by commercial and scientific divers, but its use by sport divers is likely to raise a number of concerns. Breathing oxygen at higher than one atmosphere absolute pressure is associated with seizures. A diver breathing compressed air would have to be 218 ft underwater (a depth almost never reached by sport divers) to reach this level of oxygen pressure, but a diver breathing nitrox could experience seizures at a depth of only 132 ft. In addition, the higher concentration of oxygen creates a risk of fire and explosion. Gas concentrations in a nitrox mixture must be precisely determined to ensure proper use of the special decompression tables required for nitrox. Oxygen concentration must then be rechecked before diving because variables such as gauge accuracy and temperature may not have remained constant during mixing, leading to inaccurate calculation of gas proportions. Unfortunately, these safety requirements may be too sophisticated for the ordinary diver or dive shop. It is likely that there will be an increased casualty rate with the use of these mixtures until formal training and testing protocols are instituted by the sport dive industry. Anyone interested in using nitrox should obtain formal training in its use and check the credentials and testing procedures of the vendors.[118-120]

To avoid the occurrence of the bends when flying, scuba divers who have made nondecompression dives or who have spent less than two hours underwater during the 48 hours before flying should wait at least 12 hours after their last dive before boarding a commercial aircraft. Divers who have practiced either unlimited multiday diving or who have made decompression dives should wait 24 to 48 hours before flying.[121] The cab-

ins of commercial aircraft are pressurized to an altitude of 8,000 ft, and the consequent reduced air pressure may induce decompression sickness in divers who were asymptomatic at sea level.[70,122,123] Of 270 cases of decompression sickness reported to DAN in 1987, 32 percent involved flying after diving; six divers who had been asymptomatic experienced the bends while in flight, and 11 divers became symptomatic after the flight. Seven other divers reported in this study experienced decompression sickness after riding in cars at altitudes above 5,000 ft.[87]

The CDC notes that as of 1987, no transmission of the acquired immunodeficiency syndrome (AIDS) had occurred through scuba equipment. They note, however, that there is a hypothetical risk of transmitting the virus between divers because of the use and structure of the second-stage regulator mouthpiece. They suggest a protocol for cleaning equipment to eliminate this hazard, but this approach has not been tested.[124] British worker-safety guidelines for divers do allow divers who are positive for the human immunodeficiency virus (HIV) to continue their work, noting that AIDS has not been shown to be transmitted during normal diving operations or first aid, including mouth-to-mouth resuscitation.[125]

Divers also risk being bitten by sea snakes, shellfish, or octopuses or being stung by coral, jellyfish, or poisonous fish. These hazards are discussed elsewhere [*see Chapter 28*].

Otorhinologic Problems

The most common medical problems associated with diving are difficulty in clearing the ears and trauma to the ears or sinuses after submersion.

An understanding of the regional anatomy is essential to therapy in these conditions. The opening to the eustachian tube lies posterior to the turbinate bones in the posterior nasopharynx. The openings to the maxillary and frontal sinuses are found between the turbinates in the nose. Swelling and edema of the mucous membranes overlying the turbinates frequently follow allergic rhinosinusitis, chronic infectious sinusitis, or vasomotor rhinitis and partially blocks the eustachian tube and sinus openings. This partial blockage may create problems in equalizing air pressure in the ears or sinuses during ascent or descent. If the pressure differential across the eardrum (between the air in the middle ear and the external water pressure in the auditory canal) becomes great enough, the tympanic membrane or the round or oval windows may rupture. If the pressure differential occurs across the sinus opening between the sinus and nasal passages, the sinuses will swell and bleed, filling the diver's mask with bright-red blood.

Therapy for ear or sinus blockage must be directed at the nose. Two sprays in each nostril twice a day of topical cortisone nasal sprays such as flunisolide (Nasalide) or beclomethasone (Vancenase AQ or Beconase AQ) in conjunction with a decongestant such as phenylpropanolamine (Entex LA or Dura-Vent) or an antihistamine-decongestant combination will usually relieve postdive symptoms. If the patient has had trouble with ear clearing in the past, use of a steroid nasal spray and a decongestant for one week before diving as well as immediately before each dive will usually allow adequate clearing. If the patient experiences hearing loss, vertigo, or frank blood in the middle ear after a dive, otologic referral is indicated. External otitis may occur from residual water in the external auditory canals and usually responds to topical antibiotic eardrops.

Waterslides

Waterslides provide a fast descent over a film of water through steep drops and around sharp curves. These devices have been identified as an important cause of water-related injuries (including fractures and concussions) and fatalities.[126] Such accidents account for 30 percent of all injuries related to amusement park rides.[127] Users should be cautioned about the risks.

Outbreaks of *Pseudomonas*-associated folliculitis and otitis externa have occurred in individuals after water-sliding.[128] In addition, outbreaks of giardiasis have been reported in persons using hotel waterslides.[129]

Hot Tubs

Prolonged exposure to water between 38° and 40° C can result in an increase in core temperature and cardiac output. In patients with cardiac disease, this increase may precipitate congestive heart failure or dysrhythmias. In young children, dizziness and hyperthermia may occur. A study of 24 nonpregnant young women exposed to 40° C water in a hot tub showed that the subjects reached a core temperature of 39° C (102.2° F) in 12 to 23 minutes. None of the subjects left the water before their core temperature reached 39° C, even though they were instructed to leave the water when they felt too uncomfortable to continue. Physical discomfort was therefore not a reliable measure of core temperature. The researchers recommended a time limit of 10 minutes for pregnant women because a core temperature of 39° C or higher may harm a fetus.[130] A study of 22,754 pregnant women found that exposure to heat from hot tubs and saunas or the presence of fever in the first trimester was associated with an increased risk of fetal neural tube defects. Hot-tub exposure seemed to have the greatest effect. It is recommended that women avoid using hot tubs and saunas during the first trimester of pregnancy until further data have been gathered.[131] In addition, the sitting area around the hot tub may not be chlorinated enough to kill bacteria or viruses on the surface. Folliculitis has also been documented after hot-tub exposure.[132,133]

References

1. The Pathophysiology and Treatment of Drowning and Near-Drowning. Charles C Thomas, Publisher, Springfield, Illinois, 1971
2. JAMA 260:380, 1988
3. MMWR 34:281, 1985
4. JAMA 260:390, 1988
5. Am J Dis Child 144:663, 1990
6. Pediatrics 86:1067, 1990
7. J Fla Med Assoc 77:679, 1990
8. Pediatrics 75:789, 1985
9. MMWR 37(SS-1):27, 1988
10. S Afr Med J 78:418, 1990
11. JAMA 263:1952, 1990
12. Am J Dis Child 136:777, 1982
13. NZ Med J 97:777, 1984
14. MMWR 41:329, 1992
15. Pediatr Rev 10:5, 1988
16. Arch Intern Med 145:50, 1985
17. JAMA 253:557, 1985
18. J Electrocardiol 23:235, 1990
19. Arch Pathol Lab Med 109:176, 1985
20. Anaesthesia 30:364, 1975
21. JAMA 255:2905, 1986
22. Textbook of Advanced Cardiac Life Support. American Heart Association, 1987, p 227
23. Ann Emerg Med 10:476, 1981
24. Anesthesiology 30:414, 1969
25. Emerg Med Serv 10:63, 1981
26. Emergency 13:45, 1981
27. Emerg Med Serv 10:58, 1981
28. Emerg Med Serv 11:93, 1982
29. Lancet 1:1275, 1975
30. JAMA 243:1250, 1980
31. Intensive Care Med 16:336, 1990
32. MMWR 32:576, 1983
33. Undersea Biomedical Research 18:193, 1991
34. Undersea Biomedical Research 18:181, 1991
35. Ann Intern Med 110:888, 1989
36. Arch Neurol 47:468, 1990
37. Medicine (Baltimore) 68:218, 1989
38. Ann Emerg Med 19:1390, 1990
39. Pediatrics 86:586, 1990
40. J Trauma 22:544, 1982
41. Crit Care Med 9:536, 1981
42. Pediatrics 59:364, 1977
43. J Am Coll Emerg Physicians 8:176, 1979
44. Am J Dis Child 135:1006, 1981
45. Can Anaesth Soc J 27:172, 1980
46. Neurology 40:820, 1990
47. JAMA 260:377, 1988
48. J Pediatr 117:179, 1990
49. Arch Intern Med 140:775, 1980
50. Aviat Space Environ Med 62:1063, 1991
51. 9th International Symposium on Underwater and Hyperbaric Physiology. Underwater and Hyperbaric Medical Society, Bethesda, Maryland, 1987, p 95
52. Aviat Space Environ Med 60:964, 1989
53. J Appl Physiol 64:719, 1988
54. Surg Clin North Am 68:775, 1988
55. J Emerg Med Serv 10:32, 1983
56. Alaska Med 24:106, 1982
57. Postgrad Med 88:55, 1990
58. Diving Accident Management—Forty-first Undersea and Hyperbaric Medical Society Workshop, Durham, North Carolina, January 1990, p 88
59. Ann Emerg Med 20:896, 1991
60. Ann Emerg Med 14:339, 1985
61. Aviat Space Environ Med 59:630, 1988
62. Ann Intern Med 89:519, 1978
63. Ann Emerg Med 13:994, 1984
64. Ann Surg 195:492, 1982
65. Am J Emerg Med 6:475, 1988
66. Ann Emerg Med 19:1093, 1990
67. Ann Emerg Med 19:1335, 1990
68. Ann Emerg Med 19:204, 1990
69. J Trauma 31:1247, 1991
70. J Hyperbaric Med 4:23, 1989
71. Undersea Biomed Res 11:407, 1984
72. J Am Board Fam Pract 1:194, 1988
73. Medical Examination of Sport Scuba Divers, 2nd ed. Medical Seminars, Inc, San Antonio, 1986
74. Fitness to Dive. Undersea and Hyperbaric Medical Society, Bethesda, Maryland, 1987
75. SPUMS Journal 21(2):70, 1991
76. Undersea Biomedical Research 19(2):73, 1992
77. Alert Diver 5(4):10, 1990
78. The SPUMS Diving Medical, Appendix B. The South Pacific Underwater Medicine Society, Victoria, Australia, March 1992
79. NZ Med J 89:472, 1979
80. J Am Coll Emerg Physicians 5:355, 1976
81. Lancet 2:1193, 1974
82. Lancet 1:62, 1989
83. Br Med J 284:1014, 1982
84. Undersea Biomed Res 15:377, 1988
85. 18th Annual Undersea Hyperbaric Medical Society Pacific Chapter Meeting, Nov 1–2, 1990
86. Acta Anaesthesiologica Italica 42(suppl 2):137, 1991
87. Alert Diver 5:1, 1989
88. SPUMS 18:90, 1988
89. Ann Emerg Med 16:535, 1987
90. SPUMS Journal 21(3):133, 1991
91. U.S. Navy Diving Manual. Department of the Navy, Washington, DC, 1989
92. Diving Accident Management—Forty-first Undersea and Hyperbaric Medical Society Workshop, Durham, North Carolina, January 1990, p 194
93. Undersea Biomedical Research 18(3):157, 1991
94. Diving Accident Management—Forty-first Undersea and Hyperbaric Medical Society Workshop, Durham, North Carolina, January 1990, p 38
95. Respir Physiol 71:299, 1988
96. Proceedings of Biomechanics of Safe Ascent Workshop. American Academy of Underwater Sciences. Costa Mesa, California, 1989, p 65
97. Proceedings of the XV Annual Meeting of the European Undersea Biomedical Society (EUBS), Eilat, Israel, 1989
98. Proceedings of Biomechanics of Safe Ascent Workshop. American Academy of Underwater Sciences, Costa Mesa, California, 1989, p 143
99. SPUMS Journal 21(3):135, 1991
100. Lancet 1:513, 1989
101. EUBS Proceedings: Joint Meeting on Diving and Hyperbaric Medicine. Amsterdam, The Netherlands, 1990, p 14
102. UHMS Gulf Coast Chapter Joint Annual Conference and Scientific Sessions, Birmingham, Alabama, April 1990
103. Alert Diver 5:1, 1989
104. EUBS proceedings of the XVII Annual Meeting on Diving and Hyperbaric Medicine, Crete, Greece, September 29 to October 3, 1991, p 241
105. EUBS XIV (European Underwater Biomedical Society), 1988
106. Pressure 19(5):1, 1990
107. N Engl J Med 326:30, 1992
108. Undersea Biomed Res 16:21, 1989
109. MMWR 29:69, 1980
110. Journal of Hyperbaric Medicine 5:163, 1990

111. Journal of Hyperbaric Medicine 5:159, 1990
112. SPUMS Journal 21(4):204, 1991
113. SPUMS Journal 22(1):24, 1992
114. Undersea Journal Fourth Quarter:8, 1990
115. Proceedings of Biomechanics of Safe Ascent Workshop. American Academy of Underwater Sciences. Costa Mesa, California, 1989, p 79
116. Skin Diver, June:68, 1992
117. Alert Diver Feb/Mar:1, 1990
118. Alert Diver Nov/Dec:1, 1991
119. Pressure 21(1):1, 1992
120. Pressure 20(1):1, 1991
121. 39th Undersea and Hyperbaric Medical Society Workshop. Undersea Hyperbaric Medical Society, Bethesda, Maryland, 1989
122. Chest 92:81, 1988
123. JAMA 247:1007, 1982
124. Pressure 20(3):11, 1991
125. Pressure 21(1):11, 1992
126. MMWR 35:429, 1986
127. MMWR 33:379, 1984
128. MMWR 32:425, 1983
129. Pediatr Infect Dis J 7:91, 1988
130. N Engl J Med 323:835, 1990
131. JAMA 268:882, 1992
132. Infect Control 6:418, 1985
133. Am J Med 79:10, 1985

Acknowledgment

Text under "Treatment of Near-Drowning" (pages 652–654) and "Treatment of Hypothermia" (pages 655–656) excerpted from "Standards and Guidelines for Cardiopulmonary Resuscitation (CPR) and Emergency Cardiac Care (ECC)," in *The Journal of the American Medical Association* 255:2905, 1986. ©1986 American Medical Association.

26 Carbon Monoxide Poisoning and Smoke Inhalation

EDWARD RUBENSTEIN, M.D.

Carbon Monoxide Poisoning

It is estimated that about 10,000 persons each year in the United States experience carbon monoxide poisoning.[1] During 1988, there were 878 unintentional deaths and 2,637 suicides by carbon monoxide poisoning.[2]

A dramatic and steady decrease in the number of unintentional deaths from carbon monoxide poisoning occurred during the 10-year period from 1979 to 1988, when the number of deaths fell from 1,513 to 878 a year. Of these deaths, 57 percent were caused by exposure to motor vehicle exhaust (83 percent of the vehicles were stationary). The remaining unintentional deaths were related to stoves or fireplaces, which used coal, kerosene, or wood as fuel; to the combustion of natural gas fed by pipeline; to the combustion of liquefied petroleum gas in mobile containers; and to various industrial processes.

Unintentional carbon monoxide poisoning has also resulted from improper use or maintenance of gas lamps, ovens, and stoves in poorly ventilated recreational vehicles.[3] In this setting, the risk of intoxication increases at higher altitudes as the atmospheric partial pressure of oxygen falls, contributing to hypoxemia in the victim and to impaired fuel consumption and increased carbon monoxide production by the appliance. Children riding under closed canopies or tarpaulins in the back of pickup trucks are at significant risk for severe poisoning if there is a leak in the exhaust system or if the tailpipe is located at the rear rather than at the side of the truck.[4] Poisoning has also been caused by the use of gasoline-powered resurfacing equipment in inadequately ventilated indoor ice-skating rinks[5] and by the indoor use of industrial machinery. A number of accidental poisonings in motels have also been reported.[6] The rate of unintentional deaths is about three times higher in males than in females, with the largest number occurring in persons 15 to 24 years of age. There is marked seasonal variation: four times as many deaths occur in January as in July.[7]

The striking decrease in the rate of unintentional deaths has been attributed to changes in automobile design and engineering standards, which have resulted in more than a 90 percent decrease in carbon monoxide emission since 1968.[2] In addition, improved heating and cooking appliances and better building ventilation are believed to have contributed to the lower rates of unintentional carbon monoxide poisoning.

Contrary to the pattern of unintentional deaths, the annual number of suicides attributed to carbon monoxide poisoning increased steadily from 2,329 in 1979 to 3,161 in 1987; the number declined to 2,637 in 1988. Except for a slight increase during March, April, and May, there has been no seasonal variation in the suicide rate. Males account for 71 percent of suicides. The age-specific death rates have been highest for those 35 to 44 years of age, followed by those 45 to 54 years of age.[7]

In 1990, elevated blood levels of carboxyhemoglobin were detected in 26 anesthetized patients in three hospitals in Georgia, Illinois, and North Carolina.[8] The source of the carbon monoxide in these cases has not been identified, although the possibility of contamination of an anesthetic gas or of a chemical interaction between a gas and a carbon dioxide absorbent is under study. Physicians who have witnessed similar episodes of carbon monoxide poisoning should report them to the Centers for Disease Control and Prevention (404-639-3407).

The major pathophysiological disturbance in cases of carbon monoxide poisoning is tissue hypoxia. Tissue hypoxia occurs as a consequence of the extraordinary avidity of carbon monoxide (more than 200 times that of oxygen) for hemoglobin. Carbon monoxide not only displaces oxygen from hemoglobin but also interferes with the release of oxygen to the tissues.

Carbon monoxide poisoning is often rapidly fatal. Without an emission-control device, lethal concentrations of the gas can accumulate inside a car or a small garage in 15 to 30 minutes.[9]

Clinical Manifestations

The clinical manifestations of carbon monoxide poisoning depend primarily on the duration and intensity of the exposure.[10] Sudden high concentrations of carboxyhemoglobin in the blood result in rapid loss of consciousness, coma, seizures, and death. When poisoning is slow, a sequence of influenzalike symptoms usually ensues: a throbbing headache and irritability develop, followed by dizziness, weakness, impaired vision, ataxia, nausea, vomiting, syncope, and eventually unconsciousness. In cases of intoxication involving a group of individuals, symptoms may be mistaken for those of food poisoning.[11] Such variables as physical activity, preexisting anemia, vascular disease, and the state of respiratory function influence the severity of poisoning. Cherry-red discoloration of the skin appears in only a minority of victims. Flame-shaped superficial retinal hemorrhages may call attention to the diagnosis in subacute poisoning.[12]

Mild disturbances are associated with blood concentrations of carboxyhemoglobin of about 20 percent. Severe syndromes occur when 30 to 50 percent of the hemoglobin molecules are saturated with carbon monoxide. Blood concentrations of carboxyhemoglobin that are higher than 50 percent are often fatal. Metabolic acidosis that occurs despite the presence of hyperventilation ($Pco_2 < 40$ mm Hg) is an ominous sign.[13]

Heavy smokers may have carboxyhemoglobin levels in the range of seven to 10 percent.

Occult Poisoning

Headache, dizziness, new-onset or exacerbated angina, unexplained dyspnea, and a variety of influenzalike symptoms have been attributed to subacute carbon monoxide poisoning.[14,15] The prevalence of this syndrome is controversial, but carbon monoxide poisoning should be considered when risk factors exist in the home (see above) and especially when cohabitants have similar complaints. Confirmation of the diagnosis requires demonstration of elevated carboxyhemoglobin levels.

Studies of induced carboxyhemoglobinemia in nonsmoking patients with documented coronary artery disease have shown that a carboxyhemoglobin level of six percent significantly increases the number and complexity of ventricular arrhythmias (a four percent carboxyhemoglobin level did not alter ventricular arrhythmias).[16] This finding has called attention to the potential hazard of such levels, which are found in some urban dwellers and in workers in high-risk occupations, such as tunnel construction and motor vehicle traffic control.[17]

Treatment

The victim should be removed immediately from the site of exposure and given 100 percent oxygen at a high flow rate. Most patients respond to this treatment within an hour; however, if the victim exhibits respiratory depression, an endotracheal tube should be inserted as soon as possible and mechanical ventilation begun.

Severe Poisoning

Hyperbaric oxygen (HBO) therapy has been used, reportedly with impressive results, in patients with severe or prolonged poisoning.[18] However, the equipment is not widely available, and the findings of a few controlled studies comparing HBO therapy with 100 percent oxygen therapy at one atmosphere have been inconclusive.[16] Nevertheless, HBO therapy has been recommended for significant exposure for two reasons: favorable responses in uncontrolled studies have been reported, even after treatment has been delayed for seven to 16 hours after the time of rescue; and HBO can significantly reduce the half-life of carboxyhemoglobin. Suggested guidelines for such treatment are a history of unconsciousness, neuropsychiatric abnormality, cardiac instability or ischemia, or a carboxyhemoglobin level higher than 25 percent.[19,20] For children and pregnant women, HBO is indicated for a lower carboxyhemoglobin level.

Hypothermia has also been used, but its benefits are difficult to document. High doses of barbiturates, red blood cell and exchange transfusions, and asanguineous hypothermic perfusion also require further study.[18,21] Dantrolene has been used to alleviate hyperpyrexia caused by severe muscular rigidity in a patient with carbon monoxide poisoning.[22]

Carbon Monoxide Poisoning during Pregnancy

Carbon monoxide poisoning during pregnancy can result in fetal brain damage, teratogenesis, and death, even when the mother survives.[23] In one series, all six mothers survived with good outcomes, but three of the fetuses died.[21] Two of these fetuses were delivered stillborn within 36 hours, but one remained alive in utero for 20 weeks; it was nonviable, with multiple morphological abnormalities, when delivered at 33 weeks.[24]

The use of hyperbaric oxygen therapy in pregnant patients poses a therapeutic dilemma because of the hazards of abnormally high oxygen tensions to the fetus. On the basis of limited clinical experience, Van Hoesen, Camporesi, Moon, and coworkers have suggested the following guidelines[23]:

1. Administer HBO therapy if the maternal carboxyhemoglobin level is above 20 percent at any time during the exposure.

2. Administer HBO therapy if the patient has had or currently has any neurologic signs regardless of the carboxyhemoglobin level.

3. Administer HBO therapy if signs of fetal distress are present (i.e., fetal tachycardia, decreased beat-to-beat variability on the fetal monitor, or late decelerations) that are consistent with the carboxyhemoglobin level and exposure history.

4. If HBO treatment is unavailable, administer 100 percent oxygen via a tightly fitting mask for five times as long as is needed to reduce maternal carboxyhemoglobin to normal (less than five percent).

5. If the patient continues to demonstrate neurologic signs, or if signs of fetal distress are apparent 12 hours after initial treatment, additional HBO treatments may be indicated. Multiple HBO treatments have been suggested to be beneficial in severely poisoned and nonresponsive patients exposed to carbon monoxide.[25]

It should be emphasized that these recommendations are necessarily based on limited experience; further studies may lead to their modification.

Prognosis

Patients who do not respond rapidly to the initial therapy with oxygen may suffer various degrees of permanent central nervous system damage. They exhibit cognitive, personality, and neurologic disorders, some of which can develop after apparent recovery.[26] The most common sequelae are irritability, impulsiveness, moodiness, aggressiveness, and memory loss.

Bullous skin lesions, peripheral neuropathies, skeletal and cardiac muscle damage, and mesenteric and myocardial infarction may develop as a consequence of prolonged hypoxia.[27]

In a small percentage of patients, delayed neurologic sequelae appear after a lucid interval of about three weeks; this interval may range from a few days to as long as six weeks. Those most likely to be affected are elderly patients who have suffered initial deep coma. Clinical manifestations tend to fluctuate and include mental deterioration, urinary and fecal incontinence, gait and speech disturbances, mutism, tremor, and weakness. The prognosis is relatively good, with complete recovery occurring within a year in almost three fourths of patients. The cause of these delayed neurologic sequelae is not known, and there is no effective treatment.[28]

Smoke Inhalation

Fire-related respiratory injuries result from the inhalation of hot gases, carbon monoxide, or toxic fumes. The composition of toxic fumes or smoke released in a fire has changed radically because of the increasing use of synthetic materials, which has serious clinical implications.

Because air has a low heat capacity, thermal injuries are usually limited to the upper air passages; those that involve the larynx are most significant. In contrast, inhalation of high-temperature steam, which has a far greater heat capacity than air, can result in heat injury to bronchi and bronchioles.[29] Carbon monoxide poisoning should always be considered in the evaluation of fire victims, including fire fighters. It is the inhalation of noxious chemicals, however, that causes serious or fatal damage to the lungs; such damage can occur even in cases in which the respiratory system appears normal on initial examination. A victim who has inhaled smoke should be reexamined frequently or warned to return at the first sign of airway disease.

Fire fighting is associated with small, short-term decreases of three to 11 percent in some airflow indices after exposure to smoke from house fires.[30] A small subgroup of fire fighters manifest more severe, potentially clinically significant airway obstruction.

Smoke and Toxic Fumes

Smoke is a suspension of carbon particles in air and in other gases. Most of the smoke particles, which may be coated with organic acids and aldehydes, are filtered and trapped in the upper air passages; some, however, are too small to be filtered out and thus reach the lower lung structures, together with the toxic gases.

During the late 1960s, widespread use of plastic and synthetic materials in furniture, carpets, and wall coverings and in the insulation of electrical wires, cables, and switch boxes drastically changed the composition of noxious fumes. Polyvinyl chloride (PVC) has been implicated as one of the synthetic compounds that produce dangerous breakdown products on combustion.[31] At high temperatures, PVC releases a large number of degradation products, the most important of which are hydrochloric acid and carbon monoxide.[32] Hydrochloric acid is believed to be responsible for the serious pulmonary damage suffered by persons exposed to PVC smoke during a fire or during the subsequent cleanup. Other important toxic gases found in smoke include carbon dioxide, sulfur dioxide, nitrogen oxides, ammonia, low-molecular-weight alcohols and aldehydes, and hydrogen cyanide.[33] In one residential fire, methemoglobinemia was found in survivors, with methemoglobin levels as high as 19 percent.[34]

The Syndrome of Smoke Inhalation

Respiratory distress may be evident immediately after an episode of smoke inhalation or may be delayed for as long as two days. Anyone exposed to even a few breaths of choking fumes should receive medical attention, and even patients with only minor burns of the face or singed hair (e.g., scalp, facial, eyebrow, or nostril) may have respiratory difficulties.[35]

Upper air passages often show erythema or other evidence of thermal injury. Such changes appear mild at first and may lead to underestimation of the seriousness of the extent of the burn. Fiberoptic bronchoscopy may be effective for identifying supraglottic and infraglottic lesions; inhalation scintiscans have been used for the early detection of damage to the small airways.[36]

Clinical findings in victims of smoke inhalation include tachypnea, dyspnea, rhonchi, wheezes, and rales. Stridor signals laryngeal damage, pointing to the possible need for endotracheal intubation or tracheostomy. Hypoxia is common. Pulmonary edema may ensue and can be life threatening. Bacterial pneumonia is a frequent late complication.

Carbon monoxide poisoning should always be suspected in victims of smoke inhalation. Analysis of expired air with a portable electrochemical unit at the site of a fire allows rapid estimation of carboxyhemoglobin levels.[37]

In one study of victims of residential fires, markedly elevated blood levels of cyanide were found, especially in those who died.[38] This finding calls attention to the availability of a cyanide antidote kit (Eli Lilly and Company), which contains two 300 mg ampules of sodium nitrite, two 12.5 g ampules of sodium thiosulfate, and 12 ampules of amyl nitrite; the first two agents are given intravenously, and the third is inhaled.

In view of the potential role of cyanide in smoke inhalation injury, the following recommendations have been made[39]:

> [A]fter initial life-support measures, including oxygen therapy, have been provided, treatment of smoke-inhalation victims should perhaps include the collection of arterial blood samples for prompt measurement of blood gases and carboxyhemoglobin, methemoglobin, cyanide, and lactate. A 12.5-g dose of sodium thiosulfate could safely be given immediately. The amyl nitrite ampules could also be used, but this form of treatment should not be emphasized, because its use results in the formation of very little methemoglobin. If the patient remains critically ill with persistent coma, seizures, cardiac dysrhythmias, acidemia, or hypotension—all findings suggestive of cyanide intoxication—and particularly if the plasma lactate concentration is above 10 mmol per liter and the elevation cannot be explained by other factors, then sodium nitrite should be administered while the blood pressure is carefully monitored. Unfortunately, it may take more than 30 minutes to obtain the results of plasma lactate measurements, making this information, like blood cyanide measurements (which may take 5 hours to obtain), unavailable when the most important treatment decisions must be made.

Hydroxocobalamin is known to bind cyanide avidly; its efficacy in victims of smoke inhalation is currently under investigation.

Volcanism

The eruptions of Mount St. Helens that began in 1980 demonstrate that there are probably no effective interventions for the consequences of massive direct trauma or severe blast or thermal injuries related to such events. However, autopsies on 25 victims of the Mount St. Helens eruption in May 1980 revealed that many deaths were the result of asphyxia by volcanic ash. Disposable dust masks or more sophisticated devices might prevent such fatalities.[40]

Management

Smoke or thermal injuries to the face, the neck, or the upper airway pose a threat to ventilation. Immediate intubation may be required in the event of stridor, circumferential burns of the neck, full-thickness burns of the lips, or burns of the palate, the tongue, or the pharynx.[41] Tracheostomy through burned tissue should be avoided because of the increased risk of local and airway infection. Fiberoptic bronchoscopy is often helpful. Oxygen should be administered at a rate determined by blood gas monitoring. Bronchodilators, bronchial hygiene, and antibiotics are often required.

References

1. MMWR 31:529, 1982
2. US Environmental Protection Agency publication EPA-450/491-004, 1991
3. MMWR 26:6, 1977
4. JAMA 267:538, 1992
5. MMWR 33:49, 1984
6. JAMA 261:1177, 1989
7. JAMA 266:659, 1991
8. MMWR 40:248, 1991
9. N Engl J Med 272:252, 1965
10. Ann Emerg Med 11:394, 1982
11. JAMA 251:2350, 1984
12. JAMA 239:1515, 1978
13. J Trauma 16:111, 1976
14. Ann Intern Med 107:174, 1987
15. Ann Emerg Med 16:782, 1987
16. Ann Intern Med 113:343, 1990
17. Ann Intern Med 113:337, 1990
18. JAMA 246:2478, 1981
19. JAMA 263:2216, 1990
20. Br Med J 289:960, 1984
21. Surgery 75:213, 1974
22. Br Med J 296:1772, 1988

23. JAMA 261:1039, 1989
24. Ann Emerg Med 17:714, 1988
25. Hyperbaric Oxygen Therapy. Undersea and Hyperbaric Medical Society, Inc, Bethesda, Maryland, 1986, p 33
26. Br Med J 1:318, 1973
27. N Engl J Med 291:85, 1974
28. Arch Neurol 40:433, 1983
29. JAMA 251:771, 1984
30. Chest 97:806, 1990
31. JAMA 235:393, 1976
32. JAMA 236:1449, 1976
33. Environ Health Perspect 11:163, 1975
34. Vet Hum Toxicol 31:168, 1989
35. West J Med 124:244, 1976
36. J Trauma 15:641, 1975
37. JAMA 235:390, 1976
38. N Engl J Med 325:1761, 1991
39. N Engl J Med 325:1801, 1991
40. N Engl J Med 305:931, 1981
41. JAMA 246:1694, 1981

27 Heatstroke

EDWARD RUBENSTEIN, M.D.

Marked increases in core body temperature, especially if sudden, can result in tissue damage and the dangerous syndrome of heatstroke.

Epidemics of such strokes in metropolitan areas during a heat wave may kill hundreds and contribute to the death of thousands of ill persons, especially the elderly. During heat waves, heatstroke is commonest among the elderly, those of low socioeconomic status, alcoholics, individuals living on higher floors in multistory buildings, and patients taking major tranquilizers.[1]

Individual cases are usually associated with hot industrial environments, with strenuous physical exercise (cyclists, football players, long-distance runners, and military recruits being particularly at risk), or with confinement in poorly ventilated areas such as barracks, saunas, and crowded patient rooms in older nursing homes.[2]

Of the many drugs that predispose to heatstroke, the most important are anticholinergic agents, phenothiazines, tricyclic antidepressants, monoamine oxidase inhibitors, inhalation anesthetics, and succinylcholine. Heatstroke that occurs during anesthesia has been termed malignant hyperthermia.

Impaired ability to dissipate body heat is an important pathogenetic factor. Decreased cardiac output (with diminished blood flow to the skin and extremities), dehydration, and failure of the sweat mechanism increase the risk to the individual of dangerous heat accumulation.

Clinical Manifestations

Onset is usually sudden, with delirium and impaired sensorium rapidly progressing to coma. Seizures and decerebrate rigidity may ensue. Many heatstroke victims have temperatures of 41° C or higher, but some have much lower temperatures. Sweating may or may not be present. Extreme tachycardia appears initially. In prolonged episodes of heatstroke, the circulation may eventually fail, and pulmomary edema and shock may result. Hyperventilation, leading to respiratory alkalosis, is common early in the course.

Dehydration is frequently present, and hypokalemia is often noted early. Later, severe metabolic acidosis may rapidly develop. Proteinuria, microscopic hematuria, and cylindruria occur at the onset; acute renal failure may follow in severe cases. Most patients have vomiting and diarrhea. Hepatocellular damage, usually mild and transient, may lead to increased blood levels of bilirubin and liver enzymes.

Many victims develop what appears to be mild disseminated intravascular coagulation.[3] The platelet count is diminished, the fibrinogen level is depressed, and the prothrombin time is usually prolonged. Purpura, hemoptysis, bloody diarrhea, and melena are prominent features in such cases.

Muscle damage has been reported, especially in persons who have engaged in extreme physical exertion. Elevation of muscle enzyme levels and myoglobinuria confirm the presence of myopathy.

Treatment

Immediately remove the victim from the hot environment and institute measures to lower the body temperature. Some clinicians experienced in managing hyperthermia recommend spraying room-temperature water over the patient's nude body while vigorously fanning the entire body surface.[4] Others advocate applying ice packs to the neck, axillae, inguinal regions, and abdomen.[5] Total immersion in very cold water or ice may cause such intense vasoconstriction of blood vessels in the skin and in the extremities that heat loss becomes impaired.[5] The rapid administration of room-temperature intravenous fluid (1 1/30 min) has also been used to cool core structures and to rehydrate the patient.[6] Caution should be exercised to avoid fluid overload. Body temperature should be monitored, preferably with a thermistor rectal probe, to avoid excessive cooling or the reaccumulation of dangerous heat loads.[2,7]

Supportive measures include airway maintenance and the prevention of aspiration; the control of seizures and of excessive shivering, both of which seem to increase body temperature (phenothiazines have been used to suppress shivering, but their central action on thermal regulation may interfere with the endogenous responses to hyperthermia); the correction of water and electrolyte deficits; and the management of shock, of renal failure, and of disseminated intravascular coagulation. Dantrolene has been reported to be effective in the therapy of malignant hyperthermia and may also aid in preventing the condition.[8]

Other Heat Disorders

Milder disturbances, usually presenting as light-headedness or syncope, probably represent less-severe forms of heatstroke and should be regarded as a warning of possible major problems in the individual or group at risk.

Military personnel are especially prone to experience mass fainting during inspection exercises involving long periods of standing at attention under a burning sun. Vasovagal reflexes, hypovolemia secondary to dehydration, and postural hypotension are implicated in such cases.

References

1. JAMA 247:3327, 1982
2. Aviat Space Environ Med 47:280, 1976
3. Br J Haematol 52:269, 1982
4. JAMA 245:570, 1981
5. Med Lett Drugs Ther 23:63, 1981
6. Med J Aust 2:457, 1979
7. Anaesthesia 31:270, 1976
8. Anesthesiology 53:395, 1980

PETER F. WELLER, M.D.

Bites and stings are inflicted by a diversity of mammals, insects, and other organisms. The damage that follows bites and stings reflects the extent and location of inflicted trauma, the infectious agents concomitantly introduced with the bite, and, for some organisms, the toxins that are introduced with the bite or sting. This chapter considers the management of bites inflicted by animals, including humans, and the management of venomous bites and stings.

Human and Animal Bites

Infections that complicate human and animal bites arise from microbes originating either on human skin or in the mouth of the biting person or animal. Some aspects of the management of bite wounds, especially before infection is manifest, remain uncertain. Patients who present within hours of being bitten usually seek initial care or are concerned about rabies or tetanus. In these patients, bacterial infections have not yet developed. Although there is no consensus on the routine use of antibiotics for early wounds, oral antibiotic therapy against the most likely bacterial pathogens should be initiated for more than minor abrasions and lacerations, especially those involving the hand. Further medical evaluation is advised if signs of bite wound infection develop. In contrast, patients who present days after being bitten have usually developed infections within or originating from the wound. Parenteral antibiotic therapy is usually indicated; again, selection is based on the most likely bacterial pathogens. Gram's stain may not identify all responsible bacteria, but it can disclose specific bacteria that will require initial coverage. Cultures of wounds provide further information to guide subsequent antibiotic therapy.

Before initiation of local care or antibiotic therapy, Gram's stain and aerobic and anaerobic cultures should be obtained. Open wounds should be irrigated, foreign debris should be extracted, and devitalized tissue should be surgically removed. Special caution is indicated for wounds involving the hand, and the care of an experienced hand surgeon should be sought. X-rays should be obtained if there is a possibility of bone fracture, osteomyelitis, foreign bodies, or air within joint spaces. Tetanus toxoid booster should be administered to patients who have not received a booster during the previous 10 years.

Human Bites

With human bites, as with other animal bites, the likelihood and nature of complicating infections depend on the pathogenicity of oral microbes inoculated, the extent of local tissue destruction, the depth and sites of penetration (e.g., anatomic compartments within the hand), and delay in seeking care.[1] Self-inflicted bites most commonly occur on the hands or lips. Occlusional bites of others may be inflicted at any site but frequently involve the digits of the hands. Clenched-fist injuries, which occur when a clenched fist strikes the mouth of another person, often involve the metacarpophalangeal and proximal interphalangeal joints. Initial penetration or subsequent extension into the capsular spaces of joints or into closed spaces within the hand contributes to the frequency and severity of complications that arise from hand bites and clenched-fist injuries.

The microbiology of human bites reflects the oral flora of the human mouth.[1,2] Viridans streptococci are usually the most common isolates. *Staphylococcus aureus* is recovered from about 30 to 40 percent of wounds. Penicillin-resistant gram-negative organisms, such as *Hemophilus influenzae* and *H. parainfluenzae*, are infrequently isolated. Anaerobic bacteria, however, are common in human bites and include *Bacteroides*, *Fusobacterium*, and peptostreptococci.[3] *Eikenella corrodens* is an important pathogen in clenched-fist injuries.[4]

The initial antibiotic administered, guided by data from a Gram's stain, is usually penicillin. If *S. aureus* is suspected, either of the following regimens should be used: (1) amoxicillin and clavulanic acid or (2) penicillin in combination with a penicillinase-resistant penicillin (e.g., oxacillin, nafcillin, or methicillin). The resistance of anaerobes and *E. corrodens* to the penicillinase-resistant penicillins and first-generation cephalosporins dictates that these agents should not be used alone in initial therapy for human bites. *E. corrodens* is also resistant to clindamycin and metronidazole. Identification and sensitivity testing of bacteria isolated from wound cultures provide helpful data for modifying antibiotic selections.

Dog Bites

Dog bites are common in the United States. Most bites are provoked and are caused by the patient's own pet or another known dog rather than by a stray dog. Males are more commonly bitten than females. Wounds occur most frequently on the extremities, except in young children, who are more commonly bitten on the face.

The oral bacterial flora of dogs includes *Pasteurella multocida*, *S. aureus*, *S. epidermidis*, *Weeksella zoohelcum*, and gram-negative rods such as DF-2 and EF-4. Other bacteria include *S. intermedius*, *Streptococcus*, and various anaerobes.[3,5,6] Dog-bite wounds reflect this oral flora. The pathogens most commonly associated with dog bites include *P. multocida* and DF-2. DF-2, a slowly growing gram-negative bacterium that is recovered only tardily from cultures, has caused fatalities after dog bites in both asplenic patients and normal hosts.

Unlike other mammalian bites, dog bites are infrequently infected and can often be safely sutured. If the bites are minor and do not appear infected, prophylactic antibiotics are usually unnecessary.[1] Penicillin or ampicillin is usually used to treat dog bites; these agents are active against *P. multocida*, oral anaerobes, and many aerobes. Alternatively, amoxicillin and clavulanic acid can be used, which are active against these organisms and *S. aureus*. For the penicillin-allergic patient, tetracycline should be used because erythromycin is not effective against many *P. multocida* isolates. Cefuroxime axetil and the fluoroquinolones are also active against *P. multocida*; first-generation cephalosporins are not as active against this pathogen or oral anaerobes. Enteric gram-negative bacteria and *Pseudomonas* species can complicate dog-bite wounds.[6]

Cat Bites

Females are more likely to experience cat bites, and both bites and scratches can introduce oral feline flora. The most frequent bacterial pathogen is *P. multocida*, but viridans streptococci, coagulase-negative staphylococci, and anaerobes (including *Bacteroides* and *Fusobacterium*) are common in cat-bite wounds.[1,3,5] Penetration to the periosteum can result in osteomyelitis. DF-2 bacteremia has occasionally occurred from cat bites.[7] Bites and scratches can also transmit cat-scratch fever.

Other Animal Bites

In addition to the common bacteria present in the oral flora of animals, specific pathogens can be transmitted by the bites of animals. Rat bites may cause infections with *Spirillum minus*, especially in Asia, or with *Streptobacillus moniliformis*, the prinicipal agent of rat-bite fever in the United States. Bites by laboratory mice, rats, or gerbils as well as by wild mice, rats, squirrels, and carnivores that prey on these rodents can transmit *S. moniliformis*. Tularemia may be spread by cat, coyote, and squirrel bites.

Rabies is transmissible by bites of raccoons, bats, skunks, dogs, and cats in the United States and by other wild animals in other areas of the world.

Bites from Asiatic macaca monkeys, including rhesus monkeys, can transmit *Herpesvirus simiae* (monkey B virus),[8] a fatal neurotropic virus.

A variety of reptiles, insects, arachnids, and coelenterates may produce morbid or fatal envenomations. Management of snakebites, spider bites, bites and stings of other arthropods, and coelenterate stings are discussed here. Anaphylactic reactions to the venoms of hymenoptera, including bees, wasps, hornets, and yellow jackets, are considered elsewhere.

Venomous Snakebites

Of the 8,000 people who are bitten by poisonous snakes annually in the United States, only about a dozen die. Still, poisonous snakebite can be a medical emergency; it requires expeditious treatment.[9,10]

Twenty species of venomous snakes inhabit the United States. They are divided into two groups: the pit vipers (Crotalidae) and the coral snakes (Elapidae). The pit vipers, a family that includes rattlesnakes, cottonmouths (water moccasins), copperheads, pygmy rattlesnakes, and the massasaugas, are so named because they possess deep pits located between their eyes and nostrils. These pits contain heat receptors, which detect prey and guide the direction of strike. Pit vipers inhabit all regions of the United States except for Maine, Alaska, and Hawaii; coral snakes inhabit the southern and southwestern United States. Most incidents of envenomation from these two types of snakes occur between April and October. Many snakebites are experienced by individuals who do not attempt to move away from the snake; many of these persons are under the influence of alcohol.[11] In addition, exotic venomous snakes are a source of danger to those who keep and handle them.

Clinical Manifestations

Pit Viper Venom

About 20 percent of bites by pit vipers are thought not to inject venom; however, if envenomation occurs, it will result in swelling as well as pain, which is usually present and sometimes severe.

Fang marks are usually found at the site of the bite. Soon after being bitten, the victim may experience muscle fasciculations and perioral tingling and numbness accompanied by a metallic, minty, or rubbery taste. When envenomation is moderate or severe, edema progresses rapidly, and there may be lymphangitis and lymphadenopathy. Weakness, syncope, sweating, nausea, vomiting, chills, and hypotension may ensue. Paresthesias over the scalp and digits are more frequent after bites by the Eastern diamondback, timber, and Pacific rattlesnakes. Respiratory distress is more common after bites by the Mojave and Eastern diamondback rattlesnakes. Ecchymoses are frequent. Altered hemostasis may cause gingival, gastrointestinal, and urinary tract bleeding.

Coral Snake Venom

Fang marks may not be visible. Although pain may occur at the bite site, it is often mild. Swelling is not prominent, and local effects may be limited to paresthesias. Later, sometimes up to 10 hours after a bite, systemic manifestations may appear. These symptoms include drowsiness, weakness, muscle incoordination and fast ciculations, increased salivation, difficulties in swallowing and phonation, visual disturbances, respiratory distress, bulbar paralysis, convulsions, and, occasionally, hypotension.

First Aid

Snakebite requires quick response. The patient should be moved out of danger of a second bite and kept at rest with the affected part immobilized in a functional position at heart level. A broad constricting band (not a tourniquet), sufficiently tight only to impair lymphatic and superficial venous flow, should be applied proximal to the area of the bite; the limb should be splinted.[12] Incision and suction over the wound to remove venom may be ineffective. When initial procedures are complete, the patient should be transported as quickly as possible to a medical facility.

If the snake can be killed, safely and without wasting time, it should be brought along for identification. Care must be exercised because a dead snake may deliver a reflex venomous bite.

Medical Treatment

Therapy for venomous snakebites remains uncertain and controversial. There are no data from clinical studies that directly compare specific therapeutic modalities; the efficacy of various surgical approaches to wound management and the specific indications for antivenin therapy have not been determined in formal comparative studies. Antivenin is the mainstay of snakebite treatment when envenomation is appreciable. Two kinds of antivenin, made by Wyeth-Ayerst Laboratories, are commercially available in the United States—one for pit viper bites and one for Eastern coral bites. There is no antivenin for the toxin of the Arizona coral snake; however, envenomation by this species usually produces self-limiting illness.

Approaches to therapy are based in part on the initial evaluation of the patient and the extent of envenomation. Initial laboratory tests should include a complete white blood cell count, tests of coagulation parameters (prothrombin time, partial thromboplastin time, platelet count, fibrinogen), and urinalysis. In mild envenomations, local signs and symptoms such as pain, edema, erythema, bleeding, ecchymosis, and lymphangitis are limited to the bite-site area; laboratory test values will usually be normal. In moderate envenomations, local symptoms extend beyond the bite area, laboratory tests are abnormal, and systemic symptoms such as sweating, chills, nausea, vomiting, perioral or peripheral paresthesias, changes in taste sensation, hemorrhage, hypotension, or seizures are experienced. In severe envenomations, systemic manifestations are pronounced.

The species of snake also is important when assessing the likelihood of complications and the need for antivenin therapy. Copperhead and water moccasin snakebites are often mild and can be managed without antivenin.[13,14] Mild envenomations by rattlesnakes can also be managed with antivenin.[9,10,14] Moderate or severe envenomations are treated with antivenin.

The total dosage of antivenin depends on the severity of envenomation, the species of snake, and the size of the patient. For severe pit viper bites, up to 20 to 40 vials of antivenin may be required. Adequate dosage usually leads to improvement in both the local and the systemic effects.

In addition to the administration of antivenin, the wound should be cleansed and either primary or booster tetanus immunization given. Prophylaxis with antibiotics is not necessary. Because the bacterial flora of snakes may be diverse,[15] culture and antibiotic sensitivity results should guide therapy if infection develops. In severe envenomations, careful monitoring and supportive care in intensive care units are necessary. Administration of specific blood components is indicated for coagulopathy. Hypotension, respiratory insufficiency, and renal failure require appropriate critical care. Local cooling, extensive debridement and fasciotomy (except when indicated for treatment of an established compartment syndrome), and glucocorticoid administration (for reasons other than the control of hypersensitivity reactions to antivenin horse serum) may be deleterious to successful management of snakebites.[16] Fasciotomy and debridement are not routinely needed; a better outcome and preservation of muscle function occur in test animals treated with antivenin without extensive surgery.[17]

Hypersensitivity and Anaphylaxis

Antivenins are prepared from horse serum; consequently, hypersensitivity reactions to equine proteins, including anaphylaxis during treatment and serum sickness after treatment, are not unusual and should be anticipated.[18] A skin test is customarily administered; however, it is not useful, because it can yield both false positive and false negative results and because patients who need antivenin must receive it even if the test is positive. An intravenous line should be available for administering the antivenin and other medications. Anaphylaxis can usually be managed by slowing the rate of antivenin infusion, by subcutaneous administration of epinephrine, and by adjunctive glucocorticoid therapy. A serious anaphylactic reaction may require intravenous epinephrine administration.

Spider Bites

Although a variety of spiders in the United States may bite humans, only two—the widow spiders and the brown recluse spiders—are considered to have major medical importance.[19]

Widow Spider

Latrodectus mactans (the southern black widow spider) and closely related species are widely distributed. They are commonly found around houses and prefer dry, dimly lit places. Although both males and females produce potent venom, only females have fangs capable of penetrating human skin. The mature southern black widow female is shiny-black and has a red hourglass-shaped marking on its abdomen. In other species, body coloration may be gray, brown, or black and the ventral marking may be orange or red with shapes that vary from an hourglass to transverse bands or spots. Although not aggressive, the female will attack if its web is disturbed.

Clinical Manifestations

Because the bite of the widow spider resembles a pinprick, it may be overlooked. Within an hour of envenomation, generalized muscular pain and rigidity, especially in the abdomen and lower extremities,[20] develop. Pain, which increases in intensity over several hours, lasts 12 to 48 hours. Abdominal pain and rigidity may mimic an acute abdomen. Other symptoms include fever, chills, nausea, vomiting, urinary retention, sweating, and hyperactive reflexes. Respiratory distress may develop. Death may occur, most commonly in small children and in adults with cardiac or respiratory diseases.

Treatment

Administration of 10 ml of 10 percent calcium gluconate intravenously produces a prompt but transient relief of pain, a response that corroborates the diagnosis. (A similar response to calcium gluconate occurs with puss caterpillar bites, but the pain from those bites is more localized.) Pain may be further controlled with narcotic analgesics or calcium gluconate.

The precise indications for administration of horse serum antivenin are not certain. Many patients with mild envenomations can be managed without antivenin therapy, and as with snakebites, antivenin therapy is associated with anaphylactic reactions and serum sickness. Therefore, antivenin therapy for black widow envenomations can be reserved for severe systemic reactions and can be avoided for symptomatic relief of pain.[20]

Brown Recluse Spider

The brown recluse spider (*Loxosceles reclusa* and related species) is brown and has fuzzy body hair and a dark violin- or pear-shaped band on the dorsum of its thorax. This spider is not aggressive and is generally found in secluded places, either outdoors or indoors in the southern, central, and western United States.

Clinical Manifestations

Although the bite may produce a mild stinging sensation, its actual site is often inapparent. The venom is principally cytotoxic and may provoke both local and systemic reactions. Because the local reaction usually develops two to six hours after the bite, the responsible spider is usually not noticed. Mild cases, which are common, are characterized by erythema, induration, pruritus, and pain at the bite site; necrosis does not develop, and the lesion resolves in several days. In more severe envenomations, erythema is followed by the development of violaceous coloration and blisters. Necrosis ensues over the next one to two days and leads to eschar formation and ulceration. Lesions may reach 10 to 15 cm or greater.[21,22] Such lesions heal slowly over months.

Twenty-four to 48 hours after receiving the bite with severe envenomation, the patient may develop systemic reactions manifested by fever, chills, malaise, weakness, nausea, vomiting, arthralgias, and petechial morbilliform rash.[21] In persons who experience severe reactions, disseminated intravascular coagulation and hemolysis may appear; fatalities have been recorded, principally in small children.

Treatment

Optimal initial therapy for local reactions remains uncertain. Some clinicians advocate early excision of venom-containing skin, but the results of such surgery are not necessarily successful. It therefore appears prudent to withhold debridement until necrosis is well demarcated.[22] Although various regimens of systemic or intralesional glucocorticoids have been employed, no definitive data exist on their efficacy. Dapsone, 50 mg twice a day,[21] has been used. This therapy is aimed at preventing damage from infiltrating neutrophils; however, dapsone can cause agranulocytosis and methemoglobinemia. It is not known whether dapsone therapy is effective or whether its benefits outweigh its risks. Most lesions heal with mild to moderate scarring; if local necrosis is extensive, skin grafting may be necessary.

Bites and Stings of Other Arthropods

Imported Fire Ant

Two species of fire ants have been imported into the United States: *Solenopsis invicta* and *Solenopsis richteri*. Both species have now spread throughout the southeastern United States, from North Carolina to Texas.[23] Like other fire ant species, they inhabit loose mounds of dirt. If disturbed, the ants will swarm. This cooperative behavior and the ability of each ant to inflict several bites lead frequently to a multitude of stings.[24] Each bite usually causes an immediate, burning, wheal-and-flare reaction that subsides over hours. This reaction is followed by the development of a characteristic papule, which evolves during six to 24 hours into a sterile pustule 1 to 3 mm in diameter. In addition, painful, pruritic, edematous lesions, resulting from late-phase reactions, may develop over 24 to 48 hours.[25] Localized necrosis and scarring may mark the site; secondary infection, especially streptococcal, may occur. Pustular lesions are best treated by cleansing; if secondary infection develops, antibiotics should be promptly administered.[26] Local and systemic anaphylactic reactions may occur in individuals who are hypersensitive to fire ant venom. In patients in infested regions who present with anaphylaxis, unnoticed fire-ant sting sites should be sought on the toes and feet.[23] Desensitization with whole body extract should be considered for patients who exhibit anaphylactic responses.[23] Systemic reactions, including self-limiting neurologic reactions,[27] may also occur in patients presenting with a large number of bites.

Reduviid Bug

The kissing bug (*Triatoma*), which is one type of reduviid bug, is common in the southern United States. It ranges in color from black to light brown and feeds on the blood of vertebrates, usually at night. It nests in proximity to vertebrates—for example, in the chinks and cracks in household woodwork.

The bite of the kissing bug is almost painless, but if the insect is startled or disturbed as it feeds on the skin, it may inflict a piercing pain. Depending on whether the host has been sensitized, a range of tissue reactions may ensue at the bite site[28,29]: (1) papular lesions with a central punctum, (2) grouped small vesicles, at times hemorrhagic, with edema and erythema, (3) giant urticarial lesions, and (4) hemorrhagic nodular to bullous lesions of the hand or foot, occurring several days after the bite. Therapy is primarily symptomatic.

Reduviid bugs are vectors of American trypanosomiasis (Chagas' disease) and uncommonly may transmit this protozoan infection within the United States. Allergic reactions to *T. protracta*, one species of the kissing bug, can be confirmed by skin testing, and immunotherapy can prevent anaphylactic reactions.[30]

Caterpillars

Several species of caterpillars, including the buck moth caterpillar (*Hemileuca maia*), the puss caterpillar (*Megalopyge opercularis*), and the saddleback caterpillar (*Sibine stimulea*), are present in the southern United States during warm months and may cause envenomations.[31,32] These caterpillar species possess hairs or spines capable of penetrating skin and introducing venom. The most common symptoms are pain, erythema, and local swelling at the sting site.[32] Itching, blistering, and local rashes are occasionally experienced. Less common reactions include pain radiating to extremities, paresthesias, nausea and vomiting, and, infrequently, hypotension and seizures.

Urticating hairs or spines can be removed with tweezers or cellophane tape. Therapy is usually symptomatic: antihistamines for pruritus and analgesics or intravenous calcium gluconate for pain control.

Scorpion

Scorpions are insect predators that usually hunt at night. Envenomation by the common scorpion yields a generally benign local reaction. Two species, *Centruroides sculpturatus* and *C. gertschi*, found in the desert borders of Arizona, New Mexico, and California, produce venom that contains a neurotoxin.[33] The neurotoxin causes intense pain, followed by numbness, drowsiness, perinasal pruritus, and salivation. Trismus, hyperpyrexia, oliguria, pulmonary and gastrointestinal hemorrhage, and convulsions may ensue. Antivenin is the treatment of choice.

Coelenterate Stings

Organisms of the phylum Coelenterata, including jellyfish, the Portuguese man-of-war, sea hydroids, anemones, and fire corals, possess nematocysts.[34,35] Each nematocyst contains a spiral-coiled thread tipped with a toxin-bearing barb that can be ejected into the skin. The severity of the sting will depend on the number of successful discharges and on the composition of the venom. The nematocysts in the Portuguese man-of-war and jellyfish are located on tentacles that trail in the water. Contact in the water with the tentacles is the most common means of exposure to the nematocysts. Dead Portuguese man-of-war, dead jellyfish, and free nematocysts or fragments of tentacles that bear nematocysts, which may be washed onto the shore after storms, may still be capable of discharging venom. The popularity of scuba diving and snorkeling has increased the chances of contact with the nematocysts of sessile coelenterates, such as sea anemones.

Clinical Manifestations

The clinical response will depend on the nature of the venom and on the number of nematocyst envenomations.[36,37] Pain is usually the earliest symptom, ranging from a mild stinging sensation to an exquisite, intense burning. Stings from jellyfish or the Portuguese man-of-war usually cause linear, elevated, edematous, erythematous cutaneous eruptions; anemone and fire coral stings are usually punctate. Urticarial eruptions and systemic anaphylactic reactions may occur. Muscle pain, dyspnea, and vomiting may also be prominent. Hypotension and death may occur in individuals of all ages, but most commonly in children, after stings by the deadly box jellyfish, a medusalike, four-paneled jellyfish that inhabits tropical waters in the Indian and Pacific oceans, including waters off of the Australian coast.

Treatment

Tentacles adhering to the skin should be removed immediately with a gloved or protected hand to prevent further envenomation by nematocysts. Nematocysts on the skin should be inactivated with household vinegar[38,39]; for inactivating nematocysts from sea nettle, a slurry of baking soda should be used.[19] Rubbing the affected area should be avoided as should the application of alcohol or of fresh (but not salt) water because these actions will cause nematocysts to discharge. Antihistamines may relieve pruritus. If hypotension or systemic anaphylaxis develops, epinephrine should be administered. For the deadly box jellyfish, an antivenin (available from Commonwealth Serum Laboratories, Victoria, Australia) should be given; if it is used, the precautions for the management of hypersensitivity and anaphylaxis of snakebite should be observed [*see* Venomous Snakebites, Hypersensitivity and Anaphylaxis, *above*].

Other marine animals may cause serious, and at times fatal, envenomations. The bite of the blue-ringed octopus introduces tetrodotoxin, a potent neurotoxin also found in the puffer fish. No antivenin is available, and supportive therapy, especially to prevent respiratory failure, is indicated. Some species of cone shells also contain toxins that cause neuromuscular blockade; therapy is supportive to prevent respiratory failure.

Fish in the family Scorpaenidae envenomate by spines located on their dorsal, anal, or pelvic fins. Intense local pain develops at the site of envenomation. For stings by lionfish and scorpion fish, immersion of the affected site in nonscalding hot water for 30 to 90 minutes relieves the pain, presumably by destroying the heat-labile toxin.[40] The wound should be cleansed, and tetanus prophylaxis and other supportive care should be provided as necessary. An antivenin is available for scorpaenids but is generally needed only for envenomations by stonefish, which are indigenous to the Indo-Pacific region.

References

1. Ann Emerg Med 17:1321, 1988
2. Pediatr Infect Dis J 6:29, 1987
3. Rev Infect Dis 6(suppl 1):S177, 1984
4. J Hand Surg 8:563, 1983
5. Pediatr Infect Dis J 6:24, 1987
6. Ann Emerg Med 15:1324, 1986
7. Am J Med 82:621, 1987
8. J Orthop Res 8:146, 1990
9. Annu Rev Med 31:247, 1980
10. Med Lett Drugs Ther 24:87, 1982
11. Ann Emerg Med 18:658, 1989
12. Lancet 1:183, 1979
13. J Ky Med Assoc 86:61, 1988
14. J Trauma 28:35, 1988
15. J Infect Dis 140:818, 1979
16. JAMA 240:654, 1978
17. Am J Surg 158:543, 1989
18. J Trauma 28:1032, 1988
19. Postgrad Med 70:91, 1981
20. Ann Emerg Med 16:188, 1987
21. Ann Emerg Med 16:945, 1987
22. Ann Plast Surg 20:447, 1988
23. N Engl J Med 323:462, 1990
24. Pediatrics 73:689, 1984
25. J Allergy Clin Immunol 74:841, 1984
26. South Med J 74:1361, 1981
27. J Allergy Clin Immunol 70:120, 1982
28. AMA Archives of Dermatology 74:14, 1956
29. Cutis 22:585, 1978
30. J Allergy Clin Immunol 73:369, 1984
31. N Engl J Med 271:147, 1964
32. Vet Hum Toxicol 32:114, 1990
33. Postgrad Med 70:107, 1981
34. Coelentera. Poisonous and Venomous Marine Animals of the World, rev ed. Darwin Press, Princeton, New Jersey, 1978, p 87
35. Cutis 25:242, 1980
36. Ann Emerg Med 16:1000, 1987
37. Cutis 40:303, 1987
38. Med J Aust 141:851, 1984
39. South Med J 76:870, 1983
40. JAMA 253:807, 1985

29 Guidelines for the Determination of Death*

Introduction

The criteria that physicians use in determining that death has occurred should

1. Eliminate errors in classifying a living individual as dead,
2. Allow as few errors as possible in classifying a dead body as alive,
3. Allow a determination to be made without unreasonable delay,
4. Be adaptable to a variety of clinical situations, and
5. Be explicit and accessible to verification.

Because it would be undesirable for any guidelines to be mandated by legislation or regulation or to be inflexibly established in case law, the proposed Uniform Determination of Death Act appropriately specifies only "accepted medical standards." Local, state, and national institutions and professional organizations are encouraged to examine and publish their practices.

The following guidelines represent a distillation of current practice in regard to the determination of death. Only the most commonly available and verified tests have been included. The time of death recorded on a death certificate is at present a matter of local practice and is not covered in this document.

These guidelines are advisory. Their successful use requires a competent and judicious physician, experienced in clinical examination and the relevant procedures. All periods of observation listed in these guidelines require the patient to be under the care of a physician. Considering the responsibility entailed in the determination of death, consultation is recommended when appropriate.

The outline of the criteria is set forth below in boldface headings. The indented text that follows each outline heading explains its meaning. In addition, the two sets of criteria (cardiopulmonary and neurologic) are followed by a presentation of the major complicating conditions: drug and metabolic intoxication, hypothermia, young age, and shock. It is of paramount importance that anyone referring to these guidelines be thoroughly familiar with the entire documents,

*"Guidelines for the Determination of Death" is a Report of the Medical Consultants on the Diagnosis of Death to the President's Commission for the Study of Ethical Problems in Medicine and Biomedical and Behavioral Research.

The guidelines set forth in this report represent the views of the signatories as individuals; they do not necessarily reflect the policy of any institution or professional association with which any signatory is affiliated. Although the practice of individual signatories may vary slightly, signatories agree on the acceptability of these guidelines: Jesse Barber, M.D.; Don Becker, M.D.; Richard Behrman, M.D., J.D.; Donald R. Bennett, M.D.; Richard Beresford, M.D., J.D.; Reginald Bickford, M.D.; William A. Black, M.D.; Benjamin Boshes, M.D., Ph.D.; Philip Braunstein, M.D.; John Burroughs, M.D., J.D.; Russell Butler, M.D.; John Caronna, M.D.; Shelley Chou, M.D., Ph.D.; Kemp Clark, M.D.; Ronald Cranford, M.D.; Michael Earnest, M.D.; Albert Ehle, M.D.; Jack M. Fein, M.D.; Sal Fiscina, M.D., J.D.; Terrance G. Furlow, M.D., J.D.; Eli Goldensohn, M.D.; Jack Grabow, M.D.; Phillip M. Green, M.D.; Ake Grenvik, M.D.; Charles E. Henry, Ph.D.; John Hughes, M.D., Ph.D., D.M.; Howard Kaufman, M.D.; Robert King, M.D.; Julius Korein, M.D.; Thomas W. Langfitt, M.D.; Cesare Lombroso, M.D.; Kevin M. McIntyre, M.D., J.D.; Richard L. Masland, M.D.; Don Harper Mills, M.D., J.D.; Gaetano Molinari, M.D.; Byron C. Pevehouse, M.D.; Lawrence H. Pitts, M.D.; A. Bernard Pleet, M.D.; Fred Plum, M.D.; Jerome Posner, M.D.; David Powner, M.D.; Richard Rovit, M.D.; Peter Safar, M.D.; Henry Schwartz, M.D.; Edward Schlesinger, M.D.; Roy Selby, M.D.; James Snyder, M.D.; Bruce F. Sorenson, M.D.; Cary Suter, M.D.; Barry Tharp, M.D.; Fernando Torres, M.D.; A. Earl Walker, M.D.; Arthur Ward, M.D.; Jack Whisnant, M.D.; Robert Wilkus, M.D.; and Harry Zimmerman, M.D.

The preparation of this report was facilitated by the President's Commission but the guidelines have not been passed on by the Commission and are not intended as matters for governmental review or adoption.

including explanatory notes and complicating conditions.

The Criteria for Determination of Death

An individual presenting the findings in either section A (cardiopulmonary) or section B (neurologic) is dead. In either section, a diagnosis of death requires that both *cessation of functions*, as set forth in subsection 1, *and irreversibility*, as set forth in subsection 2, be demonstrated.

A. An individual with Irreversible Cessation of Circulatory and Respiratory Function Is Dead

1. *Cessation* is recognized by an appropriate clinical examination

Clinical examination will disclose at least the absence of responsiveness, heartbeat, and respiratory effort. Medical circumstances may require the use of confirmatory tests, such as an ECG.

2. *Irreversibility* is recognized by persistent cessation of functions during an appropriate period of observation and/or trial of therapy

In clinical situations where death is expected, where the course has been gradual, and where irregular agonal respiration or heartbeat finally ceases, the period of observation following the cessation may be only the few minutes required to complete the examination. Similarly, if resuscitation is not undertaken and ventricular fibrillation and standstill develop in a monitored patient, the required period of observation thereafter may be as short as a few minutes. When a possible death is unobserved, unexpected, or sudden, the examination may need to be more detailed and repeated over a longer period, while appropriate resuscitative effort is maintained as a test of cardiovascular responsiveness. Diagnosis in those first observed with rigor mortis or putrefaction may require only the observation period necessary to establish that fact.

B. An individual with Irreversible Cessation of All Funtions of the Entire Brain, Including the Brainstem, Is Dead

The "functions of the entire brain" that are relevant to the diagnosis are those that are clinically ascertainable. Where indicated, the clinical diagnosis is subject to confirmation by laboratory tests as described below. Consultation with a physician experienced in this diagnosis is advisable.

1. *Cessation* is recognized when evaluation discloses findings of a *and* b:

a. cerebral functions are absent, and...

There must be deep coma, that is, cerebral unreceptivity and unresponsivity. Medical circumstances may require the use of confirmatory studies such as EEG or blood flow study.

b. brainstem functions are absent.

Reliable testing of brainstem reflexes requires a perceptive and experienced physician using adequate stimuli. Pupillary light, corneal, oculocephalic, oculovestibular, oropharyngeal, and respiratory (apnea) reflexes should be tested. When these reflexes cannot be adequately assessed, confirmatory tests are recommended.

Adequate testing for apnea is very important. An accepted method is ventilation with pure oxygen or an oxygen and carbon dioxide mixture for 10 minutes before withdrawal of the ventilator, followed by passive flow of oxygen. (This procedure allows P_aco_2 to rise without hazardous hypoxia.) Hypercarbia adequately stimulates respiratory effort within 30 seconds when P_aco_2 is greater than 60 mm Hg. A 10-minute period of apnea is usually sufficient to attain this level of hypercarbia. Testing of arterial blood gases can be used to confirm this level. Spontaneous breathing efforts indicate that part of the brainstem is functioning.

Peripheral nervous system activity and spinal cord reflexes may persist after death. True decerebrate or decorticate posturing or seizures are inconsistent with the diagnosis of death.

2. *Irreversibility* is recognized when evaluation discloses findings of a *and* b *and* c:

a. the cause of coma is established and is sufficient to account for the loss of brain functions, and...

Most difficulties with the determination of death on the basis of neurologic criteria have resulted from inadequate attention to this basic diagnostic prerequisite. In addition to a careful clinical examination and investigation of history, relevant knowledge of causation may be acquired by computed tomographic scan, measurement of core temperature, drug screening, EEG, angiography, or other procedures.

b. the possibility of recovery of any brain functions is excluded, and...

The most important reversible conditions are sedation, hypothermia, neuromuscular blockade, and shock. In the unusual circumstance where a sufficient cause cannot be established, irreversibility can be reliably inferred only after extensive evaluation for drug intoxication, extended observation, and other testing. A determination that blood flow to the brain is absent can be used to demonstrate a sufficient and irreversible condition.

c. the cessation of all brain functions persists for an appropriate period of observation and/or trial of therapy.

Even when coma is known to have started at an earlier time, the absence of all brain functions must be established by an experienced physician at the initiation of the observation period. The duration of observation periods is a matter of clinical judgment, and some physicians recommend shorter or longer periods than those given here.

Except for patients with drug intoxication, hypothermia, young age, or shock, medical centers with substantial experience in diagnosing death neurologically report no cases of brain functions returning following a six-hour cessation, documented by clinical examination and confirmatory EEG. In the absence of confirmatory tests, a period of observation of at least 12 hours is recommended when an irreversible condition is well established. For anoxic brain damage where the extent of damage is more difficult to ascertain, observation for 24 hours is generally desirable. In anoxic injury, the observation period may be reduced if a test shows cessation of cerebral blood flow or if an EEG shows electrocerebral silence in an adult patient without drug intoxication, hypothermia, or shock.

Confirmation of clinical findings by EEG is desirable when objective documentation is needed to substantiate the clinical findings. Electrocerebral silence verifies irreversible loss of cortical functions, except in patients with drug intoxication or hypothermia. (Important technical details are provided in "Minimum Technical Standards for EEG Recording in Suspected Cerebral Death," Guidelines in EEG 1980, Section 4., American Electroencephalographic Society, Atlanta, 1980, p 19.) When joined with the clinical findings of absent brainstem functions, electrocerebral silence confirms the diagnosis.

Complete cessation of circulation to the normothermic adult brain for more than ten minutes is incompatible with survival of brain tissue. Documentation of this circulatory failure is therefore evidence of death of the entire brain. Four-vessel intracranial angiography is definitive for diagnosing cessation of circulation to the entire brain (both cerebrum and posterior fossa) but entails substantial practical difficulties and risks. Tests are available that assess circulation only in the cerebral hemispheres, namely radioisotope bolus cerebral angiography and gamma camera imaging with radioisotope cerebral angiography. Without complicating conditions, absent cerebral blood flow as measured by these tests, in conjunction with the clinical determination of cessation of all brain functions for at least six hours, is diagnostic of death.

Complicating Conditions

Drug and Metabolic Intoxication

Drug intoxication is the most serious problem in the determination of death, especially when multiple drugs are used. Cessation of brain functions caused by the sedative and anesthetic drugs, such as barbiturates, benzodiazepines, meprobamate, methaqualone, and trichloroethylene, may be completely reversible even though they produce clinical cessation of brain functions and electrocerebral silence. In cases where there is any likelihood of sedative presence, toxicology screening for all likely drugs is required. If exogenous intoxication is found, death may not be declared until the intoxicant is metabolized or intracranial circulation is tested and found to have ceased.

Total paralysis may cause unresponsiveness, areflexia, and apnea that closely simulates death. Exposure to drugs such as neuromuscular blocking agents or aminoglycoside antibiotics, and diseases like myasthenia gravis are usually apparent by careful review of the history. Prolonged paralysis after use of succinylcholine chloride and related drugs requires evaluation for pseudo cholinesterase deficiency. If there is any question, low-dose atropine stimulation, electromyogram, peripheral nerve stimulation, EEG, tests of intracranial circulation, or extended observation, as indicated, will make the diagnosis clear.

In drug-induced coma, EEG activity may return or persist while the patient remains unresponsive, and therefore the EEG may be an important evaluation along with extended observation. If the EEG shows electrocerebral silence, short latency auditory or somatosensory evoked potentials may be used to test brainstem functions, since these potentials are unlikely to be affected by drugs.

Some severe illnesses (e.g., hepatic encephalopathy, hyperosmolar coma, and preterminal uremia) can cause deep coma. Before irreversible cessation of brain functions can be determined, metabolic abnormalities should be considered and, if possible, corrected. Confirmatory tests of circulation or EEG may be necessary.

Hypothermia

Criteria for reliable recognition of death are not available in the presence of hypothermia (below 32.2° C core temperature). The variables of cerebral circulation in hypothermic patients are not sufficiently well studied to know whether tests of absent or diminished circulation are confirmatory. Hypothermia can mimic brain death by ordinary clinical criteria and can protect against neurologic damage due to hypoxia. Further complications arise since hypothermia also usually precedes and follows death. If these complicating factors make it unclear whether an individual is alive, the only available measure to resolve the issue is to restore normothermia. Hypothermia is not a common cause of difficulty in the determination of death.

Children

The brains of infants and young children have increased resistance to damage and may recover substantial functions even after exhibiting unresponsiveness on neurological examination for longer periods than do adults. Physicians should be particularly cautious in applying neurologic criteria to determine death in children younger than five years.

Shock

Physicians should also be particularly cautious in applying neurologic criteria to determine death in patients in shock because the reduction in cerebral circulation can render clinical examination and laboratory tests unreliable.

30 Acute Diabetes—Ketoacidosis and Hyperosmolar Coma

GEORGE F. CAHILL, JR., M.D.
RONALD A. ARKY, M.D.
ANDREW J. PERLMAN, M.D., Ph.D.

Differential Diagnosis

The approach to the problem of the acutely ill diabetic is one of urgency. Diagnosis in almost all patients can be made on the basis of a brief history and quick physical examination. If possible, blood should be drawn for glucose-level measurement, but obviously, therapy should not be delayed pending results. A diabetic known to be on insulin therapy who is found unconscious or was observed becoming unconscious should be considered hypoglycemic until proved otherwise. Glucose (50 ml of 50 percent glucose) or glucagon (1 mg) should be administered intravenously immediately. If a vein cannot be found, the glucagon may be injected intramuscularly or subcutaneously. Rapid bedside estimation of blood glucose levels can be made with Dextrostix, either by eye or, more accurately, by use of a commercially available colorimeter or reflectometer. A plasma or serum keto acid test should also be done at bedside. Urine, if obtainable, should be examined for glucose and keto acids.

Diabetic coma, except in infants, may be the culmination of days or even weeks of insulin deficiency, leading to ketoacidosis, hypovolemia, and vascular collapse. Hence, dehydration, poor skin turgor, soft eyeballs, hypotension, rapid pulse, and Kussmaul's hyperventilation are all typical manifestations. Sometimes, diabetic coma is the first episode of the disease, from which the diagnosis is established. Often, however, the patient is known to be an insulin-dependent diabetic and has become comatose because of failure to increase the insulin dosage to compensate for increased need; such need may be produced by infection or by other physical or emotional stresses. Ketoacidosis may develop even in the supposedly controlled diabetic as a result of insulin resistance associated with a silent myocardial infarction or with an unsuspected infection, such as cholecystitis, bronchopneumonia, urinary tract sepsis, or perinephric abscess. Most frequently, the coma is simply the result of negligence resulting from poor patient education or poor compliance with therapy.

Several metabolic states, including hyperosmolar coma, alcoholic ketoacidosis, and lactic acidosis, can simulate acutely decompensated diabetes [*see Table 1*]. The typical patient in hyperosmolar coma is elderly. Several days of dehydration associated with progressively severe hyperglycemia leads to stupor and then to coma. As in diabetic coma, the acute state is frequently initiated by bronchopneumonia or other infections, congestive heart failure, or a cerebrovascular accident. Dehydration and prerenal azotemia generally combine with nephrosclerosis to permit glucose levels to rise to about 1,000 mg/dl, and sometimes, they may reach 2,000 to 3,000 mg/dl. Kussmaul's breathing and ketoacidosis are absent. The prerenal azotemia may be associated with blood urea nitrogen levels of 40 to 80 mg/dl and serum bicarbonate (HCO_3^-) levels of 18 to 22 mEq/L.

Alcoholic ketoacidosis results from a combination of the mild ketoacidosis produced by fasting and the increased acetate formation by the liver that occurs during alcohol metabolism. Because alcohol can inhibit gluconeogenesis in the liver during fasting, ketoacidosis may be complicated by hypoglycemia, thus requiring glucose therapy. The alcoholic, especially the diabetic

Table 1 Characteristics of Diabetic Ketoacidosis
and Other Acute Syndromes

Syndrome	Duration	Patient's Appearance	Hyper-ventilation	Glucose levels	HCO_3^-	BUN
Diabetic ketoacidosis	Days*	Very sick	Present	+ + +	Low	+ to + +
Hyperglycemic hypersmolar coma	Days	Sick and obtunded or comatose	Not present	+ + + +	Normal	+ to + +
Hypoglycemia	Minutes to hours	Healthy but confused or unresponsive	Not present	Low	Normal	Normal
Lactic acidosis	Days	Variable	Present	Low to + +	Low	Normal to +
Uremic acidosis	Weeks	Sick	Present	+ to + +	Low	+ + + +
Alcoholic ketoacidosis	Days	Variable	Present	Low to + +	Low	Normal to +

*In infants, ketoacidosis may develop in 18 to 36 hours.

alcoholic, may have normal glucose levels or, more often, moderate hyperglycemia (levels of 100 to 200 mg/dl or greater). The syndrome is highly variable.

Lactic acidosis is seen most frequently in elderly patients in whom hemodynamic failure or an infection such as bronchopneumonia occurs in conjunction with impaired liver perfusion, impaired liver function, or both. Glucose levels are variable, but they are frequently elevated because the lactic acidosis often is associated with diabetes. Most patients have a combination of lactic acidosis and ketoacidosis, together with other metabolic abnormalities.

Therapy

In diabetic ketoacidosis and hyperosmolar coma,[1,2] therapy should begin even while the diagnosis is being made. In the initial stages, treatment for the two disorders is quite similar, and the aim is to establish the diagnosis and initiate therapy as speedily as possible. Once the course of the disease is changed from progressive worsening to improvement, however, therapy may proceed more slowly, letting the metabolic disorder gradually correct itself as much as possible. From the onset, a timed flow sheet should be maintained to accurately record vital signs, laboratory data, all therapies, and changes in physical and mental states.

Diagnosis is made on the basis of available history and a cursory physical examination. Patients with diabetic ketoacidosis commonly present with nausea, vomiting, and lethargy. They appear acutely sick and may complain of generalized abdominal pain and hunger. Tachycardia, hypothermia, and Kussmaul's hyperventilation are common symptoms. A large needle is inserted into as large a vein as possible and securely anchored. Blood is withdrawn, and isotonic saline, approximately 10 ml/min, is started immediately. Blood glucose and keto acid levels are rapidly estimated by using some of the blood, preferably at bedside. The remainder is then sent to the laboratory for precise glucose, bicarbonate ion, and potassium measurements. Other tests, such as those for sodium, chloride, enzymes, and hematologic indices, can be done but are of less importance. The findings of hyperglycemia and ketoacidosis together with a history of diabetes are sufficient to establish the diagnosis of diabetic ketoacidosis. Hyperglycemia without ketoacidosis, however, suggests hyperosmolar coma or a hyperglycemia–lactic acidosis syndrome. A low bicarbonate ion level without ketoacidosis suggests lactic or uremic acidosis.

Ketoacidosis

Arterial blood gas analysis for carbon dioxide pressure (P_aCO_2) and determination of arterial blood pH (pH_a) and bicarbonate ion levels should be done in the acutely ill patient with diabetic ketoacidosis who is severely dehydrated and hypotensive and shows signs of hemodynamic failure. Therapy may be redirected on the basis of these tests. Therapy, however, should never be delayed pending laboratory results in a very ill patient with diabetic ketoacidosis. Four major therapeutic agents must be considered: fluids, insulin, potassium, and alkali.

Fluids The major thrusts of therapy are to correct volume deficit and inadequate perfusion and to return metabolism from the superfasted, or hypercatabolic, state toward a normal level of activity. Saline administration, as previously indicated, serves to correct hypovolemia and inadequate perfusion; adults with ketoacidosis have an average fluid deficit of 3 to 5 L. During the first two or three hours of treatment, 750 to 1,000 ml of saline should be given hourly, provided there is urine output and no signs of cardiac failure. If severe hypernatremia is present, 0.45 percent saline is recommended. When the glucose level falls to 200 to 250 mg/dl, five percent dextrose in saline or water should be substituted.

Insulin The amount, route, and manner of insulin administration has been a subject of controversy. The intravenous infusion of an initial bolus of regular insulin (0.2 U/kg) followed by constant infusion of 0.1 U/kg/hr has been found to be a safe and effective method.[3] Intravenous infusions are best controlled by a pump that assures constant delivery and a consistent level of insulin in the blood that is adequate to suppress gluconeogenesis, lipolysis, and ketogenesis. Glucose levels should fall by at least 10 percent an hour, and a failure to do so implies a degree of insulin resistance that warrants high doses of insulin. Insulin infusion should be continued until ketones are cleared from the plasma, even if the glucose level has fallen to normal values. Older approaches to diabetic ketoacidosis that advocate hourly intravenous doses of 50 to 100 units of regular insulin or the use of subcutaneous insulin at doses of 5 to 10 U/hr after the initial intravenous bolus still have their advocates. When metabolic regulation is achieved with the constant insulin infusion technique, a subcutaneous injection of insulin should be administered as the infusion is terminated to prevent a marked rebound in the blood glucose level.

Potassium Most patients with acute or chronic metabolic syndromes, especially diabetic ketoacidosis, are potassium depleted. In acidosis, potassium leaves cells and thereby produces hyperkalemia, despite a possibly moderate or severe total-body potassium deficit. Thus, moderate hyperkalemia usually occurs with diabetic ketoacidosis. Potassium, initially in the form of potassium chloride, should be administered at a dosage of 40 mEq/hr once glucose levels begin to fall, usually about an hour after initiation of insulin therapy. If the initial potassium level is 4.5 mEq/L or less, potassium chloride, 80 mEq/L, should be added to the saline infusion while the insulin is being administered, to prevent life-threatening hypokalemia. When glucose and potassium move back into the cells as insulin exerts its metabolic effect, hypokalemia occurs and may ultimately cause arrhythmias and respiratory or cardiac failure.

Alkali The severely ill patient with ketoacidosis may die as a result of hypovolemia and circulatory collapse. Myocardial performance and peripheral compensatory processes, such as vascular tone, are diminished in patients in whom acidosis has developed. Many physicians advocate the use of alkali in all patients whose arterial pH falls below 7.1 or 7.2 or whose serum bicarbonate is below a critical level, such as 8 mEq/L. More useful than measurements of pH or the serum bicarbonate level, however, are P_aco_2 measurements. If the patient is too weak to hyperventilate sufficiently to reduce the P_aco_2 to less than 20 mm Hg and if the HCO_3^- level is less than 10 mEq/L, death is imminent and alkali administration a must. If, however, the patient is not preterminal and is hyperventilating appropriately, alkali administration is not indicated. The ketoacidosis in the severely ill patient will subside as keto acids stop being produced and those that remain in the circulation are metabolized after insulin is administered.

For those who require alkali, 40 mEq of sodium bicarbonate should be added to each liter of saline the patient receives, and the solution should be infused at a rate of about 10 ml/min. If total vascular collapse is present or imminent, volume expanders such as plasma or albumin should be administered. Elevation of the legs and administration of oxygen, as well as all the maneuvers used in the treatment of shock, are indicated. Vasoconstricting agents, however, have proved of little help and should rarely be used. Because of the tendency of alkali to exacerbate hypokalemia, arrhythmias, and other problems that commonly develop in ketoacidotic diabetics, its use should be avoided unless necessary. Again, the indication for using alkali is impending cardiovascular collapse, not the presence of the defect in fuel metabolism that is producing ketoacidosis.

Glucose As blood glucose levels fall after the initial or subsequent insulin administration and as glucosuria and urinary volume diminish, infusion with a solution of half saline and half five percent dextrose in water provides glucose to prevent hypoglycemia and free water for rehydration. Four or five hours after initiation of therapy, the patient should be able to take by mouth such fluids as fruit juices, which provide both glucose and required potassium.

Therapeutic addenda It is very important to keep at the bedside a complete flow sheet on which all information is recorded, including inputs, outputs, medications, laboratory values, and vital signs. A single-lead precordial electrocardiogram is helpful in monitoring potassium levels, even though it is a relatively crude method compared with laboratory analysis of blood. Of course, a complete initial ECG tracing is indicated to document myocardial damage.

For persistent nausea and vomiting, especially if the stomach is distended, nasogastric drainage and lavage with isotonic saline is indicated whether or not a succussion splash can be elicited. This procedure helps prevent aspiration of vomit and may help the gastrointestinal tract recompensate.

Finally, even in the most severely decompensated diabetic in vascular collapse, there is usually some urine production because of the osmotic effect of the glucose. Urine should be tested for glucose and keto acids. Blood glucose determination at the bedside is now available in many settings, however, and this rapid test can replace urinary glucose measurements in the severely compromised patient. Catheterization for urologic rather than metabolic reasons is indicated if percussion shows a distended bladder. Acute tubular necrosis is almost unknown as a sequela of diabetic ketoacidosis, and in any case, the initial therapy would not be altered, whether or not urine was being produced. Furthermore, urinary tract infection in the diabetic is notoriously intractable, and unless absolutely necessary, urethral catheterization should not be performed. Another possible adjunct to therapy is a central venous line, particularly if the patient has had myocardial disease and volume overload could occur; its use should not delay the initial therapy.

Reassessment Concurrent with therapy, the physician should search for the cause of ketoacidosis. Usually, it is rooted in poor patient education, poor compliance with therapy, or both, but other causes of an absolute or relative insulin deficiency should be considered. Among the possibilities is insulin resistance produced by infection of the urinary, biliary, or respiratory tract. A silent myocardial infarction can also cause insulin resistance, as can an infarcted bowel or pockets of inapparent infection in perinephric or periodontal spaces.

Hyperosmolar Coma

The aim of therapy is to move expeditiously at first to reverse the course of the acute disease and then to permit the imbalances to return gradually to normal. As in the treatment of patients with ketoacidosis, once the diagnosis is made, isotonic saline should be infused to maintain extracellular fluid volume, especially in the vascular space. After one or more liters of isotonic saline have been administered, hypotonic saline may be infused to prevent excessive extracellular fluid accumulation as rehydration takes place. The first 2 L are usually infused over two to three hours; thereafter, the infusion rate is slowed. Patients may require 5 L or more. Elderly patients must be monitored carefully to avoid fluid overload.

Patients in hyperosmolar coma often respond excellently to an insulin dose such as 10 units administered intravenously or subcutaneously. In some individuals, rehydration and fluid expansion by themselves result in a marked lowering of blood glucose. Occasionally, some patients may require larger doses of insulin, as in diabetic ketoacidosis, so glucose levels should be closely monitored. Potassium levels should be checked and potassium given if initial levels are low, especially if insulin is being administered. Once blood glucose levels begin to fall, five percent dextrose in saline should be infused to prevent hypoglycemia, to augment rehydration, and also to maintain extracellular fluid volume. Infusion of dextrose is especially important if the glucose levels fall too rapidly—for example, from 1,000 to 500 mg/dl in one to two hours. At this stage of therapy, potassium levels should again be closely monitored. If glucose levels fall more slowly, a solution of half saline and half five percent glucose can be given gradually for rehydration.

As in diabetic ketoacidosis, hyperglycemia helps maintain extracellular fluid volume at the expense of intracellular fluid. If glucose levels fall too quickly, extracellular fluid volume is compromised, and cellular edema may occur, especially in the brain. Hence, a conservative approach is employed once the pathological trend is reversed.

The underlying cause of the metabolic decompensation should be sought. Common causes include infection, vascular accidents, and neglect by the patient, by the patient's family, or by nursing home staff.

References

1. N Engl J Med 309:159, 1983
2. Diabetes Mellitus, Vol V. American Diabetes Association, 1981, p 195
3. Diabetes Care 3:53, 1980

ROBERT M. BLACK, M.D.

Overview of Acute Renal Failure

Acute renal failure (ARF) is a common clinical problem characterized by a relatively abrupt decline in renal function. This reduction in the glomerular filtration rate (GFR) is manifested by a rise in the plasma creatinine concentration (P_{Cr}) and often by a fall in the daily urine volume.

When ARF develops, the differential diagnosis may be expansive, including diseases that affect the renal arteries, glomeruli, tubules, or interstitium as well as disorders that obstruct the flow of urine from the kidney. Of the many conditions that can cause ARF in adults, however, two account for approximately 70 to 75 percent of all cases: reduced renal perfusion (prerenal disease) and acute tubular necrosis (ATN). Acute interstitial nephritis is another relatively common cause of ARF. Glomerulonephritis, vasculitis, and urinary tract obstruction are other disorders that may be associated with an acute fall in GFR.

Differential Diagnosis: Prerenal Disease Versus Acute Tubular Necrosis

Acute renal failure is most often the result of a fall in renal blood flow or damage to the renal tubules from a toxin or ischemia. In the former condition (prerenal disease), the kidney attempts to defend against real salt and water losses (as in true volume depletion) or perceived losses (as in advanced heart or liver disease). This response is appropriate because in both circumstances, the effective arterial blood volume (that volume of blood perfusing vital organs) is reduced.

By comparison, the renal injury characteristic of ATN limits the normal capacity of the renal tubules to conserve fluid and electrolytes. This limited ability to reabsorb sodium is caused by cell necrosis as well as by translocation of the Na^+-K^+ ATPase from the basolateral (or blood) side of intact renal tubular cells to the luminal side; the net effect of this translocation is that Na^+ is pumped from the inside of the cell to the lumen instead of into the peritubular blood.[1] These differences in renal function are of primary importance in distinguishing between the major forms of acute renal failure.

History and Physical Examination

The history and physical examination frequently reveal important diagnostic information, such as the identification of potential causes of reduced renal perfusion or ATN. When a medication is involved, the duration of drug usage is important. For example, ATN that occurs within 48 hours of the onset of antibiotic therapy is probably not caused by aminoglycoside toxicity alone. In many patients, however, one insult (e.g., hypotension) may cause either prerenal disease or ATN. It is in these circumstances that laboratory studies may be particularly useful.

Laboratory Evaluation of Acute Renal Failure

When distinguishing acute from chronic renal failure, a history of renal insufficiency, small kidney size as determined by abdominal x-ray or ultrasound examination, and anemia are the most reliable laboratory findings indicating chronicity. In contrast, when the duration of renal failure is unknown, acute and potentially reversible renal failure must be excluded. As an example, a renal ultrasound study should be performed in all individuals to detect possible urinary tract obstruction unless another cause of ARF is obvious.

There are several laboratory tests that are most commonly used to differentiate prerenal azotemia from ATN [*see Table 1*]. These

Table 1   Laboratory Findings in the Differential Diagnosis of Acute Renal Failure

Test	Finding Supportive of Prerenal Disease	Finding Supportive of ATN
BUN : P_{Cr} ratio	> 20 : 1	< 15 : 1
Increase in P_{Cr}	Variable, with downward fluctuations in some patients	Progressive: ≥ 0.5 mg/dl each day
Urinalysis	Normal, sometimes with hyaline casts	Granular and epithelial cell casts, with free epithelial cells
Urine osmolality	> 500 mOsm/kg	< 350 mOsm/kg
Urinary sodium concentration	< 20 mEq/L	> 30 – 40 mEq/L

studies are most useful in oliguric patients (urine output less than 500 ml/day), because individuals with nonoliguric ATN typically have less severe tubular damage and their laboratory findings are likely to show more overlap with the values of patients with prerenal azotemia.[2,3]

Blood Urea Nitrogen to Creatinine Ratio

Although a fall in GFR should normally cause the blood urea nitrogen (BUN) and creatinine concentrations to rise in equal proportions, exceptions to this rule are common. Creatinine is filtered at the glomerulus as well as secreted into the proximal tubule; it is not reabsorbed. Urea, on the other hand, is filtered and reabsorbed, with passive tubular urea reabsorption increasing in parallel with salt and water reabsorption. As a result of these differences, the enhanced salt and water avidity associated with prerenal states causes a disproportionate rise in the plasma ratio of BUN to creatinine. A ratio higher than 20:1 is suggestive of prerenal azotemia in the absence of a source of increased urea production, such as gastrointestinal bleeding, tissue breakdown, high protein intake, or corticosteroid therapy. A normal BUN to creatinine ratio is less useful for differentiating between prerenal azotemia and acute tubular necrosis because the expected rise in the BUN concentration in prerenal disease may be prevented if protein intake is reduced (e.g., as a result of vomit-

ing) or if urea synthesis is impaired by concurrent liver disease.

The pattern of rise of the P_{Cr} also may be useful diagnostically. In ATN, the P_{Cr} characteristically increases by at least 0.4 to 1.5 mg/dl/day, whereas much greater increments (2 mg/dl/day or more) may be observed with rhabdomyolysis. By comparison, smaller incremental increases in the plasma creatinine concentration, particularly if they are associated with occasional downward fluctuations, are more suggestive of reduced renal perfusion.[4] Transient improvements in renal blood flow are presumably responsible for the intermittent declines in plasma creatinine concentration in this setting.

Urinalysis

The urinalysis is typically normal in prerenal azotemia, with the only common finding being the presence of hyaline casts. These casts are composed of Tamm-Horsfall mucoprotein, which is normally secreted by the cells of the thick ascending limb of the loop of Henle and which precipitates in the concentrated, acidic urine that is typical of the prerenal state. In ATN, by comparison, the urine characteristically contains many dark-brown granular casts with free renal tubular epithelial cells and epithelial cell casts, although the urine may be normal in as many as 20 to 30 percent of patients.

Confusion may arise when the urine contains a few granular casts but renal sodium reabsorption is avid, a finding that suggests intact tubular function. These findings may reflect an interphase between prerenal disease and early ATN, in which some tubular damage has occurred but fluid repletion may still improve renal function. Conversely, the finding of a urine sediment containing many dark granular casts in the presence of enhanced tubular Na^+ reabsorption is typical of the icteric patient with the hepatorenal syndrome (see below).

Urine Osmolality

The normal kidney can elaborate urine with a maximum concentration greater than 1,200 mOsm/kg in states of dehydration. The capacity to perform this function is dependent on intact tubular function, particularly in the loop of Henle. In this nephron segment, NaCl and KCl are removed from the tubule lumen but water remains behind because the thick ascending limb is impermeable to water. As a result, the osmolality in the medullary interstitium surrounding the tubules increases so that in the presence of antidiuretic hormone (ADH), the urine osmolality (U_{osm}) rises as filtrate flows through the collecting tubules. A U_{osm} greater than 500 mOsm/kg, therefore, is highly suggestive of prerenal azotemia.

In comparison, extensive tubular damage, such as that which occurs in ATN, impairs the ability of the kidney to generate a high interstitial osmolality, in part because of cellular damage in the loop of Henle. As a result, the maximum U_{osm} that can be attained is reduced. Typically, the U_{osm} in ATN is approximately 300 to 350 mOsm/kg, a value that is similar to the plasma osmolality in this setting.

Despite these differences, the U_{osm} is often not helpful in identifying the cause of acute renal failure. With prolonged renal hypoperfusion, for example, proximal tubular reabsorption of solute (NaCl and urea) increases. As a result, the quantity of solute reaching the loop of Henle and more distal nephron segments is progressively reduced. Other evidence also indicates that renal ischemia can diminish function in the loop of Henle without producing overt tubular necrosis.[5] As a result of reduced solute presentation to the loop of Henle and its reduced function, both medullary solute reabsorption and interstitial osmolality are decreased. When this occurs, the maximum U_{osm} that can be generated is limited, even in the presence of ADH. As a result, a U_{osm} less than 500 mOsm/kg is not diagnostically useful, because it can be seen in patients with ATN, prerenal disease, or underlying renal disease.

Urine Sodium Concentration and Fractional Excretion of Sodium

The urine sodium concentration (U_{Na}) is often very useful in the diagnosis of acute renal failure because reduced renal perfusion is the most potent stimulus of tubular sodium reabsorption. In prerenal azotemia, the U_{Na} typically falls below 20 mEq/L, and this value is independent of dietary salt intake and of the plasma sodium concentration. A higher U_{Na} is characteristic of acute tubular necrosis.

The U_{Na} may be misleading in patients with oliguric prerenal disease and in about 10 percent of patients with acute tubular necrosis. Although sodium reabsorption is enhanced in states of reduced renal perfusion (a process that should lower the urine sodium concentration), concomitant water reabsorption in the oliguric patient results in a higher urinary sodium concentration than would otherwise be present. Thus, an individual with prerenal azotemia may occasionally have a U_{Na} of 40 mEq/L or higher in the absence of acute tubular necrosis. In this setting, calculation of the fractional excretion of sodium is particularly helpful in making the correct diagnosis because it reflects only tubular sodium reabsorption, not water handling.

The fractional excretion of sodium (FE_{Na}) is the percent of filtered sodium ($GFR \times P_{Na}$) that is excreted in the urine ($U_{Na} \times$ urine volume).

$$FE_{Na} = \frac{\text{Excreted sodium}}{\text{Filtered sodium}} \times 100$$

$$FE_{Na} = \frac{U_{Na} \times \text{volume}}{P_{Na} \times GFR} \times 100$$

$$FE_{Na} = \frac{U_{Na} \times P_{Cr}}{P_{Na} \times U_{Cr}} \times 100 \qquad (1)$$

P_{Cr} and U_{Cr} are the plasma and urinary concentrations, respectively, of creatinine in milligrams per deciliter; U_{Na} and P_{Na} are the urinary and plasma sodium concentrations, respectively, in milliequivalents per liter; and GFR = $(U_{Cr} \times \text{volume})/P_{Cr}$. In patients with normal renal function and in those with acute renal failure caused by prerenal azotemia, the FE_{Na} is usually less than one percent.

The FE_{Na} appears to be more specific than the U_{Na} or any other single laboratory test in distinguishing prerenal azotemia from ATN.[4,6] It should be used whenever reduced renal perfusion is a potential cause of acute renal failure but the U_{Na} is greater than 20 mEq/L. In this setting, an FE_{Na} less than one percent is highly suggestive of prerenal disease, whereas an FE_{Na} greater than two percent suggests ATN (assuming diuretics are not being administered). In the range of FE_{Na} values between one and two percent, there is some overlap between prerenal azotemia and ATN.[7]

Although the FE_{Na} is very useful, it is now apparent that a number of causes of acute renal failure other than prerenal disease can, on occasion, be associated with an FE_{Na} value less than one percent [see Table 2]. For example, the type of renal dysfunction that is present in the first 48 hours of the disease, at a time when the transition from prerenal disease to ATN is occurring, may be characterized by an FE_{Na} of less than one percent.[8]

In summary, there is as yet no single test that can always distinguish prerenal azotemia from acute tubular necrosis. Therefore, the proper approach to diagnosis relies on using all of the available information in the history, physical examination, and laboratory studies. Fortunately, the two disorders are generally treated similarly: supportive care with maintenance of adequate tissue perfusion.

Prerenal Disease

A reduction in renal blood flow is the most common cause of acute renal failure. The ensuing decline in tissue perfusion may result from true volume depletion or from selective renal ischemia (as in bilateral renal artery stenosis) [see Table 3]. Certain medications that have little effect on renal function under normal conditions may contribute to the decline in GFR during prerenal azotemia (see below).

The pathophysiological factors that contribute to the rise in BUN and P_{Cr} concentrations with hypovolemia are important from a diagnostic and therapeutic standpoint.[9] The release of norepinephrine and angiotensin II leads to systemic and renal vasoconstriction; this response is, in part, appropriate because it maintains the blood pressure, redirecting blood flow away from the kidney and mesentery and toward the heart and brain.

The fall in GFR that might occur as renal blood flow is reduced in this setting is offset by two mechanisms: dilation of the afferent (preglomerular) arteriole, which allows more of the systemic pressure to be transmitted to the glomerulus, and constriction

---

Table 2   **Intrinsic Causes of Acute Renal Failure***

ATN, usually nonoliguric (occurs in about 10% of cases of ATN)

ATN superimposed on chronic prerenal disease (such as advanced liver disease or heart disease)

Administration of radiocontrast media or release of heme pigments (hemoglobin or myoglobin)

Acute glomerulonephritis or vasculitis[†]

Acute interstitial nephritis

---

*Table lists causes of ARF in patients in whom the fractional excretion of sodium is < 1%.

†These disorders also may be associated with reduced renal sodium excretion.

Table 3 Causes of Prerenal Disease

True Volume Depletion
Hemorrhage

Renal losses

Gastrointestinal losses

Skin losses

Respiratory losses

Sequestration of fluid in a so-called third space (e.g., in the abdomen in acute pancreatitis or in muscle after a crush injury)

Hypotension
Septic shock

Rapid reduction in blood pressure in patients with chronic severe hypertension

*Edematous States**
Advanced heart failure

Advanced liver disease

Localized Renal Ischemia
Bilateral renal artery stenosis or unilateral stenosis in a solitary kidney

Medications

ACE inhibitors, particularly in patients with bilateral renal artery stenosis

NSAIDs, particularly in patients with an underlying reduction in renal perfusion

---

*Most individuals with edema resulting from the nephrotic syndrome appear to have a normal effective arterial blood volume, a finding supported by the observation that plasma renin activity is not elevated in these patients.

---

of the efferent (postglomerular) arteriole, which further increases the filtration pressure across the glomerular capillaries. Studies in experimental animals suggest that afferent vasodilation is mediated by a direct myogenic response, by vasodilator prostaglandins, and by tubuloglomerular feedback; in comparison, efferent vasoconstriction is mediated primarily by angiotensin II.[10] Tubuloglomerular feedback is the process by which the afferent arteriole vasodilates in response to a low distal tubular NaCl delivery, thereby helping to restore distal delivery back to normal. This process is mediated by the macula densa at the end of the thick ascending limb, which senses changes in chloride delivery.

Observations in humans have indirectly confirmed the importance of prostaglandins (afferent vasodilation) and angiotensin II (efferent vasoconstriction) in autoregulation. For example, if preglomerular vasodilation is impaired by agents that inhibit prostaglandin production (such as indomethacin), the resulting unopposed vasoconstriction of the afferent arteriole causes an abrupt decline in renal blood flow and GFR.[11] By comparison, in bilateral renal artery stenosis (in which the intrarenal pressure distal to the stenosis tends to be lower than the systemic pressure), the administration of an angiotensin-converting enzyme inhibitor can lead to acute renal failure that is presumably caused by removal of the angiotensin II–mediated constriction of the efferent arteriole.[12] A similar problem can occur in patients with congestive heart failure who have a low systemic blood pressure; in this setting, the glomerular filtration rate may fall even though the angiotensin-converting enzyme inhibitor increases cardiac output by lowering peripheral vascular resistance.[13] In both bilateral renal artery stenosis and congestive heart failure, glomerular capillary hydraulic pressure is reduced, which accounts for the major change in renal function.

The usual causes of prerenal azotemia are true volume depletion, advanced liver disease, and congestive heart failure. In many individuals, an offending medication (such as a nonsteroidal anti-inflammatory drug or an angiotensin-converting enzyme inhibitor) is a contributing factor.

Prerenal Azotemia Caused by True Volume Depletion

The presence of one of the causes of true volume depletion is usually evident from the history. A fluid loss severe enough to produce renal insufficiency should be associated with at least some of the characteristic physical findings of this disorder, including decreased skin turgor, dry mucous membranes, flat neck veins, and postural tachycardia with or without hypotension. Those patients with the clinical syndrome of hypovolemic shock also have signs of marked hypoperfusion (caused in part by intense peripheral vasoconstriction), such as cold, clammy extremities, cyanosis, agitation, confusion, and little or no urine output.

Oliguria is present in most individuals. Because the normal response to renal hypoperfusion is the retention of Na^+ and water by the kidney, oliguria is appropriate. Normal or increased urine output in a patient with renal hypoperfusion indicates that an osmotic agent (e.g., glucose or urea) or another diuretic agent is acting or that tubular dysfunction such as ATN is present.

Concurrent abnormalities in electrolyte and acid-base balance also may be seen. For example, elderly patients with diminished mental status may become hypovolemic if insensible fluid losses are not replaced. Hypernatremia results in such cases because water is lost in excess of sodium. More commonly, however, the plasma sodium concentration is normal or low in prerenal azotemic states; the combination of reduced glomerular filtration and increased secretion of antidiuretic hormone (induced by hypovolemia) promotes the retention of ingested or administered water, thereby favoring the development of hyponatremia.

The presence of a specific acid-base abnormality may help pinpoint the cause of hypovolemia. A hypokalemic, metabolic alkalosis, for example, suggests either diuretic therapy or vomiting. By comparison, metabolic acidosis may be seen with diarrhea, diabetic ketoacidosis, or shock-induced lactic acidosis.

Rapid reduction of chronic severe hypertension of any cause is another source of acute prerenal azotemia. In this condition, renal arteriolar hyperplasia is present and is an adaptive change because it protects the glomerular capillaries from the elevated systemic pressure; similar findings are seen in the arterioles in other organs. The increase in thickness of these vessels, however, impairs their ability to dilate when the blood pressure is lowered toward normal. This lack of response can result in a decrease in tissue perfusion that, in the kidney, leads to a decline in the GFR and a subsequent elevation in the plasma creatinine concentration. In general, this response is transient because continued control of the blood pressure permits arteriolar hyperplasia to regress and renal function to improve over a period of one to three months.[14] Antihypertensive medications need not be discontinued during this interval unless there has been an excessive fall in blood pressure or an unacceptably large rise in the plasma creatinine concentration.

Treatment

Therapy for true volume depletion is aimed at restoration of the normal circulating blood volume. The major questions that must be addressed are the type of fluid to be used and the rate at which it should be given. Excluding patients with hypotension, in whom isotonic saline is the solution of choice, the tonicity of the administered fluid is determined by the plasma sodium concentration. In a hypernatremic patient, the administration of hypotonic fluids should be considered in an effort to lower the plasma sodium concentration toward normal. In contrast, hypertonic (three percent) saline is indicated when the patient has symptomatic hyponatremia. (Because rapid correction of hyponatremia or hypernatremia may result in osmotic demyelination in the brain or cerebral edema, respectively, the rate of correction should proceed according to certain guidelines.) In addition, blood replacement may be required in patients with active bleeding or marked anemia.

Although colloid solutions had been preferred to isotonic saline or Ringer's lactate in hypovolemic shock because it was thought they would expand the plasma volume more effectively (by increasing oncotic pressure), controlled studies have failed to confirm this advantage in the absence of underlying hypoalbuminemia.[15,16] Moreover, the infusion of enough albumin to raise the plasma albumin concentration above normal has been associated with acute renal failure, presumably caused by a fall in the glomerular filtration rate resulting from a high glomerular capillary oncotic pressure.[17]

The type of fluid administered also depends on the plasma potassium concentration. Solutions containing dextrose should be avoided in the absence of a low glucose concentration when hypokalemia is present, because the release of insulin will drive potassium into cells and may cause the plasma potassium concentration to fall further.[18] It is also important to correct the intravascular fluid deficit before instituting insulin therapy in the patient with hypotension and severe hyperglycemia, because the high blood sugar level defends against a further fall in blood pressure by osmotically pulling water from cells.

The rate at which replacement fluids are given depends on the clinical status of the patient. As a general rule, administration of fluids at a rate of 75 to 100 ml/hr is adequate in most adults. More rapid fluid repletion may be deleterious in patients with underlying cardiac disease and is unnecessary in the absence of continued fluid loss, marked volume depletion (as occurs with uncontrolled hyperglycemia), or shock (in which 1 to 2 L of fluid may be required in the first hour until tissue perfusion improves).

The adequacy of fluid repletion can be assessed from the physical examination and by monitoring renal function. An increase in urine output and in urinary sodium excretion, for example, generally indicates the restoration of normovolemia. It takes somewhat longer to reverse the azotemia and to lower the plasma creatinine concentration. Even when the GFR has returned to normal, a finite period is still required for the retained urea and creatinine to be excreted. It is important to note that in hypovolemic shock (as in sepsis), the development of peripheral edema is not necessarily a sign of overexpansion, because it may result from dilutional hypoalbuminemia at a time when plasma volume depletion persists.[19]

Prerenal Azotemia Caused by Advanced Liver Disease

Advanced liver disease is associated with two major changes in renal function: sodium retention, initially manifested as ascites, and a progressive decline in the GFR that, in its later stages, is called the hepatorenal syndrome. Both humoral and hemodynamic factors play a primary role in the development of these problems.

Sodium Retention and Ascites

Abnormal sodium handling can be demonstrated early in the course of hepatic cirrhosis before either ascites or peripheral edema appears. Many cirrhotic patients are less able to excrete a sodium load than patients with normal hepatic function even though the plasma volume increases, the plasma creatinine level is normal, and renin secretion is appropriately suppressed.[20] Similar findings can be demonstrated in experimental models of hepatic disease. These observations suggest that at least part of the initial sodium retention represents an overflow phenomenon in which hepatic disease stimulates renal sodium reabsorption independent of any changes in systemic hemodynamics.[21,22] The initial sodium retention may be related to the increase in intrahepatic pressure that results from fibrosis-induced postsinusoidal obstruction.[23] This intrahepatic hypertension may then activate a hepatorenal reflex, leading to an elevation in renal sympathetic nerve activity. Increased renal sympathetic tone lowers renal perfusion and directly stimulates sodium reabsorption, both of which promote sodium retention and edema formation. The elevated intrasinusoidal pressure then promotes the intraperitoneal accumulation of this excess fluid as ascites.

By the time that ascites has become clinically apparent, however, a variety of additional changes have occurred that lead to decreased tissue perfusion or underfilling of the arterial circulation (rather than overflow).[21,22] These include (1) a further increase in intrasinusoidal pressure, which promotes fluid accumulation both in the peritoneum and in the dilated splanchnic venous system, (2) peripheral vasodilation, caused in part by the formation of arteriovenous fistulas (such as the spider angiomas on the skin), and (3) hypoalbuminemia, which promotes fluid movement out of the vascular space.

These changes slowly become more marked, so that increasingly severe liver disease is associated with progressively enhanced secretion of the three so-called hypovolemic hormones—renin, norepinephrine, and ADH—leading to a very low rate of sodium and water excretion.[24,25] Furthermore, the cardiac output, which is elevated early in the disease as a result of flow through the arteriovenous fistulas, often falls to a level that is below normal.[9]

Although fluid retention, induced by the fall in effective arterial blood volume, can be seen as an appropriate attempt to enhance renal perfusion, it may be difficult to appreciate how the massively edematous patient with hepatic cirrhosis can be effectively hypovolemic. One indirect proof of the presence of volume depletion has come from studies in which cirrhotic patients are immersed to the neck in warm water. In this setting, the hydrostatic pressure of the water on the lower extremities results in the redistribution of intravascular fluid from the legs to the central cardiopulmonary circulation. This increase in venous return (which is roughly equivalent to an infusion of 2 L of isotonic saline) raises the cardiac output, often resulting in a relatively marked natriuresis (in comparison to the very low baseline level of sodium excretion) and a reduction in the secretion of renin, norepinephrine, and ADH.[26] There is also a concomitant increase in atrial natriuretic peptide, which may contribute to the increase in sodium excretion in some patients.[27]

There are, however, cirrhotic patients who do not respond to water immersion.[25] These patients tend to have a greater baseline degree of effective volume depletion as evidenced by higher vasoactive hormone levels, leading to enhanced renal vasoconstriction. The net effect is a lower renal blood flow and GFR.[25]

Diagnosis

The diagnosis of advanced liver disease as the cause of ascites and, in some cases, peripheral edema is often easily made from the history and physical examination, but right-sided heart failure can produce similar findings. These two disorders can usually be differentiated at the bedside by estimation of the jugular venous pressure. The increase in venous pressure in hepatic cirrhosis occurs below the hepatic vein. As a result, the venous pressure above the liver in the external jugular vein is generally low or normal (< 5 cm of H_2O), not elevated as in heart failure. One exception to this general rule can occur in cirrhotic patients with tense ascites, in whom upward pressure on the diaphragm raises the intrathoracic pressures. The central venous pressure, however, rapidly falls when the intra-abdominal tension is relieved by removal of a small amount of ascitic fluid.[28] Other signs of chronic liver disease (e.g., spider angiomas) also may be present.

Pathogenesis of the Decrease in Renal Function

The increases in circulating norepinephrine and angiotensin II that promote sodium retention in liver disease also lead to renal vasoconstriction, a change that contributes to a progressive fall in the GFR.[29] The relatively early decline in glomerular filtration is easily missed, however, because there is often little or no rise in the BUN or plasma creatinine concentration. Decreased hepatic production of urea limits the rise in BUN, whereas malnutrition (which diminishes muscle mass) and perhaps decreased hepatic production of creatine (the precursor of creatinine) limit the rise in the plasma creatinine concentration.[30] The result is that up to one half of cirrhotic patients with plasma creatinine concentrations in the normal range (1.0 to 1.2 mg/dl) have a reduced GFR (as measured by inulin clearance), which may be as low as 15 ml/min.[30]

The progressive decline in renal function that occurs in hepatic cirrhosis is thought to be hemodynamically mediated because tubular function is intact (as evidenced by the low urine sodium concentration and a normal urinalysis)[31] and the kidneys are histologically unremarkable (as evidenced by the successful use of such kidneys for transplantation).[32]

A possible explanation for the deterioration in renal function in hepatic cirrhosis is a neurohumoral imbalance in which the level of renal vasoconstrictors is elevated at a time when renal vasodilator activity is diminished.[9] As described earlier, intrahepatic hypertension and arterial underfilling lead to a progressive rise in the activities of the sympathetic nervous and renin-angiotensin systems. This tendency to renal ischemia is, at first, partially counteracted by enhanced production of vasodilator prostaglandins and kinins.[33-35] These important protective responses, however, become impaired with more severe hepatic disease as both prostaglandin and kinin levels are diminished.[33,34,36] Such changes may reflect the importance of normal hepatic function in the production of prekallikrein (which, when activated to kallikrein, cleaves kininogen to form the potent vasodilator lysyl-bradykinin) and in the conversion of linoleic acid to arachidonic acid (the precursor of prostaglandins).[33]

The response to insertion of a peritoneovenous shunt in patients with the hepatorenal syndrome is also compatible with this hemodynamic hypothesis for the decline in renal function. The ensuing volume expansion (as ascitic fluid is reinfused into the internal jugular vein) is associated with a diminished release of renin[37] and increased atrial natriuretic peptide secretion that may contribute to the improvement in the GFR.[27,38] The peritoneovenous shunt (see below) also may reduce intrahepatic pressure (via an unknown mechanism), an effect that could decrease renal sympathetic neural tone.[39,40]

Treatment of Ascites in Liver Disease

Dietary sodium restriction and periods of rest are the mainstays of nonmedical therapy in hepatic cirrhosis with ascites. Assumption of the supine position, for example, can produce a 40 percent rise in creatinine clearance and up to a twofold increase in sodium excretion as compared with the upright position.[41] There are, however, three relatively unique considerations in the approach to fluid removal in hepatic cirrhosis: the preferential use of spironolactone, the slow rate at which fluid should be removed from patients with ascites but no peripheral edema, and the role of paracentesis.

Diuretics When diuretic therapy is indicated, spironolactone is the agent of choice. This normally weak diuretic is frequently as effective as or even more effective than conventional doses of a loop diuretic in patients with advanced disease.[42] This surprising finding may be related to differences in the mechanism of action of the various diuretics. Most loop and thiazide diuretics are highly protein bound; as a result, they enter the tubular lumen by secretion into the proximal tubule, not by glomerular filtration. Following their entry into the tubule, these agents bind to their luminal cell receptors: the Na-K-2Cl transporter in the thick ascending limb in the case of loop diuretics (such as furosemide) or the distal tubular Na-Cl carrier for thiazide diuretics. Secretion into the proximal tubule may be impaired in hepatic cirrhosis, perhaps as a result of hypoalbuminemia or of competitive or toxic inhibition by retained compounds such as bile salts. The net effect is that entry of the diuretic into the lumen and therefore the natriuretic effect of the agent are limited.[43]

Spironolactone, in comparison, is the only diuretic that does not require secretion into the lumen; it enters the collecting tubule cells from the blood side and then competes for the aldosterone receptor. As a result, its efficacy is not impaired in patients with cirrhosis. A loop diuretic (up to 240 mg of oral furosemide) can be added in those patients who do not have an adequate response to spironolactone and sodium restriction.[44]

The other advantage of spironolactone is that it is a potassium-sparing diuretic and, unlike the loop diuretics, does not cause hypokalemia. This effect is particularly desirable in hepatic cirrhosis because potassium depletion can enhance renal ammonia production and possibly precipitate hepatic encephalopathy.[45]

The rate at which fluid can safely be removed in hepatic cirrhosis depends on the presence or absence of peripheral edema. When a diuresis is induced, the fluid is initially lost from the vascular space. The ensuing fall in intravascular pressure then allows the edema fluid to be mobilized to replete the plasma volume. The rate at which this fluid is mobilized is relatively unlimited in patients with peripheral edema.[46] In comparison, patients who have only ascites can mobilize edema fluid solely via the peritoneal capillaries. The maximum rate at which this can occur is only 300 to 500 ml/day; more fluid removal with diuretics can lead to plasma volume depletion, azotemia, and the possible precipitation of the hepatorenal syndrome.

Paracentesis Given the rate limitation of diuretic therapy, it has been suggested that patients with marked or tense ascites can be treated more rapidly and more safely with paracentesis.[47-50] With this method, 3 to 6 L or more of ascitic fluid can be removed each day. Controlled studies have demonstrated that the risk of plasma volume depletion caused by the reaccumulation of ascites can be minimized by the administration of 25 to 40 g of albumin after each large-volume paracentesis has been carried out. Many patients tolerate paracentesis without albumin infusions, and it is not currently possible to identify in advance those patients who will derive benefit from albumin therapy.

A peritoneovenous shunt, which drains into the internal jugular vein and thereby translocates the ascitic fluid into the vascular space, also may be used for the treatment of refractory ascites. However, side effects occur more frequently with this modality, and the side effects are potentially more serious than those that occur with large-volume paracentesis.

Hepatorenal Syndrome

The hepatorenal syndrome represents the most advanced stage of the hemodynamic changes typical of advanced liver disease, being characterized by oliguria and a slowly progressive rise in the BUN and plasma creatinine concentration. The plasma creatinine level may increase by as little as 0.1 mg/dl each day, with intermittent periods of stabilization or even slight improvement. The onset of renal failure may be insidious or precipitated by an acute insult such as gastrointestinal bleeding or the excessive use of diuretics.

This syndrome is most often seen with advanced alcoholic cirrhosis but can also occur with other hepatic diseases, including metastatic involvement of the liver by cancer or, rarely, fulminant acute viral hepatitis.[51,52] Hepatic encephalopathy, ascites, and biochemical abnormalities such as hyperbilirubinemia, hypoalbuminemia, and a prolonged prothrombin time are also commonly present.

One form of liver disease, primary biliary cirrhosis, appears to be relatively free from these alterations in renal function.[53] Sodium retention and ascites formation are late events, and the hepatorenal syndrome is unusual in this condition. These unique findings may be related to the natriuretic and renal vasodilator properties of retained bile salts.[53]

Diagnosis

The characteristic laboratory findings in the hepatorenal syndrome are a normal urinalysis, a low U_{Na}, and an FE_{Na} of less than one percent. The diagnosis of the hepatorenal syndrome is one of exclusion, after other possible causes of acute renal failure have been eliminated. Patients with hepatic cirrhosis, for example, may develop acute tubular necrosis following aminoglycoside therapy or an episode of sepsis or hypotension. However, the history and urinary findings usually allow this disorder to be distinguished from the hepatorenal syndrome. The urinary sediment occasionally contains muddy-brown granular casts in the jaundiced patient with the hepatorenal syndrome (via an unknown mechanism), although the low FE_{Na} and the slow rise in the P_{Cr} suggest reduced perfusion rather than ATN.

The major condition that can simulate the findings in the hepatorenal syndrome is superimposed volume depletion in a cirrhotic patient resulting from the use of diuretics or from gastrointestinal bleeding.[46] Thus, the diagnosis of the hepatorenal syndrome requires the proper clinical setting and no improvement in renal function following a trial of fluid repletion.

Prognosis and Treatment

The prognosis in the hepatorenal syndrome is poor, with many patients dying within weeks of the onset of renal failure.[38] Concurrent hepatic encephalopathy is common, and death usually results from a complication of the severe liver disease such as gastrointestinal bleeding. Recovery of renal function occurs only when hepatic function improves as a result of partial resolution of the primary disease or, rarely, hepatic transplantation.[52]

Initial therapy is supportive and includes avoidance of nephrotoxins such as nonsteroidal anti-inflammatory drugs (NSAIDs).[54,55] Because these agents diminish the synthesis of vasodilator prostaglandins, they result in increased renal vasoconstriction that can lead to a decline in both the GFR and sodium excretion. Possible exceptions among the NSAIDs are sulindac and low-dose aspirin[56]; sulindac may relatively spare renal prostaglandin synthesis and, therefore, is less likely to lead to deleterious changes in renal function. Attempts to increase the effective circulating volume with saline, fresh frozen plasma, or dextran have only transiently improved renal function.[39,57]

Another modality that might, in theory, be effective is lowering angiotensin II levels with a converting enzyme inhibitor in an effort to partially reverse the renal vasoconstriction. However, patients with the hepatorenal syndrome generally have a relatively low systolic blood pressure of 90 to 100 mm Hg,[57] and angiotensin II appears necessary to maintain even this low level. Thus, decreasing angiotensin II can lead to a marked reduction in systolic blood pressure of as much as 25 mm Hg.[58]

The major therapeutic modalities that have been shown to improve renal function in the hepatorenal syndrome are insertion of a peritoneovenous shunt, initially accompanied by the administration of loop diuretics to begin the diuresis, and performance of a side-to-side portosystemic shunt, which lowers the intrahepatic pressure and diminishes ascites formation.[37,38,59]

The peritoneovenous shunt (LeVeen shunt or Denver shunt) acts by increasing fluid return to the cardiopulmonary circulation and can lead to a marked increase in sodium excretion and an improvement in renal perfusion and function.[60,61] There is, however, no evidence that peritoneovenous shunting prolongs patient survival; patients with ascites who have normal or near-normal liver function tests may survive for several years, but patients with the hepatorenal syndrome may survive for only six weeks or less.[38]

The major problem with the peritoneovenous shunt is the relatively high rate of complications, including disseminated intravascular coagulation (caused when endotoxin or other procoagulant material in the ascitic fluid enters the bloodstream), infection of the shunt (which can lead to bacteremia), variceal bleeding (resulting from volume expansion and a concurrent rise in portal venous pressure), and small bowel obstruction.[62,63]

The net effect is that the perioperative mortality can reach 25 percent in patients with advanced disease. The perioperative morbidity can be diminished if, before insertion of the shunt, there is intraoperative drainage of ascites, which is then replaced by 5 L of isotonic saline.[60,63] This regimen can minimize those complications related to massive ascites reinfusion: disseminated intravascular coagulation and increased portal pressure leading to gastrointestinal bleeding.

In general, peritoneovenous shunting is not commonly recommended for relief of ascites or the hepatorenal syndrome. At present, insertion of a peritoneovenous shunt should be considered only in the patient who fails to respond to paracentesis or who has the hepatorenal syndrome with stable hepatic function, no hepatic encephalopathy, and no recent variceal bleeding.[64]

Prerenal Azotemia Caused by Congestive Heart Failure

Congestive heart failure (CHF) is associated with two major alterations in renal function: sodium retention early in the course of the disease and a decline in glomerular filtration rate as cardiac function worsens. Neurohumoral factors and certain therapies may contribute to these problems.[65]

Sodium Retention

Sodium retention in CHF is thought to occur initially as an adaptive response to a fall in cardiac output. The decline in effective renal perfusion pressure activates both the sympathetic nervous and renin-angiotensin systems.[9,65]

In mild CHF, sympathetically mediated increases in heart rate and cardiac contractility can return the cardiac output to normal, at least at rest [*see Figure 1*]. However, enhanced renal sympathetic activity produces renal vasoconstriction and directly stimulates proximal tubular sodium reabsorption, both of which diminish sodium excretion. Thus, a usually mild limitation of the ability to excrete sodium can occur in cardiac disease even when the cardiac output is normal[66]; this defect can, however, lead to sodium retention and edema if sodium intake is excessive.

With more advanced disease, the sympathetically mediated effects on cardiac function are inadequate, and sodium retention and plasma volume expansion are required in an attempt to restore the cardiac output. These changes lead to a rise in left ventricular filling pressure that, by enhancing the end-diastolic volume, increases cardiac contractility and cardiac output toward normal

[*see Figure 1*]. At this point, the patient may be in a state of compensated heart failure in which the cardiac output is normal, sodium excretion matches intake, and the activity of the renin-angiotensin-aldosterone system returns toward normal.[67]

This compensated state, however, usually applies only at rest. Individuals with moderate CHF and a normal cardiac output at rest are often unable to increase the cardiac output adequately with exertion. The resulting decrease in tissue perfusion can lead to augmentation of the above-mentioned neurohumoral mechanisms, producing sodium retention and eventually edema.[68] In this setting, substantial improvement may result from limiting physical activity.

Severe CHF, by comparison, is associated with a persistent decline in cardiac output both at rest and with exercise. Compensatory mechanisms are unable to restore cardiac function to normal under any circumstances [*see Figure 1*].

Diagnosis

The diagnosis of congestive heart failure as the cause of peripheral edema, pulmonary edema, or both is usually apparent from the history and physical findings. From a therapeutic viewpoint, however, it is important to distinguish between the two general forms of congestive heart failure: systolic dysfunction, in which impaired contractility is the primary abnormality, and diastolic dysfunction, in which decreased compliance of the ventricular wall limits diastolic filling and therefore forward output. Diastolic dysfunction is most likely to occur with hypertensive disease and less often with ischemic heart disease.[69,70] This abnormality can be diagnosed by measurement of the ejection fraction, which is normal rather than reduced, as is the case with systolic dysfunction; when diastolic dysfunction is causing acute pulmonary edema, it may be associated with bilateral renal artery stenosis.[71]

Another laboratory test that may be helpful in assessing prognosis is measure-

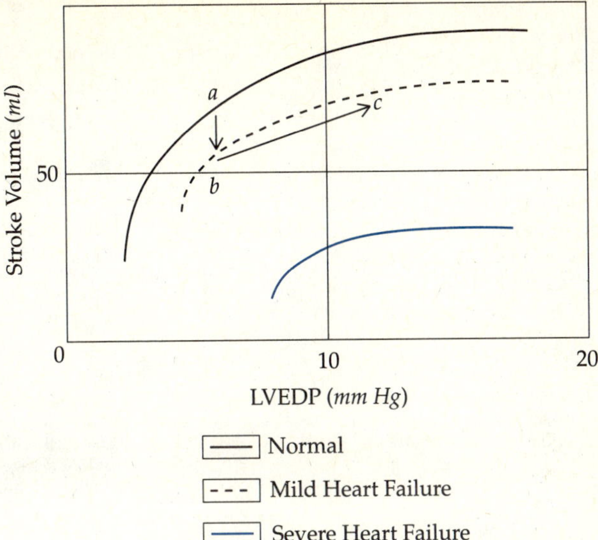

Figure 1 *Frank-Starling curves indicate the relation between left ventricular end-diastolic pressure (LVEDP), or stretch, and stroke volume, or cardiac output. The top curve depicts this relation for a normal heart. When mild congestive heart failure develops, the relation between LVEDP and stroke volume is reflected in a lower curve; that is, for a given LVEDP, the stroke volume will be lower (point b versus point a). Cardiac output can still be returned to normal by raising the LVEDP (point b to point c). As cardiac function declines in severe heart failure, however, the improvement in cardiac output achieved by increased filling pressures is markedly attenuated, leading to high pulmonary capillary pressures and pulmonary congestion or edema.*

ment of the plasma sodium concentration; otherwise unexplained hyponatremia appears to be a marker for advanced systolic dysfunction.[72] This relation of hyponatremia to cardiac function is indirect. The fall in the plasma sodium results from water retention that is primarily induced by enhanced secretion of antidiuretic hormone. The stimulus to antidiuretic hormone release in this setting is decreased perfusion; thus, renin and antidiuretic hormone levels tend to rise in parallel with increasing cardiac failure.[72,73] As a result, hyponatremia is also a poor prognostic sign; patients with hyponatremia have a shorter survival than normonatremic patients.[72]

Renal Failure

Patients with CHF also may develop acute or chronic renal failure as a result of reduced tissue perfusion. The decline in renal function is associated with the characteristic findings of prerenal disease: an elevated ratio of BUN to plasma creatinine concentration; a normal urinalysis; and a low urine sodium concentration ($U_{Na} < 20$ mEq/L) unless diuretics have recently been given.

Pathogenesis

Several different mechanisms can lead to renal failure in patients with CHF, each of which requires somewhat different therapy [*see Table 4*].

Excessive diuretic use The administration of diuretics leads to fluid loss and a reduction in intravascular pressure. These effects are beneficial because they allow pulmonary and peripheral edema to be mobilized, leading to marked symptomatic improvement. However, the decline in left ventricular filling pressure often leads to a decrease in cardiac output [*see Figure 1*].[74]

Although the resulting fall in tissue perfusion is usually not clinically important, the BUN and the plasma creatinine concentration do rise in some patients. Proper therapy at this time is to temporarily avoid further diuretic use and, if the patient has undergone excessive diuresis, to attempt cautious fluid repletion. If, however, edema persists, then vasodilator therapy may be indicated in an effort to improve cardiac function.

Nonsteroidal anti-inflammatory drugs
Although renal prostaglandins are primarily vasodilators, they do not play a major role in the regulation of renal hemodynamics in normal individuals because the basal rate of prostaglandin synthesis is relatively low. However, the release of these hormones (particularly prostacyclin and prostaglandin E_2) is enhanced by the vasoconstrictors angiotensin II and norepinephrine; secretion of these vasoconstrictors is increased in conditions of effective volume depletion, such as heart failure.[9] In this setting, vasodilator prostaglandins act to preserve renal blood flow and glomerular filtration rate by antagonizing the vasoconstrictor effects of angiotensin II and norepinephrine, particularly at the afferent arteriole.

In these patients, the fall in vasodilator prostaglandin production induced by an NSAID can lead to acute renal failure by two mechanisms: unopposed renal vasoconstriction by angiotensin II and norepinephrine and a reduction in cardiac output caused by the associated rise in systemic vascular resistance (an effect that is opposite to the beneficial decrease in cardiac afterload induced by vasodilators).[73] Thus, inhibition of prostaglandin synthesis by an NSAID can lead to reversible renal ischemia, a decline in glomerular hydraulic pressure (the major driving force for glomerular filtration), and acute renal failure.[11,75] The rise in the plasma creatinine concentration typically occurs within

Table 4 Causes and Management of Renal Failure in Patients with Congestive Heart Failure

Cause	Management
Excessive diuresis	Withhold diuretics; replete fluids cautiously, if indicated
Medications NSAIDs	Discontinue drug; consider sulindac if use of an NSAID must be continued
ACE inhibitors	Use shorter-acting drug (e.g., captopril instead of enalapril or lisinopril); reduce dosage of ACE inhibitor; reduce diuretic therapy; use alternative vasodilators (e.g., hydralazine and nitrates)
Worsening cardiac function	Consider a trial of inotropic agents or vasodilators, although renal function usually does not improve significantly with such therapy

the first three to seven days of therapy, the time required for attainment of steady-state drug levels and therefore maximum prostaglandin synthesis inhibition.[56]

As discussed earlier, there is evidence that the risk of acute renal failure is not uniform with all NSAIDs. In particular, sulindac, low-dose aspirin (studied at a dosage of approximately 40 mg/day, although somewhat higher dosages may have a similar effect), and possibly piroxicam may be safer because they are relatively sparing of renal prostaglandin synthesis.[11,56,76] With aspirin, for example, the inhibition of glomerular cyclooxygenase may only be partial and transient, in contrast to acetylation in platelets, which is irreversible. This protection, however, is not absolute, and careful monitoring is still required.

Angiotensin-converting enzyme inhibitors Angiotensin-converting enzyme (ACE) inhibitors are widely used in the treatment of congestive heart failure. These agents reduce the formation of angiotensin II, thereby decreasing both arteriolar and venous resistance. This so-called unloading effect is associated with an elevation in cardiac output, symptomatic improvement, and a 25 percent decrease in cardiovascular mortality at one to three years, attributable primarily to a slowing of the rate of progressive cardiac dysfunction.[77-79] Preliminary data in both animals and humans suggest that the administration of an angiotensin-converting enzyme inhibitor after acute myocardial infarction also may preserve cardiac function (as evidenced by an increased ejection fraction and decreased ventricular size) and possibly minimize late mortality.[80]

The administration of an ACE inhibitor together with a loop diuretic also may raise the plasma sodium concentration in patients with hyponatremia.[81] This synergism reflects the interaction between two factors:

1. Increased water delivery to the collecting tubules by the loop diuretic and by the ACE inhibitor, which acts primarily by increasing the cardiac output. The increase in cardiac output may seem paradoxical since the plasma creatinine does not fall in most patients with CHF who are treated with ACE inhibitors. It should be remembered, however, that an increase in cardiac output may permit the reduction of angiotensin II levels, which can reduce proximal tubular salt and water reabsorption. The net effect is improved renal perfusion with less efferent arteriolar vasoconstriction required to maintain the GFR.

2. Diminished water reabsorption in the collecting tubules caused both by reduced secretion of ADH (a result of the rise in cardiac output) and by ADH resistance. The diminished response to ADH appears to be mediated by two mechanisms: a diuretic-induced loss of interstitial osmolality and an increase in local prostaglandin synthesis (stimulated by the loop diuretic and possibly by the ACE

inhibitor), which block sodium reabsorption in the loop of Henle and antagonize ADH in the collecting duct.[82,83]

In view of the improvement in cardiac output and in renal blood flow, it might be assumed that the GFR would also increase. A rise in the GFR occurs in fewer than 10 percent of patients, however, and the plasma creatinine concentration actually increases in about 30 percent of patients.[13] The latter complication is most likely to occur in those settings in which maintenance of the GFR is dependent on high ambient angiotensin II levels.[13,84] Such settings include patients on high-dose diuretic therapy in whom there has been an excessive diuretic response; patients with relative hypotension who have a mean arterial pressure below 65 mm Hg; and patients with a pretreatment plasma sodium concentration below 137 mEq/L because this finding is a marker for significant neurohumoral activation.

Thus, the acute renal failure that can occur in heart failure develops by a mechanism similar to that seen in some patients with bilateral renal artery stenosis: preferential efferent arteriolar dilation with a subsequent fall in intraglomerular pressure. The baseline level of renal function can often be restored by lowering the diuretic dose. It has also been suggested that this complication is less likely to occur with a short-acting ACE inhibitor, such as captopril.[85] This observation, however, is based on a study in which relatively high doses were used; the administration of a low dose of lisinopril or enalapril (e.g., 2.5 mg/day of enalapril) as initial therapy is probably as safe as the use of captopril in most patients.[77,86] In some individuals, maintenance of the GFR may be so dependent on angiotensin II that switching to the combination of hydralazine and isosorbide dinitrate (which does not preferentially relax the efferent arteriole) may be required.[85]

It is important to note that many patients with advanced heart failure have elevations in the BUN and plasma creatinine concentrations before the institution of vasodilator therapy. This observation has potentially important therapeutic implications because the likelihood of a beneficial cardiovascular response is much lower in this setting, being less than 25 percent if the plasma creatinine concentration is more than 2.8 mg/dl as compared with 75 percent when the plasma creatinine concentration is less than 1.4 mg/dl.[87] Why patients with elevated creatinine levels do not respond well to vasodilator therapy is not well understood.

Patients with underlying renal insufficiency are also at higher risk for the development of hyperkalemia following the administration of an ACE inhibitor.[88] Advanced heart failure is associated with decreased sodium and water delivery to the potassium secretory sites in the collecting tubules. Maintenance of adequate potassium secretion in these patients is dependent on increased secretion of aldosterone. This response, however, may be partially impaired if there is diminished production of angiotensin II, because angiotensin II is the primary mediator of the hypoperfusion-induced increase in aldosterone release.

Worsening cardiac function   Worsening cardiac function is a final cause of progressive prerenal disease in CHF. In many patients, this diagnosis will be clinically apparent because of increasing cardiac symptoms or a recent myocardial infarction. In some cases, however, the evidence for a deterioration in myocardial function is somewhat masked. For example, an episode of severe coronary ischemia, without infarction, can lead to impaired cardiac contractility that persists for up to three to five days. The generation of oxygen free radicals during the period of ischemia may be responsible for the delayed recovery of cellular function in this setting (a phenomenon that has been called myocardial "stunning").[89]

In other patients, chronic ischemia can impair left ventricular function in the absence of chest pain or electrocardiographic changes.[90] This problem, which is in part adaptive because it limits myocardial oxygen requirements in the presence of diminished oxygen delivery, should be suspected in patients with ischemic heart disease in whom the severity of the heart failure is out of proportion to the apparent degree of cardiac damage. It is important to establish the diagnosis of chronic ischemia because coronary revascularization can lead to improved cardiac function.

Acute Tubular Necrosis

Acute tubular necrosis is, with prerenal disease, one of the two most common causes of acute renal failure. The characteristic tubular injury in this disorder represents a nonspecific response that can be seen with a variety of renal insults, including renal ischemia and exposure to exogenous or endogenous nephrotoxins [*see Table 5*]. The net effect is a rapid decline in renal function that, in many patients, requires a variable period of dialysis before spontaneous resolution occurs.

There are two major histologic changes in ATN: (1) tubular necrosis with sloughing of the epithelial cells and (2) occlusion of the tubular lumina by casts and by cellular debris (including the brush border of the proximal tubular cells and Tamm-Horsfall mucoprotein released from damaged cells in the thick ascending limb of the loop of Henle).[91] These changes are often patchy and may appear relatively mild in relation to the severity of the renal failure. It is important to remember, however, that many nephrons drain into a single cortical collecting tubule. Thus, obstruction of a seemingly small number of collecting tubules can lead to marked renal dysfunction.

In addition to tubular obstruction, two other factors appear to contribute to the development of renal failure in ATN: backleak of filtrate across the damaged tubular epithelia and a primary reduction in glomerular filtration. The decrease in glomerular filtration results both from arteriolar vasoconstriction (caused in part by tubuloglomerular feedback) and from mesangial contraction (which limits the surface area available for glomerular filtration).

The likelihood that ATN will develop after a given insult is often difficult to pre-

Table 5 Major Causes of Acute Tubular Necrosis

Renal Ischemia Followed by Reperfusion
  Severe prenatal disease from all causes,
    particularly hypotension during
    surgery and sepsis

Exposure to Nephrotoxins
  Aminoglycoside antibiotics

  Radiocontrast media

  Cisplatin

  Uric acid

  Heme pigments (e.g., as in
    hemoglobinuria or myoglobinuria)

  Amphotericin B

  Pentamidine

  Acyclovir

dict. Additional potentially nephrotoxic factors may be operating concomitantly (such as ischemia plus aminoglycoside administration) in some individuals but not in others, and the tubular insult may vary in severity in different individuals. For example, the reduction in GFR may be limited in one individual if there is minimal tubular obstruction by cellular debris. This clinical outcome may be manifested by a urine sediment that contains a few granular casts and little or no change in the plasma creatinine concentration or urine flow. By comparison, the same casts in another individual may cause marked tubular obstruction and extreme backleak of filtrate, thereby reducing the glomerular filtration rate dramatically.

Postischemic Acute Tubular Necrosis

Pathogenesis and Etiology

Almost any of the causes of severe prerenal disease can lead to ATN, particularly hypotension in the settings of surgery (primarily open-heart surgery or abdominal aortic aneurysm repair), sepsis, or an obstetric complication. The association with major surgery, for example, is related in part to the hemodynamic changes that often occur in this setting. Preoperative fluid depletion, anesthesia, and intraoperative fluid losses can combine to lower the GFR (by as much as 30 to 45 percent), the urine volume, and urinary sodium excretion.[92,93] Most patients are able to tolerate this transient renal ischemia without experiencing tubular injury. However, acute tubular necrosis may ensue if a further insult, such as hypotension, is added.

At first glance, it appears paradoxical that ATN develops frequently after ischemia, whereas acute myocardial infarction or stroke occurs much less commonly in states of systemic hypoperfusion. The relative frequency of postischemic ATN is particularly surprising because the kidneys receive approximately 25 percent of the cardiac output and because this high renal blood flow is accompanied by a low arteriovenous oxygen difference; blood entering the renal artery normally has a Po_2 higher than 90 mm Hg, whereas the Po_2 in venous blood leaving the kidney is higher than 40 mm Hg. The fact that ATN occurs despite high blood flow and low O_2 extraction is explained by the observation that this high oxygen tension is directed toward the cortex; in comparison, the Po_2 in the medulla is consistently in the range of 5 to 12 mm Hg [*see Figure 2*].[94,95]

Medullary hypoxemia in the resting state is a consequence of the need to concentrate the urine.[94,95] The marginal Po_2 normally present in the outer medulla poses a potential constraint on active transport by the medullary thick ascending limb of the loop of Henle. In a number of experimental conditions in which medullary hypoxemia is enhanced (such as hypotension produced by controlled hemorrhage), the zone most often damaged is the deepest portion furthest away from the vasa recta, which is the area most remote from oxygen supply. This finding is consistent with the hypothesis that O_2 diffusion away from the arterial and toward the venous branches of the vasa recta capillaries markedly diminishes O_2 supply to the deeper portion of the medulla. As a result, even a modest decrease in med-

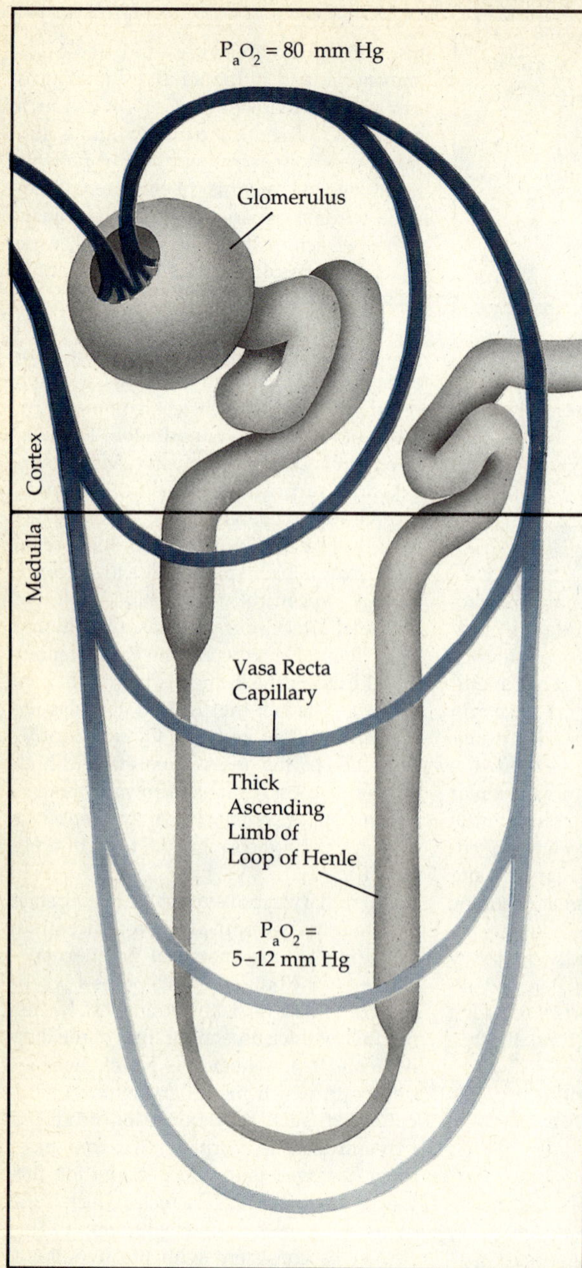

Figure 2   As a result of countercurrent diffusion of oxygen (O_2) from a higher concentration (dark blue) in the descending limb of the vasa recta capillary to a lower concentration (light blue) in the early portion of the ascending limb of this capillary, the oxygen content in the descending vasa recta progressively declines. Ultimately, the P_aO_2 in the portion of the vasa recta capillary that supplies the actively metabolizing cells of the thick ascending limb of the loop of Henle in the basal state falls to levels as low as 5 to 12 mm Hg. The net effect is that the tubular cells in this nephron region normally function in a severely hypoxemic environment, leaving them very susceptible to any further fall in oxygen delivery or any increase in energy requirements.

ullary perfusion puts these tubular cells at risk of ischemic damage.

The duration of ischemia is another important factor in both the development and the duration of ATN. In most patients, the renal failure phase lasts for seven to 21 days after the ischemic episode. However, recovery may occur within one to three days when there is only a brief period of ischemia. Some patients undergoing surgery for an abdominal aortic aneurysm, for example, require clamping of the aorta above the renal arteries, leading to total cessation of renal perfusion for 15 to 80 minutes.[93] Two hours after the operation, the GFR is reduced, and the urinary findings are typical of ATN: high urine sodium concentration, high fractional excretion of sodium, and urine osmolality similar to that in the plasma (300 to 350 mOsm/kg). By 24 hours, these parameters begin to normalize and recovery is usually complete within three days. In comparison, patients with recurrent episodes of prolonged hypotension (as may occur with persistent infection) may have continued tubular injury and persistent renal failure for weeks to months.[96]

The mechanism of tubular cell injury that leads to cell necrosis and sloughing is directly related to hypoxemic injury, a process that generates oxygen free radicals. These molecules or molecular fragments contain unpaired electrons in their outer orbital. Consequently, they are very reactive and tend to initiate chain reactions that result in irreversible chemical injury to the reacting lipid or protein, with subsequent structural damage.[97] Normally, the generation of these oxygen free radicals is limited by protective enzymes and antioxidants that are present within the cell.[98] Tubular damage may ensue if the capacity of these protective agents is exceeded.[99,100]

Under normal conditions, hypoxanthine (a breakdown product of adenosine triphosphate, or ATP) is converted to uric acid by xanthine dehydrogenase (XD), which is found exclusively in vascular endothelium and is removed by the kidneys:

$$\text{Hypoxanthine} + H_2O + NAD + \xrightarrow{XD} \text{Xanthine} + NADH + H^+$$

$$\text{Xanthine} + H_2O + NAD + \xrightarrow{XD} \text{Uric acid} + NADH + H^+$$

Ischemia and hypoxia result in several remarkable changes capable of damaging the cell; perhaps more importantly, these changes set the stage for even more dramatic developments that follow the reintroduction of oxygen (reperfusion injury). With hypoxia, cells must switch to anaerobic metabolism to continue the production of ATP. In contrast, as ATP stores are depleted, adenosine diphosphate (ADP) and adenosine monophosphate (AMP) begin to accumulate. Increased conversion of AMP to adenosine and of adenosine to hypoxanthine occurs. Concomitantly, calcium accumulates within the cell cytoplasm because calcium removal by the endoplasmic reticulum is dependent on the energy provided by ATP. The increased cytosolic calcium activates several proteases, one of which causes the irreversible transformation of XD to xanthine oxidase (XO).[99] Although this form of the enzyme is still capable of metabolizing hypoxanthine to uric acid, it uses O_2 as the electron receptor, generating oxygen free radicals ($O_2^{-}\cdot$) in the process:

$$\text{Hypoxanthine} + H_2O + 2O_2 \xrightarrow{XO} \text{Xanthine} + 2O_2^{-} + 2H^+$$

$$\text{Xanthine} + H_2O + 2O_2 \xrightarrow{XO} \text{Uric acid} + 2O_2^{-} + 2H^+$$

The reintroduction of O_2 during reperfusion drives the reaction to the right, causing production of significantly greater quantities of free radicals ($O_2^{-}\cdot$).

Thus, an imbalance between O_2 supply and demand leads to the production of reactive oxygen species that are generated at a faster rate during reperfusion. These free radicals lead to chain reactions that damage lipid and protein structures within cells, leading to cell injury and necrosis. In the kidney, this injury is most likely to occur in the rapidly metabolizing cells of the medullary thick ascending limb of the loop of Henle and portions of the proximal tubule, where it leads to sloughing that obstructs the tubule and reduces the GFR.

Prevention

Ischemia-induced ATN can be prevented in certain animal models, but it is more difficult to block in humans because the onset of the insult that leads to tubular injury (e.g., sepsis) is generally not predictable. Despite this limitation, experience from experimental models may eventually allow intervention in humans as such approaches become more refined.

Patients who are hypotensive and oliguric as a result of surgery, sepsis, or bleeding are at risk of developing postischemic ATN. In this setting, attempts have been made to preserve renal function both by protecting the cells against ischemic injury and by preventing tubular obstruction from cellular debris. In experimental animals, both loop diuretics (e.g., furosemide) and mannitol have been shown to be of benefit if given at the time of the ischemic insult.[94,101,102] These agents may have a variety of beneficial effects: (1) both can induce a diuresis, potentially washing out obstructing cellular debris and casts; (2) loop diuretics diminish active transport in the thick ascending limb, and the ensuing decrease in energy requirements protects the cell when there is a decrease in energy delivery[94]; and (3) mannitol may preserve mitochondrial function by osmotically minimizing the degree of postischemic cell swelling,[102] by causing afferent arteriolar vasodilation, and by scavenging free radicals.

Other agents have also been tried in experimental models of postischemic ATN.[103,104] The administration of either dopamine or atrial natriuretic peptide (ANP) alone appears to be without benefit, despite the ability of these agents to increase both renal blood flow and sodium excretion.[103,105] However, the administration of ANP together with dopamine to prevent hypotension[103] or with mannitol to wash out obstructing casts[106] can help preserve renal function. Calcium channel blockers can also be beneficial.[107] ANP appears to act by increasing the glomerular filtration rate via changes in arteriolar resistance,[103,106] whereas calcium channel blockers minimize the ischemia-induced entry of calcium into the cells that then leads to cellular dysfunction.[107] Infusion of glycine is also protective in experimental animals, but the mechanism of this protection is unclear.[108]

In other experimental studies, sepsis-associated ATN can be prevented when inhibitors of thromboxane synthesis are administered shortly after induction of shock.[109] These findings support a role for thromboxane in the pathogenesis of acute renal failure in this setting.

As with all animal studies, the applicability of each of these findings to humans is unproved. Uncontrolled studies have shown that patients who respond to mannitol or to furosemide and dopamine with an increase in urine output have a better outcome than those who do not respond to such therapy.[110,111] However, those who respond may simply have had less severe disease, as evidenced by a shorter duration of oliguria (less than 24 hours), a higher urine output, and a higher urine osmolality (suggesting better preservation of tubular function). Neither ANP nor calcium channel blockers have yet been evaluated in humans. Calcium blocker therapy, however, is most effective in animal models if given before or during the ischemic episode rather than after renal failure has begun.[108] Thus, its main utility in humans may be in preserving function in cadaveric renal allografts rather than minimizing the severity of postischemic ATN.

The only controlled studies in humans have been performed during established ATN, not in the early ischemic phase. In this setting, tissue perfusion has been restored and most of the tubular damage has already occurred. Therefore, it is not surprising that increasing the urine output with a loop diuretic has no effect on the severity or duration of the renal failure.[112] The loop diuretic appears to enhance the urine output in those few nephrons that are still functioning, but there is little recruitment of previously nonfunctioning nephrons. Furthermore, the high loop diuretic dose that may be required to induce a diuresis can lead to deafness, which may be permanent.[112]

In summary, the efficacy of preventive therapy in humans at risk for postischemic ATN is unproved. Nevertheless, mannitol (12.5 to 25 g given intravenously over 10 to 30 minutes) and a loop diuretic such as furosemide (working up to a maximum intravenous dose of 500 mg given over 30 minutes) can be tried in oliguric patients seen within 24 hours of the ischemic insult. Both agents are relatively safe; however, although mannitol infusions are usually well tolerated, they may cause a number of renal complications, including acute renal failure (see below). Some physicians administer furosemide together with low-dose dopamine (3 µg/kg/min) if the combination of furosemide and mannitol is ineffective.[111] Low-dose dopamine, alone, appears to increase urine output by inhibiting proximal sodium reabsorption in functioning nephrons[113]; however, the rise in urine volume is not accompanied by a large rise in GFR, because vasodilation occurs in both afferent and efferent arterioles without a net increase in glomerular capillary pressure. If any of these regimens succeed in increasing the urine output, urinary losses should be replaced to prevent further volume depletion and more renal ischemia.

Complications of Mannitol Administration

Although mannitol therapy is generally well tolerated, a variety of fluid, electrolyte, and renal complications can occur if the patient is not carefully monitored. Complications of mannitol administration may include the following:

1. Volume depletion and hypernatremia. Excreted mannitol acts as an osmotic diuretic because it does not undergo tubular reabsorption. Nonreplacement of salt and water losses can lead to volume depletion and, because free water is lost with mannitol, potentially severe hypernatremia.[114]

2. Volume expansion, hyponatremia, hyperkalemia, and metabolic acidosis. A different set of changes is seen if some of the hypertonic mannitol is retained because of underlying renal failure or because very high doses have been administered.[115,116] The ensuing rise in plasma osmolality (which can induce symptoms similar to those seen with hypernatremia) results in the osmotic movement of water out of cells. This movement of water can lead to plasma volume expansion (and possible pulmonary edema), hyponatremia, metabolic acidosis (by dilution of the plasma bicarbonate concentration), and hyperkalemia.

The rise in the plasma potassium concentration following hypertonic mannitol therapy is caused by the movement of potassium out of the cells and into the extracellular fluid via two mechanisms: (1) the rise in intracellular potassium concentration induced by water loss favors passive potassium exit through potassium channels in the cell membrane, and (2) the frictional forces between solvent (water) and solute can result in potassium being carried out through the water pores in the cell membrane (a process that is called solvent drag).

Finally, although mannitol is used in an attempt to prevent postischemic ATN, acute renal failure may be caused by an excessively high plasma mannitol concentration (> 1,050 mg/dl). Because measurement of plasma mannitol levels is not readily performed in most hospital laboratories, the concentration can be estimated using the osmolal gap. This value can be determined by subtracting the calculated plasma osmolality (P_{osm}) from the osmolality measured by the clinical laboratory.

$$\text{Calculated } P_{osm} = (2 \times Na^+) \times \frac{glucose}{18} \times \frac{BUN}{2.8}$$

Patients with marked mannitol accumulation (osmolal gap greater than 60 to 75 mOsm/kg) appear to be at highest risk for reversible acute renal failure.[116] Renal vasoconstriction appears to be of primary importance in this setting, although tubular vacuolization also may contribute.

Clinical Presentation and Course

The decline in renal function in ATN has a variable onset. It typically begins abruptly following a hypotensive episode, rhabdomyolysis, or the administration of radiocontrast media. In comparison, when aminoglycoside nephrotoxicity is the cause, the onset is more insidious, with the plasma creatinine concentration beginning to rise slowly after seven or more days of therapy. Some patients with marked prerenal disease also may have a changing course, with the urinary findings showing a gradual transition from indices typical of prerenal disease (low urine sodium concentration, low fractional excretion of sodium, and a normal urinalysis) to those typical of acute tubular necrosis (high fractional excretion of sodium and granular and epithelial cell casts in the urine).

Once renal failure begins, the BUN and plasma creatinine concentration usually rise in daily increments of 10 to 25 mg/dl and 0.5 to 2.5 mg/dl, respectively. The rise in BUN, however, can reach 50 mg/dl/day or more in hypercatabolic patients (particularly those receiving parenteral amino acid solutions); marked hyperkalemia is also more common in this setting.

Nonoliguric versus Oliguric ATN

The urine volume is variable in ATN, ranging from oliguric levels (< 500 ml/day) to normal or even above-normal levels. The maintenance of a high urine output in some patients with ATN could result from one of two factors: a less-marked decline in the GFR than in oliguric patients or a lesser degree of tubular reabsorption. In most patients, the former seems to predominate as nonoliguric ATN is associated with evidence of less severe tubular damage.[3,117] As compared with oliguric patients, patients who maintain a higher urine output tend to have a lower peak plasma creatinine concentration, a lower mortality, and a less frequent requirement for dialysis (28 percent versus 84 percent in one study).[117]

The better prognosis associated with nonoliguric ATN applies primarily to patients with spontaneous (i.e., untreated) disease. In comparison, raising the urine output with a loop diuretic in established oliguric ATN does not appear to improve the renal prognosis relative to that of untreated patients.[112] This finding reflects the fact that the diuretic acts by increasing the urine output from those few nephrons that are still functioning rather than by restoring function to damaged nephrons. In this setting, the most important variables adversely affecting outcome are deep neurologic coma, persistent hypotension, and a requirement for ventilatory support.[118]

Duration of Acute Tubular Necrosis

The renal failure phase in ischemic ATN generally lasts seven to 21 days,[96] with most patients returning to their previous baseline level of renal function. The duration, however, is highly variable and depends on the length and severity of the initial ischemic episode and on the presence or absence of recurrent ischemia.[96]

As an example, patients undergoing suprarenal aortic clamping for aortic aneurysm surgery have 20 to 80 minutes of total renal ischemia. Although clinical evidence of ATN is often present postoperatively, renal function usually returns to baseline within one to three days because the duration of ischemia is so short and because ischemia does not recur.[93,96] Similarly, the typical course of radiocontrast media–induced acute renal failure is three to five days, apparently because the renal insult is very short-lived.

In these settings of rapid recovery, it is likely that during the period of postischemic or posttoxic tubular dysfunction, the cells are morphologically normal rather than necrotic. This phenomenon, which is similar to postischemic dysfunction in the so-called stunned or hibernating myocardium, may result, at least in part, from redistribution of membrane transport proteins. Sodium is normally reabsorbed by entering the tubular cells across the luminal membrane and then being actively transported out of the cells by the Na^+-K^+-ATPase pump in the basolateral membrane. Following ischemia, however, some of these pumps may migrate from the basolateral to the luminal membrane, thereby interfering with normal ion transport [*see Figure 3*]. Recovery of function is associated with recovery of normal polarity, and the Na^+-K^+-ATPase pumps are again limited to the basolateral membrane.[1]

In comparison, patients who are persistently infected and hypercatabolic may never recover renal function.[96] In this setting, the regeneration of injured tubular cells that is required for recovery of renal function cannot be achieved. Regeneration is associated with the activation of growth response genes that are involved in cell growth.[119] This observation has potential clinical applicability because the administration of epidermal growth factor has been shown to accelerate both tubular regeneration and the recovery of renal function in postischemic and nephrotoxic acute renal failure induced in experimental animals.[120,121]

Repeated episodes of renal ischemia represent another setting in which recovery of renal function may be delayed or may not occur.[96] The kidney of a patient with ATN appears to be particularly sensitive to diminished perfusion. Normal kidneys vasodilate in the presence of ischemia as part of the normal autoregulatory response to maintain renal blood flow at near-normal levels. This response is impaired in ATN, perhaps because vascular endothelial injury inhibits the release of vasodilating substances such as prostacyclin and endothelium-derived relaxing factor (nitric oxide).[122]

Treatment

Therapy in established ATN, other than correction of the underlying problem (such as discontinuation of an aminoglycoside), is largely supportive. In particular, attention must be paid to maintenance of the fluid and electrolyte balance and of adequate nutrition. Despite optimal management, however, many patients still require a transient period of dialysis. The major indications for dialysis are marked fluid overload, severe hyperkalemia, or the presence of uremic signs or symptoms, such as pericarditis, nausea and vomiting, confusion, or bleeding in a patient with a prolonged bleeding time. On the other hand, a prolonged bleeding time may be corrected without dialysis in many patients by administering parenteral 1-desamino-8-D-arginine vasopressin (DDAVP)[123] or conjugated estrogens.[124]

The institution of prophylactic dialysis at a particular level of BUN or plasma creatinine concentration has not been shown to be of benefit as long as the BUN is less than 150 mg/dl.[125] Furthermore, dialytic therapy is associated with several potential side effects (see below).

It has also been suggested that the use of a high-calorie, low-protein diet that contains high levels of essential amino acids may minimize protein breakdown and perhaps accelerate the recovery of renal function. This theory, however, has not been generally confirmed. Only those patients with multisystem abnormalities who are likely to be hypercatabolic appear to benefit from this regimen.[126]

Whether treatment of the metabolic acidosis that frequently develops in ATN is beneficial is unclear. The usual guidelines for treating acid-base disorders should be followed. It is possible, however, that correcting the acidosis may have some deleterious effect. In at least some experimental models, acidemia appears to be protective, reducing tubular injury in the ischemic kidney, perhaps by decreasing local sodium transport and oxygen consumption.[127]

Even with the use of dialytic and dietary therapy, the mortality of all patients with ATN remains between 40 and 60 percent, with infection and the underlying disease (such as persistent postoperative hypotension) being the major causes of death.[126,128] This statistic, however, is somewhat misleading because survival is largely dependent on the patient's general health. Mortality is very high in patients with per-

a

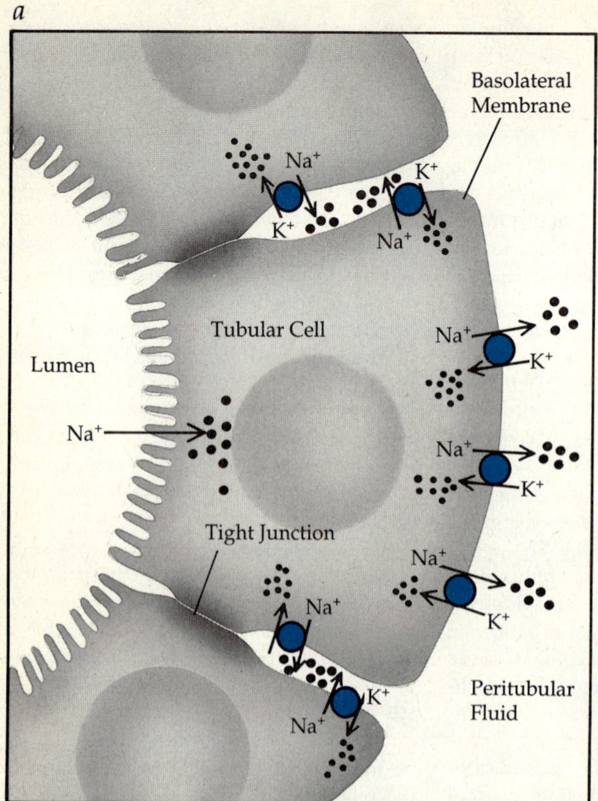

Figure 3 (a) *Under normal conditions, the Na⁺-K⁺-ATPase pump located in the basolateral membrane of the tubular cell transports sodium from the inside of the cell toward the peritubular fluid, from which it ultimately reaches the peritubular capillary. As the sodium concentration falls inside the cell, sodium can be reabsorbed from the tubular lumen. The pumping of sodium from the lumen to the peritubular side of the cell membrane requires the maintenance of sodium pumps in specific locations, a process that is dependent on intact tight junctions between the cells that limit pump migration.*

sistent multisystem involvement such as abdominal infection, pneumonia, neurologic dysfunction, and circulatory instability.[128] In comparison, the prognosis is generally excellent for ATN induced by exposure to aminoglycosides or radiocontrast media if the patient is otherwise well.

Urine Output in ARF and Effect of Dialysis

Although the glomerular filtration rate is very low in patients with renal failure, the urine output is variable. It had been thought that tubular damage that impaired the ability to reabsorb sodium and water contributed to the maintenance of an adequate urine output in this setting. It seems more likely, however, that volume expansion (caused by initial sodium retention) and a urea osmotic diuresis (as the daily urea load is excreted by fewer functioning nephrons) play a more important role in the persistent urine output. Volume expansion, for example, leads to an increase in atrial natriuretic peptide and a decrease in aldosterone, both of which promote sodium excretion despite the very low GFR.

In contrast, water intake (which usually determines the urine volume via changes in the secretion of ADH) plays a relatively small role in regulating the urine output in ATN. Patients with ATN can neither dilute nor concentrate the urine normally: the range of urine osmolality that can be achieved may vary from a minimum of 250 mOsm/kg to a maximum of 350 mOsm/kg as compared with 50 to 1,200 mOsm/kg in normal subjects. The net effect of this ADH

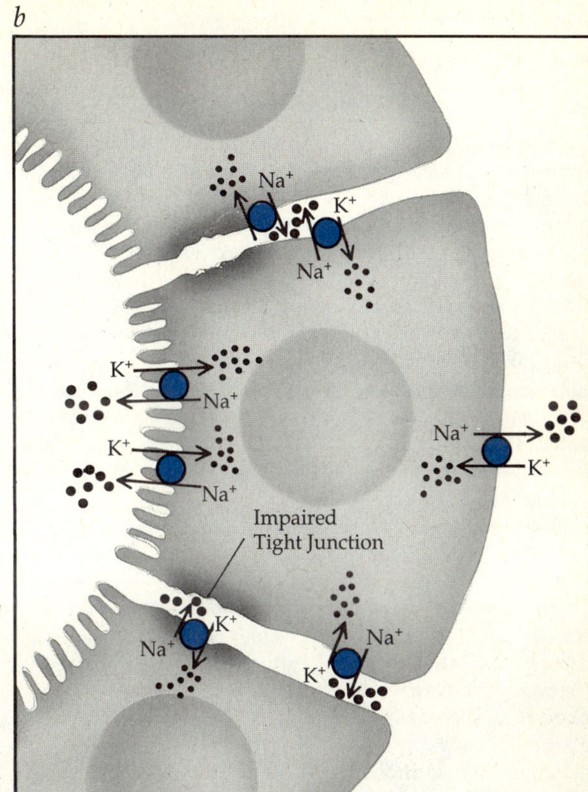

b

(b) *During renal ischemia, however, there is a loss of cell polarity. The function of the tight junctions is impaired, and sodium transporters migrate from the basolateral membrane to the luminal membrane. Transport of sodium out of the cell and into the lumen can impair the ability of the tubular cell to reabsorb sodium.*

resistance is that variations in ADH release in response to changes in water intake and plasma osmolality have relatively little effect on the urine output.

Both volume expansion and the high urea load per nephron are rapidly reversed by dialysis, which removes sodium, water, and urea. It is therefore not surprising that in many patients the urine output is markedly reduced or even ceases when dialysis is instituted.[129] This observation has raised the question of whether dialysis itself impairs renal function in patients with acute renal failure. Although there is no definitive answer to this question, it seems unlikely that dialysis has a major deleterious effect. In a patient with acute renal failure who requires dialysis, fewer than five percent of the nephrons are functioning.[130] The decline in urine output following dialysis reflects an increase in tubular reabsorption in these few nephrons. Even if the function of these nephrons became impaired (perhaps because slow flow may promote obstruction by tubular debris), this development should not delay the recovery from renal failure.

Recovery depends on the restoration of function in the 95 percent of nephrons that are currently nonfunctioning; these damaged nephrons are not likely to be adversely affected by the removal of fluid and urea by dialysis. One potential exception might be observed if fluid loss were excessive, leading to hypotension and reduced tissue perfusion. In this setting, further ischemic damage to the kidney resulting from dialysis might indeed delay the restoration of renal function.

Acute Tubular Necrosis Caused by Nephrotoxins

Aminoglycoside Nephrotoxicity

Acute renal failure caused by tubular necrosis is a relatively common complication of aminoglycoside therapy, with a rise in the plasma creatinine concentration of more than 0.5 to 1 mg/dl occurring in 10 to 20 percent of patients.[131,132] The aminoglycosides are freely filtered; almost all of the drug is then excreted, with a small amount being taken up by and stored in the tubular cells, leading to damage, particularly in the proximal tubule. Acute renal failure can occur even if drug levels are closely monitored,[133] although the risk is clearly greater in those patients with high levels.[131,132]

The number of cationic amino groups (NH_3^+) per molecule appears to be an important determinant of nephrotoxicity.[131,134] Thus, among the aminoglycosides, neomycin (six amino groups per molecule) produces the most renal injury and streptomycin (three groups per molecule) produces the least. Gentamicin (five groups), tobramycin (five groups), netilmicin (four groups), and amikacin (four groups) have intermediate toxicity.[132] Although initial reports suggested that gentamicin was more nephrotoxic than tobramycin, patients with sepsis or hypotension were excluded in these studies in an attempt to eliminate other potential causes of renal failure. In this selected population, gentamicin was more nephrotoxic, but the renal injury was mild, and the peak plasma creatinine concentration was less than 2 mg/dl in almost all patients.[133] When all patient populations are included, by comparison, there seems to be no increase in nephrotoxicity with gentamicin administration as compared with tobramycin.[135,136]

The role of molecular charge seems to be related to binding of the cationic aminoglycoside to receptors in the luminal and subcellular membranes.[131] At the luminal membrane, binding may occur by attachment to anionic phospholipids or to H^+–organic cation exchangers, either of which will promote drug entry into the tubular cell.[131,137] Once inside the cell, the drug accumulates within lysosomes, an effect that may also be mediated by the charge on the aminoglycoside. Inhibition of lysosomal phospholipases, leading to impaired lysosomal function or to the release of lysosomal enzymes into the cytosol, may then be responsible for the cellular injury induced by the aminoglycoside. Typically, renal failure does not occur until therapy has been administered for a prolonged period (at least nine to 10 doses of aminoglycoside). The delay in onset may be caused by preferential shunting and accumulation of plasma membrane components into lysosomal compartments; thus, the membranes become slowly depleted and cannot be regenerated, because the building blocks are sequestered and not recycled.

The relation of molecular charge to toxicity may have potential therapeutic implications. Experimental studies suggest that aminoglycoside nephrotoxicity can be diminished by the following measures (each of which is related to ionic charge):

1. Coadministration of a cationic molecule, such as the calcium channel blockers verapamil or nitrendipine, which may compete with the aminoglycoside for uptake into the tubular cell.[137]
2. Coadministration of polyaspartic acid, a polyanion that may bind the aminoglycoside and thereby prevent it from interacting with anionic membrane lipids.[138,139]
3. Administration of $NaHCO_3$ to alkalinize the urine because raising the pH will decrease the net positive charge on the aminoglycoside.[140]

These protective effects, which have not been studied in humans, may be mediated by reduced aminoglycoside uptake by the tubular cells or by reduced entry of the drug into lysosomes once it is within the cell. Concurrent administration of a penicillin, such as ticarcillin, also may be effective by decreasing aminoglycoside uptake[134,141]; whether the protection afforded by these agents is a result of their anionic charge, however, is unknown. An alternative may be to give higher doses of the aminoglycoside at longer dose intervals because the uptake mechanism in the proximal tubule is saturable; thus, higher individual doses may not increase renal uptake as the drug is being excreted but will be associated with less total uptake because the drug is given less often.[142]

Predisposing Factors

A number of factors have been suggested to potentiate the development of renal insufficiency in patients who are treated with an aminoglycoside. Such factors include the duration of therapy, drug dosage, reduced renal perfusion, liver disease, and concomitant cephalothin administration.

Duration of aminoglycoside therapy The development of renal insufficiency generally requires at least seven days of aminoglycoside therapy. In the presence of concurrent renal ischemia, however, the combined insults can lead to renal failure within one to two days, even though neither problem alone may be sufficient to produce tubular injury.[143]

Dose Careful monitoring of plasma levels is an important component of aminoglycoside therapy, although impaired renal function can occur even when plasma drug levels remain well within the normal range.[133] On the other hand, the risk is much higher in patients with high peak (> 10 µg/ml) concentrations. High trough concentrations (> 2 to 3 µg/ml), in comparison, are more often the result, rather than the cause, of a low glomerular filtration rate.

When estimating the gentamicin dose, it is important to remember that both muscle mass and the glomerular filtration rate decline with age; consequently, a plasma creatinine concentration of 1 mg/dl in an individual 20 years of age may represent a GFR that is two to three times greater than that of an individual 80 years of age with a similar plasma creatinine. This difference can be estimated using the following formula to calculate the creatinine clearance (C_{Cr}), which reflects the GFR[144]:

$$C_{Cr} \text{ (ml/min)} = \frac{(140 - \text{age}) \times \text{lean body weight (kg)}}{P_{Cr} \times 72}$$

The value for C_{Cr} calculated by this formula should be multiplied by 0.85 in women because a lower fraction of their body weight is composed of muscle (which is the source of plasma creatinine).

Volume depletion, hypotension, and sepsis The likelihood of cell injury depends in part on energy delivery. Thus, decreased renal perfusion enhances cell injury in the presence of a normally subtoxic dose of aminoglycoside.[145] This synergism is most prominent in the third (S3), and final, segment of the proximal tubule; this region is particularly sensitive to ischemia because it runs into the outer medulla, which normally is less well oxygenated than the renal cortex. Studies using cultured renal tubular cells suggest that furosemide, in addition to potentiating volume depletion, also potentiates gentamicin toxicity by accelerating uptake of the aminoglycoside by these cells.[146]

Liver disease Hepatic disease, particularly obstructive jaundice in which the plasma bilirubin level is more than 5 mg/dl, predisposes to aminoglycoside-associated acute renal failure.[147] The mechanism of this interaction is unknown, but either bilirubin or endotoxin (which is absorbed because of decreased bile salt entry into the intestinal lumen) may increase the sensitivity of renal tubular cells to aminoglycosides.

Concurrent cephalothin administration Initial studies suggested that cephalothin increased the nephrotoxicity of aminoglycosides.[148] However, patients with sepsis or hypotension were excluded. In this limited population, cephalothin did have a potentiating effect, but the renal injury was mild. In contrast, there seems to be no additive toxic effect when all patients are included.[132] Preliminary evidence suggests that even if there is a small risk with cephalothin, this risk does not extend to any of the other cephalosporins currently used.[149]

Clinical Manifestations and Diagnosis

ATN is a relatively common complication of therapy with the aminoglycoside antibiotics, with most damage occurring in the cells of the proximal tubule. However, the more distal nephron segments can also be affected, resulting in impaired function; decreased concentrating ability and hypomagnesemia (caused by enhanced urinary losses) are commonly seen.[150]

Most patients with aminoglycoside-induced ATN are nonoliguric (urine output > 500 ml/day), perhaps reflecting the concurrent impairment of concentrating ability.[151] The diagnosis of this disorder is made from a history of acute renal failure beginning more than five days after the institution of aminoglycoside therapy, a urine sediment that either is normal or shows granular and epithelial cell casts, and a fractional excretion of sodium higher than one percent.

Treatment

Initial therapy of aminoglycoside-induced ARF is supportive and consists of discontinuing the aminoglycoside and of maintaining the fluid and electrolyte balance. Recovery, with return of renal function to the prior baseline level, usually occurs within 21 days after cessation of aminoglycoside therapy. However, recovery may be delayed if the patient remains septic or catabolic. Irreversible injury is uncommon following acute aminoglycoside nephrotoxicity, although it may occur when the aminoglycoside therapy is prolonged, even when the agent is given in low doses.[152]

Radiocontrast Media–induced Acute Renal Failure

The administration of radiocontrast media can lead to a reversible form of acute renal failure that begins soon after the contrast agent is administered.[153-157] The mechanism by which this occurs is not well understood, but renal vasoconstriction and the generation of oxygen free radicals may be important.[158-160] As in most cases of acute tubular necrosis, the fractional excretion of sodium is generally higher than one percent; however, lower values (suggestive of intact tubular function) are not infrequently observed in this disorder.[155,158]

Predisposing Factors

Prospective studies have shown that a small rise in the plasma creatinine concentration (averaging 0.2 mg/dl) is a common occurrence after a radiocontrast study.[155] A more marked decline in renal function can occur, however, particularly in patients with one or more of the following risk factors[153-158]: (1) underlying renal insufficiency, with a plasma creatinine level exceeding 1.5 mg/dl, (2) diabetic nephropathy associated with renal insufficiency, (3) advanced heart failure, (4) high total dose of contrast media, or (5) multiple myeloma.

In general, the incidence of a rise in the plasma creatinine concentration of more than 50 percent above baseline or of more than 1 mg/dl is negligible in patients with normal renal function, even if they are diabetic.[153] It is about four to 11 percent in patients with mild to moderate renal insufficiency alone (plasma creatinine between 1.5 and 4.0 mg/dl)[153,154,156]; this risk, however, may be increased to above 40 percent by more advanced renal dysfunction, marked volume depletion, severe heart failure, or the performance of multiple contrast studies within a 72-hour period.[154] The chance of a significant rise in the plasma creatinine increases to between nine and 38 percent in patients with mild to moderate renal insufficiency and diabetes mellitus,[153,157] and it is higher than 50 percent when the baseline plasma creatinine is greater than 4 to 5 mg/dl.[158,161]

A dose-dependent risk of renal dysfunction has been demonstrated in some studies. When a low dose, variably defined as less than 125 ml or as less than 5 ml/kg (up to a maximum of 300 ml), of contrast media is compared with a higher dose, the incidence of acute renal failure may be two percent versus 20 percent in patients with renal insufficiency alone[154,157] and six percent versus 38 percent in patients with renal insufficiency and diabetes mellitus.[157]

In almost all of these patients, the decline in renal function is mild and transient and of little clinical importance. Some patients, however, have a peak rise in the plasma creatinine that can exceed 5 mg/dl, which occasionally requires acute dialysis; this rise is most likely to occur when the baseline plasma creatinine is greater than 4 mg/dl.[154,158] Persistent renal failure is rare and has been described primarily in patients with far-advanced underlying disease (i.e., the baseline plasma creatinine is usually higher than 8 mg/dl).[158,161]

Patients with multiple myeloma also may be at increased risk from a contrast study. Prior dehydration (which promotes the intratubular precipitation of filtered light chains) and a possible interaction between the light chains and the contrast agent may be important in this setting.[162]

Prevention and Therapy

The best treatment of contrast-induced renal failure is prevention. The use, if possible, of ultrasonography or CT scanning without contrast is preferable, particularly in high-risk patients. Furthermore, lower doses of contrast should be used,[154,157,158] and repetitive studies that are closely spaced should be avoided. If possible, volume depletion should be corrected and nonsteroidal anti-inflammatory drugs should be discontinued before the initiation of contrast studies because both of these factors can increase renal vasoconstriction.

In addition to these preventive measures, there is suggestive evidence that hydration with mannitol (250 ml of a 20 percent mannitol solution administered beginning one hour after the contrast study) may offer some protection to high-risk patients.[158,163] Furosemide also may be protective in some animal models.[164,165] One study in which low-dose dopamine (2.5 µg/kg/min) was administered to 60 pa-

tients with chronic renal failure beginning at the onset of arteriography and continuing for 12 hours indicated that this measure reduced the incidence of contrast-induced acute renal failure.[166] Newer and much more expensive nonionic agents have not been shown to be less nephrotoxic than the standard contrast media when tested in patients with relatively normal renal function. A possible benefit may exist in high-risk patients.[156,158,167]

Platinum-induced Acute Renal Failure

Platinum-based compounds are effective chemotherapeutic agents that are also nephrotoxic.[168] Cisplatin, for example, leads to a cumulative decline in renal function. Approximately 25 to 35 percent of patients will develop a mild and partially reversible fall in GFR after the first course of therapy. The incidence and severity of renal failure increase with subsequent courses, eventually becoming irreversible. As a result, discontinuing therapy is generally indicated in those patients who experience a progressive rise in the plasma creatinine concentration. Preliminary studies suggest that carboplatin may be less toxic to the kidney than cisplatin; however, carboplatin appears to be more toxic to the bone marrow, particularly by inducing thrombocytopenia.[168,169]

The pathogenesis of cisplatin nephrotoxicity involves tubular cell injury. Within the kidney, the late S3 segment of the proximal tubule is most prominently affected, but the distal nephron also may be involved. Cisplatin is a potent tubular toxin, particularly in a low chloride environment such as the cell interior. In this setting, the chloride groups in the *cis* position of the cisplatin molecule are replaced by water molecules; this reaction is followed by the formation of highly reactive hydroxyl radicals that appear to produce injury by binding to nucleophilic sites on DNA.[168]

In addition to the rise in the plasma creatinine concentration, potentially irreversible hypomagnesemia resulting from urinary magnesium wasting occurs in over one half of patients treated with cisplatin.[170]

Subjects with normal renal function are able to make the urine virtually magnesium free once the plasma magnesium concentration falls below 1.5 mg/dl (the plasma magnesium level is 1.7 to 2.1 mg/dl).[171] Thus, a fractional excretion of magnesium (FE_{Mg}) higher than 2.5 percent is indicative of some component of magnesium wasting in this setting.[172] The value for FE_{Mg} can be calculated from a formula similar to that for the fractional excretion of sodium:

$$FE_{Mg} = \frac{U_{Mg} \times P_{Cr}}{(0.7 \times P_{Mg} \times U_{cr})} \times 100$$

The terms U_{Mg} and U_{Cr} refer to the urine concentrations (from a random specimen) of magnesium and creatinine, respectively, and P_{Mg} and P_{Cr} designate their plasma concentrations. The plasma magnesium concentration is multiplied by 0.7 because only about 70 percent of the circulating magnesium is free (i.e., not bound to albumin) and therefore able to be filtered across the glomerulus.

The urine output typically remains above 1,000 ml/day in such patients (unless renal failure is advanced), with a urine osmolality that is similar to that of the plasma. This concentrating defect probably reflects platinum-induced damage to the loop of Henle (where the countercurrent gradient that is required for urinary concentration is established) or the collecting tubules (the site of action of antidiuretic hormone).

Cisplatin may produce a different form of ARF when given together with bleomycin: a thrombotic microangiopathy with features of the hemolytic-uremic syndrome or thrombotic thrombocytopenic purpura. This disorder presumably reflects direct vascular injury with secondary platelet activation. Onset of renal failure may be abrupt or insidious; in the latter setting, it can develop months after therapy has been withdrawn. The diagnosis of this form of nephrotoxicity is suggested by the concurrent presence of a microangiopathic hemolytic anemia and thrombocytopenia. In experimental animals, I.V. glycine infusions protect against cisplatin nephrotoxicity, but this therapy is untested in humans.[172]

Prevention

There is evidence that the nephrotoxicity associated with cisplatin or carboplatin therapy can be diminished by vigorous hydration (250 ml of isotonic saline an hour) and perhaps by giving the drug in a hypertonic solution (such as 250 ml of three percent saline).[168,173] The high chloride concentration provided by hypertonic saline solutions may minimize the formation of the highly reactive platinum compounds that produce tubular injury (see above), whereas either the isotonic or the hypertonic solution may reduce the uptake of cisplatin by the renal tubular cells (by increasing the flow of filtrate).

Patients with intraperitoneal tumors may be treated with intraperitoneal cisplatin or carboplatin to achieve high local drug levels. Intravenous thiosulfate has been given concurrently so that it can react covalently with and bind to the platinum that enters the systemic circulation. The resulting complex has no systemic or renal toxicity and also has no antitumor effect[168,174]; thus, only the intraperitoneal drug remains active.

Heme-induced Acute Tubular Necrosis

Acute renal failure can be induced by the release of heme pigments, as occurs with myoglobinuria resulting from rhabdomyolysis and hemoglobinuria resulting from intravascular hemolysis.[175-177] The renal failure in this setting is caused by multiple factors, including obstructing intratubular heme pigment casts, pigment- and iron-induced cell toxicity (which may deplete ATP stores[178]), constriction and dilation of the afferent and efferent arterioles, respectively,[179] and volume depletion resulting from fluid sequestration in damaged muscle.

The most common causes of rhabdomyolysis are trauma (including ischemic muscle damage after a drug overdose), alcoholism, seizures, and exertional heat-stroke, particularly in physically unfit subjects or those with sickle cell trait.[175,180-182] Less frequent etiologies of rhabdomyolysis are hypokalemia, hypophosphatemia, cocaine intoxication, human immunodeficiency virus (HIV) infection or the administration of zidovudine (also known as azidothymidine, or AZT), the neuroleptic malignant syndrome, and the use of an inhibitor of 3-hydroxy-3-methylglutaryl coenzyme A (HMG-CoA) reductase (such as lovastatin) to treat hypercholesterolemia.[180-187] The risk of rhabdomyolysis is low when lovastatin is used alone, but it can be as high as 30 percent when the agent is given with cyclosporine and five to eight percent when it is given with gemfibrozil.[186,187]

Marked overproduction of hemoglobin or myoglobin typically leads to red or brown urine, unless pigment excretion is limited because of a low glomerular filtration rate or because the pigment is cleared from the plasma by extrarenal mechanisms.[180] These compounds, however, have different and diagnostically important effects on the color of the plasma. Hemoglobin is relatively poorly filtered because of its large size (molecular weight, 69,000 for the tetramer and 34,000 for the dimer) and because of protein binding to haptoglobin. As a result, hemoglobin reaches a relatively high total concentration in the plasma (before excretion in the urine), giving a red or brown tint to the normally straw-colored plasma. Myoglobin, in comparison, is a monomer (molecular weight, 17,000) and is not protein bound; consequently, it is rapidly filtered and excreted, and thus, the plasma retains its normal color when myoglobin is overproduced unless renal failure limits myoglobin excretion.

Patients with rhabdomyolysis typically present with the triad of pigmented granular casts in the urine, a red to brown color of the urine supernatant, and a marked elevation in the plasma level of creatine kinase. Other cellular elements also may be released, commonly resulting in hyperkalemia, hyperphosphatemia, and hypocalcemia (caused both by calcium phosphate precipitation in damaged muscle and calcium entry into the ischemic muscle cells); hyperuricemia and a rapid increase in the

plasma creatinine concentration are also observed.[175,180] In contrast to the findings in most other forms of acute tubular necrosis, the fractional excretion of sodium is often less than one percent, a finding that may reflect the primacy of tubular obstruction rather than tubular necrosis.[188]

Treatment and Prevention

Treatment is most effective if begun early; with rhabdomyolysis caused by crush injury, for example, therapy can be initiated before the crush is relieved and therefore before the heme pigment has been released into the circulation.[175,189] There are two major modalities that may prevent or minimize the severity of acute renal failure in this setting:

1. Hydration with isotonic saline, both to enhance renal perfusion (thereby minimizing ischemic injury) and to increase the urine output to wash out obstructing casts.

2. A forced alkaline-mannitol diuresis because raising the urine pH to more than 6.5 can markedly diminish the renal toxicity of myoglobin and hemoglobin. Alkalinization of the urine may increase the solubility of heme pigments and minimize the conversion of hemoglobin to the more toxic methemoglobin.[176,177]

There is a potential risk to alkalinization because it can promote the precipitation of calcium phosphate and can lower the ionized calcium concentration. The net effect is likely to be beneficial, however, if therapy is begun early.[175]

The aim of initial treatment is to maintain the urine output at about 300 ml/hr until pigmenturia has ceased. In the first six to 12 hours after hydration has been initiated following a crush injury, most patients with rhabdomyolysis will be in markedly positive fluid balance as a result of fluid sequestration into damaged muscle.[175] This hydration regimen is less likely to be effective and may lead to symptomatic fluid overload if it is begun after this initial period when the renal failure may already be established.[175]

One last problem that is unique to rhabdomyolysis-induced acute renal failure is the development of hypercalcemia during the recovery phase in approximately 20 to 30 percent of patients.[190,191] In part, this problem results from the mobilization of calcium that has been deposited in the injured muscle.[192] Both correction of hyperphosphatemia (resulting from the rise in glomerular filtration rate) and an unexplained increase in 1,25-dihydroxyvitamin D_3 also contribute to this response.[190] To minimize this complication, the administration of calcium should be avoided during the renal failure phase unless the patient has symptomatic hypocalcemia or severe hyperkalemia.

Acute Uric Acid Nephropathy

There are three different types of uric acid renal disease: uric acid nephrolithiasis, chronic urate nephropathy, and acute uric acid nephropathy. Chronic urate nephropathy is a form of chronic renal failure induced by the deposition of sodium urate crystals in the medullary interstitium. This deposition leads to a secondary inflammatory response (similar to that seen with microtophus formation elsewhere in the body), eventually leading to interstitial fibrosis and chronic renal failure. Although urate nephropathy was seen in the past in patients with tophaceous gout, both tophus formation and particularly urate nephropathy are currently rare.[193] There are patients who have chronic renal insufficiency, a bland urine sediment, and hyperuricemia out of proportion to the degree of renal insufficiency, findings compatible with urate nephropathy. However, in the great majority of these patients, lead intoxication appears to be the primary problem.[194-196]

Acute uric acid nephropathy (UAN), in comparison, is characterized by acute oliguric or anuric renal failure caused by uric acid precipitation within the tubules.[197] UAN most often is the result of overproduction and oversecretion of uric acid in patients with lymphoma, leukemia, or a myeloproliferative disease (such as polycythemia vera), particularly after chemotherapy or radiation has induced rapid cell lysis. Less frequent causes of UAN include tissue catabolism resulting from seizures or from treatment of solid tumors; primary overproduction of uric acid, as occurs in the rare syndrome of hypoxanthine-guanine phosphoribosyltransferase deficiency; or hyperuricosuria resulting from decreased uric acid reabsorption in the proximal tubule, as can occur with a Fanconi-like syndrome.[197,198]

UAN is typically associated with no symptoms referable to the urinary tract, although flank pain can occur if there is renal pelvic or ureteral obstruction. The diagnosis should be suspected when otherwise unexplained acute renal failure develops in any of the above settings in association with marked hyperuricemia (plasma uric acid concentration generally higher than 15 mg/dl). In most other forms of acute renal failure, the plasma uric acid concentration is less than 12 mg/dl, except for prerenal disease in which there is an increase in sodium and urate reabsorption in the proximal tubule.

The urinalysis in UAN may show many uric acid crystals, but it can be relatively normal when there is no output from the obstructed nephrons. Overexcretion of uric acid can be documented in many patients by the finding of a uric acid to creatinine ratio (mg/mg) higher than 1.0 on a random urine specimen; in comparison, the value is less than 0.60 to 0.75 in most other forms of acute renal failure.[199]

Release of other intracellular constituents also occurs when there is marked tissue breakdown, possibly leading to hyperkalemia, hyperphosphatemia, and hypocalcemia (caused by the deposition of calcium phosphate in tissues). In some individuals, precipitation of calcium and phosphate in the renal tubules can induce acute renal failure, independent of uric acid precipitation.[200]

Prevention and Treatment

The ideal therapy for UAN is prevention. Patients about to receive chemotherapy or radiation for a cancer with a rapid cell turnover should be pretreated with allopurinol (initially with higher than normal doses of

600 to 900 mg/day) plus fluid loading to maintain a high urine output (more than 2.5 L/day) with or without sodium bicarbonate for urinary alkalinization (urine pH of about 6.5). In an alkaline urine, uric acid will be converted to the more soluble urate salt, thereby diminishing the tendency to uric acid precipitation. Even with optimal prophylaxis, however, the degree of cell lysis is so great that acute renal failure will still develop in some patients.[197]

Therapy of early renal failure consists of administering allopurinol (if it has not already been given) and attempting to wash out the obstructing uric acid crystals with a loop diuretic and fluids. Careful monitoring is essential, however, because retention of the administered fluid may cause volume overload leading to pulmonary edema. Hemodialysis to remove the excess circulating uric acid should be used in those patients in whom a diuresis cannot be induced. The prognosis for complete recovery is excellent if treatment is initiated rapidly.

The role of urinary alkalinization with acetazolamide and sodium bicarbonate is less clear. Experimental studies suggest that hydration with saline alone is as effective as alkalinization in minimizing uric acid precipitation.[201] Even when bicarbonate is administered, it may be difficult to raise the urine pH in the patient with acute renal failure. Alkalinization also has the potential disadvantage of promoting calcium phosphate deposition in patients with marked hyperphosphatemia.

Amphotericin B Nephrotoxicity

Amphotericin B is used in the treatment of life-threatening fungal infections. Its administration, however, is frequently associated with renal functional impairment that may be manifested by a rise in the plasma creatinine concentration, urinary potassium wasting and hypokalemia, urinary magnesium wasting and hypomagnesemia, metabolic acidosis caused by type 1 (or distal) renal tubular acidosis, and polyuria resulting from nephrogenic diabetes insipidus.[202-204] However, not all patients develop renal failure, and long-term therapy (i.e., longer than one year) may not result in a decline in renal function.[205]

The fall in GFR induced by amphotericin B may exceed 50 percent and is associated with concurrent renal vasoconstriction. These changes are manifested clinically by an elevation (above baseline) in the plasma creatinine concentration of up to 2.5 mg/dl.[202,206] The fall in GFR usually begins within the first two weeks of therapy. More severe renal failure resulting from the administration of amphotericin B alone is uncommon even with continued therapy but can occur with diuretic-induced volume depletion or the concurrent administration of another nephrotoxin, such as an aminoglycoside antibiotic.[203] The likelihood of renal disease is also dose dependent, with the risk of renal dysfunction being relatively low at dosages of less than 0.5 mg/kg/day.[207]

The mechanism by which these changes occur is incompletely understood. It has been proposed that the tubular changes induced by amphotericin B may play an important role, perhaps by activating the tubuloglomerular feedback system. Under most circumstances, increased sodium reabsorption by the macula densa cells in the early distal tubule leads to a reduction in the GFR.[208] This feedback is physiologically appropriate because the increase in NaCl entry usually reflects increased NaCl delivery out of the proximal tubule; reducing the GFR lowers distal delivery back toward normal, thereby preventing excessive NaCl losses.

In comparison, amphotericin B interacts with membrane sterols, thereby increasing membrane permeability, a process that may activate the tubuloglomerular feedback system.[202,209] Within the macula densa cells in the early distal tubule, the ensuing increase in entry can activate the feedback system, causing a reduction in the GFR.[202,206]

The increase in membrane permeability induced by amphotericin B is also thought to account for the electrolyte abnormalities that may be seen in patients receiving this drug. The increased permeability can promote distal potassium secretion down the favorable concentration gradient between the cell and the tubular lumen[210]; it can also diminish net hydrogen secretion. A urine pH of 5.0, for example, represents a hydrogen ion concentration that is more than 200 times greater than that in the extracellular fluid. An increase in tubular permeability will promote the back-diffusion of secreted hydrogen ions, thus limiting acid excretion.[211,212]

The net effect of these changes is that both hypokalemia and metabolic acidosis are commonly seen and are caused by potassium loss and hydrogen retention, respectively.[210-212] Resistance to antidiuretic hormone and decreased net magnesium reabsorption also may occur, possibly leading to polyuria and polydipsia and hypomagnesemia.[204] Unlike the decline in GFR, these signs of tubular dysfunction do not appear to be ameliorated by volume expansion.[213]

The nephrotoxicity associated with amphotericin B is usually reversible with discontinuation of therapy.[206,214] However, renal dysfunction can recur if treatment is reinstituted.[214]

Prevention and Treatment

The hypothesis that tubuloglomerular feedback may be activated by amphotericin B has led to the use of saline loading because volume expansion reduces the sensitivity of this system. Studies in both humans and animals have shown that saline loading can protect against or ameliorate the amphotericin B–induced decline in GFR.[202,206,213] It has not been proved, however, that this beneficial effect is related to tubuloglomerular feedback.

Studies suggest that the incidence and severity of these renal abnormalities can be minimized by administering amphotericin B in phospholipid vesicles (liposomes).[215] The liposomes may be preferentially distributed to the reticuloendothelial system, where amphotericin B can be transferred directly to trapped fungi, thereby diminishing its delivery to other cholesterol-containing cells such as those in the renal tubules. Despite initially favorable findings, further

observations on a larger number of patients are required before the role of this therapy can be more accurately defined.[216]

In addition, observations in animals suggest that a calcium channel blocker given shortly before and again after amphotericin B administration protects against nephrotoxicity.[217] The precise mechanism of this effect and its potential application to humans are unclear.

Pentamidine-induced Acute Renal Failure

Pneumonia caused by *Pneumocystis carinii* in patients with acquired immunodeficiency syndrome (AIDS) is often treated with relatively high doses of intravenous pentamidine. In this setting, reversible acute renal failure is a relatively common complication, occurring in more than 25 percent of patients in some series.[218,219] A decline in renal function can also rarely occur with aerosolized pentamidine therapy.[220]

The mechanism by which pentamidine produces acute renal failure is unclear, but a direct nephrotoxic effect, leading to acute tubular necrosis, is probably involved. As is the case with other tubular toxins (such as the aminoglycosides, cisplatin, and amphotericin B), pentamidine can also induce urinary magnesium wasting, leading to hypomagnesemia and hypocalcemia.[221] In contrast to the effect of these other tubular toxins (with which hypokalemia is commonly seen), pentamidine has produced hyperkalemia, which may be related to the severity of the renal failure.[218]

Discontinuation of pentamidine leads to recovery of renal function, although such recovery may not occur for several weeks.[218,221] Persistence of pentamidine in the renal parenchyma after the cessation of therapy probably contributes to the delay in improvement.[218]

Patients who develop pentamidine nephrotoxicity should be treated, when necessary, with alternative agents such as trimethoprim-sulfamethoxazole. Retreatment with pentamidine should be avoided if possible because renal failure can recur.[218]

Acyclovir-induced Acute Renal Failure

Acute renal failure is a not uncommon complication of therapy with intravenous acyclovir, which is usually given in a dose of 500 mg/m^2. Acyclovir is primarily excreted in the urine and has a relatively low solubility. Thus, bolus intravenous therapy, particularly if the patient is not well hydrated, can lead to the deposition of acyclovir crystals in the tubules, resulting in intratubular obstruction and foci of interstitial inflammation.[222]

Renal function typically begins to deteriorate soon after therapy is initiated. Patients may complain of nausea and flank or abdominal pain at this time, presumably induced by the urinary tract obstruction.[222] In some cases, birefringent needle-shaped acyclovir crystals can be seen in the urine when a specimen is viewed under polarized light.

The decline in renal function may be severe, with the plasma creatinine concentration occasionally exceeding 8 mg/dl. However, complete recovery typically occurs within four to nine days after withdrawal of acyclovir.

It is likely that most cases of acyclovir nephrotoxicity can be prevented by prior hydration (with the urine output maintained at a level higher than 75 ml/hr) and slow infusion of the drug over the course of one to two hours. Patients who develop acute renal failure can usually be safely rechallenged, if necessary, by limiting the dose of intravenous acyclovir to 250 mg/m^2 or less.[222]

A complication similar to that produced by acyclovir can be induced by other drugs that can also precipitate in the tubules, including sulfonamide antibiotics such as sulfadiazine or sulfamethoxazole (commonly used to treat toxoplasmosis in AIDS patients), high doses of vitamin C, which is partially metabolized to oxalate, and high doses of methotrexate.[223-226] When ARF develops as a result of methotrexate toxicity, bone marrow suppression is more likely to occur.

References

1. Am J Physiol 256:F430, 1989
2. Ann Intern Med 89:47, 1978
3. Am J Kidney Dis 6:71, 1985
4. Am J Med 71:916, 1981
5. Arch Intern Med 140:907, 1980
6. Clin Nephrol 13:73, 1980
7. Am J Med 77: 699, 1984
8. Am J Nephrol 6:450, 1986
9. Ann Intern Med 113:155, 1990
10. Kidney Int 25:53, 1984
11. Kidney Int 32:1, 1987
12. Lancet 1:225, 1984
13. Ann Intern Med. 106:346, 1987
14. Circulation 40:893, 1969
15. Surgery 89:434, 1981
16. Surgery 89:525, 1981
17. Am J Med 87:359, 1989
18. Intensive Care Medicine, 2nd ed. Little, Brown & Co, Boston, 1991, p 794
19. Ann Intern Med 93:723, 1980
20. Gastroenterology 81:205, 1981
21. Kidney Int 23:303, 1983
22. Ann Intern Med 105:573, 1986
23. J Clin Invest 72:1594, 1983
24. N Engl J Med 307:1552, 1982
25. Kidney Int 30:417, 1986
26. Kidney Int 24:788, 1983
27. Gastroenterology 99:766, 1990
28. Am J Med 59:165, 1975
29. Am J Med 49:175, 1970
30. Am J Med 82:945, 1987
31. Ann Intern Med 94:198, 1981
32. N Engl J Med 280:1367, 1969
33. Kidney Int 26:72, 1984
34. Gastroenterology 90:274, 1986
35. Gastroenterology 97:1304, 1989
36. Gastroenterology 73:1114, 1977
37. Kidney Int 15:54, 1979
38. Kidney Int 30:736, 1986
39. Am J Med 82:427, 1987
40. Gastroenterology 80:119, 1981
41. Br Med J 292:1351, 1986
42. Gastroenterology 84:961, 1983
43. Gastroenterology 92:294, 1987
44. Ann Intern Med 114:886, 1991
45. Gastroenterology 51:1046, 1966
46. Gastroenterology 90:1827, 1986
47. Gastroenterology 93:234, 1987
48. Gastroenterology 94:1493, 1988
49. Hepatology 8:207, 1988
50. Ann Intern Med 112:889, 1990
51. Pathophysiology of Renal Disease, 2nd ed. McGraw-Hill Book Co, New York, 1987, p 63
52. Br Med J 2:338, 1978
53. Kidney Int 29:598, 1986
54. Gastroenterology 90:182, 1986
55. Am J Kidney Dis 8:351, 1986
56. Ann Intern Med 112:568, 1990
57. J Clin Invest 46:1894, 1967
58. Kidney Int 9:511, 1976
59. Gastroenterology 82:790, 1982
60. N Engl J Med 321:1632, 1989
61. J Hepatol 9(suppl 1):S86, 1989
62. Am J Surg 139:125, 1980
63. Ann Surg 201:488, 1985
64. N Engl J Med 321:1675, 1989
65. Kidney Int 3:1402, 1987
66. Am J Physiol 245:H98, 1983
67. J Clin Invest 57:1606, 1976
68. Circ Res 31:881, 1972
69. Am J Cardiol 55:1032, 1985
70. N Engl J Med 312:277, 1985
71. Lancet 2:551, 1988
72. Circulation 73:257, 1986
73. N Engl J Med 310:347, 1984
74. Circulation 37:900, 1968
75. N Engl J Med 319:761, 1988

76. J Clin Invest 69:1366, 1982
77. N Engl J Med 316:1429, 1987
78. Am Heart J 115:1085, 1988
79. JAMA 259:539, 1988
80. N Engl J Med 319:80, 1988
81. Ann Intern Med 100:777, 1984
82. Am J Cardiol 58:300, 1986
83. Kidney Int 32:845, 1987
84. J Am Coll Cardiol 10:837, 1987
85. N Engl J Med 315:847, 1986
86. J Am Coll Cardiol 13:1240, 1989
87. Ann Intern Med 104:147, 1986
88. Am J Med 73:719, 1982
89. Am J Physiol 252:H566, 1987
90. J Am Coll Cardiol 8:1467, 1986
91. Medicine 58:362, 1979
92. N Engl J Med 270:1373, 1964
93. J Clin Invest 73:329, 1984
94. Kidney Int 26:375, 1984
95. Am J Kidney Dis 13:253, 1989
96. N Engl J Med 314:97, 1986
97. Mayo Clin Proc 63:390, 1988
98. Kidney Int 38:282, 1990
99. N Engl J Med 312:159, 1985
100. Nephron 49:9, 1988
101. Am J Physiol 241:F556, 1981
102. Am J Physiol 247:F365, 1984
103. Kidney Int 40: 21, 1991
104. Kidney Int 37:171, 1990
105. Kidney Int 37:1148, 1990
106. Am J Physiol 258:F1266, 1990
107. Kidney Int 32:313, 1987
108. Am J Physiol 259:F80, 1990
109. Am J Kidney Dis 13:114, 1989
110. Am J Med Sci 259:168, 1970
111. Nephron 37:39, 1984
112. Clin Nephrol 15:90, 1981
113. Ann Intern Med 115:153, 1991
114. N Engl J Med 272:1116, 1965
115. Am J Med 42:648, 1967
116. Medicine (Baltimore) 69:153, 1990
117. N Engl J Med 296:1134, 1977
118. Nephron 51:307, 1989
119. J Clin Invest 85:766, 1990
120. J Clin Invest 84:1757, 1989
121. Am J Physiol 259:F438, 1990
122. J Clin Invest 82:532, 1988
123. N Engl J Med 308:8, 1983
124. N Engl J Med 315:731, 1986
125. Clin Nephrol 25:249, 1986
126. Arch Intern Med 138:950, 1978
127. Kidney Int 34:791, 1988
128. Am Heart J 113:1138, 1987
129. Kidney Int 7:103, 1975
130. J Lab Clin Med 98:21, 1981
131. Kidney Int 33:900, 1988
132. Ann Intern Med 100:352, 1984
133. N Engl J Med 302:1106, 1980
134. Am J Kidney Dis 8:292, 1986
135. Am J Med 80(suppl 6B):119, 1986
136. Am J Nephrol 3:11, 1983
137. J Pharmacol Exp Ther 251:937, 1989
138. J Infect Dis 159:945, 1989
139. Am J Physiol 258:C1141, 1990
140. Kidney Int 37:1492, 1990
141. Antimicrob Agents Chemother 27:897, 1985
142. Clin Pharmacol Ther 45:22, 1989
143. Kidney Int 38:459, 1990
144. Nephron 16:31, 1976
145. Am J Physiol 254:F574, 1988
146. Nephron 53:138, 1989
147. Am J Med 85:47, 1988
148. Lancet 2:604, 1978
149. Am J Med 80(suppl 6B):119, 1986
150. Nephron 23:50, 1979
151. Arch Intern Med 136:1101, 1976
152. J Lab Clin Med 112:694, 1988
153. N Engl J Med 320:143, 1989
154. Ann Intern Med 104:501, 1986
155. Ann Intern Med 110:119, 1989
156. N Engl J Med 320:149, 1989
157. Am J Med 86:649, 1989
158. Kidney Int 36:730, 1989
159. Am J Physiol 258:F115, 1990
160. Journal of the American Society of Nephrology 1:596, 1990
161. Ann Intern Med 86:56, 1977
162. Kidney Int 27:46, 1985
163. Arch Intern Med 141:1652, 1981
164. Kidney Int 36:730, 1989
165. Am J Kidney Dis 14:377, 1989
166. Radiology 176:651, 1990
167. Am J Kidney Dis 13:189, 1989
168. Am J Kidney Dis 8:368, 1986
169. Ann Intern Med 110:409, 1989
170. Ann Intern Med 90:929, 1979
171. Am J Kidney Dis 8:164, 1986
172. Kidney Int 40:273, 1991
173. Ann Intern Med 100:19, 1984
174. Ann Intern Med 97:845, 1982
175. N Engl J Med 322:825, 1990
176. Am J Physiol 256:F446, 1989
177. Lab Invest 60:619, 1989
178. Kidney Int 39:111, 1991
179. J Clin Invest 84:1967, 1989
180. Medicine (Baltimore) 61:141, 1982
181. Kidney Int 23:888, 1983
182. Ann Intern Med 115:99, 1991
183. N Engl J Med 313:163, 1985
184. N Engl J Med 319:673, 1988
185. N Engl J Med 322:1098, 1990
186. N Engl J Med 318:47, 1988
187. JAMA 264:71, 1990
188. Arch Intern Med 144:981, 1984
189. Arch Intern Med 144:277, 1984
190. J Clin Endocrinol Metab 63:137, 1986
191. N Engl J Med 305:117, 1981
192. Am J Med 89:523, 1990
193. Kidney Int 30:280, 1986
194. N Engl J Med 304:520, 1981
195. Kidney Int 26:319, 1984
196. N Engl J Med 309:17, 1983
197. Arch Intern Med 133:349, 1974
198. Am J Med 84:153, 1988
199. Arch Intern Med 138:612, 1978
200. Clin Nephrol 22:47, 1984
201. J Clin Invest 58:681, 1976
202. Arch Intern Med 148:2389, 1988
203. Ann Intern Med 61:175, 1964
204. Am J Med 77:471, 1984
205. Am J Med 85:591, 1988
206. Am J Med 75:476, 1983
207. Am J Med 87:547, 1989
208. Kidney Int 38:577, 1990
209. Kidney Int 22:626, 1982
210. Am J Med 46:154, 1969
211. Pflugers Arch 413:280, 1989
212. Kidney Int 30:546, 1986
213. Am J Kidney Dis 11:313, 1988
214. Arch Intern Med 147:593, 1987
215. Arch Intern Med 149:2533, 1989
216. Arch Intern Med 149:2402, 1989
217. Journal of the American Society of Nephrology 2:98, 1991
218. Am J Med 87:260, 1989
219. Ann Intern Med 109:280, 1988
220. Lancet 1:1271, 1989
221. Am J Med 89:380, 1990
222. Am J Med 84:1067, 1988
223. Br Med J 2:172, 1978
224. Am J Kidney Dis 12:72, 1988
225. Cancer Treat Rep 61:695, 1977
226. Ann Intern Med 100:530, 1984

Acknowledgments

Table 1 Adapted from *Clinical Problems in Nephrology*, by B. D. Rose and R. M. Black. Little, Brown & Co., Boston, 1988, p. 140. Used by permission.

Figure 1 Janet Betries.

Figures 2 and 3 Dana Burns.

Reproduced by special arrangement with
WILLIAM M. BENNETT, M.D., and SUZANNE K. SWAN, M.D.
[Adapted in part from *Drug Prescribing in Renal Failure: Dosing Guidelines for Adults*, 2nd ed., by W.M. Bennett, G.R. Aronoff, T.A. Golper, et al. American College of Physicians, Philadelphia, 1991]

The various categories of drugs appear as follows:

Antimicrobial Agents (pages 730–739)
Analgesics (pages 739–741)
Sedatives, Hypnotics, and Drugs Used in Psychiatry (pages 741–745)
Cardiovascular and Antihypertensive Agents (pages 745–754)
Miscellaneous Agents (pages 754–763)

Antimicrobial Agents

Drug	Elimination and Metabolism	Method	Adjustment for Renal Failure			Removed by Dialysis	Toxic Effects and Remarks (GT — group toxicity; GR — group remarks)
			GFR (ml/min)				
			>50	10–50	<10		
Aminoglyco-sides*†							*GT: all agents in this group nephrotoxic and ototoxic; rarely cause respiratory paralysis †GR: need usual loading doses in renal failure patients; blood levels best guide to therapy; concurrent penicillin administration may result in subtherapeutic blood levels
Amikacin	R	D* I	60–90 12	30–70 12–18	20–30 24	Yes (He, P)	GT; GR *D and I methods are combined
Gentamicin	R	D* I	60–90 8–12	30–70 12	20–30 24	Yes (He, P)†	GT; GR; absorption of 50% of intraperitoneal dose in 6-hr continuous ambulatory peritoneal dialysis (CAPD) exchange; poor clearance from blood to peritoneum in CAPD *D and I methods are combined †May add 5 mg to each liter of peritoneal dialysate to obtain satisfactory serum levels
Netilmicin	R	D* I	60–90 8–12	30–70 12	20–30 24	Yes (He, P)	GT; GR *D and I methods are combined
Tobramycin	R	D* I	60–90 8–12	30–70 12	20–30 24	Yes (He, P)†	GT; GR *D and I methods are combined †May add 4–5 mg to each liter of peritoneal dialysate to obtain satisfactory serum levels

Antimicrobial Agents (continued)

Drug	Elimination and Metabolism	Method	Adjustment for Renal Failure			Removed by Dialysis	Toxic Effects and Remarks (GT — group toxicity; GR — group remarks)
			GFR (ml/min)				
			>50	10–50	<10		
Antifungal drugs Amphotericin B	Non-R	I	24	24	24–36†	No (He, P)	Nephrotoxic; renal tubular acidosis; hypokalemia; renal failure; nephrogenic diabetes insipidus *Terminal phase half-life equals 15 days because of drug movement from a slowly equilibrating compartment †Ineffective for renal parenchymal infection
Fluconazole	R	D	Unch	50–100	25	Yes (He)*	May increase blood cyclosporine levels *Patients on peritoneal dialysis should receive 50–100 mg daily
Flucytosine	R	I	6	12–24	24–48	Yes (He, P)*	Hepatic dysfunction; marrow suppression more common in azotemic patients; either D or I method is applicable *Dose of 20–30 mg/kg needed after hemodialysis
		D	50	30–50	20–30		
Itraconazole	H	D	Unch	Unch	Unch	No (He, P)	—
Ketoconazole	H	D	Unch	Unch	Unch	No (He)	May increase blood cyclosporine levels
Antimycobacterial drugs Clofazimine	Non-R	D	Unch	Unch	Unch	No (He, P)	—
Ethambutol	R	I	24	24–36	48	Yes (He, P)	Decreased visual acuity; peripheral neuritis may mimic uremia

Abbreviations used in table:

R — renal
H — hepatic

I — interval extension method of dosage adjustment; data units are hours between maintenance doses
D — dose reduction method of dosage adjustment; data units are percent of usual maintenance dose

Unch — unchanged
He — hemodialysis
P — peritoneal dialysis

ESRD — end-stage renal disease
GFR — glomerular filtration rate

Antimicrobial Agents (continued)

Drug	Elimination and Metabolism	Method	Adjustment for Renal Failure				Toxic Effects and Remarks (GT — group toxicity; GR — group remarks)
			GFR (ml/min)			Removed by Dialysis	
			>50	10–50	<10		
Isoniazid	H* (R)	D	Unch	Unch	66–75	Yes (He, P)	*Genetic variation in hepatic acetylation. Adjustment for renal failure values apply to slow acetylators.
	—	—	—	—	—	—	—
Pyrazinamide	H	D	Unch	Unch	50–100	Yes (He)	Hyperuricemia
Rifampin	H	I	Unch	Unch	Unch	No (He)	May cause acute renal failure (toxic or immunologic), potassium wasting, and other tubular defects
Antiviral agents Acyclovir	R	I	8	24	48	Yes (He)	CNS toxicity in patients with renal failure; may cause acute renal failure if injected rapidly intravenously
2',3'-Dideoxy-cytidine (ddC)	R	D*	Unch	50–75	25–50	?	*Recommendations for dosage reduction method based on limited clinical data
2',3'-Dideoxy-inosine (ddI)	H (R)	D*	Unch	75–100	50–75	?	Hyperuricemia *Recommendations for dosage reduction method based on limited clinical data
Foscarnet	R	D	50–100	15–50	Avoid	Yes (He)	Nonoliguric acute renal dysfunction is common
Ganciclovir	R	I	12–18	18–24	24	Yes (He)	Neutropenia may be more common if drug accumulates
Vidarabine	R (H)	D	100	100	75	Yes (He)	50% of active hypoxanthine metabolite is excreted by the kidney
Zidovudine (AZT)	H (R)	D	100	75	50	Yes (He)	Inactive metabolite accumulates in renal failure

Antimicrobial Agents (continued)

Drug	Elimination and Metabolism	Method	Adjustment for Renal Failure			Removed by Dialysis	Toxic Effects and Remarks (GT — group toxicity; GR — group remarks)
			GFR (ml/min)				
			>50	10–50	<10		
Cephalosporins*							*GT: agents in this group may enhance nephrotoxicity if given in combination with aminoglycoside antibiotics, diuretics, and volume depletion; rare allergic interstitial nephritis; well absorbed from peritoneal fluid in CAPD, but transfer from blood to peritoneum is generally poor; some agents may cause bleeding in patients with renal failure
Cefamandole	R	I	6	6–8	12	Yes (He)	GT
Cefazolin	R	I	8	12	24–48	Yes (He); No (P)	GT; ineffective for urinary tract infections when GFR <10 ml/min
Cefixime	R (H)	I	12	12	24	No (He, P)	GT
Cefmenoxime	R	I	6–8	8–12	12–24	Yes (He)	GT
Cefoperazone	H	I	Unch	Unch	Unch	No (He, P)	GT; administer drug after dialysis
Cefotaxime	R (H)	I	6–8	8–12	12–24	Yes (He); No (P)	GT *Half-life of desacetyl active metabolite 10 hr in ESRD
Cefotetan	R	D	Unch	50	25	Yes (He); No (P)	GT
Cefoxitin	R	I	8	8–12	24–48	Yes (He); No (P)	GT; may raise serum creatinine levels by interference with autoanalyzer methods
Ceftazidime	R	I	8–12	24–48	48–72	Yes (He, P)	GT
Ceftizoxime	R	I	8–12	36–48	48–72	Yes (He)	GT

Abbreviations used in table:

R — renal
H — hepatic

I — interval extension method of dosage adjustment; data units are hours between maintenance doses
D — dose reduction method of dosage adjustment; data units are percent of usual maintenance dose

Unch — unchanged
He — hemodialysis
P — peritoneal dialysis

ESRD — end-stage renal disease
GFR — glomerular filtration rate

Antimicrobial Agents (continued)

Drug	Elimination and Metabolism	Method	Adjustment for Renal Failure			Removed by Dialysis	Toxic Effects and Remarks (GT — group toxicity; GR — group remarks)
			GFR (ml/min)				
			>50	10–50	<10		
Ceftriaxone	R (H)	D	Unch	Unch	Unch	No (He, P)	GT; associated with cholelithiasis
Cephalexin	R	I	6	6–8	6–12*	Yes (He)	GT *Need usual doses to treat urinary tract infections
Cephapirin	R (H)	I	6	6–8	12	Yes (He); No (P)	GT
Cephradine	R	D	Unch	50	25	Yes (He, P)	GT
Chloroquine*	R (H)	D	Unch	Unch†	50‡	No (He)	Excretion enhanced in alkaline urine *Refers only to dose for malarial infection †150 mg/day ‡If prolonged treatment is necessary, cut dose to 50–100 mg/day
Cilastatin	R (H)	D	Unch	50	Avoid	Yes (He)	—
Clavulanic acid	R	D	Unch	Unch	50–75	Yes (He)	Combined with amoxicillin or ticarcillin for clinical use
Clindamycin	H (R)	D	Unch	Unch	Unch	No (He, P)	Pseudomembranous enterocolitis may cause volume depletion
Imipenem	R (H)	I D	6 100	8 75	12 50	Yes (He)	Combine with cilastatin, a dipeptidase inhibitor that has similar kinetics to imipenem, to prevent renal inactivation

Drug	Elimination and Metabolism	Method	Adjustment for Renal Failure			Removed by Dialysis	Toxic Effects and Remarks (GT — group toxicity; GR — group remarks)
			GFR (ml/min)				
			>50	10–50	<10		
Macrolides							
Clarithromycin	H (R)	D	Unch	Unch	50–75	?	Increases theophylline serum levels; hepatotoxicity reported in animal models
Erythromycin	H (R)	D	Unch	Unch	50–75	No (He, P)	*Doubled in ESRD; may be ototoxic in renal failure
Metronidazole*	H (R)†	D	Unch	Unch	50	Yes (He); No (P)	Neurotoxic (vestibular); gastrointestinal symptoms may mimic uremia *Recommendations pertain to bacterial infections †Active metabolites have long half-life in ESRD
Monobactams							
Aztreonam	R	D	Unch	50–75	25	Yes (He); No (P)	—
Carumonam	R	D* / I	Unch / Unch	Unch / 12–24	50 / 24	Yes (He)	*D and I methods are combined
Nitrofurantoin	Non-R (R)	D	Unch	Avoid*	Avoid*	Yes (He)	Peripheral sensory neuropathy caused by accumulation of metabolites; excretion enhanced in alkaline urine; may elevate blood urea nitrogen (BUN) and urinary creatinine levels spuriously *Ineffective when GFR <20–30 ml/min

Antimicrobial Agents (continued)

Abbreviations used in table:

R — renal
H — hepatic

I — interval extension method of dosage adjustment; data units are hours between maintenance doses
D — dose reduction method of dosage adjustment; data units are percent of usual maintenance dose

Unch — unchanged
He — hemodialysis
P — peritoneal dialysis

ESRD — end-stage renal disease
GFR — glomerular filtration rate

Antimicrobial Agents (continued)

Drug	Elimination and Metabolism	Method	GFR (ml/min)			Removed by Dialysis	Toxic Effects and Remarks (GT — group toxicity; GR — group remarks)
			>50	10–50	<10		
Penicillins*							*GT: agents in this group may cause allergic interstitial nephritis; seizures and coagulopathy at high blood levels
Amoxicillin*	R (H)	I	6	6–12	12–16†	Yes (He); No (P)	GT *Same data apply for amoxicillin esters (bacampicillin, hetacillin, pivampicillin, talampicillin) †High doses needed to treat urinary tract infections in ESRD
Ampicillin	R (H)	I	6	6–12	12–16*	Yes (He); No (P)	GT; contains 3 mEq Na$^+$/g *High doses needed to treat urinary tract infections in ESRD; adverse reactions more common in renal failure
Azlocillin	R (H)	I	4–6	6–8	8	Yes (He); No (P)	GT; contains 2.7 mEq Na$^+$/g
Carbenicillin	R (H)	I	8–12	12–24	24–48*	Yes (He); No (P)†	GT; may inactivate aminoglycosides; acidosis at high blood levels; contains 4.7 mEq Na$^+$/g; can cause hypokalemic alkalosis *Ineffective for treating urinary tract infections when GFR <15 ml/min †May be added to peritoneal dialysate
Cloxacillin	R (H)	D	Unch	Unch	Unch	No (He)	GT
Dicloxacillin	R (H)	I	Unch	Unch	Unch	No (He)*	GT *May be added to peritoneal dialysate
Mezlocillin	R (H)	I	4–6	6–8	8	Yes (He, P)	GT; elimination is dose dependent; contains 1.9 mEq Na$^+$/g
Nafcillin	H (R)	D	Unch	Unch	Unch	No (He)	GT; dose must be reduced in combined hepatic and renal failure to avoid high serum levels and coagulopathy

Adjustment for Renal Failure

Drug	Elimination and Metabolism	Method	Adjustment for Renal Failure			Removed by Dialysis	Toxic Effects and Remarks (GT — group toxicity; GR — group remarks)
			GFR (ml/min)				
			>50	10–50	<10		
Antimicrobial Agents (continued)							
Penicillin G	R (H)	D I	Unch 6–8	75 8–12	25–50 12–16	Yes (He); No (P)*	GT; upper limit of 4–6 million U/day in severe renal failure; false positive urine protein reactions with biuret reagent and sulfosalicylic acid; potassium salt has 1.7 mEq K^+/million units *May be added to peritoneal dialysate
Piperacillin	R (H)	I	4–6	6–8	8	Yes (He)	GT; contains 1.9 mEq Na^+/g; elimination is dose dependent
Ticarcillin	R	I	8–12	12–24	24–48	Yes (He, P)	GT; remarks same as carbenicillin; contains 5.2 mEq Na^+/g
Pentamidine	R	I	24	24–36	48	No (He, P)	Nephrotoxic *Tissue uptake extensive
Pyrimethamine	Non-R* (H)	D	Unch	Unch	Unch	?	*Metabolites excreted in urine for weeks because of tissue storage
Quinolones Ciprofloxacin	R (H)	I D	Unch Unch	12–24 75	24 50	No (P) Yes (He)	Poorly absorbed if taken with antacids or phosphate binders
Lomefloxacin	R (H)	D	Unch	50–100	50	No (He, P)	—
Norfloxacin	H (R)	D	Unch	12–24	Avoid	No (He)	—
Ofloxacin	R	I	Unch	24	24–36	No (He)	—
Pefloxacin	H	D	Unch	Unch	Unch	No (He)	—

Abbreviations used in table:

R — renal
H — hepatic

I — interval extension method of dosage adjustment; data units are hours between maintenance doses

D — dose reduction method of dosage adjustment; data units are percent of usual maintenance dose

Unch — unchanged
He — hemodialysis
P — peritoneal dialysis

ESRD — end-stage renal disease
GFR — glomerular filtration rate

Antimicrobial Agents (continued)

Drug	Elimination and Metabolism	Adjustment for Renal Failure					Toxic Effects and Remarks (GT — group toxicity; GR — group remarks)
		Method	GFR (ml/min)			Removed by Dialysis	
			>50	10–50	<10		
Temafloxacin	R	D, I*	Unch	400 mg q.d.[†]	400 mg q.d.[†]	No (He)	*D and I methods are combined †Give patients with $C_{Cr} > 40$ ml/min a loading dose of 800 mg
Sulbactam	R	I	Unch	8–12	12–18	Yes	Combined with ampicillin for clinical use
Sulfisoxazole	R (H)	I	6	8–12	18–24[†]	Yes (He, P)	Rare crystalluria *Binding to plasma proteins decreased in ESRD †If high urine level desired, normal intervals required
Teicoplanin	R	I	24–36	36–48	48–72	No (He, P)	Rare ototoxicity
Tetracyclines*†							*GT: agents in this group may potentiate acidosis, increase catabolism, raise serum phosphorus levels and BUN †GR: phosphate binders may retard absorption; not useful for urinary tract infections if GFR <20 ml/min
Doxycycline	R (H)	I	12	12–18	18–24	No (He, P)	Group drug of choice for extrarenal infections
Tetracycline	R (H)	I	8–12	12–24	24*	No (He, P)	GT; GR *Avoid if possible

Drug	Elimination and Metabolism	Adjustment for Renal Failure					Toxic Effects and Remarks (GT — group toxicity; GR — group remarks)
		Method	GFR (ml/min)			Removed by Dialysis	
			>50	10–50	<10		
Antimicrobial Agents (continued)							
Trimethoprim-sulfamethox-azole (T-S)	T: R (H) S: H (R)	I	12	18	24‡§	Yes (He); No (P)	*Half-life reduced in alkaline urine †Binding to plasma proteins decreased in ESRD ‡May cause increase in serum creatinine levels in patients with creatinine >2 mg/dl; this may reflect secretory competition with creatinine or a nephrotoxic reaction §May achieve adequate urine concentration in patients with low GFR using normal doses; hematologic side effects caused by antifolate action
Vancomycin	R	I	24–72	72–240	240	No (He, P)	Ototoxic at levels of 80–100 µg/ml; best guide to therapy is serum level before next dose; elimination variable in renal failure; can be used intraperitoneally in CAPD
Analgesics							
Narcotics and narcotic antagonists*							*GT: agents in this group may cause excessive sedation and respiratory depression
Butorphanol	H	D	Unch	Unch	Unch	?	GT
Codeine	H (R <16%)	D	Unch	Unch	50–75	No (He)	GT
Fentanyl	H	D	Unch	Unch	Unch	?	GT

Abbreviations used in table:

R — renal
H — hepatic

I — interval extension method of dosage adjustment; data units are hours between maintenance doses
D — dose reduction method of dosage adjustment; data units are percent of usual maintenance dose

Unch — unchanged
He — hemodialysis
P — peritoneal dialysis

ESRD — end-stage renal disease
GFR — glomerular filtration rate

Analgesics (continued)

| Drug | Elimination and Metabolism | Adjustment for Renal Failure | | | | | Toxic Effects and Remarks (GT — group toxicity; GR — group remarks) |
| | | Method | GFR (ml/min) | | | Removed by Dialysis | |
			>50	10–50	<10		
Meperidine	H (R <10%)*†	D	Unch	Unch	Unch	No (He)	GT *Excretion increased 20%–30% in acid urine †Active metabolites with longer half-life than normal accumulate in renal failure (may result in seizures)
Methadone	H (R <21%)*	D	Unch	Unch	50–75†	No (He, P)	GT *Excretion increased in acid urine †Accumulation of metabolites of uncertain significance; fecal elimination increased in ESRD
Morphine	H (R <12%; GI <10%)	D	Unch	Unch	50–75	No (He)	GT; active metabolite morphine-6-glucuronide may accumulate
Naloxone	H	D	Unch	Unch	Unch	?	GT
Pentazocine	H (R <12%)	D	Unch	Unch	Unch	?Yes (He)	GT
Nonnarcotic analgesics Acetaminophen	H	I	4	6	8*	Yes (He)†; No (P)	Overdoses result in nephrotoxicity caused by a reactive metabolite; drug is major metabolite of phenacetin *Metabolites accumulate †Half-life reduced 50% during dialysis; dialysis major route of excretion in anephric patients

	Drug	Elimination and Metabolism	Method	Adjustment for Renal Failure			Removed by Dialysis	Toxic Effects and Remarks (GT — group toxicity; GR — group remarks)
				GFR (ml/min)				
				>50	10–50	<10		
Analgesics (continued)	Acetylsalicylic acid	H (R)*	I	4	4–6	Avoid	Yes (He, P)	Nephrotoxic in overdoses; may decrease GFR when renal blood flow is prostaglandin dependent; antiplatelet, gastrointestinal effects add to uremic symptoms *Maximal excretion in alkaline urine
Sedatives, Hypnotics, and Drugs Used in Psychiatry	Antidepressants							
	Amoxapine	H	D	Unch	Unch	Unch	?	—
	Bupropion	H	D	Unch	Unch	Unch	?	—
	Fluoxetine	H*	D	Unch	Unch	Unch	No (He)	*Pharmacologically active metabolite with long half-life
	Paroxetine	H	D	Unch	Unch	50–75	?	Marked individual variability in pharmacokinetic properties
	Barbiturates*							*GR: may increase osteomalacia in hemodialysis patients; half-life decreases with chronic therapy because of hepatic microsomal enzyme induction; hemodialysis more effective than peritoneal dialysis in overdoses; charcoal hemoperfusion best for massive overdoses; all agents in this group may cause excessive sedation

Abbreviations used in table:

R — renal
H — hepatic

I — interval extension method of dosage adjustment; data units are hours between maintenance doses
D — dose reduction method of dosage adjustment; data units are percent of usual maintenance dose

Unch — unchanged
He — hemodialysis
P — peritoneal dialysis

ESRD — end-stage renal disease
GFR — glomerular filtration rate

Drug	Elimination and Metabolism	Method	Adjustment for Renal Failure				Toxic Effects and Remarks (GT — group toxicity; GR — group remarks)
			GFR (ml/min)			Removed by Dialysis	
			>50	10–50	<10		
Phenobarbital	H (R 30%)	I	Unch	Unch	12–16	Yes (He, P)	GR; up to 50% of drug excreted unchanged in alkaline diuresis
Secobarbital	H	D	Unch	Unch	Unch	No (He, P)	GR
Benzodiazepines*							*GT: all agents in this group may cause excessive sedation or encephalopathy, or both, in chronic hemodialysis patients
Alprazolam	H	D	Unch	Unch	Unch	?	GT
Chlordesmethyl-diazepam	H	D	Unch	Unch	50–75	No (He)	Increased unbound fraction in ESRD; marked decrease in V_D in ESRD
Chlordiaze-poxide	H (R)*	D	Unch	Unch	Unch	No (He)	GT *Active metabolite excreted by kidney
Clonazepam	H	D	Unch	Unch	Unch	?	GT
Clorazepate	H (R)	D	Unch	Unch	Unch	?	GT
Clozapine	H	D	Unch	Unch	Unch	No*	Agranulocytosis in 1%–2% *No data available, but V_D precludes removal by dialysis
Diazepam	H (R,* GI†)	D	Unch	Unch	Unch	No (He)	GT *Active metabolite desmethyl-diazepam excreted by kidney †Enterohepatic circulation exists
Flurazepam	H (R)*	D	Unch	Unch	Unch	No (He)	GT *First-pass hepatic metabolism; excretion routes and half-life pertain to active metabolites
Lorazepam	H	D	Unch	Unch	50	No (He)	GT
Midazolam	H	D	Unch	Unch	Unch	No (He)	GT *Protein binding decreased in ESRD

Sedatives, Hypnotics, and Drugs Used in Psychiatry (continued)

Sedatives, Hypnotics, and Drugs Used in Psychiatry (continued)

Drug	Elimination and Metabolism	Method	Adjustment for Renal Failure			Removed by Dialysis	Toxic Effects and Remarks (GT — group toxicity; GR — group remarks)
			GFR (ml/min)				
			>50	10–50	<10		
Prazepam	H (R)	D	Unch	Unch	Unch	?	GT
Triazolam	H	D	Unch	Unch	Unch	?	GT
Buspirone	H	D	Unch	Unch	50–75*	Yes (He)	*Active metabolite accumulates
Haloperidol	H (R, GI)	D	Unch	Unch	Unch	No (He, P)	May cause hypotension, excessive sedation
Lithium carbonate	R	D	Unch	50–75	25–50	Yes (He, P)†	Nephrogenic diabetes insipidus; nephrotic syndrome; renal tubular acidosis; chronic interstitial fibrosis; toxicity when serum levels are >1.2 mEq/L; serum levels 12 hr after a dose should be measured periodically; toxicity enhanced and drug clearance reduced by volume depletion, nonsteroidal anti-inflammatory drugs, and diuretics; excretion enhanced by NaHCO$_3$, acetazolamide, aminophylline, and osmotic diuretics *Plasma half-life does not reflect extensive tissue accumulation †Plasma levels rise after dialysis as re-equilibration with tissue stores occurs

Abbreviations used in table:

R — renal
H — hepatic

I — interval extension method of dosage adjustment; data units are hours between maintenance doses
D — dose reduction method of dosage adjustment; data units are percent of usual maintenance dose

Unch — unchanged
He — hemodialysis
P — peritoneal dialysis

ESRD — end-stage renal disease
GFR — glomerular filtration rate

Drug	Elimination and Metabolism	Adjustment for Renal Failure				Toxic Effects and Remarks (GT — group toxicity; GR — group remarks)
		Method	GFR (ml/min)		Removed by Dialysis	
			>50	10–50	<10	
Phenothiazines*						
Chlorpromazine	H	D	Unch	Unch	Unch[†]	No (He, P)	*GT: all agents in this group are anticholinergic; may cause urinary retention, orthostatic hypotension, confusion, and extrapyramidal symptoms; characteristic acute toxic psychosis; > 800 mg/day of thioridazine causes retinitis; prototype chlorpromazine GT *Very large volume of distribution after oral dose †May need to decrease dose and increase interval if excessive sedation occurs
Tricyclic antidepressants*						
Amitriptyline	H* (R <5%)	D	Unch	Unch	Unch[†]	No (He, P)	*GR: all agents in this group are anticholinergic and may cause urinary retention; may decrease hypotensive effects of guanethidine, clonidine, and methyldopa; enterohepatic circulation and genetic variation in metabolism exist; increased excretion in acid urine (total remains small); smoking, alcohol, and sedatives induce metabolism; neuroleptics and advanced age inhibit metabolism; may cause excessive sedation; physostigmine indicated for life-threatening overdose GR *Metabolized to nortriptyline †Reported to stimulate weight gain and appetite in dialysis patients

Drug		Elimination and Metabolism	Adjustment for Renal Failure					Toxic Effects and Remarks (GT — group toxicity; GR — group remarks)
			Method	GFR (ml/min)			Removed by Dialysis	
				>50	10–50	<10		
Sedatives, etc. (continued)	Desipramine	H (R <5%)	D	Unch	Unch	Unch	No (He, P)	GR
	Doxepin	H	D	Unch	Unch	Unch	No (He, P)	GR
	Imipramine	H* (R <5%)	D	Unch	Unch	Unch	No (He, P)	GR *Metabolized to desipramine
	Nortriptyline	H (R <5%)	D	Unch	Unch	Unch	No (He, P)	GR
Cardiovacular and Antihypertensive Agents	Adrenergic modulators and blockers*							*GR: blood pressure best guide to dose and interval
	Clonidine	R	D	Unch	Unch	50–75	No (He)	GR; may potentiate CNS depressant effects of alcohol, barbiturates, and sedatives; rebound hypertension can occur when drug is abruptly withdrawn; tricyclic antidepressants decrease efficacy
	Doxazosin	Non-R	D	Unch	Unch	Unch	No (He, P)	GR; renal patients may be sensitive to small doses
	Guanabenz	Non-R	D	Unch	Unch	Unch	?	GR
	Guanfacine	H	D	Unch	Unch	Unch	No (He)	*Decreased renal clearance matched by extrarenal disposition

Abbreviations used in table:

R — renal
H — hepatic

I — interval extension method of dosage adjustment; data units are hours between maintenance doses
D — dose reduction method of dosage adjustment; data units are percent of usual maintenance dose

Unch — unchanged
He — hemodialysis
P — peritoneal dialysis

ESRD — end-stage renal disease
GFR — glomerular filtration rate

| Drug | Elimination and Metabolism | Adjustment for Renal Failure | | | | | Toxic Effects and Remarks (GT — group toxicity; GR — group remarks) |
| | | Method | GFR (ml/min) | | | Removed by Dialysis | |
			>50	10–50	<10		
Methyldopa	R* (H 18%–48%)	I	6	9–18	12–24†	Yes (He, P)	GR; orthostatic hypotension; retroperitoneal fibrosis; prolonged hypotension from active metabolites retained in severe renal failure; hepatitis *Renal excretion more important with I.V. drug administration †Retention of active metabolites in severe renal failure
Prazosin	H (R)	D	Unch	Unch	Unch†	No (He, P)	GR; may produce profound hypotension with first dose †May get response to lower dose in ESRD
Terazosin	R (H)	D	Unch	Unch	Unch	?	GR
Angiotensin-converting enzyme inhibitors*							*GR: particularly useful for treatment of malignant or unilateral renovascular hypertension; effect magnified by natriuretic agents or sodium depletion
Benazepril	H* (R)	D	Unch	25–100	25–50	No (He)	GR; hyperkalemia *Active moiety, benazeprilat, is hepatic metabolite and renally excreted
Captopril	R (H)	D I	Unch 8–24	Unch 24–72	50 71–108	Yes (He)	GR; blood pressure best guide to dose and interval; proteinuria; nephrotic syndrome; granulocytopenia; hyperkalemia

Cardiovascular and Antihypertensive Agents (continued)

| Drug | Elimination and Metabolism | Method | Adjustment for Renal Failure | | | Removed by Dialysis | Toxic Effects and Remarks (GT — group toxicity; GR — group remarks) |
| | | | GFR (ml/min) | | | | |
			>50	10–50	<10		
Enalapril	H*	D	100	75–100	50	Yes (He)	GR *Active moiety, enalaprilat, is formed by hepatic ester hydrolysis and is renally excreted; hyperkalemia
Fosinopril	H 50% R 50%	D	Unch	Unch	75*	No (He, P)	GR *Avoid administering to patients with concurrent liver disease and ESRD
Lisinopril	R	D	100	75	25–50	Yes (He)	GR; hyperkalemia
Perindopril	R*	D† I†	50–100 Unch	25–100 Unch	25 48	Yes (He)	GR *Active moiety, perindoprilat, is hepatic metabolite and renally excreted †D and I methods may be combined
Quinapril	H* (R)	D	Unch	50–75	25–50	No (He, P)	GR; hyperkalemia *Active moiety, quinaprilat, is hepatic metabolite and renally excreted
Ramipril	H*	D	100	50–75	25–50	Yes (He)	GR *Active moiety, ramiprilat, is formed in the liver
Antiarrhythmic agents*							*GR: in this group, blood levels best guide to therapy; half-life may be prolonged in heart disease or with reduced hepatic blood flow, or both
Amiodarone	H	D	Unch	Unch	Unch	No (He)	GR; thyroid dysfunction; peripheral neuropathy; hepatic dysfunction; pulmonary fibrosis

Abbreviations used in table:

R — renal
H — hepatic

I — interval extension method of dosage adjustment; data units are hours between maintenance doses
D — dose reduction method of dosage adjustment; data units are percent of usual maintenance dose

Unch — unchanged
He — hemodialysis
P — peritoneal dialysis

ESRD — end-stage renal disease
GFR — glomerular filtration rate

Cardiovascular and Antihypertensive Agents (continued)

Drug	Elimination and Metabolism	Method	GFR (ml/min)			Removed by Dialysis	Toxic Effects and Remarks (GT — group toxicity; GR — group remarks)
			>50	10–50	<10		
Bretylium	R (Non-R 20%)	D	Unch	25–50*	Avoid*	?	GR; poorly tolerated when used to control blood pressure *No specific data in ESRD
Cibenzoline	R	D* I	Unch 6–12	66–100 12–24	66 24	No (He)	GR *D and I methods are combined
Disopyramide	R and H	I	Unch	12–24	24–40	No (He)	GR; active metabolite
Flecainide	H (R)	D	Unch	Unch	50–75	No (He)	GR; renal excretion enhanced in acid urine
Lidocaine	H* (R <20%)	D	Unch	Unch	Unch	No (He)	GR: half-life dependent on hepatic blood flow; active metabolite *Excretion enhanced in acid urine
Mexiletine	H (R)	D	Unch	Unch	50–75	Yes (He); No (P)	GR; renal excretion markedly enhanced in acid urine
Procainamide	R* (H 7%–24%)	I	4	6–12	8–24	Yes (He)†	GR; may induce lupus nephritis *Renal excretion of active metabolite N-acetylprocainamide †May be able to treat poisoning with hemodialysis
Propafenone	H	D	Unch	Unch	Unch	No (He, P)	*Depends on acetylator phenotype
Quinidine	H* (R 10%–50%)	I	Unch	Unch	Unch	Yes (He, P)†	GR; active metabolite; may cause lupuslike syndrome; increases plasma digoxin and possibly digitoxin *Excretion enhanced in acid urine †Hemodialysis with low potassium bath may be effective for poisoning
Beta blockers*							*GR: blood pressure best guide to dose and interval
Acebutolol	R (H)	D	Unch	50*	30–50*	No (He)	GR *Active metabolite with long half-life accumulates

Cardiovascular and Antihypertensive Agents (continued)

Drug	Elimination and Metabolism	Method	Adjustment for Renal Failure			Removed by Dialysis	Toxic Effects and Remarks (GT — group toxicity; GR — group remarks)
			GFR (ml/min)				
			>50	10–50	<10		
Atenolol	R	D I	Unch 24	50 48	25 96	Yes (He); No (P)	GR; significant accumulation in ESRD
Betaxolol	H	D	Unch	Unch	50	No (He, P)	GR
Carteolol	R	D	Unch	50	25	?	GR
Celiprolol	Non-R	D	Unch	Unch	50–75	?	GR; has alpha-adrenergic receptor blocking action, which minimizes peripheral vasoconstriction
Esmolol	Non-R	D	Unch	Unch	Unch	?	Suitable for critical care situations; rapidly hydrolyzed by red blood cell esterases
Labetalol	H	D	Unch	Unch	Unch	No (He)	GR
Metoprolol	H	D	Unch	Unch	Unch	Yes (He)	GR *Hypotension effect lasts 24 hr
Nadolol	R	D	Unch	50	25	Yes (He)	GR; significant accumulation in ESRD
Pindolol	H (R)	D	Unch	Unch	Unch	?	GR
Propranolol	H*	D	Unch	Unch	Unch†	No (He)	GR; metabolites may accumulate; metabolites spuriously increase bilirubin by interference with assay *Clearance depends on hepatic flow; p.o. dose <30 mg extracted by normal liver; decreased hepatic extraction in ESRD †Complex biexponential pharmaco-kinetics in ESRD; blood levels best guide; less frequent doses needed during chronic therapy

Abbreviations used in table:

R — renal
H — hepatic

I — interval extension method of dosage adjustment; data units are hours between maintenance doses
D — dose reduction method of dosage adjustment; data units are percent of usual maintenance dose

Unch — unchanged
He — hemodialysis
P — peritoneal dialysis

ESRD — end-stage renal disease
GFR — glomerular filtration rate

Drug	Elimination and Metabolism	Method	Adjustment for Renal Failure			Removed by Dialysis	Toxic Effects and Remarks (GT — group toxicity; GR — group remarks)
			GFR (ml/min)				
			>50	10–50	<10		
Sotalol	R	D	Unch	30	15–30	Yes (He)	GR
Timolol	H	D	Unch	Unch	Unch	No (He)	GR
Calcium blocking agents*							*GR: associated with headache, flushing, and dizziness in patients with renal disease
Amlodipine	H	D	Unch	Unch	Unch	No (He, P)	GR
Diltiazem	H	D	Unch	Unch	Unch	No (He)	GR; active metabolites
Felodipine	H	D	Unch	Unch	Unch	No (He)	GR
Isradipine	H	D	Unch	Unch	75	?	GR
Nicardipine	H	D	Unch	Unch	Unch	No (He)	GR
Nifedipine	H	D	Unch	Unch	Unch	No (He)	GR; may cause edema
Nimodipine	H	D	Unch	Unch	Unch	No (He, P)	GR; lowers blood pressure in 5% of patients
Nitrendipine	H	D	Unch	Unch	Unch	No (He)	GR
Verapamil	H	D	Unch	Unch	50–75	No (He)	GR; active metabolites
Cardiac glyco-sides*							*GR: agents in this group add to uremic gastrointestinal symptoms; serum level best guide to dosage; equations, nomograms, and computer programs available; usual clinical practice is to reduce size of dose when renal failure is present; toxicity enhanced by dialysis removal of potassium and magnesium
Digitoxin	H* (R)	D	Unch	Unch	50–75	No (He, P)	GR; serum level may rise if quinidine given *Converted to digoxin (8%); conversion increased in ESRD

Drug	Elimination and Metabolism	Adjustment for Renal Failure					Toxic Effects and Remarks (GT — group toxicity; GR — group remarks)
		Method	GFR (ml/min)			Removed by Dialysis	
			>50	10–50	<10		
Digoxin	R (Non-R 15%–40%)*	D I	Unch 24	25–75 36	10–25† 48	No (He, P)†‡	GR; radioimmunoassay may overestimate serum levels in ESRD; variable bioavailability; clearance decreased by hypokalemia, spironolactone, quinidine, and verapamil *Volume of distribution and total body clearance decreased in ESRD †Serum level 12 hr after dose best guide in ESRD; decrease loading dose by 50% in ESRD ‡Serum level transiently decreased by dialysis; myocardial level decreased by uremia; charcoal hemoperfusion may be useful in massive overdoses
Ouabain	R	I	12–24	24–36	36–48	No (He, P)	GR
Diuretics*							*GR: all agents are natriuretic and may produce extracellular fluid volume depletion
Amiloride	R	D	Unch	50*	Avoid*	?	*Hyperkalemia common with GFR <30 ml/min (diabetics especially susceptible); may produce hyperchloremic metabolic acidosis

Cardiovascular and Antihypertensive Agents (continued)

Abbreviations used in table:

R — renal
H — hepatic

I — interval extension method of dosage adjustment; data units are hours between maintenance doses
D — dose reduction method of dosage adjustment; data units are percent of usual maintenance dose

Unch — unchanged
He — hemodialysis
P — peritoneal dialysis

ESRD — end-stage renal disease
GFR — glomerular filtration rate

Cardiovascular and Antihypertensive Agents (continued)

Drug	Elimination and Metabolism	Method	GFR (ml/min)			Removed by Dialysis	Toxic Effects and Remarks (GT — group toxicity; GR — group remarks)
			>50	10–50	<10		
Bumetanide	R (H)	D	Unch	Unch	Unch	No (He)	GR; ototoxic, particularly in combination with aminoglycosides; may augment aminoglycoside nephrotoxicity; rare allergic interstitial nephritis; high doses useful in ESRD; cramps common with high doses; clearance unchanged in ESRD; gynecomastia; muscle weakness
Chlorthalidone	R (Non-R)*	I	24	24	48	?	GR *Enterohepatic circulation exists
Furosemide	R (H)	D	Unch	Unch	Unch*	No (He)	GR; uncommon allergic interstitial nephritis; ototoxic, particularly in combination with aminoglycosides; may augment aminoglycoside nephrotoxicity *High doses useful in ESRD
Indapamide	R	D	Unch	Unch	Unch	No (He)	GR
Metolazone	R	D	Unch	Unch	Unch	No (He)	GR; high doses may be useful in ESRD; gynecomastia and impotence simulate that seen in ESRD; may produce hyperchloremic metabolic acidosis
Spironolactone	H (R)*	I	6–12	12–24†	Avoid†	?	GR *Metabolites are pharmacologically active and excreted by kidney †Hyperkalemia common with GFR <30 ml/min (diabetics especially susceptible)
Thiazides*	R	D	Unch	Unch†	Avoid†	?	GR; hyperuricemia *Prototype chlorothiazide †Ineffective when GFR <30 ml/min

<table>
<tr><td rowspan="4">Drug</td><td rowspan="4">Elimination
and
Metabolism</td><td colspan="5">Adjustment for Renal Failure</td><td rowspan="4">Toxic Effects and Remarks
(GT — group toxicity;
GR — group remarks)</td></tr>
<tr><td rowspan="3">Method</td><td colspan="3">GFR (ml/min)</td><td rowspan="2">Removed by
Dialysis</td></tr>
<tr><td>>50</td><td>10–50</td><td><10</td></tr>
<tr></tr>
<tr><td colspan="8">Cardiovascular and Antihypertensive Agents (continued)</td></tr>
<tr><td>Triamterene</td><td>H (R)</td><td>I</td><td>12</td><td>12†</td><td>Avoid*</td><td>?</td><td>GR; folic acid antagonist; may cause renal calculi
†Hyperkalemia common with GFR <30 ml/min (diabetics especially susceptible)</td></tr>
<tr><td>Inotropic agents
Amrinone
Milrinone</td><td>
R (H)
R</td><td>
D
D</td><td>
Unch
Unch</td><td>
Unch
Unch</td><td>
50–75
25–50</td><td>
?
?</td><td>
—
—</td></tr>
<tr><td>Nitrates*

Nitroglycerin

Isosorbide
dinitrate</td><td>

H

H</td><td>

I

I</td><td>

Unch

Unch</td><td>

Unch

Unch</td><td>

Unch

Unch</td><td>

?

?</td><td>*GR: renal blood flow may drop if mean arterial pressure is excessively decreased in ESRD
GR; sublingual pharmacological effect lasts 15–30 min
GR; metabolized to pharmacologically active compounds</td></tr>
<tr><td>Vasodilators*

Hydralazine</td><td>

H (Non-R)</td><td>

I</td><td>

8</td><td>

8</td><td>

8–16 (fast);
12–24 (slow)</td><td>

No (He, P)

No (He, P)</td><td>*GR: blood pressure best guide to dose and interval
GR; may induce lupus nephritis</td></tr>
</table>

Abbreviations used in table:

R — renal   I — interval extension method of dosage adjustment; data units are hours between maintenance doses

H — hepatic   D — dose reduction method of dosage adjustment; data units are percent of usual maintenance dose

Unch — unchanged

He — hemodialysis

P — peritoneal dialysis

ESRD — end-stage renal disease

GFR — glomerular filtration rate

Drug	Elimination and Metabolism	Adjustment for Renal Failure					Toxic Effects and Remarks (GT — group toxicity; GR — group remarks)
		Method	GFR (ml/min)			Removed by Dialysis	
			>50	10–50	<10		
Cardiovascular and Antihypertensive Agents (continued)							
Minoxidil	H	D	Unch	Unch	Unch	Yes (He)	GR; may produce fluid retention, pericardial effusion, and T wave changes; prolonged hypotension may occur
Sodium nitro-prusside	Non-R	D	Unch	Unch	Unch*	Yes (He)†	GR; toxic metabolite—thiocyanate—accumulates, producing hypothyroidism, seizures, and coma; careful monitoring required to prevent wide swings in blood pressure *Need to monitor thiocyanate levels to keep <10 mg/dl; half-life for thiocyanate is 1 wk †Thiocyanate dialyzable
Miscellaneous Agents							
Antiasthmatic agents							
Cromolyn	R (H)	D	Unch	Unch	Unch	?	—
Terbutaline	H* (R)	D†	Unch	50	Avoid	?	*Large first-pass effect; I.V. or subcutaneous doses cleared by renal excretion †Recommendations for I.V. doses only; oral doses unchanged
Theophylline	H	D	Unch	Unch	Unch	Yes (He, P)	May add to uremic gastrointestinal symptoms; seizures at high blood levels
Anticoagulants*							*GT: agents in this group should be carefully titrated to achieve therapeutic effects; may potentiate uremic bleeding
Heparin	Non-R	D	Unch	Unch	Unch	No (He, P)	GT

Cardiovascular and Antihypertensive Agents (continued)

Drug	Elimination and Metabolism	Method	Adjustment for Renal Failure				Toxic Effects and Remarks (GT — group toxicity; GR — group remarks)
			GFR (ml/min)			Removed by Dialysis	
			>50	10–50	<10		
Streptokinase	—	D	Unch	Unch	Unch	?	GT
Urokinase	—	D	Unch	Unch	Unch	?	GT
Warfarin	H (R)*	D	Unch	Unch	Unch	No (He)	GT *Metabolites with anticoagulant properties are excreted renally
Antidiabetic agents							
Chlorpropa-mide	R (H)	I	24	Avoid*	Avoid*	No (P)	Impairs renal water excretion *Prolonged hypoglycemia in azotemic patients
Glipizide	H	D	Unch	Unch	Unch	?	—
Glyburide	H	D	Unch	Unch	Unch	?	—
Insulin	H (R)	D	Unch	75*	50*	?	*Dosage dependent on blood glucose level
Tolbutamide	H (R)	D	Unch	Unch	Unch	No (He)	May impair water excretion
Antihistamines							
Cetirizine	R	D	Unch	75	50	No (He)	—
Diphenhydra-mine	H* (R <4%)	I	6	6–9	9–12	?	May cause excessive sedation; anticholinergic; may cause urinary retention *50% of oral dose metabolized in first pass through liver
Terfenadine	H	D	Unch	Unch	Unch	?	—

Abbreviations used in table:

R — renal
H — hepatic

I — interval extension method of dosage adjustment; data units are hours between maintenance doses

D — dose reduction method of dosage adjustment; data units are percent of usual maintenance dose

Unch — unchanged
He — hemodialysis
P — peritoneal dialysis

ESRD — end-stage renal disease
GFR — glomerular filtration rate

Drug	Elimination and Metabolism	Adjustment for Renal Failure					Toxic Effects and Remarks (GT — group toxicity; GR — group remarks)
		Method	GFR (ml/min)			Removed by Dialysis	
			>50	10–50	<10		
Antineoplastic and immuno-suppressive agents*							*GT: agents in this group cause marrow depression, which adds to uremic bleeding and risk of infection
Azathioprine	H	D I	Unch 24	Unch 24	75 36	Yes (He) ?	GT; acute renal failure reported; allopurinol increases drug activity
Bleomycin	R	D	Unch	Unch	50	No (He)	GT; pulmonary toxicity, including fibrosis; hypertension and dysuria reported; toxicity enhanced in renal failure
Busulfan	H	D	Unch	Unch	Unch	?	GT; may cause hemorrhagic cystitis
Carboplatin	R	D	Unch	75	50	Yes (He)	GT; nephrotoxic (less than cisplatin)
Cisplatin	R (Non-R)	D	Unch	75	50	Yes (He)*	GT; nephrotoxic (effect potentiated by other nephrotoxins and modified or prevented by hydration); renal Mg^{++} wasting noted *Dialysis only effective first 3 hr after dose
Cyclophos-phamide	H (R)	I D	12 Unch	12 Unch	18–24 50–75	Yes (He) ?	GT; hemorrhagic cystitis, bladder fibrosis, and bladder carcinoma; sterility; alopecia; inappropriate antidiuretic hormone secretion reported
Cyclosporine	H	D	Unch	Unch	Unch	No (He, P)	Nephrotoxic, hepatotoxic; hypertension with seizures and hirsutism reported
Doxorubicin	H* (R)	D	Unch	Unch	75	No (He)	GT; cardiac toxicity may add to uremic cardiomyopathy; acute renal failure and nephrotic syndrome reported *Half-life of metabolites, 32 hr

Miscellaneous Agents (continued)

| Drug | Elimination and Metabolism | Method | Adjustment for Renal Failure | | | Removed by Dialysis | Toxic Effects and Remarks (GT — group toxicity; GR — group remarks) |
| | | | GFR (ml/min) | | | | |
			>50	10–50	<10		
Etoposide	H	D	Unch	75	50	?	—
5-Fluorouracil	H (R)	D	Unch	Unch	Unch	Yes (He)	GT
Idarubicin	Non-R (H)	D	Unch	Unch	Unch	?	Leukopenia often dose-limiting; cardiotoxicity has been reported but may occur less frequently with idarubicin than with other anthracyclines
Ifosfamide	R (H)	D	Unch	50	50	?	Nephrotoxic; hemorrhagic cystitis reduced by concomitant sulfhydryl compound (MESNA)
Melphalan	H (R 13%)	D	Unch	Unch	Unch	?	GT
Methotrexate	R	D	Unch	50	Avoid	Yes (He); No (P)	GT; folate deficiency; nephrotoxic (precipitates in renal tubules); vigorous hydration and alkalinization may prevent nephrotoxicity
Mithramycin	R	D	Unch	75	50	?	GT; cumulative nephrotoxicity; occasional acute renal failure; decreased Ca^{++}, K^+, PO_4 noted
Plicamycin	R	D	Unch	75	50	?	GT; cumulative nephrotoxicity
Semustine (Methyl-CCNU)	R	D	Unch	Unch	Avoid*	?	GT *Dose-related nephrotoxicity (for >1,500 mg/m^2)
Tamoxifen	H	D	Unch	Unch	Unch	?	—

Abbreviations used in table:

R — renal
H — hepatic

I — interval extension method of dosage adjustment; data units are hours between maintenance doses
D — dose reduction method of dosage adjustment; data units are percent of usual maintenance dose

Unch — unchanged
He — hemodialysis
P — peritoneal dialysis

ESRD — end-stage renal disease
GFR — glomerular filtration rate

Miscellaneous Agents (continued)

| Drug | Elimination and Metabolism | Method | Adjustment for Renal Failure | | | Removed by Dialysis | Toxic Effects and Remarks (GT — group toxicity; GR — group remarks) |
| | | | GFR (ml/min) | | | | |
			>50	10–50	<10		
Vinblastine	H	D	Unch	Unch	Unch	?	GT; vinca alkaloids may cause inappropriate antidiuretic hormone secretion; nephrotoxicity reported
Vincristine	H	D	Unch	Unch	Unch	?	GT; neurotoxicity can add to uremic neuropathy; inappropriate antidiuretic hormone secretion reported
Corticosteroids*							*GT: all agents in this group increase catabolism and aggravate azotemia, sodium retention, hypertension, and glucose intolerance
Cortisone	H	D	Unch	Unch	Unch	No (He)	GT
Dexamethasone	H	D	Unch	Unch	Unch	?	GT
Hydrocortisone	H	D	Unch	Unch	Unch	?	GT
Methylprednisolone	H	D	Unch	Unch	Unch	Yes (He)	GT
Prednisolone*	H	D	Unch	Unch	Unch	No (He)	GT *Dose- and age-dependent pharmacokinetics
Prednisone	H	D	Unch	Unch	Unch	Yes (He)	GT; metabolized to prednisolone
H$_2$-receptor blockers							
Cimetidine	R (H)	D	100	75	50	No (He, P)	May increase serum creatinine level and decrease creatinine clearance (because of inhibition of renal tubular secretion) without change in GFR; can cause confusion in patients with renal or hepatic disease, or both; acute renal failure reported

Miscellaneous Agents (continued)

Drug	Elimination and Metabolism	Method	GFR (ml/min)			Removed by Dialysis	Toxic Effects and Remarks (GT — group toxicity; GR — group remarks)
			>50	10–50	<10		
Famotidine	R	D	100	75	50	No (He)	—
Ranitidine	R (H)	D	Unch	75	50	Yes (He)	—
Hyperlipoprotein-emia agents							
Cholestyramine	Not absorbed	D	Unch	Unch	Unch	—	Hyperchloremic metabolic acidosis can occur
Gemfibrozil	R (fecal)	D	Unch	Unch	Unch	No (He, P)	—
Lovastatin	H	D	Unch	Unch	Unch	?	Rhabdomyolysis reported in transplant patients
Pravastatin	H (R)	D	Unch	Unch	50–75	?	May cause muscle necrosis or rhabdomyolysis; in patients with ESRD or on cyclosporine, administer low doses and use caution
Probucol	Fecal	D	Unch	Unch	Unch	?	—
Neurologic agents							
Bromocriptine	H	D	Unch	Unch	Unch	?	May cause orthostatic hypotension; digital vasospasm at higher doses
Carbamazepine	H (R)*	D	Unch	Unch	75	No (He)	May cause inappropriate antidiuretic hormone secretion; active metabolites excreted renally *Other anticonvulsants and long-term therapy induce metabolism and shorten half-life

Abbreviations used in table:

R — renal
H — hepatic

I — interval extension method of dosage adjustment; data units are hours between maintenance doses

D — dose reduction method of dosage adjustment; data units are percent of usual maintenance dose

Unch — unchanged
He — hemodialysis
P — peritoneal dialysis

ESRD — end-stage renal disease
GFR — glomerular filtration rate

Miscellaneous Agents (continued)

Drug	Elimination and Metabolism	Method	Adjustment for Renal Failure			Removed by Dialysis	Toxic Effects and Remarks (GT — group toxicity; GR — group remarks)
			GFR (ml/min)				
			>50	10–50	<10		
Carbidopa	H	D	Unch	Unch	Unch	?	
Levodopa	Non-R (R)*	D	Unch	Unch	Unch	?	*May darken urine; active and inactive metabolites excreted in urine
Phenytoin	H (R)	D	Unch	Unch	Unch	No (He)	May cause folate deficiency; interstitial nephritis reported
Valproic acid	H	D	Unch	Unch	Unch	No (He, P)	May cause hepatotoxicity
Neuromuscular blocking agents*							*GR: aminoglycosides, hypokalemia, acidosis, and hypermagnesemia may enhance neuromuscular blocking effects
Atracurium	Non-R	D	Unch	Unch	Unch	?	GR; can be used safely in renal failure
Doxacurium	R (H)	D	Unch	50–75	25–50	?	Prolonged neuromuscular blockade in ESRD
Neostigmine	R (Non-R)*	I	6	6	12–18	?	GR; active metabolites accumulate in ESRD *ESRD patients may have low cholinesterase levels prolonging drug action; bladder atony
Pancuronium	R (H)	D	Unch	Unch	Avoid*	?	GR; recurarization may occur up to 24 hr after dose *Active metabolites accumulate in ESRD
Pyridostigmine	R*†	D	Unch	Unch	Unch	?	GR *Renal excretion decreased by basic drugs †ESRD patients may have low cholinesterase levels prolonging drug action; bladder atony

Miscellaneous Agents (continued)

Drug	Elimination and Metabolism	Method	Adjustment for Renal Failure			Removed by Dialysis	Toxic Effects and Remarks (GT — group toxicity; GR — group remarks)
			GFR (ml/min)				
			>50	10–50	<10		
Succinylcholine	Non-R*	D	Unch	Unch	Unch†	?	GR *Renal excretion of active metabolites †Acute hyperkalemia should be anticipated in ESRD
Tubocurarine	R (H)	D	Unch	Unch	Unch*	?	GR; considered neuromuscular blocking agent of choice in ESRD *Large or repetitive doses may prolong drug effects; recurarization may occur
Vecuronium	Non-R	D	Unch	Unch	Unch	?	GR; can be used safely in renal failure
Rheumatologic agents*							*GT: agents in this group add to uremic bleeding and gastrointestinal symptoms; nonsteroidal anti-inflammatory drugs in this group may be associated with renal dysfunction secondary to prostaglandin inhibition; nephrotic syndrome, interstitial nephritis, and hyperkalemia reported
Allopurinol	R*	I D	8 Unch	8–12 75	12–24 50	?	GT; syndrome of worsening renal function, eosinophilia, fever, and skin desquamation; rare xanthine stones *Renal excretion of active metabolite—oxypurinol—which causes toxicity syndrome

Abbreviations used in table:

R — renal
H — hepatic

I — interval extension method of dosage adjustment; data units are hours between maintenance doses
D — dose reduction method of dosage adjustment; data units are percent of usual maintenance dose

Unch — unchanged
He — hemodialysis
P — peritoneal dialysis

ESRD — end-stage renal disease
GFR — glomerular filtration rate

| Drug | Elimination and Metabolism | Method | Adjustment for Renal Failure | | | Removed by Dialysis | Toxic Effects and Remarks (GT — group toxicity; GR — group remarks) |
| | | | GFR (ml/min) | | | | |
			>50	10–50	<10		
Colchicine	R (H)	D	Unch	Unch*	50*	No (He)	GT *Avoid prolonged use if GFR <50 ml/min; reversible myoneuropathy with drug retention
Etidronate	R (bone)	D	Unch	Unch	Avoid	?	Can cause elevated serum creatinine
Fenoprofen	H	D	Unch	Unch	Unch	No (He)	GT
Gold sodium thiomalate	R	D	Unch	Avoid	Avoid	No (He)	GT; nephrotoxic: can cause proteinuria and membranous glomerulonephritis
Ibuprofen	H	D	Unch	Unch	Unch	No (He)	GT; may cause sodium retention and decreased GFR
Indomethacin	H (R <15%)	D	Unch	Unch	Unch	No (He)	GT; acute renal failure reported; antidiuretic; sodium retention; decreases effect of loop diuretics; probenecid may increase serum levels
Ketoprofen	H	D	Unch	Unch	Unch	?	GT
Naproxen	H	D	Unch	Unch	Unch	No (He)	GT; sodium retention; half-life prolonged by probenecid; can reduce GFR
Piroxicam	H	D	Unch	Unch	Unch	?	GT
Probenecid	R*	D	Unch	Avoid†	Avoid†	?	GT *Renal excretion dependent on urine flow and pH †Ineffective
Sulindac	H (R)	D	Unch	Unch	50	?	GT

Miscellaneous Agents (continued)

Drug	Elimination and Metabolism	Method	Adjustment for Renal Failure			Removed by Dialysis	Toxic Effects and Remarks (GT — group toxicity; GR — group remarks)
			GFR (ml/min)				
			>50	10–50	<10		
Other drugs							
Digoxin Immune Fab	H	D	Unch	Unch	Unch	?	Rebound of digoxin level delayed in ESRD patients (96 hr vs. 48 hr); very limited pharmacokinetic data available
Goserelin	Non-R	D	Unch	Unch	Unch	?	—
Granisetron	Non-R	D	Unch	Unch	Unch	No	
Metoclopramide	R (H)	D	Unch	75	50	?	—
Octreotide	R (H)	D	Unch	Unch	50–75	?	—
Ondansetron	H	D	Unch	Unch	Unch	?	No studies in patients with renal impairment have been conducted; may cause elevation of aminotransferase and bilirubin
Penicillamine	R	D	Unch	75	25	Yes (He)	Reversible, rapidly progressive glomerulonephritis; nephrotic syndrome; interstitial nephritis; proteinuria, which is usually reversible
Pentoxifylline	R	D	Unch	Unch	50–75	?	—
Recombinant human erythropoietin	H	D	Unch	Unch	Unch	No	Lower doses required when using subcutaneous dosing

Abbreviations used in table:

R — renal
H — hepatic

I — interval extension method of dosage adjustment; data units are hours between maintenance doses
D — dose reduction method of dosage adjustment; data units are percent of usual maintenance dose

Unch — unchanged
He — hemodialysis
P — peritoneal dialysis

ESRD — end-stage renal disease
GFR — glomerular filtration rate

 Dialysis and Transplantation

NINA E. TOLKOFF-RUBIN, M.D.

Hemodialysis

Principles of Hemodialysis

When a failing kidney can no longer adequately excrete waste products, regulate acid-base balance, and maintain sodium and water homeostasis, dialysis should be instituted. The major goals of dialysis are to adjust the solute concentration of the blood and to remove excess fluid. The methods for accomplishing renal replacement therapy are hemodialysis and peritoneal dialysis. Other methods must be employed to substitute for the endocrine functions of the kidney.

In hemodialysis, solute removal occurs predominantly by diffusion, which is the movement of solutes (e.g., urea or potassium) from the blood compartment to the dialysate compartment across a semipermeable membrane. The clearance of a particular solute depends on various factors[1,2]:

1. Membrane surface area: the net flux of a solute increases as membrane surface area increases.
2. Membrane permeability for the solute: permeability is dependent on the specific characteristics of the membrane.
3. Concentration gradient between blood and dialysate fluid: the greater the concentration gradient, the more rapidly diffusion occurs.
4. Blood and dialysate flow rates: blood and dialysate normally flow in opposite directions (countercurrent flow) to maintain a maximal gradient for diffusion across the dialysis membrane.
5. Molecular size: clearance is higher for smaller molecules and lower for larger molecules.

The movement of solute across a semipermeable membrane can also occur by ultrafiltration.[2] As plasma water moves across the dialysis membrane, there is a bulk movement of solute along with the water. This process, called convective mass transfer, occurs because frictional forces between solvent and solute, called solvent drag, pull solute molecules through the membrane as water flows through. In this process, solute removal is not dependent on concentration gradients between the blood and dialysate.

Although the convective transfer of solutes is minimal during conventional hemodialysis, this mode plays a larger role in the new, extremely permeable high-flux dialyzers that have high ultrafiltration rates.[2]

Fluid removal occurs by ultrafiltration. In conventional hemodialysis, excessive extracellular fluid can be removed by applying positive pressure to the blood compartment or negative pressure to the dialysate compartment. The sum of these two pressures is called the transmembrane pressure. One of the major determinants of the ultrafiltration rate is the ultrafiltration coefficient of the dialyzer. This number indicates how much water can be removed from the blood during a given period at a specific transmembrane pressure.

Until recently, the physician determined the transmembrane pressure required to achieve a specified weight loss during the course of a hemodialysis run by referring to the specific ultrafiltration coefficient of the available dialyzer. The new ultrafiltration control devices on modern dialysis machines can be programmed for a desired weight loss, and the machine will continually adjust the transmembrane pressure across the dialysis membrane according to blood flow rate and dialysate pressures to remove the appropriate volume.

Dialysis and ultrafiltration usually proceed together. However, it has been observed that separating ultrafiltration from dialysis (i.e., sequential ultrafiltration and dialysis) permits faster and more efficient removal of fluid.[3-5] This process is better tolerated by patients and results in less hypotension, cramping, nausea, and vomiting. It appears that during isolated ultrafiltration, despite a decrease in cardiac output and stroke volume, systemic vascular resistance increases; consequently, blood pressure remains stable. In contrast, if vigorous ultrafiltration is attempted during diffusive dialysis, the decrease in cardiac output and stroke volume is frequently accompanied by a reduction in systemic vascular resistance and a fall in blood pressure.[3-5]

The greater hemodynamic stability observed during isolated ultrafiltration is not well understood but may reflect the fact that the serum osmolality remains constant during ultrafiltration, allowing for refilling of the vascular space.[3-5] In contrast, the serum osmolality falls during hemodialysis, leading to fluid movement into the cells as well as into the dialysate solution.

Whatever the reason, the separation of ultrafiltration and dialysis is a clinically important technique in caring for critically ill patients with volume overload and hemodynamic instability.

Vascular Access

One of the initial obstacles to the widespread application of dialysis on a long-term basis was the difficulty in attaining repeated access to the circulation. A major advance came with the development of the arteriovenous shunt by Quinton, Dillard, and Scribner in 1960.[6] This device consists of external silastic cannulas inserted into the radial artery and cephalic vein and connected by a piece of Teflon tubing. This form of access enables immediate and repeated hemodialyses. Although shunts are still used for some patients with acute renal failure, this form of access is now used infrequently because it requires surgical placement (sacrificing a peripheral artery and vein) and because it is associated with a significant risk of clotting, dislodging, bleeding, and infection.[7] For temporary access in patients with acute or chronic renal failure who require hemodialysis, the percutaneous placement of double-lumen catheters in either the femoral, internal jugular, or subclavian vein by a modified Seldinger technique is now the preferred approach.[8] These catheters provide immediate, repeated, and convenient access to the circulation, generally allowing blood flows of greater than 200 ml/min. Potential complications of subclavian line placement include the development of pneumothorax, bleeding, arterial laceration, brachial nerve injury, subclavian stenosis, and line sepsis.[7]

One of the major advances in vascular access for chronic renal failure patients came with the introduction of the arteriovenous (AV) fistula in 1966 by Brescia and Cimino.[9] This technique involves the surgical anastomosis of the radial artery and cephalic vein subcutaneously, with subsequent arterialization of the superficial forearm veins. Because the AV fistula generally requires time to "mature," that is, for the vessels to become large enough to permit adequate blood flow, this access cannot be used immediately and must be placed at least eight weeks before it will be required. Therefore, vascular access should be constructed by the time the serum creatinine level reaches 8 mg/dl. Because the fistula is internal, there is less risk of trauma, bleeding, and infection. Although the fistula remains the best method of access for chronic-maintenance hemodialysis patients,[7,10] prosthetic grafts may be required for vascular access in patients with failed fistulas and in elderly patients or diabetics with small blood vessels.[7]

Hemodialyzers

The modern dialysis machine consists of the dialyzer (i.e., the dialysis membrane), a pump that regulates blood-flow rate, and a dialysate solution delivery system. In addition, there are a series of safety monitors that continuously determine arterial and venous pressures, the conductivity of the dialysate solution, and water temperature. These monitors also check for blood leaks or air within the extracorporeal circuit.

The hollow-fiber dialyzer is the most frequently used type. It consists of thousands of parallel capillary tubes. Blood flows through the tubes, and dialysate flows around them. The advantages of this dialyzer are its small priming volume, low leak rate, predictability of clearance and ultrafiltration, ease of reuse, efficiency, and low cost.[1]

The dialyzer membrane is the critical component of the dialysis system. There are three considerations when evaluating dialysis membranes: performance (permeability), biocompatibility, and price.[11] Conventional dialysis membranes are made of cuprophane or cellulose acetate. These membranes have excellent small-molecule clearance but poor middle-molecule clearance. It is well established that cuprophane and other regenerated cellulose membranes activate complement via the alternative pathway, leading to transient leukopenia, with trapping of leukocytes in the pulmonary vasculature and impaired oxygen exchange (see below).[12] Occasional anaphylactic reactions involving fever, chest pain, respiratory distress, and circulatory collapse also have been reported with cuprophane and regenerated cellulose membranes.[11] Reuse of cellulose membrane dialyzers appears to decrease these first-use symptoms and improve biocompatibility.[13] It has also been demonstrated that cuprophane membranes may stimulate the generation of interleukin-1 (IL-1), either directly by activating adhering monocytes or indirectly by complement activation, with release of C5a.[14,15] It has been postulated that interleukins may be responsible for several acute and chronic symptoms observed in patients dialyzed with regenerated cellulose membranes (e.g., hypotension and β_2-microglobulin accumulation).[16]

More-permeable membranes made of polycarbonate, polyacrylonitrile (PAN), and polymethyl methacrylate are now available. These membranes not only have a high diffusive clearance for larger molecules and higher ultrafiltration rates but also are less likely to induce complement activation and its consequences, appear to be less thrombogenic, and may have a lower incidence of first-use reactions, such as sneezing, itching, and shortness of breath.[11]

The potential long-term benefits of high-flux, high-permeability membranes remain to be determined. Although these very efficient membranes reduce dialysis time (certainly a perceived benefit from the patient's standpoint) and increase the clearance of middle molecules, such as β_2-microglobulin,[11] they are considerably more expensive and require meticulous ultrafiltration control.[9]

Long-term studies are necessary to determine whether these membranes decrease the occurrence of neuropathy and whether removal of β_2-microglobulin improves or prevents dialysis-related arthropathies (i.e., carpal tunnel syndrome and amyloid deposition) that can incapacitate long-term dialysis patients (see below).[11]

Anticoagulation

Standard dialysis membranes activate not only the complement cascade but also the clotting mechanism. Anticoagulation is necessary to avoid the clotting of blood within the dialyzer system. For chronic maintenance hemodialysis, systemic anticoagulation with heparin is generally performed during treatment, either by repeated boluses or constant infusion along with monitoring of the whole blood partial thromboplastin time or activated clotting time (ACT).[17] A number of protocols[18-21] have been developed to decrease the risk of systemic anticoagulation in high-risk patients who require hemodialysis, such as those with pericarditis or gastrointestinal bleeding or patients in the postoperative period, who are at high risk for bleeding.

Regional heparinization has been used, whereby heparin is infused in the arterial line and protamine is infused in the venous line to neutralize the heparin. Because protamine has a shorter half-life in the body than heparin, some free heparin may circulate hours after dialysis is terminated, even if an extra dose of protamine is given at the end of the run. This complication is called heparin rebound.[17,18] Fractional low-dose heparinization, using small boluses of heparin and targeting the ACT to 30 seconds above control, has also been used.[1,2,17] However, despite these efforts to minimize the risk of bleeding, there is a 15 to 19 percent incidence of major bleeding complications in high-risk hemodialysis patients.[18] Although prostacyclin[19] has successfully replaced heparin in acute hemodialysis patients, the routine long-term use of this drug is not feasible because of the close hemodynamic monitoring required. Protocols using citrate anticoagulation have been reported,[20] but this method is complicated and difficult to perform.

So-called heparin-free dialysis is making other anticoagulation regimens obsolete in patients at high risk for bleeding.[17,21] The critical elements of this technique include heparin priming of the extracorporeal circuit, maintaining high blood-flow rates, and periodic saline flushes. Using this heparin-free dialysis protocol, clotting of the dialyzer will occur in approximately five to eight percent of cases.[21] However, this level is acceptable because it outweighs the danger of bleeding associated with heparin administration in high-risk patients.

Dialysate Solutions

The dialysate solution is a balanced salt solution with an appropriate buffer. Most dialysis equipment now uses a dialysate concentrate that is diluted 1:34 with water that is purified by reverse osmosis to remove potentially harmful trace elements, such as aluminum, copper, and fluoride. The sodium concentration of the dialysate generally ranges from 135 to 140 mEq/L. Higher dialysate sodium concentrations are used to counteract the hypotension, muscle cramping, nausea, vomiting, and headache that are often seen with rapid fluid shifts.[22] The higher sodium concentration appears to improve tolerance to dialysis by preventing sudden, precipitous falls in serum osmolality.[4,22]

The standard potassium concentration in the dialysate solution is 2.0 mEq/L, but this concentration may be varied to suit the individual requirements of the patient. Because rapid removal of potassium is likely to induce arrhythmias, close cardiac monitoring is necessary, particularly if the patient is receiving a digitalis preparation.

Either acetate or bicarbonate buffer is added to the dialysate solution to correct the metabolic acidosis of uremia. In the original dialysis system, bicarbonate was used as the buffer, and CO_2 was bubbled into the system to prevent the precipitation of relatively insoluble calcium and magnesium salts. To avoid these technical and practical problems on a large scale, acetate was substituted for bicarbonate in commercial dialysate concentrates.

Acetate is metabolized in the body via the Krebs cycle to generate bicarbonate. This reaction takes place predominantly in the liver and muscle. Although normal individuals can metabolize large amounts of acetate (approximately 300 mEq/hr), the influx of acetate may often greatly exceed this capacity during hemodialysis.[23] Simultaneously, acetate will accumulate in the blood and bicarbonate will be lost to the dialysate solution. This process occurs in patients dialyzed on large-surface-area dialyzers at high blood-flow and high dialysate-flow rates and becomes particularly important in critically ill patients with sepsis, lactic acidosis, diabetes, or liver failure. Under these conditions, the normal metabolic pathways for removal of acetate are markedly impaired, and the influx of acetate from the dialysate solution overwhelms the body's capacity to utilize it.[22,23] As a result, patients develop acetate intolerance, a condition manifested by exacerbation of metabolic acidosis, nausea, vomiting, cramping, headache, and marked hemodynamic instability.[22-29] The instability may be caused by the vasodilator and myocardial depressant properties of acetate; increased acetate levels may therefore be poorly tolerated in patients with a precarious cardiac status.[26,27]

Dialysate solutions containing acetate may contribute to the hypoxemia of dialysis. The Po_2 may drop by 15 to 30 mm Hg during hemodialysis.[30] Although this decrease may not be significant in the stable patient on long-term hemodialysis, it can be critically important in patients with underlying coronary or lung disease, in which this fall in Po_2 can precipitate the need for intubation.

Two factors contribute to dialysis-related hypoxemia: the membrane and the dialysate bath.[23,30] As noted previously, the dialysis membrane activates the complement cascade, which leads to white blood cell aggregation, sequestration of white cell emboli in the lungs, and hypoxia.[12] This phenomenon, which generally appears within 15 minutes of initiating dialysis, is much more common with unsubstituted cuprophane membranes than with synthetic membranes and appears to be diminished by reuse of the dialyzer.[11,22] When an acetate dialysate solution is used in hemodialysis, blood passing through the dialyzer loses CO_2 to the dialysate solution, resulting in hypocapnia. This decrease leads to hypoventilation to maintain the blood Pco_2, thus exacerbating hypoxemia.[22,30] In contrast, the Pco_2 remains constant in a bicarbonate bath, where there is constant generation of CO_2.[30]

Bicarbonate dialysis may therefore be preferred for specific patients. Solutions containing bicarbonate are more effective than those containing acetate in correcting metabolic acidosis in critically ill patients and in patients on high-permeability dialyzers; in addition, better hemodynamic stability can be achieved with bicarbonate dialysis, allowing higher ultrafiltration rates.[27-30] The risk of dialysis-induced hypoxemia is also diminished with a bicarbonate bath.[30] Double-blind studies[28,29] have shown that for both chronic hemodialysis patients and acutely ill patients, hemodialysis with a solution containing bicarbonate is associated with a reduction in the frequency of such dialysis-related symptoms as nausea, vomiting, headaches, and cramping compared with acetate dialysis. Moreover, results of postdialysis task-performance tests are worse after acetate dialysis as compared with bicarbonate dialysis.[28,29]

Bicarbonate dialysate solutions in the new commercially available liquid concentrate form are preferred for acute care and for use with highly permeable, high-flux dialysis membranes with large surface areas. However, bicarbonate dialysis is considerably more expensive and requires a complex dual-concentrate delivery system. There have also been a number of reports of bacterial contamination with the liquid concentrate form.[31]

Indications for Hemodialysis

There are five major indications for instituting hemodialysis: uremia, hyperkalemia, volume overload, acidosis, and uremic pericarditis. The most common indications for hemodialysis therapy are the manifestations of the uremic syndrome, such as nausea, vomiting, anorexia, increasing fatigue, or changes in mental status (lethargy, confusion, seizures, or coma). Although most physicians usually initiate dialysis when the blood urea nitrogen (BUN) level is greater than 125 mg/dl, the presence of symptoms and signs of the uremic syndrome is more important than BUN and creatinine levels.

Hyperkalemia is another indication for initiating hemodialysis, particularly in the presence of ECG changes, oliguria, severe hypercatabolism, or failure of conservative therapy. These conservative methods include reduction of dietary potassium to 2 g/day, administration of oral ion exchange resins, or the short-term administration of glucose, insulin, or bicarbonate.

Hemodialysis is also indicated for patients with fluid overload that is unresponsive to diuretics. Emergency ultrafiltration may be required in patients with pulmonary edema or severe volume-dependent hypertension. Detection of a pericardial friction rub, which indicates the presence of uremic pericarditis, is another indication for starting dialysis. Frequently, patients with severe metabolic acidosis require initiation of hemodialysis therapy to remove sufficient fluid to allow for further administration of sodium bicarbonate.

Table 1　Toxin Removal by Hemodialysis and Hemoperfusion

Drug	Toxic Level	Procedure	Signs and Symptoms
Salicylates	80 mg/dl	Hemodialysis	Persistent respiratory alkalosis and anion-gap metabolic acidosis CNS toxicity
Lithium	2.5–3.5 mEq/L	Hemodialysis	Ataxia, coma, convulsions Arrhythmias, hypotension
Phenobarbital	10 mg/dl	Hemodialysis or hemoperfusion	Sedation, coma
Methanol	> 50 mg/dl	Hemodialysis[*]	Metabolic acidosis with increased anion gap from formic acid accumulation Osmolar gap (31 mOsm for 100 mg/dl of methanol) Visual disturbances
Ethylene glycol (antifreeze)	50 mg/dl	Hemodialysis[*]	Metabolic acidosis with increased ion gap and osmolar gap Oxalate crystals in urine
Theophylline	30–40 μg/ml	Hemoperfusion (preferred) or hemodialysis	Cardiac arrhythmias CNS toxicity: seizures, agitation, coma
Glutethimide	4 mg/dl	Hemoperfusion	Hypotension, circulatory collapse CNS depression, coma
Methaqualone	4 mg/dl	Hemoperfusion	CNS toxicity

[*]Additional procedure: ethanol infusion to compete for alcohol dehydrogenase, which decreases metabolism of methanol to formic acid and metabolism of ethylene glycol to oxalic acid (loading dose, 6 g/kg; maintenance infusion, 70–140 mg/kg/hr); alternative agent is 4-methylpyrazole, an alcohol dehydrogenase inhibitor (experimental).

Acute institution of hemodialysis is also indicated in drug intoxications by low-molecular-weight, water-soluble compounds such as methanol, ethylene glycol, lithium carbonate, and salicylate [*see Table 1*].[1,2,32] In contrast, lipid-soluble drugs such as glutethimide, methaqualone, and barbiturates are best removed by hemoperfusion.[32]

Hemoperfusion Hemoperfusion is a technique that involves adsorption of the potential toxin on a column of activated microencapsulated charcoal. Hemoperfusion is the treatment of choice for patients with severe theophylline overdoses, although hemodialysis may be somewhat effective if hemoperfusion is not available.[32]

Like hemodialysis, hemoperfusion requires the establishment of vascular access, a pump to move blood through a cartridge, and systemic anticoagulation. Previously, two major problems with hemoperfusion were embolization of charcoal granules and the severe bleeding caused by the adsorption of platelets. The cartridges now available have obviated these complications. Nonetheless, bleeding, hypotension, and hypocalcemia can occur.[32]

Complications During Hemodialysis

Dialysis Disequilibrium

Patients with acute or chronic renal failure who begin hemodialysis with markedly elevated BUN levels are at risk for dialysis disequilibrium.[33-36] This syndrome is manifested by varying degrees of nausea, vomiting, restlessness, headache, lethargy, muscle twitching, confusion, and, on occasion, generalized seizures.[34] Many factors contribute to dialysis disequilibrium, but a sudden increase in the volume of brain water appears to be the major pathological process. During vigorous hemodialysis, when the plasma osmolality and urea level are rapidly lowered, the plasma becomes hypotonic with respect to brain tissue, resulting in cerebral edema.[34,35]

In addition, despite the fact that dialysis corrects systemic metabolic acidosis, a paradoxical acidosis develops in the cerebrospinal fluid.[36] Acidosis occurs because CO_2 diffuses more rapidly than bicarbonate across the blood-brain barrier. As a result, the cerebrospinal fluid and the brain intracellular pH remain low. This decrease in pH appears to alter the binding of certain intracellular cations, increasing the osmotic gradient from the brain to blood and causing subsequent cerebral edema.[34,36]

Because the disequilibrium syndrome occurs most often during rapid, aggressive hemodialysis, the most important principle is prevention: the initiation of slower and shorter but more frequent dialysis treatments at lower blood-flow rates will avoid the initial rapid fall in serum osmolality.[34-36] The incidence of disequilibrium can also be minimized by the use of a dialysate with a high sodium concentration and the administration of intravenous mannitol (1 g/kg) over the course of dialysis.[37] Mannitol, an osmotically active agent, will counteract the effect of rapidly lowering the BUN level, thereby maintaining serum osmolality at a relatively constant level. There are no controlled studies demonstrating the efficacy of anticonvulsants in the prophylaxis of dialysis disequilibrium.

Hypotension

The development of hypotension is the major complication of hemodialysis for both stable and acutely ill patients.[2,22,30,33,38,39] Hypotension most often results from excessive ultrafiltration and volume depletion; it responds to saline infusion, regulation of the ultrafiltration rate, and appropriate adjustment of the patient's weight.[38] As previously noted for patients who are hemodynamically unstable, the use of isolated ultrafiltration without dialysis allows more rapid and efficient fluid removal without hypotension by maintaining stable serum osmolality and systemic vascular resistance.[3-5]

Although a reduction in extracellular fluid volume remains the most common cause of hypotensive episodes in dialysis patients, a fall in blood pressure can occur whenever the body's vasoconstrictive mechanisms are impaired. Such impairment can result from the effect of antihypertensive medications taken before the run, the effect of acetate-containing dialysate solutions, and the presence of autonomic neuropathy, particularly in diabetics, which impairs the alpha-receptor response.[2,22,30,33] Dialysis may remove norepinephrine and epinephrine mediators that are critical to the vasoconstrictor response.[22] Hypotension may also be part of the first-use syndrome seen with cuprophane or cellulose acetate membranes (see above).[30]

Hemorrhage, acute myocardial ischemia, arrhythmias, sepsis, and pericardial effusion must be excluded as the cause of hypotension in any patient who does not respond readily to volume replacement.[2,22] Any patient who becomes increasingly unstable on dialysis without an obvious source should undergo cardiac ultrasonography to exclude tamponade, which can be an acute, potentially life-threatening complication.

Air Embolus

A number of technical problems can complicate the hemodialysis procedure: hemolysis from the incorrect dialysate solution or high temperature,[40-42] sepsis from a contaminated dialysate solution,[2,40] water contamination,[43] or hemorrhage from blood leaks.[2] However, the most devastating technical complication is an air embolus. If it is not recognized and treated immediately, an air embolus can lead to death.[2,30,40] Air detectors on dialysis machines significantly decrease the possibility that air in the blood circuit will reach the patient. If air is detected, a relay switch automatically clamps the venous line and shuts off the blood pump. Despite this safeguard, however, the increased use of subclavian catheters for temporary dialysis access and repeated attachment and disconnection of lines for administration of intravenous fluids can introduce a small amount of air into the bloodstream.

The signs and symptoms of an air embolus depend on the position of the patient.[40] If the patient is sitting upright in a chair, air entering the bloodstream will travel up the jugular vein to the brain. Neurologic deficits, seizures, and loss of consciousness may occur. If the patient is supine, the air will pass to the right ventricle, where it foams and can lead to arrhythmias and impaired myocardial function. The patient may complain of marked agitation, severe dyspnea, cough, and chest pain. On auscultation, a peculiar churning sound may be heard.[22,40]

Immediate treatment is critical. The patient should be positioned on the left side, with head and chest lower than the abdomen, to trap air in the right ventricle. In addition, 100 percent oxygen should be administered by face mask or endotracheal tube.[23,30,40]

Prevention is equally important. Vented glass bottles should not be used during dialysis; all intravenous fluids should be administered from collapsible bags. An air detector should always be present on the venous line, and the administration of intravenous fluids through the dialysis machine should be closely supervised.

Long-term Complications

Anemia

Pathogenesis Anemia remains one of the major long-term problems in individuals undergoing dialysis. More than 25 percent of patients require transfusions, and most individuals become disabled by weakness and marked fatigability.[44] It is now well recognized that decreased erythropoietin production is the major factor contributing to the anemia of chronic renal failure.[44] However, a number of other factors related to the dialysis procedure may contribute to this condition. Iron deficiency may occur in dialyzed patients as a result of gastrointestinal bleeding, blood sampling, or loss of blood into the dialyzer or at fistula sites.[2] Folate deficiency may also occur because this vitamin is lost during dialysis. Because folate is required for erythropoiesis, its replacement is necessary.

Dialysis-related hemolysis, although rare, can contribute to large decreases in serum hematocrit levels. Hemolysis can be caused by several factors, including copper[45] and chloramine contamination of the water supply,[46,47] overheated or hypotonic dialysate solution,[41,42] and formaldehyde contamination.[48]

A number of dialysis patients in the United States have died of copper-induced acute hemolysis. This situation has occurred when ionized copper was leached from copper tubing in the inflow dialysis fluid circuit.[43] Copper contamination should be suspected in any patient who presents with skin flushing, chills, vomiting, abdominal cramps, and diarrhea during dialysis.[40]

Chloramine, which is often added to city water supplies to decrease bacterial contamination, can lead to methemoglobinemia and acute hemolysis.[43,46,47] Deionization of the water supply or neutralization of the dialysis fluid with ascorbic acid can prevent complications from chloramine.[43,46,47]

Formaldehyde, which is used to sterilize dialysis equipment, has been implicated in the anemia of dialysis patients. Formaldehyde inhibits red blood cell glycolysis, leading to hemolysis.[48] Some investigators have found hemolysis to be associated with the development of red blood cell antibodies, and they have postulated that the prolonged exposure of red blood cells to residual formaldehyde trapped in the dialyzer during reuse is the most likely cause.[49]

Aluminum toxicity, either from aluminum contamination of the water supply or through the use of phosphate-binding agents, has been associated with microcytic anemia in chronic dialysis patients with normal iron stores.[50] It is thought that aluminum interferes with iron uptake by red blood cells, causing a relatively intracellular deficiency of iron and microcytic anemia.[44,50] This condition responds to deferoxamine chelation therapy.[50]

Some investigators have suggested that the hyperparathyroidism that occurs secondary to chronic renal failure may contribute to the anemia seen in hemodialysis patients.[51-53] It is thought that excess parathyroid hormone inhibits erythropoiesis by replacing bone marrow with fibrous tissue (osteitis fibrosa).[54] In some cases, subtotal parathyroidectomy can lead to decreased red blood cell mass.[54]

Although these dialysis-related factors play a role in the pathogenesis of anemia in specific cases, the major factor responsible for the hypoproliferative anemia of dialysis patients is decreased erythropoietin production.[44,55]

Until recently, the therapy for anemia in the patient with end-stage renal disease has been rather limited and directed toward associated conditions, such as iron deficiency anemia and aluminum toxicity, and toward the removal of potential toxins from the dialysate.[44,55] Androgens have been administered to some patients to increase erythropoiesis and appear to be moderately effective.[56,57] Androgens are thought to stimulate both renal and extrarenal production of erythropoietin, but the response rate with these drugs is variable and unpredictable. Nandrolone decanoate can be administered in doses of 200 to 300 mg intramuscularly each week. Liver function abnormalities are a frequent complication of these drugs. In addition, androgens may produce virilizing effects.[57]

Transfusions have been the main treatment for symptomatic anemia in dialysis patients, particularly in those with angina, congestive heart failure, or severe symptoms of weakness and increased fatigability. However, transfusions have many potential consequences.[58]

One drawback is the risk of transmitting viral infections, such as hepatitis, cytomegalovirus, and the human immunodeficiency virus (HIV). Although screening programs have significantly decreased the risk of transmission of hepatitis B and HIV, the incidence of hepatitis C has remained high. The transfusion-associated risk of hepatitis C is approximately one per 125 exposures and can lead to chronic active hepatitis and cirrhosis.[59] New screening procedures for hepatitis C virus will most likely decrease this problem.

Another transfusion-related problem in the hemodialysis population is the attendant risk of iron overload, with the potential for liver dysfunction, hemosiderosis, increased skin pigmentation, and cardiomyopathy.[58,60] It has also been suggested that excess iron may stimulate the growth of fungi such as *Candida*, gram-negative bacteria such as *Pseudomonas*, and gram-positive bacteria such as *Listeria monocytogenes*.[58,61] A third problem is that transfusions increase the risk of sensitizing potential transplant patients to histocompatibility antigens, as a result of exposure to the HLA antigens on white blood cells.[58]

The most important and significant addition to the treatment of the anemia of chronic dialysis patients is recombinant human erythropoietin, which was approved in 1989 for clinical use. A number of studies[44,62-66] indicate that erythropoietin effectively corrects the anemia of hemodialysis patients when iron deficiency anemia, folate deficiency, aluminum toxicity, infection, and blood loss are excluded.[63] The hematocrit increases in a dose-dependent manner; doses between 100 and 150 U/kg appear sufficient to raise the hematocrit to normal levels.[63] In the absence of blood loss, the need for periodic transfusions has been virtually eliminated with the administration of erythropoietin. An additional benefit in some dialysis patients has been correction of the bleeding time to normal.[66]

Many investigators describe increased well-being, decreased fatigue, and improvements in neurobehavioral function, cognitive function, sexual function, quality of life, and cardiopulmonary performance with erythropoietin administration.[62-65,67-70]

Iron replacement therapy may be required to meet the demands of stimulated erythropoiesis in patients with decreased iron stores. Maintenance of the transferrin saturation level above 20 percent or a ferritin level greater than 150 units should ensure an adequate iron supply for most patients.[44] (The transferrin saturation level is defined as serum iron/total iron binding capacity × 100 percent.) In addition, erythropoietin may effectively reduce iron levels in patients with iron overload and hemosiderosis.

Although a preliminary report[63] suggested a possible rise in predialysis serum creatinine, BUN, and potassium levels in patients treated with erythropoietin, further studies using both conventional and high-flux dialyzers have not demonstrated significant increases.[71,72]

The findings in the preliminary reports probably reflected increased protein and potassium intake that resulted from increased appetite and sense of well-being rather than from diminished dialytic clearances. However, the fact that two patients in the initial study[63] had severe, recurrent episodes of hyperkalemia and that one patient apparently died of hyperkalemia reinforces the need for meticulous dietary supervision.

A number of potential adverse effects have been noted.[62-65]

A rise in blood pressure has been well documented, requiring either initiation of antihypertensive therapy or additional antihypertensive medication in up to 30 to 40 percent of dialysis patients treated with erythropoietin.[62-65,73] This rise may be caused by increases in peripheral vascular resistance, which are mediated by active arteriolar vasoconstriction that occurs as anemia-dependent vasodilatation is corrected.[74] Alternatively, increases in viscosity may play a role.[75] The

hypertensive effect does not necessarily preclude the administration of erythropoietin to dialysis patients. Rather, slow introduction of the drug is recommended, aiming for a rise in hematocrit of one percent a week.

Seizures have been noted in dialysis patients with hypertensive encephalopathy and in those with only moderate hypertension.[62,63] Seizures have not been observed in nonuremic patients treated with erythropoietin. It is not known whether seizures are drug related or are related to the underlying uremia and its treatment.[63,65]

Initial trials with erythropoietin also found an increased incidence of vascular access thrombosis in association with the progressive rise in hematocrit.[63] Although this finding has not been observed in subsequent multicenter trials when the target hematocrit has been maintained below 35 percent,[65] mean hourly heparin requirements have increased in some patients receiving erythropoietin who were undergoing conventional or high-flux dialysis.[65,76,77] This finding suggests that increased clotting occurs within dialyzers in association with the use of erythropoietin. This issue requires extensive investigation.

There are a number of critical, unresolved questions about erythropoietin usage in dialysis patients.[64]

1. Is intravenous or subcutaneous administration the best and most cost-effective route, and what is the optimal dosage schedule?

2. What is the optimal rate of increase in the hematocrit, and what is the ideal target hematocrit? A hematocrit between 30 and 33 percent rather than 35 percent may achieve the beneficial therapeutic effects without incurring hypertension and seizures.

3. What are the long-term consequences of erythropoietin? Specifically, does the increase in hematocrit and blood viscosity lead to a significant increase in vascular thrombosis, hypertension, and acceleration of atherosclerosis? Will raising the hematocrit and blood viscosity change

the effectiveness and adequacy of dialysis, especially with high-flux dialyzers?

Long-term studies are currently under way to answer these questions.

Hemodialysis-Related Amyloidosis

Long-term hemodialysis patients (those who undergo hemodialysis for more than seven years) manifest unique musculoskeletal syndromes, such as carpal tunnel syndrome, arthropathy, and pathological fractures, that do not appear to be caused by hyperparathyroidism or the accumulation of aluminum.[78] A unique variety of amyloid has been isolated from the tissues of these patients. The term hemodialysis-related amyloidosis is used to describe the constellation of clinical findings.[78,79]

The amyloid isolated from the synovium and bone of dialysis patients stains positively for Congo red, exhibits an apple-colored birefringence under polarized light, and manifests the twisted β-pleated sheet configuration on x-ray crystallography, but its chemical structure is quite different from the amyloid protein of primary or secondary amyloidosis.[78,79]

In the hemodialysis-related amyloid syndrome, the protein subunit appears to be β_2-microglobulin.[78,79] This protein is normally present on all cell membranes (except for red blood cells) and comprises the β chain of the HLA class I molecule required for cell-cell recognition. β_2-Microglobulin is largely metabolized and cleared by the kidney, and the plasma concentration of β_2-microglobulin is markedly elevated in dialysis patients.[79]

A number of investigators have noted a relation between the β_2-microglobulin level and the chemical composition of the dialysis membrane.[78,79] Predialysis serum levels of β_2-microglobulin in patients dialyzed with cuprophane membranes are only slightly higher than those in patients dialyzed with polyacrylonitrile membranes. However, during the course of a dialysis treatment, the serum β_2-microglobulin level is reduced with a synthetic membrane but can actually increase when a cuprophane membrane is used.[11,79] The cuprophane membrane can activate the complement system, with the subsequent generation of IL-1, leading to increased stimulation and synthesis of β_2-microglobulin.[14]

Preliminary clinical trials suggest that the synthetic membranes, which are less likely to activate complement, may prevent hemodialysis-related amyloidosis.[11] Carefully controlled studies are required before these very expensive membranes are routinely employed.

Aluminum Toxicity

Normally, the kidney is the major route of excretion of aluminum, which enters the body by oral or parenteral routes.[80] In the dialysis population, where renal excretion of aluminum and other solutes is impaired, the major sources of aluminum are the water supply used to prepare the dialysate solution and orally administered aluminum-containing phosphate binders.[80-82]

Aluminum toxicity in the dialysis patient takes a variety of forms: dialysis encephalopathy, vitamin D–resistant osteomalacia, and a microcytic anemia.[80,81]

Dialysis encephalopathy Dialysis encephalopathy is a distinctive clinical syndrome that was first described by Alfrey and colleagues in 1976.[83] Patients present with subtle changes in personality, reduction in short-term memory, and slurring of speech, which initially occurs toward the end of dialysis and eventually persists. Myoclonic spasms of the face, arms, legs, and trunk may become apparent. Major seizures, often leading to progressive deterioration in mental status and global dementia, may occur. The EEG can exhibit a distinctive pattern: episodic bursts of high-voltage spike activity on a background of slow wave activity. No specific pathological features have been found on microscopic examination of the brain in these patients.[80,81,83]

A number of lines of evidence have implicated aluminum toxicity as the cause of the syndrome.[80,81,83] First, the aluminum concentration in the brain gray matter of dialysis patients dying of dialysis encephalopathy has been found to be higher than that in dialysis patients dying of other causes. Second, a number of epidemiological studies have demonstrated that in areas with clusters of cases of dialysis encephalopathy, there were high concentrations of aluminum in the water used to prepare the dialysate. When aluminum was removed from the water by reverse osmosis or deionization, the number of cases significantly decreased.[80,81,83] Third, deferoxamine chelation therapy reduces neurologic toxicity and subsequently reduces serum aluminum levels (see below).[80,81,83-85] Renal transplantation, which restores the normal excretion of aluminum, also reduces symptoms.[86]

Skeletal toxicity Aluminum accumulation can also cause a vitamin D–resistant osteomalacia.[80,81] This skeletal syndrome is characterized by low parathyroid hormone (PTH) levels, mildly increased calcium levels, proximal myopathy, and pathological fractures. Bone biopsy demonstrates markedly decreased bone formation, with deposition of aluminum along the trabecular surface.[81,87] The accumulation of aluminum at the calcification front may inhibit the deposition of calcium and phosphorus.[87] Evidence implicating aluminum as the potential cause of this skeletal syndrome comes from epidemiological studies and is similar to the evidence noted for dialysis encephalopathy. High aluminum concentrations were demonstrated in the water supply that was used to prepare dialysate solutions, and improvement in the skeletal syndrome was noted with removal of aluminum from the water supply[80,81,85] and treatment with deferoxamine.[87]

Microcytic anemia Aluminum accumulation has also been shown to produce a microcytic anemia in humans with adequate iron stores and normal ferritin levels.[88,89] Aluminum appears to interfere with iron utilization, a defect that can be reversed with deferoxamine chelation therapy.[81]

Diagnosis In patients undergoing dialysis, monitoring of serum aluminum levels twice a year is recommended, particularly if the patient is taking aluminum-containing phosphate binders.[90] Samples must be stored in stoppered plastic tubes that have been pretested for the amount of aluminum they release.[90] The normal serum aluminum concentration is less than 10 µg/L, as measured by atomic absorption spectroscopy, whereas in most dialysis patients, serum aluminum concentrations range from 30 to 100 µg/L; concentrations over 100 µg/L are usually associated with clinically significant accumulation in bone or brain.[81,90]

Although serum levels appear to reflect exposure to aluminum and may be useful indicators of toxicity, such levels have a limited correlation with total body aluminum load; that is, serum levels may be normal even though levels in the soft tissue and brain are elevated.[81,90] It has therefore been suggested that a deferoxamine challenge is a better indicator of the amount of aluminum deposited in tissues than is the baseline serum aluminum level.[90,91] This test should be performed in all dialysis patients who have signs or symptoms suggestive of aluminum toxicity. The deferoxamine challenge is considered positive when the increment in serum aluminum exceeds 200 µg/L.[90,91]

Treatment Purification of the water used for dialysis by means of reverse osmosis or deionization has virtually eliminated the epidemics of dialysis encephalopathy previously observed.[80,81,89] Periodic testing is essential to ensure that the water treatment system is functioning properly.[90] At present, most cases of aluminum overload result from the ingestion of aluminum-containing phosphate binders. All efforts should be made to discontinue these drugs and to replace them with calcium-containing preparations.[81,92]

Clearance via hemodialysis is minimal because aluminum is tightly bound to protein.[93] Therefore, if toxicity occurs, deferoxamine therapy should be instituted. This chelating agent binds aluminum, forming a deferoxamine-aluminum complex. It can be administered intravenously (2 g) at the end of a hemodialysis session or intraperitoneally in an overnight dwell in peritoneal dialysis patients.[90] The deferoxamine-aluminum complex can be removed by hemodialysis or peritoneal dialysis. Accelerated removal of the complex can be achieved by using a charcoal hemoperfusion cartridge in series with the dialyzer.[94] A number of studies have demonstrated improvement in aluminum-related bone disease after six months of deferoxamine therapy. Bone biopsy specimens have shown decreased aluminum staining, increasing bone formation, and increased osteoblastic and osteoclastic activity.[87,95-97]

Unfortunately, a number of side effects have been observed with deferoxamine.[90] The drug must be administered cautiously over half an hour during the end of the run, and vital signs must be carefully monitored for signs of acute hypotension. Retinal and auditory toxicity have been observed with long-term administration. In addition, increased susceptibility to mucormycosis and *Yersinia* sepsis has been reported with the use of this drug.[98-100] Also, deferoxamine may precipitate or exacerbate dialysis encephalopathy.[90]

Adequacy of Dialysis

There is no standardized method of evaluating the adequacy of dialysis. Most patients are dialyzed empirically on the basis of clinical assessment, decrease in symptoms, and a general sense of well-being.[2,33] A number of factors, however, are clearly important in determining what degree of hemodialysis is necessary.[98] These factors include the generation rate of uremic toxins, residual renal function, protein intake, and body weight of the patient, in addition to dialysis-related factors such as the clearance rate of the dialyzer, dialysis time, and frequency of treatment.[33] A number of models for assessing the adequacy of dialysis have been proposed.

In the early 1970s, it was postulated that molecules of middle molecular weight were responsible for the toxic effects of uremia, and efforts were made to optimize therapy to increase their clearance. There is currently little evidence to support this theory, and it is generally thought that uremic symptoms correlate best with the level of urea and other small molecules.[33]

The blood urea level in the patient on intermittent hemodialysis is dependent on two processes: the decrease that occurs during the dialysis treatment and the increase that occurs during the interdialytic period. Any model that looks at the adequacy of dialysis has to consider both aspects and must include the patient's protein intake and nutritional status.

Uremic kinetic modeling is one method currently used to determine the adequacy of dialysis.[101,102] This approach uses the urea clearance per treatment, normalized to the volume of urea distribution (KT/V, where K = the urea clearance of the dialyzer, T = the treatment time, and V = the volume of distribution of urea). Utilizing this model, the National Cooperative Dialysis Study[101] suggested that urea was an excellent marker for measuring the adequacy of dialysis. Specifically, those patients with a KT/V less than 0.8 had a higher probability of death, hospitalization, and withdrawal from dialysis for medical reasons than those with a KT/V between 0.9 and 1.5.

The search for reliable methods to assess the adequacy of dialysis has become increasingly important as high-flux dialysis becomes more popular and efforts are directed toward shortening dialysis time.

Mortality

Hemodialysis has emerged during the past two decades as a safe, effective method of treating patients with end-stage renal disease. Mortality now averages five to eight percent a year for patients between 20 and 50 years of age.[33] Of course, this figure varies with age and underlying disease; for example, fewer than 25 percent of diabetics undergoing hemodialysis for chronic renal failure survive five years.[33] Cardiovascular complications remain the major cause of death, particularly stroke and myocardial infarction, which arise from long-standing hypertension and vascular disease. Infection and loss of access to the vascular system are also significant.[2,33] Discontinuation of hemodialysis is increasingly becoming a cause of death, which indicates that even though dialysis may successfully keep patients alive, quality of life may be significantly impaired for many patients, with marked restrictions in diet and travel and an inability to return to work.[33,103]

Peritoneal Dialysis

Peritoneal dialysis is an alternative form of renal replacement therapy and is performed by introducing dialysate solution containing glucose (dextrose) into the peritoneal cavity. Toxic waste products and excess fluid move from the blood into the dialysate solution by diffusion and ultrafiltration across the peritoneal membrane.[104] In peritoneal dialysis, osmotic ultrafiltration is achieved by adding increasing concentrations of glucose to the dialysate solution. The osmotic pressure generated by the glucose draws water from the blood and tissues into the dialysate.[104] With time, glucose is absorbed from the peritoneal cavity; thus, the osmotic effect is transient. In contrast to hemodialysis, in which membrane pore size almost completely restricts passage of molecules greater than 1,300 daltons, in peritoneal dialysis some transport of larger molecules, even proteins, occurs.

Peritoneal dialysis has been a well-established technique for the treatment of acute renal failure for more than two decades. This modality has been particularly useful for critically ill patients because it avoids the marked swings in blood pressure and chemical fluctuations caused by hemodialysis. Moreover, peritoneal dialysis can be safely performed in patients at high risk for bleeding because it avoids the use of heparin.[104] Only recently, however, has continuous ambulatory peritoneal dialysis (CAPD) emerged as a viable method for the treatment of patients with end-stage renal failure.

In CAPD, dialysate solution is infused from collapsible plastic bags into the abdominal cavity, where it remains, or dwells, for a given period and is then drained. Generally, three to five exchanges are performed daily, with an overnight dwell. Although numerous peritoneal catheters are now available, the one devised by Tenckhoff remains the most widely used.

Continuous ambulatory peritoneal dialysis has a number of medical and psychological advantages over hemodialysis for long-term therapy[104]:

1. Peritoneal dialysis does not require vascular access; avoidance of the potential risks and complications of vascular access is particularly important in children and in patients with severe atherosclerosis or diabetes. Anticoagulation is not required.

2. Peritoneal dialysis is a slower, more gentle procedure; therefore, it avoids precipitous changes in biochemical parameters, and dialysis disequilibrium is much less likely to occur.

3. Hemodynamic shifts are significantly reduced during peritoneal dialysis; therefore, this procedure is much better tolerated by children and by elderly individuals with angina or precarious cardiac status.

4. Peritoneal dialysis can improve the patient's quality of life. The technique can be performed at home, providing patients with a greater sense of independence and participation. The diet can be more liberal with respect to protein, salt, potassium, and fluid intake. The hematocrit tends to be higher in chronic peritoneal dialysis patients; therefore, there is less need for transfusion.[104] In addition, with the use of new automated cyclers, dialysis can be performed at night while the patient sleeps, thereby avoiding any interruption of work or school schedule.

5. Peritoneal dialysis is the preferred mode of therapy for children because, in addition to the reasons mentioned above, CAPD obviates the need for fistula sticks and, most importantly, enables growth.[104]

Complications

Peritoneal dialysis is contraindicated in anyone who cannot safely perform the procedure without contamination because of poor vision, lack of manual dexterity, or multiple abdominal surgical procedures and adhesions. Moreover, despite its many advantages, peritoneal dialysis has a number of potential complications, including technical problems with catheter placement or malfunction, failure of dialysis fluid to infuse or drain, dialysate leaks, alterations in peritoneal membrane permeability, and infection (see below).[104]

There are other potential problems of chronic peritoneal dialysis[104,105]:

1. Protein loss results from the high permeability of the peritoneal membrane.
2. Glucose absorption from the dialysate can lead to weight gain and exacerbate problems with diabetic blood glucose control.
3. Long-term metabolic consequences, including hyperlipidemia.
4. Increased intra-abdominal pressure from indwelling dialysate, which can lead to abdominal hernia.
5. Finally, and of most concern, the technique must be performed four to five times every day, thus interfering with daily activities. This requirement results in high dropout rates (15 to 20 percent) in the first year.[104]

CAPD is therefore not a panacea. However, this modality is an excellent alternative for children and the elderly and provides an alternative therapy for all patients with end-stage renal disease. Long-term studies that compare survival rates of patients receiving CAPD with those of patients on hemodialysis are needed.

Infection

Infection can occur at the catheter exit site, in the catheter tunnel, or within the peritoneal cavity. Exit-site infections are generally caused by organisms commonly found on the skin (*Staphylococcus aureus* or *S. epidermidis*) and should be treated aggressively to avoid contiguous contaminations of the cuff or tunnel. Tunnel infections may present with fever, pain, and swelling along the subcutaneous catheter tract. Frequently, in addition to antibiotic treatment, catheter removal becomes necessary to eradicate the infection.[104,105]

Peritonitis is the most serious infectious problem associated with long-term peritoneal dialysis.[104-107] The incidence is about one episode of peritonitis per patient per year, although it varies from 0.22 to four episodes per patient per year.[104] The first sign of peritonitis is a cloudy dialysate containing more than 100 polymorphonuclear leukocytes/mm^3, with or without abdominal pain, tenderness, or fever.[107] A Gram's stain and culture should be performed on the dialysate. Bacteriologic identification of the organism is critical for treatment. More than 70 percent of cases of peritonitis are caused by gram-positive organisms; the principal organisms are *S. epidermidis* and *S. aureus*. Twenty-five percent of the episodes of peritonitis are caused by gram-negative organisms, and fewer than five percent are caused by fungi or anaerobic bacteria.[103-109]

The previously reported high incidence of culture-negative peritonitis (up to 20 percent of cases) most likely resulted from inadequate processing of the dialysis fluid. Bacteriologic diagnosis may be significantly improved by culturing dialysate on blood culture media.[110]

A number of antibiotic protocols have been proposed to treat peritonitis in CAPD patients [*see Figure 1*].[107] Most treatment regimens use a combination of drugs given intravenously or intraperitoneally that empirically treat the most common organisms (*S. epidermidis*, *S. aureus*, and gram-negative organisms).[103-109] Frequent peritoneal lavage is no longer recommended. After several exchanges to decrease the inflammatory response and relieve abdominal pain, regular CAPD dwells are resumed. It may be necessary to add heparin (500 U/L dialysate) to decrease fibrin formation.[109]

Fungal peritonitis presents a therapeutic challenge.[109,111-113] Yeast species are the most common fungi, and *Candida* species are pre-

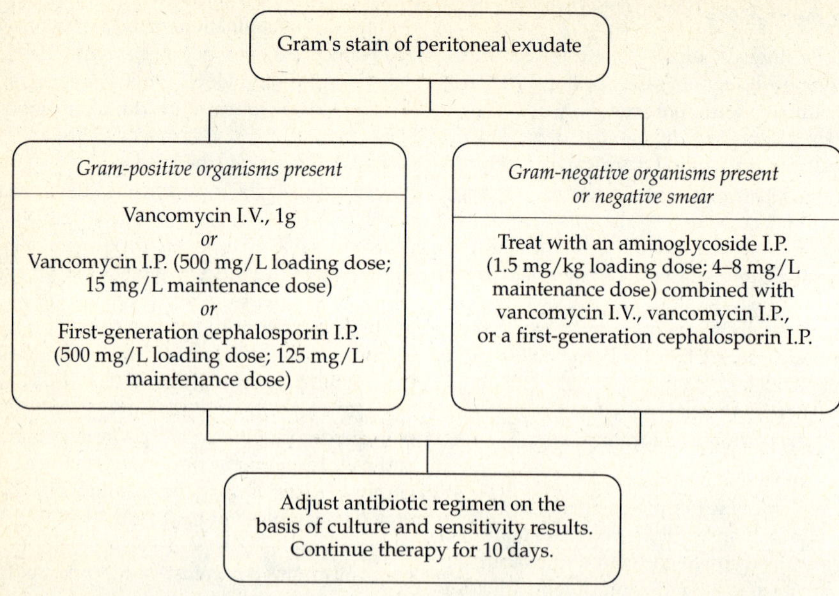

Figure 1   This flowchart illustrates the approach to a peritoneal dialysis patient with peritonitis.

dominant; filamentous fungi are occasionally observed. Although a cure rate of approximately 60 percent has been reported with amphotericin B (1.5 to 2.0 g total dose), catheter removal is generally required to eradicate colonization of the catheter lumen with hyphae, and there is a high rate of relapse after antifungal therapy is withdrawn.[111] Two cases of *Candida* peritonitis have been successfully treated with fluconazole.[114] If these results are confirmed, a more convenient oral form of antifungal therapy is on the horizon. In both cases, catheter removal was also required. Notably, both patients were able to successfully resume CAPD after therapy, without development of peritoneal adhesions.[114]

Occasionally, fecal peritonitis may occur as a result of perforation of a diverticulum or the appendix or from ischemic colitis. Fecal peritonitis should be suspected when cultures show polymicrobial infection with more than one species of gram-negative bacteria or anaerobes. Treatment involves not only the appropriate antibiotics (including anaerobic coverage) but also surgical exploration to determine the site of perforation.

Renal Transplantation

During the past two decades, renal transplantation has evolved from an experiment in human biology to an established therapy for end-stage renal disease. When successful, renal transplantation offers patients the best chance to resume normal lives and achieve full rehabilitation. However, despite technical advances and improvements in graft and patient survival, two serious and interrelated problems remain: rejection and infection. When an individual receives a renal allograft from either a living donor or a cadaver, the body recognizes the tissue as foreign and an immune response is initiated. To suppress the rejection mechanism, immunosuppressive medications are required. Although these drugs are administered in an attempt to prevent rejection, they also suppress the body's defenses against infection. Thus, transplantation requires a continued effort to induce acceptance of the graft without paralyzing the body's immune system.

It must be realized in transplantation that it is better to sacrifice a kidney in the presence of overwhelming rejection than to sacrifice a patient to overimmunosuppression. That is, rather than endanger a patient's life with continued high-dose immunosuppression, it is safer to resume dialysis and hope for a successful transplant in the future. This approach has reduced mortality after one year to less than five percent for patients receiving a kidney from a living, related donor and to less than 10 percent for those receiving a transplant from a cadaver donor—an impressive accomplishment.[115]

There has also been a striking improvement in allograft survival during the past five years. The results of living, related donor organ transplantation have remained excellent (85 to 95 percent graft survival at the end of one year, depending on the degree of genetic compatibility), but the most exciting result is the improvement in cadaver allograft survival. In 1983, cadaver graft survival was 61 percent after one year.[116] In 1989, with the use of steroid-sparing protocols and the administration of cyclosporine at our institution, cadaver graft survival was 80 to 83 percent at the end of one year. These improved patient survival rates support the idea that transplantation is an excellent alternative modality, in the carefully selected patient (see below), for the treatment of end-stage renal disease.

Recipient Evaluation

The potential transplant recipient must be carefully evaluated and must meet the following criteria: established end-stage renal disease without any potentially reversible component, no evidence of active infection that could be exacerbated by immunosuppression, and no evidence of active malignant disease. Psychiatric evaluation is also important to establish motivation, compliance, and absence of ongoing alcohol or substance abuse. Noncompliance is one of the major causes of long-term allograft loss.[117,118]

Most transplant recipients are between 15 and 50 years of age, but these age boundaries continue to be extended to include the very young (younger than two years) as well as those older than 65 years who are otherwise medically stable. In fact, excellent results and rehabilitation have been reported in older patients.[119]

The preoperative evaluation requires a thorough workup to exclude comorbid conditions, such as cardiac or pulmonary disease, that would significantly increase the risk of surgery. In addition, it is critical to rule out any potential problems that might be exacerbated by immunosuppressive therapy. For example, for patients with asymptomatic peptic ulcer disease who have no evidence of bleeding, surgery is no longer recommended before transplantation because of the availability of H_2 blockers. However, patients with active diverticular disease should undergo colectomy before transplantation to avoid the risk of perforation or intra-abdominal abscess caused by steroid therapy after renal transplantation.

In the past, bilateral nephrectomy was frequently performed before transplantation to control hypertension. With the availability of more powerful antihypertensive agents, particularly the angiotensin-converting enzyme (ACE) inhibitors, this procedure is rarely necessary. Generally, the only patients who should undergo nephrectomy before transplantation are those with active kidney infection (e.g., polycystic kidney disease or chronic pyelonephritis with reflux nephropathy) whose infection cannot be adequately eradicated with antibiotics. Patients with sequestered, smoldering infection are at risk for significant postoperative sepsis.

It is critical to examine the anatomy of the lower urinary tract before transplantation to determine whether reflux is present. This information may guide the surgical approach—that is, whether to perform a pyeloureterostomy using the patient's native ureter or to insert a ureteral implant (ureteroneocystostomy), tunneling the new ureter into the recipient's bladder. Pyeloureterostomy has two advantages: it is nonrefluxing, and the bladder need not be invaded, allowing faster removal of the indwelling bladder catheter. Because the native ureter is used for this anastomosis, rejection of the ureter and associated ischemia and necrosis are avoided.[120] On occasion, a kidney has been attached to a functioning ileal loop of a patient with a poorly functioning bladder.

Although the information may not always be available, it is helpful to know the underlying disease that led to renal insufficiency. For example, in patients with Goodpasture's syndrome, it is important to wait until the anti–glomerular basement membrane (anti-GBM) antibody titer becomes negative before attempting transplantation to avoid recurrent disease within the allograft.[121,122] It is generally recommended that patients with lupus erythematosus become clinically and serologically quiescent (a condition described as burned out) before renal transplantation is performed.[123,124] A number of primary glomerular diseases can also recur in the renal allograft. These include focal glomerular sclerosis, membranous glomerulonephritis, and membranoproliferative nephropathy.[121-123,125] Although these diseases do not necessarily preclude transplantation and do not invariably lead to graft loss, it is important that a transplant candidate be informed of the risk of recurrence.

Antibody titers against varicella-zoster virus (VZV), cytomegalovirus (CMV), hepatitis B, and human immunodeficiency virus should be obtained before transplantation. An immunosuppressed patient who is seronegative for VZV is at considerable risk for fulminant varicella, with interstitial pulmonary infiltrates and pancreatitis, when exposed to this virus. Therefore, until a vaccine becomes available, transplant patients who are seronegative for VZV should be informed of this risk and should receive varicella-zoster immune globulin (VZIG) at transplantation. However, VZIG is only about 75 percent effective; careful clinical follow-up is essential because VZIG may attenuate the rash without affecting lethal

visceral dissemination. The intravenous administration of high doses of acyclovir can be lifesaving; if this therapy is initiated early in the clinical course, it can prevent fulminant pancreatitis and disseminated intravascular coagulation.[126]

Transplant recipients who are seronegative for CMV are also at high risk for serious CMV infection (manifested as a febrile mononucleosis-like illness, leukopenia, pneumonia, or hepatitis) from a seropositive donor. Seropositive recipients are also at risk for CMV infection, from either the reactivation of latent virus or the acquisition of a different strain of virus from a seropositive donor. Anti-CMV antibodies do not confer protection. Recent studies have suggested that there is a potential benefit to prophylactic administration of intravenous CMV hyperimmune globulin[127] or prophylactic antiviral therapy (high-dose oral acyclovir administration, 3.2 g/day)[128] in patients at risk for primary CMV infection.

If a patient comes from an area where parasitic infections such as *Strongyloides* or *Schistosomiasis* are endemic, stool specimens should be examined for ova and parasites. If these infections are identified, patients should be treated for the diseases before transplantation. A number of fatal cases of disseminated *Strongyloides* infection have been reported in immunosuppressed renal transplant patients.[126,129]

The tuberculosis status of an individual should be ascertained by tuberculin skin test using appropriate controls and by chest x-ray. Patients with a positive skin test and a negative chest x-ray can be carefully followed postoperatively for signs of reactivation. If a patient has radiographic evidence of tuberculosis and a positive skin test, a year-long course of isoniazid prophylaxis should be instituted starting one month after transplantation. Liver function and cyclosporine levels should be carefully monitored.[126]

Tissue Typing

One critical element of the pretransplant evaluation is tissue typing.[116,130,131] The first step is determination of the patient's blood group because the recipient must receive a transplant from a blood group–compatible donor to avoid irreversible allograft rejection. The Rh factor need not be compatible. Histocompatibility testing is then performed to assess the degree of genetic compatibility, or matching, between donor and recipient. This procedure entails using peripheral blood lymphocytes to serologically define the HLA phenotype of an individual.

The HLA antigens are the major transplantation antigens; their structure is determined by a complex of genes located on the sixth chromosome at a site termed the major histocompatibility complex. These genes code for two classes of HLA antigens, which are glycoproteins found on the surface of all cells. Class I HLA antigens (HLA A, B, and C) can be detected on most cells and appear to be the primary targets for antibody- and cell-mediated reactions against transplanted tissues.[130] In contrast, class II HLA (HLA DR) antigens are restricted to B cells, monocytes, and parenchymal cells that have been activated. They appear to be involved in immune recognition and the regulation of immune responsiveness.

HLA matching is of great importance when assessing family members as kidney donors. Transplantation of organs between identical twins, who are immunogenetically identical, requires no immunosuppression; success is only limited by technical complications or by some other disease process. Transplantation from a living, related donor who is not an identical twin can be divided into two categories: transplantation from an HLA-identical sibling, which has a success rate of approximately 95 percent at one year, and transplantation from a non-HLA identical relative, which has a success rate of 85 to 90 percent at one year. Thus, the degree of match is an important consideration when choosing the appropriate donor from among several candidate family members.

The importance of HLA matching for cadaver donor transplantation is controversial.[116,130-134] Because graft survival has improved with the administration of cyclosporine, some transplant centers have questioned the practicality of HLA matching and sharing organs between centers because this approach imposes a longer wait for a kidney as well as a greater risk that the kidney will not be functional when it is shipped a long distance after procurement. However, many reports suggest that HLA matching, particularly for the DR and B loci, is beneficial even in cyclosporine-treated patients. HLA matching appears to improve long-term survival of grafts from cadaver donors.[132-134]

For all potential renal transplant recipients, however, it is important to determine and carefully monitor their level of pre-sensitization to HLA antigens. Blood transfusions, pregnancy, or a previous failed transplant can all result in the formation of antibodies to HLA antigens, which can produce immediate allograft destruction (hyperacute rejection).[116,130,131] To monitor an individual's level of sensitization, monthly serum specimens are screened against a standard panel of T cells that express a wide range of HLA antigens. If the patient is sensitized to more than 50 percent of the panel, the individual is considered to be highly sensitized. It is then important to define the HLA antigens to which the individual has been sensitized so that they can be avoided in a potential donor. The level of presensitization, however, may decrease. This often occurs when transfusions can be avoided (i.e., through the administration of erythropoietin) and sufficient time passes. Recent evidence suggests that patients can successfully receive grafts from donors despite previous reactions to their T or B cells as long as sera from the past three to six months lack donor-specific T cell antibodies.[135,136]

Even when the level of sensitization does not fall, successful transplantation can still be accomplished using the following two steps: precisely define the HLA antigens to which the recipient is sensitized, so that these antigens can be avoided, and use a very sensitive crossmatch technique. In a crossmatch, cells from the potential donor are mixed with serum recently obtained from the recipient and complement. A positive T cell crossmatch, which is demonstrated by cell lysis, indicates the presence of HLA antibodies in the serum of the recipient that are directed against the donor. A positive crossmatch is an absolute contraindication to transplantation. The significance of a positive B cell crossmatch, in contrast, is controversial.

Donor Selection

One third of the kidneys transplanted in the United States come from living, related donors; the rest are from cadaver sources. Because of the enhanced degree of genetic compatibility, the survival rates of grafts from living, related donors are higher, and it may be possible to reduce postoperative immunosuppression in such cases. Another advantage of transplanting a kidney from a living, related donor is that surgery can be planned at a time that is optimal for both donor and recipient.

The decision to transplant a kidney from a living, related donor requires meticulous attention not only to the medical evaluation and histocompatibility but also to the psychological and ethical issues. Organ donation is a unique situation; a healthy individual undergoes surgery that poses a small but real risk for the benefit of someone else. Although organ donation is voluntary, it is the responsibility of the transplantation team to ensure that there is no coercion by the recipient or family. Moreover, the donor needs to recognize that even though most living, related allografts have excellent survival, there is no guarantee that a transplanted kidney will work and rejection may occur.

Potential donors must be ABO compatible, have excellent general health with normal blood pressure and normal renal function, have no contraindications to general anesthesia or surgery, and show a willingness to undergo nephrectomy. Death of a donor is rare, and serious treatable complications (e.g., wound infections, phlebitis, pulmonary emboli, and urinary tract infections) occur in only two to three percent of cases.[137] Long-term follow-up of donors (20 years or longer) has documented a slight elevation in the rate of protein excretion but no significant increase in the incidence of renal disease.[138,139] Long-term psychiatric follow-up of related donors has demonstrated improved self-esteem and favorable long-term adjustment.[140]

Although the success rate of cadaver transplantation has improved, the available donor pool remains limited. For example, the waiting time for an unsensitized patient with blood group O in New England is now generally longer than one year, and a patient who is highly sensitized may have to wait significantly longer. There is a need for improved availability of organs.

Because of the shortage of cadaver donors, a number of centers have used living, unrelated donors, such as spouses, in carefully selected cases.[141] Intensive psychiatric and medical evaluations are required. In these cases, transplantation has generally been preceded by donor-specific transfusions and immunosuppression of the recipient to avoid the risk of sensitization.[142] A graft survival rate of 85 to 90 percent at one year has been achieved with this protocol.[143]

Factors Influencing Graft Survival

Blood Transfusions

The effect of blood transfusions on allograft survival remains controversial. In the early 1970s, blood transfusions were generally withheld because of the risk of hepatitis B transmission unless the patient became extremely symptomatic (i.e., fatigue and weakness from anemia) or developed angina or congestive heart failure. However, a number of studies demonstrated that multiple transfusions before transplantation improved graft survival by 15 to 20 percent.[132,144-146] These results led to a variety of intentional transfusion protocols designed to optimize what is called immunologic preconditioning. There has been no agreement on the mechanism by which the beneficial effect of transfusion is induced or how much blood is required to achieve this effect. It has been speculated that the improvement in allograft survival that results from transfusions may be mediated by the induction of T cell unresponsiveness or the production of blocking antibodies. Other researchers have postulated that transfusions work by a selection effect rather than by an active immunologic effect.[146]

However, blood transfusions pose risks. Despite screening procedures for hepatitis B and HIV, the potential remains for other transfusion-related infections, particularly from hepatitis C and cytomegalovirus. In addition, there is the significant risk that a transplant candidate may become sensitized (i.e., develop anti-HLA antibodies) as a result of exposure to histocompatibility antigens on white blood cell fragments.

Data from a large multicenter study[147] of transplant patients receiving cyclosporine suggest that pretransplant blood transfusions may no longer have as great an impact on graft survival as previous immunosuppressive protocols. Thus, although some centers still advocate the use of intentional transfusions (particularly transfusions from living, related donors who do not share a haplotype or from living, unrelated donors), it is our general policy to transfuse patients only if medically indicated. The number of transplant recipients who have not received transfusions is bound to increase with the greater availability of erythropoietin. The impact of reduced transfusions on graft survival needs to be evaluated.

Rejection Rejection of a renal allograft is mediated by both humoral and cellular mechanisms.[148,149] Acute humoral rejection (hyperacute rejection) is generally an overwhelming, irreversible process that occurs when kidneys are transplanted into recipients who have preformed cytotoxic antibodies against ABO or HLA antigens of the donor allograft. The kidney may become swollen and blue from microvascular thrombosis and stop functioning while the patient is still on the operating table. No combination of immunosuppressive drugs is capable of reversing this rapid process.

This lesion is best prevented by careful attention to blood group matching and the crossmatch procedure.

A more chronic form of humoral rejection can also occur that leads to slow but usually inexorable graft loss. Antibody is generally directed against the vascular endothelium of the renal allograft, and the condition is usually refractory to therapy.

In contrast, acute cellular rejection, a process predominantly characterized by tubulointerstitial inflammation, responds to treatment with immunosuppressive agents. Clinical manifestations of acute rejection may include fever, graft swelling or tenderness, oliguria, and increases in BUN and serum creatinine levels.

Both humoral and cellular rejection result from the activation of specific clones of recipient T cells (CD8$^+$ cytotoxic T cells and CD4$^+$ helper T cells) directed against donor histocompatibility antigens (class I and class II). An elaborate amplification process occurs as graft antigens interact with recipient T cells and macrophages, stimulating the production of lymphokines, IL-1, and interleukin-2 (IL-2). These factors stimulate clonal proliferation of T cells and activation of B cells and macrophages.[148,149] Specific immunosuppresive agents can block this cascade at distinct points.

Immunosuppressive Therapy

Glucocorticoids

The glucocorticoid prednisone has been the cornerstone of immunosuppressive therapy for renal transplantation. In addition to producing nonspecific immunosuppressive and anti-inflammatory effects, glucocorticoids are thought to act by blocking the transcription of IL-1, thus preventing transmission of the signal that normally leads to T cell activation.[148,150] Glucocorticoids also inhibit the migration of monocytes and macrophages to the sites of inflammation.

However, long-term steroid therapy is fraught with complications. Prednisone causes a general suppression of host defenses, which predisposes to infection, particularly viral and fungal infection. Steroids have numerous metabolic effects: they may exacerbate hypertension, induce hyperglycemia, produce marked weight gains and changes in facial appearance, delay wound healing, irritate gastric mucosa, and lead to subcapsular cataracts. In addition, they may possibly cause psychiatric disturbances, such as mood swings, hallucinations, insomnia, and psychoses. Many transplant patients suffer from renal osteodystrophy, which can be aggravated by high-dose steroid treatment and can lead to aseptic necrosis of the hips and knees. A myopathy may also result from long-term, high-dose steroid therapy. Because most steroid side effects tend to be dose related, current immunosuppressive protocols reduce steroid dosage to a minimal baseline level. This concern is particularly important in children, whose growth may be retarded unless the steroid dose can be tapered.

Azathioprine

Azathioprine has been another mainstay of immunosuppressive therapy since the initiation of renal transplantation.[116,150] Maintenance dosages range from 75 to 125 mg/day orally. Azathioprine is a derivative of the antimetabolite 6-mercaptopurine and inhibits both DNA and RNA synthesis and blocks the cellular proliferation of T cells.[150] The most common complication of azathioprine is leukopenia. This condition is generally reversible and dose dependent. The dosage of azathioprine is therefore adjusted according to the total white blood cell count; therapy is postponed when the white blood cell count falls below $3,000/mm^3$. The simultaneous administration of allopurinol and azathioprine must be avoided or the dose of azathioprine must be drastically reduced, because allopurinol blocks azathioprine metabolism and may lead to fatal bone marrow suppression. Other potential toxicities of azathioprine include thrombocytopenia, anemia, abnormal liver function tests (generally an obstructive pattern), and an increased incidence of squamous cell carcinoma and lymphoma.

Cyclosporine

The administration of cyclosporine, a unique cyclic endecapeptide derived from a fungal metabolite, has revolutionized renal and all other types of solid-organ transplantation.[151] Numerous clinical trials have shown a striking improvement in renal allograft survival in patients treated with cyclosporine and prednisone as compared with patients treated with azathioprine and prednisone.[151-157] At our own institution, recipients of cadaver transplants treated with prednisone and cyclosporine currently have an 83 percent graft survival rate after one year and a patient survival rate of 94 percent.

Cyclosporine has also reduced the morbidity of transplantation as well as the length of initial hospitalization and the rate of readmission.[158] In addition, the use of cyclosporine has permitted reductions in steroid doses and steroid-related side effects; the prednisone dosage can now be safely decreased to 20 mg/day at the end of the first week after transplantation. Before cyclosporine became available, six months would pass before the dose of prednisone could be reduced to this level.

Cyclosporine is a highly lipophilic agent that is insoluble in water and can be administered in oral or intravenous form. The oral solution is mixed in an olive oil vehicle and is generally administered in chocolate milk. A formulation of cyclosporine in gelatin capsules has become available. Anaphylactic reactions to the intravenous solutions have been reported and have ranged from mild flushing and hypertension to hypotension, crushing chest pain, dyspnea, and respiratory distress. However, these reactions are thought to be primarily caused by the solvent (castor oil–based) or by rapid infusion rates. As a result, slow constant infusion rather than bolus administration is recommended when intravenous administration is essential.[151]

Cyclosporine is metabolized in the liver by the cytochrome P_{450} system and excreted through the biliary tract. There are marked individual variations in the pharmacokinetics of the drug. The monitoring of cyclosporine drug levels by radioimmunoassay or high-performance liquid chromatography has been recommended[151] to maintain minimum serum levels within a so-called therapeutic window of 100 to 250 ng/ml. However, the correlation between blood levels and clinical status has been inconsistent, and toxicity may occur with allegedly normal blood levels. In an attempt to individualize cyclosporine dosage schedules, pretransplant pharmacokinetic profiling has been suggested,[159] although this has not been widely adopted.

Coadministration of drugs that interact with the cytochrome P_{450} system clearly affect cyclosporine levels.[151] For example, cytochrome P_{450} inhibitors such as erythromycin, oral contraceptives, and calcium channel blockers increase cyclosporine levels. Diltiazem appears to have a greater inhibitory effect than nicardipine or verapamil. Nifedipine has no effect. Some investigators have suggested combining erythromycin and cyclosporine to achieve therapeutic blood levels of cyclosporine at a lower dose of the drug, thereby decreasing cost.[160] In contrast, agents that induce cytochrome P_{450} enzymes, such as rifampin, phenobarbital, phenytoin, carbamazepine, and valproate, decrease cyclosporine levels and increase the risk of rejection.[151,161]

A number of other drug interactions have been reported. Rhabdomyolysis and acute myoglobinuric renal failure have been noted in several cardiac transplant patients receiving lovastatin, with or without gemfibrozil, and cyclosporine.[162,163] In addition, various drugs that either are nephrotoxic or influence renal hemodynamics can aggravate cyclosporine nephrotoxicity. These drugs include amphotericin B, nonsteroidal anti-inflammatory agents, radiocontrast agents, and aminoglycosides. Moreover, several reports suggest that the use of high-dose trimethoprim-sulfamethoxazole promotes significant elevations in serum creatinine levels when used with cyclosporine.[164]

It must therefore be recognized that the addition of any new drug to the medication regimen of a patient on cyclosporine may be hazardous, leading to a higher incidence of either rejection or drug-induced toxicity. It is critical, therefore, to monitor renal function studies and cyclosporine levels.

Cyclosporine is unique in that it selectively inhibits the immune process that is related to the rejection response. Specifically, cyclosporine appears to inhibit the production of T cell growth factors, particularly the release of IL-2 and interferon gamma from activated helper T cells, thus decreasing the signal for T cell activation and clonal expansion of helper, inducer, and cytotoxic T cells.[151] Cyclosporine appears to spare suppressor T cells (CD8$^+$ cells) as well as T cell–independent, antibody-mediated B cell responses. One of the major advantages of cyclosporine immunosuppression is that it achieves its immunosuppressive effect without bone marrow suppression; granulocyte function remains intact.

Complications Despite the significant impact of cyclosporine administration on renal allograft survival, the drug remains extremely expensive (approximately $7,000 for the first year of treatment), and it has a number of important side effects. Nephrotoxicity is a major complication of cyclosporine administration, and it has three distinct patterns[116,149,151,161,165]: acute (immediate posttransplant dysfunction), subacute (early posttransplant dysfunction), and chronic (interstitial fibrosis).

An acute decline in glomerular filtration rate may occur immediately after the transplant procedure or during the first week after transplantation. This acute form of cyclosporine nephrotoxicity has been reported to occur more frequently when the kidney has undergone prolonged ischemia at body temperature or prolonged preservation or when completion of the renovascular anastomosis required at least 45 minutes. In these settings, cyclosporine tends to delay resolution of acute tubular necrosis. As a result, several groups administer antilymphocyte sera or monoclonal antibody prophylactically to patients with initial delayed

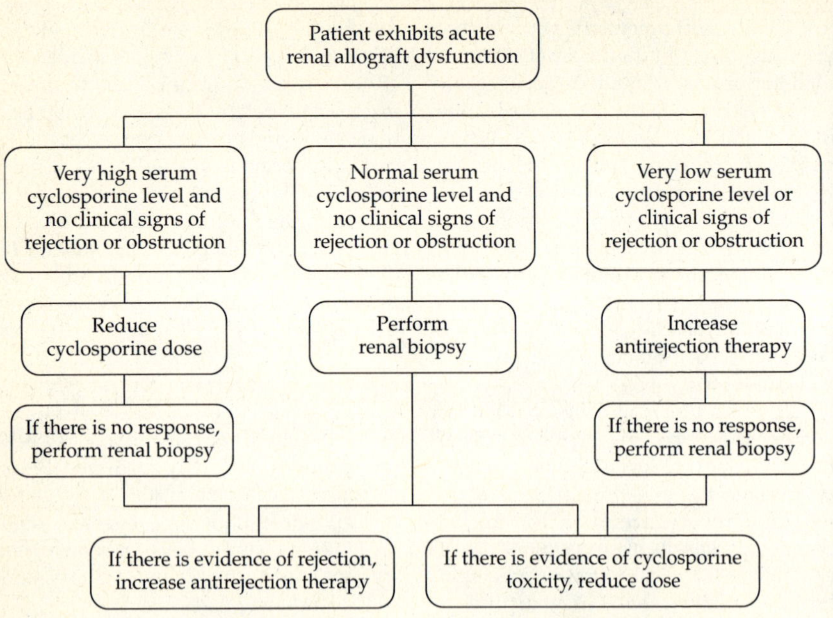

Figure 2   *This flowchart illustrates the diagnostic approach to renal allograft rejection.*

graft function to avoid exposing them to cyclosporine. Once oliguria resolves, cyclosporine maintenance therapy is begun[166]; alternatively, cyclosporine is initiated at doses that are lower than usual once a reasonable urine output is established.

Subacute cyclosporine nephrotoxicity is frequently seen in the first few weeks or months after renal transplantation, and it is often unclear whether the renal allograft dysfunction results from acute cellular rejection or cyclosporine toxicity. Renal biopsy is often necessary to guide therapy [*see Figure 2*]. Although there are no histologic features pathognomonic of cyclosporine toxicity, the diagnosis is based on the presence of tubular lesions (vacuolization), atrophy, edema, and microcalcifications and the absence of an acute cellular infiltrate that is characteristic of acute rejection. Other clinical signs of acute cyclosporine toxicity include hyperkalemia, hypertension, tremors, seizures, hirsutism, gingival hypertrophy, and breast fibroadenomas. Both immediate and early forms of cyclosporine nephrotoxicity generally respond well to a reduction in cyclosporine dose.

A less common presentation of cyclosporine nephrotoxicity is renal vasculopathy.[167,168] This form of toxicity presents with rapid deterioration in renal function and a histologic picture similar to that seen with the hemolytic-uremic syndrome: intimal proliferation, fibrin deposition, and thrombotic occlusion in the arcuate and intralobular arteries of the renal cortex. Thrombocytopenia and a microangiopathic hemolytic anemia may also occur. The renal failure is usually progressive, despite discontinuation of cyclosporine.

A chronic form of cyclosporine nephrotoxicity has also been recognized and is characterized by chronic interstitial fibrosis and a slow but progressive decline in renal function. This process has been observed not only in renal transplant patients but also in heart transplant recipients[169] and patients with uveitis who were treated with cyclosporine.[170] It is unclear how great an impact chronic cyclosporine toxicity has on long-term renal allograft function. Clearly, the risk of chronic cyclosporine nephrotoxicity will need to be carefully balanced with the risk of rejection; approximately 15 percent of renal transplant patients reject the graft when switched from cyclosporine to azathioprine.

A number of experimental studies have clarified the hemodynamic basis of acute and subacute forms of cyclosporine nephrotoxicity. Cyclosporine increases renovascular resistance, which leads to decreases in renal blood flow and glomerular filtration rate and to systemic hypertension. Vasoconstriction tends to be dose dependent and reversible after discontinuation or reduction in the dose of cyclosporine. The exact mechanism by which vasoconstriction occurs is unclear, but it appears that the renin-angiotensin system and the atrial natriuretic hormone response are normal. Because increased vasoconstriction occurs even in denervated renal allografts, a major role for the sympathetic nervous system cannot be implicated.[151] Studies suggest that endothelin, a vasoconstrictive peptide produced by endothelial cells, may mediate the vasoconstrictive response induced by cyclosporine.[171]

Several investigators have suggested that cyclosporine alters the balance of eicosanoid production.[172,173] A decrease in prostacyclin synthesis and an increase in thromboxane A_2 production lead to renal vasoconstriction and proliferation of vascular smooth muscle in the intima. Work in animals has suggested that by decreasing thromboxane production, fish oils may decrease cyclosporine toxicity.[174] Studies are currently under way to evaluate the potential benefit of administering cyclosporine in a fish oil vehicle.

One of the most disturbing findings of early cyclosporine research was the extraordinarily high rate of lymphomas, which usually occurred soon after transplantation.[175,176] However, reduction of the dosage of cyclosporine (to 12 to 15 mg/kg) has decreased both toxicity and the incidence of lymphoproliferative disease. Recent experience with lower cyclosporine dosages suggests that the incidence of lymphoproliferative disease is no greater than that observed with other immunosuppressive agents.[176] The lymphoproliferative syndromes that develop appear to be related to the total immunosuppressive experience (the net state of immunosuppression) rather than to high doses of cyclosporine. Most patients who are now developing lymphoproliferative syndromes have received cyclosporine, azathioprine, prednisone, and treatment for acute rejection, particularly with an antilymphocyte antibody preparation.

The role of Epstein-Barr virus (EBV) in the development of cyclosporine-associated B cell lymphomas is becoming increasingly apparent.[126] Cytotoxic T cells are normally responsible for the surveillance and destruction of EBV-infected B cells. Cyclosporine impairs this surveillance mechanism, leading to the proliferation of virus-infected cells. These cells appear to undergo a cytogenetic change, with progression from polyclonal proliferation to the emergence of a monoclonal stage. The nature of the clonality of these tumors has therapeutic implications. In some EBV-related polyclonal tumors, treatment with high-dose acyclovir[177] and reduction in overall immunosuppression have led to remission.[178] However, the response rate to this treatment has been extremely poor for monoclonal tumors, even when patients are treated with surgery, radiotherapy, or chemotherapy.

Because of the cost, toxicity, and malignant potential of cyclosporine, new agents are desirable. Preliminary reports suggest that the addition of the prostaglandin E_1 analogue misoprostol to cyclosporine and prednisone may prevent acute allograft rejection.[179] In addition, two new macrolides, FK506 and rapamycin, show promise as immunosuppressive drugs.[180,181] The mechanism of action of FK506 appears to be similar to that of cyclosporine; FK506 also prevents IL-2 production, which is critical for lymphocyte activation and proliferation.[182] Cyclosporine and FK506 bind to distinct peptidyl prolyl isomerases, which are intracellular enzymes that promote protein folding.[183,184] Rapamycin, a fungal macrolide structurally similar to FK506, also appears to inhibit T cell activation.[181] The results of ongoing clinical trials with these agents hold considerable interest.

Treatment of Acute Rejection

Glucocorticoids

A number of regimens are available for the treatment of acute rejection, which typically presents as fever, graft swelling or tenderness, decreased urine output, or elevated BUN and creatinine levels. An inflammatory cell infiltrate is seen on a biopsy specimen.

High-dose, pulse glucocorticoid therapy (500 mg to 1 g of methylprednisolone I.V. for three consecutive days) is the established treatment for acute cellular rejection. All other antirejection protocols have been evaluated against this regimen.[185]

Glucocorticoids reverse rejection by blocking the release of lymphokines from activated macrophages and lymphocytes, which inhibits antigen-stimulated proliferation of T cells. Specifically, steroids inhibit IL-1 release, which in turn decreases IL-2 production.[116,185]

The major problem associated with repeated high-dose, pulse steroid therapy is its contribution to immunosuppression and increased patient susceptibility to infection. Other potential complications include hyperglycemia, hypertension, avascular necrosis, peptic ulcer disease, and psychiatric disturbances.

Creatinine elevation that occurs 10 days to two weeks after transplantation is generally treated with a pulse dose of methylprednisolone (500 mg) and a reduction in cyclosporine dose, particularly if there are clinical signs of cyclosporine toxicity, such as hyperkalemia, hypertension, or an elevated minimum level of cyclosporine, as measured by radioimmunoassay. A persistent elevation in the creatinine level, however, generally prompts a renal allograft biopsy to more precisely evaluate the etiology of renal dysfunction; the results of the biopsy often suggest alternative therapies that provide more specific antirejection activity and, at the same time, minimize steroid doses.[185]

Antilymphocyte Sera

Polyclonal anti–T cell antibodies such as antilymphocyte globulin (ALG) and antithymocyte globulin (ATG) have been successfully used as potent immunosuppressive agents in the treatment of acute rejection[185] and in prophylactic therapy to avert rejection.[166] The sera are generally prepared by injecting human lymphocytes or thymocytes into horses, goats, or rabbits. The IgG fraction is then separated from the collected serum.

These preparations need to be administered intravenously through a central line. Although anaphylactic reactions have been exceedingly rare, allergic reactions (e.g., fever and chills and myalgia) are common, and premedication with steroids, antihistamines, and acetaminophen is generally required. Hemolytic anemia, thrombocytopenia, and serum sickness have been reported with the polyclonal antilymphocyte preparations. Antilymphocyte sera contain nonspecific antibodies to T and B cell antigens and to irrelevant antigens. These antibodies most likely account for many of the allergic manifestations seen with antilymphocyte sera.[185]

Antilymphocyte sera are preparations pooled from several different animals, so each batch of antiserum has a different potency and toxicity. Moreover, there is a lack of reliable in vitro tests to determine the immunosuppressive potential of the polyclonal sera.

Immunologic monitoring of T cell levels in peripheral blood has proved most useful in the management of the patients receiving ATG as primary treatment for allograft rejection. A reduction of T cell levels to less than 10 percent of the pretreatment value has correlated well with improvement in allograft function. The usual dose of ATG ranges from 10 to 15 mg/kg body weight/day, and it is given for seven to 10 consecutive days.[185]

Studies of antilymphocyte sera administered in combination with cyclosporine show an unacceptable incidence of neoplasia and viral and opportunistic infections; therefore, at our institution, we omit cyclosporine and reduce the level of azathioprine during ATG therapy.[186]

Monoclonal Antibodies

The application of hybridoma technology has led to the production of pure, monoclonal, antilymphocyte antibodies in large quantities. Monoclonal antibody therapy has many advantages over polyclonal sera, including precisely defined specificity, minimized lot-to-lot variability, and the ability to administer much less foreign protein.[187]

OKT3 is the only commercially available monoclonal antibody that has demonstrated efficacy for acute rejection. It has been administered to patients who are receiving prednisone, azathioprine, or prednisone and cyclosporine.[185,187,188] OKT3 specifically reacts with the CD3 antigen-recognition structure of human T cells and blocks the T cell effector function that is involved in allograft rejection.[185] Because it reacts only with T3, OKT3 has an absolute specificity for late thymocytes and mature T cells.

Most reactions occur after administration of the first dose. A number of side effects have been noted, including chills and fever, nausea, vomiting, diarrhea, rash, pruritus, headache, and photophobia.[185,189] Of particular concern have been episodes of life-threatening acute pulmonary edema. These episodes all occurred in oliguric renal transplant patients who had significant weight gains in the week before drug administration. Patients with marginally compensated left ventricular function before OKT3 treatment may be pushed into frank failure during the acute syndrome of chills and fever that may follow the injection. A chest x-ray is mandatory before instituting OKT3 therapy. If the patient has fluid overload and is oliguric, dialysis should be instituted before OKT3 therapy is begun to avoid cardiac decompensation.

Because most reactions occur after the first injection, it is safe to administer OKT3 on an outpatient basis after the third infusion. Bolus intravenous injections of 1 to 10 mg are given into a peripheral vein.[185] Diarrhea and the symptoms of aseptic meningitis (headache, fever, and photophobia) have been seen in the latter part of the treatment course.

The two major limitations of OKT3 therapy are subsequent rejection episodes in perhaps 50 percent of patients despite treatment and the development of antimurine antibodies, which in some cases prevents a second course of OKT3 therapy. An increased incidence of lymphoproliferative disorders (i.e., EBV-related lymphomas) has been noted in cardiac transplant patients treated with OKT3.[190] As seen with ATG therapy (see above), this disturbing result occurred in highly immunosuppressed patients (i.e., in those who are receiving azathioprine, cyclosporine, and prednisone). It is our policy to omit or markedly reduce the level of cyclosporine during OKT3 therapy.[187]

Animal studies and early human trials suggest that another monoclonal antibody directed against the IL-2 receptor may effectively prevent rejection of renal allografts.[182,191-193] In contrast to OKT3, this monoclonal antibody specifically reacts only with activated T cells, thus sparing T cells not involved in the rejection response. The monoclonal antibody against the IL-2 receptor appears to have fewer side effects than rabbit antithymocyte globulin.[193] This information is preliminary, and additional studies are needed.

Long-term Complications

The major cause of death in the transplant patient is infection. Cardiac disease, hepatic dysfunction, and malignant disease, particularly squamous cell carcinoma and lymphoma, assume a more prominent position five years after transplantation.[194,195]

Specific infections occur during three distinct time periods.[126] In the first month after transplantation, patients generally suffer from two types of infection: those acquired from transfusions before transplantation, such as hepatitis B and hepatitis C, and typical postoperative infections, such as aspiration pneumonia, wound infection, or line-related sepsis. Opportunistic infections are unusual during this period; their occurrence suggests an excessive nosocomial hazard. Epidemics of invasive aspergillosis, Legionnaires' disease, and gram-negative pneumonia, caused by aerosolization of these organisms within the hospital environment, have been reported among transplant patients in the first month.[126]

The second period of infection occurs between one and six months after transplantation. The patient is at the highest risk for opportunistic infection during this period because the duration and degree of immunosuppressive therapy have had a profound effect on host defenses. Immunosuppression and rejection lead to the appearance of herpesviruses, especially cytomegalovirus (CMV) and Epstein-Barr virus (EBV). These viruses significantly depress host defenses, increasing the net state of immunosuppression. Infections caused by opportunistic pathogens such as *Pneumocystis carinii, Listeria monocytogenes*, and the various fungi typically occur during this period.

Urinary tract infections also occur during this period and lead to a high rate of transplant pyelonephritis and bacteremia. Prophylactic trimethoprim-sulfamethoxazole therapy (160 mg of trimethoprim and 800 mg of sulfamethoxazole), begun when the Foley catheter is removed and continued for four to six months, decreases the incidence of the serious, early form of gram-negative urinary tract infection from 34 percent to essentially zero percent.[126,196] In patients allergic to sulfonamide, trimethoprim or ciprofloxacin can be safely substituted.

The third period of infection begins six months after transplantation. The common problems during this period are the following:

1. Those resulting from chronic viral infections that have progressed because of the chronic state of immunosuppression— for example, chorioretinitis from CMV, progressive hepatitis B, hepatocellular carcinoma from hepatitis B, or EBV-associated lymphoproliferative disease.
2. Infectious diseases similar to those seen in the general community. These conditions are most often seen in patients on minimal immunosuppression with good renal function.
3. Opportunistic infections, which generally occur in patients with poor allograft function who have undergone too much immunosuppression.

Rejection and infection are now regarded as two sides of the same problem. Any intervention that permits reduction of immunosuppressive therapy will be associated with a lower rate of infection. Alternatively, strategies that decrease the incidence of infection permit the use of more intensive immunosuppression. Great strides have been made in preventing infections arising from technical complications and excessive nosocomial hazards. For example, the incidence of aspergillosis has been reduced dramatically at our institution by the installation of high-efficiency particulate air (HEPA) filtration units. The availability of acyclovir has provided symptomatic improvement for patients with active herpes simplex virus infection. The use of prophylactic antifungal agents such as nystatin and clotrimazole has prevented *Candida* overgrowth of the oropharynx and gastrointestinal tract of patients receiving high-dose immunosuppression and antimicrobial agents. The present challenge is the development of strategies for the clinical management of CMV and fungal infections.

References

1. Acute Renal Failure, 2nd ed. Churchill Livingstone, New York, 1988, p 767
2. The Kidney, 3rd ed. WB Saunders Co, Philadelphia, 1986, p 1791
3. Clin Nephrol 9:156, 1978
4. Nephron 27:134, 1981
5. Kidney Int 17:801, 1980
6. Trans Am Soc Artif Intern Organs 6:104, 1960
7. Handbook of Dialysis. Little, Brown & Co, Boston, 1988, p 40
8. Am J Kidney Dis 2:474, 1983
9. N Engl J Med 275:1089, 1966
10. Access Surgery. George A. Bogden & Son, Inc, Ridgewood, NJ, 1983, p 1
11. Seminars in Dialysis 2:7, 1988
12. N Engl J Med 296:769, 1977
13. Handbook of Dialysis. Little, Brown & Co, Boston, 1988, p 99
14. Kidney Int 33:29, 1988
15. J Exp Med 156:912, 1982
16. Blood Purif 6:164, 1988
17. Handbook of Dialysis. Little, Brown & Co, Boston, 1988, p 87
18. Kidney Int 16:513, 1979
19. N Engl J Med 304:934, 1981
20. N Engl J Med 308:258, 1983
21. Kidney Int 31:1351, 1987
22. Diseases of the Kidney, 4th ed. Little, Brown & Co, Boston, 1988, p 3281
23. Artif Organs 6:370, 1982
24. Artif Organs 6:410, 1982
25. Artif Organs 6:421, 1982
26. Trans Am Soc Artif Intern Organs 23:399, 1977
27. Artif Organs 8:411, 1984
28. Proc Clin Dial Transplant Forum 10:220, 1980
29. Ann Intern Med 88:332, 1978
30. Handbook of Dialysis. Little, Brown & Co, Boston, 1988, p 106
31. Contrib Nephrol 62:24, 1988
32. Handbook of Dialysis. Little, Brown & Co, Boston, 1988, p 437
33. Diseases of the Kidney, 4th ed. Little, Brown & Co, Boston, 1988, p 3323
34. The Kidney, 3rd ed. W B Saunders Co, Philadelphia, 1986, p 1731
35. Kidney Int 4:177, 1973
36. J Clin Invest 58:306, 1976
37. Ann Intern Med 86:554, 1977
38. Am J Kidney Dis 2:290, 1982
39. Kidney Int 11:21, 1978
40. Replacement of Renal Function by Dialysis, 2nd ed. Martinus Nilhoff Publishers, 1983, p 611
41. Journal of Dialysis 1:447, 1977
42. Ann Intern Med 73:443, 1970
43. Nephron 46:1, 1987
44. Kidney Int 35:134, 1989
45. Ann Intern Med 73:409, 1970
46. Nephron 13:427, 1974
47. Clin Nephrol 10:105, 1978
48. N Engl J Med 294:1416, 1976
49. Kidney Int 12:59, 1977
50. Kidney Int 27:128, 1985
51. Am J Med 63:755, 1977
52. J Clin Invest 67:1263, 1981
53. Arch Intern Med 139:889, 1979
54. Arch Intern Med 138:1650, 1978
55. Kidney Int 28:1, 1985
56. Ann Intern Med 78:527, 1973
57. N Engl J Med 291:1046, 1975
58. Semin Nephrol 9:30, 1989
59. N Engl J Med 304:989, 1981
60. N Engl J Med 304:319, 1981
61. Am J Med 79:397, 1985
62. Lancet 2:1175, 1986
63. N Engl J Med 316:73, 1987
64. Semin Dial 2:87, 1989
65. Kidney Int 35:229, 1989
66. Lancet 2:1227, 1987
67. Seminars in Dialysis 2:81, 1989
68. Semin Nephrol 9:22, 1989
69. Kidney Int 33:248, 1988
70. Kidney Int 33:238, 1988
71. Kidney Int 33:219, 1988
72. Kidney Int 33:239, 1988
73. Br Med J 295:1017, 1987
74. Q J Med 25:175, 1956
75. Lancet 1:97, 1988
76. Seminars in Dialysis 2:80, 1989
77. Seminars in Dialysis 2:78, 1989
78. Seminars in Dialysis 2:4, 1988
79. Kidney Int 35:567, 1989
80. N Engl J Med 310:1113, 1984
81. Diseases of the Kidney, 4th ed. Little, Brown & Co, Boston, 1988, p 3371
82. N Engl J Med 296:1389, 1977
83. N Engl J Med 294:184, 1976
84. Ann Intern Med 88:502, 1978
85. Lancet 2:29, 1983
86. Br Med J 2:740, 1977
87. Kidney Int 31:1344, 1987
88. Proc Eur Dial Transplant Assoc 17:226, 1980
89. N Engl J Med 306:654, 1982
90. Handbook of Dialysis. Little, Brown & Co, Boston, 1988, p 397
91. Ann Intern Med 101:775, 1984
92. N Engl J Med 320:1140, 1989
93. Kidney Int 29(suppl):S100, 1986
94. Am J Kidney Dis 13:308, 1989
95. Kidney Int 35:1371, 1989
96. Diseases of the Kidney, 4th ed. Little, Brown & Co, Boston, 1988, p 3035
97. N Engl J Med 311:140, 1984
98. Ann Intern Med 107:678, 1987
99. Clin Nephrol 29:261, 1988
100. Nephron 49:169, 1988
101. Kidney Int 23(suppl):S101, 1983
102. Kidney Int 28:526, 1985
103. N Engl J Med 312:553, 1985
104. Diseases of the Kidney, 4th ed. Little, Brown & Co, Boston, 1988, p 3235
105. The Kidney, 3rd ed. W B Saunders Co, Philadelphia, 1986, p 1847
106. Ann Intern Med 92:7, 1980
107. Rev Infect Dis 9:604, 1987
108. Peritoneal Dial Bull 7:55, 1987
109. Handbook of Dialysis. Little, Brown & Co, Boston, 1988, p 252
110. Am J Kidney Dis 13:184, 1989
111. Seminars in Dialysis 2:190, 1989
112. Am J Nephrol 5:169, 1985
113. Am J Kidney Dis 9:66, 1987
114. Am J Med 86:825, 1989
115. US Renal Data System 1989: Annual Data Report. RS Renal Data System Coordinating Center (NIH contract No. N01-DK-8-2234)
116. The Kidney, 3rd ed. W B Saunders Co, Philadelphia, 1986, p 1941
117. XII International Congress of the Transplantation Society, Book II, 1988, p 128
118. Am J Psychiatry 146:972, 1989
119. Arch Surg 110:1107, 1975
120. Ann Surg 196:588, 1982
121. Transplantation 34:237, 1982
122. Am J Kidney Dis 12:85, 1988
123. Ann Intern Med 94:444, 1981
124. Transplantation 46:703, 1988
125. Transplantation 47:595, 1989
126. Clinical Approach to Infection in the Compromised Host, 2nd ed. Plenum Publishing Corp, New York, 1988, p 557
127. N Engl J Med 317:1049, 1987
128. N Engl J Med 320:1381, 1989
129. Medicine (Baltimore) 57:527, 1978
130. Contemporary Issues in Nephrology. Churchill Livingstone, New York, 1989, p 1
131. Contemporary Issues in Nephrology. Churchill Livingstone, New York, 1989, p 21
132. N Engl J Med 311:675, 1984
133. Transplant Proc 19:641, 1987
134. Transplantation 45:410, 1988
135. Lancet 2:1240, 1982
136. Transplant Proc 17:113, 1985

137. Contemporary Issues in Nephrology. Churchill Livingstone, New York, 1989
138. Mayo Clin Proc 60:367, 1985
139. Kidney Int 29:1072, 1986
140. Psychonephrology 2: Psychological Problems in Kidney Failure and Their Treatment. Plenum Publishing Corp, New York, 1983, p 275
141. N Engl J Med 314:914, 1986
142. Transplantation 34:352, 1982
143. Transplant Proc 20:1074, 1988
144. N Engl J Med 299:799, 1978
145. Clinical Kidney Transplants 1985. UCLA Tissue Typing Laboratory, Los Angeles, 1985, p 73
146. Organ Transplantation and Replacement. J B Lippincott Co, Philadelphia, 1988, p 151
147. Transplant Proc 20:1069, 1988
148. Diseases of the Kidney, 4th ed. Little, Brown & Co, Boston, 1988, p 3177
149. Contemporary Issues in Nephrology. Churchill Livingstone, New York, 1989, p 45
150. Contemporary Issues in Nephrology. Churchill Livingstone, New York, 1989, p 97
151. N Engl J Med 321:1725, 1989
152. Lancet 2:1323, 1978
153. Lancet 2:57, 1982
154. N Engl J Med 309:809, 1983
155. N Engl J Med 318:1499, 1988
156. Ann Intern Med 101:667, 1984
157. N Engl J Med 310:148, 1984
158. N Engl J Med 321:1086, 1989
159. Transplantation 46:631, 1988
160. Transplantation 43:263, 1987
161. Ann Intern Med 99:851, 1983
162. N Engl J Med 381:47, 1988
163. N Engl J Med 318:46, 1988
164. Transplantation 36:204, 1983
165. Kidney Transplant Rejection: Diagnosis and Treatment. Marcell Dekker, New York, 1986, p 424
166. Transplantation 43:85, 1987
167. N Engl J Med 305:1392, 1981
168. Surgery 98:54, 1985
169. N Engl J Med 311:699, 1984
170. N Engl J Med 314:1293, 1986
171. J Am Soc Nephrol 1:76, 1990
172. Cyclosporine. Grune & Stratton, Orlando, Florida, 1984, p 182
173. Transplantation 43:282, 1987
174. Transplantation 43:271, 1987
175. Lancet 1:788, 1984
176. Transplantation 43:32, 1987
177. Ann Surg 198:356, 1983
178. Lancet 1:583, 1984
179. N Engl J Med 322:1183, 1990
180. Lancet 2:1000, 1989
181. Lancet 2:227, 1989
182. N Engl J Med 322:1224, 1990
183. Nature 341:755, 1989
184. Nature 341:758, 1989
185. Contemporary Issues in Nephrology. Churchill Livingstone, New York, 1989, p 129
186. Transplantation 31:143, 1981
187. N Engl J Med 313:337, 1985
188. Am J Kidney Dis 11:90, 1988
189. Am J Kidney Dis 11:112, 1988
190. N Engl J Med 323:1723, 1990
191. J Exp Med 162:358, 1985
192. Am J Kidney Dis 14(suppl 2):54, 1989
193. N Engl J Med 322:1175, 1990
194. Organ Transplantation and Replacement. J B Lippincott Co, Philadelphia, 1988, p 481
195. Kidney Int 37:1363, 1990
196. Rev Infect Dis 4:614, 1982

Acknowledgments

Figure 1 Janet Betries. Modified from "CAPD Related Peritonitis Management and Antibiotic Therapy Recommendations," by W. F. Keane, E. D. Everett, R. N. Fine, et al, in *Peritoneal Dialysis Bulletin* 7:55, 1987. Used by permission.

Figure 2 Janet Betries.

ROBERT W. P. CUTLER, M.D.

Spinal Cord Disorders

Herniation of Intervertebral Disks

The intervertebral disk acts as a shock absorber between vertebral bodies. It can be damaged by trauma or degenerative changes. Nerve root compression results when the nucleus pulposus protrudes through the posterolateral aspect of the anulus fibrosus. Occasionally, a large central protrusion of the disk occurs. A protrusion in the cervical or thoracic region will produce signs of spinal cord compression; if it is in the lumbar region, it will produce signs of cauda equina compression.

Cervical Disk Disease

Lateral herniation of cervical disks usually occurs at the C5-6 or C6-7 intervertebral space [*see Figure 1*]. A C5-6 disk rupture compresses the sixth cervical root and causes pain in the outer aspect of the upper arm and forearm and in the thumb, weakness of the biceps muscle, and reduction of the biceps reflex. A C6-7 disk rupture compresses the seventh cervical root and causes pain in the shoulder blade and back of the arm and in the index and middle fingers, weakness of the triceps muscle, and a reduction of the triceps reflex. In either case, coughing, sneezing, and straining commonly aggravate the symptoms. These symptoms also occur when osteophytes compress the nerve roots in the intervertebral foramina.

Conservative therapy should be tried first. Patients should be instructed to wear a cervical collar for as many hours of the day as they can tolerate it. The collar is generally uncomfortable at first. It must be firm and adjusted to stretch the neck—loose-fitting or felt collars are not very helpful. Patients who do not show improvement may be treated at home with cervical traction while in a sitting position. An over-the-door traction apparatus is used, and the patient exerts a pulling force of 10 to 20 lb for 30 minutes three times a day. Conservative treatment is usually successful; those patients whose symptoms do not improve may require surgery.

Lumbar Disk Disease

In one half of cases of lumbar disk disease, a history of trauma is obtained at the onset of neurologic symptoms; often, the trauma is trivial. The most common sites for disk protrusion are the L4-5 and L5-S1 intervertebral spaces [*see Figure 1*]. Both herniations produce low back pain, which radiates down the posterior and lateral aspects of the thigh and calf. The L4-5 disk compresses the L5 nerve root. Paresthesia and sensory loss occur in the lateral aspect of the calf, the medial dorsal surface of the foot, and the three medial toes. Foot dorsiflexion may be weak. The L5-S1 compresses the S1 nerve root. Sensory loss occurs in the lateral and plantar aspects of the foot and the two lateral toes. The ankle jerk is depressed or absent, and plantar flexion of the foot and toes may be weak.

Pain from lumbar herniation is aggravated by movement of the back, increased intraspinal pressure (coughing, Valsalva maneuver, jugular vein compression), or stretching of the sciatic nerve (straight leg raising, Lasègue's sign). These mechanical signs help to distinguish herniated disk disorders from peripheral nerve disorders, such as diabetic mononeuritis.

Conservative therapy consists of absolute bed rest in a supine position on a firm

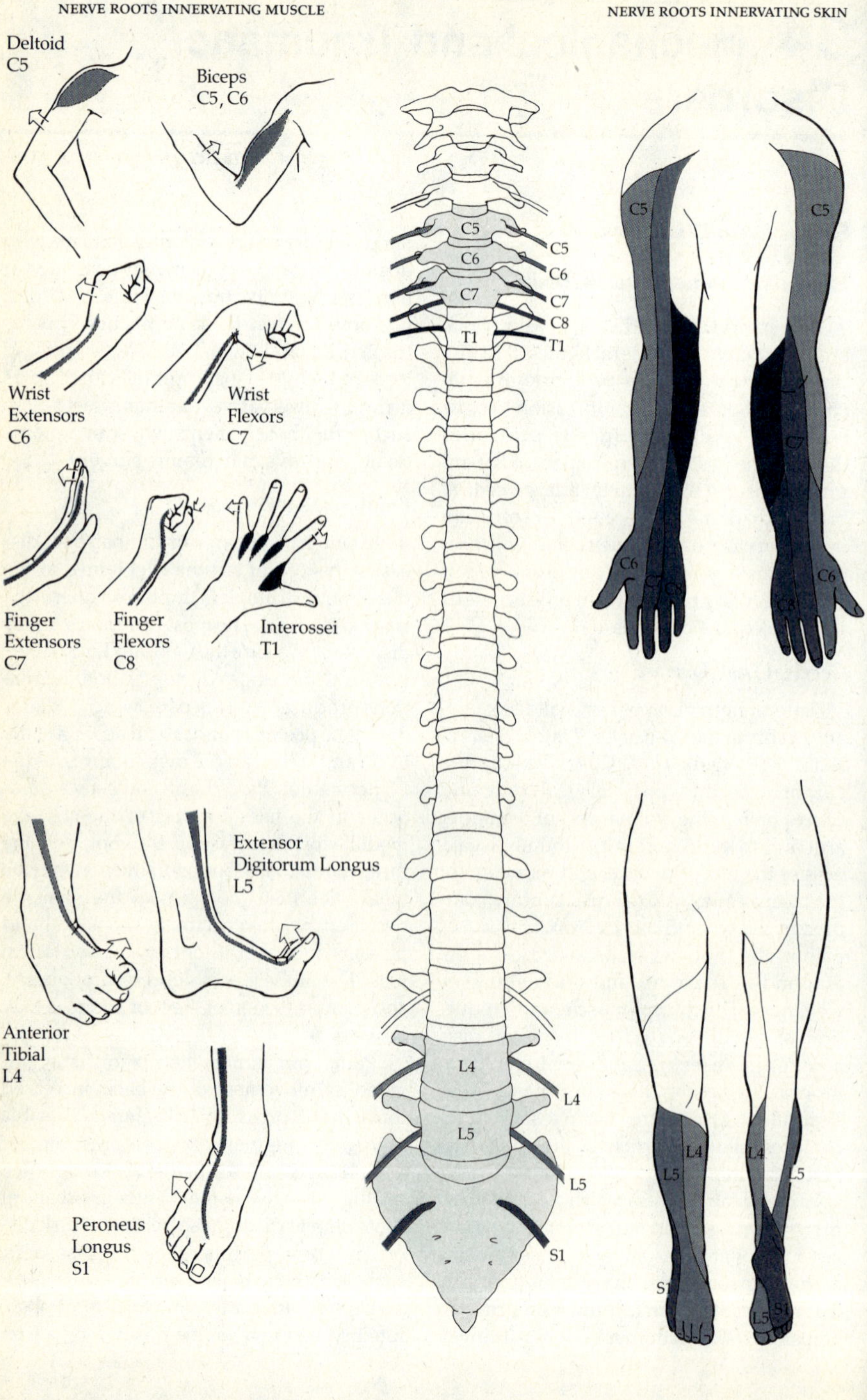

NERVE ROOTS INNERVATING MUSCLE
Deltoid
C5
Biceps
C5, C6
Wrist
Extensors
C6
Wrist
Flexors
C7
Finger
Extensors
C7
Finger
Flexors
C8
Interossei
T1
Anterior
Tibial
L4
Extensor
Digitorum Longus
L5
Peroneus
Longus
S1
C5
C6
C7
C8
T1
C5
C6
C7
C8
T1
L4
L5
L4
L5
S1
NERVE ROOTS INNERVATING SKIN
C5
C5
C6
C7
C8
C8
C6
L4
L5
L4
L5
S1
L5
S1

mattress with a board between the bed-springs and mattress. Heat, analgesics, and muscle relaxants such as diazepam, 5 to 10 mg by mouth q.i.d, are useful. Patients generally respond to this therapy within a few days, and most are ambulatory within two or three weeks. Pelvic traction is rarely helpful.

If there is no neurologic deficit and if symptoms do not abate during an extended period of observation (e.g., three weeks or longer) and the diagnosis has been confirmed radiographically, spinal surgery (laminectomy or microdiskectomy) or chymopapain chemonucleolysis should be considered. CT scanning and myelography have a high rate of diagnostic accuracy, but neither technique is infallible.[1]

Chymopapain for lumbar disk disease has been widely used since its approval by the FDA in 1982. Chymopapain is injected into the disk, where it enzymatically digests the chondromucoprotein of the nucleus pulposus. Complication rates for the first 85,000 treated patients were relatively low, but serious complications did occur. The most common complication was anaphylaxis, which was observed in about one percent of patients and resulted in three deaths.[2] Other serious neurologic complications, such as paraplegia and subarachnoid hemorrhage, also occurred. Many neurosurgeons have been disappointed with the results of the procedure and have therefore abandoned it.[3] Others have reported favorable outcomes in 10-year follow-up reviews, in which about 75 percent of patients had relief from pain and were able to return to full employment—results comparable with those reported for surgery.[2,4] Chymopapain nucleolysis, if unsuccessful, does not preclude a subsequent operation.

Claudication of the Cauda Equina

Osteophyte formation, disk degeneration, and anterior protrusion of the ligamenta flava in the lower spine can distort and narrow the lumbar spinal canal and cause intermittent claudication of the cauda equina.[5] The disorder usually begins in persons 40 to 70 years of age and almost exclusively affects men. Patients typically complain of tingling paresthesias in the buttocks and lower extremities that develop after standing or walking. The paresthesias are relieved by sitting or remaining stationary. Many patients also complain of exercise-induced weakness or polyradicular pains in the legs. Neurologic signs are often minimal; they include absent or depressed knee and ankle jerks and Lasègue's sign. Computed tomography is the definitive radiologic procedure for defining the extent of spinal cord distortion. Laminectomy, usually at multiple levels, provides long-term relief of symptoms for most patients.[5]

Cervical Fracture-dislocation

Trauma from motor vehicle and sports accidents is the most common cause of cervical vertebral fracture-dislocation. Occasionally, rheumatoid arthritis of the spine leads to spontaneous dislocation of the C1 vertebra on the C2 vertebra and produces a clinical syndrome of progressive spastic quadriparesis, painless sensory loss in the arms, and pain in the back of the head.[6] Some patients experience symptoms of lower

---

Figure 1   *The site of a cervical or lumbar disk herniation can be identified based on the location of muscle weakness, the site of pain and sensory loss, and the impairment of deep tendon reflexes. Disks that herniate are most commonly those between vertebral bodies C5-6, C6-7, L4-5, and L5-S1. Lateral herniation of the disk will compress the lower nerve root in each case. For example, lateral herniation of the C5-6 disk will compress the C6 nerve root and cause weakness of the biceps muscle and wrist extensors; pain or sensory loss, or both, in the outer aspect of the forearm and thumb; and a reduction of the biceps reflex. A lateral herniation of the L4-5 disk will compress the L5 nerve root and cause weakness of the extensor muscles of the foot and sensory disturbance in the lateral aspect of the lower leg and medial dorsal surface of the foot. The dermatome maps may vary in different individuals.*

brain stem dysfunction. Patients may suddenly become quadriplegic if the head is severely flexed or extended. The spinal symptoms result from a combination of cord compression and ischemic necrosis of the central gray matter secondary to occlusion of branches of the anterior spinal artery. Spinal roentgenograms, tomography, and myelography aid in establishing the diagnosis. Patients with cervical fracture-dislocation are treated by immediate immobilization and head traction. The halo-thoracic brace appears to provide adequate immobilization and allows early rehabilitation therapy.[7]

Because of the salutary effects of steroids in the treatment of experimental cord injury in animals, it has become widespread practice to administer steroids to patients with spinal cord injury. However, results of the first National Acute Spinal Cord Injury Study (NASCIS 1) indicated that there was no convincing evidence to support this practice. Methylprednisolone, given in a dosage of 1,000 mg/day for 10 days, showed no more benefit than a conventional regimen of the drug (100 mg/day for 10 days).[8] Unfortunately, a placebo-treated group was not included in this study. More recently, in NASCIS 2—a randomized, double-blind, placebo-controlled trial involving 487 patients—even higher dosages of methylprednisolone were given, and the effects of naloxone were also studied.[9] Results of the trial demonstrated that methylprednisolone, given intravenously as a bolus of 30 mg/kg body weight followed by an infusion of 5.4 mg/kg/hr for 23 hours, improved neurologic recovery to a modest degree if given within the first eight hours after injury. Naloxone, given intravenously in a bolus of 5.4 mg/kg body weight followed by an infusion of 4.0 mg/kg/hr for 23 hours, did not appear to be beneficial.

Cervical Spondylosis

Cervical spondylosis is a very common disorder that leads to osteophyte formation and degenerative disk disease. The cause is uncertain, but trauma, diabetes, and advancing age are related factors. The disorder produces narrowing of the spinal canal and compression of the spinal cord in addition to nerve root compression by bony spurs in the intervertebral foramina. Cord compression is more likely to occur in persons with congenital narrowing of the spinal canal. Cervical spondylosis is the most common cause of cervical myelopathy that develops after middle age. The spinal cord dysfunction results from mechanical compression by transverse osteophytes and from ischemic infarction secondary to bony compression of spinal arteries.[10]

In general, symptoms develop insidiously after 50 years of age. Neck pain and radicular pains in the shoulders and arms are accompanied by signs of sensory impairment, weakness, wasting, and loss of upper extremity reflexes. Fasciculations may be as prominent as in amyotrophic lateral sclerosis, but sensory loss contradicts that diagnosis. The process is seldom symmetrical. Later, motor and sensory signs appear in the lower extremities. The gait becomes slow, stiff legged, and unsteady; the tendon reflexes are increased; and there is loss of position and vibration sensations. Sphincter disturbances are uncommon. This constellation of symptoms and signs in middle-aged or elderly patients strongly suggests cervical cord compression from spondylosis.

X-rays of the spine usually reveal osteoarthritic changes, but bony changes correlate poorly with neurologic symptoms. Advanced arthritic changes may be seen in asymptomatic persons. Myelography is generally more helpful and shows cord compression in the anteroposterior plane and radiographic-dye interruption at intervertebral disk spaces [*see Figure 2*].

The course is quite variable. Often, symptoms are mild and do not progress. Such cases are best treated conservatively with a cervical collar and intermittent traction as necessary. Elderly patients often experience progression of symptoms and more serious neurologic impairment. Surgery should be recommended to arrest progression of myelopathic symptoms in

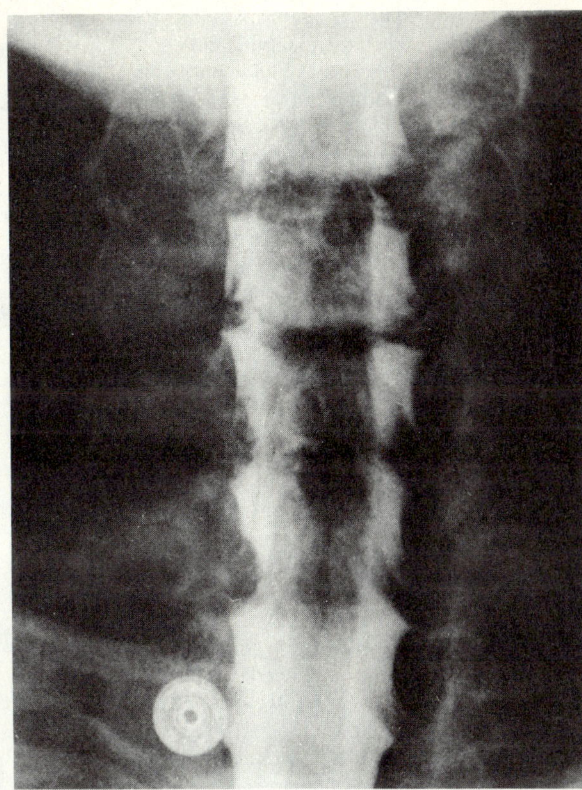

Figure 2 *Cervical myelogram of a 62-year-old man with weakness and numbness of both hands and a spastic gait shows midline cervical disks that interrupt the column of dye at several levels. Cervical cord compression was found at operation.*

patients whose general condition is satisfactory. One review of surgical techniques and outcomes showed that about 85 percent of patients may achieve satisfactory results.[11]

Head Trauma

Head trauma is a major public health problem. Yearly, about half a million people in the United States are hospitalized for head injuries. Most of these injuries are sustained in accidents involving motor vehicles or in industrial mishaps.

The evaluation of patients with severe head injuries has been greatly enhanced by use of the Glasgow Coma Scale (GCS) [*see Table 1*]. The GCS provides an effective, simple, and reproducible method of assessing the degree of coma and brain damage. It has clarified prognosis: about 50 percent of pa-

tients with GCS scores of 8 or less die or remain in a vegetative state.[12] The type of injury is also an important determinant of outcome in patients with low GCS scores. For example, patients with acute subdural hematomas have a poorer prognosis than patients with diffuse contusion injuries. Age is another important determinant; mortality in children with severe head injuries is much lower than that in adults.[12]

Steps that must be taken immediately in the emergency management of serious head injuries are proper immobilization of the head and neck, endotracheal intubation, and artificial ventilation. CT scanning should be performed as quickly as possible. Increased intracranial pressure should be treated with intravenous mannitol, 1.5 to 2.0 g/kg, and with controlled hyperventilation to lower

Table 1 Glasgow Coma Scale

Test	Response	Score
Eye opening	Spontaneous	4
	To speech	3
	To pain	2
	None	1
Best verbal response	Oriented	5
	Confused	4
	Inappropriate	3
	Incomprehensible	2
	None	1
Best motor response (arm)	Obedience to commands	6
	Localization of pain	5
	Withdrawal response to pain	4
	Flexion response to pain	3
	Extension response to pain	2
	None	1

the P_aco_2 to about 25 mm Hg. Some clinicians recommend high-dose barbiturate (pentobarbital or thiopental) infusions as well.[13] Although administration of dexamethasone has been advocated for treatment of head trauma and increased intracranial pressure, results of prospective randomized studies do not confirm the value of this approach. High-dosage dexamethasone, 100 mg/day for the first several days, neither reduced intracranial pressure nor affected the long-term outcome of patients with severe head injury.[14]

Two important complications of head trauma are epidural hematoma and subdural hematoma. CT scanning has greatly facilitated their identification.

Epidural hematoma results from arterial bleeding into the space between the skull and dura. The cause is usually rupture of a meningeal artery associated with skull fracture. Classically, the patient loses consciousness immediately after a head injury but regains consciousness and remains awake for a variable time. In the large series of patients studied by Jamieson and Yelland, however, only one third of patients exhibited this clinical sequence; one quarter of the group never lost consciousness, and one quarter never regained consciousness.[15] Headache, hemiparesis, pupillary dilatation, and bradycardia develop rapidly, usually within a few hours after injury. Occasionally, these symptoms are delayed five to seven days. If epidural hematoma is suspected, burr holes should be placed at the site of skull fracture immediately; time must not be wasted on diagnostic procedures.

Subdural hematoma may develop acutely after head injury when veins bridging the space between the dura and arachnoid rupture. Alternately, it may be subacute or chronic, evolving over days to weeks. Spontaneous subdural hematomas may occur in patients on long-term dialysis or on anticoagulant therapy or in patients who have had a ventricular shunt; usually, the presenting complaint is headache. Drowsiness and obtundation, which may fluctuate markedly from hour to hour, are characteristic findings. Lateralizing neurologic signs of hemiparesis, hemianopsia, and language disturbances eventually result.

The prognosis is poor for patients in a coma induced by subdural hematoma; death or serious disability occurs in 90 percent of cases.[12] There is some evidence that evacuation of the clot within four hours of injury improves survival.[16]

References

1. JAMA 251:1192, 1984
2. J Neurosurg 62:662, 1985
3. JAMA 256:317, 1986
4. J Neurosurg 65:1, 1986
5. Brain 101:211, 1978
6. Ann Neurol 3:144, 1978
7. J Neurosurg 58:508, 1983
8. J Neurosurg 63:704, 1985
9. N Engl J Med 322:1405, 1990
10. Brain 109:259, 1986
11. J Neurol Neurosurg Psychiatry 49:353, 1986
12. J Neurosurg 56:19, 1982
13. Ann Neurol 6:194, 1979
14. J Neurosurg 64:81, 1986
15. J Neurosurg 29:13, 1968
16. N Engl J Med 304:1511, 1981

Acknowledgments

Figure 1 Carol Donner. Data adapted from "Aids to the Investigation of Peripheral Nerve Injuries," in *Medical Research Council War Memorandum*, No. 7, rev. 2nd ed. Her Majesty's Stationery Office, London, 1943, pp. 47–48; and from *Orthopaedic Neurology*, by Stanley Hoppenfeld. J.B. Lippincott Company, Philadelphia, 1977, p. 32. Used by permission.

Table 1   Data adapted from "Adding Up the Glasgow Coma Score," by G. Teasdale, G. Murray, L. Parker, et al, in *Acta Neurochirurgica Supplementum (Vienna)* 28:13, 1979. Used by permission.

35 Central Nervous System Infections

MORTON N. SWARTZ, M.D.
PETER O'HANLEY, M.D., Ph.D.

Overview

Central nervous system infections are frequently life-threatening and under certain conditions constitute medical emergencies that require prompt and accurate diagnosis. Fortunately, advances in methods of diagnosis and treatment developed during the past 20 years have significantly improved the prognoses associated with many of these illnesses. Computed tomography yields prompt and specific information and is especially useful in the diagnosis of brain abscess. The ability of magnetic resonance imaging (MRI) to discriminate between densities of fluid and solid is even greater than that of the CT scan, and MRI may eventually prove to be the diagnostic test of choice for evaluating CNS infections. Several chemotherapeutic agents, both antibacterial (e.g., the third-generation cephalosporins) and antiviral (e.g., acyclovir), have improved the prognoses of many of these infections. New diagnostic methods supplement rather than supplant cerebrospinal fluid studies. Cerebrospinal fluid studies frequently provide important initial information needed for clinical and microbiological diagnosis; when such studies are not definitive, they serve at least to focus the differential diagnosis.

In addition, advances in the understanding of the pathogenic and pathophysiological mechanisms that underlie bacterial meningitis have led to the development of adjunctive strategies for managing this disease. For example, the local and systemic production of inflammatory cytokines, such as interleukin-1 (IL-1), interleukin-6 (IL-6), and tumor necrosis factor (TNF), in response to bacterial meningitis has been found to be correlated with mortality. The use of adjunctive dexamethasone therapy in infants and children who are suffering from bacterial meningitis has reduced the incidence of long-term neurologic sequelae in such patients. The benefit from corticosteroid therapy is believed to be related to the inhibition of inflammatory cytokine synthesis and secretion by host stromal cells. Dexamethasone therapy, however, has not been shown to reduce the mortality associated with bacterial meningitis.

Pyogenic central nervous system diseases, which include the bacterial meningitides and parameningeal infections, are discussed in detail below. Also included are discussions on shunt infections and amebic meningitis and meningoencephalitis.

Acute Pyogenic Meningitis

Etiologic Agents

The identity of the bacterial agent in pyogenic meningitis is frequently suspected on the basis of epidemiological and clinical clues. The first and perhaps most important clue is a patient's age because there are striking correlations between the common types of bacterial meningitis and the age groups they afflict [*see Table 1*]. Epidemiological studies now suggest that three fourths of the estimated 25,000 new cases of bacterial meningitis that occur annually in the United States develop in children younger than 12 years. The epidemiology and etiology of pyogenic meningitis are quite similar in industrialized nations and developing countries. The only major exception is that enteric organisms, such as *Salmonella* species, account for a higher frequency of bacterial meningitis in developing countries than in industrialized nations.[1]

Table 1 Frequency of Bacterial Causes of Meningitis by Age Group

	Neonates (One Month or Younger)	Children (One Month to 15 Years)	Adults (Older Than 15 Years)
Streptococcus pneumoniae	0–5%	10%–20%	30%–50%
Neisseria meningitidis	0–1%	25%–40%	10%–35%
Hemophilus influenzae	0–3%	40%–60%	1%–3%
Streptococci (other than *S. pneumoniae*)	20%–40%[*]	2%–4%	5%
Staphylococci	5%	1%–2%	5%–15%
Listeria	2%–10%	1%–2%	5%
Gram-negative bacilli	50%–60%[†]	1%–2%	1%–10%

[*]Almost all streptococcal isolates in neonatal meningitis are group B.

[†]Of all the organisms causing neonatal meningitis, both gram-positive and gram-negative, *Escherichia coli* accounts for approximately 40 percent of isolates.

The principal bacteria responsible for neonatal meningitis are gram-negative bacilli (most commonly, *Escherichia coli* strains bearing the K1 capsular antigen) and group B streptococci.[2] Group B streptococci have become an increasingly prevalent cause of neonatal meningitis and in some instances have surpassed *E. coli* in frequency. *Hemophilus influenzae* type B meningitis is the most common form of bacterial meningitis in children and mainly affects those who are two months to three years of age.[2] The appearance of *H. influenzae* meningitis in adults is so unusual that its presence still suggests predisposing anatomic or immunologic defects that have permitted circumvention of the barrier normally provided by serum bactericidal mechanisms.

The most common bacterial causes of adult meningitis are *Streptococcus pneumoniae* and *Neisseria meningitidis*. Meningococcal meningitis is the only kind of bacterial meningitis that occurs in outbreaks, usually in susceptible populations in close living quarters, such as recruits living in military barracks or residents of a crowded urban area. Secondary cases of *H. influenzae* meningitis, however, have been found in close contacts of affected children, such as family members and day care center contacts.[3]

Certain clinical conditions predispose to specific types of bacterial meningitis. The conditions that predispose to pneumococcal meningitis are acute otitis media and mastoiditis (30 percent of cases), pneumonia (10 to 25 percent), nonpenetrating head injury (five to 10 percent), CSF rhinorrhea or otorrhea (five percent), acute sinusitis (occasionally), alcoholism and cirrhosis of the liver (10 to 25 percent of adult patients in urban hospitals with pneumococcal meningitis), sickle cell anemia, and defects in host defenses such as congenital or acquired immunoglobulin deficiencies and asplenic states.

S. pyogenes meningitis is now uncommon but occasionally appears as a complication of acute otitis media, mastoiditis, or sinusitis.

Other bacteria are infrequently involved in cases of meningitis. *Listeria monocytogenes* is an occasional cause of meningitis in the neonate. Its involvement in adult cases has been increasing primarily among those who are immunosuppressed (which account for 70 percent of cases of *L. monocytogenes* meningitis in adults)[4] and in patients who have underlying neoplastic disease.[5] *L. mono-cytogenes* resembles a diphtheroid organism, both on Gram's stain and in culture, and can easily be mistaken for a contaminant.

Isolation of an anaerobic organism from the CSF is rare and strongly suggests intraventricular leakage of a brain abscess or the presence of a parameningeal focus of infection.

Staphylococcus aureus meningitis is associated with neurosurgical procedures, penetrating cranial trauma, staphylococcal bacteremia and endocarditis, immunosuppressive therapy, and underlying neoplastic disease.[5] Meningitis complicating ventriculoatrial or ventriculoperitoneal shunting procedures is usually caused by *S. aureus* or *S. epidermidis*.[6]

Gram-negative bacillary meningitis (caused by *E. coli, Enterobacter, Klebsiella, Proteus, Serratia,* or *Pseudomonas* species) is usually a nosocomial infection and affects neurosurgical patients, immunosuppressed patients (including the elderly), patients who have neoplastic disease, and neonates.[4,5,7,8]

The specific bacterial agent is not identified in five to 10 percent of patients with pyogenic meningitis. Simultaneous mixed meningitis is rare and is found most often in neonates, particularly in association with a neuroectodermal defect, and occasionally in older patients after a penetrating head injury.

Pathogenesis

Infecting organisms may enter the meninges in several ways: (1) via the bloodstream in systemic bacteremia, (2) by direct ingress from the upper respiratory tract (skull fracture, congenital dural defect, or eroding sequestrum in mastoid) or from the body surface (neuroectodermal defect), (3) through intracranial passage via nasopharyngeal venules, (4) by direct spread from an adjacent focus of infection (sinusitis or intraventricular leakage of a brain abscess), or (5) by introduction of organisms at the time of a neurosurgical operation or diagnostic procedure (lumbar puncture). Bacteremia is the most frequent source of infection. Organisms are often demonstrable in the bloodstream in the very early stages of the three most common types of bacterial meningitis beyond the neonatal period: those caused by *H. influenzae, N. meningitidis,* and *S. pneumoniae*.[9] Disruption of the integrity of the leptomeninges, by trauma to the head or spine or even by performance of a lumbar puncture during a bacteremic episode, enhances the opportunity for organisms to enter the CSF and initiate meningeal infection. Once meningeal infection becomes established, it quickly extends throughout the subarachnoid space; the presence of ventriculitis can be demonstrated at the time of admission in at least 70 percent of neonates who are diagnosed as having meningitis.[10]

Clinical Features

Most cases of *H. influenzae, N. meningitidis,* and *S. pneumoniae* meningitis are preceded by upper respiratory tract infection, otitis media, or pneumonia. The onset is usually acute and develops over the course of 24 to 36 hours with fever, generalized headache, vomiting, and stiff neck. In some instances, the onset is less acute, extending over three to five days. Myalgias (particularly in meningococcal disease) and backache are common. Once meningitic signs are evident, the infection progresses rapidly, producing confusion, obtundation, and, ultimately, coma. Indications of leptomeningeal inflammation (drowsiness, stiff neck, and Kernig's and Brudzinski's signs) are almost always present.

The usual manifestations of meningitis may be partially obscured in an elderly person who has underlying congestive heart failure or pneumonia and is obtunded and hypoxic. Similarly, a neonate with meningitis may have decreased appetite, fever, irritability, lassitude, and vomiting but may not exhibit either stiff neck or bulging fontanelles. Such patients should be examined carefully for meningitic signs, and if any question about the presence of meningitis remains, the cerebrospinal fluid should be examined.

Neurologic Findings and Complications

Cranial nerve dysfunction Cranial nerve dysfunction involving primarily the third, fourth, sixth, or seventh nerve appears in 10 to 20 percent of patients with bacterial meningitis. These palsies usually disappear within some weeks after recovery. Sensorineural hearing loss, which is sometimes permanent, has been reported after bacterial meningitis, but it is not a complication of viral meningitis. Hearing loss is a more frequent sequela of meningococcal meningitis than of the other two common types of primary pyogenic meningitis (i.e., meningitis caused by *H. influenzae* or *S. pneumoniae*).

Focal cerebral signs Hemiparesis, dysphasia, and hemianopsia occur in about 15 percent of patients with pyogenic meningitis. These focal cerebral signs are often secondary to occlusive vascular inflammation; they may appear early in the course of the infection or, paradoxically, later when the meningeal process is subsiding. Similar cerebral signs may be caused by postictal changes (Todd's paralysis) but usually persist for no more than a few hours. The persistence of significant focal cerebral findings suggests the presence of a complicating cerebral arteritis, cortical venous thrombophlebitis, or an associated mass lesion (e.g., a subdural effusion, cerebral abscess, or subdural empyema).

Focal or generalized seizures Twenty to 30 percent of patients who have bacterial meningitis experience focal or generalized seizures. Seizures may be caused by focal cerebral injury or by such readily reversible conditions as high fever and hypoglycemia (in infants), acute brain swelling, or penicillin neurotoxicity. Neurotoxicity results when large doses of penicillin are administered in the presence of some degree of renal failure. Development of myoclonic jerking of the face and extremities before the onset of overt seizure activity suggests the diagnosis. As with focal cerebral findings, seizures caused by occlusive vascular changes may occur early in the disease course; they can

also appear five to 10 days later, during the recovery phase.

Acute cerebral edema Occasionally, bacterial meningitis results in acute brain swelling associated with CSF pressures of 450 mm H_2O or more. Elevation of pressure to this level may occur in the absence of an associated mass lesion. Such pressures may result in seizures, third nerve palsies, hypertension, bradycardia, and coma. CSF pressures in this range may also lead to a temporal lobe or cerebellar pressure cone, especially in the period after a lumbar puncture. Prompt treatment is necessary to forestall these complications.

The acute brain swelling of pyogenic meningitis does not usually produce papilledema. The presence of papilledema suggests the coexistence of an independent or complicating space-occupying suppurative intracranial process, such as a brain abscess or subdural empyema. Cerebral edema, subdural effusion (in the infant), hydrocephalus, cortical vein thrombophlebitis, and loculated ventriculitis may all cause persistence or late onset of obtundation or coma. Marked central hyperpnea is often a sign of severe bacterial meningitis and is caused mainly by increased CSF levels of lactic acid.

Ten to 20 percent of patients with bacterial meningitis experience residual neurologic abnormalities after resolution of the acute infection. Less obvious alterations in behavior and cognitive function are important potential late sequelae of meningitis in infants and young children; proper assessment of these changes will require extensive prospective studies.

Findings Specific to Certain Meningitides

Delirium Delirium and maniacal behavior may occur occasionally with any type of bacterial meningitis but appear most frequently with meningococcal infections, perhaps because such infections tend to be associated with cerebral edema. It is important to emphasize that these same manifestations may be present in other types of infections of the central nervous system, such as encephalitis or temporal lobe abscess.

Indolent course The presence of *L. monocytogenes* meningitis is suggested by an indolent course that lasts some days or weeks before hospitalization in a patient whose cerebrospinal fluid shows a mild neutrophilic pleocytosis ($\leq$ 1,000 cells/mm^3).

Exanthem A maculopetechial or purpuric rash in a patient with meningitis usually signifies the presence of meningococcal infection. *N. gonorrhoeae* is very rarely the cause of such skin lesions. Infrequently, petechial and purpuric skin lesions develop in the course of *S. pneumoniae* bacteremia and meningitis, reflecting disseminated intravascular coagulation.

Multiple skin lesions almost identical to those observed in patients with meningococcemia occur rarely in patients with acute *S. aureus* endocarditis. Meningitic signs and a CSF neutrophilic pleocytosis may also develop in such patients and are caused by embolic cerebral infarction rather than by bacterial meningitis. Usually, one or two of the numerous skin lesions are purulent purpura; staphylococci can be demonstrated on Gram's stain of the aspirated contents of the purulent centers of such lesions.

The maculopetechial rash of echovirus aseptic meningitis (particularly type 9, which has been responsible for extensive outbreaks) may be mistaken for the rash of meningococcal meningitis. This type of viral meningitis may produce an early and marked CSF neutrophilic pleocytosis (up to 1,000 or more cells/mm^3, of which as many as 70 to 80 percent are neutrophils). The rash in meningococcal meningitis may involve the face and neck but only after it has already extensively covered other parts of the body. In echovirus type 9 meningeal infection, the rash involves the face and neck early in the course of the exanthem, before other parts of the body are significantly involved. When any question about the diagnosis remains after initial examination of the CSF, the most prudent course is to treat for bacterial (meningococcal) infection.

Laboratory Diagnosis

CSF Examination

Although the CSF changes of bacterial meningitis resemble those of various other infections of the CNS, there are subtle differences that provide an important element in differential diagnosis.

Three basic patterns, or profiles, of CSF findings can be distinguished: (1) purulent [*see Table 2*], (2) lymphocytic with a normal glucose level [*see Table 3*], and (3) lymphocytic with a low glucose level [*see Table 4*]. The purulent profile is characterized by a polymorphonuclear leukocytic pleocytosis, often a low glucose level (< 50 to 60 percent of the simultaneous blood glucose concentration), and an elevated protein concentration. Both lymphocytic profiles are characterized by a pleocytosis (usually < 1,000 lymphocytes/mm^3) and a normal or only mildly elevated protein level.

The foregoing categorization necessarily involves some overlap. For example, *L. monocytogenes* meningitis is usually characterized by a purulent CSF profile, but occasionally in infants and rarely in adults, it is associated with a lymphocytic–low glucose CSF profile. Likewise, early tuberculous or cryptococcal meningitis usually produces a lymphocytic–normal glucose CSF profile, whereas subsequent examinations reveal a progressive lowering of CSF glucose.

Cell count The CSF cell count [*see Table 5*] in the majority of cases of untreated bacterial meningitis ranges from 100 to 5,000 cells/mm^3, of which more than 80 percent are neutrophils.[11] Cell counts of 50,000 cells/mm^3 or higher are occasionally observed in primary bacterial meningitis, but such a marked pleocytosis also suggests the possibility of intraventricular rupture of a cerebral abscess. Sometimes, a grossly clear CSF containing only five to 10 neutrophils/mm^3 is observed in patients with meningitis and underlying granulo-

Table 2   Neutrophilic–Low Glucose (Purulent) CSF Profile

	Infectious Cause	*Noninfectious Cause*
Common	Bacterial meningitis	—
Uncommon	Viral meningitis* (in very early phase only)	Chemical meningitis
	Certain parameningeal infections	Exogenous (e.g., contrast media, detergents used in cleaning needles)
	Subdural empyema* (usually produces lymphocytic-normal glucose profile)	Endogenous (release of material into CSF from tumors: dermoids, craniopharyngiomas)
	?Early brain abscess at bacterial cerebritis stage*	Unusual diseases*
	Cerebral abscess with leakage or rupture into ventricle	Initial phase of Mollaret's meningitis
	Embolic cerebral infarction* (bacterial endocarditis)	Behçet's syndrome
	Amebic meningoencephalitis	Hypersensitivity meningitis
	Tuberculous meningitis (only very early in the disease and only in a small percentage of cases)	Drug-induced* (sulfonamides, tolmetin, ibuprofen, isoniazid)
	Acute hemorrhagic leukoencephalitis	

*Glucose level in CSF usually normal.

cytopenia or in patients with early *H. influenzae* or *N. meningitidis* meningitis. Rarely, in an elderly or granulocytopenic patient with pneumococcal meningitis, the CSF may be grossly turbid but contain few, if any, leukocytes; the cloudiness stems from the presence of enormous numbers of pneumococci. The prognosis for these patients is extremely poor.

Eosinophils may be found in the CSF under a variety of circumstances.[12] Eosinophilic meningitis characteristically has been associated with infection by *Angiostrongylus cantonensis*, the rat lungworm, which has a peculiar tropism for the human nervous system. *A. cantonensis* appears to be indigenous to Southeast Asia and tropical areas of the Pacific Basin; it has also been detected in patients in Cuba. CSF eosinophilia has also been reported in cases of CNS cysticercosis, the fungal meningitides (caused by *Coccidioides immitis*, *Candida albicans*, or *Aspergillus*), and, rarely, in cases of viral meningitis (coxsackieviral and lymphocytic choriomeningitis). The introduction of foreign materials, such as rubber catheters, into the ventricular system for CSF shunting can also lead to CSF eosinophilia, as can neoplastic infiltration of the leptomeninges by lymphoma or leukemia.

Glucose More than half of patients with bacterial meningitis have CSF glucose levels of 40 mg/dl or lower (< 50 to 60 percent of the simultaneous fasting blood glucose level) [*see Table 5*]. A normal CSF glucose concentration, however, is not inconsistent with a diagnosis of bacterial meningitis.

The primary importance of the CSF glucose determination is not in aiding diagnosis of the average case of acute pyogenic meningitis (which can usually be diagnosed on the basis of the Gram's stain of the CSF and the CSF cell count). Rather, the CSF glucose level is most useful in distinguishing chronic meningitides marked by hypoglycorrhachia—such as those that are caused by *Listeria*, *Nocardia*, *Actinomyces*, *Cryptococcus*, or *Coccidioides* organisms—from parameningeal infections and viral aseptic meningitides, which do not lower CSF glucose levels.[13]

Table 3   Lymphocytic–Normal Glucose CSF Profile

	Infectious Cause	Noninfectious Cause
Common	Viral meningitis or encephalitis Postinfectious encephalomyelitis	
Uncommon	Partially treated pyogenic meningitis caused by common bacteria Parameningeal infections (brain abscess, subdural empyema, epidural abscess) Fungal and tuberculous meningitis (early) Parasitic disease (trichinosis, toxoplasmosis, cysticercosis) Whipple's disease	Neoplastic meningitis (cerebral or metastatic tumors) Uveoencephalitides (Vogt-Koyanagi syndrome, Harada's syndrome) Systemic lupus erythematosus Primary cerebral granulomatous arteritis

The basis for the hypoglycorrhachia associated with diffuse meningeal inflammation is probably twofold: (1) increased glycolysis mainly in the cells of adjacent brain and spinal cord tissue and to a lesser extent in the neutrophils in the CSF and (2) inhibition of the membrane-carrier system, which transports glucose from the circulation to the CSF.

Protein   Patients with bacterial meningitis usually have CSF protein concentrations higher than 120 mg/dl [*see Table 5*]. Occasionally, levels of 1,000 mg/dl or greater are observed, suggesting actual or impending subarachnoid block secondary to meningitis.

Chemical and enzymatic changes   Elevated levels of CSF lactic acid in the range of 35 to 700 mg/dl are characteristic of pyogenic or tuberculous meningitis[14]; lactic acid concentrations lower than 35 mg/dl are usually found in the CSF of patients with aseptic meningitis and parameningeal infections. Unfortunately, CSF lactic acid levels in aseptic and pyogenic meningitis overlap to some extent, and thus, lactic acid determination is probably of no greater value than the usual parameters (i.e., CSF leukocyte count, glucose level, and protein level) in the differential diagnosis of meningitis.[15] Elevated CSF lactate levels correspond to low CSF glucose levels. Increased glycolysis in

Table 4   Lymphocytic–Low Glucose CSF Profile

	Infectious Cause	Noninfectious Cause
Common	Tuberculous meningitis Fungal meningitis (cryptococcal, coccidioidal, or *Histoplasma* meningitis)	
Uncommon	Partially treated pyogenic meningitis caused by common bacteria Bacterial meningitis caused by certain organisms uncommonly implicated in meningitis: *Listeria monocytogenes, Leptospira interrogans, Treponema pallidum* (acute syphilitic meningitis) Viral meningitis (in 10% of cases of mumps meningitis, occasionally in lymphocytic choriomeningitis, rarely in echoviral meningitis)	Neoplastic meningitis Sarcoidosis of the meninges

Table 5   CSF Findings in Intracranial Infections

	Pressure (mm H_2O)	Cell Count (WBCs/mm^3)	Glucose (mg/dl)	Protein (mg/dl)	Demonstration of Organism in CSF
Normal values	90–180	0–5 lymphocytes	50–175 (at least 50% of simultaneous serum glucose)	15–40	—
Bacterial meningitis	200–300	100–5,000; neutrophils usually > 80%	Reduced (< 40)	100–1,000	Organism seen on Gram's stain (80% of cases); recovered on culture (80%–90% of cases)
Brain abscess	180–300	10–200 lymphocytes	Normal	70–400	—
Brain abscess with leak into ventricle	200–300	3,000–100,000 neutrophils	Reduced (< 40)	200 –> 500	Organism, often an anaerobe, seen on culture and smear
Subdural empyema	200–300	10–2,000 lymphocytes (neutrophils predominate when empyema is associated with bacterial meningitis or neurosurgery)	Normal; reduced if meningitis is also present	50–500	—
Cerebral epidural abscess	180–250	10–300 lymphocytes	Normal	50–200	—
Septic thrombophlebitis of cortical veins	180–250	10–300; mild neutrophilic predominance	Normal	50–200	—
Tuberculous meningitis	180–300	Usually < 500 lymphocytes	Reduced (< 40)	100–200, but up to 1,000 if CSF block is present	If *Mycobacterium tuberculosis* is not found in lumbar CSF, cisternal tap may reveal the organism
Cryptococcal meningitis	180–300	10–200 lymphocytes	Reduced (<40)	50–200	Organism recovered on culture; cryptococcal antigen also present

	Pressure (mm H₂O)	Cell Count (WBCs/mm³)	Glucose (mg/dl)	Protein (mg/dl)	Demonstration of Organism in CSF
Viral meningitis	90–200	10–300 lymphocytes; may be > 1,000 in echoviral and mumps meningitis and in lymphocytic choriomeningitis (LCM); early echoviral meningitis may show up to 80% neutrophilic predominance	Normal; occasionally slightly reduced in mumps meningitis and LCM	50–100	LCM virus and herpesvirus type 2 isolated from CSF (enteroviruses isolated from stool)
Viral encephalitis	180–300	0–500 lymphocytes	Normal	50–100	Virus not recovered from CSF (herpes simplex virus isolated from brain biopsy)

adjacent cerebral tissue and in cellular infiltrates in the leptomeninges may possibly account for high CSF lactic acid concentrations.

The activity of certain enzymes that are normally present in low levels in the CSF, such as lactic dehydrogenase and muramidase, is markedly increased in patients with bacterial or fungal meningitis. The activity of these enzymes is only mildly elevated in patients with viral meningitis. The elevated enzyme levels apparently correlate with the neutrophilic pleocytosis and probably add little information that would be helpful in diagnosis.

Bacteriologic findings Definitive diagnosis requires isolation of the causative organism or demonstration of its characteristic antigen. The implicated bacterium can be demonstrated on a Gram's stain of the CSF in about 80 percent of cases of bacterial meningitis. The bacteria that are most likely to be missed on Gram's stain are meningococci and *Listeria* organisms.[16]

Insufficient decolorization of the slide or failure to recognize certain properties of particular organisms may result in errors in interpretation of Gram's stains of the CSF. For example, *H. influenzae*, a gram-negative bacillus that stains a little more darkly at each pole than in the middle, might be mistaken for a gram-positive diplococcus. The latter, however, is considerably larger. *Acinetobacter calcoaceticus* and *Pasteurella multocida*, which are rare causes of pyogenic meningitis, may be very pleomorphic. Either one may be mistaken on smear for mixtures of gram-negative bacilli and *Neisseria*.

Pneumococcus is the most likely bacterial agent involved whenever gram-positive diplococci are seen in the CSF, even when admixed with gram-positive cocci in short chains. Enterococcus, which resembles pneumococcus on Gram's stain, rarely causes meningitis. Enterococcal meningitis is usually found in the clinical settings of urinary tract infection, cirrhosis, abdominal sepsis, or recent neurosurgery.[17] Identification of enterococcus is important because effective antimicrobial therapy requires the combined administration of an aminoglycoside and either penicillin G or ampicillin.

Penicillin-allergic patients with enterococcal meningitis can be treated with a combination of an aminoglycoside and vancomycin.

Definitive identification of pneumococci can be made by the capsular swelling (quellung) reaction. This test, which uses pooled pneumococcal antisera, can be performed only when sufficient numbers of organisms are present in the CSF. It is especially useful when a Gram's stain of the CSF leaves some question as to the identity of the gram-positive coccus. Failure to demonstrate capsular swelling suggests that the organism is some streptococcal species other than *S. pneumoniae*. Initially, this situation warrants penicillin-aminoglycoside therapy until the results of blood and CSF cultures are forthcoming. Together, Gram's stains of the CSF, CSF cultures, and blood cultures yield enough information to permit determination of the bacterial etiology in about 90 percent of cases of bacterial meningitis.

Special immunologic and miscellaneous procedures for bacteriologic diagnosis The three most common bacterial meningitides, those caused by *H. influenzae*, *N. meningitidis*, and *S. pneumoniae*, are associated with mean CSF bacterial concentrations ranging from 10^5 to 10^7 organisms/ml.[18] This quantity of organisms introduces envelope polysaccharide antigens into the CSF in amounts sufficient to be detectable by counterimmunoelectrophoresis (CIE) and the latex agglutination test. These procedures have been used most extensively in the rapid diagnosis (i.e., one to two hours) of *H. influenzae* meningitis. CIE has been helpful in the rapid diagnosis of pneumococcal and meningococcal (groups A, B, C, and Y) meningitis as well, and it can be used to detect *E. coli* K1 capsular antigen and group B streptococcal antigen in neonatal meningitis.

The bacterial capsular antigens of the three common etiologic agents in primary bacterial meningitis can be successfully identified in 60 to 80 percent of cases.[19-21] The reliability of these immunoprecipitin techniques depends heavily on the activity of the antisera employed. False positive results occasionally arise from cross-reactions. For example, certain *E. coli* capsular antigens cross-react with antisera to *H. influenzae* type B and group B meningococcal antigens. Because the bacterial etiology can be established in about 90 percent of cases of bacterial meningitis by more traditional microbiological means, CIE is not essential for diagnosis. It serves as an important adjunct, however, permitting early diagnosis in cases in which no organisms are seen on smear or in which cultures remain negative because of prior antibiotic therapy. Even in cases in which the morphology of the organism is revealed by Gram's stain, CIE is useful because it permits definitive identification of the agent.

The limulus test of CSF is a rapid, fairly sensitive method for diagnosing purulent meningitis caused by endotoxin-containing organisms such as *E. coli* and other Enterobacteriaceae, *H. influenzae*, and *N. meningitidis*.[21-23] Various limitations, however, have served to relegate this test primarily to the realm of research.

Gas-liquid chromatographic analysis of fatty acids and carbohydrates drawn from the CSF of patients with bacterial meningitis shows promise as an effective means of identifying the involved bacterial agent.[24]

Other Laboratory Studies

Blood cultures Bacteremia is demonstrable in 80 percent of cases of *H. influenzae* meningitis, 50 percent of cases of pneumococcal meningitis, and 30 to 40 percent of cases of *N. meningitidis* meningitis.[9]

Respiratory tract cultures Cultures of the upper respiratory tract are not helpful in establishing the identity of the etiologic agent in a given patient with pyogenic meningitis. *S. pneumoniae* may be isolated as frequently from the nasopharynx of patients with meningococcal meningitis as from those with pneumococcal meningitis (25 to 30 percent of patients).

Serum electrolytes Hyponatremia occurs in patients in whom the syndrome of inappropriate antidiuretic hormone (SIADH) secretion complicates a course of bacterial, fungal, or tuberculous meningitis. After dehydration has been corrected, the serum creatinine determination serves as the basis for adjustment of penicillin dosage in the presence of renal dysfunction; penicillin overdose may result in hyperkalemia and seizures.

Radiologic studies Roentgenograms of the chest, air sinuses, and mastoids should be performed at an appropriate time after institution of antimicrobial therapy because infections in these areas are frequently associated with meningitis in older children and adults.

Radionuclide or CT scanning should be performed without delay when history, clinical setting, or physical findings suggest the presence of a suppurative intracranial collection, such as a brain abscess or subdural empyema. Meningitis itself induces the following changes on the CT scan: contrast enhancement of the leptomeninges and ventricular lining, widening of the subarachnoid space, and patchy areas of diminished density in the cerebrum from cerebritis and necrosis.[25,26] CT scanning may also be helpful in evaluating the patient with a prolonged course or deteriorating clinical status and in detecting suspected complications, such as sterile subdural collections or empyema, ventricular enlargement secondary to communicating or obstructive hydrocephalus, ventriculitis or ventricular empyema (as revealed by ventricular wall enhancement), or cerebral infarction caused by arteritis or cortical vein thrombophlebitis.

Differential Diagnosis

Because the clinical features of meningeal inflammation, that is, headache, fever, stiff neck, and obtundation, are common to various types of meningitis and to other forms of infection of the CNS, CSF findings are important elements in the development of the differential diagnosis [*see Table 5*].

Particular attention should be given to the patient with meningitic signs, an atypical neutrophilic CSF pleocytosis, a normal CSF glucose level, and no demonstrable organisms on a Gram's stain of the CSF smear. The differential diagnosis in such a case includes certain treatable diseases that require management different from that of pyogenic meningitis. A parameningeal infection such as an epidural abscess, a subdural empyema, or a brain abscess might be suspected in a patient with these findings who also has a chronic ear, sinus, or lung infection. Isolation of anaerobic organisms from the CSF is highly suggestive of parameningeal infection. Anaerobes may enter the CSF via intraventricular leakage of a cerebral abscess; they may also reach the CSF through extension of infection from a focus of osteomyelitis or from an epidural abscess. Focal cerebral signs may be an indication of a space-occupying intracranial infection; they may also appear during the course of bacterial meningitis as a result of occlusive vascular injury. When focal cerebral signs develop, the history should be searched for any neurologic symptoms antedating the onset of the acute meningitis.

Bacterial endocarditis may present with prominent meningitic symptomatology and CSF pleocytosis. Such a presentation is either the result of frank meningitis caused by pyogenic organisms or the result of sterile embolic cerebral infarctions produced by normally nonpyogenic organisms, such as viridans streptococci. Careful auscultation for cardiac murmurs and a search for peripheral signs of endocarditis (petechiae, splenomegaly, or Osler's nodes) should be carried out.

Trace amounts of disinfectants or detergents can be inadvertently introduced into the CSF during performance of a lumbar puncture from use of improperly washed syringes or needles. Such a lapse in technique can result in exogenous chemical meningitis. CSF findings in exogenous chemical meningitis may include a neutrophilic pleocytosis and hypoglycorrhachia. Obviously, when meningitis occurs within one or two days of a lumbar puncture, the possibility of a bacterial etiology from contamination (e.g., with *Pseudomonas* or coliform organisms) is a most important consideration until ruled out by bacteriologic studies. Iatrogenic meningitis from lumbar puncture procedures, however, is exceedingly rare. It is most likely to occur in patients who have bacteremia at the time of the procedure.[27]

Endogenous chemical meningitis results from leakage into the subarachnoid space of the contents of an intracranial tumor, such as a craniopharyngioma or an epidermoid tumor of the posterior fossa. CSF changes consist of a neutrophilic or lymphocytic pleocytosis and hypoglycorrhachia. Birefringent material, such as keratinized material from an epidermoid tumor or the material from a craniopharyngioma, might be seen under polarized light microscopy in cases of endogenous chemical meningitis.

Nonneurologic Complications

Shock

Shock developing early in the course of acute bacterial meningitis is usually the consequence of intense bacteremia (meningococcemia) rather than of the meningitis itself. The pathogenesis of human septic shock is complex. When microorganisms are killed by antibiotics, they liberate toxins directly or indirectly, and these toxins can cause myocardial depression and endothelial damage.[28,29] Also, bacterial products can stimulate production of inflammatory cytokines (e.g., IL-1, IL-6, TNF) and other endogenous mediators (e.g., platelet activating factor [PAF], arachidonic acid metabolites, kinins, complement, and endorphins) that can contribute to the pathophysiological alterations in bacterial meningitis.[28] Bacterial meningitis is characterized by locally increased permeability of the blood-brain barrier, cerebral edema, and intracranial hypertension.[29,30] In addition, there is decreased systemic vascular resistance and increased cardiac output. Management involves the measures ordinarily used to treat septic shock [see Chapter 1].

Coagulation Disorders

Coagulopathies of varying severity may accompany bacteremias and hypotension in patients with meningitis; mild forms consist only of thrombocytopenia. Clinical and laboratory findings consistent with disseminated intravascular coagulation are seen in patients with more severe illness. Because these abnormalities usually subside with control of infection, their presence alone does not warrant heparin therapy unless active bleeding supervenes [see Chapter 14].

Septic Complications

Early treatment of the initiating infection has rendered acute bacterial endocarditis a very rare complication of pneumococcal meningitis and bacteremia. When endocarditis does ensue, it usually involves the aortic valve and may not become evident until some days after completion of antibiotic therapy for meningitis. Septic arthritis secondary to the three common types of pyogenic meningitis, that is, those caused by *H. influenzae*, *N. meningitidis*, and *S. pneumoniae*, may develop from the accompanying bacteremia early in the course of the nervous system infection.

Prolonged Fever

Most patients with pneumococcal, meningococcal, or *H. influenzae* meningitis become afebrile within two to five days of the start of appropriate antibiotic therapy; occasionally, however, fever continues beyond eight to 10 days or recurs after having disappeared. Prolonged or recurrent fever accompanied by headache, focal cerebral signs, and obtundation suggests that antimicrobial therapy has been inadequate; another possibility is that a neurologic complication such as cortical vein thrombophlebitis, ventriculitis, ventricular empyema, subdural effusion, or subdural empyema has developed. Reevaluation of CSF findings, including Gram's stains and cultures, is essential. Persistent fever in a patient whose clinical course and CSF findings show progressive improvement may be indicative of drug fever.

A serum sickness–like syndrome, consisting of fever, arthritis, and pericarditis, occurs three to six days after the start of antibiotic treatment in about 10 percent of patients with meningococcal meningitis. Synovial and pericardial fluids are serosanguineous and sterile in contrast to the purulent infected effusions that can sometimes be found at both sites earlier in the course of the infection. Pericardial effusions are usually not hemodynamically significant, but careful monitoring of the patient's cardiovascular status is nevertheless indicated. Salicylates or other anti-inflammatory agents provide symptomatic relief. Immunopathologic study of synovial lesions has suggested that immune complex formation is involved in their pathogenesis.

Treatment

General Aspects of Antibiotic Treatment

Most antibiotics employed in the therapy for bacterial meningitis, with the exception of chloramphenicol, do not readily penetrate the normal blood-brain barrier. The presence of meningitis enhances the entry of penicillin and some other antimicrobial agents into the CSF and allows successful therapy with these drugs in large parenteral doses. Antibiotics should be administered intravenously in divided doses at intervals that provide high concentration gradients across the meninges. Dosage should not be tapered with clinical improvement, because the normalization of the blood-brain barrier that accompanies resolution of the infection reduces attainable antibiotic levels in the CSF.

The absence of intrinsic opsonic and bactericidal activity in infected CSF indicates the need for bactericidal rather than bacteriostatic agents in the treatment of bacterial meningitis.[31] Although they are effective in vitro against many species that are capable of causing meningitis, clindamycin, erythromycin, and first- and second-generation cephalosporins (including cefamandole) should not be used in bacterial meningitis, because effective bactericidal levels cannot be predictably achieved in the CSF.

Intrathecal therapy Intrathecal therapy is not needed for treatment of uncompli-cated cases of the three common types of bacterial meningitis, which can be treated with drugs that enter the CSF in bactericidal quantities (i.e., the penicillins and chloramphenicol). Chloramphenicol is bactericidal against *H. influenzae, N. meningitidis,* and *S. pneumoniae* in concentrations that are readily achieved in the CSF, but it is only bacteriostatic against enteric gram-negative bacilli. Adjunctive intrathecal therapy with an aminoglycoside antibiotic is often employed in meningitis caused by resistant enteric gram-negative bacilli, *Pseudomonas aeruginosa,* and enterococci (see below).

Duration of therapy The standards for duration of therapy have not been critically evaluated by clinical trials.[32] Treatment of common bacterial meningitides for longer than 14 days is not usually necessary in the otherwise immunocompetent patient,[32] but therapy for meningitis caused by *L. monocytogenes* or Enterobacteriaceae should be prolonged for at least 21 days. The criteria for minimal duration of therapy must always be based on the patient's response to therapy. Repeat CSF examination should be performed 24 to 48 hours after the start of antibiotic therapy if progress seems unsatisfactory or if the etiology remains uncertain. Meningococcal meningitis should be treated until the patient remains afebrile for five to seven days. With prompt and satisfactory response to antibiotics, it may not be necessary to repeat the CSF examination at the end of therapy. Patients with *H. influenzae* meningitis should be treated for at least seven days after they have become afebrile. Again, a follow-up CSF examination may not be necessary in patients who show rapid and complete clinical recovery.

Patients with pneumococcal meningitis should probably be treated for 10 to 14 days. Prolonged therapy is necessary in the presence of an underlying mastoiditis. When mastoidectomy is required, it should be performed toward the end of the course of therapy but while the patient remains under continuing antibiotic coverage. Occasionally, a patient will present with pneumococcal meningitis and acute mastoiditis in the form of an acute bone abscess with a subperiosteal collection (Bezold's abscess). The swollen, red, tender fluctuant area of the mastoid requires surgical drainage, but mastoid surgery should be delayed for 24 to 48 hours after the start of antibiotic therapy, if possible, even if the abscess is pointing. The delay allows time for achieving bactericidal levels of penicillin in the meninges and CSF and for bringing the acute meningeal infection under control.

Specific Antimicrobial Therapy

Bacterial meningitis is a life-threatening medical emergency that requires prompt initiation of antimicrobial therapy based on examination of the Gram's stain of CSF sediment [*see Table 6*]. A serious but common error in managing a patient with suspected meningitis is delay in performing a diagnostic lumbar puncture and in starting antibiotic therapy.[33] If clinical assessment does not suggest the presence of an intracranial mass lesion [*see* Parameningeal Infections, Brain Abscess, *below*], lumbar puncture need not be delayed until a head CT scan has been completed. Antibiotic therapy should never be delayed in cases of suspected bacterial meningitis. When imaging studies are needed to exclude an intracranial mass before a lumbar puncture is performed, it is recommended that antibiotics be initiated after blood has been obtained for culture. The choice of antibiotics depends on the pathogen suspected on the basis of such criteria as the patient's age and the clinical setting. The scan and the lumbar puncture may be done while the patient is receiving this empirical therapy. If a diagnostic lumbar puncture is performed after a mass lesion has been excluded by CT scan and the Gram's stain results reveal the presence of bacterial types not covered by the initial empirical therapy, the regimen can then be altered to kill these organisms. Animal models of meningitis suggest that such initial empirical therapy will not affect the subsequent CSF culture results if the spinal fluid is sampled within two to three hours of the start of antibiotic therapy.[33]

Clinical and experimental evidence suggests that optimal chemotherapy for bacterial meningitis requires that the CSF concentration of the antibiotic be severalfold greater than the in vitro minimal bactericidal concentration (MBC) for the pathogen. Other principles that should guide therapy for meningitis include the following: (1) the antibiotic must be capable of killing the pathogen, (2) the pathogen must be shown to be highly susceptible to the selected antibiotic, as measured by quantitative dilution studies (e.g., in vitro CSF killing levels or in vitro MBC tests), (3) because the antibiotic must reach local concentrations sufficient to kill the pathogen, the selected agent must readily penetrate into the infected CSF or, if not, be directly instilled into the CSF by intrathecal or intraventricular injection, and (4) foci of suppurative parameningeal infection must be drained whenever the procedure can be performed without causing serious neurologic damage. The extent to which various antibiotics penetrate into the CSF during meningitis differs [*see Table 7*]. In general, antibiotic levels are higher in the CSF of children and neonates with meningitis than in adults with meningitis.

The presence of local leukocytes, especially neutrophils, is probably necessary for the infected meninges to become permeable to antibiotics. For example, limited experience suggests that antibiotics, such as vancomycin, that tend to accumulate in the CSF of otherwise healthy adults with bacterial meningitis do not show similarly enhanced CSF kinetics in neutropenic leukemia patients with documented bacterial meningitis. Therefore, it is recommended that serial CSF drug level measurements or serial CSF bacterial killing studies be performed in severely neutropenic patients to document the effectiveness of antibiotic therapy. Otherwise, serial intrathecal or intraventricular injections of the antibiotics must be performed.

The third-generation cephalosporins usually reach CSF levels that are at least 10 times the MBC against the common Enterobacteriaceae that cause meningitis (e.g.,

Table 6 Antibiotic Therapy for Bacterial Meningitis of Known Etiology

Organism	Antibiotic	Preferred Therapy		Optional Adjunctive Therapy for Adults (24-hour dose)	Alternative Therapy for Adults (24-hour dose)
		Adults (24-hour dose)	Children (24-hour dose)		
Steptococcus pneumoniae	Penicillin G[a]	24 million units I.V.	300,000 units/kg I.V.	—	Chloramphenicol 4–6 g I.V. *or* Third-generation cephalosporin[b]
Streptococcus Groups A and B	Penicillin G[a]	24 million units I.V.	300,000 units/kg I.V.	—	Third-generation cephalosporin[b] *or* Chloramphenicol 4–6 g I.V.
Group D (enterococci)	Penicillin G[a] *and* Gentamicin[c]	24 million units I.V. 5 mg/kg I.V. and intrathecally	300,000 units/kg I.V. 5.0–7.5 mg/kg I.V. or I.M.[d]	Gentamicin 2–4 mg intrathecally[e]	Vancomycin 2 g I.V. *and* Gentamicin 5 g/kg I.V.
Staphylococcus aureus (methicillin sensitive)	Nafcillin[a]	12 g I.V.	200–300 mg/kg I.V.	—	Vancomycin 2 g I.V.
Staphylococcus aureus (methicillin resistant)	Vancomycin	2 g I.V.	30–45 mg/kg I.V.	—	Trimethoprim-sulfamethoxazole (TMP-SMZ): 10–20 mg/kg I.V. (TMP); 50–100 mg/kg I.V. (SMZ)

Table 6 (Continued)

Organism	Antibiotic	Preferred Therapy		Optional Adjunctive Therapy for Adults (24-hour dose)	Alternative Therapy for Adults (24-hour dose)
		Adults (24-hour dose)	Children (24-hour dose)		
Listeria monocytogenes	Penicillin[a] *or* Ampicillin	24 million units I.V. 12–14 g I.V.	300,000 units/kg I.V. 300–400 mg/kg I.V.	Gentamicin 5 mg/kg I.V.	Either chloramphenicol 4–6 I.V. *or* Trimethoprim-sulfamethoxazole: 10–20 mg/kg I.V. (TMP); 50–100 mg/kg I.V. (SMZ) *plus* Gentamicin 5 mg/kg I.V.
Hemophilus influenzae (β-lactamase negative)	Ampicillin	12–14 g I.V.	300–400 mg/kg I.V.[d]	—	Chloramphenicol 4 g I.V. *or* Third-generation cephalosporin[b]
Neisseria meningitidis	Penicillin G[a]	24 million units I.V.	300,000 units/kg I.V.	—	Chloramphenicol 4 g I.V. *or* Third-generation cephalosporin[b]
Escherichia coli, Klebsiella, Proteus, and similar organisms	Third-generation cephalosporin[b] *and* Gentamicin	See below[b] 5 mg/kg I.V. and intrathecally	See below[b] 5.0–7.5 mg/kg I.V. or I.M.[d]	Gentamicin 4–10 mg intrathecally[e]	—

Table 6   (Continued)

Organism	Antibiotic	Preferred Therapy		Optional Adjunctive Therapy for Adults (24-hour dose)	Alternative Therapy for Adults (24-hour dose)
		Adults (24-hour dose)	Children (24-hour dose)		
Pseudomonas	Gentamicin[c] and Ceftazidime	5–6 mg/kg I.V. and intrathecally 4–6 g I.V.	5.0–7.5 mg/kg I.V. or I.M.[d] 90–150 mg/kg I.V.	Gentamicin 4–10 mg intrathecally,[e] intracisternally, or intraventricularly	—

[a]Penicillins should be given in divided doses every 2–4 hr in adults and every 4 hr in infants and young children.

[b]Third-generation cephalosporins that are recommended for meningitis include cefotaxime and ceftriaxone. Ceftazidime should be reserved for documented *Pseudomonas aeruginosa* infections or infections in which multidrug-resistant organisms are isolated. Adult parenteral doses are 8–12 g/day for cefotaxime, 2 g/day for ceftriaxone, and 4–6 g/day for ceftazidime. Pediatric parenteral doses are 100–200 mg/kg/day for cefotaxime; a 75 mg/kg loading dose and then 100 mg/kg/day for ceftriaxone; and 60 to 300 mg/kg/day for ceftazidime.

[c]Administered in divided doses every 8 hr. Dose should be adjusted for reduced renal function and to achieve therapeutic serum level; I.V. infusion should be administered cautiously.

[d]7.5 mg/kg/24 hr in children up to 2 yr of age.

[e]In 5–10 ml of CSF or in a volume of sterile saline comparable to the 5–10 ml of CSF removed from an adult for analysis. (A smaller volume is used in an infant.) Injection should be given slowly over 10 min.

Table 7   Relative Penetration of Antibiotics into CSF in Adults with Meningitis

Agent	24-Hour Dose	Mean Concentration (µg/ml)		CSF Penetration (%)
		Serum	CSF	
Penicillin G	20 million units I.V.	10–30	0.5–1.5	5
Ampicillin	8–12 g I.V.	30–50	3–6	15
Nafcillin	8–12 g I.V.	30–50	1–3	5
Vancomycin	2 g I.V.	30	3–4	10
Chloramphenicol	4–6 g I.V.	30	5–10	30
Gentamicin	5 mg/kg I.V.	6–10	1–2	20
Sulfadiazine	4 g I.V.	40–60	20–40	50–80
Trimethoprim	10 mg/kg I.V.	5–8	2–3	30
Cephalothin	8–12 g I.V.	30–50	< 0.5	< 1
Cefuroxime	4.5 g I.V.	100	6–16	10
Ceftriaxone	1–2 g I.V.	75–150	1.3–18.0	2–5
Cefotaxime	8–12 g I.V.	75–100	5–15	5
Ceftazidime	4–6 g I.V.	15–56	4.1–7.2	13–27

Note: from data provided by Merle A. Sande, M.D.

E. coli, Klebsiella species, and *Proteus mirabilis*), a level that appears to be needed to cure meningitis.[34] It is questionable, however, whether these agents when used alone can achieve 10-fold MBC levels in the CSF against such organisms as *Pseudomonas, Flavobacterium, Enterobacter, Serratia,* and *Acinetobacter* species.

The appearance of penicillinase-producing *H. influenzae* type B strains that are highly resistant to ampicillin (about 10 percent of isolates in the United States) has required a shift in the focus of initial management of this form of meningitis. Chloramphenicol is now mandatory in the therapy for *H. influenzae* meningitis until the isolate has been demonstrated to be ampicillin susceptible in vitro. There does not appear to be any antagonism between the antibacterial effects of chloramphenicol and of ampicillin against *H. influenzae.* For this reason, and because rare strains of *H. influenzae* resistant to either ampicillin or chloramphenicol alone have been isolated, many pediatricians use both drugs initially until susceptibility testing is performed and then discontinue chloramphenicol if the organism is demonstrated to be susceptible to ampicillin.

There is an emerging problem, however, that might necessitate a reappraisal of this therapeutic strategy. Some strains of *H. influenzae* have now been found to be resistant to both ampicillin and chloramphenicol. Resistance to ampicillin is caused by β-lactamase production, whereas chloramphenicol resistance is associated with acetyltransferase production.[35,36] Although such resistant strains are currently rare in the United States, epidemiological data suggest that they may account for as many as 25 percent of the clinical isolates of *H. influenzae* within the next decade. Therefore, the newer third-generation cephalosporins (i.e., cefuroxime, cefotaxime, and moxalactam) might be the agents of choice in the near future because they have been shown to be as effective as standard therapy for *H. influenzae* meningitis in neonates and are not inactivated by bacterial enzymes.[37]

A patient with *S. aureus* meningitis should be treated with a penicillinase-resistant penicillin such as nafcillin because 80 to

90 percent of *S. aureus* isolates are resistant to penicillin G.

Enterococcal meningitis requires the use of intravenous penicillin or ampicillin supplemented by parenterally administered gentamicin [*see Table 6*]. When lumbar puncture reveals an organism that resembles an enterococcus, an immediate intrathecal dose of gentamicin (4 to 8 mg for an adult) should be considered. Furthermore, if a patient fails to respond promptly to parenteral therapy with penicillin and gentamicin, continued adjunctive intrathecal gentamicin may be given.

The Special Problem of Gram-Negative Bacillary Meningitis

The antibiotics that have commonly been used parenterally in the treatment of gram-negative bacillary meningitis are ampicillin, chloramphenicol, and the aminoglycosides. The results of treatment, however, have been far from satisfactory: mortality ranges from 30 to 60 percent.[38,39] The use of ampicillin as primary therapy for this form of meningitis is limited by the fact that about 30 percent of strains of gram-negative bacilli that cause neonatal meningitis and the majority of isolates from adults with meningitis are ampicillin resistant. Chloramphenicol also has some drawbacks in addition to its potential toxicity in neonates. Although the minimum inhibitory concentrations (MIC) of chloramphenicol for many gram-negative bacilli (2 to 6 µg/ml) are achievable in the CSF, minimum bactericidal concentrations are generally so much higher (> 60 µg/ml) that they are not attainable in the CSF.[40] Antagonism of the bactericidal effect of gentamicin by chloramphenicol has been observed in a rabbit model of *P. mirabilis* meningitis.[41] This antibiotic combination results in an antibacterial effect comparable to the bacteriostatic effect of chloramphenicol alone against this organism. The significance of this antibiotic antagonism in the clinical situation is unclear, except in patients with granulocytopenia.

Adjunctive intrathecal antibiotic therapy has come into use in gram-negative bacillary meningitis for two reasons: (1) parenteral administration of gentamicin and tobramycin yields low (< 1 µg/ml) and inconsistent levels in the CSF and (2) patients treated only with systemic agents have a high mortality. The high mortality associated with neonatal gram-negative bacillary meningitis, however, has not been reduced by the addition of lumbar intrathecal administration of gentamicin to parenteral therapy with ampicillin and gentamicin.[2] Unfortunately, the ventricles are common sites of infection in bacterial meningitis, and little of the antibiotic introduced intrathecally in the lumbar area reaches the ventricular system: the unidirectional circulation of the CSF inhibits drug entry. Adjunctive intraventricular administration of gentamicin either via a ventriculostomy reservoir or by percutaneous injection would circumvent this obstacle. However, a controlled study of neonates with gram-negative bacillary meningitis demonstrated a higher mortality among infants who received intraventricular gentamicin along with systemic antibiotics (42.9 percent) than among those who received systemic antibiotics alone (12.5 percent).[10] This finding suggests that intraventricular therapy with gentamicin is harmful in neonates with gram-negative bacillary meningitis.

By contrast, adjunctive intraventricular administration of amikacin via a Rickham reservoir (1 to 5 mg at 24-hour intervals) has been employed with some success after neurosurgical procedures in neonates with gram-negative bacillary meningitis and ventriculitis.[42] Important in the success of intraventricular amikacin therapy is the achievement of high peak ventricular levels of antibiotic (up to 100 µg/ml) and maintenance levels of at least five to 10 times the MIC of amikacin for the infecting organism; maintenance levels are achieved by daily adjustment of intraventricular dosages. Careful and constant monitoring of ventricular and CSF aminoglycoside levels is essential; this monitoring ensures that therapeutic yet nontoxic levels of the drug are maintained.

Table 8   CSF Bactericidal Index Based on MBCs of the Infecting Organisms and CSF Drug Concentrations

Organism	Cefotaxime	Ceftizoxime	Ceftriaxone	Cefoperazone	Ceftazidime	Moxalactam
Group B streptococci	10–60	10–60	10–60	5–20	2–10*	2–5*
Escherichia coli	10–100	10–50	10–100	2–25†	10–100	10–100
Streptococcus pneumoniae	10–60	10–50	10–100	5–50	2–20*	2–5*
Hemophilus influenzae	10–200	10–200	10–300	5–40	10–100	10–300
Neisseria meningitidis	10–200	10–200	10–300	10–20	10–100	10–300
Klebsiella species	10–200	10–100	10–100	2–50†	10–100	10–200
Pseudomonas species	<10*	<10*	<10*	<10*	2–10*	<10*

Note: see reference 44.   *Not uniformly adequate.   †Not adequate if strain is TEM β-lactamase type.

At present, the adjunctive use of lumbar intrathecal aminoglycoside (e.g., gentamicin) is recommended in children and adults with gram-negative bacillary meningitis (other than *H. influenzae* meningitis) because of the high overall mortality associated with this disease when it is treated with parenteral antibiotics alone.[7,8] Parenteral administration of third-generation cephalosporins unaccompanied by intrathecal use of an antibiotic represents an attractive prospect for successful treatment of gram-negative bacillary meningitis. The median MBC of third-generation cephalosporins for most enteric gram-negative bacilli and *H. influenzae* is less than 0.5 to 2.0 μg/ml. Perhaps the most important therapeutic advantage of third-generation cephalosporins lies in the treatment of meningitis.[43] These drugs are becoming the agents of choice for the common gram-negative bacillary meningitides because they can achieve CSF concentrations that exceed by 10-fold the MBC for various bacterial species that commonly cause meningitis [*see Table 8*].[34] The precise role of the third-generation cephalosporins in the treatment of other cases of bacillary meningitis is being evaluated in ongoing clinical studies.[44-54] A number of clinical trials support their efficacy in the treatment of cases of meningitis that are caused by various bacterial agents [*see Table 9*] and that occur in different age groups.[37]

Several general guidelines have been proposed regarding the use of the newer cephalosporins in the treatment of bacterial meningitis: (1) final selection of the antibiotic or antibiotics for the treatment of bacterial meningitis should be based on which drug or drugs have the greatest bactericidal activity for the causative agent, as determined by the MBC, (2) a CSF bactericidal titer should be performed to demonstrate that the use of a selected cephalosporin is appropriate, (3) for gram-negative bacillary meningitis in adults, it is recommended that one of the newer cephalosporins be administered parenterally together with an aminoglycoside that is administered both parenterally and intrathecally (this combination is superior to former regimens that employed aminoglycosides and chloramphenicol with or without ampicillin), (4) the newer cephalosporins do not offer any advantage over penicillin G in the treatment of group B streptococcal meningitis, (5) cefotaxime, moxalactam, ceftriaxone, and ceftizoxime appear to be as effective as chloramphenicol or ampicillin in the treatment of *H. influenzae* meningitis, (6) cefotaxime and ceftriaxone appear to be equal to penicillin G or chloramphenicol in the treatment of meningococcal and pneumococcal meningitides, and either might be considered as a replacement for chloramphenicol in the penicillin-allergic patient, (7) meningitis caused by *Pseudomonas, Acinetobacter, Enterobacter,* or *Serratia* organisms cannot be successfully treated with third-generation cephalosporins alone, and (8) meningitis caused by *Listeria,* staphylococci, or streptococcal isolates other than group B or *S. pneumoniae* should not be treated with third-generation cephalosporins, which lack activity against these organisms.

Although there are few clinical studies that compare the efficacy of different antibiotic regimens for bacterial meningitis, two recent studies evaluated different regimens for the treatment of this disorder in children. One study evaluated ceftriaxone versus cefuroxime,[53] and the other study compared four commonly used antibiotic regimens: cefotaxime, ceftriaxone, ampicillin, and chloramphenicol.[54] The first report suggests that ceftriaxone is superior to cefuroxime, and the benefits of milder hearing loss and more rapid sterilization of the CSF with ceftriaxone outweigh its potential biliary tract toxicity.[53] The second report indicates

Table 9   Third-Generation Cephalosporins Effective in Sepcific Types of Meningitis

Causative Organism	Agents Used Successfully
Neisseria meningitidis	Cefotaxime, ceftizoxime, ceftriaxone
Hemophilus influenzae (including ampicillin-resistant strains)	Cefotaxime, ceftizoxime, ceftriaxone
Streptococcus pneumoniae	Cefotaxime, ceftizoxime, ceftriaxone
Group B streptococci	Cefotaxime, ceftriaxone
Escherichia coli	Cefotaxime, ceftizoxime, ceftriaxone, cefoperazone
Proteus species	Cefotaxime, ceftriaxone
Salmonella species	Cefotaxime

Note: see reference 44.

that cefotaxime, ceftriaxone, ampicillin, and chloramphenicol produce very similar results in terms of such parameters as clinical recovery, normalization of laboratory indices, adverse reactions, sequelae, and mortality. However, the investigators in this study concluded that (1) chloramphenicol is not the preferred agent in such cases because of occasional clinical failures that might be related to delayed sterilization of the CSF and (2) bacterial resistance might be a problem with ampicillin. They found cefotaxime and ceftriaxone to be equally acceptable for the treatment of bacterial meningitis in children because there is no difference in clinical outcome or sequelae with these agents.[54] Extensive clinical experience with aztreonam, imipenem, or quinolones in the treatment of bacterial meningitis is lacking.

Treatment of Bacterial Meningitis of Unknown Etiology

Treatment of bacterial meningitis of unknown etiology should be initiated in patients seriously suspected of having bacterial meningitis if an etiologic agent is not identified on examination of a Gram's stain of CSF sediment or if performance of a lumbar puncture must be delayed (because the patient must be transported to another facility or a CT scan must be performed because of a suspected intracranial mass lesion).

Treatment is directed at the most likely etiologic organisms based on the age of the patient and available clinical clues [*see Table 10*].

Meningitis in neonates may be caused by a wide range of enteric gram-negative bacilli and gram-positive organisms, such as group B streptococci or *Listeria*. Such a variety of organisms necessitates the use of combined therapy with drugs such as ampicillin and either gentamicin or a third-generation cephalosporin such as cefotaxime. In children, antibacterial therapy is aimed at the three organisms most commonly responsible for childhood bacterial meningitis: *H. influenzae, N. meningitidis,* and *S. pneumoniae.* A combination of ampicillin and chloramphenicol is most frequently employed.

Table 10   Initial Antibiotic Therapy of Meningitis of Unknown Etiology

Age Group	Preferred Therapy		Alternative Therapy	
	Antibiotic	24-Hour Dose	Antibiotic	24-Hour Dose
Neonate (1 mo of age or younger)	Ampicillin* *and either* Gentamicin† *or* Third-generation cephalosporin†	100–200 mg/kg I.V. 5.0–7.5 mg/kg I.V. or I.M. See below‡	Chloramphenicol *and* Third-generation cephalosporin‡	25–50 mg/kg I.V. See below‡
Child	Ampicillin* *and* Chloramphenicol *or* Third-generation cephalosporin‡	400 mg/kg I.V. 100 mg/kg I.V. See below‡		
Adult	Ampicillin* *or* Penicillin G*	12–14 g I.V. 24 million units I.V.	Chloramphenicol *or* Third-generation cephalosporin‡	4 g I.V. See below‡
Immunocompro-mised adult (e.g., older than 60 yr with cirrhosis or neoplastic disease)	Ampicillin* *and* Third-generation cephalosporin‡ *and* Gentamicin†	12–14 g I.V. See below‡ 3–5 mg/kg I.V. and intrathecally§	Trimethoprim (TMP)-sulfamethoxazole (SMZ) *or* Chloramphenicol *and* Third-generation cephalosporin‡ *and* Gentamicin†	10–20 mg/kg I.V. (TMP) 50–100 mg/kg I.V. (SMZ) 4 g I.V. See below‡ 3–5 mg/kg I.V. and intrathecally§
Postcraniotomy patient	Nafcillin* *and* Third-generation cephalosporin‡ *and* Gentamicin†	12 g I.V. See below‡ 3–5 mg/kg I.V. and intrathecally§	Vancomycin *and* Third-generation cephalosporin‡ *and* Gentamicin†	2 g I.V. See below‡ 3–5 mg/kg I.V. and intrathecally§

*Ampicillin or penicillin should be given in divided doses: every 4 hr in infants, young children, and adults; every 12 hr in the first week of life, and every 8 hr in the next 3 wk. When staphylococcal infection is suggested by the clinical setting or Gram's stain of the CSF, nafcillin should be employed [*see Table 6*]. All doses of ampicillin should be adjusted for reduced renal function to avoid penicillin-induced seizures.

†Gentamicin should be given at 12-hr intervals during the first week of life and thereafter at 8-hr intervals, unless renal function is reduced.

‡Third-generation cephalosporins recommended for treatment of meningitis include cefotaxime or ceftriaxone. Ceftazidime should be reserved for treatment of documented *Pseudomonas aeruginosa* infections or infections in which multidrug-resistant organisms are isolated. Pediatric parenteral doses are 100–200 mg/kg/day for cefotaxime; a 75 mg/kg loading dose and then 100 mg/kg/day for ceftriaxone; and 60–300 mg/kg/day for ceftazidime. Adult parenteral doses are 8–12 g/day for cefotaxime; 2 g/day for ceftriaxone; and 4–6 g/day for ceftazidime.

§Intrathecal gentamicin (4 mg q 12 hr or 5–10 mg q 24 hr) should also be given to any adult suspected of having gram-negative meningitis.

However, because third-generation cephalosporins have been effective against the common childhood bacterial meningitides, an agent such as cefuroxime, cefotaxime, ceftriaxone, or ceftazidime is now being recommended by some authorities as the preferred or alternative therapy for meningitis of unknown etiology in children.

S. pneumoniae meningitis and *N. meningitidis* meningitis are the meningitides that most commonly affect adults, but the incidence of invasive *H. influenzae* infection in adults is on the rise. Ampicillin, therefore, is the antibiotic of choice in bacterial meningitis of unknown etiology in the adult because it is effective against *S. pneumoniae* and *N. meningitidis* as well as more than 90 percent of *H. influenzae* strains. Chloramphenicol is still an appropriate alternative choice for patients allergic to penicillin. It has also been recommended that a third-generation cephalosporin, such as cefotaxime or ceftriaxone, be used as an alternative antibiotic in the empirical therapy for meningitis of unknown etiology in adults. The incidence of uncommon types of meningitis in certain clinical settings has increased, such as meningitis caused by *S. aureus* in postcraniotomy patients and meningitis caused by gram-negative bacilli or *Listeria* in patients who are immunocompromised because of advanced age, neoplastic disease, or cirrhosis. Broader initial antibiotic therapy is warranted in the management of patients with these conditions.

Nonantibiotic Aspects of Treatment

Steroid therapy Dexamethasone has been recommended as adjunctive therapy for bacterial meningitis in children.[30] The data convincingly demonstrate that children treated with corticosteroids experience less hearing loss than those treated with placebo. The beneficial effect of dexamethasone is probably related to inhibition of IL-1. By preventing production of this cytokine, the stimulation of the cascade of other inflammatory mediators is blocked. There are no convincing clinical data to warrant the use of corticosteroids as adjunctive therapy in bacterial meningitis in adults; further clinical trials are needed.

Increased intracranial pressure Acute cerebral edema is an occasional complication of bacterial meningitis, and patients sometimes present with initial CSF pressures of more than 400 or 500 mm H_2O. These pressures may be associated with the development of a temporal lobe or cerebellar pressure cone, particularly in the period after a lumbar puncture.[55] An intravenous infusion of mannitol is required to reduce the mechanical threat posed by such CSF pressures. In adults, 100 g of mannitol is administered as 500 ml of a 20 percent solution over a period of 20 to 60 minutes. Thereafter, control of brain swelling is continued as needed by the administration of mannitol, corticosteroids, or both. Dexamethasone sodium phosphate is a commonly employed corticosteroid preparation. In adults, 10 mg of the drug is given intravenously initially, followed by 4 mg every six hours until the symptoms of brain swelling subside, and the dose is then tapered. Marked cerebral edema is the only indication for corticosteroid use in the treatment of acute bacterial meningitis. The adverse effects of corticosteroid use on pyogenic infections do not appear to pose a clinical problem when the meningitis is caused by an organism such as *N. meningitidis* or *S. pneumoniae*. These meningitides are readily treated with highly effective bactericidal β-lactam antibiotics.

Fluid restriction (to levels of 1,200 to 1,400 ml daily in adults) is indicated initially in bacterial meningitis to minimize the occurrence of cerebral edema. Other possible factors contributing to cerebral edema should be minimized, including hypoxia that may be secondary to an associated pneumonia or to a complicating aspirational event. All patients with cerebral edema should be managed in an intensive care unit.

Seizures Treatment of seizures should be vigorous and include the use of anticonvulsant drugs. Constant nursing attention is essential to prevent aspiration and hypoxia. For acute control of a seizure, diazepam may be administered slowly for several minutes intravenously (5 to 10 mg in adults; 1 mg per year of age to a maximum of 10 mg in children). For subsequent maintenance therapy, phenytoin is given intravenously until oral medication can be safely administered.

Certain complications have resulted from the concomitant administration of antibiotics and antiseizure medications. For example, coadministration of phenytoin and chloramphenicol can lead to potentially toxic serum levels of chloramphenicol. Phenytoin appears to delay glucuronidation of chloramphenicol by competing for the hepatic enzymes that carry out this process.[37] Another problem may arise if phenobarbital is used to control or prevent seizures in patients who are receiving chloramphenicol for meningitis. Because phenobarbital induces hepatic glucuronidative enzymes, the conversion of chloramphenicol to its inactive glucuronide form is accelerated, resulting in subtherapeutic concentrations of this drug. Thus, chloramphenicol should not be used to treat patients who have liver disease or who are receiving other drugs that are metabolized by the liver, especially antiseizure medications, unless the chloramphenicol serum level is carefully monitored.

Chemoprophylaxis

Meningococcal meningitis is the only type of bacterial meningitis that occurs in epidemic form. Close contacts of an index case, such as other household members, infants in day care centers, or military recruits, are at increased risk for meningococcal disease; casual contacts, such as schoolmates, do not appear to be at risk. Hospital personnel in close initial patient contact (e.g., during nasotracheal suctioning or mouth-to-mouth resuscitation) are at increased risk, but personnel who come into contact with the patient after institution of respiratory precautions and antibiotic therapy are not. Chemoprophylaxis is indicated only for such initial close contacts. Sulfonamides, once widely employed in chemoprophylaxis, should no longer be used for that purpose; approximately 25 percent of meningococcal isolates are now sulfonamide resistant. Rifampin is the drug of choice (600 mg orally every 12 hours for two days or 600 mg orally every day for four days in adults). About 50 percent of secondary cases among close contacts occur at least five days after onset of the disease in the index case. This fact prompts consideration of the use of meningococcal bivalent vaccine (groups A and C), as an adjunct to chemoprophylaxis, for extending protection if chemoprophylaxis is unsuccessful.

Secondary cases of systemic *H. influenzae* type B infections may occur in close household and day care center contacts of an initial case of *H. influenzae* meningitis. The risk for household contacts younger than 12 months is six percent; for those younger than four years, it is 2.1 percent.[3] The risk of severe *H. influenzae* disease among household contacts appears to be 585 times greater than the age-adjusted risk in the general population.

Various drugs, including ampicillin, trimethoprim-sulfamethoxazole, and cefaclor, have been tested but were found ineffective in eradication of nasopharyngeal carriage of *H. influenzae* type B.[56] In several preliminary studies, rifampin (20 mg/kg daily for four days) has been successful in eradication of carriage.[56] Although information on the efficacy of rifampin is incomplete, many experts recommend that this drug be used for prophylaxis when two or more cases of invasive *H. influenzae* type B disease occur in an enclosed population. Chemoprophylaxis is then given to the contact and index cases. In addition, three *H. influenzae* type B polysaccharide protein conjugate vaccines, HbOC (HibTITER), PRP-OMP (PedvaxHIB), and PRP-D (ProHIBIT), are licensed for use in children 15 months of age or older.[57-59] Two of these vaccines, HbOC and PRP-OMP, were approved by the FDA in 1990 for administration to infants beginning at two months of age. However, because of the time required to generate an immunologic response, vaccination should not be used after exposure to prevent secondary cases of *H. influenzae* type B infection. Universal immunization of infants with HbOC or PRP-OMP, including those attending day care centers, should substantially reduce the occurrence of primary cases of *H. influenzae* type B disease in such facilities.[59]

Recurrent Meningitis

The most common and important cause of recurrent meningitis is bacterial infection. Other causes must be considered when microbiological studies do not implicate a bacterial agent [*see Table 11*].

Recurrent Bacterial Meningitis

Recurrent episodes of bacterial meningitis are most frequently the result of anatomic defects that permit ingress of organisms into the subarachnoid space. Congenital defects of the neural tube, particularly of its spinal end, result in persistent dermal sinuses or meningoceles. Such anatomic defects can precipitate meningitis or recurrent meningitis in the neonate and young child. Pericranial CSF fistulas are the most common anatomic defects that lead to meningitis in older children and adults. The fistulas are situated in (1) the cribriform plate, (2) the paranasal sinuses, and (3) the temporal bone.

CSF fistulas are conveniently categorized as traumatic (accidental or surgical) and nontraumatic. Traumatic fistulas may result from recent or remote skull fractures through the cribriform plate, paranasal sinuses, or petrous ridge of the temporal bone. Nontraumatic fistulas are divided into high-pressure and normal-pressure types. Nontraumatic high-pressure fistulas usually result from obstructive hydrocephalus secondary to posterior fossa tumors, basilar arachnoiditis, or other obstructive causes. Distinguishing high-pressure fistulas from normal-pressure fistulas is important. Repair of the defect is the initial step in managing a normal-pressure fistula, whereas implantation of a CSF shunt or removal of the obstruction to CSF flow is the first step

---

Table 11 Causes of Recurrent Meningitis

*Bacterial Meningitis**
  Predisposing anatomic defects
    Congenital: meningomyeloceles, dermal sinuses
    Traumatic: skull fractures through cribriform plate or petrous ridge
    Postoperative: craniotomy, transsphenoidal hypophysectomy
    Tumors: direct invasion through the dura
    Empty sella syndrome
  Parameningeal infections*
    Mastoiditis, sinusitis, osteomyelitis of skull
  Immunologic defects*
    Immunoglobulin deficiencies: congenital or acquired (e.g., myeloma)
    Asplenic state: splenectomy or functional asplenia (e.g., sickle cell anemia)
    Complement deficiencies: C6, C7, C8 deficiency

Endogenous Chemical Meningitis
  Tumors†
    Craniopharyngioma, epidermoid cyst

Unusual Nonbacterial Recurrent Meningitides
  Mollaret's meningitis†
  Behçet's syndrome†
  Drug hypersensitivity†
    Sulfonamides, ibuprofen
  Systemic lupus erythematosus†
  Uveoencephalitides‡ (Vogt-Koyanagi syndrome, Harada's syndrome)

---

*Neutrophilic CSF pleocytosis.
†Either neutrophilic or lymphocytic CSF pleocytosis.
‡Lymphocytic CSF pleocytosis.

---

in managing a high-pressure fistula after treatment of the meningitis.[60]

By far, the most frequently implicated organism in recurrent meningitis is *S. pneumoniae*. In one large series, 11 percent of patients with pneumococcal meningitis had more than one attack, whereas only 0.5 percent of patients with meningitis from other bacterial species had recurrences.[61] Different studies have implicated *S. pneumoniae* in 66 to 83 percent of cases of recurrent meningitis after skull fracture.[11,62] *H. influenzae* and *N. meningitidis* are less frequent causes of recurrent bacterial meningitis. Enteric gram-negative bacilli and *P. aeruginosa* are rarely implicated in recurrent meningitis, except in patients with penetrating or open head wounds.

CSF rhinorrhea may arise from a defect in the cribriform plate or a pericranial sinus. CSF rhinorrhea may also result from a defect in the temporal bone, when fluid exits via the middle ear and eustachian tube into the nasopharynx. Fluid may flow from one or both nostrils when the nose is in a dependent position.

CSF otorrhea occurs when there is a leak into the middle ear associated with perforation of the tympanic membrane. A CSF leak may not develop for many years in the setting of a congenital or acquired defect until a vigorous cough or sneeze presumably ruptures an attenuated, tense leptomeningeal membrane.

CSF rhinorrhea may subside during the course of acute bacterial meningitis. For this reason, it is important to check all patients who have either an initial or recurrent episode of bacterial meningitis for CSF rhinorrhea at the onset of the illness and again after recovery. Symptoms associated with CSF rhinorrhea include a salty taste in the back of the throat and frequent swallowing caused by extra liquid entering the pharynx from above. Loss of sense of smell is a symptom of cribriform plate leakage. Fluid loss into the middle ear from the mastoid produces hearing loss and a sense of fullness in the ears. Fluid and air bubbles may be seen behind the eardrum on otoscopic examination.

Rhinorrhea of an otic or sphenoid origin may be observed only in the lateral recumbent or prone position; a brow-down position is used to demonstrate rhinorrhea from the cribriform plate and ethmoid and frontal sites. Visual fields should be checked because they are often abnormal when pituitary tumors or cysts are the cause of CSF rhinorrhea; they are normal in the atrophic type of empty sella syndrome.

The fluid from CSF rhinorrhea, unlike nasal mucus, does not stiffen a handkerchief on drying. Cerebrospinal fluid has a glucose content of 50 to 70 mg/dl; it has a chloride content of about 120 mEq/L, which is higher than that of blood. Glucose oxidase test paper (Tes-Tape) and Dextrostix are unreliable in distinguishing CSF from nasal mucus or lacrimal fluid. The best method of determining whether a clear nasal secretion is CSF is to analyze it for glucose and chloride content. The fluid is simply collected by taping a tube to the patient's nose while he or she is in an appropriate position.

Studies aimed at defining a possible anatomic defect are indicated in a patient who experiences recurrent bacterial meningitis, with or without CSF rhinorrhea. Skull, mastoid, and sinus films and polytomography are helpful in delineating these defects. Such studies may show air within the cranial cavity, opacification or air-fluid levels in a sinus, and skull fractures. CT head scanning should be performed in cases of nontraumatic CSF leak to seek possible causes of high-pressure leaks. Direct verification of the leak exit site is essential for the required surgical correction because the exit site indicates the region in which the leak originates (temporal bone, sphenoid sinus, cribriform plate, or other structure). Radiolabeled (^{131}I, ^{99m}Tc) albumins are used in cisternography and in detection of CSF on cotton pledgets placed in the nose, oropharynx, and ear canals. Some physicians prefer to use the dye fluorescein to detect leaking CSF. With the aid of ultraviolet light, fluorescein-stained CSF absorbed onto cotton pledgets can be visualized directly and immediately. In contrast, use of radiolabeled albumins is accompanied by a delay necessary for counting radioactive samples. Fluorescein has other advantages. In the presence of CSF otorrhea, it actually stains the tympanic membrane. It also may be used intraoperatively, and the fluorescein-stained fluid may serve as a guide to the origin of the leak.

Most cases of posttraumatic rhinorrhea or otorrhea subside within two weeks of the trauma. Surgical repair is indicated when (1) there has been a prior leak and one or more episodes of meningitis, (2) leakage is profuse and does not slacken during the two weeks after acute trauma, and (3) leakage persists for more than six weeks after the trauma.[60] The value of prophylactic administration of penicillin in the prevention of bacterial, particularly pneumococcal, meningitis in patients with a CSF leak has not been prospectively studied in a controlled fashion. A retrospective study of a total of 402 cases found no significant decrease in the frequency of meningitis in those patients with a CSF leak who were receiving antibiotic prophylaxis.[63] Although the use of prophylactic penicillin may possibly be of value in the immediate posttraumatic period (if dosages are sufficient to eliminate nasopharyngeal colonization with *S. pneumoniae*), prolonged use would be expected to increase the likelihood of later infection by resistant organisms. Posttraumatic staphylococcal meningitis has occurred in patients receiving penicillin prophylaxis.

Surgical repair by placement of fat, fascia, or muscle grafts is generally indicated for nontraumatic leaks, large CSF leaks, leaks that do not cease spontaneously in four to six weeks, and leaks through infected bone. New transsinus approaches have been developed by otolaryngologists for operative treatment of leaks through the frontal sinuses, cribriform plate, and sphenoid sinuses, thereby obviating the necessity for a major craniotomy in patients with these defects.[60]

Chronic Meningitis

Chronic meningitis is defined as meningeal inflammation that persists for more than four weeks without clinical improvement. Occasionally, meningitis may persist for months or even years. The CSF profile is usually of the lymphocytic–normal glucose or lymphocytic–low glucose type, but rarely do neutrophils predominate. This prolonged illness, although uncommon, presents a difficult problem in differential diagnosis.[64] The differential diagnosis of chronic meningitis requires a consideration of the various conditions and microorganisms that may be responsible for this disorder [*see Table 12*]. The most important causes of chronic meningeal inflammation, because of their therapeutic implications and frequencies, are three infections: tuberculous meningitis, cryptococcal meningitis, and parameningeal infections [*see* Parameningeal Infections, *below*].

The clinical course of coccidioidal, *Histoplasma*, or blastomycotic meningitis resembles that of cryptococcal meningitis. Epidemiological considerations, evidence of involvement of lungs and other organs, serologic studies, and CSF cultures provide the means of distinguishing among these entities.

Infections of CSF Shunts

Infections have occurred in as many as 25 percent of patients who have undergone CSF ventriculovenous shunting for the treatment of hydrocephalus; the frequency of infection is lower with ventriculoperitoneal shunts.[6] The manifestations of infection include low-grade fever, nausea, vomiting, headache, and signs of increased intracranial pressure. The last finding suggests shunt malfunction. Infections that develop shortly after shunt placement manifest themselves through erythema or drainage at an incisional site along the course of the shunt. Bacteremia is common in patients with infected ventriculovenous shunts because of direct communication between the shunt and the bloodstream. Meningitic signs and CSF neutrophilic pleocytosis are present in about one third of patients with infected shunts.

S. epidermidis isolates (usually methicillin-resistant strains) account for more than 50 percent of CSF shunt infections.[6] For this reason, vancomycin is the antibiotic of choice for empirical therapy until results of cultures and antibiotic-susceptibility tests are available.[65] *S. aureus* and streptococci are also common isolates in CSF shunt infec-

---

Table 12 Causes of the Syndrome of Chronic Meningitis

Lymphocytic Pleocytosis

Bacterial causes

    Actinomyces, Nocardia, Brucella, syphilis, leptospirosis, tuberculosis

Fungal causes

    Cryptococcus, Candida species, coccidioidomycosis, histoplasmosis, blastomycosis

Viral causes

    Lymphocytic choriomeningitis, mumps, enteroviruses in patients with agammaglobulinemia

Parasitic causes

    Cysticerosis, echinococcosis, toxoplasmosis, trichinosis

Parameningeal infections

    Brain abscess, subdural empyema, epidural abscess, major dural venous sinus phlebitis

Hypersensitivity to contrast material (e.g., that used in myelography)

Brain neoplasms

    Primary: glioblastoma, glioma, cerebral dysgerminoma, epidermoid tumors, craniopharyngioma, medulloblastoma, meningeal sarcoma

    Metastatic: melanoma; stomach, breast, or lung cancer; leukemia; lymphoma

Miscellaneous: sarcoid, Behçet's syndrome, uveoencephalitides (Vogt-Kayanagi syndrome, Harada's syndrome), Mollaret's meningitis, superficial meningeal hemosiderosis, primary cerebral granulomatous arteritis, systemic lupus erythematosus, Whipple's disease, chronic lymphocytic meningitis of unknown etiology

Neutrophilic Pleocytosis

Bacterial etiologies

    Actinomyces, Nocardia

---

riod of four to six weeks. For ventriculoperitoneal shunt infections, the administration of antibiotic therapy plus externalization of the peritoneal catheter has frequently been curative (e.g., in one series, 10 of 11 patients were successfully treated using this approach).[65] In most cases, however, it has been necessary to remove the shunt as well. Once the infection has been eradicated, placement of a new shunt in a different location can be performed.

Acute Primary Amebic Meningitis and Meningoencephalitis

Etiology, Pathogenesis, and Pathology

Primary amebic meningoencephalitis is caused by free-living amebas (principally *Naegleria*, but also *Acanthamoeba*), which are widespread in nature. Infection by *Naegleria* is acquired by swimming in freshwater ponds and lakes, mainly in the southern United States. The amebas enter through the nasal mucosa and spread to the CNS via the olfactory nerves. The organisms initially cause an acute purulent meningitis but then rapidly spread beyond the leptomeninges to cerebral tissue, where they produce an acute hemorrhagic necrotizing encephalitis.[66]

The pathogenesis of meningoencephalitis caused by *Acanthamoeba* species is not well understood. In general, this form of amebic infection tends to be subacute or chronic in its onset and course. *Acanthamoeba* meningitis occurs frequently in immunosuppressed or debilitated patients. It is often associated with multiple hemorrhagic necrotic granulomatous abscesses of the brain, especially in midline and posterior fossa structures.

Clinical Features

Primary amebic meningoencephalitis caused by *Naegleria* strikes children and young adults in the summer. Five or six days elapse between contact with amebas and onset of symptoms, which include bifrontal headache, high fever, and nausea and vomiting. Olfactory abnormalities and dysgeusia are frequent symptoms, and meningeal

tions; Enterobacteriaceae species are sometimes associated with ventriculoperitoneal shunt infections. The diagnosis of shunt infection is established by isolation of organisms from blood and cerebrospinal fluid. Shunt infections are occasionally treated successfully with antibiotics alone for a pe-

signs appear rapidly. Neurologic findings include bizarre behavior, diplopia, ataxia, seizures, and coma. If the illness is not treated or if treatment is unsuccessful, it progresses rapidly to death in three to 11 days.

Laboratory Findings

The CSF in patients with *Naegleria* meningoencephalitis contains numerous erythrocytes and shows a polymorphonuclear leukocytic pleocytosis of 300 to 10,000 cells/mm³. The CSF glucose level is low. Careful examination of unstained CSF in a counting chamber will reveal amebas that are not visible on Gram's stain. By contrast, the CSF of patients with *Acanthamoeba* meningoencephalitis usually does not contain inflammatory cells or amebas.

Treatment

No satisfactory chemotherapy exists for primary amebic meningitis or meningoencephalitis, regardless of whether the infection is acute, subacute, or chronic. The antifungal agent amphotericin B is the most effective drug currently available for treating primary amebic meningoencephalitis caused by *Naegleria*. Of more than 100 cases that have been reported, only four patients have survived, and all four had received amphotericin B. In addition, even in cases that proved fatal, amphotericin B appeared to have eradicated the amebas from the CNS and the CSF.[67] Amphotericin B is generally administered intravenously in a dosage of 1 mg/kg daily. Whether it is absolutely necessary to give the drug intrathecally as well has not been established, but administration by both routes is recommended if there are no contraindications. There is anecdotal experience suggesting that miconazole, tetracycline, or rifampin therapy may also supplement amphotericin B therapy for this generally fatal infection. Because only 25 cases of *Acanthamoeba* meningitis or meningoencephalitis have been reported, there has not been sufficient clinical experience to evaluate adequately the various modalities that have been employed in the empirical treatment of this disease. Flucytosine, miconazole, polymyxin B, and sulfamethazine have all proved ineffective in the treatment of CNS infections caused by *Acanthamoeba*.

Parameningeal Infections

The parameningeal infections are a group of localized pyogenic infections that are found adjacent to the meninges. They are capable of producing meningitic signs and a CSF pleocytosis, thus mimicking bacterial, viral, or fungal meningitis. This group of infections consists of brain abscess, subdural empyema, cerebral epidural abscess, spinal epidural abscess, and septic thrombophlebitis of the cortical veins and dural venous sinuses. Osteomyelitic infections of the cranium and of the walls of the nasal air sinuses are also classified as parameningeal infections because such infections extend to the periosteal and epidural areas.

Brain Abscess

Etiology, Pathogenesis, and Pathology

The bacteriology of brain abscess is highly varied. Examination of Gram's stains of material aspirated at the time of surgical drainage is essential to selection of antimicrobial therapy. Multiple bacterial species, both aerobic and anaerobic, are found in 25 to 50 percent of brain abscesses, particularly those of otogenous origin.[68] Anaerobes have been recovered from 37 to 88 percent of brain abscesses[69,70] and appear to be the major etiologic agents, particularly in those brain abscesses associated with chronic infections of the ear and paranasal sinuses.[71] The most common anaerobic isolates in descending order of frequency are anaerobic streptococci, *Bacteroides*, *Veillonella*, *Propionibacterium*, and *Actinomyces*. *B. fragilis* is the most common anaerobic isolate in otogenous temporal lobe abscess.[72] *S. aureus* is most commonly isolated from brain abscesses in the setting of recent penetrating head trauma or craniotomy. Species belonging to the family Enterobacteriaceae, particularly *Proteus*, are most commonly associated with brain abscesses of otogenous origin and those that follow penetrating head trauma or neurosurgery. *Clostridium perfringens* has caused brain abscesses that followed combat wounds.

Various streptococci, particularly some of the microaerophilic strains, are often found in cerebral abscesses associated with cyanotic congenital heart disease. Occasionally, *Nocardia asteroides* and *Hemophilus aphrophilus* are isolated from brain abscesses.

Brain abscesses resulting from direct extension of contiguous infection are found adjacent to the initiating extracerebral site of infection (e.g., mastoid or frontal sinus). Abscesses developing from retrograde venous spread of infection may be located some distance from the primary focus but remain within the area of venous drainage. For example, a chronic ear infection can extend along veins of the inner ear through diploetic vessels of the skull and from there pass through intracranial venous channels into the cerebrum. Hematogenous brain abscesses are usually located in the distribution of the middle cerebral artery.

Brain abscess begins as a poorly demarcated area of bacterial encephalitis that undergoes liquefaction necrosis during several weeks. Several satellite abscesses may develop in communication with the principal cavity. Multiple small brain abscesses, too small to be drained surgically, may occur in the course of acute *S. aureus* endocarditis. In a few patients, CT head scanning has allowed identification of as many as six or more cryptogenic abscesses, presumably of hematogenous origin.

Once formed, some abscesses develop a thick capsule in the succeeding weeks or months; other abscesses continue to enlarge by spreading through the central white matter, sometimes penetrating the ventricular wall to produce acute meningitis. When bacterial meningitis and cerebral abscess coexist, the meningitis is almost always a result of intraventricular spread of the abscess.

Predisposing Factors

Thirty to 50 percent of brain abscesses are secondary to an adjacent focus of infection. Examples of such foci are chronic otitis media and mastoiditis, paranasal sinusitis, oral and dental infections, face and scalp infections, osteomyelitis of the skull, penetrating head injuries, and craniotomy wound infections.[72,73] Another third of brain abscesses are hematogenous in origin, arising from a pleuropulmonary focus (lung abscess, bronchiectasis, or empyema), a cardiac lesion (*S. aureus* endocarditis, congenital right-to-left shunts), or distant foci of infection (burns or pelvic infection). The remaining brain abscesses are cryptogenic.

Subacute and chronic otitis media and mastoiditis Ear disease remains the single most important predisposing condition in brain abscesses. The inferior aspect of the temporal lobe is the most frequent site of otogenous brain abscess. The ipsilateral cerebellar hemisphere is a common site of abscess, particularly in children. Abscesses may develop simultaneously in both locations.

Infections of the paranasal sinuses Exacerbation of chronic frontal or ethmoidal sinusitis often predisposes to rhinogenous frontal lobe abscess. Spread of infection from osteomyelitis of the posterior wall of the frontal sinus may cause simultaneous epidural abscess, frontal lobe abscess, and subdural empyema.

Infections of the face and skull Brain abscesses secondary to facial infections develop through an intervening septic thrombophlebitis.

A missile injury to the skull can introduce a bone spicule, a metal fragment, or other exogenous material into devitalized brain, where it can serve as a nidus for infection. Such an infection may develop immediately or only after a protracted period (as long as 20 years in some cases). At times, the initial trauma seems trivial and is overlooked. A childhood accident in which a pencil point or piece of stick penetrated the orbital wall might come to light years later when a recent-onset seizure disorder is found to be caused by an encapsulated frontal lobe abscess that contains a piece of graphite or a wood fragment.[74]

Clinical Features

Brain abscesses can occur at any age. They most frequently develop during the first five decades of life: peak incidences are found in preadolescence and in the productive years of adulthood.[72] Brain abscesses are rare in infancy even in patients with cyanotic congenital heart disease. Approximately 32 cases of brain abscesses in infants younger than three months have been reported in the 20th century. About half were caused by enteric gram-negative bacilli (*E. coli, Proteus,* and *Citrobacter*).[75] Brain abscesses in infants younger than three months often reach great size because of the expandable skull and are frequently diagnosed by chance during a diagnostic or therapeutic ventricular tap.

The clinical presentation of brain abscess is often that of an expanding mass lesion with obtundation, headache, seizures, and focal neurologic findings. Fever and the epiphenomena of infection are absent in almost half of cases. The course may extend for several weeks or even months, suggesting a diagnosis of cerebral neoplasm. Hematogenous abscess is often marked by a fulminant course with high fever, ending fatally within five to 15 days. In a few patients, initial symptoms resemble those of a cerebrovascular accident. Occasionally, the presence of a mild CSF lymphocytosis and focal neurologic findings in a patient with cerebral abscess can lead to an incorrect diagnosis of multiple sclerosis. Prominent psychiatric features in frontal lobe abscesses have suggested diagnoses of hysteria and schizophrenia. About 15 percent of patients with brain abscess have clinical features suggestive of a viral or fungal meningitis (mild meningitic signs and lymphocytic CSF pleocytosis, which results from contiguity of the abscess to the subarachnoid space) or features suggestive of a pyogenic meningitis (nuchal rigidity and neutrophilic CSF pleocytosis secondary to leakage of abscess into the ventricular space). The presence of any of the preceding clinical presentations in a patient with chronic ear, sinus, or pleuropulmonary disease or with a right-to-left shunt suggests a diagnosis of a cerebral abscess. Occasionally, such latent otogenous temporal lobe abscesses become clinically evident shortly after mastoidectomy for chronic otitis media.[76]

Headache, sometimes generalized but often localized to the side of the abscess, is the most common initial symptom of brain abscess. It may develop insidiously or suddenly. If attention is not paid to a recent change in location or intensity, it may be inappropriately attributed to a preexisting ear or sinus infection. The development of unexplained headaches in a child with cyanotic congenital heart disease strongly suggests a brain abscess.

Manifestations of increased intracranial pressure such as somnolence, vomiting, and sixth and third nerve palsies are common; papilledema is a relatively late finding, observed in less than half of cases.

In a small group of patients, an initial preabscess stage of suppurative encephalitis or bacterial cerebritis may be suspected on the basis of clinical findings: prominent headache, localized neurologic manifestations, fever, and mild CSF pleocytosis (either lymphocytic or neutrophilic) appearing in the setting of chronic ear disease or a similar predisposing process. Fever and other symptoms may abate over a few days only to recur and progress as the intracranial effects of the newly established abscess become evident. Successful antibiotic therapy without surgery has been reported in a few instances in which an early presumptive diagnosis was made.[77] Serial CT head scanning has enabled visualization of the evolution of cerebritis to a localized encapsulated abscess and, likewise, resolution of presumed cerebritis with early institution of antibiotic therapy.[78,79] A few patients with multiple surgically inaccessible abscesses have been treated successfully with antibiotics alone; complete resolution of the multiple infected foci was shown by sequential CT scanning.[80]

Temporal lobe abscess Most temporal lobe abscesses are otogenous. Involvement of the dominant temporal lobe may cause a nominal or a Wernicke's aphasia (inability to read, write, or understand spoken words). Either a homonymous superior quadrantic or a hemianoptic field defect may be a feature of temporal lobe abscess; the passage of the optic radiation through the inferior portion of the temporal lobe produces these features. A field defect may also be the only sign of abscess in the nondominant temporal lobe. Involvement of the pyramidal tracts is uncommon; the only motor deficit may be a slight contralateral faciobrachial monoparesis. The temporal lobe may suddenly herniate through the tentorium, producing bilateral pyramidal tract signs, ipsilateral pupillary dilatation, and coma. When surgical drainage of an otogenous temporal lobe abscess does not result in clinical improvement, the presence of a coexistent cryptic cerebellar abscess should be suspected.

Cerebellar abscess Cerebellar abscesses represent 25 to 33 percent of otogenous brain abscesses. Headache, usually suboccipital, is almost always present. Fever, stiff neck, and symptoms of increased intracranial pressure may be the only other manifestations. Focal neurologic signs may be evident as well. Ataxia, with veering to the side of the lesion, might be present. Nystagmus is common and is usually coarser when the patient looks toward the side of the lesion. Ipsilateral incoordination of arm and leg movements can often be elicited along with an intention tremor. Poor truncal control, increased tendency to fall, and dysarthria suggest a lesion in the vermis. Brain stem compression may develop, rapidly producing contralateral or bilateral pyramidal tract signs. Cerebellar abscesses are less likely to be encapsulated and tend to progress more quickly than cerebral abscesses.

Frontal lobe abscess About 40 percent of brain abscesses are located in the frontal lobes and are associated with frontal and ethmoidal sinusitis.[72] Impaired intellectual function, poor judgment, inattention, and even mutism may be prominent findings. Grasp, suck, and snout reflexes can often be elicited. Focal or generalized seizures occur in about 25 percent of patients; a common seizure pattern involves turning of the head and eyes to the side opposite the lesion. Contralateral hemiparesis occurs when the abscess is large or when it is located in the posterior aspect of the frontal lobe.

Parietal lobe abscess Most parietal lobe abscesses are hematogenous in origin. Occasionally, large otogenous temporal lobe abscesses extend into the parietal lobe. Anteriorly located parietal lesions produce impairment of position sense, of two-point discrimination, and of stereognosis. Focal, sensory, and motor seizures may be accompanying features. Deep posteriorly located parietal lesions result in homonymous hemianopsia, visual inattention to simultaneous bilateral visual field stimulation, and impaired opticokinetic nystagmus. An abscess situated in the region where the dominant temporal, parietal, and occipital lobes come together can produce Gerstmann's syndrome: acalculia, finger agnosia, difficulty in distinguishing right from left, and agraphia.

Brain stem abscess Very rarely, pyogenic infection establishes itself in the brain stem as an abscess or as an acute tegmental encephalitis.[81] Such infections are usually hematogenous. Brain stem abscesses usually involve streptococci or staphylococci; tegmental encephalitis has been produced by *L. monocytogenes*, *Mycoplasma pneumoniae*, and *Toxoplasma gondii*. Clinical manifestations include fever, vomiting, headache, facial weakness, dysphagia, multiple other cranial nerve palsies, and hemiparesis. Early in the course, CSF findings may be normal or show a small lymphocytic or neutrophilic pleocytosis; CSF cultures are negative. Thus, the clinical picture and CSF findings of a brain stem abscess may mimic those of a viral brain stem encephalitis.

Brain abscess presenting as apparent meningitis Occasionally, the first recognized symptoms in a patient with a brain abscess are fever, headache, and stiff neck, which together suggest a diagnosis of meningitis. Focal neurologic signs may be minimal or overlooked. The picture suggestive of meningitis may occur during the early bacterial encephalitis phase of brain abscess or later, when an established abscess leaks or ruptures into the ventricular system. In the early pre-abscess stage, the CSF may show a pleocytosis of a few to several hundred cells (lymphocytes only or a mixture of neutrophils and lymphocytes) and a normal glucose concentration. The possibility of an early brain abscess should be considered in a patient with chronic ear or sinus disease in whom a clinical picture resembling meningitis develops.

Meningitic signs are more prominent when an abscess leaks into a lateral ventricle. The isolation of an anaerobic organism or of several different organisms from the CSF should suggest either such leakage or the presence of a meningitis caused by extension of infection from some other parameningeal focus. Rupture of a large abscess into a ventricle is accompanied by high fever, coma, and a marked CSF polymorphonuclear leukocytic pleocytosis ($\geq$ 50,000 cells/mm^3). Lumbar puncture is contraindicated when brain abscess is thought to be present because of the danger of subsequent transtentorial herniation.

Laboratory Findings

Computed tomographic scanning CT is a highly sensitive method for detecting brain abscesses 1.0 cm or greater in diameter[82]; it can sometimes detect lesions as small as 0.6 cm. Focal lesions can be picked up by radionuclide scanning and angiography, but CT has the distinct advantage of providing detailed anatomic definition of the lesion, such as its location and size.

CT scanning yields important information about the mass effects of the lesion as well as the underlying pathological process. Plain scans usually show large low-density areas corresponding to the lesion.

The scan performed with injection of contrast media commonly reveals a sharply circumscribed, circular, lucent area that is surrounded by a ringlike zone of increased density (contrast enhancement), which in turn is surrounded by a peripheral zone of decreased density. The central lucent area, obviously, corresponds to the abscess. The ringlike zone of increased density represents either a true capsule or a surrounding area of increased vascularity. The peripheral zone of decreased density represents edema. Occasionally, contrast enhancement demonstrates what appears to be a dense nodule.

A brain abscess caused by *Toxoplasma gondii* in an immunosuppressed patient produced a picture on CT scan identical to that produced by pyogenic abscess.[83] Other lesions that have a similar appearance on CT scan and might thus mimic an abscess are cerebral metastases, glioblastomas, granulomas, hemorrhagic infarctions, hematomas, and changes caused by recent surgery.[82] Detection of gas bubbles within a lesion on CT scan when there has been no recent surgery or cranial trauma is diagnostic of an abscess.

Although radionuclide scanning and angiography can detect most focal lesions, these techniques do not distinguish between a focal suppurative cerebritis and a solitary encapsulated abscess. This important distinction can be made on the basis of the appearance, density, and enhancement of the lesion on CT scan.[78,82] CT is of particular value in the definition of multiple abscesses. It is also valuable in following the resolution of an abscess, especially when the condition has been treated by aspiration rather than excision. CT scanning is more sensitive than radionuclide scanning for detecting posterior fossa abscesses. It is important to recognize that administration of corticosteroids in treatment of cerebral edema can alter a scan by markedly reducing contrast enhancement, thereby producing a scan suggestive of cerebritis when, in fact, a well-formed abscess may actually be present.

Until more convincing and extensive clinical studies are available, the value of MRI over CT scanning in detecting brain abscesses is unknown. However, because MRI has greater sensitivity than CT scanning for soft tissue variations and does not require the administration of contrast agents, it may ultimately become the method of choice for detecting CNS infections.

Radionuclide scanning When CT is not available, radionuclide (^{99m}Tc) brain scanning may be used instead because it can detect well over 80 percent of lesions. However, the findings are relatively nonspecific and do not provide many clues about underlying pathology, that is, whether it is an abscess, cerebritis, or neoplasm. False negative scans may occur with lesions smaller than 2 cm in diameter and with parasellar and posterior fossa lesions. The latter lesions may be obscured by artifacts produced by overlying vessels. Very rarely, an abscess undetected by CT with contrast enhancement is delineated, but not identified specifically as an abscess, by ^{99m}Tc radionuclide scanning.[84]

Cerebral angiography Cerebral angiography can identify the presence and general extent of an avascular mass but usually cannot precisely locate the lesion or identify it as an abscess.[82] A ring blush (a ringlike zone of contrast enhancement), which represents either an actual capsule or a zone of increased vascularity, is visible in only 20 percent of cases. Where CT has become available, it has supplanted angiography for the detection of suppurative intracranial collections.

CSF examination A pleocytosis of a few to several hundred cells per cubic millimeter (mainly lymphocytes), a normal glucose level, an elevated protein concentration, and an elevated pressure characterize the CSF in brain abscess [*see Table 5*]. Examination of the CSF is required when the clinical presentation is suggestive of meningitis. Because of the potential hazard involved in performing a lumbar puncture in the presence of elevated intracranial pressure, however, other studies should be undertaken first if brain abscess is seriously considered as a diagnosis.

Diagnosis

Diagnosis of cerebral abscess is based on the clinical picture (i.e., the presence of a predisposing focus of infection, neurologic findings, and CSF findings) with radiologic confirmation by CT scan or, when it is not available, by the combination of radionuclide scan and cerebral angiography. The appearance of a mass lesion in the absence of fever and a source of infection may indicate the presence of tumor, subdural hematoma, or intracerebral hemorrhage. CT can aid in distinguishing among these processes within the limitations previously noted. In a patient with fever and an intracerebral mass, with or without a predisposing primary site of infection, the differential diagnosis includes other parameningeal infections (subdural empyema, epidural abscess, and thrombophlebitis of the major dural venous sinuses and cortical veins), embolic strokes in patients with bacterial endocarditis, mycotic aneurysms with leakage, acute localized necrotizing viral encephalitis (usually the result of herpes simplex), acute hemorrhagic leukoencephalitis, and certain parasitic diseases (cerebral toxoplasmosis and cerebral cysticercosis).

Treatment

Early diagnosis and prompt antibiotic and usually surgical therapy are crucial in the management of an established brain abscess. Cerebral edema is controlled with intravenous mannitol and dexamethasone, particularly during the perioperative period. The antibiotic management of brain abscess initially involves the selection of a drug based on available knowledge of the bacterial flora of the predisposing site of infection or on ancillary information such as a blood culture. Antibiotic choice may be modified after surgery is performed, based on results of a Gram's stain and culture of the abscess.

In view of the frequency with which various streptococci, *Bacteroides*, and Enterobacteriaceae are implicated in brain abscess, initial treatment in the adult in the absence of specific bacteriologic clues calls for intravenous penicillin G (12 to 20 million units daily), a third-generation cephalosporin such as ceftriaxone (1 to 2 g daily), and metronidazole (15 mg/kg I.V. initially, followed by 7.5 mg/kg every six to eight hours), all in divided doses. *S. aureus* is the suspected etiologic agent in brain abscess after craniotomy or penetrating head injury and during the course of *S. aureus* endocarditis. In treatment of suspected *S. aureus* brain abscess, a penicillinase-resistant penicillin such as nafcillin or oxacillin (9 to 12 g daily in divided doses) is substituted for penicillin G. In the penicillin-allergic patient, vancomycin (2 g daily), aztreonam (6 to 8 g daily), or chloramphenicol (4 g daily) or a combination of these agents can be substituted as necessary for β-lactam antibiotics. Antibiotic treatment should be continued for three to four weeks after surgery. Intravenous metronidazole alone has been used successfully in a small number of patients for treatment of *Bacteroides fragilis* meningitis and brain abscess. The usual dosage is 15 mg/kg initially, followed by 7.5 mg/kg every six hours.

Surgical treatment of brain abscess consists of aspiration or total excision. Aspiration is in wider use today than it was a decade ago, primarily because of the advent of CT. CT scanning techniques provide for preoperative detection of secondary loculi and frequent postoperative monitoring of lesions. Emergency excision of the abscess is indicated whenever the formation of a cerebellar pressure cone becomes evident[85]; an enlarged pupil and bilateral extensor plantar responses are obvious manifestations of pressure cone formation. Excision rather than aspiration is indicated for cerebellar abscesses because the small capacity of the posterior fossa increases the likelihood of coning. Most authorities suggest that brain abscesses that appear with ring enhancement on CT scanning should be drained by aspiration and, if necessary, by surgical excision.

A small number of cases of bacterial cerebritis, defined by clinical criteria and CT, have been successfully treated with antibiotics alone, rather than with a combination of antibiotics and surgery.[77,79] An essential element in this approach is the use of sequential CT scans to follow the course of the lesion. In one study, seven from a group of 20 patients with brain abscesses (defined by the presence of a ringlike zone of contrast enhancement on CT scan) were successfully treated in this manner without surgery. All seven patients had small abscesses.[78] A few patients with multiple (as many as eight to 10) abscesses, some of which were deeply placed in inaccessible areas such as the thalamus, have been successfully treated with a six- to eight-week course of antibiotics.

Surgery is indicated in a patient being treated for cerebritis or a small cerebral abscess by antibiotics alone when (1) the patient shows depressed sensorium or signs of increased intracranial pressure, (2) the patient fails to show marked clinical improvement within a week of the start of antimicrobial therapy, or (3) sequential CT scans show an increase in the size of the abscess.[79] After treatment, a residual enhancing focus may remain at the original site of an abscess for two to four months or longer. However, this finding per se does not necessitate further antibiotic administration.

Prognosis

When left untreated, a brain abscess usually causes death either by producing a tentorial or foramen magnum pressure cone or by rupturing into a ventricle. Very rarely, an abscess may become chronic during the course of several years, developing firm encapsulation and even calcification; a seizure disorder may be the only indication of its presence.

The mortality from brain abscess has declined steadily. It fell from more than 60 percent to about 40 percent after the advent of antibiotic therapy. By the early 1970s, mortality had declined still further to about 25 percent.[85] With the introduction of CT, mortality has now shrunk to five to 15 percent, excluding postcraniotomy cases.[78,85] Seizures are common sequelae of brain abscesses, and most patients should receive anticonvulsants for several years after treatment.

Subdural Empyema

Pathogenesis and Pathology

Subdural empyema is usually a complication of paranasal sinusitis. It results either from direct extension of the sinus infection or from retrograde septic thrombophlebitis of mucosal veins extending to dural vessels. Mastoiditis is much less often a precursor of subdural empyema than it once was. Other factors predisposing to subdural empyema include penetrating head wounds and intracranial surgery, bacteremic infection of preexisting subdural hematoma or rarely of the normal subdural space, and primary pyogenic meningitis.[86-88]

Once subdural pus develops, it spreads widely over the cerebrum and along the falx. Occasionally, the collection is predominantly along the falx, and this is evident on CT scan. Most fatal cases of subdural empyema are complicated by septic thrombophlebitis of cortical veins and venous infarction of adjacent cerebral cortex; an ipsilateral temporal pressure cone may ensue as the terminal event.

Etiology

Anaerobic organisms such as *Peptostreptococcus*, *Bacteroides*, and *Fusobacterium* have been isolated, both separately and in mixed culture, from about 40 percent of rhinogenic subdural empyemas.[88] Various aerobic streptococci have also been implicated. Postcraniotomy infections are most often caused by *S. aureus* or Enterobacteriaceae species.

Clinical Findings

The presence of generalized headache, very high fever, vomiting, and stiff neck in a patient with an acute exacerbation of chronic sinusitis is an indication of intracranial spread of infection. The rapid onset of obtundation, hemiparesis, and focal or generalized seizures in this context suggests the development of subdural empyema as well as pyogenic meningitis or cerebral abscess. Hemianesthesia, hemianopsia, and dysphasia are additional signs of empyema, occurring when the empyema overlies the dominant hemisphere. These findings are caused either by compressive effects of the purulent collection or by cerebral infarction secondary to cortical vein thrombophlebitis. As intracranial pressure increases, palsies of the third and sixth cranial nerves, papilledema, and coma supervene. If subdural empyema is not diagnosed and treated early, the course becomes rapidly fatal.

Laboratory Findings

A peripheral leukocytosis is commonly present. Lumbar puncture is contraindicated in subdural empyema because of the increased risk of transtentorial herniation. If CSF is examined because of suspicion of meningitis, it will show cell counts from 10 to 1,000 cells/mm^3, with a lymphocytic or neutrophilic predominance.

Skull films usually exhibit evidence of sinusitis, mastoiditis, or osteomyelitis. CT is the most helpful noninvasive diagnostic technique. A subdural empyema emerges as an elliptical area of decreased density abutting on the dura and compressing adjacent brain and ventricle. Contrast enhancement reveals a thin, relatively dense margin. Carotid angiography should be performed when the clinical findings suggest a subdural empyema but the CT scan is negative. In the presence of subdural empyema, angiography shows a mass effect with inward displacement of meningeal vessels and a contralateral shift of the anterior cerebral arteries.

Diagnosis

When the clinical picture just described develops in a patient with sinusitis, subdural empyema is a likely diagnosis. The differential diagnosis includes bacterial meningitis, brain abscess, acute encephalitis, and acute hemorrhagic leukoencephalitis. CT, carotid angiography, or both will establish the diagnosis.

Treatment

Treatment of subdural empyema requires prompt surgical drainage by multiple burr holes or craniotomy. Surgical treatment of the underlying sinusitis or mastoiditis is deferred until the acute intracranial infection is under control. Knowledge of the predisposing source of infection initially guides antibiotic management. Later, management is modified on the basis of bacteriologic findings at surgery. When an underlying sinusitis or a mastoiditis is present, therapy is designed to cover polymicrobial aerobic and anaerobic bacterial pathogens, especially *Bacteroides* species, anaerobic streptococci, and Enterobacteriaceae. Previously recommended regimens included a combination of intravenous penicillin and intravenous chloramphenicol (20 million units of penicillin G plus 4 g of chloramphenicol, in divided doses daily). The current recommendation for initial empirical treatment of subdural empyema in adults is a combination of intravenous penicillin G, a third-generation cephalosporin such as ceftriaxone, and metronidazole, all administered in high doses. Empirical antibiotic treatment of a postcraniotomy subdural empyema before the results of bacteriologic study are available might reasonably consist of a combination of a penicillinase-resistant penicillin such as nafcillin, a third-generation cephalosporin such as ceftriaxone, and gentamicin to provide coverage of *S. aureus* and Enterobacteriaceae.

Cranial Epidural Abscess

A cranial epidural abscess consists of a collection of pus or granulation tissue situated between the inner table of the skull and the dura. It is commonly a result of direct spread of infection from paranasal sinusitis, especially in the frontal sinus, where the infection may penetrate the posterior wall. Cranial epidural abscess may also arise from spread of infection from mastoiditis, osteomyelitis of the skull, craniotomy wound in-

fection, or penetrating head injury. Such abscesses are usually limited in size by the close adherence of the dura to the skull. Anaerobic organisms (such as *Peptostreptococcus, Bacteroides*, or *Fusobacterium*) or facultative streptococci are usually involved in empyemas secondary to sinusitis or mastoiditis. Occasionally, a hyperacute frontal sinusitis develops in conjunction with Pott's puffy tumor and a simultaneous cranial epidural abscess, all of which are caused by *S. aureus*. Cranial epidural abscesses that develop after penetrating head trauma or craniotomy are usually caused by *S. aureus* or Enterobacteriaceae species.

The symptoms of cranial epidural abscess primarily consist of those of the underlying sinusitis, mastoiditis, or osteomyelitis. In addition, a slight nuchal stiffness may be present. The size of the collection is rarely sufficient by itself to cause increased intracranial pressure or focal neurologic signs. A moderate-sized collection resulting from osteomyelitic destruction of the posterior wall of the frontal sinus may produce a high fever. On CT scan, an epidural collection may resemble a subdural collection, except that an epidural abscess can spread across the midline. Spread of indolent infection from the mastoid along the petrous ridge can produce Gradenigo's syndrome (lateral rectus muscle paralysis from paresis of the sixth cranial nerve and temporoparietal pain from involvement of fifth cranial nerve sensory fibers).

The CSF in a patient with a cranial epidural abscess is sterile and contains a few to several hundred lymphocytes per cubic millimeter [*see Table 5*]. Often, the finding of an epidural abscess is an incidental observation at the time of sinus or mastoid surgery or at the time of surgical drainage of an associated brain abscess or subdural empyema. Initial antibiotic therapy is based on knowledge of the likely infecting organisms in the antecedent sinusitis, mastoiditis, or other source of infection. Some small epidural infections are probably eradicated by antibiotic therapy alone.

Spinal Epidural Abscess

Spinal epidural abscesses are uncommon, but the potential for permanent neurologic damage in their wake makes early diagnosis and prompt therapy of extreme importance. The primary site of involvement is more frequently the thoracic spine rather than the lumbar or cervical spine.[85] About half of spinal epidural abscesses are acute purulent collections; in such cases, the interval between the onset of symptoms and the performance of surgery is less than two weeks. The balance consists of chronic granulating masses, the course of which can be protracted for weeks to months before the diagnosis is made and surgery performed.

Anatomy, Pathogenesis, and Pathophysiology

Most spinal epidural abscesses are situated in the posterior epidural space. The average span of an abscess is four or five vertebral segments, but it can extend over as many as 11 to 22 segments.[89] Infection is usually derived from one of three sources: (1) the bloodstream (30 percent of cases), particularly from the skin or upper respiratory tract, (2) vertebral osteomyelitis (50 percent of cases), which is derived from the usual bacteremias and from retrograde spread of infection originating in the pelvis and genitourinary tract via Batson's plexus, and (3) contiguous infection (20 percent of cases), such as psoas abscess or operative wound infection. A history of back trauma can be elicited in about 30 percent of cases. Epidural abscesses produce destructive changes in the spinal cord by a combination of compressive effects and impaired circulation to the cord.

Etiology

S. aureus is the bacterium most commonly involved in spinal epidural abscess.[89,90] Various streptococci are occasionally implicated. Gram-negative bacilli are isolated from about 20 percent of cases.

Clinical Features

Heusner's description in 1948 of the four phases of an epidural abscess still holds: spinal ache, root pain, weakness, and paralysis.[90] The spinal ache starts at the affected level of the spine. Initially, percussion tenderness over the involved area may be elicited; meningismus and paraspinal muscle spasm may also be present. Root pains radiating from the involved area of the spine develop one or two days after onset of ache. Fever is usually an accompanying feature. Occasionally, the overlying soft tissues become edematous. Reflex abnormalities can be elicited by this time. They consist of decreased tendon reflexes in the lower extremities when the abscess is at the level of the cauda equina and of increased reflexes and extensor plantar responses when the abscess is over the spinal cord. If left untreated at this stage, the process progresses to the stage of motor weakness, which manifests itself, on the average, four to five days after the onset of root pain. Ascending numbness with a sensory level and impaired bladder and bowel control accompany motor weakness. Recognition of the nature of the process by the time weakness appears is critical. Progression to irreversible paralysis often occurs within 24 hours unless surgical drainage is undertaken at once.

Fever and leukocytosis are often absent in the patient with chronic epidural abscess. Spinal ache is severe; root pains follow within a week of onset of ache and become persistent. Neck flexion causes paresthesias described as electric shock sensations in the extremities (Lhermitte's sign); paresthesias also arise spontaneously.

Laboratory Findings

Only those patients with the acute form of spinal epidural abscess have a peripheral leukocytosis. CSF findings are those characteristic of parameningeal infection: zero to several hundred leukocytes per cubic millimeter (consisting of neutrophils and lymphocytes, approximately equal in number), a normal glucose content, and an elevated protein level of 300 to 700 mg/dl.

Introduction of a spinal needle into the lumbar area in the presence of a lumbar epidural abscess can readily produce bacterial meningitis. For this reason, spinal puncture or myelography should be done by lateral cervical puncture under fluoroscopic control if lumbar involvement is suspected. Even if lumbar involvement does not seem primary, lumbar puncture should be performed cautiously because of the propensity of spinal epidural abscesses to extend over many spinal segments. Spinal puncture should be executed with intermittent aspiration of any collection on reaching the epidural space. This precaution allows the spinal needle to be withdrawn short of penetration of the dura, in the presence of an epidural abscess.

Radiographs of the spine demonstrate vertebral osteomyelitis before surgery in 60 percent of patients whose abscesses are secondary to vertebral body osteomyelitis; most are patients with the chronic form of the disease. Myelograms are uniformly abnormal, showing complete block in most instances and partial block in the remainder. CT, particularly with third-generation machines, is useful in the delineation of the site of an epidural abscess.

Diagnosis

Diagnosis of spinal epidural abscess is based on history, neurologic findings, and myelographic results. The differential diagnosis includes a variety of processes. Meningitis may produce diffuse back pain, but headache is usually the principal complaint; localized vertebral tenderness is a symptom of vertebral osteomyelitis. Acute transverse myelopathy can cause back pain, weakness, and paralysis; back pain, however, afflicts only a minority of patients as an initial symptom. The course is extremely rapid: paralysis occurs within 72 hours or less of onset of myelopathy. The myelogram is usually normal. Vertebral osteomyelitis may present with back pain or root signs; vertebral collapse and displacement may produce spinal cord compression. Radiologic changes provide the clue. An extruded disk may cause similar symptoms, but the CSF findings are usually normal. Interruption of the vascular supply of the cord may result

from shock, vasculitis, or dissecting aortic aneurysm. Vascular interruption may mimic epidural abscess by producing a similar picture of paralysis. The course of vascular interruption is more rapid, however, and early backache and root pain are not features. Intraspinal tumors may present in a fashion similar to that of a chronic epidural abscess; myelography is necessary to distinguish between the two.

Treatment

Laminectomy should be carried out at once in any patient who has a clinical picture consistent with spinal epidural abscess and a myelogram that reveals a spinal block or epidural mass. Laminectomy should include exposure and drainage of the full extent of the abscess, or as close to it as possible, and full decompression of the spinal cord. Blood cultures should be obtained before the start of antibiotic therapy. Material obtained at operation should be examined by Gram's stain and cultured to provide guidance in altering antibiotic management. A chronic abscess that is found to be a granulating epidural mass should be histologically examined for the presence of tuberculosis or tumor. If there are no obvious predisposing infected foci to provide a clue as to bacterial etiology, a penicillinase-resistant penicillin such as nafcillin should be employed initially. However, if gram-negative bacteria are seen on the Gram's stain of the clinical specimen, a third-generation cephalosporin, such as ceftriaxone, plus gentamicin should be given parenterally. Epidural abscess should be treated with parenteral antibiotics for three to four weeks after surgical drainage. Concomitant vertebral osteomyelitis warrants antibiotic treatment for a total of six to eight weeks.

Septic Thrombophlebitis of Major Cerebral Venous Sinuses

Spread of infection from cranial epidural abscess, subdural empyema, or infected extracranial veins may result in septic thrombophlebitis of the major dural venous sinuses. The cavernous, lateral, and superior longitudinal sinuses are most frequently involved.

Cavernous Sinus Thrombophlebitis

Cavernous sinus thrombophlebitis occurs most commonly as a complication of infection in the nose, upper lip, or upper face. It occasionally develops from spread of contiguous infection in the sphenoid or posterior ethmoid air sinuses. The majority of these infections are caused by *S. aureus*. The prevalence of cavernous sinus thrombophlebitis has decreased markedly since the advent of antibiotics.

Local findings initially include frontal venous congestion, orbital and perinasal edema, ptosis, chemosis, and proptosis.[91] These findings are initially unilateral but become bilateral as the phlebitis extends to the opposite cavernous sinus. Ensuing paresis of the third, fourth, and sixth cranial nerves, which pass through the cavernous sinus, produces total ophthalmoplegia. The pupils usually dilate, and pupillary reactions are often absent. Involvement of the trigeminal nerve produces eye pain and frontal hyperesthesia. Retinal veins become engorged; retinal hemorrhages and papilledema follow late in the course. Bacteremia accompanied by metastatic skin lesions and abscesses elsewhere may supervene. CSF findings are consistent with a minimal meningeal reaction secondary to a parameningeal focus.

Orbital cellulitis and abscess are the principal conditions to be excluded in the differential diagnosis. They arise chiefly as complications of paranasal sinusitis. Ultrasound studies of the orbit and orbital venography may be helpful in distinguishing between these processes and cavernous sinus thrombophlebitis. Rhinocerebral phycomycosis may present with a similar clinical picture, but it is usually found in the setting of poorly controlled diabetes mellitus. It is associated with early development of black necrotic lesions of the nasal turbinates.

Lateral Sinus Thrombophlebitis

This form of dural venous sinus thrombophlebitis is almost always a complication of mastoiditis. Aerobic streptococci, anaerobes, and staphylococci are the most commonly implicated bacterial agents. The clinical picture is that of an underlying ear infection, including high fever and chills and manifestations of increased intracranial pressure. Postauricular tenderness, venous engorgement, and edema signal involvement of the mastoid emissary vein; extension into the neck with jugular vein involvement may occur. Papilledema is a common feature of lateral sinus thrombophlebitis. Focal neurologic findings are usually absent except in cases in which the phlebitis extends in a retrograde fashion into the veins of the cerebral cortex. Rarely, the phlebitis extends to the jugular bulb, where it produces palsies of the ninth, 10th, and 11th cranial nerves. Cerebrospinal fluid changes consist of an elevated pressure and an elevated cell count ranging from a few to several hundred cells per cubic millimeter. The CSF glucose level is normal, and no bacteria are present.

Superior Sagittal Sinus Thrombophlebitis

The superior sagittal sinus is less frequently involved in septic thrombophlebitis than the cavernous and lateral sinuses. Bacterial meningitis, contiguous osteomyelitis, and peridural infection are initiating foci of infection. Pelvic infections can be initiating sites as well, leading to spread via the vertebral veins. Spread of infection from the lateral and cavernous sinuses may also result in superior sagittal sinus phlebitis.

Thrombosis of only the anterior portion of the sinus is often asymptomatic. Thrombosis of the posterior portion of the sinus elevates intracranial pressure. Extension of the thrombophlebitis to cortical veins may cause infarction of the underlying cortex. Focal seizures, sometimes involving one and then the other side of the body, may ensue. Hemiparesis, hemianopsia, aphasia, and conjugate deviation of the eyes may also follow. The superior and medial surfaces of the cerebral hemispheres are most likely to be the sites of hemorrhagic venous infarctions; therefore, weakness and sensory changes tend to be evident in the lower extremities.

The CSF findings are similar to those found in lateral sinus thrombophlebitis. Thrombosis can be demonstrated on the venous phase of a cerebral arteriogram or by a radionuclide cerebral flow study.

Treatment of Dural Sinus Thrombophlebitis

Treatment of dural sinus thrombophlebitis consists of appropriate antimicrobial therapy in high dosages, combined with surgical drainage and removal of infected bone and extradural or intrasinus abscesses. A penicillinase-resistant penicillin, such as nafcillin, should be included in the initial antibiotic regimen because a penicillinase-producing strain of *S. aureus* may be involved. Anticoagulants should not be employed, because the risk of hemorrhage complicating venous cerebral infarction is too great. The prognoses for cavernous and lateral sinus thrombophlebitis are reasonably good if the disease is detected early and treated intensively. Otitic hydrocephalus may remain after the resolution of lateral sinus phlebitis; this complication is more likely to develop when occlusion occurs on the right because the right sinus is usually larger and more important for venous drainage than the left sinus.

References

1. Rev Infect Dis 12:128, 1990
2. J Pediatr 89:66, 1976
3. N Engl J Med 301:122, 1979
4. Rev Infect Dis 2:207, 1980
5. Medicine (Baltimore) 52:563, 1973
6. J Infect Dis 131:543, 1975
7. Yale J Biol Med 50:31, 1977
8. Current Clinical Topics in Infectious Diseases, Vol 1. McGraw-Hill Book Co, New York, 1980, p 68
9. N Engl J Med 272:725, 1965
10. Lancet 1:787, 1980
11. Rev Infect Dis 2:725, 1980
12. Ann Intern Med 91:70, 1979
13. Medicine (Baltimore) 63:379, 1984
14. J Infect Dis 137:384, 1978
15. J Infect Dis 139:529, 1979
16. West J Med 140:433, 1984
17. Arch Intern Med 136:883, 1976
18. N Engl J Med 296:433, 1977
19. J Clin Microbiol 5:405, 1977
20. J Clin Microbiol 10:519, 1979
21. J Pediatr 88:706, 1976
22. N Engl J Med 289:931, 1973
23. JAMA 235:617, 1976
24. J Infect Dis 140:453, 1979
25. Arch Neurol 37:137, 1980
26. J Pediatr 96:820, 1980
27. N Engl J Med 305:1079, 1981
28. Ann Intern Med 113:227, 1990
29. Pediatr Infect Dis J 8:904, 1989
30. N Engl J Med 319:964, 1988
31. J Lab Clin Med 95:362, 1980
32. Pediatr Infect Dis J 9:2, 1990
33. Rev Infect Dis 10:365, 1988
34. Am J Med 71:507, 1981
35. Pediatr Infect Dis J 2:352, 1983
36. Antimicrob Agents Chemother 25:706, 1984
37. Am J Med 79(suppl 2A):47, 1985
38. J Infect Dis 143:293, 1981
39. Am J Med 71:199, 1981
40. Antimicrob Agents Chemother 16:13, 1979
41. J Infect Dis 137:251, 1978
42. J Infect Dis 143:141, 1981
43. J Infect Dis 155:403, 1987
44. Bacterial Meningitis. Churchill Livingstone, Inc, New York, 1985, p 203
45. Antimicrob Agents Chemother 23:191, 1983
46. J Antimicrob Chemother 10(suppl C):141, 1982
47. Pediatr Infect Dis J 5:402, 1986
48. Lancet 1:1241, 1983
49. Pediatr Infect Dis J 5:416, 1986
50. Pediatr Infect Dis J 5:408, 1986
51. Antimicrob Agents Chemother 25:40, 1984
52. Pediatr Infect Dis J 5:293, 1986
53. N Engl J Med 322:141, 1990
54. Lancet 1:1281, 1989
55. Ann Neurol 7:524, 1980
56. Current Clinical Topics in Infectious Disease, Vol 3. McGraw-Hill Book Co, New York, 1982, p 218
57. Bacterial Meningitis. Churchill Livingstone, Inc, New York, 1985, p 123
58. MMWR 40(RR-12):1, 1991
59. MMWR 40(RR-1):1, 1991
60. Current Clinical Topics in Infectious Disease, Vol 3. McGraw-Hill Book Co, New York, 1982, p 254
61. Am J Med Sci 264:319, 1972
62. Ann Intern Med 72:869, 1970
63. J Neurosurg 33:312, 1970
64. Medicine (Baltimore) 55:341, 1976
65. Rev Infect Dis 9:595, 1987
66. Ann Intern Med 74:923, 1971
67. Bacterial Meningitis. Churchill Livingstone, Inc, New York, 1985, p 219
68. Br Med J 2:981, 1977
69. Anaerobic Bacteria: Role in Disease. International Conference on Anaerobic Bacteria, Center for Disease Control, 1972. Charles C Thomas, Publisher, Springfield, Illinois, 1974, p 309
70. Am J Med 35:682, 1963
71. Anaerobic Bacteria in Human Disease. Academic Press, Inc, New York, 1977, p 155
72. Am J Med 54:201, 1973
73. Ann Intern Med 82:571, 1975
74. N Engl J Med 288:674, 1973
75. J Pediatr 93:86, 1978
76. Transactions of the American Laryngology, Rhinology, and Otology Society, 1964, p 120
77. JAMA 218:1542, 1971
78. Radiology 135:663, 1980
79. Ann Intern Med 91:87, 1979
80. Ann Neurol 3:474, 1978

81. Ann Neurol 7:371, 1980
82. Radiology 121:641, 1976
83. Am J Med 67:711, 1979
84. Arch Intern Med 138:628, 1978
85. Q J Med 46:389, 1977
86. Am J Med 53:85, 1972
87. Medicine (Baltimore) 54:485, 1975
88. Am J Med 58:99, 1975
89. N Engl J Med 293:463, 1975
90. N Engl J Med 239:845, 1948
91. Bull Johns Hopkins Hosp 109:68, 1961

Acknowledgments

Table 7 From data provided by Merle A. Sande, M.D., University of California at San Francisco.

Tables 8, 9 From "Use of Cephalosporins in the Treatment of Bacterial Meningitis," by H. C. Neu, in *Bacterial Meningitis*, edited by M. A. Sande, A. L. Smith, and R. K. Root. Churchill Livingstone, Inc., New York, 1985, p. 203. Used by permission.

 Cerebrovascular Diseases

ROBERT W. P. CUTLER, M.D.

Epidemiology

There are approximately 750,000 new cases of stroke each year in the United States. No age group is spared. Stroke accounts for 250,000 deaths annually and ranks third, behind heart disease and cancer, among all causes of adult death. Nearly 50 percent of patients hospitalized for neurologic care have cerebrovascular disease. The residual disability is often considerable. In the long-term follow-up provided by the Framingham study, 16 percent of stroke survivors remained institutionalized, 31 percent needed assistance in self-care, and 71 percent had decreased vocational function.[1] The incidence of stroke has declined nearly 50 percent over the past three decades, particularly in elderly persons. It is likely that treatment of hypertension, by far the most important predisposing factor for stroke, is at least partially responsible for this decline. Other major predisposing factors are age, heart disease, diabetes mellitus, and race. It has long been known that the incidence of stroke is higher in blacks than in whites, which has been attributed to the higher rates of hypertension and diabetes mellitus among blacks. Stroke is the most important factor in the difference in mortality between blacks and whites. Recent epidemiological data derived from the First National Health and Nutrition Examination Survey suggest that even after adjustments for age, hypertension, and diabetes mellitus, the incidence of stroke remains higher in blacks than in whites.[2]

Preventable risk factors are gradually being revealed through multivariate analyses of data collected during prospective studies of large cohorts of men and women. Such analyses control for age, race, hypertension, and diabetes. The most important preventable factors are cigarette smoking and alcohol consumption. Several studies have shown that the risk of ischemic stroke is two to four times higher in smokers than in nonsmokers, for both men and women. The risk of cerebral hemorrhage, either parenchymatous or subarachnoid, is particularly striking: smokers have a 10-fold greater risk of cerebral hemorrhage than nonsmokers.[3-5] Most importantly, cessation of smoking markedly reduces the risk of stroke. A similar increased risk of hemorrhagic stroke is associated with alcohol consumption, although the risk of ischemic stroke appears to be reduced from normal in persons who are light to moderate drinkers (< 24 g/day).[6-8]

Another reported risk factor for hemorrhagic stroke is a low serum cholesterol level. The Multiple Risk Factor Intervention Trial, in which 350,000 middle-aged men were followed for a six-year period, disclosed a threefold increase in deaths from intracranial hemorrhage in men who were hypertensive and had serum cholesterol levels below 160 mg/dl. By contrast, the risk of ischemic stroke was positively correlated with an elevated serum cholesterol level.[9]

It is important for the physician to ascertain the presence of other known risk factors (e.g., use of oral contraceptives,[10] presence of antiphospholipid antibodies,[11] hypercoagulable states,[10] atrial fibrillation,[12] orthostatic hypotension,[13] migraine headache,[14] mitral valve prolapse,[10] or substance abuse[15]) and to apply preventive measures when possible.

Cerebral Blood Flow and Metabolism

The brain has a very high metabolic rate and a limited store of energy substrates. Glucose is essentially the sole metabolic substrate, and the brain cannot survive prolonged deprivation of glucose and oxygen. Although the brain constitutes only two percent of body weight, it receives 15 percent of the cardiac output of blood and requires 25 percent of the oxygen and 70 percent of the glucose consumed by the body.

Under normal conditions, the rate of blood flow to an area of the brain is directly related to the rate of metabolism in that region. Increases in cerebral blood flow have been found in the expected regions during the performance of manual tasks and mental activity and during focal cortical seizures. This coupling of blood flow and metabolism is often lost in acute cerebrovascular disease; that is, the flow rate may be high when the metabolic rate is low (luxury perfusion). In most conditions in which brain function is depressed, however, there is a reduction in both blood flow and oxygen utilization.

Normally, the rate of blood flow to the entire brain is relatively constant, and it does not change in response to alterations in mean systemic blood pressure over a range of 50 to 150 mm Hg. This phenomenon, known as autoregulation, protects the brain from the effects of hypotension and from cerebrovascular hemorrhage caused by excessive intravascular pressure. Autoregulation is largely controlled by small arterioles, but the mechanisms involved are poorly understood.[16] The rapidity of an autoregulatory response suggests a vascular smooth muscle response, perhaps related to the periarteriolar accumulation of vasoactive metabolites such as adenosine. The blood carbon dioxide tension is also an important regulator of cerebral blood flow, which increases linearly with rising partial pressure of CO_2 (P_aCO_2).

A state of regional vasomotor paralysis occurs in focal cerebral ischemia resulting from stroke, with loss of autoregulation and responsiveness to inhaled CO_2. In the center of the infarct, blood flow is greatly reduced or absent, whereas at its margin, maximum vasodilatation results from the lactic acid formed during anaerobic glycolysis. This marginal region of increased flow is often the site of edema formation. When CO_2 is inhaled or a cerebral vasodilator such as papaverine is administered to patients with focal infarction, only the vessels in normal areas of the brain dilate, resulting in an intracerebral steal of blood away from the infarcted zone. Conversely, when hypocapnia is induced, blood may be shunted toward the infarcted zone (inverse steal syndrome). A general impairment of autoregulation may also appear in patients with chronic hypertension.

The metabolic events that accompany brain hypoxia and ischemia include a fall in adenosine triphosphate (ATP) content, a rise in acid metabolites and free fatty acids, and marked alterations in transmembrane ion fluxes. The depletion of cellular energy stores is accompanied by cellular release of the excitatory amino acid glutamate. It is now known that glutamate, acting as a so-called excitotoxin, mediates both acute and delayed changes in ion transport in neurons through activation of the N-methyl-D-aspartate (NMDA) receptor. The acute change, measured in minutes, consists of neuronal uptake of sodium, chloride, and water. The delayed change, measured in hours, consists of calcium influx, secondary free radical generation, and cell death. The recent elucidation of these NMDA receptor–mediated events has led to important new strategies for the treatment of ischemic stroke.[17] Selective NMDA antagonists substantially reduce neuronal damage in rats in which either focal or global ischemia is induced, and partial protection is conferred even when the antagonist is administered after the ischemic insult.[18,19]

Cerebral Transient Ischemic Attacks

The designation of cerebral transient ischemic attacks (TIAs) refers to episodes of neurologic dysfunction that develop suddenly, last five minutes to several hours (never more than 24 hours), and clear completely. Symptoms that develop during an attack generally point to disturbances of circulation in either the carotid or the vertebrobasilar arterial systems (see below). The peak age for the development of TIAs is 60 to 70 years. The incidence of stroke in patients with TIAs is not precisely known. In general, if untreated, about one third of patients with TIAs will suffer a completed stroke, one third will continue to have TIAs without infarction, and one third will have a spontaneous remission.

It is believed that transient ischemic attacks result largely from thromboembolism; aggregated platelets and debris from ulcerated atheromatous plaques in the extracranial carotid artery are two common types of emboli. The transient nature of the attack is explained by the rapid fragmentation and dissolution of these microemboli. Other sources of emboli include vegetations on heart valves, valvular prostheses, and clots associated with atrial fibrillation. Transient hypotension, mechanical kinking of vessels during rotation of the head, compression by osteophytes, and cardiac arrhythmias play less important roles in precipitating TIAs.

It is important, although not always possible, to distinguish attacks of carotid insufficiency from those of vertebrobasilar insufficiency because the prognosis and treatment for the two types of attacks are quite different. Symptoms of vertebrobasilar insufficiency rarely result from shunting of blood from the posterior to the anterior circulation in patients with normal vertebral arteries who have stenosis or occlusion of one or both carotid arteries. Treatment of the carotid artery disease may possibly be beneficial in such cases.

Carotid Artery Syndrome

Transient ischemia of the retina or of a cerebral hemisphere causes carotid artery syndrome. These events rarely occur together. Retinal ischemia, from reduced blood flow or microembolization in the ophthalmic branch of the internal carotid artery, causes transient blackout of vision (amaurosis fugax). Patients often feel as though a shade has been pulled down over one eye. Funduscopy may show refractile cholesterol emboli (Hollenhorst plaques) or whitish platelet emboli in retinal arteries.

Cerebral hemisphere ischemia produces the sudden onset of such symptoms as contralateral monoparesis or hemiparesis, localized tingling numbness, hemianopic visual loss, or aphasia. Loss of consciousness is very rare. The rapidity of onset of symptoms helps distinguish transient ischemic attacks from focal seizures, which are commonly characterized by a so-called march of symptoms from distal to proximal parts. Episodes of loss of consciousness should also suggest the diagnosis of seizure or Adams-Stokes syndrome.

By definition, a transient ischemic attack leaves no neurologic sequelae. In many cases, however, a neurologic deficit may last longer than 24 hours, eventually clearing within one or two weeks. The more prolonged syndrome is referred to as a reversible ischemic neurologic deficit and, from the viewpoints of pathophysiology and treatment, should not be distinguished from TIAs.

Findings on neurologic examination of patients with TIAs are generally normal. Vascular examination may reveal reduced carotid or temporal artery pulsations or the presence of a bruit, commonly located over the carotid bifurcation. A bruit over the carotid artery suggests arterial stenosis; however, false positive bruits are heard in 10 percent of persons examined, and a large percentage of persons with proven carotid stenosis do not have bruits. A careful search should be made for microemboli in retinal vessels. In some instances of carotid occlusive disease, the sympathetic fibers will be involved, and Horner's syndrome is present.

Vertebrobasilar Artery Syndrome

The characteristic symptomatology of vertebrobasilar artery syndrome is referable to the posterior portions of the brain—the occipital lobes and brain stem. In this syndrome, bilateral disturbance of vision results from insufficiency of the posterior cerebral arteries that supply the visual cortex. Visual symptoms are described as dim, gray, or blurry vision; total blindness may even occur transiently. Another common visual complaint is diplopia caused by the transient disturbance of conjugate gaze. Attacks of vertigo, unsteadiness, nausea, and vomiting point to circulatory disturbances either in the labyrinth or in the vestibular nuclei of the medulla. Other brain stem symptoms are slurring dysarthria, dysphagia, perioral numbness, and weakness or paresthesias of all four limbs.

So-called drop attacks, in which there is a sudden loss of postural tone in the legs, are also characteristic of basilar insufficiency. The patient abruptly falls to the ground, often landing on his or her knees. Careful inquiry reveals there is no loss of consciousness—the patient remembers striking the ground and attempting to rise almost at once, distinguishing the attack from simple syncope or an Adams-Stokes syndrome heart block.

It is likely that many, if not all, cases of transient global amnesia are related to vertebrobasilar artery insufficiency. This syndrome, which affects men much more frequently than women, is characterized by the abrupt development of memory loss and confusion. During the attack, there is retrograde amnesia for a variable period; self-identity is generally preserved. The episode subsides in a period of minutes to several hours; as it subsides, the period of retrograde amnesia gradually shortens until amnesia remains only regarding the period of the attack. This gap in memory is permanent. It is believed that ischemia of portions of the temporal lobes or thalamus supplied by posterior cerebral arteries is responsible for this disturbance.

In contrast to patients with carotid artery insufficiency, those with vertebrobasilar attacks more often describe a relation between symptoms and abrupt changes in posture. In those cases, one commonly finds postural hypotension or a relatively low blood pressure for the patient's age. In addition, the vertebral artery may be compressed by osteophytes of the cervical spine, and movements of the head, particularly hyperextension, may aggravate the compression. Occasionally, in vertebrobasilar insufficiency, a bruit may be heard over the subclavian artery, and x-rays of the cervical spine may show calcification of the vertebral arteries.

The transient nature of the neurologic disturbance points to a vascular disorder, in contrast to diseases in which symptoms are more persistent, such as multiple sclerosis and acoustic neuroma. Basilar artery migraine would be expected to occur in younger patients. Vestibular neuronitis and Ménière's disease may be diagnosed from appropriate findings on audiometry and caloric testing.

Subclavian Steal Syndrome

Symptoms of claudication of an exercised arm accompanied by the symptoms of vertebrobasilar insufficiency constitute the subclavian steal syndrome. If the subclavian or innominate artery becomes occluded and the major cranial vessels remain patent, reversal of blood flow in the ipsilateral vertebral artery may occur [*see Figure 1*]. The hemodynamic changes are accentuated during use or exercise of the arm on the affected side.

A bruit may be heard over the subclavian artery, and a significant difference (> 20 mm Hg) in systolic blood pressure may be found in the two arms. A delay of 30 milliseconds or longer in pulse wave propagation in the brachial artery on the involved side, recorded by a Doppler ultrasound detector, is said to correlate with reversed vertebral artery blood flow.[20]

Laboratory Investigation of Transient Ischemic Attacks

Laboratory investigation is recommended for patients in whom the diagnosis of TIAs is in doubt or in whom endarterectomy is contemplated. The definitive procedure is cerebral arteriography, but a number of noninvasive tests are available with which to assess the adequacy of cerebral circulation. The carotid bifurcation may be visualized by B-mode ultrasonography unless there is near or complete occlusion of the artery. Atherosclerotic plaques, ulcerations, and luminal competency may be assessed anatomically by ultrasonography. A more complete picture of the degree of arterial stenosis and its functional significance may be achieved by including a Doppler ultrasound examination to measure red blood cell flow velocity. Oculoplethysmography, a noninvasive technique for measuring pressure in the ophthalmic artery, is also useful for determining whether a hemodynami-

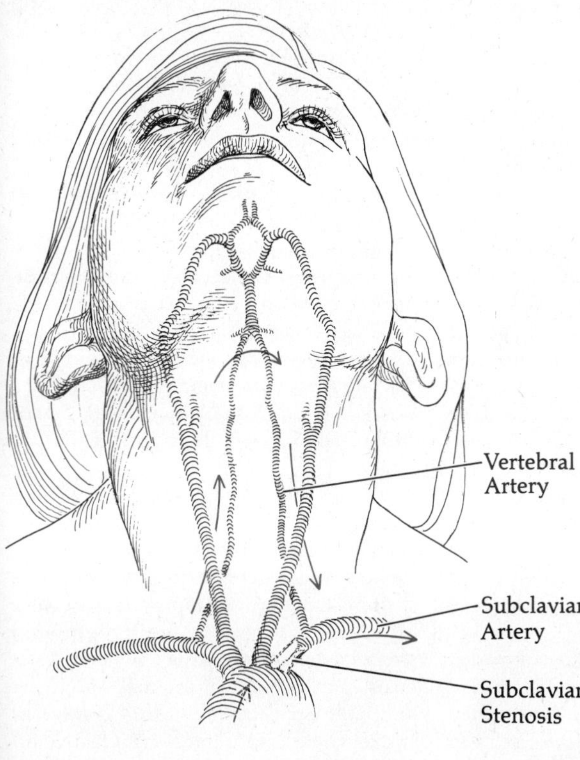

Figure 1 *Stenosis of the left subclavian artery has caused reversal of blood flow in the patent ipsilateral vertebral artery. Arrows indicate the pattern of blood flow through the cerebral circulation that is characteristic of the subclavian steal syndrome.*

cally significant degree of carotid stenosis is present. Finally, transcranial Doppler ultrasonography, a newer technique that employs lower ultrasound frequencies (1 to 2 MHz) than are used in the neck (2 to 10 MHz), has been valuable for detecting hemodynamically significant stenosis in the major intracranial arteries at the base of the skull and for assessing patterns of collateral blood flow.[21]

Cerebral arteriography, carried out via a femoral artery catheter, is the procedure of choice. In one large prospective study, the rate of permanent stroke from cerebral arteriography was 0.4 percent and was more likely to occur in older patients with diabetes.[22] Advances in magnetic resonance imaging (MRI) of major brain arteries are occurring rapidly, and this technique shows promise of largely supplanting conventional methods of arteriography.

If clinical circumstances suggest that the heart may be the source of emboli, then echocardiography should be performed. Such circumstances might include evidence of transient ischemia in the distribution of more than one artery, cardiac arrhythmias, physical signs of mitral valve prolapse, or symptoms and signs of bacterial or marantic endocarditis.

Two-dimensional contrast echocardiography may also detect a patent foramen ovale through which a venous clot may paradoxically embolize to the brain. In an echocardiographic study of 60 stroke patients who were younger than 55 years, a patent foramen ovale was present in 54 percent of patients with no identifiable cause for their strokes, compared with only 10 percent of normal volunteers.[23] A septal defect should prompt a search for silent venous thrombosis; closure of the septal defect should be considered in younger patients.[24]

Treatment of Transient Ischemic Attacks

The mainstays of treatment of TIAs are carotid endarterectomy and pharmacotherapy designed to prevent platelet aggregation.[25,26] In addition, maintenance of good general health, particularly cessation of smoking, is important. Establishing the value of therapy for cerebrovascular disease is time-consuming and expensive, requiring cooperative prospective trials that are often international in scope.[27] Even such trials may fail to provide proof of the value of a given treatment. For instance, aspirin has been used for TIA in eight major cooperative trials, with results ranging from marginal to highly significant efficacy in the prevention of stroke. The guidelines for therapy suggested below cannot be considered definitive.

Carotid Endarterectomy

Carotid endarterectomy is performed at a rate of more than 100,000 operations annually in the United States. The efficacy of the procedure has been difficult to assess in an era in which the incidence of stroke, both fatal and nonfatal, has been declining. Risk factor reduction and the use of antiplatelet agents have confounded the issue. The findings of several clinical trials appear to support the use of endarterectomy in patients with 70 percent or greater narrowing of an internal carotid artery.[28-30] The North American Symptomatic Carotid Endarterectomy Trial, involving 50 centers in the United States and Canada, compared the efficacy of endarterectomy with that of medical therapy alone for stroke prevention in a group of 659 patients who had suffered a recent hemispheric or retinal transient ischemic attack or nondisabling stroke. The first results indicated that endarterectomy produced a significant reduction of risk at two years for any ipsilateral stroke (nine percent versus 26 percent) and for major or fatal ipsilateral stroke (2.5 percent versus 13.1 percent). All patients, including the control subjects, re-

ceived optimal medical therapy, including antiplatelet agents.[28]

Similar results were reported by the European Carotid Surgery Trial. In a group of 778 symptomatic patients with severe stenosis (70 to 99 percent narrowing), 7.5 percent of those randomly assigned to surgery suffered an ipsilateral stroke or death within 30 days; according to life-table estimates, the risk of ipsilateral stroke during the following three years for the surgical group was 2.8 percent, compared with 16.8 percent for the patients who were treated medically.[29] Thus, despite an increased incidence of stroke in the immediate postoperative period, there was a significant reduction in the risk of stroke in the ensuing three years in the surgical group.

A third trial, the Veterans Affairs Cooperative Studies Program, involved 16 university-affiliated Veterans Affairs Medical Centers. There were 189 patients with transient ischemic attacks, transient monocular blindness, or recent small completed strokes; all had greater than 50 percent stenosis of the ipsilateral internal carotid artery. After a mean follow-up of 11.9 months, stroke or crescendo transient ischemic attacks occurred in 7.7 percent of endarterectomized patients, versus 19.4 percent of control subjects. The benefit of surgery was more marked in those with greater than 70 percent stenosis.[30]

In none of these studies did endarterectomy appear to be of benefit in patients with less than 70 percent stenosis. The results of long-term follow-up studies of patients in these clinical trials are awaited. Levy has concluded, "Endarterectomy adds a little—but not a lot. It is useful to a small proportion of patients but can subject persons who are not eligible for endarterectomy to the risks of angiography. The benefits are temporary. Endarterectomy can improve the quality of life for a small number of carefully selected patients by preventing a recurrence of stroke for 2 years."[31]

One study, in which an expert panel based its judgments on data that were available before these three recent studies, rated the indications for endarterectomy and concluded that the procedure was warranted in only one third of operated cases.[32] The indications for endarterectomy in patients with TIA, on which there was expert consensus, were high-grade (70 to 99 percent) ipsilateral carotid stenosis, large carotid wall ulcerations, and recurrent attacks while the patient was receiving medical therapy. In addition, the panel agreed that endarterectomy was appropriate for asymptomatic patients who were at high risk for stroke because of severe ipsilateral stenosis and contralateral carotid occlusion. The procedure should be performed in a tertiary care center, where the surgical mortality and morbidity from stroke are expected to be less than three or four percent.[33]

Most authorities agree that carotid endarterectomy is not indicated in patients with TIAs that are referable to the basilar-vertebral system, in patients with significant deficits from prior strokes, or in patients in whom a stroke is evolving. Extracranial-intracranial bypass surgery has been shown to be ineffective in preventing stroke and may exacerbate neurologic dysfunction.[34]

Medical Therapy

The cumulative results of trials of aspirin therapy provide evidence that aspirin is effective in reducing the risk of recurrent TIAs and stroke. It is recommended for patients who are not suitable candidates for endarterectomy. Although the dosage employed in various trials has differed, it is likely that 300 mg of aspirin taken once daily is an effective antithrombotic dose.[35] The use of dipyridamole confers no additional advantage.[36] A newer platelet antiaggregant, ticlopidine, has been studied in two major trials[37,38] and has been found to be somewhat more effective than aspirin in the prevention of strokes, although it is more toxic. Anticoagulation therapy, employing either heparin or warfarin, is not indicated in the treatment of TIA.

Concomitant Coronary Artery Disease

The principal cause of death among patients with TIAs is myocardial infarction. In fact, TIA may be a more frequent warning of heart attack than is angina pectoris. For this reason, it is prudent to carefully assess the cardiac status of patients with TIAs, especially before the recommendation of carotid endarterectomy, which appears to carry a higher risk in patients with coronary artery atherosclerosis.

The converse risk (i.e., the risk of stroke in patients undergoing coronary artery bypass grafting) continues to be debated.[39,40] Most studies report a frequency of stroke of approximately two percent after bypass surgery. Risk factors include carotid bruits, prolonged cardiopulmonary bypass time, postoperative atrial fibrillation, congestive heart failure, and a history of TIAs.[40] Many vascular surgeons advocate combined carotid endarterectomy and coronary bypass surgery for patients with high-grade (> 90 percent) carotid stenosis.

Asymptomatic Carotid Bruit

Several studies have begun to clarify the risks associated with the presence of a carotid bruit that is disclosed on physical examination but is not associated with neurologic symptoms. In a prospective study from the Mayo Clinic of 566 patients with asymptomatic cervical bruits, the one-year stroke or TIA rate was 2.5 percent, compared with a rate of 0.7 percent in a population-based control group without bruits.[41] This rate was similar to that for all patients with asymptomatic bruits in a report from Toronto.[42] In this investigation, patients were also studied by carotid Doppler ultrasonography; the risk of stroke or TIA was directly related to the severity or progression of carotid artery stenosis and reached 5.5 percent annually in those with greater than 75 percent stenosis. Another study revealed that the risk of stroke or TIA was 5.2 percent annually in patients who had an asymptomatic bruit associated with a hemodynamically significant carotid obstruction, as defined by oculopneumoplethysmography.[43] In each of these studies, excess mortality associated with cardiovascular disease was found in the groups with carotid bruits.

Employment of Doppler ultrasonography and oculopneumoplethysmography should allow the physician to define more clearly the risk of ischemic stroke in patients who have asymptomatic bruits. Sequential studies may disclose expanding atherosclerotic plaques that signify a high risk.[44] Unfortunately, however, bruits can be heard in only one third of patients who have moderate to severe carotid artery stenosis that is angiographically proven.[45]

Ischemic Stroke

Etiology and Evolution

An ischemic stroke may result from either embolic or thrombotic occlusion of an intracerebral artery, a distinction that is often difficult to make on clinical grounds. Nearly 50 percent of patients with stroke have had one or more premonitory TIAs.

Symptoms from cerebral embolism develop rapidly, often becoming maximal within a few seconds. Headache on the affected side is common, and focal seizures may occur. The diagnosis is strongly supported by the presence of conditions that predispose to embolus formation, such as mitral stenosis, atrial fibrillation, endocarditis, or mitral valve prolapse. In addition to dislodged thrombi, emboli may also consist of fat, tumor cells, and air or nitrogen bubbles.

Symptoms from cerebral thrombosis generally evolve over minutes or hours. Occasionally, the stroke progresses stepwise over days or weeks. Recognition of this variability in evolution is important because it dictates a commonsense policy that patients with ischemic stroke be hospitalized until the process has stabilized.

Factors leading to the development of cerebral arterial thrombosis fall mainly into two categories:

1. Disorders of cranial blood vessels. By far, the most common cause of cerebral thrombosis is atherosclerosis, very often associated with hypertension, diabetes mellitus, and coronary artery or peripheral vascular disease. Inflammatory blood vessel disorders, which occur in syphilis, tuberculosis, temporal arteritis, or collagen vascular disease or as a result of radiation injury, may also predispose to thrombus formation. Trauma to the head and neck may cause thrombosis of major arteries.

2. Disorders of the cardiovascular system. Stroke may follow systemic hypotension from myocardial infarction, heart block, shock, surgical anesthesia, or too vigorous treatment of chronic hypertension.

Other less common causes of cerebral arterial thrombosis are hematologic diseases associated with thromboses. Such disorders include polycythemia vera, sickle cell anemia, disseminated intravascular coagulation, and thrombotic thrombocytopenic purpura. Exogenous agents, such as oral contraceptives and ε-aminocaproic acid (EACA), and metabolic disorders, such as homocystinuria, have also been known to be occasionally associated with cerebral thrombosis.

Common Clinical Syndromes

Middle Cerebral Artery Thrombosis

The middle cerebral artery is the most frequent site of intracranial vascular thrombosis [*see Figure 2*]. When the main trunk is occluded, infarction of a large portion of the cerebral hemisphere will result, producing hemiplegia, hemianesthesia, homonymous hemianopsia, and a deviation of the head and eyes toward the side on which the lesion is located. When branches of the artery are involved, neurologic deficit will be less profound; motor and sensory impairment will be greater in the face and arm than in the leg.

Anterior Cerebral Artery Thrombosis

Thrombosis of the anterior cerebral artery is a less common condition, which characteristically produces a more profound degree of impairment in the leg than in the face and arm. Urinary incontinence and primitive reflexes (sucking and grasping) are often present. If both anterior cerebral

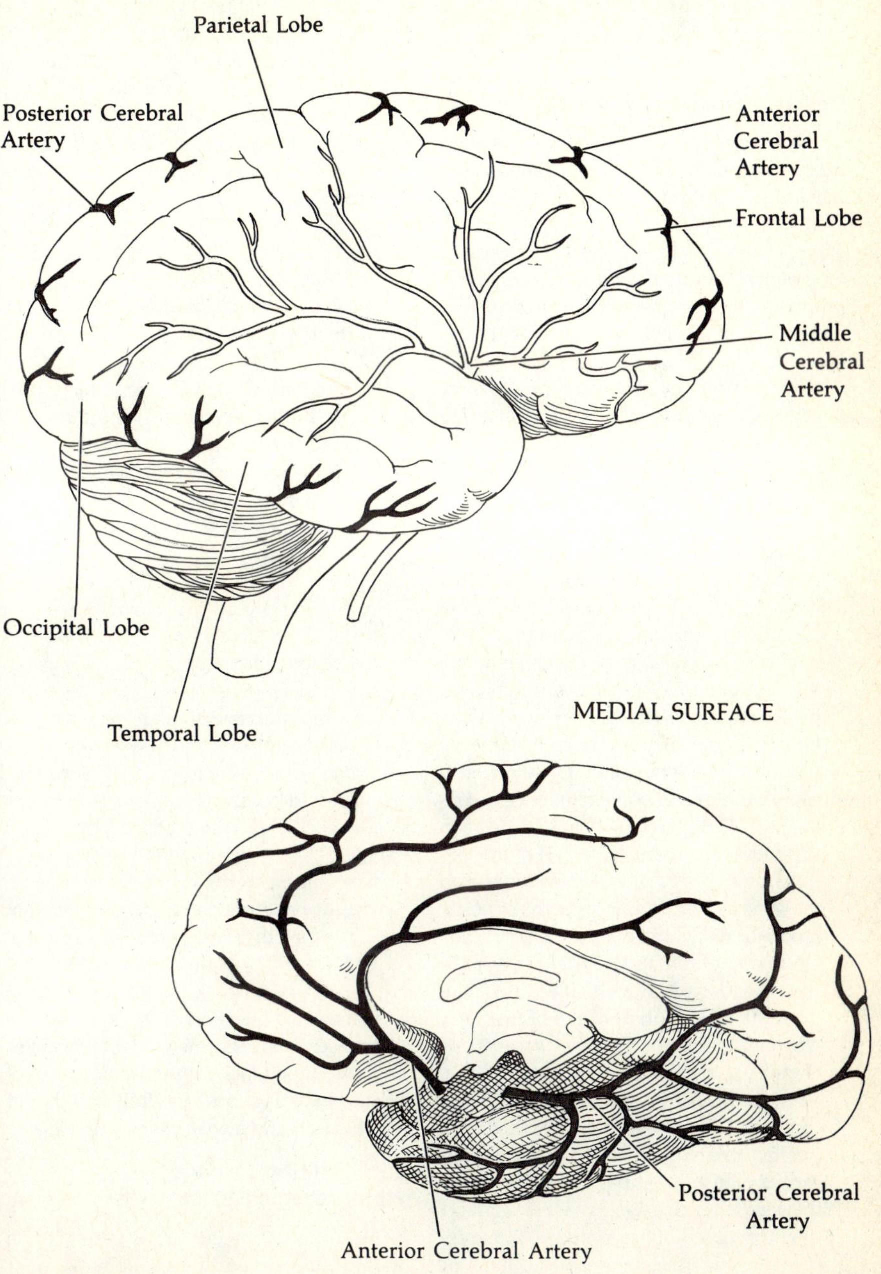

Figure 2 *The middle cerebral artery (blue), the posterior artery (light gray), and the anterior cerebral artery (dark gray) supply blood to the cerebral hemispheres.*

arteries arise from a single trunk, then occlusion of the trunk may lead to bilateral parasagittal infarction and a state of anarthria with paraplegia.

Vertebrobasilar Artery Thrombosis

The symptoms and signs of disturbance of the posterior circulation are more often attributable to blockage of one or more branches than to occlusion of the main trunk. Knowledge of the vascular supply and neuroanatomy of the brain stem will be most helpful in pinpointing the source of the disturbance; a few principles and examples are given.

1. Occlusion of paramedian arteries. Midline structures are involved, including, at different levels, cranial nerves III (oculomotor), IV (trochlear), VI (abducens), and XII (hypoglossal); pyramidal motor tracts; the medial lemniscus, which carries proprioceptive sensation; and the medial longitudinal fasciculus, which connects various cranial nerve nuclei. The hallmark of brain stem infarction is ipsilateral cranial nerve palsy with contralateral hemiplegia. Infarction of the midbrain produces partial ophthalmoplegia and contralateral hemiplegia. Infarction of the pons, depending on the level, produces ipsilateral paralysis of conjugate gaze or internuclear ophthalmoplegia, contralateral hemiplegia, and loss of position and vibratory senses. Infarction of the medulla produces paralysis of the tongue on the same side and paralysis of the opposite limbs; the face is spared.
2. Occlusion of circumferential arteries. In these syndromes, involvement is of the dorsolateral quadrant of the brain stem. Depending on the level, structures included are cranial nerves V (trigeminal), VII (facial), VIII (vestibular and cochlear divisions), IX (glossopharyngeal), and X (vagus); the spinothalamic tract, which carries pain and temperature sensations; the cerebellar peduncles, which contain fibers involved in the coordinated movements of the limbs; and central fibers of the sympathetic nervous system. Symptoms and signs of lateral brain stem in-

farction vary with the level of the lesion.

The most frequently encountered syndrome is the lateral medullary (Wallenberg) syndrome, which results from occlusion of the vertebral artery or posterior inferior cerebellar artery. Symptoms on the ipsilateral side are impaired sensation over the face, paresis of the palate and vocal cords with dysphagia and dysphonia, ataxia of the limbs, nystagmus, and Horner's syndrome. On the contralateral side, there is loss of pain and temperature senses in the limbs and trunk.

3. Occlusion of the internal auditory artery, a branch of the basilar artery or of the anterior inferior cerebellar artery, produces sudden ipsilateral deafness, vertigo, unsteadiness, and vomiting. The syndrome may resemble Ménière's disease, but the deafness resulting from arterial occlusion is permanent.

Lacunar Syndromes

A number of clinical syndromes that are attributed to small areas of infarction (lacunes), resulting from atheromatous occlusion of deep penetrating branches of the major cerebral arteries, have been described. Four relatively distinctive syndromes are pure motor hemiplegia, the dysarthria-clumsy-hand syndrome, pure sensory stroke, and homolateral ataxia with crural paresis. It has been thought that these small strokes require no treatment. Computed tomography has demonstrated, however, that the clinical syndromes are often the result of large infarctions, rather than lacunar infarcts, and neuropathologic examination has raised the question of embolization in some cases. It is recommended that the management of patients with the syndromes of lacunar infarcts should be similar to that of patients with transient ischemic attacks.

Cerebral Hemorrhage (Hemorrhagic Stroke)

Bleeding may occur in the parenchyma of the brain or within the subarachnoid space; the former is most often caused by hypertension, and the latter usually indicates a ruptured aneurysm. In the presence of moderate to severe hypertension, small penetrating arterioles may rupture deep within the brain, causing a hematoma that displaces brain structures. Common sites in the cerebral hemisphere are the putamen and thalamus. In the posterior fossa, the pons and cerebellum are preferred sites. The onset of symptoms is less abrupt than it is when an embolism occurs: an evolution over several hours is characteristic.[46] Headache, vomiting, and altered states of consciousness are common symptoms.

With hemorrhage deep in the cerebral hemisphere, flaccid hemiplegia, dense hemianesthesia, and hemianopsia are present. The eyes are tonically deviated toward the injured side of the brain. With thalamic hemorrhage, the eyes may be deviated downward. Stupor, coma, and decerebrate rigidity may result from large shifts or extension of blood into the ventricles.

In pontine hemorrhage, there is paralysis of conjugate gaze, marked pupillary miosis, and flaccid quadriplegia. Eye movements cannot be induced by ice-water irrigation of the auditory canals (caloric testing), nor does rotation of the head induce eye movements (doll's-eye responses).

Cerebellar hemorrhage leads to headache, vomiting, unsteadiness of gait, and collapse. Examination may reveal nuchal rigidity, ipsilateral paresis of conjugate gaze or skew deviation, dysarthria, reduced corneal reflex, and peripheral facial weakness. Frank ataxia is surprisingly uncommon.

Management of Stroke

Acute Phase

General therapeutic measures should include ensurance of an open airway, hydration with intravenous fluids, and judicious treatment of hypertension.[47] Because of the risk of vomiting and aspiration, patients with severe hemispheric or brain stem strokes should be given nothing orally during the acute phase. Appropriate steps should be taken to evaluate and treat coexisting cardiac or other systemic disease.

Arteriography and endarterectomy are not indicated during the acute phase of a major stroke. If possible, computed cranial tomography should be performed to distinguish ischemic infarction from hemorrhage, a distinction that is often difficult to make clinically. A lumbar puncture does not improve the accuracy of diagnosis.

A number of important and innovative studies of acute pharmacological intervention for stroke are planned or under way. Each interventional drug must be administered during the acute phase of an ischemic stroke, requiring more rapid transport to and triage by emergency medical facilities. Although one study showed that only 42 percent of stroke patients reached a university hospital within 24 hours, another reported that the time from stroke onset to initiation of treatment was 90 minutes.[48,49]

The newer therapeutic approaches include administration of agents to prevent or promote dissolution of clots (e.g., heparinoids[50] and tissue plasminogen activator[49]) and agents to prevent ischemic neuronal death (e.g., calcium channel blockers[51] and NMDA antagonists[52]). Until trials of these agents have demonstrated their efficacy, aspirin should be administered if it is not contraindicated by comorbid states.

The primary prevention of cardiogenic brain emboli is discussed under Cardiovascular Medicine [see Chapters 3 and 5].

In 1986, the National Conference sponsored by the American College of Chest Physicians and the National Heart, Lung and Blood Institute issued the following recommendations concerning the use of anticoagulant therapy in patients with recurrent cerebral emboli: "For the prevention of recurrent bland (aseptic) emboli to the brain, it is recommended that heparin followed by warfarin therapy, at a dose that prolongs the prothrombin time to an INR of 3.0 to 4.5 (1.5 to 2.0 times the control prothrombin time using rabbit-brain thromboplastin), be instituted in nonhypertensive patients with small to moderate-sized embolic strokes in whom a computed tomographic scan done 24 hours or more after stroke onset documents the absence of spontaneous hemorrhagic transformation. Anticoagulant therapy should be postponed several days in patients with large embolic strokes or severe hypertension (who are prone to late hemorrhagic transformation). Anticoagulant therapy should be postponed 18 days in patients with embolic strokes complicated by hemorrhagic transformation.

"In native valve endocarditis, anticoagulants are not recommended for the primary prevention of stroke. If a cardiogenic brain embolus does occur, and if a CT scan confirms the absence of hemorrhagic transformation and arteriography confirms the absence of mycotic aneurysm, the recommendations for bland emboli apply.

"In mechanical and prosthetic valve endocarditis, it is recommended that the prior anticoagulant therapy be continued. If a cardiogenic brain embolus does occur, it is recommended that anticoagulants be stopped for 48 hours and a CT scan and arteriography be performed. If the CT scan confirms the absence of hemorrhagic transformation and arteriography confirms the absence of mycotic aneurysm, the recommendations for bland emboli apply." Decisions regarding the use of antithrombotic therapy should be based on a consideration of comorbid states and the overall status of the patient.

It is difficult to predict which patients will suffer secondary brain hemorrhage after cardioembolic stroke. Data indicate that large infarct size increases the risk of this complication. Spontaneous hemorrhagic transformation may be missed by CT examination performed at an early stage, that is, within 12 hours of stroke onset. Initiation of anticoagulation therapy at this early stage may lead to clinical worsening in patients predisposed to spontaneous hemorrhagic transformation.

Recurrent cerebral emboli in patients with nonrheumatic atrial fibrillation can be prevented through the use of long-term warfarin therapy at a dose adjusted to maintain the prothrombin time at 1.2 to 1.5 times the control value.[53]

Surgical evacuation of hematomas should be weighed in noncomatose patients with cerebellar hemorrhage and in patients with superficial cerebral hematomas causing progressive signs of temporal lobe herniation.

Recovery Phase

Physical therapy should be started as soon as possible to prevent contractures. Special attention should also be paid to the urinary and digestive systems; bladder problems include urinary retention with infection or incontinence that leads to macerated skin and decubitus ulcer. Condom or catheter drainage, frequent turning, and water mattresses will help alleviate these problems. Fecal impaction may lead to agitation, tachycardia, and fever—manifestations that are often misdiagnosed as sepsis. Insights into the management of stroke patients are provided in the personal account of Howell.[54]

Prognosis

The ultimate prognosis depends largely on the extent of brain tissue damage. In massive cerebral hemorrhage, nearly 80 percent of patients succumb during the acute illness; the mortality is far lower in patients with ischemic stroke. In the peri-ictal period, cerebral edema accounts for one third of the deaths, and cardiac or pulmonary failure is responsible for the other two thirds.

Subarachnoid Hemorrhage

Bleeding into the cerebrospinal fluid may occur in a variety of instances. Conditions to consider include ruptured congenital or mycotic aneurysm, extension from parenchymatous hemorrhage, primary bleeding disorders, leukemia, anticoagulation therapy, hemorrhagic encephalitis, and hemorrhage from a tumor or arteriovenous malformation, including one in the spinal canal. Ruptured congenital aneurysm accounts for the majority of cases. There are several common intracranial sites at which aneurysms form [see Figure 3].

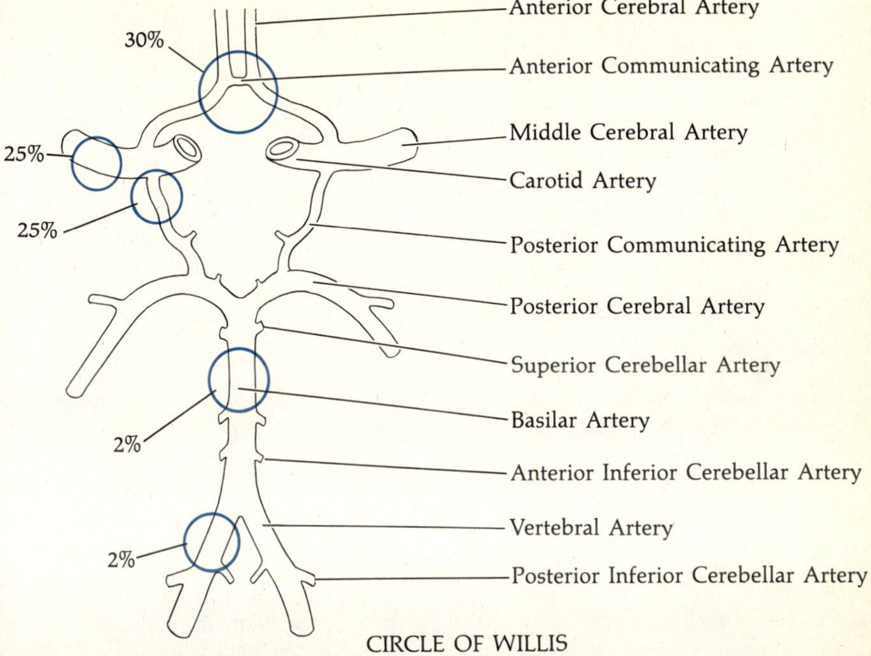

Figure 3 *Most cerebral aneurysms occur in or near the circle of Willis. Fifty percent occur in the middle cerebral artery and in the posterior communicating artery. The region where the anterior communicating artery joins the anterior cerebral arteries accounts for another 30 percent. Additional sites are the basilar artery and the vertebral artery. Colored circles mark common aneurysm sites.*

Aneurysm may occur at any age; middle age is the most common time for rupture. The probability of rupture is small when the aneurysm is less than 1 cm in diameter.[55] Approximately 50 percent of patients will experience a warning leak before aneurysm rupture.[56] The leak generally occurs a few days to one month before the catastrophic event and produces abrupt-onset headache, nausea and vomiting, photophobia, meningism, and, occasionally, focal neurologic signs that depend in character on the location of the aneurysm. The diagnosis is rarely made until frank rupture of the aneurysm, when the patient presents with a sudden violent headache (the worst ever experienced), followed rapidly by confusion and agitation, collapse, and coma. There may be no focal neurologic signs. Nuchal rigidity and other signs of meningeal irritation will be present, and the finding of grossly bloody spinal fluid under increased pressure will confirm the diagnosis. Hypertension often develops, and subhyaloid hemorrhages are commonly seen in the fundus. Fever and leukocytosis result from meningeal irritation. Hyperglycemia and glycosuria may appear transiently. Xanthochromia develops in the spinal fluid within four hours, which distinguishes subarachnoid hemorrhage from traumatic spinal tap.

On occasion, large aneurysms will produce focal neurologic signs that lead to a correct diagnosis before rupture. Aneurysms of the intracavernous portion of the carotid artery may compress adjacent cranial nerves III, IV, and VI, leading to various degrees of ophthalmoparesis and ptosis. The carotid artery may also compress the ophthalmic division of cranial nerve V, causing pain and hypalgesia over the forehead. Aneurysms of the posterior communicating artery may compress the nearby third nerve. Aneurysms of the basilar artery may produce symptoms of vertebrobasilar insufficiency, tic douloureux, or facial spasm.

There are two major complications of subarachnoid hemorrhage from a ruptured aneurysm: rebleeding and cerebral vasospasm. Both occur with a peak incidence between the first and second week after the primary event. Vasospasm with cerebral ischemia is now recognized as the most prevalent and serious complication and the major cause of death. Vasospasm occurs in approximately one third of patients. It is most likely to develop in patients who are receiving antifibrinolytic drugs and in those in whom CT scans reveal thick, focal collections of subarachnoid blood.[57] Cerebral ischemia is also seen more frequently in patients with hyponatremia, another common complication of subarachnoid hemorrhage probably related to inappropriate secretion of antidiuretic hormone and elevated levels of plasma atrial natriuretic factor.[58,59]

When a diagnosis of subarachnoid hemorrhage is made, angiography and subsequent neurosurgical treatment should be performed as soon as the patient's condition permits, with the goal of preventing rebleeding. Medical management consists of measures to prevent or ameliorate vasospasm and cerebral ischemia. A CT scan should be performed to assess the risk of vasospasm. The CT scan will also reveal the presence of secondary hydrocephalus, which may require treatment.[60] Transcranial Doppler ultrasonography is also useful in predicting impending vasospasm; an increase in flow velocity in the middle or posterior cerebral arteries on the order of 200 cm/sec is a forewarning of cerebral ischemia.[21]

Several studies have now confirmed the value of nimodipine in reducing the risk of vasospasm.[61,62] This lipophilic calcium channel blocker appears to have a predilection for dilating cerebral blood vessels, and it is given at a dose of 60 mg every four hours for 21 days. Hypervolemic hemodilution using plasma expanders, with a goal of reducing the hematocrit to about 35 percent and raising the central venous pressure to 10 to 12 mm Hg, has also been advocated.[63] Transluminal angioplasty has been reported to restore intracranial vessel diameter and improve neurologic function. Antifibrinolytic therapy, in vogue in the early 1980s, has been implicated as a causative factor in cerebral ischemia and has not been effective in reducing the incidence of rebleeding. It is no longer recommended.

The ultimate outcome in well-managed cases of ruptured aneurysm is still unsatisfactory: less than half of patients who were initially considered to be good risks experience a complete recovery.[64]

Arteriovenous malformations (AVMs) of the brain, although congenital, usually go undetected until adult years. In most series, the mean age of presentation is about 35 years. Approximately 50 percent of patients will present with intracerebral or intraventricular hemorrhage; recurrence of hemorrhage may be expected at any time thereafter. An annual rate of recurrent hemorrhage of four percent was found in a population-based study of virtually all patients with known AVMs in Finland.[65] In this series, combined annual mortality and severe neurologic morbidity was 2.7 percent. These annual rates remained constant over a mean follow-up period of 24 years. Angiographic features that appear to predict hemorrhage from an AVM are a periventricular or intraventricular location and a system of drainage through central rather than superficial veins.[66] Accessible lesions may be removed surgically or treated by intravascular embolization techniques.[67] Lesions not amenable to these approaches may be treated by stereotactic heavy-charged particle radiation. In a series at Stanford, the obliteration rate three years after radiation ranged from 100 percent for small ($< 4\,\text{cm}^3$) lesions to 70 percent for large ($> 25\,\text{cm}^3$) lesions.[68] Disadvantages of this form of treatment are the occurrences of either delayed radionecrosis of white matter or rebleeding from malformations undergoing obliteration in approximately 20 percent of patients.

Hypertensive Encephalopathy

Hypertensive encephalopathy generally develops in response to rapid elevation of systemic blood pressure and is thought to result from failure of autoregulation of cerebral blood flow. The syndrome is most commonly encountered in patients with chronic hypertension. In such patients, a diastolic blood pressure of 150 mm Hg is often required to produce symptoms, whereas patients with acute hypertension (e.g., from eclampsia, glomerulonephritis, or drugs) may become symptomatic with a diastolic pressure of 100 mm Hg.[69] There is rapid development of confusion and toxic delirium, often accompanied by myoclonic twitching or convulsion, which may progress to a state of stupor or coma. Focal neurologic signs, such as aphasia, hemiparesis, or cortical blindness, may be present. There is a prodrome of increasingly severe headaches, which are characteristically occipital and are worse in the early morning. These features resemble those of headaches caused by increased intracranial pressure. Examination reveals elevation of diastolic blood pressure, retinal hemorrhages and exudates, papilledema, and focal neurologic signs.

Treatment consists of rapid lowering of blood pressure. Sodium nitroprusside is the drug of choice. It is recommended that during the first hour of treatment, the mean arterial blood pressure should be reduced by 20 to 25 percent or to a diastolic level of 100 mm Hg, whichever is higher.[69] Increased intracranial pressure may result from cerebral edema and should be treated with dexamethasone, 4 mg intravenously every six hours. Generalized convulsions should be treated with phenytoin, 500 to 1,000 mg intravenously, at a rate of 50 mg/min.

Cerebral Arteritis

Inflammatory intracranial arteritis may be seen in patients with giant cell arteritis, collagen vascular disease, herpes zoster, Hodgkin's disease, sarcoidosis, syphilis, tuberculosis, or the acquired immunodeficiency syndrome (AIDS).[70] It may also occur as a primary neurologic illness known as isolated angiitis of the central nervous system.[71] This uncommon condition usually begins with a waxing-and-waning encephalopathic syndrome of headaches, confusion, and intellectual decline, which progresses in weeks or months to include focal events related to cerebral or spinal infarction. The diagnosis is aided by cerebral angiography, which reveals multifocal segmental narrowing of medium-sized arteries, and by leptomeningeal biopsy, which reveals a mononuclear cell infiltrate. Establishing the diagnosis of isolated angiitis of the central nervous system is important because vigorous immunosuppression provides successful therapy. Recommended treatment consists of prednisone, 40 to 60 mg, and cyclophosphamide, 100 to 150 mg, daily orally. Treatment is continued until the patient is symptom free for at least one year.

Giant Cell Arteritis

Giant cell arteritis is by far the most important inflammatory arteritis affecting the nervous system. It deserves special emphasis because blindness is a frequent complication in untreated cases. Blindness and the various neurologic complaints (neuropathy, TIA, vertigo, and depression) associated with active disease may be prevented by adequate doses of prednisone.[72,73] The disease, also known as temporal arteritis, affects elderly persons of either sex but is somewhat more common in women. It rarely begins before 50 years of age and has an annual incidence of 17 per 100,000 in the population of individuals older than 50 years.

Early symptoms of systemic illness are low-grade fever, anorexia with weight loss, fatigue, and depression. Headache, usually nonspecific in character, occurs in most cases and is frequently the symptom for which medical assistance is sought. At times, patients have more specific complaints of scalp tenderness or painful nodules. The syndrome of polymyalgia rheumatica refers to symptoms of muscle and joint stiffness and pain, most prominently located in the shoulder and hip girdles. True weakness is rarely present. Many patients complain of claudication of the jaw muscles while chewing or talking. This striking symptom is often considered pathognomonic of giant cell arteritis.

These systemic symptoms are commonly present for weeks or months before the diagnosis is made. Unfortunately, the nature of the illness often goes unsuspected until the patient loses vision in one eye. Visual loss generally occurs abruptly and without pain. It results from ischemic optic neuritis from obliterative arteritis of branches of the ophthalmic artery. In a small percentage of cases, visual loss is bilateral.

Physical examination may disclose tender nodular swellings of arteries in the scalp. Bruits may sometimes be heard over the carotid and femoral arteries and the abdominal aorta. Optic disk edema is present for the first few days after onset of blindness; optic atrophy eventually develops.

The most important screening test is measurement of the erythrocyte sedimentation rate (ESR), which is elevated in a great many cases. A mild anemia is found in 40 percent of cases. Serum α-globulins and fibrinogen are often elevated, but these changes are not specific.

Once giant cell arteritis is suspected, treatment with prednisone should be started at a daily dosage of 40 to 60 mg orally. A generous portion of the temporal artery should be biopsied, and a histologic study should then be performed to confirm the diagnosis.

Symptomatic improvement should be observable within a few days; the ESR will return to normal within one or two weeks. Loss of vision is irreversible. The duration of treatment is somewhat arbitrary, but recurrences are common when prednisone is discontinued prematurely. It has been suggested that a gradual reduction in dose be attempted when the clinical and laboratory signs of inflammation have completely subsided and that a maintenance dosage be continued for a minimum of six to eight months.[74]

References

1. N Engl J Med 293:954, 1975
2. JAMA 264:1267, 1990
3. N Engl J Med 318:937, 1988
4. JAMA 259:1025, 1988
5. Arch Intern Med 149:2053, 1989
6. JAMA 255:2311, 1986
7. N Engl J Med 315:1041, 1986
8. N Engl J Med 319:267, 1988
9. N Engl J Med 320:904, 1989
10. Arch Intern Med 146:73, 1986
11. Ann Neurol 25:221, 1989
12. N Engl J Med 323:1556, 1990
13. Neurology 39:30, 1989
14. Arch Neurol 47:458, 1990
15. N Engl J Med 323:699, 1990
16. Stroke 15:413, 1984
17. Ann Intern Med 110:992, 1989
18. Ann Neurol 27:606, 1990
19. Ann Neurol 27:612, 1990
20. N Engl J Med 302:1349, 1980
21. Neurology 40:696, 1990
22. Stroke 18:997, 1987
23. N Engl J Med 318:1148, 1988
24. N Engl J Med 323:1698, 1990
25. N Engl J Med 317:1505, 1987
26. Ann Intern Med 111:660, 1989
27. Arch Neurol 47:441, 1990
28. N Engl J Med 325:445, 1991
29. Lancet 337:1235, 1991
30. JAMA 266:3289, 1991
31. JAMA 266:3332, 1991
32. N Engl J Med 318:721, 1988
33. Arch Neurol 44:651, 1987
34. JAMA 257:2043, 1987
35. Br Med J 296:316, 1988
36. Stroke 16:406, 1985
37. Lancet 1:1215, 1989
38. N Engl J Med 321:501, 1989
39. Stroke 16:797, 1985
40. N Engl J Med 319:1246, 1988
41. Stroke 21:984, 1990
42. N Engl J Med 315:860, 1986
43. JAMA 258:2704, 1987
44. J Am Coll Cardiol 12:1515, 1988
45. Arch Neurol 46:418, 1989
46. J Neurosurg 72:195, 1990
47. Arch Intern Med 146:66, 1986
48. JAMA 263:65, 1990
49. Ann Intern Med 111:449, 1989
50. Neurology 39:262, 1989
51. N Engl J Med 318:203, 1988
52. Ann Neurol 25:398, 1989
53. N Engl J Med 323:1505, 1990
54. Br Med J 289:35, 1984
55. N Engl J Med 304:696, 1981
56. Br Med J 301:190, 1990
57. Neurology 37:1586, 1987
58. Ann Neurol 27:106, 1990

59. Stroke 19:1119, 1988
60. Arch Neurol 46:744, 1989
61. N Engl J Med 308:619, 1983
62. J Neurosurg 68:505, 1988
63. Stroke 18:365, 1987
64. J Neurosurg 60:909, 1984
65. J Neurosurg 73:387, 1990
66. Radiology 176:807, 1990
67. Neurosurgery 26:570, 1990
68. N Engl J Med 323:96, 1990
69. N Engl J Med 323:1177, 1990
70. Arch Neurol 45:514, 1988
71. Neurology 39:167, 1989
72. Neurology 38:352, 1988
73. Am J Med 89:67, 1990
74. Medicine (Baltimore) 50:1, 1971

Acknowledgments

Figures 1 through 3   Carol Donner.

A portion of the text under "Management of Stroke" (page 855) has been excerpted from "Cerebral Embolism," by D. G. Sherman, M. L. Dyken, M. Fisher, et al, in *Chest* 89(suppl 2):82S, 1986. Reprinted by permission.

GEORGE P. CANELLOS, M.D.

Many medical emergencies that confront patients with cancer can be treated successfully if they are recognized and treated promptly. The complications described here arise from a wide variety of malignant conditions originating in different primary sites; however, the successful treatment of these various emergencies is to a large extent independent of the cancer that is involved.

Superior Vena Cava Obstruction

Acute or subacute obstruction of the superior vena cava (SVC) is a complication of progressive tumor growth in the right anterior-superior region of the mediastinum. The SVC is particularly vulnerable to obstruction because of its anatomic location: it is confined by the sternum and the right main bronchus, and it is surrounded by the lymph nodes that drain the right side of the thoracic cavity and the lower part of the left side of the chest. In addition, the SVC is thin walled and has a low venous pressure. Obstruction is caused either by compression of the SVC by tumorous lymph nodes or by direct invasion of the vessel wall by the neoplasm, both of which can result in thrombosis. Thrombosis is seen in one third to one half of patients with SVC obstruction examined at postmortem.

About 85 percent of the cases of SVC obstruction are caused by carcinoma of the lung; almost half of such cases are due to small cell undifferentiated lung cancer, a tumor that characteristically originates centrally and invades locally.[1] However, SVC obstruction occurs in only three to eight percent of patients who have lung cancer. Approximately 10 to 15 percent of cases of SVC obstruction are caused by malignant lymphoma, usually large cell non-Hodgkin's lymphoma.

Nonneoplastic causes of SVC obstruction include idiopathic sclerosing mediastinitis, primary venous thrombosis, and thrombus formation and fibrosis around a central venous catheter, especially in patients who have pacemakers.[2]

Diagnosis

SVC obstruction can be recognized by shortness of breath, which is the most common presenting feature, and by edema of the face, trunk, or upper extremities. Edema of the face and tachypnea occur in one third to one half of patients. Chest pain, cough, and dysphagia, which are caused by edema of the deeper structures of the chest, such as the esophagus, trachea, and bronchi, are less common presenting symptoms. Hoarseness may result from edema of the vocal cords. The increase in cerebral venous pressure can induce somnolence, nausea, syncope, headache, convulsions, and coma. The patient is likely to have distention of neck veins and collateral veins in the chest wall. Other symptoms include cyanosis and Horner's syndrome (anhidrosis, ptosis, miosis, and enophthalmos caused by paralysis of the cervical sympathetic nerves).[2,3] Spinal cord compression is often associated with superior vena cava obstruction (see below).

The clinical diagnosis of SVC obstruction is usually obvious and requires little further investigation. A chest x-ray visualizes the obstruction in almost all patients with the condition. Tomography or CT scanning is rarely needed for visualizing the right superior mediastinum. Additional diagnostic procedures are required, however, to determine the histopathologic type of the cancer, which dictates the choice of therapy for the SVC obstruction. Most patients with SVC obstruction have lung cancer, and the procedures used to detect lung cancer—sputum cytologic studies, bronchoscopy, and bronchial washings—will also identify the cause of SVC obstruction in 70 percent of cases. Invasive techniques such as venography, bronchoscopy, and mediastinoscopy can be hazardous for patients with raised venous pressure and should be deferred until after the SVC obstruction is relieved.[2,3] A thoracotomy can definitively establish the diagnosis once symptoms are relieved.

Management

The histopathologic type of the tumor determines the mode of treatment. Patients whose SVC obstruction is caused by lymphoma or small cell carcinoma of the lung can be treated initially with combination chemotherapy; the injections must not be given into obstructed arm veins. Irradiation should be used when the histopathologic type of the tumor is uncertain or when the obstruction must be rapidly relieved. Patients with SVC obstruction caused by lymphoma require lower doses of irradiation and achieve higher response rates than do those whose obstruction is caused by other malignant disorders. Irradiation for SVC obstruction caused by lymphoma is usually given in two or four high-dose fractions (2,000 to 4,000 rads).[4] Symptoms are completely resolved in at least 75 percent of lymphoma patients and in 20 percent of lung cancer patients. Symptoms are relieved in 75 percent of patients in three to four days and in almost 90 percent in seven days. An objective response can take up to 14 days; some improvement occurs during the first week of irradiation.[3,4]

Patients refractory to irradiation may have thrombosis of the SVC and require thrombolytic therapy or surgical diversion of the venous system. Surgical diversion, however, involves considerable morbidity and mortality and should only be used as a last resort.

Spinal Cord Compression

Spinal cord compression in patients with neoplastic disease is a medical emergency that requires prompt diagnosis and therapy to prevent neurologic damage. In more than 95 percent of cases, compression is caused either by extension of a metastatic lesion located in a vertebral body, which is usually associated with breast, prostate, or lung cancer or with multiple myeloma; by direct metastatic spread via the presacral venous plexus, which is associated with prostate and gastrointestinal tumors; or by direct extension of a tumor through the intervertebral foramina from paraspinous lymph nodes, which is associated with lymphomas. Most cases of spinal cord compression occur in the upper thoracic segment, which is the largest component of the spine.[5]

The quartet of symptoms that typically characterize spinal cord compression is pain, weakness or paralysis, autonomic dysfunction, and sensory loss. Such symptoms can develop months or years after the initial diagnosis of cancer. Prodromal symptoms such as central back pain, with or without a radicular component, may be present for weeks. Radicular pain occurs more commonly when cervical or lumbrosacral regions of the spinal cord are compressed than when the thoracic region is affected. When the compression does involve the thoracic region, the radicular pain is usually bilateral.

Pain from a herniated disk can be differentiated from pain due to spinal cord compression by having the patient lie flat: this position usually eases pain from a herniated disk but worsens pain from an epidural tumor. In addition, weakness, sensory loss, and autonomic dysfunction are less common presenting features of a herniated disk.

Compression of the upper thoracic segment is often associated with compromise of the uniquely vulnerable vascular supply of the spinal cord, which results in infarction. Metastases to upper cervical vertebrae can cause weakness in the upper extremities and can lead to respiratory failure. Metastases to the conus medullaris and cauda equina may cause saddle-type anesthesia, which leads to loss of urethral, rectal, and vaginal sensation and of bowel and bladder function. Patients who develop bowel and bladder dysfunction have a particularly poor prognosis; the majority of these patients become paraparetic or paraplegic. Sensory changes that evolve to loss of sensation are observed prior to the development of paraplegia.

Diagnosis

The diagnosis of spinal cord compression must be confirmed by radiographic studies because clinical examination usually underestimates the degree of compression. An x-ray of the spinal column visualizes abnormalities such as erosion of the pedicles, vertebral body collapse, and paraspinal masses in more than three quarters of patients[6]; about 15 percent of patients will have no osseous abnormality. Myelography is essential for planning proper therapy because it can visualize epidural deposits and the upper and lower limits of the compression; however, lumbar puncture can increase paresis in about 10 percent or less of patients and may require immediate surgical intervention. A CT scan of the spine can confirm bone destruction visualized by roentgenography, and it may be the only diagnostic technique that can be used when myelography is contraindicated, such as when the patient is allergic to the imaging dye.

Management

High doses of steroids (60 mg prednisone or 16 mg dexamethasone), which are administered daily or as needed, are used to reduce the acute swelling of the spinal cord and to reduce postoperative or postradiation edema.

The appropriate local therapy, either irradiation or surgery, is determined by the histologic classification of the tumor, the location and duration of the spinal block, the rapidity of the development of symptoms, and the extent of neurologic impairment. Patients who have slowly developing or minimal neurologic symptoms, an incomplete block (as detected by myelography), or involvement of the cauda equina by itself can be treated with radiation therapy alone. Laminectomy followed by irradiation should be performed for all other patients with spinal cord obstruction; however, it is not clear whether surgery and irradiation are superior to irradiation alone for most patients. Irradiation might be sufficient therapy for cord compression caused by tumors that are especially responsive to radiation therapy, such as lymphomas.

Patients who are likely to respond to local treatment include those who are ambulatory at the outset of therapy, those whose symptoms progress slowly (longer than three days) without complete compression of the cord, those who retain sphincter tone, and those whose lesions are in the distal thoracic segment (T5 to T12). Surgery is more successful for lower than for upper thoracic regions. Patients who develop paraplegia or prolonged loss of sphincter tone respond poorly to treatment; less than 10 percent of such patients regain ambulation. Almost half of patients who have compressive lesions in vertebrae T5 to T12 regain ambulation, compared with 25 percent of those with compressive lesions in vertebrae T1 to T4.[5]

Chemotherapy may complement surgery or irradiation but should not be used as a primary treatment. A rare form of paraplegia that is seen in oncology practice is a necrotizing myelopathy following intrathecal administration of methotrexate or cytarabine. One pathologic abnormality caused by such treatment is microvascular obstruction in the white matter of the cord.[7]

Other Neurologic Complications

Expanding metastatic tumors within the brain or surrounding structures commonly complicate the course of lung and breast cancer and carcinomas of unknown etiology. The incidence of metastases to the brain is increasing, perhaps because of improvements in the management of other systemic metastases with agents that cannot cross the blood-brain barrier, as in the case of small cell lung cancer. Brain metastases can occur late in the course of disease, but they can also be the presenting feature, as in occult lung cancer.

The frontal lobe of the cerebrum is the most common site of involvement, followed by the temporal, parietal, and occipital lobes. The most common presenting features include impaired mental function, lethargy, loss of motor function, focal neurologic defects, and seizures.

Other complications involving the CNS include meningeal carcinomatosis and paraneoplastic syndromes. The most common symptoms of meningeal carcinomatosis include headache, cranial neuropathy, and stiff neck. Paraneoplastic syndromes are usually chronic. Very rarely, acute cerebral embolism develops in cancer patients as a result of nonbacterial thrombotic (marantic) endocarditis, which occurs in patients with carcinoma of the pancreas, stomach, lung, and other organs and tissues.[8]

Diagnosis

The CT scan is the most useful diagnostic test for detecting metastatic brain tumors, except in cases of meningeal carcinomatosis or lymphomatosis. In these two instances, spinal fluid analysis for tumor cells or for elevated protein and glucose is usually diagnostic; cytologic findings are less likely to be positive for carcinomatosis than for lymphomatosis. Caution is required when performing a spinal tap in patients with increased cranial pressure—sudden reduction of spinal fluid pressure could result in herniation of the cerebellum through the foramen magnum, which can result in fatal compression of the brainstem.

Management

Treatment of acute increased intracranial pressure caused by a neoplasm is treated by (1) maintaining airway and intravenous access, (2) restricting the extent of hydration, (3) administering large doses of steroids, such as 20 to 40 mg of methylprednisolone and 16 mg of dexamethasone, and (4) by administering an anticonvulsant, such as phenytoin. A marked increase in intracranial pressure and clinical deterioration necessitate more aggressive dehydration therapy using diuretics and intravenous administration of hypertonic mannitol.

Radiation therapy is the usual palliative treatment of intracranial lesions. Palliative doses, typically 3,000 rads administered over two weeks, reduce or eliminate headaches in half of patients and reduce motor defects in about one third. When the brain is the only site of metastatic disease, higher doses are justified because they may prolong survival. The functional status of the patient, extent of CNS involvement, and sensitivity of the tumor to irradiation determine whether a patient will respond to irradiation. Even so, approximately one half of patients receiving radiation therapy will develop fatal recurrences of their CNS tumor within 20 to 40 weeks.[9]

Surgery may be appropriate for patients with only one metastatic lesion that is located in either accessible or so-called silent areas of the brain and when systemic disease is absent or under good control with therapy. Intrathecal administration of chemotherapeutic agents rather than surgery is required when the meninges are involved. Methotrexate (up to 20 mg), cytarabine (100 mg), and rarely, thiotepa are the only antitumor agents that can be administered intrathecally. These agents are administered twice weekly until the spinal fluid is cleared of malignant cells. The use of an Ommaya reservoir may be necessary for administering the drugs into the cerebral subarachnoid space.

Craniospinal irradiation may be required for meningeal carcinomatosis. However, meningeal carcinomatosis is more difficult to manage than hematologic neoplasms that have spread to the meninges because the former is less sensitive to irradiation and chemotherapeutic agents.

Hypercalcemia

Hypercalcemia of malignancy was first recognized in the 1920s and has emerged as the most common cause of hypercalcemia among hospitalized patients; most patients with primary hyperparathyroidism, the other main cause of hypercalcemia, are asymptomatic and are diagnosed as outpatients. Hypercalcemia can produce serious morbidity in the course of some malignant diseases such as carcinomas of the breast and lung, epidermoid cancers of the head and neck and of the esophagus, multiple myeloma, and hypernephroma[10,11]; it occurs most commonly in patients with multiple myeloma (in 20 to 30 percent of patients). Hypercalcemia can appear abruptly and, unless reversed, can be fatal.

Two mechanisms are responsible for hypercalcemia of malignancy. In one mechanism, local osteolytic activity is induced by the presence of metastatic tumor cells in bone; this complication is especially seen in patients with breast cancer or multiple myeloma. In the second mechanism, hypercalcemia is mediated by humoral factors that have not been definitively characterized (see below); this second form, which is termed ectopic humoral hypercalcemia, is seen in patients with squamous cell cancer of the head and neck, bladder and ovarian cancers, hypernephroma, and rarely, lymphoma. Both mechanisms induce bone resorption and mobilization of skeletal calcium by activating the osteoclast. Rates of normal mineralization of bones and osteoblastic activity are also reduced.

Ongoing research has sought to define the factors mediating humoral hypercalcemia. Factors that have been considered include osteoclast-activating factors, calcitriol, prostaglandins, and parathyroid hormone; however, the evidence supporting parathyroid hormone and prostaglandins is scant or controversial.[12-17]

The rapid onset of hypercalcemia and the high serum calcium levels seen in patients with neoplastic disease result in nausea, vomiting, anorexia, lethargy, confusion, stupor, and coma. The symptoms of primary hyperparathyroidism, such as renal calculi, band keratopathy, pruritus, hypertension, and GI symptoms, are not often present in hypercalcemia of malignancy.

A secondary effect associated with hypercalcemia mediated by an osteolytic tumor involves interference with the urinary concentrating mechanism, which results in polyuria, dehydration, reduced glomerular filtration rate, and reduced renal calcium excretion. Immobilization and hypophosphatemia increase the release of skeletal calcium.

Management

The aim of therapy is to decrease calcium mobilization from bone and to increase urinary calcium excretion; the degree of therapy is determined by the serum level of calcium: the greater the calcium level, the more intense the therapy. In addition, the specific therapy is determined by the histologic type of the tumor and the clinical status of the patient. Plasma volume, which is usually depleted in patients with hypercalcemia, can be restored, and urinary flow can be increased by hourly infusion of 200 to 300 ml of saline; serum potassium and magnesium levels must be monitored during the infusion.

Mild hypercalcemia ($\leq$ 12.5 mg/dl) in asymptomatic patients can be controlled by ambulation and oral hydration with 3 l of saline a day. Moderately symptomatic patients who have serum calcium levels between 12.5 and 14.0 mg/dl require 3 to 6 l of saline a day. Hydration alone will reduce the serum calcium level by 2 to 3 mg/dl in 24 to 48 hours.[18]

After hydration, moderately symptomatic patients should be treated with furosemide, 40 to 80 mg every 12 to 24 hours, to augment urinary calcium loss caused by saline infusion. When no response to furosemide is seen by 24 hours, either calcitonin (4 MRC units/kg, subcutaneously every six to 12 hours) or plicamycin (I.V. infusion of 25 μg/kg in 50 ml of five percent dextrose over three hours) should be administered. Other adjuvant measures include glucocorticoids (40 to 60 mg prednisone/day) in patients who have hematologic neoplasms or, possibly, breast cancer, for their direct antitumor effect. Prostaglandin synthesis inhibitors, as noted, are rarely useful. Dialysis may be considered for patients who are refractory to treatment and whose renal function is deteriorating. Diphosphonates, which are potent inhibitors of osteoclastic bone resorption, effectively reduce or prevent hypercalcemia of malignancy when administered orally or parenterally; however, the more active, parenterally administered derivatives, dichloromethylene diphosphonate (Cl_2MDP) and aminohydroxypropylidene diphosphonate (ADP), are not yet available in the United States.[19,20]

Long-term management of hypercalcemia entails restriction of calcium and vitamin D intake, mobilization, and in some cases, oral phosphate therapy: usually, phosphate preparations containing 500 to 1,500 mg/day of elemental phosphorus are given in divided doses in patients with serum phosphate levels less than 2.5 to 3.0 mg/dl. Intravenous administration of phosphate is hazardous, however, because of the risk of massive calcium phosphate deposition in tissues.[21] A reduction of the tumor burden is required for all patients to effect durable control of hypercalcemia.

Renal Complications

Renal complications of neoplastic disease are caused either by direct invasion of the kidney by the tumor or by damage from tumor products or chemotherapeutic agents.

Tumor Invasion

Acute renal failure is an unusual complication of renal invasion by a tumor. Gradual deterioration of renal function occurs more commonly and is seen occasionally in patients with acute lymphoblastic leukemia or non-Hodgkin's lymphoma; it is usually caused by bilateral invasion by the tumor. Radiographic studies demonstrate enlarged kidneys, and autopsy examination commonly reveals renal infiltration in such patients; however, infiltration rarely leads to renal failure or even gradual deterioration of renal function. Renal infiltration may respond to antitumor therapy.[22]

Extensive retroperitoneal cancer can lead to ureteral obstruction and, secondarily, to uropathy and uremia, especially when obstruction occurs bilaterally; uremia caused by ureteral obstruction commonly leads to death in patients with advanced cancer of the cervix and, occasionally, with other types of tumors. Surgical ureteral diversion, followed by pelvic irradiation, when possible, is the standard treatment of ureteral obstruction; however, use of such vigorous therapy should be tempered by consideration of the condition and prognosis of the patient.

Tumor Products

Renal failure is a complication of plasma cell myeloma that follows from glomerular damage caused by light-chain fragments (Bence Jones proteins) and from precipitation of immunoglobulin components within the renal tubules [*see Chapter 16*]. Dehydration and acidification of the urine are the most likely predisposing factors. Treatment involves adequate hydration (including nocturnal supplements) and long-term alkalinization of the urine. In addition, careful hydration is necessary during intravenous urography to decrease the likelihood of renal failure.

Acute hyperuricemic nephropathy was formerly a complication of hematologic neoplasms, especially when treatment of the tumor killed a large number of tumor cells. Currently, administration of 300 to 800 mg/day of allopurinol, in combination with hydration and urinary alkalinization, has effectively prevented serious renal damage from the precipitation of uric acid crystals within the renal tubules, medulla, and collecting ducts. Because allopurinol inhibits the conversion of xanthine to uric acid, allopurinol administration can occasionally lead to renal failure by causing the formation of xanthine stones. Hydration and alkalinization can prevent this complication, however, because xanthine is more soluble in alkaline urine.

Hypercalcemia can also lead to renal failure [*see* Hypercalcemia of Malignancy, *above*]. Although renal calculi and interstitial calcification are rarely seen in acute-onset hypercalcemia, these complications follow from chronic hypercalcemia.

Chemotherapeutic Agents

The use of some antitumor agents, such as methotrexate, cisplatin, streptozocin, mitomycin, and nitrosoureas, and the use of irradiation have been associated with renal failure. Methotrexate, which is excreted mainly by the kidneys, can precipitate in the renal tubules when administered in high doses; hydration and alkalinization can prevent precipitation. The diminishing role of high-dose methotrexate in the treatment of neoplastic diseases has reduced the problem of methotrexate nephrotoxicity, except in rare circumstances such as the treatment of osteogenic sarcoma. Of the commonly used antineoplastic agents, cisplatin carries the greatest risk of producing renal damage.[23] Cisplatin causes lesions primarily in the proximal tubule, which involves degeneration of tubular cells, thickening of basement membranes, and tubular necrosis. Toxicity is dose related and occurs seven to 14 days after administration. Hydration therapy before administration and avoidance of large boluses have reduced renal toxicity substantially.

Acute hemorrhagic cystitis is a rare complication of cyclophosphamide therapy; it has been seen in patients undergoing either long-term, low-dose oral or high-dose intravenous therapy. Urinary metabolites of cyclophosphamide such as acrolein are also toxic to the bladder mucosa. Cystitis can be prevented, especially in patients receiving high-dose therapy, by the coadministration of thiol compounds such as *N*-acetyl-L-cysteine or sodium 2-mercaptoethanesulfonate (MESNA). Closed bladder drainage with constant irrigation to reduce the concentration of metabolites can be used for treatment in certain patients.[24]

Tumor Lysis Syndrome

Tumor lysis syndrome is caused by the sudden, massive release of cellular constituents following cytolysis of a tumor mass. The predominant compounds released that lead to complications are precursors to uric acid, such as purines; potassium, which is the principal intracellular cation; and phosphate, which is present both as an inorganic salt and covalently bound to various organic molecules.

The tumor lysis syndrome occurs most often following treatment of hematologic neoplasms such as acute lymphoblastic leukemia and Burkitt's lymphoma[25,26] and occasionally following treatment of myeloproliferative diseases and non-Hodgkin's lymphomas. Solid tumors are rarely complicated by the tumor lysis syndrome, except for tumors that are sensitive to chemotherapy or radiation therapy, such as Ewing's sarcoma and small cell carcinoma.

The electrolyte imbalances of the tumor lysis syndrome can lead to serious medical complications. Hyperkalemia (> 6 mEq/l) can cause life-threatening arrhythmias in patients with compromised renal function. Hyperphosphatemia (> 10 mg/dl) can lead to secondary hypocalcemia by causing deposition of calcium phosphate at extraskeletal sites[27]; in addition, the consequent hypocalcemia increases the risk of fatal ventricular arrhythmias from hyperkalemia[28] and can cause neuromuscular symptoms such as cramps and tetany. Hyperuricemia (> 10 mg/dl) [*see* Renal Complications, *above*] and azotemia (elevated blood urea nitrogen and serum creatinine) can also occur.

Renal failure, convulsions, and arrhythmias can usually be prevented by careful hydration and correction of dehydration prior to initiating antineoplastic therapy. Hemodialysis should be considered as an emergency measure if, despite all precautions, the tumor lysis syndrome develops.[29] Infusion of calcium may be required if hypocalcemia becomes symptomatic.

Acute Respiratory Complications

Acute onset of dyspnea is the primary symptom of compromised pulmonary function that can be caused by malignancy or antitumor therapy[30]; it can be caused directly or develop as a consequence of congestive heart failure (as seen after treatment with doxorubicin), cardiac tamponade, or leukostasis. Factors likely to influence the risk of pulmonary toxicity due to antineo-plastic drugs include the total dose administered, the concomitant use of other agents or irradiation, a history of pulmonary disease, and the age of the patient.

Interstitial Pneumonitis

Bleomycin-induced interstitial pneumonitis and fibrosis are the most commonly encountered respiratory complications of antineoplastic therapy; they appear in three to six percent of patients treated with bleomycin and are lethal in less than one percent. Toxicity rarely occurs when the total dose is less than 150 units/m^2, except in patients who are treated with more than one antineoplastic agent. The pneumonitis can appear either as acute diffuse interstitial pneumonitis or as subtle, evolving pulmonary insufficiency; the complications can appear even after cessation of the drug. Other drugs and treatments that can cause interstitial pneumonitis and fibrosis include mitomycin, methotrexate, alkylating agents such as the nitrosoureas (e.g., carmustine), and radiation therapy. Administration of steroids following radiation therapy can result in the development of pneumonitis in rare cases.[31]

The usual symptoms of interstitial pneumonitis include the insidious onset of a nonproductive cough, dyspnea, tachypnea, diffuse rales, and occasionally, fever that appears four to 10 weeks after the start of antineoplastic therapy. A biopsy of the lung shows alveolar damage, organizing interstitial pneumonitis, loss of type I pneumocytes, and proliferation of fibroblasts and type II pneumocytes. X-rays visualize diffuse linear densities in the lower lung fields.[32,33]

Incipient toxicity can be detected by measuring the diffusion capacity of the lung for carbon monoxide (D_{Lco}) or by a gallium-67 scan of the lung. A drop in D_{Lco} greater than 25 percent warrants withdrawal of the drug. The gallium scan can detect early stages of pneumonitis that are not detected on the x-ray; however, the diffuse uptake of the radionuclide is not specific for bleomycin-induced pneumonitis.

The clinical and radiographic features of antineoplastic agent–induced interstitial pneumonitis are difficult to distinguish from pneumonia caused by *Pneumocystis carinii*; biopsy of the lung may be required to rule out *P. carinii* pneumonia.[34]

Administration of steroids is the only available treatment for drug- or radiation-induced pneumonitis, and their effectiveness has not been determined. Although steroids may reverse the acute effects, interstitial and alveolar fibrosis are irreversible.

Leukostatic Pneumopathy

Respiratory failure caused by intravascular leukostasis may occur during the course of acute or chronic granulocytic leukemia.[35-37] Blast cell leukocytosis (> 100,000 cells/mm^2) is usually also present in such patients. Dyspnea and hypoxemia are thought to be caused by an excess of nondeformable myeloblasts, which obstruct capillaries and continue to proliferate within the occluded vessels, leading to septal and alveolar edema.

The symptoms of leukostatic pneumopathy are usually promptly reversed by appropriate antileukemic therapy; however, less than 10 percent of patients do not respond to therapy and succumb to respiratory failure. Leukapheresis and systemic chemotherapy can both rapidly reduce the large number of blast cells.

Acute Cardiac Complications

Pericardial effusion caused by malignancy, most often by direct invasion of the pericardium, can lead to tamponade, sudden reduction in cardiac output, and circulatory collapse. The severity of the tamponade is directly proportional to the rapidity of fluid accumulation[38]; the fluid can be bloody and have a high protein concentration. The only specific test for malignant invasion of the pericardium is positive cytologic findings. In most studies, lung cancer has been found to be the most common cause of pericardial tamponade. Cardiac tamponade is rarely the presenting manifestation of a malignant tumor. The symptoms vary from extreme anxiety to cough, hoarseness, and dysphagia. Pericardial effusion is discussed elsewhere in greater detail [*see Chapter 6*].

Radiation pericarditis is caused by irradiation to a large volume of the heart; it can occur during or many months after therapy has been terminated.[39]

Cardiotoxicity occurs in one to five percent of patients treated with doxorubicin who are receiving a total dose of up to 500 mg/m^2; congestive heart failure usually occurs within a month of cessation of therapy and rarely develops after three years following treatment. Very high doses of cyclophosphamide (> 180 mg/kg), administered alone or with other antineoplastic agents, can lead to acute lethal carditis.[40]

The optimal treatment of neoplastic pericardial tamponade is prompt removal of fluid followed by surgical placement of a pericardial window. Radiotherapy may be useful for reducing the size of the pericardial metastasis in previously untreated patients who have radiosensitive tumors. Intrapericardial instillation of tetracycline or antineoplastic agents has resulted in long-term control of pericardial fluid accumulation.[41]

Hematologic Complications

Most hematologic complications of malignant disease result either from the slow infiltration and replacement of bone marrow by tumor cells or from marrow-suppressive therapy [*see Chapter 15*]. Hematologic cancers are the most common cause of such complications, although some solid tumors, especially metastatic breast cancer, can lead to hematologic complications such as pancytopenia preceded by myelophthisic anemia (leukoerythroblastosis).

Another complication, acute hemolytic anemia, occurs during the course of some lymphoproliferative disorders such as chronic lymphocytic leukemia and small cell lymphocytic lymphoma.[42-44] The anemia usually has an autoimmune basis (i.e., Coombs' positive) and requires prompt institution of steroid therapy. Splenectomy is needed in those rare cases that are refractory to steroids.

An unusual form of microangiopathic hemolytic anemia (MAHA) has been associated with advanced microvascular metastatic disease, especially when there has been extensive pulmonary vascular replacement. This syndrome occurs frequently in patients with adenocarcinoma, usually in those with adenocarcinoma of the gastrointestinal tract. Coagulation studies reveal disseminated intravascular coagulation in only a few patients.[42] Schistocytes in the peripheral blood, hemolysis, reticulocytosis, and anemia occur as preterminal events unless the condition is reversed by chemotherapy.[43] A condition similar to thrombotic thrombocytopenic purpura has been seen in patients receiving antineoplastic chemotherapeutic agents such as mitomycin, cisplatin, bleomycin, and vinca alkaloids.[45-48] Histopatholgic studies reveal thrombi and intimal hyperplasia in the microvasculature and capillary cells with atypical nuclei, thrombi, and fibrin deposits within the glomeruli. This condition is commonly fatal and should be treated rigorously by plasma exchange.

References

1. Cancer 57:847, 1986
2. Mayo Clin Proc 56:407, 1981
3. Semin Oncol 5:123, 1978
4. Cancer Treat Rev 12:209, 1985
5. Semin Oncol 5:135, 1978
6. Cancer 55:2839, 1985
7. Cancer 50:42, 1982
8. Am J Med 54:23, 1973
9. Int J Rad Oncol Biol Phys 6:1, 1980
10. Medicine (Baltimore) 59:262, 1980
11. Cancer 52:2261, 1983
12. N Engl J Med 310:1718, 1984
13. N Engl J Med 309:257, 1983
14. Ann NY Acad Sci 230:240, 1974
15. Ann Intern Med 100:1, 1984
16. N Engl J Med 303:1377, 1980
17. N Engl J Med 309:325, 1983
18. Am J Med 74:475, 1983
19. N Engl J Med 308:1499, 1983
20. Lancet 2:907, 1985
21. Am J Med 74:421, 1983
22. Semin Oncol 5:155, 1978

23. Am J Med 65:307, 1978
24. Cancer Principles & Practice of Oncology. JB Lippincott, Philadelphia, 1985
25. Lancet 1:10, 1973
26. Am J Med 62:283, 1977
27. N Engl J Med 289:1335, 1973
28. Cancer 39:2290, 1977
29. Am J Med 648:486, 1980
30. Oncologic Emergencies. Grune & Stratton, Inc, New York, 1981
31. Ann Intern Med 86:81, 1977
32. Cancer Treat Rev 10:221, 1983
33. JAMA 235:1117, 1976
34. Cancer 55:453, 1985
35. Cancer 51:1808, 1983
36. Am J Med 79:43, 1985
37. Cancer 50:2763, 1982
38. Cancer 45:1697, 1980
39. Semin Oncol 5:181, 1978
40. Arch Intern Med 141:758, 1981
41. J Clin Oncol 2:631, 1984
42. Ann Intern Med 79:368, 1973
43. Medicine (Baltimore) 58:377, 1979
44. Cancer 48:1738, 1981
45. Cancer 45:2252, 1980
46. Eur J Cancer Clin Oncol 20:905, 1984
47. Ann Intern Med 101:41, 1984
48. Cancer Treat Rep 67:429, 1983

38 Respiratory Failure

JAMES W. LEATHERMAN, M.D.
ROLAND H. INGRAM, JR., M.D.

Pathophysiology of Respiratory Failure

Respiratory failure is the inability of the respiratory system to provide adequate oxygenation of the arterial blood with or without adequate elimination of carbon dioxide. It may result from various primary or secondary disorders of the airways, lung parenchyma, chest wall (i.e., skeletal structures and respiratory muscles), and neural processes involved in breathing.

Arterial hypoxemia resulting from a right-to-left intracardiac shunt or low inspired oxygen tension in ambient air is excluded from this definition of respiratory failure because the defect is not in the integrated respiratory system. Tissue hypoxia caused by anemia, reduced cardiac output, or poisoning with carbon monoxide or cyanide is also excluded. These causes of tissue hypoxia require specific interventions that are different from ventilation support and improvement of lung function, which are the cornerstones of management of defects in the respiratory system.

Arterial Hypoxemia

An abnormally low arterial oxygen tension for any given alveolar oxygen tension ($P_{A}O_2$), that is, an increased alveolar-arterial difference in oxygen (A-aDo_2), is often present in patients with lung disease. However, significant desaturation of arterial blood occurs only when arterial oxygen tension levels fall below 60 mm Hg. Hence, from a therapeutic standpoint, arterial hypoxemia is defined as an arterial oxygen tension less than or equal to 60 mm Hg.

Ventilation-perfusion (V_{A}/Q)mismatch, intrapulmonary right-to-left shunting, and alveolar hypoventilation are the most important causes of low arterial oxygen tension ($P_{a}O_2$). In the presence of an increased arterial carbon dioxide tension ($P_{a}CO_2$), calculation of the alveolar-arterial difference in oxygen tension ($P_{A}O_2 - P_{a}O_2$) is helpful in determining whether hypoxemia is caused entirely by hypoventilation (e.g., respiratory muscle weakness or depressed ventilatory drive) or by the combination of hypoventilation and V_{A}/Q imbalance (e.g., chronic obstructive lung disease). With pure hypoventilation, the alveolar-arterial oxygen gradient (A-aDo_2) is normal, but when there is a (V_{A}/Q) mismatch or an intrapulmonary shunt, the A-aDo_2 gradient is increased. The A-aDo_2 gradient is measured by subtracting the measured $P_{a}O_2$ from the calculated $P_{A}O_2$. At sea level and without supplemental oxygen, the $P_{A}O_2$ is equal to $150 - [P_{a}CO_2 \times 1.25]$, assuming a respiratory exchange ratio of 0.8. The normal A-aDo_2 gradient is no higher than 15 mm Hg; it may be higher in the elderly. A second use of the A-aDo_2 gradient is to uncover an occult V_{A}/Q disturbance, signifying an abnormality in the lung when the measured $P_{a}O_2$ is normalized by hyperventilation. For example, a $P_{a}O_2$ of 90 mm Hg and $P_{a}CO_2$ of 20 mm Hg would represent a significant V_{A}/Q abnormality, as evidenced by the calculated A-aDo_2 gradient of 36 mm Hg.

Increasing the fraction of inspired oxygen ($F_{I}O_2$) can be expected to improve arterial oxygenation in all conditions except significant (≥ 30 percent) right-to-left shunting. In fact, the change in $P_{a}O_2$ that occurs in response to various $F_{I}O_2$ values allows the shunt to be estimated as a percent of cardiac output, assuming normal values for the mixed venous oxygen content and arterial carbon dioxide tension [*see Figure 1*]. It is noteworthy that with a shunt of 30 percent or greater, the $P_{a}O_2$ rises little if any with increasing $F_{I}O_2$. In contrast, a comparison of varying degrees of V_{A}/Q imbalance illus-

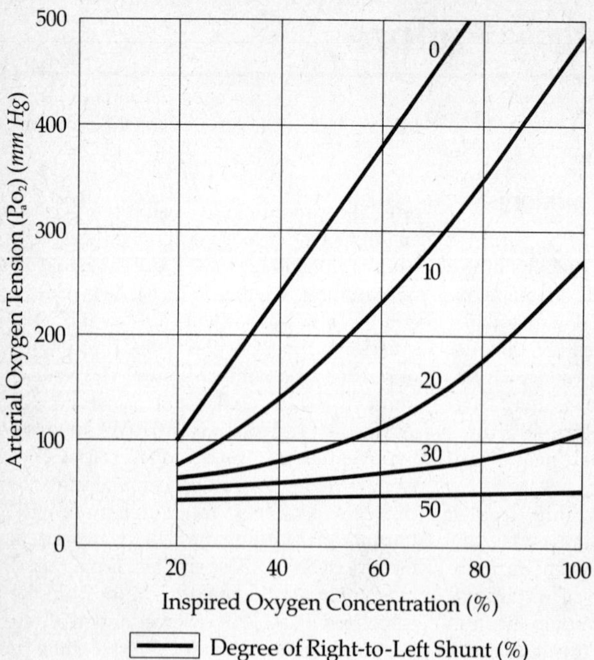

Figure 1 The oxygen concentration of inspired gas is plotted against arterial oxygen tension (P_aO_2) for right-to-left shunts ranging from 0 to 50 percent of cardiac output. The arterial-venous oxygen content difference is assumed to be normal. Note that with right-to-left shunts in excess of 30 percent, there is virtually no increase in P_aO_2 with oxygen enrichment of inspired gas.

trates that the rise in P_aO_2 with oxygen therapy is appreciable even with a severe V_A/Q mismatch [*see Figure 2*]. These differing responses to oxygen are important in treating the major types of respiratory failure.

The compensatory mechanisms for hypoxemia vary depending on whether the process is acute or chronic. In acute hypoxemia, three compensatory mechanisms come into play. First, ventilation increases in direct proportion to the degree of arterial oxygen desaturation, a physiologic response that reflects an attempt to increase both alveolar and arterial oxygen tension by decreasing carbon dioxide tension.[1] Second, pulmonary arteriolar constriction occurs as the degree of alveolar hypoxia increases. This mechanism reflects an attempt to decrease perfusion of hypoxic alveolar regions and to send mixed venous blood to better oxygenated alveoli.[2] However, the mechanism fails when all alveoli are hypoxic. Third, sympathoadrenal activity intensifies with increases in pulse rate and cardiac output in an attempt to increase the overall rate of oxygen delivery to tissues.[3] In chronic hypoxemia, there is more time for the body to compensate for the oxygen deficiency. Thus, in patients with long-term hypoxia, erythrocyte mass increases, which enhances the oxygen-carrying capacity of the blood.[4]

The arterial oxygen tension levels at which ventilatory and cardiovascular compensatory mechanisms come into operation vary enormously among individuals, but as a rough guideline, compensation begins in acute hypoxia when P_aO_2 levels fall to about 60 mm Hg and in chronic hypoxia when levels are at about 50 mm Hg. Below these levels of hypoxemia, adverse effects may occur: mental acuity may be diminished, with initial agitation followed by somnolence, and renal function may be impaired, with diminished glomerular filtration and sodium retention.[5] At levels below 25 to 30 mm Hg, compensatory mechanisms fail: tissue hypoxia and cellular damage ensue; further impairment of consciousness occurs, even to the point of stupor and convulsions; and at levels below 20 mm Hg, hypoxia causes central respiratory depression [*see Figure 3*].[6]

Hypercapnia

Hypercapnia is defined as an arterial carbon dioxide tension of 45 mm Hg or greater. Hypercapnia results from a level of alveolar ventilation that is below that needed to adequately eliminate the amount of carbon dioxide produced by metabolism ($\dot{V}co_2$). One cause of hypercapnia is a reduced minute ventilation (V_E). Minute ventilation can be decreased because of deficient central chemoreceptor activity or inability of the respiratory system to respond to such activity. Such a situation may result from various CNS and neuromuscular disorders. It may also arise during compensation for metabolic alkalemia, unless the concomitant fall in P_aO_2 reaches a level that stimulates ventilation despite alkalemia.

A second cause of hypercapnia is a decrease in alveolar ventilation that is not accompanied by a decrease in minute ventilation [*see Figure 4*]. In this instance, the proportion of wasted ventilation, defined as the ratio of the dead space volume (V_D) to the tidal volume (V_T), is increased. An increased V_D/V_T ratio can result from a breathing pattern characterized by small tidal volumes and high frequency, so that a disproportionate amount of overall ventilation is delivered to anatomical dead space. An increased V_D/V_T ratio can also be caused by pulmonary disorders that lead to overventilation of many regions relative to their perfusion (physiologic dead space).

Because of the enormous ventilatory reserve of the normal respiratory system, increased $\dot{V}co_2$ alone never causes hypercapnia. However, with decreased $\dot{V}_E$ or an increased V_D/V_T ratio, an increase in $\dot{V}co_2$

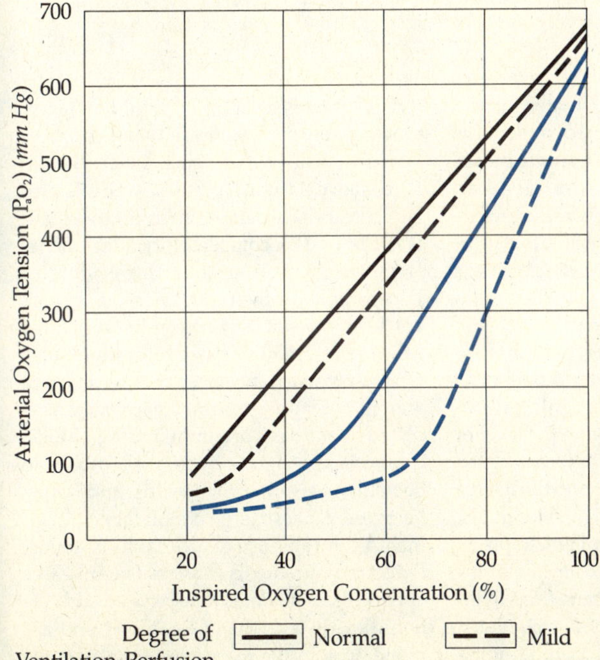

Figure 2   *Isopleths depict the effects of varying inspired oxygen concentrations on arterial oxygen tension (P_aO_2) for various degrees of ventilation-perfusion ($\dot{V}_A/\dot{Q}$) mismatch. In contrast to the negligible effect on P_aO_2 of oxygen enrichment in patients with severe right-to-left shunting [see Figure 1], oxygen enrichment in patients with ventilation-perfusion mismatches results in large increases in P_aO_2.*

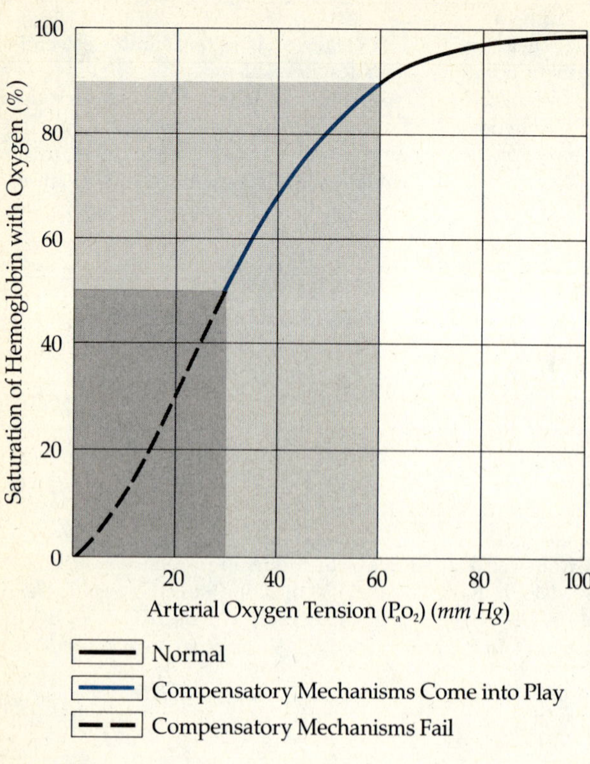

Figure 3　*Three ranges of oxygenation are indicated on the oxygen-hemoglobin dissociation curve. At arterial oxygen tension (P_aO_2) levels greater than 60 mm Hg, the level of saturation of hemoglobin with oxygen is 90 percent or greater, and although the alveolar-arterial difference in oxygen ($A\text{-}aDO_2$) may be abnormal, there is no significant hypoxemia. When P_aO_2 levels are between 60 mm Hg (90 percent saturation) and 30 mm Hg (50 percent saturation), compensatory mechanisms come into play; in addition, adverse clinical effects occur. At P_aO_2 levels less than 30 mm Hg, compensatory mechanisms fail and clinical impairment is severe.*

can contribute significantly to hypercapnia.[7] Increased V_{CO_2} in hospitalized patients is usually a result of infection, trauma, burns, or other major stresses that lead to hypermetabolism. Also, delivery of nutrients (especially carbohydrates) with a caloric value far in excess of resting energy needs can lead to increased V_{CO_2}.[8] Finally, agitation, myoclonus, or other causes of muscle activity can increase V_{CO_2} and contribute to hypercapnia in the compromised patient.

Symptoms and signs related to hypercapnia depend not only on the level of P_aCO_2 but also on the rate of increase of the P_aCO_2 level, which in turn relates to the degree of compensatory adjustment of blood pH, and on the effects of concomitant hypoxia. Acute rises in P_aCO_2 are associated with increased cerebral blood flow, elevations in intracranial pressures, headaches, and, rarely, papilledema. Manifestations include agitation, coarse tremor, slurred speech, and as-

terixis.[9] Acute elevation in P_aCO_2 to 80 to 90 mm Hg may cause confusion and occasionally convulsions and coma. In contrast, a P_aCO_2 above 100 mm Hg may be well tolerated if hypercapnia develops slowly and acidemia is minimized by compensatory adjustments. It is worth noting that the effects of hypercapnia on the central nervous system are fully reversible, whereas hypoxia may cause permanent damage to brain tissue.

The presence and severity of hypoxemia and hypercapnia cannot be reliably predicted on the basis of clinical findings alone. Cyanosis as a sign of hypoxemia proves to be neither sensitive nor specific, and it may be present because of circulatory impairment in the absence of arterial hypoxemia. Direct measurements of arterial blood gases are necessary to determine oxygen and carbon dioxide tensions in the blood and are mandatory in the management of patients with acute respiratory failure.

Principles of Management of Respiratory Failure

The three major principles of management of respiratory failure in order of urgency are (1) assurance of an unobstructed airway that allows free passage of gases and removal of secretions, (2) restoration of oxygenation of arterial blood, and (3) maintenance or restoration of sufficient ventilation to eliminate metabolically produced carbon dioxide so that blood pH returns close to the physiologic range. The ease with which these principles are served and the determination of reasonable clinical and functional end points depend primarily on the type of disease process and the presence or absence of chronic abnormalities in gas exchange. For instance, initial management of acute upper airway obstruction (e.g., angioedema of the glottis) or chronic upper airway obstruction (e.g., tracheal stenosis) requires utilization of only the first principle, that is, reestablishment of the airway through nasotracheal or orotracheal intubation or via tracheostomy. More often, however, acute management of respiratory failure requires more extensive intervention: all three principles of management must be utilized to support gas exchange until the underlying disease process improves either spontaneously or as a result of treatment.

Assurance of Airway Patency

Airway obstruction may develop in any patient with a depressed consciousness. Obstruction develops because of decreased tone and lack of inspiratory activity of upper airway muscles and because of failure to eliminate secretions from the nasopharynx, oropharynx, and infraglottic airways.

Simple measures such as pushing the mandible forward or putting the patient in a lateral decubitus position may alleviate obstruction caused by relaxed upper airway muscles. Occasionally, oropharyngeal or nasopharyngeal artificial airways are needed, especially when frequent suctioning of secretions is required. If there is a likelihood that the patient will vomit, however, endotracheal intubation (via the nasal or oral route) using an inflatable cuff is required to protect the airway from aspiration of gastric

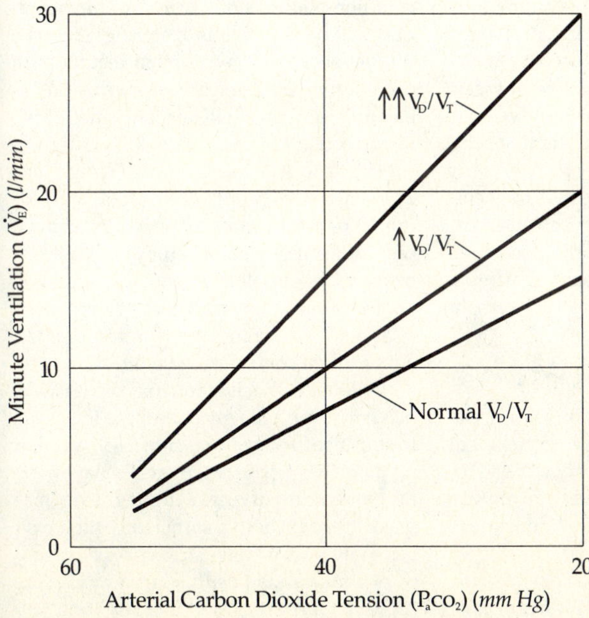

Figure 4   The arterial carbon dioxide tension (P_aCO_2) is plotted against minute ventilation ($\dot{V}_E$). By assigning a constant rate of CO_2 production, wasted ventilation ratio (V_D/V_T) isopleths of varying values are shown, ranging from normal (approximately 0.30) to abnormal (0.30 to 0.50) to highly abnormal (>0.50). Increases or decreases in minute ventilation are inversely related to changes in P_aCO_2. As V_D/V_T becomes increasingly abnormal, a much greater minute ventilation is needed to maintain P_aCO_2 values in the normal range. Thus, alveolar hypoventilation with high $\dot{V}_E$ results if V_D/V_T is abnormal.

contents. Tracheostomy is urgently required only if there is glottic or infraglottic anatomic obstruction or if, for other reasons, endotracheal intubation cannot be performed (e.g., because of severe trauma to the oropharynx). Endotracheal intubation is desirable in a patient with depressed consciousness if bronchial secretions are voluminous and viscid and if less invasive measures (e.g., an artificial oropharyngeal airway) do not permit adequate suctioning to eliminate such secretions. Tracheal intubation using an inflatable cuff for a seal is necessary for most forms of mechanical ventilatory support (see below).

Both endotracheal intubation and tracheostomy can injure the airway. Endotracheal intubation can cause laryngeal stenosis or vocal cord paralysis[10] and, if the nasotracheal route is used, sinusitis. Tracheostomy may be complicated by stomal bleeding and infection. Both types of tracheal intubation can lead to the serious sequela of tracheal stenosis or tracheomalacia as a consequence of ischemic injury to the tracheal wall from the inflatable cuff. The latter complications have been markedly reduced since the advent of high-volume, low-pressure cuffs, and risk during prolonged intubation can be further reduced by avoiding excess cuff volume. There does not seem to be any major advantage or disadvantage of prolonged (as long as several weeks) translaryngeal intubation instead of early tracheostomy. However, because tracheostomy may be associated with improved patient comfort and more effective secretion removal, the need for mechanical ventilation beyond two to three weeks is a reasonable indication for tracheostomy.

Restoration of Arterial Oxygen Level

Restoration of oxygenation of arterial blood may require only oxygen enrichment of the inspired air. The goal should be a P_aO_2 of 60 mm Hg or higher (≥ 90 percent oxygen saturation of hemoglobin) for acute hypoxemia and a P_aCO_2 of 50 mm Hg or higher for chronic hypoxemia with hypercapnia. The danger of giving excess-

ive oxygen, beyond that needed to achieve these goals, is twofold. First, prolonged exposure to high concentrations of oxygen (i.e., > 50 to 60 percent) can lead to lung injury. Second, in the presence of chronic hypoxemia and hypercapnia, respiratory drive may be mediated in large part by hypoxemia; and rapid normalization of P_aO_2 by the overzealous administration of oxygen can lead to respiratory depression, hypercapnia, and coma.

Supplemental oxygen may be administered to spontaneously breathing patients via nasal cannulas, loose-fitting masks, or a T-piece fitting on the free end of an endotracheal tube. Nasal cannulas and loose-fitting masks, the most commonly used noninvasive techniques, seldom provide inspired oxygen concentrations greater than 40 to 50 percent. Even though a higher concentration (i.e., 60 to 100 percent) may be delivered through the tubing that connects the oxygen source to the patient, entrainment of room air at the face mask will dilute the concentration of oxygen that is actually delivered to the trachea to 50 percent or less, especially if the patient is hyperventilating. Hence, common methods of oxygen supplementation will be effective in restoring adequate P_aO_2 levels only if hypoxemia results from mild or moderate ventilation-perfusion imbalances, and they will be totally ineffective in correcting hypoxemia caused by significant right-to-left shunting [*see Figures 1 and 2*]. Fractional oxygen concentrations exceeding 40 percent can be achieved by using a cascade arrangement whereby high flows of oxygen are supplied through a large-volume face mask or an inspiratory reservoir bag. Such an arrangement minimizes the entrainment of air during inspiration.

If high levels of inspired oxygen (80 to 90 percent) have been given and the P_aO_2 level is still insufficient (< 60 mm Hg), another noninvasive technique is available: an arrangement involving a tight-fitting face mask in which both a sufficiently high oxygen flow and a downstream resistor produce continuous positive airway pressure (CPAP). CPAP serves to increase lung volume, which in turn results in opening of previously closed alveoli (decreased intrapulmonary right-to-left shunting) and better ventilation of previously underventilated alveoli (improvement in ventilation-perfusion imbalance). The major drawback of this method is that if the patient vomits, there is an increased risk of aspiration because of the tight fit of the face mask.

Mechanical Ventilatory Support

If adequate oxygenation cannot be provided by noninvasive means or if there is progressive hypoventilation and hypercapnia with respiratory acidosis, it is necessary to provide mechanical ventilatory support. Mechanical ventilatory support can be provided by devices that produce intermittent positive pressure at the airway opening or by devices that intermittently create a negative pressure around the chest wall. Use of negative pressure ventilators, such as the iron lung, is generally restricted to cases involving neuromuscular weakness or chest wall deformity.

There are two basic types of positive pressure ventilation. The most commonly used mode is volume-cycled ventilation, which provides a fixed tidal volume and in which inflation pressure is the dependent variable. A pressure limit is set so that when inflation pressure exceeds this value, a so-called pop-off valve prevents further gas flow to the patient. This valve prevents potentially dangerous overinflation of alveoli and functions as an alarm, warning of a change in the pressure required to deliver the preset tidal volume (see below). The second type of positive pressure ventilation is pressure-cycled ventilation, which provides gas flow at a preset pressure. With this pressure-preset mode of ventilation, tidal volume is the dependent variable.

During volume-cycled ventilation, the pressure required to deliver the preset tidal volume is termed the peak airway pressure. The peak airway pressure can be subdivided into the pressure required to overcome flow-resistive properties of the airway and external apparatus and the pressure required to overcome the elastic properties of the lung and chest wall [*see Figure 5*]. At breathing frequencies used in the clinical setting, the elastic properties of the lungs and chest wall are the major determinants of the pressure that is required to deliver a given tidal volume. The pressure required to overcome only the elastic recoil force of the lungs and chest wall (i.e., plateau, or static, pressure) is measured by interrupting flow at full inspiration. The plateau pressure is a close approximation of the alveolar pressure. The static compliance of the respiratory system is computed by dividing the tidal volume delivered to the patient by the plateau pressure. Normally, this value is higher than 60 ml/cm H_2O.

High alveolar pressures may impede venous return, leading to decreases in cardiac output and blood pressure, and may increase the risk of barotrauma (e.g., pneumothorax, pneumomediastinum, and subcutaneous emphysema). Hence, it is advisable to adjust tidal volume and breathing frequency to minimize alveolar (plateau) pressure while maintaining alveolar ventilation and arterial oxygenation.

With volume-cycled ventilation, a large increase in peak inflation pressure signals a change in the pressure required to overcome flow-resistive or elastic forces so that the preset tidal volume can be delivered. When an increase in peak pressure is associated with a similar increase in plateau pressure, the problem is localized to the lung parenchyma or chest wall rather than the airways. This pattern may be seen with worsening of pulmonary edema, tension pneumothorax, mainstem intubation, and a large region of atelectasis. In contrast, airway problems (e.g., kinking of the endotracheal tube, mucous plugs, or bronchospasm) typically produce a large increase in peak pressure with little change in plateau pressure.[11]

Airway problems can produce an increase in plateau pressure if the reduction in expiratory flow is sufficient to cause an incomplete exhalation of the tidal volume. With both positive pressure and negative pressure ventilators, exhalation is passive

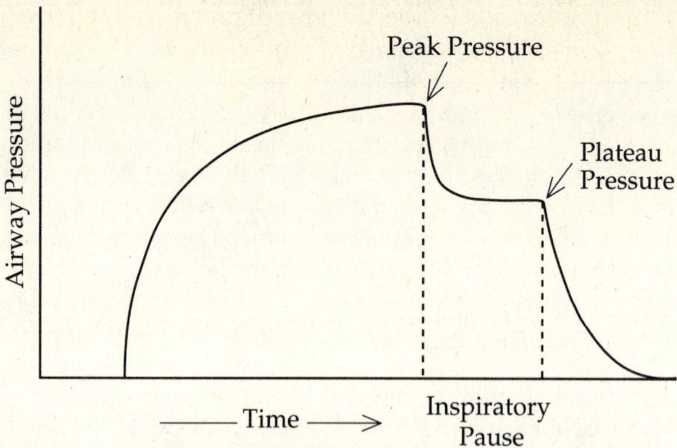

Figure 5 *In volume-cycled, positive pressure ventilation, the total pressure required to overcome flow-resistive and elastic forces and deliver the preset tidal volume is termed the peak airway pressure. The plateau pressure is the pressure required to keep the lung and chest wall inflated with the preset tidal volume during a brief period in which there is no flow (inspiratory pause). The difference between the peak and plateau pressures is a reflection of the flow-resistive component of ventilation and is increased when airway resistance or inspiratory flow rate is increased. The plateau pressure is a function of lung and chest wall compliance and is unaffected by airway resistance and inspiratory flow rate unless increased resistance to expiratory flow or reduction in inspiratory flow rate results in failure to exhale the full tidal volume (gas trapping).*

and is provided by the elastic recoil of the inflated lungs and chest wall. The rate at which exhalation occurs depends on the flow resistance of the airways: a high resistance, such as that seen in patients with chronic airway obstruction or asthma, will prolong exhalation. If the subsequent tidal volume is delivered before exhalation is complete, positive airway pressure will be maintained throughout the respiratory cycle, with a resultant increase in end-expiratory lung volume.[12] One can correct for this effect by decreasing the ventilator rate, thereby allowing more time for exhalation.

For volume-cycled ventilation, two primary modalities are used: assist-control ventilation and synchronized intermittent mandatory ventilation (SIMV) [*see Figure 6*]. In the assist-control mode, a breath is delivered at the preset tidal volume every time the patient creates a small negative deflection in proximal airway pressure (–1 to –2 cm H_2O) by inspiratory muscle activity. In this mode, the preset respiratory rate is in effect a backup rate, guaranteeing that the patient will receive a predetermined number of ventilator-delivered breaths even if inspiratory efforts cease. SIMV allows the patient to breathe at a spontaneous rate and tidal volume while at the same time a certain minute ventilation is delivered from the ventilator. The circuit is modified to provide an ample flow of gas for spontaneous breathing and also to allow periodic mandatory breaths synchronous with the patient's inspiratory efforts to be delivered from the ventilator. The assist-control mode has certain advantages in that it requires minimal respiratory effort from the patient, reduces oxygen consumption, and rests respiratory muscles that may be fatigued. Putative advantages of SIMV include the exercising of respiratory muscles, the lowering of mean intrathoracic pressure, the prevention of respiratory alkalemia, and improved patient-ventilator coordination. Recent evidence has shown that the respiratory muscles continue to perform considerable work during assist-control breathing, especially when minute ventilation is increased.[13] Also, it has been shown that a change from assist-control ventilation to SIMV does not correct respiratory alkalemia caused by respiratory overdrive.[14]

Positive end-expiratory pressure (PEEP) can be added to intermittent positive pressure ventilation using any of the modes described above. Positive pressure applied during spontaneous breathing is referred to as continuous positive airway pressure, or CPAP.

Management of Respiratory Failure in Specific Clinical Settings

Hypoxemic and Hypercapnic Respiratory Failure

Combined hypoxemic and hypercapnic respiratory failure arises when minute ventilation is low or when minute ventilation is high but ventilation-perfusion abnormalities are severe [*see Figures 2 and 4*].

Respiratory failure in the setting of diminished minute ventilation often arises

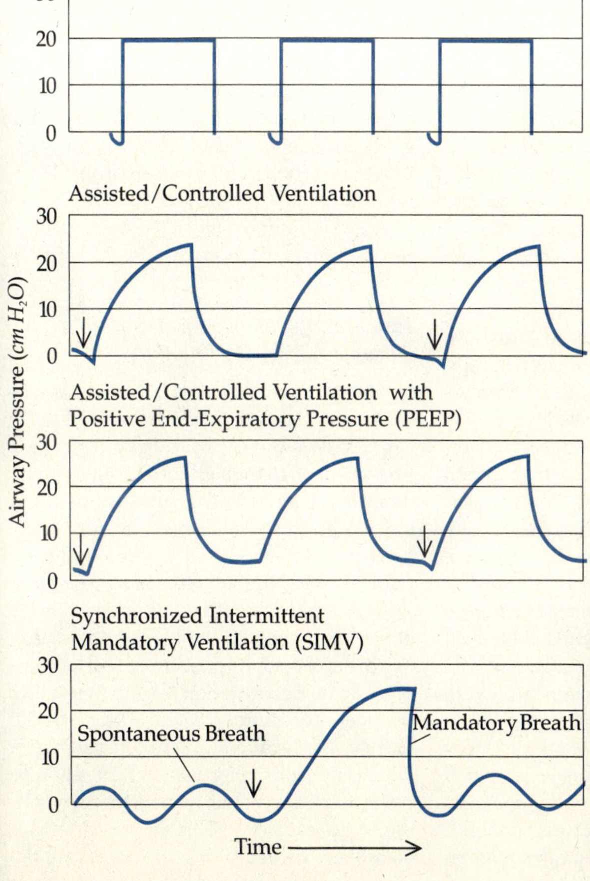

Figure 6 *Pressures measured at the endotracheal tube are shown as a function of time to illustrate the effects of various modes of pressure-preset (top panel) or constant tidal volume (bottom three panels) mechanical ventilation. Supra-atmospheric pressures have positive values, whereas subatmospheric pressures have negative values. Arrows indicate initiation of inspiration by the patient, which triggers the ventilator to deliver an assisted breath.*

because of a defect in the respiratory pump. The defect may originate in the central nervous system (e.g., narcotic or sedative overdose), the anterior horn cells of the CNS (e.g., poliomyelitis), the peripheral nerves (e.g., Guillain-Barré syndrome), the neuromuscular junctions (e.g., myasthenia gravis), or the muscles themselves (e.g., muscular dystrophy). In such patients, mechanical ventilation can be achieved with low inflation pressures. Oxygen enrichment of the inspired air is not necessary unless a secondary intrapulmonic process (e.g., pneumonia or atelectasis) is present.

Severe upper airway obstructions (e.g., angioedema of the glottis) or extreme abnormalities of the chest wall (e.g., flail chest) also cause a diminution in minute ventilation. Hypoxemic and hypercapnic respiratory failure results even when neuromuscular function is intact. Removal or bypass of the obstructive process is the only treatment required for upper airway obstruction. Mechanical ventilation is required for flail chest: as in other forms of respiratory failure associated with diminished minute ventilation, mechanical ventilation can be accomplished with minimal inflation pressures and oxygen requirements.

Chronic and severely restrictive chest wall processes such as kyphoscoliosis also produce hypoxemic and hypercapnic respiratory failure. Respiratory failure in such cases is chronic and is associated with acute periods of clinical worsening. Mechanical ventilatory support may require higher than normal inflation pressures, and because ventilation-perfusion abnormalities are usually present, modest oxygen enrichment of the inspired air is required as well. The chronic mechanical load on the respiratory muscles that is imposed by the stiffened chest wall can lead to respiratory muscle fatigue, which can be relieved by periodic mechanical ventilatory support in the absence of an acute major insult.[15] Such patients may benefit from nocturnal ventilatory support provided by use of an intermittent negative pressure ventilator (e.g., cuirass-type thoracoabdominal shell) or by positive pressure ventilation by nose mask. Such support serves not only to rest the respiratory muscles but also to prevent sleep-related decreases in blood oxygen levels and elevations in blood carbon dioxide levels.

It is important to remember that chronic hypoxemia and hypercapnia result in alterations of the respiratory control mechanisms that lead to diminished ventilatory responsiveness to acute changes in blood gases.[16] For instance, patients with persistently elevated levels of arterial carbon dioxide tension have blunted responsiveness of the medullary respiratory centers to hypercapnia and therefore have an increased dependence on hypoxemia as a stimulus for increased ventilation. As a result, removal of the hypoxic drive to breathing by correction of the P_aO_2 to normal with overzealous oxygen administration can lead to severe depression of the drive to spontaneous breathing.[17] Hence, when long-term abnormalities are present, the goal during episodes of acute worsening is to restore blood values to the chronic level, not to expected normal values. This caveat is especially important in the management of acute exacerbations of chronic airway obstruction.

Respiratory Failure in Patients with Chronic Airway Obstruction

Patients with severe chronic airway obstruction are often hypoxemic and hypercapnic on a long-term basis and adapt, albeit precariously, to their abnormal state. Acute deterioration may be triggered by the added stress of endobronchial infection, use of sedatives, onset of dehydration-electrolyte imbalance, muscular weakness, pneumothorax, congestive heart failure, or a major exposure to air pollutants. The worsening hypoxemia and hypercapnia that accompany acute deterioration lead to increasing dyspnea, cor pulmonale, sleep disruption, and sometimes alterations in consciousness. Depressed consciousness in turn leads to retention of secretions and further worsening of gas exchange. This vicious circle can be broken by identifying and rectifying the processes that have precipitated the acute deterioration and by providing support to improve gas exchange while the underlying problems are being approached.

Arterial blood gas analysis is crucial to the proper assessment and management of acute exacerbations. During severe episodes, the use of indwelling arterial cannulas for frequent sampling of arterial specimens and continuous blood pressure monitoring are usually required. The first therapeutic priority is to administer oxygen if the patient's P_aO_2 level is less than 50 mm Hg while breathing air. Oxygen must be given in modest concentrations to raise the P_aO_2 level to above 50 mm Hg, but the P_aO_2 level should not be raised to much greater than 60 mm Hg, because excessive levels of arterial oxygen might remove the hypoxic drive and lead to increasing hypercapnia, somnolence, or even coma or seizures.

The most reliable way to control the F_IO_2 is with a Venturi mask, which provides a set F_IO_2 independent of the oxygen flow rate. A reasonable starting value for the F_IO_2 is 0.24, which increases the partial pressure of inspired oxygen (P_IO_2) by approximately 21 mm Hg over the partial pressure of oxygen in air. A 10 to 15 mm Hg elevation in P_aCO_2 is common when oxygen is given to patients with chronic airway obstruction and does not represent a failure of controlled oxygen therapy, provided there is not a critical reduction in blood pH (e.g., < 7.2). Once oxygenation has improved, the major therapeutic goals are promotion of bronchopulmonary drainage by encouragement of cough, administration of inhaled bronchodilators and systemic corticosteroids, and treatment of underlying endobronchial infection. There is probably no added benefit to giving theophylline to patients with chronic airway obstruction who are receiving the above medications.[18]

Tracheal intubation and mechanical ventilatory support are required if increasing hypercapnia and stupor develop because of excessive oxygen administration, worsening airway obstruction, respiratory muscle fatigue, or inadvertent use of sedatives (which should be avoided). A value for P_aCO_2 at which intubation and mechanical ventilation become necessary cannot be specified, because the degree of chronic renal compensation will vary among individual patients. In general, ventilator support should be considered in patients with chronic airway obstruction if hypercapnia is severe enough to cause profound acidemia (pH ≤ 7.2) or to induce somnolence that interferes with effective cough and cooperation with medical care. Recently, use of positive pressure ventilation via nose mask, without endotracheal intubation, has been used successfully in the management of patients with exacerbations of chronic airway obstruction who may otherwise have required intubation.[19]

The goal of ventilatory support is to reestablish P_aO_2 and P_aCO_2 values at chronic levels rather than to attempt to restore these values to normal. Overventilation may result in alkalemia accompanied by cardiac dysrhythmias or grand mal seizures. To achieve the desired P_aCO_2 level, the appropriate ventilator settings for tidal volume and respiratory frequency are determined primarily by trial and error, that is, by choosing initial settings, measuring the resultant P_aCO_2, and making adjustments accordingly. Typical initial settings in chronic obstructive lung disease are a tidal volume of 10 ml/kg at 10 breaths/min. During the period of mechanical ventilatory support, continued bronchopulmonary drainage and bronchodilator therapy are necessary, often in combination with antibiotics. Mechanical ventilatory support should be withdrawn once the underlying cause of deterioration has sufficiently diminished and the patient can once again sustain ventilation independently.

Respiratory Failure in Patients with Adult Respiratory Distress Syndrome

Hypoxemic respiratory failure in the setting of diffuse alveolar damage with noncardiogenic pulmonary edema has a mortality of 50 to 60 percent, even when treatment is aggressive.

The initial steps in the treatment of a patient with respiratory failure and ARDS who cannot otherwise be adequately oxygenated are endotracheal intubation and ventilatory support with volume-cycled ventilation. F_IO_2 values should be sufficiently high to maintain P_aO_2 levels in the range of 60 to 80 mm Hg. An initial tidal volume of 10 ml/kg is recommended. Higher tidal volumes (12 to 15 ml/kg) have commonly been used in ARDS, but these higher volumes could lead to overdistention of certain alveoli with resultant barotrauma, especially when PEEP has been used to increase end-expiratory lung volume (see below). Measurements of static compliance may help in the determination of appropriate tidal volume. High tidal volumes that are associated with reduced compliance should be avoided because they may cause alveolar overdistention and barotrauma. Also, barotrauma risk may be lessened by adjusting the tidal volume so that a marked elevation in plateau pressure (e.g., > 35–40 cm H_2O) is avoided.[20] In general, tidal volume should be determined by assessing lung mechanics rather than by measuring arterial blood gases; adjustments in minute ventilation are made by altering the respiratory rate. The backup respiratory rate should be sufficient to guarantee adequate minute ventilation if the patient's intrinsic rate is decreased by therapeutic sedation or paralysis.

PEEP improves oxygenation by preventing alveolar collapse at end-expiration, thereby increasing lung volume. PEEP does not reduce the amount of extravascular lung water. PEEP is indicated in cases in which high F_IO_2 values fail to oxygenate arterial blood. In addition, because PEEP may lessen the risk of oxygen toxicity by allowing a lower F_IO_2 to be given, it is indicated in cases in which high concentrations of inspired oxygen ($F_IO_2 > 0.5$) are required for a prolonged period. The lowest PEEP associated with improved oxygenation should be used because high levels of PEEP produce a fall in cardiac output and increase the incidence of barotrauma (e.g., pneumothorax, pneumomediastinum, and subcutaneous emphysema).[21] Furthermore, very high levels of PEEP can actually decrease oxygenation of arterial blood by overdistending open alveoli, thereby compressing the capillaries surrounding these alveoli and shunting more blood to those alveoli that remain closed.

ARDS is characterized by increased capillary permeability. Hence, any increase in capillary pressure further magnifies the flux of liquid and protein into the interstitial spaces and alveoli.[22] Keeping the capillary pressure as low as possible can slow the rate of functional deterioration. Physical findings and portable chest radiographs are exceedingly poor in assessing pulmonary vascular congestion in such patients. Accurate estimates of pulmonary capillary pressure require the passage of a flow-directed, balloon-tipped (Swan-Ganz) catheter into the pulmonary artery, an invasive procedure associated with a number of complications.

If there is deterioration of lung function (as indicated by decreasing compliance and worsening oxygenation) and if the blood pressure and urinary output indicate that cardiac output is adequate, a trial of diuretics combined with a decrease in the amount of intravenous liquids being given should precede pulmonary arterial catheterization.[23] When ARDS is associated with hypotension and jugular venous pressure is normal or increased, the administration of dopamine may be appropriate. However, as a rule, patients with moderate to severe ARDS who have concomitant hypotension or oliguria can be managed physiologically with the aid of a pulmonary arterial catheter; knowledge of wedge pressure, cardiac output, and vascular resistances can then be used to tailor therapy with fluid, PEEP, inotropes, or vasopressors.

It is important to note that technical errors in measurements of the pulmonary capillary wedge pressure can lead to therapeutic errors.[24] Thus, careful calibration of the catheter-transducer system and assurance of the wedge position are necessary before measurements are taken and therapy is begun. In general, to minimize continued leakage of fluid into the lungs, a therapeutic goal in ARDS is to achieve the lowest possible pulmonary capillary wedge pressure consistent with adequate cardiac output and blood pressure. Many factors affect the relation between the wedge pressure and left ventricular preload (e.g., myocardial ischemia, left ventricular hypertrophy, PEEP, and high levels of endogenous or exogenous catecholamines). One patient may have optimal preload at a wedge pressure of 8 mm Hg, whereas a second patient may be relatively hypovolemic at a wedge pressure of 18 mm Hg. Thus, for each individual, it is necessary to define the wedge pressure that gives adequate preload; wedge pressure should be compared with thermodilution-measured cardiac output and blood pressure during the manipulation of intravascular volume by diuretics or volume challenges.

Gastrointestinal Bleeding

In all forms of respiratory failure, the risk of upper gastrointestinal bleeding is increased. In the setting of ARDS complicated by consumptive coagulopathy, there is the added risk of bleeding from nonocclusive, diffuse ischemic necrosis of the bowel. Prophylactic use of H_2-receptor antagonists or sucralfate reduces the risk of upper gastrointestinal bleeding.[25]

Nutritional Support

Nutrition should not be neglected in the acute management of respiratory failure.[8] For patients with acute exacerbations of chronic obstructive pulmonary disease (COPD), nutritional support should be initiated if, after a few days of ventilatory assistance, the patient has not improved sufficiently to allow extubation. Such patients are rarely hypermetabolic and generally require only modest caloric intake (25 to 30 kcal/kg/day) to meet tissue energy needs. Avoidance of overfeeding with carbohydrates is important because of the increased amount of carbon dioxide that is produced when excess carbohydrates undergo lipogenesis. Patients with ARDS are generally hypermetabolic and seldom are able to be extubated within a few days. Thus, nutritional support should be started promptly with caloric intake that is higher than normal (e.g., 30 to 35 kcal/kg/day or higher). The adequacy of caloric intake may be assessed by nitrogen balance studies and measurements of oxygen consumption.[26]

Withdrawal of Mechanical Ventilatory Support

Improvement in the gas exchange function of the lungs, restitution of ventilatory drive, and diminution in the excess mechanical load on respiratory muscles allow the process of withdrawal of mechanical ventilatory support to begin. Several numerical values for $A\text{-}aDo_2$, spontaneous tidal volume, vital capacity, and the maximum voluntary inspiratory pressures that can be generated have been proposed as guidelines to begin the withdrawal process. So-called weaning parameters (tidal volume, negative inspiratory force, vital capacity, and minute ventilation) are most useful for predicting failure of spontaneous ventilation. If these parameters are grossly abnormal, they clearly predict failure, even when the patient has clinically improved. The most important criterion for deciding whether a patient can be safely extubated is that the alert and cooperative patient tolerates a trial of spontaneous ventilation without excessive tachypnea, tachycardia, or obvious respiratory distress. Breathing at high frequency and low tidal volume is usually predictive of an inability to undergo extubation safely.[27]

When the patient is ready for withdrawal trials, two choices are available: (1) synchronized intermittent mandatory ventilation [*see* Principles of Management of Respiratory Failure, *above*], which allows spontaneous breathing and diminishing numbers of mandatory breaths per minute until the patient is breathing unassisted, (2) intermittent trials with mechanical support totally removed (through the use of a T-piece), or (3) use of decreasing levels of pressure-support ventilation. No convincing data indicate that any one method is preferable. The process of withdrawal may be needlessly prolonged by the SIMV method if small adjustments in the SIMV rate are made only infrequently, such as once a day. Correction of the underlying condition that necessitated ventilatory support is much more important to successful intubation than is the method of weaning.

Several processes may interfere with the withdrawal of mechanical ventilatory support. The first is the administration of higher than needed concentrations of inspired oxygen, resulting in too high a P_aO_2 level, or adjustment of ventilator settings at excessive frequencies and tidal volumes, resulting in too low a P_aCO_2 level. These ill-advised measures diminish potential spontaneous ventilatory drive, and as a result, severe hypoventilation may occur, leading to a rapid fall in the P_aO_2 level and a rapid rise in the P_aCO_2 level when mechanical support is removed. While the patient is being supported mechanically, the aim should be to achieve blood gas values that the patient is capable of maintaining on his or her own.

A second process that can interfere with successful withdrawal from ventilatory support is the development of acid-base or electrolyte disturbances (e.g., metabolic alkalemia and hypokalemia). Such disturbances often result from diuretic therapy or nasogastric suction. Sufficient chloride and potassium replacement can avert this problem.[28] Similarly, profound phosphate depletion can cause muscle weakness; phosphate disturbances should therefore be prevented or corrected.[29]

A third process that can interfere with withdrawal from ventilatory support is the use of sedatives, tranquilizers, or narcotic analgesics, all of which depress ventilatory drive. Careful evaluation of patient medications and, if possible, discontinuance of all such agents should aid in avoiding this problem.

Fourth, if excess secretions and bronchospasm are present, failure to perform bronchopulmonary drainage or to administer bronchodilators during the withdrawal period will interfere with the ability to attain a self-supporting status.

Fifth, in the setting of ARDS, worsening of oxygenation when the patient is off the ventilator might indicate progressive alveolar collapse. Such collapse can be avoided or remedied by the use of CPAP [*see* Principles of Management of Respiratory Failure, *above*] rather than by the reinstitution of the mechanical ventilator.

Fatigue of respiratory muscles can occur during the withdrawal period while the patient is breathing spontaneously.[30] Elements that can contribute to the early onset of fatigue of the inspiratory muscles include disuse atrophy, inadequate nutritional status, lowered cardiac output, electrolyte disturbances, and increasing mechanical loads imposed by alveolar collapse, hyperinflation, excessive airway secretions, or bronchospasm. The consequence of respiratory muscle fatigue is a decline in the volume of a tidal breath. Hence, alveolar hypoventilation and carbon dioxide retention ensue. Physical findings indicative of diaphragmatic fatigue include a paradoxic inward movement of the abdominal wall during inspiration in the supine patient.

Management of respiratory muscle fatigue is dependent on detection and alleviation of the many factors that can contribute to it. There are reports that theophylline infusions may help to reverse fatigue,[31] but because evidence of clinical benefit is lacking, theophylline should be administered for this indication only after the other treatable factors have been rectified. Digoxin and beta agonists have also been shown to alter respiratory muscle fatigue patterns in experiments in animals, but the ultimate utility, if any, of these agents in humans remains to be assessed.[32,33]

References

1. Am Rev Respir Dis 109:345, 1974
2. Progress in Respiration Research 5:156, 1970
3. J Appl Physiol 22:1124, 1967
4. J Appl Physiol 21:73, 1966
5. Clin Sci 37:327, 1969
6. Am J Med 70:1247, 1981
7. Crit Care Med 19:916, 1991
8. JAMA 257:3094, 1987
9. Medicine (Baltimore) 35:389, 1956
10. Am J Med 70:65, 1981
11. Crit Care Med 4:173, 1976
12. Am Rev Respir Dis 126:166, 1982
13. Am Rev Respir Dis 134:902, 1986
14. Am Rev Respir Dis 132:1071, 1985
15. Am Rev Respir Dis 135:1049, 1987
16. Seminars in Respiratory Medicine 3:76, 1981
17. Thorax 41:897, 1986
18. Ann Intern Med 107:305, 1987
19. N Engl J Med 323:1523, 1990
20. Chest 100:494, 1991
21. N Engl J Med 292:284, 1975
22. J Clin Invest 67:409, 1981
23. Am J Cardiol 47:963, 1981
24. Am Rev Respir Dis 128:319, 1983
25. Ann Intern Med 106:562, 1987
26. Chest 98:682, 1990
27. N Engl J Med 324:1445, 1991
28. Am J Med 38:172, 1965
29. N Engl J Med 313:420, 1985
30. Am Rev Respir Dis 119(suppl 2, no 2):93, 1979
31. Am Rev Respir Dis 127:148, 1983
32. J Appl Physiol 61:1767, 1986
33. J Appl Physiol 56:922, 1984

Acknowledgments

The previous (4/88) version of this subsection was written by Roland H. Ingram, Jr., M.D., and Christopher H. Fanta, M.D.

Figures 1 to 4   Al Miller.

Figures 5 and 6   Janet Betries.

39 Disorders of Acid-Base Metabolism

EUGENE D. ROBIN, M.D.

Clinical Approach to Acid-Base Disorders

Patients with disorders affecting many different organ systems show abnormalities of acid-base metabolism. Because the diagnosis and treatment of these abnormalities commonly produce important therapeutic gains for the patient, every physician who cares for seriously ill patients needs to have a working knowledge of acid-base disturbances.

The enormous clinical importance of acids and bases is related to several factors. Acids and bases affect the chemical behavior of water.[1] Because most chemical reactions within the body take place in water solutions, changes in the concentration of acids or bases have significant chemical effects. Because hydrogen ions are highly mobile charged particles, changes in their concentration ultimately affect the distribution of such ions as sodium, potassium, and chloride in the cell environment. Changes in hydrogen ion concentration are important because such changes produce conformational changes in proteins that influence their biochemical activity and affect normal cell function. Enzymes exhibit optimal activity within a narrow range of pH.

Hydrogen ions are produced or used in reactions involving energy metabolism, biosynthesis, biodegradation, and detoxification. Consequently, changes in the hydrogen ion concentration decisively influence these reactions.

A number of physiologic functions are influenced by hydrogen ion concentration. For example, increasing the concentration leads to the following changes: (1) increased pulmonary vascular resistance,[2] (2) decreased flow resistance in many systemic vascular beds,[3] (3) decreased myocardial contractility,[4] and (4) decreased association between hemoglobin and oxygen.[5] Because the hydrogen ion concentration plays such a key role in biochemical and physiologic functions, it is closely regulated. Thus, severe changes of concentration are incompatible with normal function and, indeed, with life itself.

Quantifying Acid-Base Metabolism

Both diagnosis and therapy of acid-base disturbances require a quantitative treatment of changes in acid-base variables. For this purpose, the expression first derived by Henderson and Hasselbalch is generally used:

$$pH = pK + log \frac{[HCO_3^-]}{\alpha CO_2 \times P_{CO_2}} \qquad (1)$$

The value of pK is constant at a given body temperature and at a given osmolality. In plasma at 37° C, pK equals 6.10. The P_{CO_2} is the partial pressure of carbon dioxide; $[HCO_3^-]$ is the bicarbonate ion concentration. The value αCO_2 refers to the solubility of carbon dioxide in plasma. At a given temperature and osmolality, αCO_2 is also constant, and in plasma at 37° C, it equals 0.03 mmole of carbon dioxide per millimeter Hg P_{CO_2}.

Because acid-base status is usually assessed by measuring arterial plasma, equation 1 can be rewritten as:

$$pH_a = 6.10 + log \frac{[HCO_3^-]_a}{0.03 P_a CO_2} \qquad (2)$$

There is now an expression with three unknowns, pH_a (arterial pH), $P_a CO_2$ (arterial P_{CO_2}), and $[HCO_3^-]_a$ (arterial $[HCO_3^-]$), and two constants, pK and αCO_2. In clinical medicine, it is customary to measure pH_a and P_aco_2 directly. The former is measured by a pH glass electrode and the latter by a specialized Pco_2 electrode. Once these two values are known, the bicarbonate ion concentration is calculated.

In a normal person, the arterial pH averages about 7.40, ranging between 7.35 and 7.45. The P_aco_2 normally averages about 40 mm Hg, with a range between 36 and 42. When the average values for pH_a and P_aco_2 are substituted in equation 2, a normal bicarbonate concentration is found to be 24 mEq/l plasma (range 24 to 28):

$$7.40 = 6.10 + \log \frac{24}{0.03 \times 40} \tag{3}$$

Several characteristics of equation 2 should be emphasized. It should be noted that the value of arterial pH depends on the ratio of bicarbonate concentration to Pco_2 rather than on the individual value of each. (The ratio of $[HCO_3^{-2}]$ to 0.03 Pco_2 is normally 20:1.) Thus, if there is a primary disturbance associated with an increase in Pco_2, the degree of change in pH will depend on the change not only in Pco_2 but also in bicarbonate concentration. If the increase in bicarbonate concentration is proportional to the change in Pco_2, then pH will be unchanged. In all acid-base disturbances, compensatory processes operate to maintain arterial pH at a relatively constant value by appropriate changes of Pco_2 or of bicarbonate concentration. Thus, the direction of compensatory changes in various acid-base disturbances can be predicted. For example, if a patient has a primary acid-base disturbance characterized by a decrease in the numerator of equation 2, the compensatory processes will operate to decrease the denominator.

The effectiveness of compensatory mechanisms at maintaining a normal pH varies for the different acid-base disturbances. In respiratory acidosis, compensatory changes are not sufficient to restore pH to normal. Thus, a patient with primary re-

spiratory acidosis who has a normal pH must have an additional complicating acid-base disturbance. A normal pH does not mean normal compensation. In clinical circumstances, there are frequently mixed acid-base disturbances, and thus patients show combinations of disturbed acid-base metabolism. At times, the complicating disorders affect pH in the same direction and, under other circumstances, in opposite directions.

Inspection of equation 2 reveals the possibility of four classes of primary acid-base disturbances. In the first group of disorders, collectively called respiratory acidosis, there is a primary increase in the P_aco_2. The second type of abnormality, respiratory alkalosis, is marked by a primary decrease in the P_aco_2. In the third type, metabolic acidosis, there is a primary decrease in bicarbonate concentration. The fourth group, associated with a primary increase in bicarbonate concentration, is termed metabolic alkalosis.

Respiratory Acidosis

Respiratory acidosis occurs as a result of abnormally high P_aco_2. The value of arterial Pco_2 varies directly with changes in the metabolic production of carbon dioxide and indirectly with the amount of alveolar ventilation, as shown in equation 4:

$$P_aco_2 = C \cdot \frac{\dot{V}CO_2}{\dot{V}_A} \tag{4}$$

In this equation, C is a constant, $\dot{V}CO_2$ is the amount of carbon dioxide produced in milliliters per unit time, and $\dot{V}_A$ is the alveolar ventilation in liters per unit time.

In disease states, primary increases in P_aco_2 typically result from abnormally low carbon dioxide excretion by the lung, or alveolar hypoventilation. In one form of this disorder, termed global alveolar hypoventilation, the lungs themselves are normal. The term global means that all alveoli within the lung share the same degree of hypoventilation and thus experience a similar rise in alveolar P_{CO_2}. In such cases, alveolar ventilation may be depressed by a reduction in neurogenic respiratory drive caused by an overdose of sedative agents, disorders of neuromuscular control of the respiratory muscles, or intrinsic disturbances of the respiratory muscles.

Regional alveolar hypoventilation is the most common form of this disorder and is the result of regional disturbances of pulmonary mechanics within the lung. When these abnormalities are severe enough to produce net alveolar hypoventilation, P_aCO_2 rises. This form of alveolar hypoventilation is usually responsible for carbon dioxide retention in patients with pulmonary disease.

Sequence of Changes

When alveolar hypoventilation is present, carbon dioxide tensions increase because the metabolism generates more carbon dioxide than the lungs excrete. It should be noted that P_{CO_2} increases not only in arterial plasma but also in venous and capillary blood and, indeed, in all the body water in perfused organs. Because most cell membranes are highly permeable to carbon dioxide gas, an increase in blood P_{CO_2} is accompanied by an increase in P_{CO_2} in cellular water in the brain, liver, heart, and other organs.

The increased P_{CO_2} in mixed venous blood raises the concentration gradient for carbon dioxide between mixed venous blood and alveolar air, leading to increased carbon dioxide excretion. As a result of the altered gradient, a point is reached at which all the carbon dioxide that is generated metabolically is excreted by the lung. The P_{CO_2} in blood and various body fluids thus stabilizes, although at a higher value than before the development of alveolar hypoventilation.

As carbon dioxide accumulates in blood and other body fluids, it becomes hydrated as follows:

$$CO_2 + H_2O \rightleftarrows H_2CO_3 \rightleftarrows H^+ + HCO_3^-$$

The initial effect of a rise in P_{CO_2} is an increase in hydrogen ion concentration, that is, a decrease in pH. The degree to which pH falls depends not only on the degree of the P_{CO_2} increase but also on the direction and degree of change in bicarbonate concentration.

Mechanisms of Change in Bicarbonate Concentration

As P_{CO_2} increases, a secondary increase in bicarbonate that limits the change in pH is produced by two mechanisms. One of these involves the buffering of carbonic acid by blood and body buffers:

$$H_2CO_3 + OH^- \rightleftarrows HCO_3^- + H_2O$$

The buffering of H_2CO_3 has several features, one of which is that buffering produces an increase of bicarbonate concentration within seconds after a rise in P_{CO_2}. Thus, the buffer response reflects the changes seen in acute respiratory acidosis. Another feature is that buffering takes place in all compartments of body water. Therefore, the rise in bicarbonate concentration involves not only the blood but also intracellular water. Third, the increased bicarbonate concentration evoked by buffering is moderate in magnitude. For every 10 mm Hg increase in P_{CO_2} above 40 mm Hg, there is about a 1 mEq/l increase in bicarbonate concentration.[6] Thus, as P_{CO_2} increases from 40 to 80 mm Hg, bicarbonate concentration rises from 25 to 29 mEq/l; this increase still leaves the plasma and body fluids quite acidic. Finally, the degree of buffering is essentially the same in all patients with no other acid-base abnormalities.

The second mechanism that produces an increase in bicarbonate concentration involves the response of the kidney to increased P_{CO_2} concentrations. As P_{CO_2} is increased in the blood, renal tubular cells augment their hydrogen ion excretion. Such increased excretion leads to increased reabsorption of bicarbonate into the blood, raising the plasma bicarbonate concentration.

This renal mechanism has several important characteristics. First, it operates more slowly than the buffer mechanism. Maximal changes in bicarbonate produced by increases in P_{CO_2} require some 48 to 72 hours to develop after the primary increase in P_{CO_2}. Addition of the renal response to the buffer response brings about the changes of bicarbonate concentration in chronic respiratory acidosis.[7] A second characteristic is that most of the increase in bicarbonate concentration occurs in plasma and extracellular fluid and not intracellular water, because bicarbonate ion, unlike CO_2 gas, passes across most cell membranes rather slowly. A third characteristic is that the quantitative contribution of the renal response is substantially greater than that produced by buffering. For a 10 mm Hg increase in P_{CO_2}, there is approximately a 2 mEq/l increase in plasma bicarbonate. Thus, of the total increase in bicarbonate evoked by increases in P_{CO_2}, approximately 65 percent occurs as a result of renal tubular activity and only 35 percent is related to buffering. The amount of bicarbonate ion added to blood by the kidney for a given increase in P_aCO_2 varies little from patient to patient, and deviations from this value (2 Eq/l for a 10 mm Hg increase in P_{CO_2}) reflect complicating acid-base disturbances. The sum total of the increased bicarbonate concentration produced by the renal response and by buffering (about 3 mEq/l for each 10 mm Hg increase in P_aCO_2) is insufficient to normalize arterial pH. As a result, uncomplicated respiratory acidosis is always associated with lowering of pH.[8]

Complicating Metabolic Acid-Base Disturbances

It is not uncommon for patients with primary respiratory acidosis to experience either complicating metabolic acidosis or metabolic alkalosis. With complicating metabolic acidosis, the increase in bicarbonate concentration produced by a given increase in P_aCO_2 is less than the minimal one found when the condition is not present. Indeed, with severe metabolic acidosis, plasma bicarbonate concentrations may actually fall. For each 10 mm Hg increase in P_aCO_2, the minimal increase in bicarbonate produced by buffering alone is 1 mEq/l. Thus, patients with respiratory acidosis who show less than a 1 mEq/l increase in bicarbonate concentration have complicating metabolic acidosis.

Complicating metabolic acidosis, when present in patients with carbon dioxide retention, usually results from either renal insufficiency or lactic acidosis. Renal insufficiency is found in patients with chronic lung disease that is severe enough to produce cor pulmonale and right ventricular failure. As a result, renal perfusion falls, tubular acidification mechanisms become inadequate, and complicating metabolic acidosis ensues. Lactic acidosis is most commonly found under circumstances associated with severe right ventricular failure, sharp reductions in cardiac output, and decreased hepatic perfusion. Tissue hypoxia leads to increased lactate production, whereas hepatic hypoperfusion leads to decreased lactate removal. As a result, there is a marked increase in blood lactate concentration, which sharply lowers plasma pH and decreases bicarbonate concentration.

Complicating metabolic alkalosis (commonly called posthypercapnic alkalosis) may be diagnosed by finding that the increase in bicarbonate concentration for a given increase in P_aCO_2 exceeds the maximal one found when the condition is not present. A greater than 3 mEq/l increase in bicarbonate concentration for each 10 mm Hg increase in P_aCO_2 indicates the presence of complicating metabolic alkalosis.

Four common problems may cause complicating metabolic alkalosis. One of these is iatrogenic and occurs when hospitalized patients with marked elevations of P_{CO_2} are put on mechanical ventilators. Because the effectiveness of mechanical ventilators in increasing CO_2 excretion is high, plasma and whole-body P_{CO_2} may decrease rapidly. The rate at which bicarbonate ion can be excreted by the kidney, however, is relatively slow. Therefore, although the P_{CO_2} is brought down rapidly, the bicarbonate concentration does not decrease proportionately, and the patient may have an elevated bicarbonate concentration for any given P_{CO_2}. This form of alkalosis may produce disastrous consequences. The marked increase in pH may result in neuromuscular instability, convulsions, coma, and death. It is therefore necessary to bring Pco_2 down relatively slowly in patients who are maintained on mechanical ventilators. In some cases, it may be necessary to add more dead space to the ventilator system or to use carbon dioxide–enriched gas mixtures to prevent a rapid and sharp decrease in Pco_2 and a rise in pH.

A second cause of complicating metabolic alkalosis is chloride ion deficiency. This deficiency is related to a decrease in chloride intake and absorption as well as to an increase in urinary excretion of chloride. When plasma chloride is decreased, renal bicarbonate reabsorption tends to be more efficient, thereby giving rise to metabolic alkalosis.

Potassium deficiency, the third cause of complicating metabolic alkalosis, is common in carbon dioxide retention. If cellular potassium stores are inadequate, renal hydrogen ion excretion leads to metabolic alkalosis. Finally, diuretic agents that depress proximal sodium reabsorption in the kidney may increase the amount of sodium in the distal tubule, raising hydrogen ion excretion and leading to metabolic alkalosis [*see* Metabolic Alkalosis, *below*].

Treatment

Uncomplicated respiratory acidosis is treated by measures designed to normalize alveolar ventilation. In many circumstances, this objective can be accomplished by treating the underlying pulmonary disease. In cases of acute respiratory failure, it may be necessary to use mechanical ventilation. Complicating metabolic acidosis may require not only treatment of the underlying abnormality but also additional therapy with bicarbonate, at least in cases in which the decrease in plasma pH is severe.

Metabolic alkalosis can usually be controlled by an adequate intake of potassium chloride. In patients with life-threatening metabolic alkalosis causing major hemodynamic or neurologic abnormalities, carbonic anhydrase inhibitors are useful.

Respiratory Alkalosis

Respiratory alkalosis comprises those disorders characterized by a primary decrease in Pco_2. Primary respiratory alkalosis always occurs as a result of alveolar hyperventilation. The conditions associated with alveolar hyperventilation are pulmonary parenchymal disease (originating from reflexes or hypoxemia), pulmonary vascular disease, liver disease, fever, endotoxemia, pregnancy, midbrain lesions, hyperventilation syndrome (psychogenic), and salicylate intoxication.

It is often not appreciated that pulmonary parenchymal disease may be associated with low as well as high Pco_2. The most common cause of alveolar hyperventilation in pulmonary disease is a reflex stimulation of the central nervous system originating from disordered lung or chest wall mechanics. Arterial hypoxemia is another important cause of respiratory alkalosis. Alveolar hyperventilation in this circumstance occurs mainly because reductions in arterial Po_2 evoke impulses in the peripheral chemoreceptors—the carotid body and aortic bodies. Abnormalities of the pulmonary vasculature are also able to evoke alveolar hyperventilation. Although the specific mechanism is not known, this association suggests that the lung vasculature possesses receptors that stimulate the central nervous system and thereby increase ventilation.

Severe liver disease is frequently associated with alveolar hyperventilation. Indeed, an important sign of impending hepatic coma is the presence of a low Pco_2 and an appropriately high pH.[9]

Fever commonly produces an increase in ventilation that is disproportionately high for the increase in metabolism caused by the fever. As a result, Pco_2 tends to be low.

Patients in septic shock, particularly when it is associated with endotoxemia, often show alveolar hyperventilation.

Low values of Pco_2 develop approximately three weeks after the inception of pregnancy, and alveolar hyperventilation is maintained for several weeks after term. The cause of the hyperventilation is possibly related to high progesterone or progesteronelike activity in the tissues.[10]

Profound hyperventilation is an important sign of lesions in the midbrain and is most commonly found after acute vascular injury of the brainstem.[11]

In a significant number of cases, respiratory alkalosis develops as a result of the so-called hyperventilation syndrome, which has a psychogenic basis. This disorder affects men as well as women and may be associated with chronic hyperventilation as well as with acute, paroxysmal hyperventilation.

Intoxication by various drugs may lead to respiratory alkalosis. For example, salicylate intoxication produces direct stimulation of the respiratory center and leads to severe respiratory alkalosis initially. As the disorder progresses, metabolic acidosis may develop.

Sequence of Changes

As ventilation removes more carbon dioxide than the metabolism produces, there is a decrease of P_{CO_2} in the blood and other compartments of body fluids. Consequently, mixed venous P_{CO_2} is reduced, and the gradient for excretion of CO_2 in the lung becomes smaller. Ultimately, the metabolic production and pulmonary excretion of CO_2 become balanced at a lower P_{CO_2} level throughout the body fluids. The reduction in P_{CO_2} leads to a lower carbonic acid concentration and, therefore, an increase in pH.

The increase in pH is related not only to the level of reduced P_{CO_2} but also to changes in bicarbonate concentration. Three processes tend to decrease bicarbonate concentration as P_{CO_2} becomes reduced. One of these is buffering. As pH rises, blood and body buffers react with bicarbonate ion as follows:

$$HCO_3^- + H^+ \rightarrow H_2O + CO_2$$

The second mechanism involves a sharp rise in pH that augments the activity of the key enzyme in anaerobic glycolysis and thereby increases the rate of lactic acid generation.

Both these processes operate quickly and are found in acute respiratory alkalosis. They reduce bicarbonate concentrations in the plasma by about 1.5 mEq/l for each 10 mm Hg decrease in P_aCO_2.

The third process is renal: decreased P_{CO_2} leads to a reduction of net hydrogen ion excretion by the kidney. As a result, hydrogen ion reabsorption increases and plasma bicarbonate concentration decreases. The renal mechanism requires 48 to 72 hours for maximal effect and is found in chronic respiratory alkalosis. The renal mechanism reduces bicarbonate concentration in the plasma by about 3 mEq/l for each 10 mm Hg decrease in P_aCO_2. Thus, the greatest reduction in bicarbonate concentration evoked by respiratory alkalosis amounts to about 4.5 mEq/l for each 10 mm Hg decrease in P_aCO_2.[12]

In acute respiratory alkalosis, the net effects of buffering and lactic acid generation are insufficient to lower plasma pH to normal levels. In chronic respiratory alkalosis, however, the compensatory mechanisms lower plasma bicarbonate proportionately to the reduction in P_{CO_2}, and plasma pH tends to be high normal or normal. Thus, unlike respiratory acidosis, chronic respiratory alkalosis is usually associated with a normal pH.

The most common concurrent acid-base disturbance in respiratory alkalosis is complicating metabolic alkalosis [*see* Metabolic Alkalosis, *below*]. This condition can be diagnosed by finding a reduction in bicarbonate less than 4.5 mEq/l for each 10 mm Hg change in P_aCO_2 in the chronic state. Its mechanisms do not differ from those seen in respiratory acidosis. Specific treatment directed at the low P_{CO_2} itself is generally not indicated, and therapy is for the underlying disorder.

Metabolic Acidosis

Metabolic acidosis is defined as a group of disorders [*see Table 1*] characterized by a primary decrease in bicarbonate concentration.

The ingestion of preformed hydrogen ion occurs rarely. Normally, it follows the

Table 1 Causes of Metabolic Acidosis

Ingestion or administration of preformed acid
  Mineral acid ingestion
  Rhubarb poisoning (oxalic acid)

Acid metabolized from exogenous substances
  Ammonium chloride $\rightarrow$ urea + H$^+$
  Methyl alcohol $\rightarrow$ formic acid
  Ethylene glycol $\rightarrow$ oxalic acid
  Sulfur $\rightarrow$ sulfate + H$^+$

Disturbances of endogenous acid metabolism
  Lactic acidosis
  Diabetic ketoacidosis

Renal acidosis
  Reduction of nephron mass
  Renal tubular acidosis

Hypoaldosteronism
Hyperparathyroidism
Extrarenal bicarbonate loss

accidental, suicidal, or therapeutic use of strong acids. Green rhubarb contains high concentrations of oxalic acid. The ingestion of this plant by infants has reportedly led to high levels of oxalic acid in body fluids and overwhelming metabolic acidosis.

There are several substances that can cause severe metabolic acidosis when they are ingested because they are metabolized to hydrogen ion. Ammonium chloride in large doses is metabolized to urea and hydrogen ion. Methyl alcohol, which is occasionally ingested when it is mistaken for ethanol, is metabolized to formic acid. Ethylene glycol, which is found in antifreeze, may be ingested under a variety of circumstances; one of its metabolic products is oxalic acid, which accumulates in body fluids [*see Chapter 23*]. Chronic metabolic acidosis may be associated with the ingestion of elemental sulfur.[13] Sulfur, used as a home remedy for various ailments, is reduced to sulfide by colonic organisms and is oxidized to sulfate with the release of hydrogen ions.

A variety of endogenous metabolic disturbances can lead to the accumulation of high concentrations of various organic acids. In this category, the two most common and important disorders by far are lactic acidosis[12] and diabetic ketoacidosis.

Lactic Acidosis

Etiology

In lactic acidosis, lactic acid, which is the end product of glycolysis, accumulates in the blood and tissues. The subsequent depletion of body buffers leads to substantial reductions in pH. Four mechanisms regulate blood lactate levels: the rate of lactate generation; the rate of lactate transport from tissues to plasma and from plasma to the liver, where lactate is utilized; the rate of lactate utilization, which occurs largely but not exclusively in the liver; and the rate of lactate excretion by the kidney. Only the first three mechanisms are important clinically. Ordinarily, they operate to produce a normal blood lactate concentration of approximately 1 mEq/l. Three factors regulate the rate of lactate generation:

1. Oxygen availability. As adenosine triphosphate (ATP) generation from oxidative phosphorylation decreases, cells respond with a higher rate of glycolysis, which increases lactate concentrations in the tissues and, ultimately, in the blood.
2. pH. Increases in pH raise the activity of phosphofructokinase, the rate-limiting enzyme of glycolysis. As pH increases, so does the activity of the enzyme, and more lactate is formed.
3. Oxidation-reduction state. Oxidation-reduction potentials are an important determinant of the rate at which glucose is metabolized to lactate.

The rate of lactate utilization also depends on several factors, including the availability of oxygen in liver cells—the oxidation of lactate is an oxygen-requiring process; the degree of hepatic perfusion—decreases in liver perfusion limit the quantity of lactate presented to liver cells; and the functional capacity of hepatocytes—alterations of hepatocyte function may impair lactate oxidation. Disorders producing lactic acidosis can be classified on the basis of these considerations [*see Table 2*].

Increased generation of lactate is most commonly caused by reduced tissue perfusion, as occurs in shock or cardiac arrest. When perfusion is reduced, the oxygen supply to various tissues becomes inadequate and glycolysis is enhanced. Generalized convulsive states may be caused by raised blood lactate concentrations resulting from the increased glycolysis that occurs in exercising muscle.

Large tumor masses, such as leukemias, lymphomas, and extensive visceral metastatic disease, may increase lactate generation. Many tumor cells have an increased rate of glycolysis even when oxygen is in high supply. Thus, tumor-associated rates of lactate generation may occasionally cause lactic acidosis.

In cyanide poisoning, ATP formation depends on anaerobic glycolysis; thus, there is a greatly increased rate of lactate generation, resulting in lactic acidosis.[14] Carbon monoxide poisoning limits oxygen supply and is associated with substantial increases in the rate of lactate production.

The drinking of alcohol leads to modest elevations in blood lactate concentrations. Occasionally, severe alcoholism, particularly when it occurs under conditions of caloric depletion, is associated with marked increases in blood lactate concentrations. The precise mechanism of the increase in lactate is not known, but ethanol probably competes for electrons in the liver. Lactic acidosis of alcoholism is therefore possibly caused by decreased utilization rather than increased generation of lactate.

Decreased hepatic removal of lactate is the second major cause of increased lactate levels in blood. Hepatic oxidation of lactate can be decreased by any form of severe liver failure, which may be related to reduced hepatic perfusion, hepatocyte failure, or replacement of hepatocytes by a tumor or other infiltrating tissue.

Table 2   Causes of Lactic Acidosis

Increased generation of lactate
  Decreased tissue perfusion
    Shock
    Cardiac arrest
  Increased skeletal muscle activity
    Convulsive states
  Large tumor masses
  Cyanide poisoning
  Carbon monoxide poisoning
  Alcoholism (possibly causes decreased utilization of lactate)

Decreased utilization of lactate
  Phenformin intoxication
  Liver failure
    Reduced hepatic perfusion
    Hepatocyte failure
    Hepatocyte replacement (e.g., by tumor)
  Diabetes mellitus

Lactic acidosis X
Factitial lactic acidosis

Nearly every patient with diabetic ketoacidosis has a moderate elevation of blood lactate concentration. True lactic acidosis, however, is rare in diabetes mellitus; when present, its cause is not clear. It may occur in the absence of shock or other overt precipitating events and may be related to decreased utilization of lactate.

The term lactic acidosis X had been used for many years to describe a condition in which overwhelming lactic acidosis occurred without obvious cause.[15] Patients with this condition were a mixed group whose acidosis developed in the absence of shock, liver failure, or tissue hypoxia. Since the time of that description, similar patients (formerly classified as having lactic acidosis X) have been classified as belonging to one of the etiologic categories described above. The term, however, has been retained, and a rare case is seen for which this designation is appropriate.

So-called factitial lactic acidosis can occur when blood (usually with a high white cell count) that is drawn for blood gas analysis is stored for relatively long periods of time at room temperature. Such conditions can lead to lactic acid generation by both red cells and white cells. Subsequent analysis of the blood reveals a markedly low pH and a high lactate concentration. Of course, the lactic acidosis is in the blood in the syringe and not in the patient; therefore, this form of lactic acidosis requires recognition rather than treatment.

Sequence of Changes

As lactic acid accumulates in the blood, the first stage of the process is compensated acidosis. During this stage, each 1 mEq lactic acid is stoichiometrically buffered by 1 mEq bicarbonate according to the following equation:

$$BHCO_3 + HLAC \rightleftarrows B\ Lactate + H_2O + CO_2$$

The patient experiences alveolar hyperventilation, and changes in arterial pH are not dramatic at this point.

As lactic acid continues to accumulate, a state of uncompensated acidosis develops, blood buffers are depleted, and arterial pH rapidly falls.

In the third stage, a so-called alkaline overshoot may develop. This condition occurs when the metabolic abnormality that originally produced the lactic acidosis is reversed. As the reversal occurs, lactate is transported to the liver, where it is oxidized, as shown in the following equation:

$$Lactate + H_2CO_3 + 3\ O_2 \rightarrow 3\ CO_2 + HCO_3^-$$

Each 1 mEq lactate that is oxidized gives rise to 1 mEq bicarbonate.

If the patient has been treated so that the sum of lactate and bicarbonate concentrations exceeds 25 mEq/l (the normal bicarbonate concentration), the bicarbonate concentration following oxidation of lactate will be higher than normal, and the patient may experience metabolic alkalosis. For exam-ple, a patient with a blood lactate concentration of 15 mEq/l and a plasma bicarbonate concentration of 10 mEq/l may be treated so as to raise the plasma bicarbonate concentration to 25 mEq/l. After the underlying metabolic abnormality is corrected, the 15 mEq/l of lactate will be converted to 15 mEq/l bicarbonate, and the final bicarbonate concentration can be as high as 40 mEq/l.

Diagnosis

The possibility that lactic acidosis is present should be considered in the differential diagnosis of severely acidotic patients, particularly those who have a known precipitating condition. In contrast to patients with diabetic ketoacidosis, patients with lactic acidosis have only moderate hyperglycemia or may even have hypoglycemia. Ketones are low or absent in the urine and blood.

A so-called anion gap will be found. The term anion gap refers to the negative charges in plasma that are not accounted for by chloride ion, bicarbonate ion, and protein. The sum of positively charged ions in the plasma must be equal to the sum of negatively charged ions. An anion gap indicates that the number of negative ions from such normal sources as chloride, bicarbonate, and protein does not equal the observed number of positive charges contributed by sodium and potassium. To calculate the anion gap, the sodium and potassium ion concentrations are first added to get an estimate of positive charge. Next, the negative charge is estimated by summing the chloride concentration, the bicarbonate concentration, and 20 mEq/l—this last constant allows for negative charges on protein, phosphate, and sulfate [see Table 3]. In the presence of organic acidosis, such as lactic acidosis, the organic ion will account for some of the negative charges required for electroneutrality.

It is important to recognize that not only lactate ion but any organic anion will give rise to a significant anion gap.[16] Once the anion has been identified as lactate, however, calculations of the anion gap may be used to follow the progress of the patient. The most specific way of diagnosing lactic acidosis is

Table 3 Calculation of Anion Gap

	Positive Charges (mEq/l)		Negative Charges (mEq/l)		Anion Gap
Normal	Na^+ K^+ Total	140 5 ___ 145	Cl^- HCO_3^- Protein⁻, phosphate⁻, and sulfate⁻ Total	100 25 20 145	145 - 145 = 0 mEq/l
Organic (lactic) acidosis	Na^+ K^+ Total	140 5 ___ 145	Cl^- HCO_3^- Protein⁻, phosphate⁻, and sulfate⁻ Total	95 10 20 125	145 - 125 = 20 mEq/l

to measure blood lactate concentrations directly. This rate is a fairly simple measurement, made by an enzymatic technique.

Alterations in the acid-base status of the plasma may affect the magnitude of the anion gap independently of increases in lactate (organic acid) concentrations.[17] For example, alkalosis increases and acidosis decreases the net negative charge on plasma proteins. Alkalosis is therefore associated with an increase in the calculated anion gap, whereas acidosis decreases this gap. Thus, in patients with metabolic alkalosis, organic anion accumulation should not be diagnosed merely on the basis of an increased anion gap.

Treatment

The underlying cause of lactic acidosis should be treated if possible. Thus, in patients with lactic acidosis that results from shock, cardiac arrest, or convulsions, treatment must be directed toward the correction of these underlying conditions.

In addition, bicarbonate should be given to raise the serum bicarbonate concentration. Before the amount of bicarbonate needed can be assessed, a quantitative estimate of the lactic acid transfer rate must be obtained. This rate is estimated by giving a specified amount of bicarbonate during a known period of time and noting the effect on plasma bicarbonate concentration. In the absence of increased lactic acid transfer to the plasma and of renal excretion of bicarbonate, 100 mEq bicarbonate infused during a one-hour period should raise the serum bicarbonate concentration by about 3 mEq/l.

The use of insulin in diabetics with significant lactic acidosis reportedly reduces the need for bicarbonate and greatly decreases mortality.[18]

Unnatural D-Lactic Acidosis

D-Lactic acid is an optical isomer of lactic acid: unlike L-lactic acid, it is produced by microorganisms but not by animals. Some patients with the short bowel syndrome may experience D-lactic acidosis as a result of increased production of D-lactic acid by certain intestinal bacteria. D-Lactic acid is not metabolized by human L-lactate dehydrogenases and can be excreted only by the kidneys. Accumulation of D-lactic acid in the gut followed by systemic absorption leads to metabolic acidosis, which can develop whether or not large amounts of *Lactobacillus* tablets have been ingested.[19]

The diagnosis of D-lactic acidosis should be suspected in a patient with the short bowel syndrome who shows central nervous system dysfunction, dehydration, and Kussmaul's breathing in the absence of a known cause of metabolic acidosis. The symptoms of patients who have D-lactic acidosis are disproportionately severe for the degree of acidosis, which suggests that D-lactate itself may produce abnormalities independent of the decrease in pH.

Specific diagnosis requires the direct identification and measurement of D-lactic acid in plasma. D-Lactate dehydrogenase is employed in the enzymatic analysis of lactic acid. The anion gap tends to be high normal because plasma chloride concentrations are high in patients with this disorder. Severe D-lactic acidosis, however, produces a sharply increased anion gap. In the absence of suitable analytic methods, a presumptive diagnosis should be made on clinical grounds.

Therapy includes hydration, use of oral vancomycin or a nonabsorbable antibiotic such as neomycin, and a sharp reduction in oral carbohydrate intake.

Diabetic Ketoacidosis

It has been generally accepted that the decrease in the plasma bicarbonate concentration in diabetic ketoacidosis is balanced by the sum of the plasma concentrations of the beta-hydroxybutyrate and acetoacetate anions (pure anion-gap acidosis). Several studies indicate, however, that diabetic patients show a broad spectrum of forms of metabolic acidosis, ranging from pure anion-gap acidosis to pure hyperchloremic acidosis. Consequently, the plasma organic acid concentrations cannot be reliably estimated from the calculated anion gap.[20] The status of renal function evidently determines which form of acidosis develops—hyperchloremic or anion-gap acidosis. Patients with pure diabetic hyperchloremic acidosis recover more slowly than those with pure anion-gap acidosis. It not clear whether other forms of acute organic acid metabolic acidosis, such as lactic acidosis, show such variable acid-base patterns.

Primary treatment is insulin and fluid replacement, not bicarbonate. Insulin reverses the metabolic abnormality and returns the patient's acid-base status to normal. Bicarbonate should not be given unless the patient's pH is less than 7.1; even then, the amount of administered bicarbonate should be limited until the metabolic abnormality is reversed by treatment with insulin, water, electrolytes, and glucose.

Heritable Metabolic Abnormalities

Heritable metabolic abnormalities also cause endogenous organic acid accumulation.[21] There are effective therapies for some of these rare diseases.

One such disorder includes the methylmalonic acidemias, which are composed of six biochemically distinct mutant classes marked by varying abnormalities. Affected children have an autosomal recessively inherited deficiency of methylmalonyl coenzyme A (CoA) mutase. Methylmalonyl CoA mutase catalyzes the conversion of L-methylmalonyl CoA to succinyl CoA and requires cobalamin as a cofactor molecule.[22]

The clinical picture consists of life-threatening or lethal metabolic acidosis marked by the accumulation of large amounts of ketones and methylmalonic acid in the blood, urine, and cerebrospinal fluid. Some patients will respond to pharmacologic doses of cobalamin vitamers by showing dramatic clinical and chemical improvement. The response to therapy depends on the nature of the biochemical defect in the methylmalonyl CoA mutase.[22]

Renal Acidosis

Acidosis commonly develops in patients with kidney disease. There are two etiologic forms of renal acidosis. One form involves a widespread reduction in nephron mass in the absence of specific renal tubular lesions. This form is seen in glomerulonephritis, chronic pyelonephritis, and vascular lesions of the kidney. As the nephron mass declines, the ability of the kidney to excrete hydrogen ion in the form of ammonium ion and titratable acidity also decreases. Renal excretion of free hydrogen ions, however, is only partially impaired, so that urinary pH remains acid until late in the course of the disease.[23]

The other form, renal tubular acidosis,[24] is characterized by specific abnormalities of renal tubular acidification mechanisms. It may be inherited or acquired; a number of drugs can cause this abnormality. When the site of the defect is at the level of the proximal tubule, the acidosis appears to result from a partial failure of bicarbonate reabsorption. Renal acidosis may also be caused by a distal tubular defect. In such cases, the distal tubule cannot develop an appropriate hydrogen ion gradient between extracellular fluid and tubular urine; this deficiency raises the urine pH to a level too high for the patient's acid-base status.

Patients with hypoaldosteronism usually have metabolic acidosis. In such patients, elevated urine pH may be caused by hyperkalemia, which decreases the excretion of ammonium in the urine and thus interferes with renal acidification.[25]

Patients with hyperparathyroidism tend to show high plasma chloride and low plasma bicarbonate concentrations, even in the absence of renal disease.[26] Parathyroid hormone appears to increase directly the tubular reabsorption of chloride ion. Consequently, bicarbonate reabsorption is depressed, and metabolic acidosis (usually mild) develops. The loss of body fluids rich in bicarbonate ion, as occurs during severe diarrhea in young children, may also lead to metabolic acidosis.

Sequence of Changes in Metabolic Acidosis

In metabolic acidosis, as bicarbonate concentrations decrease, three compensatory mechanisms become operative. One is the titrating of hydrogen ion by blood and body buffers. Buffers present in bone play a particularly important role in this process; in fact, chronic metabolic acidosis is commonly associated with loss of bone mass.

The second mechanism is enhanced excretion of hydrogen ion, in the form of both ammonium and titratable acidity, in urine with a low pH. Patients whose metabolic acidosis is related to underlying kidney disease cannot compensate in this manner.

The third mechanism involves an increase in alveolar ventilation in response to the change in plasma pH. The consequent decrease in Pco_2 tends to maintain an almost normal pH. The decrease in Pco_2 is biphasic. In acute metabolic acidosis, reductions in pH stimulate the peripheral chemoreceptors to evoke hyperventilation. The resultant drop in Pco_2, however, inhibits the central chemoreceptors, which respond rapidly to changes in Pco_2 but rather slowly to alterations in blood hydrogen ion and bicarbonate ion. The intensity of the ventilatory response is therefore blunted by the initial fall in Pco_2. In chronic metabolic acidosis, the respiratory center develops an increased sensitivity to CO_2, leading to a further increase in alveolar ventilation. The relationship between the primary reduction in bicarbonate ion and the secondary drop in Pco_2 appears quite reproducible from patient to patient.

In most patients with metabolic acidosis, the Pco_2 drops by about 1.1 mm Hg for each mEq/l reduction in plasma bicarbonate concentration.[27] The major complicating acid-base disturbance is respiratory acidosis, caused by abnormalities of pulmonary carbon dioxide exchange. Such patients show less than a 1.1 mm Hg fall in Pco_2 for each 1 mEq/l decrease in serum bicarbonate ion concentration.

Treatment depends on the underlying cause of the metabolic acidosis. The administration of base, usually in the form of bicarbonate, is a commonly employed approach [*see* Lactic Acidosis *and* Diabetic Ketoacidosis, *above*].

Metabolic Alkalosis

Metabolic alkalosis, characterized by a primary increase in plasma bicarbonate concentration, has several causes [*see* Table 4].[28] Prolonged, excessive ingestion of base in absorbable antacid preparations is a rare cause of metabolic alkalosis.

Vomiting and gastric drainage result in the loss of hydrochloric acid, sodium chloride, and potassium chloride and lead directly to metabolic alkalosis. Potassium deficiency and reduction of the extracellular volume accentuate the degree of metabolic alkalosis. Congenital alkalosis with diar-

Table 4 Causes of Metabolic Alkalosis
Excessive ingestion of base
Extrarenal loss of acid
Vomiting, gastric suction, or gastric fistula
Congenital alkalosis with diarrhea
Renal tubular dysfunction
Chloride deficiency
Potassium deficiency
Increased distal sodium delivery
?Hyperaldosteronism
Metabolic conversion of organic acids to bicarbonate (alkaline overshoot)
Contraction of blood volume
Excessive increase in plasma bicarbonate concentration in response to rise in P_aCO_2 (posthypercapnic metabolic alkalosis)

rhea, found at birth, is marked by a profuse watery stool and metabolic alkalosis; stool chloride is higher than stool sodium plus potassium, and urinary chloride excretion is reduced or absent. The main defect appears to be an inability of the ileum to reabsorb chloride ion actively, which leads to an excessive loss of hydrogen ion in the stool.

In a variety of circumstances, the kidney excretes more hydrogen ion than is appropriate for the acid-base status of the plasma, thus causing renal tubular alkalosis. In chloride deficiency, bicarbonate ion reabsorption may be increased. Potassium deficiency leads to excessive hydrogen ion excretion, probably by an ion exchange mechanism. Increased delivery of sodium ion to the distal tubule (e.g., following the use of diuretics that inhibit proximal sodium reabsorption) raises potassium ion and hydrogen ion excretion. Hyperaldosteronism increases sodium ion reabsorption by the distal tubule, which may raise hydrogen ion excretion. Studies indicate, however, that hyperkalemia in hypoaldosteronism produces metabolic acidosis by suppressing the excretion of ammonium

ion; therefore, hyperaldosteronism may not be a cause of renal tubular alkalosis.

Posthypercapnic metabolic alkalosis and metabolic alkalosis caused by the hepatic oxidation of organic acids to bicarbonate ion have already been described. Use of diuretics in edematous patients may cause contraction alkalosis by accelerating excretion of sodium chloride without producing a matching loss of sodium bicarbonate. In such cases, metabolic alkalosis may develop without net loss of hydrogen ions or gain of negative ions.

Sequence of Changes

As plasma pH increases and bicarbonate concentrations rise in metabolic alkalosis, several compensatory changes occur. The accumulated base is partially neutralized by blood and body buffers. In nonrenal forms of metabolic alkalosis, excretion of hydrogen ion may decrease. In acute metabolic alkalosis, the urinary pH tends to be high, whereas in persistent metabolic alkalosis, urinary pH tends to decline. (Acid urine in conjunction with high plasma pH is frequently described as paradoxic aciduria.) A major compensatory change is the ventilatory depression caused by the high plasma pH. In acute conditions, a decrease in the neural output from the carotid and aortic bodies is presumably responsible for this depression of ventilation. A chronically high pH may depress the sensitivity of the respiratory center. Some patients show a relatively appropriate respiratory response to metabolic alkalosis, whereas others may have a relatively normal P_{CO_2}. In any case, the respiratory compensation is always incomplete, and metabolic alkalosis is the most poorly compensated acid-base disorder because the plasma pH is always elevated.

Measurement of Acid-Base Variables and Clinical Overview

Effect of Temperature

Core body temperature varies between 64.4° F (18° C) in hypothermic anesthesia and 105.8° F (41° C) in severe hyperpyrexia. Although blood pH and P_{CO_2} change as temperature does, both values are measured at 98.6° F (37° C). Thus, most authorities maintain that the measured arterial pH and P_{CO_2} values should be corrected for changes in body temperature, especially in cases of profound hypothermia, in which temperature deviation may be significant. In hyperpyrexia, however, deviation of body temperature from normal is small; hence, correction of pH and P_{CO_2} seldom affects management.

Effect of Severe Illness

Conventional measurement of acid-base variables relies on the assumption that at a given temperature, the dissociation constant of carbonic acid (pK'_a) and the solubility of CO_2 (αP_{CO_2}) do not vary. Yet this assumption may not be true in acutely ill patients, and a calculation of $[HCO_3^-]$ based on these values may then be erroneous. In such cases, total plasma CO_2 measurement, which is independent of pK'_a and αP_{CO_2}, should be used.[29]

These considerations and the impact of temperature on acid-base variables (see above) raise a fundamental issue. Conventional clinical practice assumes that acid-base changes result from $[HCO_3^-]$ alterations (largely regulated by the kidney) or from P_{CO_2} alterations (largely regulated by ventilation). Several other mechanisms, however, probably also cause plasma pH changes in vivo. Such factors include alterations in H^+ activity (increased or decreased binding of H^+ to proteins), in pK'_a, or in αP_{CO_2} (CO_2-binding dependent). Alterations in the latter two variables depend on osmolality, temperature, and other factors. Consequently, changes in organ function or cell function may occur independently of changes in ventilation or renal function.

Summary of Acid-base Metabolism

An organized approach to the interpretation of acid-base abnormalities can be formulated based on the observed pattern of changes in such variables as pH, P_{CO_2}, and $[HCO_3]$ [*see Figure 1*]. The degree and direction of change in these variables differ for the primary acid-base disturbances [*see Table 5*]. In a few patients, however, the mixture of acid-base disturbances is too complex for this analytic approach; this approach is also not applicable to patients in whom acid-base variables are rapidly changing. The approach, however, should permit the accurate diagnosis of more than 90 percent of isolated acid-base disturbances.

The first judgment to be made is whether the arterial pH is low (less than 7.35), high (greater than 7.45), or normal (between 7.35 and 7.45). If it is low, then respiratory acidosis and metabolic acidosis must be considered. In respiratory acidosis, the P_{CO_2} and bicarbonate concentrations are high; in metabolic acidosis, the P_{CO_2} and bicarbonate concentrations are low. If the bicarbonate concentration is less than normal (below 25 mEq/l) or not appropriately high in patients with respiratory acidosis, complicating metabolic acidosis must also be present. Some patients with a high P_{CO_2} experience complicating metabolic alkalosis while still maintaining low pH values. If patients with metabolic acidosis do not have an appropriately low P_{CO_2}, complicating respiratory acidosis (the most common additional acid-base abnormality in such patients) must be present.

If the pH of the patient is high, there are two possible abnormalities: acute respiratory alkalosis or metabolic alkalosis. Patients with acute respiratory alkalosis will have a low P_{CO_2} and a low serum bicarbonate concentration. If the bicarbonate concentration is not appropriately low, the patient has complicating metabolic alkalosis (the most common complicating disorder in this group of patients). The presence of metabolic alkalosis is indicated by a high P_{CO_2} and a high bicarbonate concentration. However, some patients with metabolic alkalosis do not have substantial elevations of P_{CO_2}, and some patients with the combination of respiratory acidosis and complicating metabolic alkalosis may have elevated pH values.

If the pH is normal, there are four possibilities. The first, the absence of an acid-base

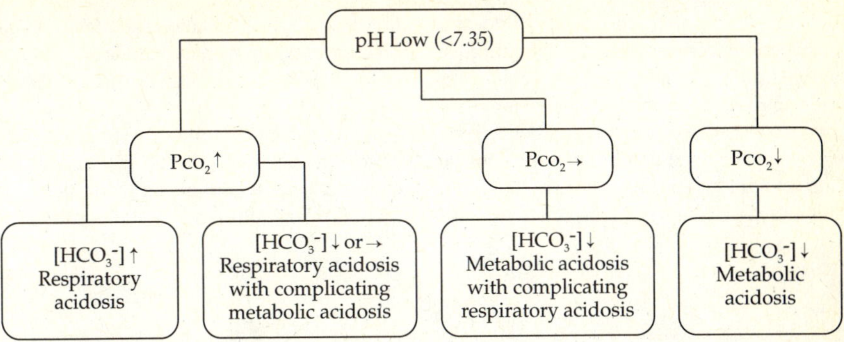

Some patients with a very high Pco$_2$ and complicating metabolic alkalosis may have a low pH.

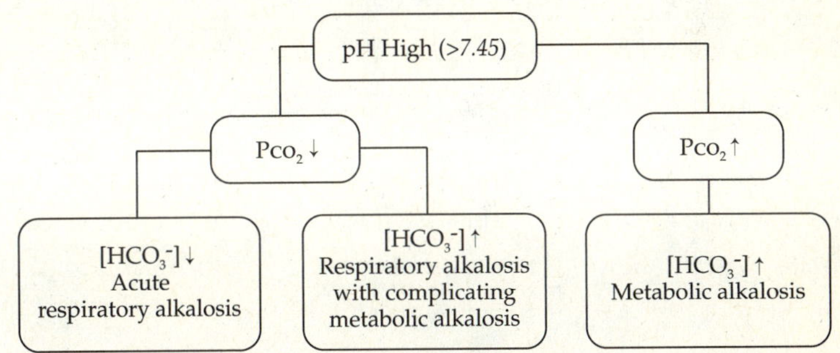

Some patients with respiratory acidosis complicated by metabolic alkalosis may have a high pH.

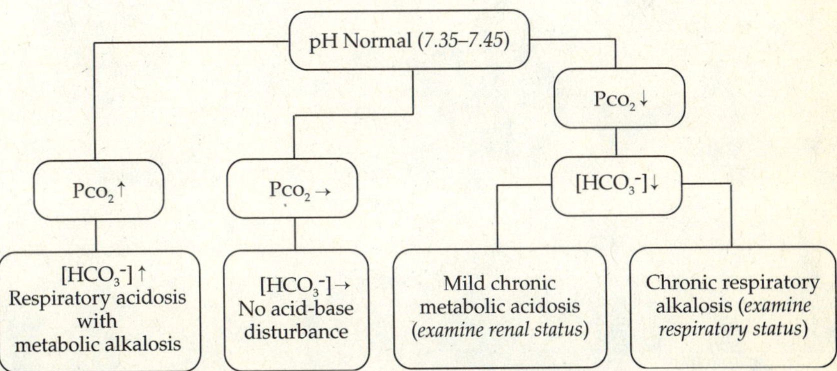

Figure 1   *Illustration presents a diagnostic approach to common acid-base disturbances. Fluctuations in* Pco$_2$ *and* [HCO$_3^-$] *and the associated abnormalities observed at different pH levels are shown.*

disturbance, is indicated by a normal Pco$_2$ and bicarbonate concentration. The second possibility, chronic respiratory alkalosis, is suggested by a low Pco$_2$ and low bicarbonate concentration. Patients with the third possibility, mild chronic metabolic acidosis, however, may also show a low P_{CO_2} and bicarbonate concentration. To distinguish between chronic respiratory alkalosis and mild chronic metabolic acidosis, the physician may need to look at the patient's renal or respiratory status. Finally, a normal pH and a high P_{CO_2} and bicarbonate concentration may be present in patients with respiratory acidosis and metabolic alkalosis. As indicated previously, however, low and high pH values have also been found in this patient group.

Once the nature of the acid-base disturbance has been established, the search for causes can begin and the appropriate treatment can be instituted.

References

1. Fundamentals of Acid-Base Regulation, 4th ed. Blackwell Scientific Publications, Oxford, 1972
2. Circulation 35:1019, 1967
3. J Clin Invest 40:31, 1961
4. Mechanisms of Contraction of the Normal and Failing Heart, 2nd ed. Little, Brown & Co, Boston, 1976
5. Adv Protein Chem 4:407, 1948
6. J Clin Invest 44:291, 1965
7. J Clin Invest 32:972, 1953
8. N Engl J Med 280:162, 1969
9. Trans Assoc Am Physicians 88:202, 1975
10. J Clin Endocrinol Metab 14:522, 1954
11. Breathing: Hering-Breuer Centenary Symposium on Breathing, 1969. Churchill Livingstone, New York, 1970
12. Am J Med 30:840, 1961
13. N Engl J Med 297:869, 1977
14. Arch Intern Med 137:1051, 1977
15. N Engl J Med 293:468, 1975
16. N Engl J Med 297:814, 1977
17. N Engl J Med 300:1421, 1979
18. Ann Intern Med 87:591, 1977
19. N Engl J Med 306:1344, 1982
20. N Engl J Med 307:1603, 1982
21. N Engl J Med 295:310, 1976
22. N Engl J Med 308:857, 1983
23. Medicine (Baltimore) 44:263, 1965
24. N Engl J Med 281:1405, 1969
25. N Engl J Med 294:361, 1976
26. Ann Intern Med 79:566, 1973
27. Ann Intern Med 66:312, 1967
28. Kidney Int 1:306, 1972
29. N Engl J Med 306:864, 1982

40 Systemic Lupus Erythematosus

DWIGHT R. ROBINSON, M.D.

Systemic lupus erythematosus (SLE) varies greatly in clinical manifestations, mode of presentation, and course. The course of this chronic multisystemic inflammatory disease may range from benign to fatal. No cure is available, but medical measures often ameliorate the symptoms of SLE.

The incidence is not precisely known. An annual incidence of about seven cases per 100,000 was found in two major studies.[1] Ninety percent of SLE cases occur in women; black females are affected more often than white females. The first symptoms usually appear between 15 and 25 years of age.

Clinical Manifestations

A clinical presentation of fever, rash, and arthritis in a young female should raise the possibility of SLE. Patients may also present with acute hemolytic anemia, thrombocytopenic purpura, or pericarditis. Remission usually occurs, and a symptom-free interval of several years may follow. Eventual recurrence in a variety of forms is likely. The severity ranges from a mild illness with negligible morbidity to an acute illness simultaneously involving many organs. The course is unpredictable; involvement of the kidneys or central nervous system is probably an unfavorable prognostic sign.

Several factors may precipitate exacerbation: infections, physical or emotional stress, sunlight, surgery, pregnancy, and certain drugs. Illness may recur without apparent cause. Patients have an increased susceptibility to bacterial infections. Corticosteroid treatment and the presence of renal disease[2,3] further increase the risk posed by ordinary pathogens as well as by opportunistic bacteria and fungi. Patients treated with immunosuppressive drugs have an increased incidence of herpes zoster (an incidence of 21 percent in one series), but the infection seldom becomes disseminated.[4]

Fever

Fever occurs in the majority of SLE patients. It is usually low grade but may be extreme in a so-called lupus crisis. Often, evidence of multisystemic involvement accompanied by high fever is seen during such a crisis, but fever may also be an isolated manifestation.[1,5] Fever caused by SLE should be distinguished from that caused by a superimposed infection. Serious infections, including life-threatening bacteremias, are common in SLE. Shaking chills, neutrophilic leukocytosis, and normal levels of anti-DNA antibodies are more often associated with fever caused by bacterial infections than with fever caused by active systemic lupus erythematosus.[6]

Skeletal Disorders

Arthritis, one of the most common manifestations of SLE, occurs in about 90 percent of patients. It commonly involves arthralgia, overt swelling and effusions, and morning stiffness. The arthritis is symmetric and polyarticular, frequently affecting the hands, wrists, elbows, knees, and ankles. The arthritic episodes are usually intermittent, lasting from hours to months followed by varying periods of remission. Chronic joint deformity (often a swan-neck deformity or an ulnar deviation, similar to deformities seen in rheumatoid arthritis) develops in about 30 percent of patients. In rare cases, x-ray or pathologic examination demonstrates evidence of cartilage or bone destruction.[1]

Tendinitis may develop. Achilles, patellar, or hand tendons rarely rupture, but when they do, such ruptures usually occur in patients treated with corticosteroids.[1,7] Another form of skeletal involvement is osteonecrosis, or avascular necrosis, which may either be asymptomatic or cause severe pain. Large joints, usually more than one at a time, are most commonly affected, especially the hips and knees. Osteonecrosis is a known complication of corticosteroid therapy, but this disorder may also occur as part of the disease process of systemic lupus erythematosus.[5,8,9]

Synovial fluid analysis does not show evidence of inflammation, despite the inflammatory appearance of the joints on physical examination. The leukocyte count is usually less than 3,000/mm^3, in contrast to the higher count in rheumatoid arthritis. The fluid is viscous and contains good mucin precipitates. Glucose levels are similar to those in serum. Histologic synovial tissue study reveals only minor evidence of inflammation, in contrast to the intense inflammatory reaction characteristic of rheumatoid arthritis. Mild joint infiltration by lymphocytes and plasma cells and some evidence of edema and fibrinoid necrosis are usually the only histologic synovial findings in SLE.[1,7]

Skin Lesions

Skin lesions are frequent and are often an important diagnostic clue.[1,5] Most typical is an erythema over the nasal and malar areas of the face. This so-called butterfly rash may be the first manifestation of the disease. The rash is usually transient, often accompanies flare-ups, and subsides without residua. Alternatively, it may become chronic and exhibit areas of atrophy, follicular plugging, telangiectasia, pigmentation, or depigmentation. The SLE rash may take other forms, including a patchy erythema, with or without scaling, that appears on the extremities, trunk, and face. Other common lesions are erythematous patches around the fingertips, palms, and periungual areas, usually accompanied by telangiectasia at the borders of the fingernails. These finger lesions, also seen in other connective tissue diseases, are not diagnostic.

Alopecia frequently accompanies flare-ups in other systems. It often occurs in the form of diffuse thinning of hair on a normal scalp, but the scalp may also be affected by chronic erythema, scaling, and atrophy. In the absence of chronic changes in the scalp, the hair loss, which may be quite extensive, is usually reversible. Ulcerations of the mouth or lips—usually small, erythematous, shallow, painful areas—may be seen. Purpura accompanies thrombocytopenia, as expected, but it may also occur with normal platelet counts as a result of small-vessel vasculitis.

There is hyperkeratosis with keratin plugging of hair follicles and of sweat and sebaceous glands. In addition, acanthosis (diffuse hyperplasia and proliferation of the prickle cell layer) and degenerative changes of the basal cell layer can be demonstrated. There may also be lymphocytic infiltration of the dermis and fibrinoid necrosis of dermal collagen bundles. Immunofluorescent examination of biopsy specimens characteristically reveals immunoglobulin and complement components at the dermal-epidermal junction.[1]

Renal Dysfunction

Patients with systemic lupus erythematosus usually manifest some degree of renal involvement. Urinalysis may show proteinuria, pyuria, hematuria, and granular or red cell casts. More severe renal involvement can result in hypoalbuminemia, other features of the nephrotic syndrome, or a decreased glomerular filtration rate, leading to nitrogen retention, electrolyte disturbance, and acidosis.[1,10]

The most benign lesion of lupus nephritis is minor mesangial change, probably present in most or all lupus patients [*see Table 1*], but this lesion has no significant morbidity. The focal proliferative form of the renal lesion is also benign and often resolves spontaneously. Membranous glomerulonephritis is characteristically accompanied by some or all elements of the nephrotic syndrome. Remissions are common, as are relapses, and slowly progressive renal failure may develop. Diffuse proliferative nephritis is the most serious form, often associated with some renal insufficiency and hypertension. However, the class of renal pathology changes with time in more than half of patients with documented

Table 1   Pathologic Findings in Lupus Nephritis

	Light Microscopy	Electron Microscopy	Immunofluorescence	Characteristic Clinical Features
Mesangial lupus nephritis	Mild or absent mesangial widening, or mesangial hypercellularity	Mesangial electron-dense deposits	IgG, C3, and sometimes IgA and IgM staining in mesangial regions	Either no abnormalities or minimal proteinuria, hematuria
Focal pro-liferative nephritis	Segmental pro-liferation of glomerular tufts. Some degree of glomerular sclerosis, mesangial widening, small epithelial crescents	Mesangial, subepithelial, subendothelial, and basement membrane electron-dense deposits	IgG and C3 granular deposits in mesangial regions and glomerular capillary walls	Proteinuria, hematuria
Membranous lupus nephritis	Uniform thickening of peripheral capillary loops in glomeruli. Some mesangial cell proliferation and sclerosis. No epithelial crescents	Subepithelial and mesangial electron-dense deposits	IgG, C3, and some-times IgM in fine granular deposits out-lining capillary walls	Proteinuria, nephrotic syndrome; sometimes hematuria, hypertension
Diffuse pro-liferative nephritis	Proliferative changes involv-ing most or all glomeruli. Epithelial crescents or sclerosis. Possible necro-tizing vasculitis	Extensive electron-dense deposits	Diffuse granular staining for IgG, IgM, and C3	Proteinuria, hema-turia, renal insuf-ficiency; often nephrotic syndrome, hypertension

renal disease, a fact that limits the prognostic value of renal biopsy.[11]

Deterioration of renal function during a one-year period in patients with systemic lupus erythematosus has been predicted by certain specific biopsy findings. The charac-teristic findings include extensive glomeru-lar sclerosis and, on electron microscopy, the absence of subendothelial deposits.[12,13]

Nervous System Disorders

Some involvement of the nervous system occurs in about one half of patients,[1,14] fre-quently entailing a variety of psychologic changes. Reactive depressions are common. A functional psychosis with thought and mood disturbances characteristic of schizo-phrenia may occur, but manifestations sug-gesting organic psychosis are more common. The latter include deterioration of intellectual capacity, memory loss, and dis-orientation. Psychoses may be a complica-tion of corticosteroid therapy, although it is well established that psychologic problems are often a manifestation of the disease itself. In addition, these psychoses are associated with seizures and other evidence of neurologic involvement. The seizures are often of the grand mal type, although focal seizures have been described.

Neurologic changes include signs of pyramidal tract involvement. These disturbances, along with spastic paralysis, sometimes result from a typical cerebrovascular accident. Cranial nerve deficits commonly affect the seventh nerve (inducing facial weakness) and the extraocular motor nerves (inducing ptosis or diplopia). Peripheral neuropathies are uncommon; they may take the form of either sensory or mixed sensorimotor deficiencies. Rarely, there may be asymmetric multiple sites of peripheral nerve involvement, presenting a picture of mononeuritis multiplex, which is seen in many necrotizing vasculitis syndromes. Other infrequent neurologic abnormalities include ataxia, chorea, scotomas, aseptic meningitis, and spinal cord lesions.

Central nervous system manifestations are typically transient. Psychoses, seizures, hemiplegias, diplopia, and other findings often clear dramatically, except in the unusual case of irreversible pathology, such as severe intracerebral hemorrhage. It is difficult to determine whether therapy with corticosteroids or other drugs influences the outcome of CNS involvement, but spontaneous improvement does occur.

Neurologic examination reveals few changes not detected on physical examination. Even with rather extensive neurologic changes, lumbar puncture may be normal or may reveal elevation of protein levels and mild pleocytosis. Electroencephalograms are occasionally abnormal, whereas radioisotopic brain scans are usually normal. In fact, evidence of intracranial mass defects on scanning procedures suggests a complication such as an intracerebral infection or lymphoma, especially when such defects are found during corticosteroid and cytotoxic drug therapy.

The pathology of CNS involvement is often remarkable for the paucity of histologic findings despite severe clinical manifestations. The most frequent finding is a mild, perivascular inflammatory cell infiltrate; a true necrotizing vasculitis in the brain is unusual. Microinfarcts, often multiple, are common. An apparent increase in the frequency of CNS infections may be linked to the use of corticosteroid and cytotoxic drug therapy.[15]

Neuropsychiatric manifestations may appear at any time but usually occur early, often within the first year. They are normally accompanied by evidence of SLE in other organ systems. CNS involvement has been said to indicate a poor prognosis, but a large-scale study demonstrated 94 percent survival after five years and 93 percent survival after 10 years following evidence of CNS disease.[14] Lupus psychosis was strongly associated with antiribosomal P protein in one study.[16]

Cardiac Involvement

Pericarditis, which causes chest pain and friction rub, is the most common cardiac manifestation.[1] Small effusions may occur, but pericardial tamponade is rare. Myocarditis is much less common than pericarditis. Myocarditis may resemble a cardiomyopathy, resulting in ventricular arrhythmias and congestive heart failure.[17,18] Libman-Sacks endocarditis, a noninfectious endocarditis that is characterized by small verrucous vegetations near the rings of the heart valves, is common. These lesions are usually asymptomatic, but rarely, they are complicated by thromboembolism, infective endocarditis, or valvular dysfunction. Coronary artery disease and myocardial infarction may be related to coronary vasculitis in SLE patients, but these conditions more commonly result from atherosclerosis, which may be accelerated by glucocorticoid therapy.[17,18]

Pulmonary Involvement

Pleuritic chest pain, another common manifestation, may be mild or severe and may be accompanied by friction rubs and pleural effusions. Pleural fluid analysis usually reveals an exudate containing protein concentrations greater than 3 g/dl; transudates may also be observed. Concentrations of mononuclear leukocytes may range up to several thousand cells per cubic millimeter. Pleural fluid glucose levels are usually similar to blood glucose levels in SLE patients; in contrast, pleural fluid glucose levels are reduced in rheumatoid arthritis patients.

Parenchymal lung involvement may manifest as bacterial pneumonia, pulmonary infarcts, uremic pneumonitis, or pulmonary edema caused by congestive heart failure. Chronic diffuse interstitial pneumonitis may also occur, causing exertional dyspnea and cyanosis; the results of pulmonary function tests tend to show a restrictive pattern.[1]

Lupus pneumonia is usually acute and characterized by dry cough, dyspnea, and hypoxemia; pulmonary hemorrhage may result. Radiologic findings consist of infiltrates that are usually most prominent at the lung bases. Pathologic findings include interstitial fibrosis, vasculitis, and pleuritis.[19,20]

Pulmonary hypertension has been reported with increasing frequency. Patients present with exertional dyspnea and less commonly with chest pain. The pathologic findings in SLE are similar to those in idiopathic pulmonary hypertension except that pulmonary artery vasculitis may be present in SLE.[21]

Gastrointestinal Disturbances

Anorexia, nausea, vomiting, and abdominal pain are common; often, no cause can be found. Mesenteric vasculitis may lead to intestinal infarcts and perforations. Pancreatitis may be associated with corticosteroid therapy in some patients.[1]

Liver Disease

Liver enlargement and minor abnormalities in liver function tests are seen occasionally in SLE but are usually erythema of little clinical significance. Liver biopsies reveal only minor, nonspecific changes.[1,6] Chronic hepatitis rarely occurs.[1] SLE has been reported in a few patients with primary biliary cirrhosis.[22]

Disorders Associated with Antiphospholipid

Antiphospholipid antibodies are present in a significant number of SLE patients, although most persons with such antibodies do not have SLE. These antibodies lead to abnormal values of phospholipid-dependent coagulation tests, including the activated partial thromboplastin time and the Russell viper venom time. The fact that these abnormal values are not corrected by normal plasma, however, indicates that the abnormality in SLE serum results from an antibody and not from a deficiency of a clotting factor. Antiphospholipid antibodies may be detected by several assays that are not equivalent [*see Chapter 14*]; these include the lupus anticoagulant test, the anticardiolipin assay, the standard test for syphilis (STS), the activated partial thromboplastin time, and the Russell viper venom time. Whether antiphospholipid antibodies are detected in a specific patient depends on which assay is used. For instance, one patient may test positive for these antibodies on one assay and negative on another, whereas a second patient may have opposite findings. The most frequently positive test is the anticardiolipin assay, which is positive in up to 40 percent of SLE patients. Results utilizing several assays indicate that antiphospholipid antibodies are present in 35 to 50 percent of SLE patients.[23-25]

Although a few patients may have a bleeding tendency, the risk of hemorrhage in patients with the lupus anticoagulant is low, even after surgery. Paradoxically, this autoantibody is associated with recurrent venous and arterial thrombosis.[23-26] Thrombosis involves several regions of the vasculature and may result in various vascular syndromes, including strokes, myocardial infarction, peripheral arterial occlusion, peripheral venous thrombosis with pulmonary embolization, and renal vein thrombosis.

Antiphospholipid Antibodies and Pregnancy

Fertility is normal in patients with SLE. Earlier studies concluded that pregnancy induced flares in disease activity in SLE, but a controlled prospective study found no evidence of exacerbation of disease during pregnancy.[27] SLE patients as well as other patients with antiphospholipid antibodies encounter specific obstetric problems (e.g., platelet counts are decreased but usually not to less than 70,000/mm^3). More significant is the association of antiphospholipid antibodies with fetal death after the first trimester. Placental thrombosis and infarction have not been consistently observed, and the cause of fetal loss remains uncertain. Premature birth is also associated with the lupus anticoagulant, but early spontaneous abortion is not. SLE patients who are pregnant may also experience abrupt onset of hypertension, edema, and proteinuria that is indistinguishable from pregnancy-induced hypertension and that is independent of the presence of antiphospholipid antibodies. Midtrimester fetal death is usually associated with either antiphospholipid antibodies or pregnancy-induced hypertension.[23,27,28]

The neonatal lupus syndrome consists of transient cutaneous lupus lesions and less frequently transient thrombocytopenia, anemia, and hepatic involvement. The most serious manifestation of neonatal lupus is congenital heart block, which is usually complete and often permanent; congenital heart block may be responsible for fatalities in the neonatal period. Mothers and their affected infants almost always have autoantibodies to ribonucleoprotein—usually to Ro (also termed SS-A) and, less commonly, to La (also termed SS-B) or U$_1$RNP [*see* Laboratory Findings, Antinuclear Antibodies, *below*].[27,29] The long-term prognosis for infants surviving the neonatal period is good; however, those infants with heart block may require permanent pacing.[30] Although only about one half of the mothers of affected infants have mild symptoms of autoimmune disease at the time of delivery, almost all of these mothers will eventually experience mild symptoms.[30]

The risk of neonatal lupus in infants or mothers who have anti-Ro antibodies is unknown, but the neonatal lupus syndrome appears to affect only a small percentage. However, the risk of neonatal lupus in pregnancies following the birth of an affected child has been reported to be 25 percent.[30] The presence of anti-Ro antibodies does not appear to increase the risk of early spontaneous abortion.[24,30]

There are insufficient data to support the prophylactic use of either glucocorticoids or anticoagulants in patients with abnormal levels of antiphospholipid antibodies. Most SLE patients with elevated levels of antiphospholipid antibodies have no related pathologic findings.[25] However, long-term anticoagulant therapy has been recommended for patients with antiphospholipid antibodies and recurrent thrombosis.[23]

Miscellaneous Disorders

Myopathy may develop, followed by weakness of proximal muscle groups and elevation of the serum creatine kinase level. The elevated CK level and the pathologic changes in involved muscle may be identical to those seen in polymyositis, but at times, vacuolar degeneration of muscle fibers is the rule.[1]

Generalized lymphadenopathy appears frequently, and splenomegaly is found in about 20 percent of patients. Characteristic onion-scale lesions, consisting of concentric layers of perivascular fibrous tissue, are often found in the spleen.[1]

Sjögren's syndrome, which affects the salivary and lacrimal glands, with associated keratoconjunctivitis sicca may develop in a few patients. It is less common in SLE than in rheumatoid arthritis and has been seen in SLE patients with nondeforming erosive arthritis.[1]

Laboratory Findings

Anemia is frequent and may be the result of hemolysis or chronic disease, or both. Leukopenia, rarely severe, is also common; the total leukocyte count is usually above 2,000/mm^3. The differential leukocyte count is usually normal, in contrast to the count in Felty's syndrome. Thrombocytopenia is frequent but is clinically significant only when the platelet count is reduced to less than 50,000/mm^3. Severe thrombocytopenia associated with purpura and other bleeding manifestations may occur, requiring vigorous treatment. Mild thrombocytopenia may become more significant in the presence of the lupus anticoagulant or SLE inhibitor [*see Chapter 14*]. The latter agent rarely causes clinical bleeding unless other hemostatic defects are present. Circulating anticoagulants may cause prolongation of prothrombin and partial thromboplastin times. Occasionally, however, the results of these tests are normal, and in such cases, special laboratory procedures are required to detect the circulating anticoagulants in SLE patients.[1]

Patients with circulating anticoagulants usually demonstrate a biologic false positive test for syphilis. False positive serologic tests for syphilis occur in about 25 percent of patients with SLE. Such reactions result from antibodies that react to the antigenic material used in the serologic tests for syphilis (Wassermann, Hinton, Kahn, and similar tests). False positive reactions can be distinguished from true positive reactions by the absence of antibody reaction to a specific treponemal antigen (in a fluorescent treponemal antibody absorption test).[1]

Antinuclear Antibodies

Some of the most characteristic of the numerous autoantibodies in SLE are the antinuclear antibodies (ANA).[31,32]

More than 90 percent of patients with SLE have positive antinuclear antibody tests. However, the test is also positive in several other conditions and in some elderly patients who are without apparent disease. Although a repeatedly negative test makes the SLE diagnosis unlikely, five to 10 percent of patients in whom the diagnosis is well established will test negatively. Most ANA-negative patients have circulating antibodies to the cytoplasmic antigens Ro and La and to single-stranded DNA. Such patients usually have photosensitive dermatitis, a low incidence of renal and central nervous system involvement, and a good prognosis.[33]

The lupus erythematosus (LE) cell factor, an antibody to deoxyribonucleoprotein, reacts with damaged cell nuclei to form a hematoxylin body, a homogeneous mass of nuclear material that has a characteristic histologic appearance. A polymorphonuclear leukocyte that has phagocytized such a hematoxylin body is called a lupus erythematosus cell. The hematoxylin bodies may also be detected in tissue sections. The use of LE cell tests on peripheral blood has been largely replaced by other tests for antinuclear antibodies.

Antibodies to many antigenic determinants in cell nuclei have been described in autoimmune diseases, and typical patterns of antibody responses have been seen in some disorders. Several antinuclear antibodies have been characterized, but these antibodies are directed against a limited number of potential antigenic epitopes in the nucleus. These epitopes are found in three different nuclear structures: the chromatin, the small nuclear ribonucleoprotein (snRNP), and the Ro particle. Chromatin, a major component of cell nuclei, consists of DNA and histones. Antibodies to DNA and to histones are found in SLE but also occur in other autoimmune diseases. Anti-DNA antibodies may be directed against denatured single-stranded DNA or against native double-stranded DNA, but the latter are quite specific for SLE. Antibodies to one or more histones occur in most SLE patients; the strongest responses are directed against histones H1 and H2B. Patients with antibodies to DNA usually also have antibodies to histones.[34]

Cells contain RNA in four forms: messenger RNA, ribosomal RNA, transfer RNA, and a heterogeneous group of small RNA molecules. Each of these RNAs associates with specific proteins to form ribonucleoproteins. Because ribonucleoproteins are soluble in aqueous buffers, they have also been referred to as extractable nuclear antigens (ENA). A variety of ribonucleoproteins may be recognized by autoantibodies, but the predominant antibodies present in SLE are anti-U_1RNP, anti-Sm, and anti-Ro. These antibodies all recognize determinants on snRNPs. Anti-Sm antibodies are specific for

SLE. Patients with anti-Sm antibodies almost always have antibodies to U_1RNP as well, but the converse is not true.[34] High titers of antibodies to U_1RNP are associated with mixed connective tissue disease.[35]

The protein La binds to many species of snRNP and carries an epitope recognized by anti-La antibodies. Anti-La antibodies are almost always accompanied by anti-Ro antibodies, but anti-Ro antibodies may occur without anti-La antibodies. Neither anti-Ro nor anti-La antibodies are specific for SLE. These antibodies are often seen in patients with Sjögren's syndrome and other autoimmune disorders.[34]

Complement

Reduction in complement (C) serum levels has been cited as evidence of increased consumption of complement components during immune complex formation and tissue damage.[31,32] Some of the reductions in serum complement components may be caused by decreased synthesis rather than increased consumption; however, complement consumption is definitely increased in SLE. C3, in particular, and immunoglobulin may be seen with immunofluorescent techniques as localized clumps in the renal glomeruli and other damaged tissues.[5,32] Moreover, properdin has been detected in the glomeruli of lupus patients, indicating that the alternative pathway participates in complement activation.[32]

Activation of the classical complement pathway can be demonstrated clinically by a reduced level of total hemolytic complement (CH50). Alternatively, complement activation can be determined by immunochemical measurement of the C3 component. The hemolysis method requires functioning levels of all complement components. However, because several components can be present in excess in SLE patients, reductions in some components (e.g., a reduction of up to one half in C3 level) may occur without causing an abnormality in the hemolysis assay. A wide variety of diseases resulting in inflammation and tissue necrosis cause elevations in serum levels of several complement components and other plasma proteins that are acute-phase reactants. A few diseases, including SLE, certain forms of glomerulonephritis, and acute serum sickness, are associated with reduced levels of serum complement components.[32,36]

Serum complement components are not always reduced in active SLE. In one study, SLE patients with active extrarenal disease had higher levels of CH50, C4, and C3 and lower levels of circulating immune complexes than did patients with active renal disease. Anti-DNA antibodies did not distinguish the two groups.[36]

Several kindreds have been described with hereditary deficiency of the C2 component. Homozygous family members have undetectable or very low levels, whereas heterozygous individuals have about half the normal level. About one third of C2 deficiency homozygotes have been found to have SLE or a similar syndrome that may represent a partially expressed disease. Moreover, even the C2 deficiency heterozygotes were found to have an increased incidence of SLE. It seems unlikely, however, that significant abnormality in complement function would result from the 50 percent reduction in C2 level seen in heterozygous individuals, especially because the normal amount of serum C2 is thought to be in excess of the amount required for hemolytic complement activity. Instead, the gene for C2 may be in linkage disequilibrium with an immune response gene. This linked deficiency is thought to be associated with the abnormal immune functions in SLE.[37]

Lupus Band Test

The lupus band test uses immunofluorescent techniques to detect immunoglobulins and complement components at the dermal-epidermal junction. A lupus band is observed in nonlesional skin in about 80 percent of patients with active SLE and in 30 to 40 percent of those with inactive disease. All lupus skin lesions yield positive band tests, but a positive test in either lesional or nonlesional skin is not entirely specific for SLE.[1]

The terminal complement complex, or membrane attack complex, composed of C5b, C6, C7, C8, and C9, has been detected in the active skin lesions of patients with SLE and discoid lupus. The absence of this complex from uninvolved skin suggests it is a mediator of inflammatory skin lesions.[38]

Pathogenesis

SLE appears to be a disorder of immunologic regulation that causes a loss of tolerance; resulting autoimmune reactions against host antigens lead to inflammation and damage to vascular and other tissues.[32] There are many mechanisms that can cause disordered immunity; for example, a T cell deficiency, such as decreased activity of suppressor T cells, might lead to excessive B cell expression. The etiology remains unknown, but the most popular candidate is an infectious, probably viral, agent that disrupts the suppressor T cell population. Patients with SLE exhibit some evidence of decreased cellular immunity. Delayed skin hypersensitivity can be impaired, and evidence of decreased T cell function can be seen in vitro; antilymphocyte antibodies have been shown to be present in these patients, and this abnormality may be related to the observed lymphocytopenia and T cell hypofunction.[32]

The picture, however, has grown more complicated. Measurements using monoclonal antibodies have shown that not all SLE patients manifest a deficiency of suppressor T cells. Instead, ratios of helper to suppressor T cells varied widely among SLE patients when compared with those ratios in a population of normal control subjects.[39] In addition, a deficiency in a specific subset of helper T cells (also termed CD4$^+$ T cells) has been identified in some SLE patients. Two subsets of CD4$^+$ T cells with different functions have been recognized: the 4B4 and the 2H4 subsets. The 4B4 subset responds to soluble antigens and induces B cells to secrete immunoglobulin. The 2H4 subset (formerly called the juvenile rheumatoid arthritis subset because of the presence of antibodies to the subset in patients with

juvenile rheumatoid arthritis) induces CD8$^+$ T cells to express T suppressor cell functions, including the suppression of antibody synthesis. SLE patients with active renal disease have reduced numbers of the 2H4 subset of CD4$^+$ T cells, a finding that may be associated with deficient suppressor T cell function in these patients.[40,41]

Several observations indicate that sex hormones may significantly influence the pathogenesis of SLE. The frequency of SLE in females, the adverse effects of estrogens in both men and women with the disease, and the beneficial effects of androgens in murine lupus support this concept. Levels of several active androgens are reduced in female SLE patients, especially in those with active disease, probably because of abnormalities in hormone metabolism in SLE.[42]

Genetic factors are important in SLE. The incidence of the disease in first-degree relatives of lupus patients is about one percent. A higher percentage of first-degree relatives have a positive antinuclear antibody test; in general, studies have reported an incidence that ranges from four to 14 percent. However, increased frequencies of positive antinuclear antibody tests are found in nonconsanguineous as well as in consanguineous relatives, which suggests that environmental factors may also be involved in the disease. The high concordance of SLE in monozygotic twins, approximately 60 percent, and the lower concordance in dizygotic twins indicate that genetic factors contribute to SLE susceptibility. Also lending support for a genetic component in SLE are the associations of the histocompatibility antigens HLA-B8 and HLA-DR3 with spontaneous SLE and HLA-DR4 with SLE induced by hydralazine.[43]

A plausible hypothesis for the pathogenesis of SLE incorporates several factors. There is evidence supporting the existence of a genetic predisposition to the disease that leads to excessive B cell activation. Excessive B cell activation may result from one or several mechanisms, including an intrinsic B cell defect, a defect in helper T cells that leads to abnormal B cell stimulation, or a defect in suppressor T cells that results in a failure to control B cell proliferation. Activation of B cells may be triggered by exogenous or endogenous factors, including chemicals, drugs, viruses, or bacterial antigens. The individual manifestations of disease may be determined by genetic or other factors that favor the activation of specific classes of autoantibody-producing cells.[44]

In human SLE, circulating immune complexes have been suggested as the cause of tissue injury in many organ systems. The antigen most frequently implicated is native DNA, which can be found along with complement components and immunoglobulins in diseased kidneys.[27] Clearance of circulating immune complexes is facilitated by their attachment to the CR1 receptors, about 90 percent of which are present on erythrocytes. These receptors function in part to transport circulating immune complexes to the reticuloendothelial system, where they are degraded. The number of CR1 receptors on erythrocytes is an inherited trait, and individuals in the normal population may have high, intermediate, or low numbers of receptors. Studies of restriction fragment length polymorphisms (RFLPs) of DNA indicate that inheritance of CR1 complement receptors is similar in SLE patients and in normal control subjects. Thus, the reduced levels of CR1 receptors in SLE patients is not a genetic susceptibility trait.[45,46]

Therapy

The treatment of systemic lupus erythematosus is controversial. Because the disease has such a highly variable course and because symptom patterns differ greatly among different patients, the response to treatment is difficult to evaluate. In the absence of carefully controlled drug trials, recommendations for therapy must, unfortunately, be based on less objective criteria.[5,7,47]

Periods of bed rest are indicated for patients with evidence of active SLE.[5,7] Physical and emotional stress adversely affects the course of the disease[7]; stresses such as surgery, infections, and pregnancy should be avoided.

Exposure to sunlight should also be avoided; about one third of SLE patients are photosensitive.[1] Sunlight appears to cause flare-ups of systemic manifestations as well as skin disease. When sun exposure is unavoidable, patients should use sunscreens that contain aminobenzoic acid (PABA) and that have high protective factor (PF) ratings. These preparations contain both PABA ester and benzophenones or other combinations of agents that block both the erythema spectrum and the long-wavelength spectrum of ultraviolet light.

Because of evidence that estrogens may exacerbate SLE, only oral contraceptives containing minimal doses of estrogens should be used. Barrier contraception is preferable to either oral contraceptives or intrauterine devices.[27]

Salicylates

Anti-inflammatory therapy with full doses of aspirin is indicated in many patients who have active SLE, especially in individuals with fever, arthritis, pleurisy, or pericarditis.[5,7,47] Aspirin should be taken in doses slightly below the toxicity threshold. Use of buffered or enteric-coated preparations may circumvent the frequent gastrointestinal side effects of aspirin; taking the medication with meals may also be helpful. The total daily dose will vary—as much as 6 g/day may be required in younger adults. Most adult patients will require between 3.6 and 4.8 g/day, but patients older than 65 years frequently require lower doses. Side effects other than gastritis are unusual. Some patients with active SLE may experience aspirin-induced hepatitis. Its manifestations are usually limited to elevated levels of serum aminotransferase and, sometimes, alkaline phosphatase and are rapidly reversible once salicylates are stopped. Antiplatelet effects of aspirin are rarely of clinical significance, unless other coagulation disorders are also present. Salicylates should probably be avoided in the case of severe thrombocytopenia and in the presence of renal disease.

Antimalarial Drugs

Chloroquine and hydroxychloroquine have proved useful in controlling certain SLE manifestations, especially skin rashes and probably arthralgia and arthritis. These drugs should be given in doses of 200 to 500 mg; adverse effects are infrequent under these conditions. Gastrointestinal side effects may occur. Vision may blur as a result of cycloplegia or corneal deposits; this effect is reversible. The most serious side effect is an irreversible retinopathy, which may lead to blindness. This risk is minimal, especially if the treatment does not exceed one year.[32] Skeletal muscle myopathy, cardiomyopathy, and peripheral neuropathy may follow long-term therapy with chloroquine and hydroxychloroquine.[48,49]

Corticosteroids and Cytotoxic Drugs

Glucocorticoids often dramatically suppress many SLE manifestations.[47] Despite their wide use in SLE, their effects on survival remain unknown, and the indications for their use are often unclear. Patients without life-threatening manifestations of SLE who have arthralgias, skin rash, fatigue, low-grade fever, and pleuritic pain may be managed conservatively with rest, salicylates, and an antimalarial drug. It is usually best to avoid the potential toxicity of corticosteroids when dealing with these symptoms. More threatening manifestations, such as severe hemolytic anemia or thrombocytopenia, are indications for corticosteroid therapy.

A lupus crisis with high fever, prostration, and other symptoms may also require corticosteroids. Fever, arthritis, skin rash, pleurisy, pericarditis, and certain other manifestations can respond dramatically. It may be difficult, however, to reduce the dose without precipitating a flare-up. Patients may then be faced with the serious toxicity of long-term corticosteroids. Attempts to reduce toxicity with alternate-day dosage schedules have often been unsatisfactory in SLE and other rheumatic diseases because symptoms often recur on drug-free days.[47]

Treatment of Renal Disease

Treatment of lupus renal disease also remains controversial. There has been no satisfactorily controlled trial comparing corticosteroid-treated patients with untreated patients. It has not been proved that corticosteroids alter the ultimate course or outcome of glomerulonephritis in SLE.[47] Nonetheless, it seems reasonable to carry out a limited course of prednisone in patients with diffuse proliferative or membranous glomerulonephritis. The risk of serious complications in long-term therapy suggests that it is unwise to treat with more than 40 to 60 mg of prednisone a day in divided doses for more than three months. After this initial three-month course, the dosage should be reduced gradually, over several weeks, to levels of 10 to 15 mg/day.

Long-term randomized trials of prednisone combined with oral cyclophosphamide and oral azathioprine demonstrated only marginal benefits compared with prednisone administered alone in moderate doses.[50,51] A regimen of intermittent intravenous cyclophosphamide plus low doses of prednisone, however, reduced the frequency of end-stage renal failure and produced less serious toxicity than either high-dose prednisone alone or prednisone combined with daily oral doses of cytotoxic drugs.[52] The severity of chronic histologic changes on renal biopsy was correlated with the development of progressive renal failure. Furthermore, patients in whom the severity of these changes was of an intermediate degree were most likely to respond to immunosuppressive therapy; those with mild, chronic changes appeared not to require therapy, and those with the most severe changes were unresponsive.[53,54]

Total lymphoid irradiation reportedly improved the course of lupus nephritis in an uncontrolled study of 15 patients who had been refractory to previous treatment with glucocorticoids and cytotoxic drugs.[55] Severe side effects were not observed among the patients in this study, but a subsequent report described fatal complications and no clinical benefits in two other patients with refractory SLE who were also treated with total lymphoid irradiation.[56] Therefore, the role of this modality in the treatment of systemic lupus still remains to be established. Plasmapheresis has been used with corticosteroid and cytotoxic drug regimens, but the effectiveness of this approach has not yet been determined.[47]

End-stage renal disease (ESRD) in SLE is now effectively managed with long-term hemodialysis and transplantation. In two studies, long-term hemodialysis was associated with reduced severity of both renal and nonrenal disease. Despite gradual withdrawal of immunosuppressive therapy, some patients recovered from renal failure and were able to stop receiving dialysis. Deaths were infrequent and were usually related to high-dose corticosteroid therapy. Renal transplantation is well tolerated. The long-term clinical course of patients with ESRD caused by SLE resembles that of end-stage renal disease produced by other causes.[57,58]

Treatment of CNS Disease

The basis for therapeutic decisions regarding central nervous system lupus is even more tenuous.[47] Many apparently serious CNS complications resolve spontaneously, making evaluation of therapy difficult. Although no objective evidence is available, some authorities believe that CNS lupus responds to corticosteroids; yet, extremely high doses of steroids will almost certainly lead to serious complications, especially if administered for long periods.

Prognosis

The prognosis for a patient with SLE is difficult to determine. Renal failure, heavy proteinuria, and anemia are poor prognostic signs. Mortality is higher in patients of low socioeconomic status, but increased mortality shows no independent predilection for persons of a particular race or ethnic origin.[59]

The most frequent causes of death are active renal disease (often accompanied by involvement of other systems) and infections. The prognosis of SLE appears to be improving, however, and more than 80 percent of patients with diffuse proliferative glomerulonephritis, the most severe form of renal involvement, survive longer than five years.[1] Factors associated with progression to irreversible renal failure are young age, male gender, elevated serum creatinine, and renal histologic changes of glomerular and interstitial sclerosis and tubular atrophy as revealed by kidney biopsy.[60] Death caused by complications of CNS disease[14] and myocardial infarction are infrequent. Malignancy is rare.[61]

Drug-Induced Systemic Lupus Erythematosus

In many patients, clinical and laboratory manifestations of SLE develop in association with certain drugs. In some, the drug appears to give rise to a symptom complex identical to that of SLE, whereas in others, an incomplete form may develop. Criteria proposed for drug-induced SLE are (1) clinical criteria similar to those proposed for the diagnosis of spontaneous SLE, (2) administration of the drug prior to the onset of symptoms, usually continuously, for periods of three weeks to two years, and (3) clinical signs and symptoms that reverse promptly on removal of the drug. Clinical symptoms usually begin to resolve within days, although some laboratory signs may not resolve for months or even years.[62]

A wide variety of therapeutic agents has been implicated in the drug-induced lupus syndrome [*see Table 2*]; a causal relationship, however, has not been clearly established for all of these agents. Drugs that most frequently cause the SLE syndrome are hydralazine and procainamide; practolol and penicillamine may also be in this higher-risk group. Less frequently implicated are isoniazid, hydantoin anticonvulsants, ethosuximide, and trimethadione. Thiouracil and related compounds and phenothiazines rarely cause the syndrome. Neither sulfonamides nor oral contraceptive agents have any proved tendency to cause systemic lupus erythematosus, although the association has been reported.[62]

The clinical picture is similar to that of spontaneous SLE, except that drug-induced

Table 2 Drugs Implicated in Systemic Lupus Erythematosus

Degree of Risk	Agent
High	Antihypertensives Hydralazine

	Antiarrhythmics
	  Procainamide
	  Practolol (beta-adrenergic
	    blocking agent)

	Chelating agents Penicillamine
Moderate	Antitubercular drugs Isoniazid

	Anticonvulsants
	  Hydantoins: phenytoin,
	    mephenytoin
	  Oxazolidinediones:
	    trimethadione
	  Succinimides: ethosuximide

Low	Antithyroid drugs
	  Thiourea derivatives
	  Psychotropic drugs
	  Phenothiazine derivatives

Undefined	Oral contraceptive agents
	  Estrogen-progestin
	    combinations
	Sulfonamides

SLE is generally milder and renal complications are less frequent.[5,62] Drug-induced SLE is more frequent in women than in men. Patients tend to be of middle age or older, probably because many of the drugs are most often used by persons in these age groups.

The incidence of the SLE syndrome in patients exposed to drugs is uncertain, but the fully developed form is probably present in one percent or less, even among those exposed to high-risk drugs such as procainamide and hydralazine. Other patients experience isolated or limited symptoms, such as arthralgias, that may be manifestations of SLE. Positive antinuclear antibody test results, usually unaccompanied by symptoms of SLE, are observed in more than 50 percent of patients exposed to high-risk drugs. Antibodies to native DNA, present in 50 percent or more of patients with spontaneous SLE, are generally not found in patients with drug-induced SLE; tests for these two types of antibodies help to make the distinction.[62]

The frequency of manifestations of SLE in patients taking drugs such as hydralazine or procainamide makes it unlikely that these drugs act solely by unmasking an underlying diathesis. Host factors may be important; however, individuals in whom the complete syndrome develops may have an innate predisposition. Susceptibility to the SLE syndrome that has been induced by hydralazine or procainamide is related to the patient's acetylator phenotype. Both drugs are metabolized by the hepatic N-acetyltransferase system. Patients who are genetically slow acetylators metabolize the drugs more slowly than patients who are rapid acetylators. During therapy with either hydralazine or procainamide, positive antinuclear antibody test results are observed sooner and the SLE syndrome occurs more frequently in patients who are slow acetylators than in those who are rapid acetylators.[5,63]

Discoid Lupus

Chronic discoid lupus is a limited form of lupus erythematosus characterized by superficial inflammation of the skin. The typical skin lesion initially appears raised, papular, and erythematous and then becomes atrophic, hyperpigmented, or depigmented. Late stages are associated with hair loss, follicular scaling and plugging, telangiectasia, and atrophy. Lesions are usually distributed as irregular plaques on the face, scalp, upper arms, or chest. Sunlight often aggravates the condition.[64]

Most discoid lupus patients have normal serologic test results and no evidence of systemic involvement; however, an unpredictable minority will acquire the systemic disease. Discoid lesions are also commonly observed with SLE.[1]

Corticosteroids, injected intralesionally or applied topically, or oral antimalarials are usually effective in discoid lupus.[64]

Mixed Connective Tissue Disease

Patients have been described who exhibit clinical features that suggest several rheumatic diseases and who do not easily fit into any diagnostic category. Such patients have features suggestive of systemic lupus, erythematosus, scleroderma, and polymyositis, justifying a separate rheumatic category: mixed connective tissue disease (MCTD). High titers of antibodies to extractable nuclear antigens also distinguish these patients from patients with other rheumatic diseases.[65]

The clinical features of MCTD are diverse.[65] The age range is five to 80 years, and 80 percent of patients are female. Almost all patients have arthralgias, and about two thirds have an arthritis resembling rheumatoid arthritis, although it is usually nondeforming. Swelling of the fingers develops because of increased skin collagen and edema; this condition may progress to the chronic changes of scleroderma with telangiectasia and is usually limited to the hands. Rashes resembling those of SLE or polymyositis may be present. Esophageal dysfunction consists of decreased amplitude of both lower sphincter pressure and peristalsis in the lower two thirds of the esophagus, although in most patients these findings are not associated with symptoms.

Evidence of pulmonary disease, such as decreased diffusing capacity, is also common but is usually not associated with symptoms. Occasionally, more extensive disease may lead to exertional dyspnea associated with pulmonary infiltrates on chest x-rays, pleural disease, and sometimes, pulmonary hypertension. Pericarditis is occasionally seen.

Myositis consists of a proximal myopathy with tenderness and weakness, elevated levels of muscle enzymes, abnormal electromyograms, and pathologic muscle changes on biopsy. All of these changes are similar to those seen in polymyositis.

Renal disease is uncommon in patients with MCTD and is often mild when present. Kidney biopsies have shown mesangial change, focal nephritis, and diffuse membranous nephritis. Immunofluorescent stains have identified granular deposits of IgG, C3, and C4 in the glomerular basement membrane.

Neuropsychiatric abnormalities may be more common than previously suspected, occurring in one half of patients in one series.[65] Trigeminal neuralgia is the most common neurologic finding. Rare problems are transient confusion, cerebral infarction, aseptic meningitis, and seizures. Aseptic meningitis in MCTD responds to corticosteroids. Other disorders include peripheral neuropathy and psychosis.

Abnormal laboratory findings commonly include elevated sedimentation rates, leukopenia, and diffuse hypergammaglobulinemia. In rare cases, there is significant Coombs'-positive hemolytic anemia and thrombocytopenia. Rheumatoid factor tests are positive in about one half of patients.

Serologic tests for antinuclear antibodies provide the most helpful diagnostic findings in patients with MCTD. A high titer of fluorescent antinuclear antibody of the speckled pattern is usually present and tends to remain constant regardless of disease activity. The most typical finding is a strongly positive test for antibody to an RNP antigen [*see* Laboratory Findings, Antinuclear Antibodies, *above*]. Serum containing antibody to RNP antigen alone is most commonly seen in MCTD. Anti-RNP antibodies, however, are not entirely specific for MCTD.[34]

MCTD is not firmly established as a distinct clinical entity; in fact, it may represent part of the spectrum of SLE.[66] However, CNS disease, renal disease, antibodies to DNA, low serum complement levels, positive LE cells, and antibodies to Sm antigen are all common in SLE and uncommon in MCTD.[65,66]

The course of MCTD is variable and, in some patients, chronic. Features that suggest SLE, scleroderma, and polymyositis may appear simultaneously, or different features of the disease may unfold over many months or years. Corticosteroid therapy for MCTD has apparently been reasonably successful, although there have been no controlled trials to date. Mild symptoms may respond to nonsteroidal anti-inflammatory drugs. Abnormalities in pulmonary and esophageal function tests have improved with corticosteroid therapy.

Systemic Nodular Panniculitis

Systemic nodular panniculitis, also called Weber-Christian disease, defines a syndrome that may exist by itself or may accompany SLE or pancreatic disease.[1,67,68] The syndrome is characterized by recurrent attacks of crops of painful, red, tender subcutaneous nodules, most commonly located on the legs and buttocks. The outbreaks are accompanied by fever, leukocytosis, and eosinophilia. Attacks are self-limited, lasting two to three weeks. Slightly depressed pigmented areas may remain. In severe disease, any area of the body may be involved except the face; there may also be extracutaneous sites of involvement, such as the mesentery. In a variant of this disease, the lesions may undergo liquefaction and drain white, viscous material consisting of necrotic adipose tissue. Localization of the inflammatory nodules in periarticular areas leads to apparent acute arthritis of one or more joints, but studies of synovial fluids or synovial tissues are lacking.

Studies of the subcutaneous lesions reveal infiltration by neutrophils and eosinophils accompanied by leukoclastic changes and variable degrees of fat cell necrosis; histiocytes, foam cells, and giant cells surround the necrotic fat cells.

Differential Diagnosis

Panniculitis associated with SLE also presents as inflammatory subcutaneous nodules that may progress to chronic depressed lesions with drainage of necrotic fat.

Histologic features of lupus panniculitis include subcutaneous lymphocytic infiltration, vasculitis, and deposition of complexes in vessel walls. Although erythema nodosum is also characterized by tender red nodules, its clinical and histologic features differ from those of systemic nodular panniculitis. Systemic nodular panniculitis may be distinguished from nodular vasculitis in that the lesions of nodular vasculitis are chronic, slightly tender, firm subcutaneous nodules that usually occur on the back of the legs. They tend to progress to ulceration and scarring.[67]

Systemic nodular panniculitis may be accompanied by pancreatitis or by pancreatic adenocarcinoma, especially in males.[68]

Nonsteroidal anti-inflammatory drugs and corticosteroids are sometimes used as therapy for systemic nodular panniculitis, but the efficacy of these groups of drugs has not been proved.[67,68]

Sjögren's Syndrome

Sjögren's syndrome is a chronic inflammatory autoimmune disease of the exocrine glands that is frequently associated with other autoimmune diseases.[69,70] More than 90 percent of patients are women who are older than 50 years, although the syndrome may occur in children and young adults. It is estimated that between two and three million individuals in the United States have the disease. However, the exact prevalence is unknown because the symptoms of the syndrome may be subtle and thus may remain undiagnosed. Approximately 10 to 15 percent of patients with rheumatoid arthritis and a smaller number of patients with other rheumatic diseases (e.g., systemic lupus erythematosus and scleroderma) have clinical evidence of Sjögren's syndrome; other patients with rheumatic diseases remain asymptomatic, and evidence of Sjögren's syndrome is apparent only on histologic examination.

Clinical Manifestations

The most frequent clinical manifestations are those arising from the sicca syndrome, which consists of keratoconjunctivitis sicca (dry eyes) caused by lacrimal gland involvement and xerostomia (dry mouth) caused by salivary gland involvement.[69,70] Symptoms of the sicca syndrome may develop either slowly and insidiously or rapidly. When the onset is rapid, episodic parotitis may accompany the disease. Keratoconjunctivitis causes a sensation of a foreign body in the eyes, a variable accumulation of thick secretions near the inner canthus of the eyelids, decreased tearing, redness, and photophobia. A film of thickened secretions over the cornea may interfere with vision, and excessive dryness may cause corneal ulceration and serious loss of vision.

Salivary insufficiency leads to difficulty in chewing. Swallowing food may require frequent ingestion of water or other liquids while eating. Severe dental caries and breakdown of dental restorations may develop. Less commonly, dryness of the upper respiratory tract and tracheobronchial tree may cause epistaxis, hoarseness, bronchitis, or pneumonia. Parotid gland enlargement occurs in about one half of patients.

Many other manifestations may be present in patients with Sjögren's syndrome. Dryness of the skin and genital mucous membranes is described. Involvement of nonexocrine organs may lead to autoimmune thyroiditis, cranial and peripheral neuropathies, and myositis. Findings attributable to Sjögren's syndrome also include acute or chronic pancreatitis, biliary cirrhosis with antimitochondrial antibodies, and various renal tubular disorders, including renal tubular acidosis, nephrogenic diabetes insipidus, or the complete Fanconi's syndrome. Glomerulonephritis occurs infrequently. In one study, neuropsychiatric abnormalities were found in a majority of patients with Sjögren's syndrome in the absence of any associated rheumatic disease.[71] Psychiatric findings included depression and personality disorders without serious functional impairment. Neurologic abnormalities included mild cognitive defects, focal electroencephalographic discharges, and entrapment neuropathies. The high frequency of subtle neurologic disease suggests that the psychiatric abnormalities are of organic origin. These findings differ from the neuropsychiatric abnormalities of systemic lupus erythematosus, the most common of which are psychoses and seizures. In one study, the neuropsychiatric abnormalities in patients with Sjögren's syndrome frequently resembled those in patients with multiple sclerosis.[72] An increased frequency of hypersensitivity reactions to various drugs also occurs in patients with Sjögren's syndrome.

Rheumatoid arthritis, usually the classic type, occurs in about one half of patients with Sjögren's syndrome. Other patients may acquire a mild, nonerosive inflammatory arthritis of the knees and elbows. Polymyositis, SLE, and scleroderma may be associated with Sjögren's syndrome. Raynaud's phenomenon occurs with or without other rheumatic diseases. Associated vasculitic syndromes may involve either medium-sized vessels, as in polyarteritis nodosa, or small vessels, sometimes with hyperglobulinemia or cryoglobulinemia.

Pathologic Findings

The major and minor salivary glands, lacrimal glands, and other exocrine glands of the respiratory and gastrointestinal tracts and of the vagina are infiltrated with both T and B cells and plasma cells.[69,70] There is atrophy of the glandular secretory acinar tissue and of some of the cells that line the salivary ducts. Proliferation of the epimyoepithelial cells in ducts gives rise to characteristic clusters called epimyoepithelial islands. The lobular architecture is usually not severely distorted, unless changes of pseudolymphoma or malignant lymphoma occur (see below).

Laboratory Abnormalities

Salivary flow rates can be measured to determine if a patient has Sjögren's syndrome.[69,70] Lemon juice is placed on the tongue to stimulate the flow of saliva; the saliva is then collected from the orifice of the parotid duct in specialized cups. Flow rates of less than 0.5 ml a minute are found in Sjögren's syndrome. Abnormalities of the major salivary glands can also be determined by secretory sialography. In this technique, radiographs of the parotid ducts are obtained after small amounts of radiopaque contrast media have been injected into the orifice of the parotid ducts. Typical findings include distortion of the normal arborization pattern of the parotid ducts and reduced emptying of contrast media from the ducts. Alternatively, salivary function may be estimated by scintigraphy, which measures the uptake and release of the radionuclide technetium-99m pertechnetate after stimulation of the salivary glands. Finally, the diagnosis of Sjögren's syndrome should be confirmed by histologic study of the minor salivary glands obtained by biopsy of the lower lip; this procedure quantitates the lymphocytic infiltrate and distortion of the architecture of the minor salivary glands.

The erythrocyte sedimentation rate is usually elevated, and hypergammaglobulinemia is common. Rheumatoid factors, which are antibodies to IgG globulins, are present in more than 90 percent of patients with Sjögren's syndrome. A high percentage of the rheumatoid factors in these patients share a common structural feature not often present in rheumatoid factors observed in patients with other diseases. Monoclonal antibodies identify a common cross-reactive idiotype on the variable segment of *k*-type immunoglobulin light chains in the rheumatoid factors in Sjögren's syndrome.[73] Moreover, B cells that give rise to cells producing this class of rheumatoid factors selectively accumulate in the salivary gland lesions but are not present in synovial tissues or blood. It is possible that the presence of this idiotype identifies clones of B cells that have an increased frequency of undergoing neoplastic transformation, and this finding may account for the association of non-Hodgkin's lymphoma with Sjögren's syndrome (see below).

Antinuclear antibodies, which usually demonstrate a homogeneous or speckle pattern on immunofluorescence, are present in about 70 percent of patients. Antibodies to the nucleoprotein antigen SS-B, which is also called La, are found in the majority of patients, and antibodies to SS-A antigen, or Ro, are present in about one half of patients. When Sjögren's syndrome is associated with rheumatoid arthritis, antibodies to SS-A and SS-B are seen in less than 10 percent of patients. Various other autoantibodies have been identified, but each is present in only a minority of patients, illustrating the general (non–organ-specific) nature of autoimmunity in Sjögren's syndrome. These include antibodies to gastric parietal cells, thyroid, smooth muscle, pancreatic cells, and mitochondria. Antibodies to salivary duct epithelium antigens may be present in patients with Sjögren's syndrome but usually only in association with rheumatoid arthritis.

Evidence for a genetic basis for susceptibility is found in an increased prevalence of the histocompatibility antigen HLA-DR3 and the HLA supertype MT2 (DRw52).[74] Sjögren's syndrome in men is also associated with an increased prevalence of MT2 but a normal prevalence of DR3. Clinical features of the syndrome are similar in men and women, but men have a lower incidence of positive tests for rheumatoid factor and antibodies to SS-A.[74]

Therapy

Sjögren's syndrome should usually be managed conservatively.[69,70] Artificial tear preparations are usually effective for keratoconjunctivitis sicca. Complications such as corneal ulceration require intensive ophthalmologic attention. Mucolytic agents may be required for removal of inspissated secretions, and antibiotics are indicated for local infections. Xerostomia is usually managed with increased and frequent oral intake of fluids, although artificial saliva preparations are sometimes useful. Oral candidiasis may require topical mycostatin. Careful dental hygiene is important, including conscientious oral rinsing, dental brushing and flossing, plaque control programs, fluoride applications, and reduced sucrose ingestion. Increased humidity and saline nasal solutions may be helpful. Associated rheumatic diseases should be managed as they would be when they do not coexist with Sjögren's syndrome. Usually, steroids and cytotoxic drugs are not indicated for uncomplicated Sjögren's syndrome.

Lymphoma Associated with Sjögren's Syndrome

Lymphoid infiltration of salivary tissue is constant in Sjögren's syndrome. The development of lymphoma may be suspected when the lymphoproliferation becomes extreme, leading to prominent, firm salivary gland enlargement. In addition, lymphoid hyperplasia may develop in extrasalivary sites, including regional lymph nodes near the face and neck as well as those in distant areas. Infiltration of lymphocytes into other organs, such as the lung or kidney, may lead to dysfunction of those organs. Extensive lymphoid proliferation, referred to as pseudolymphoma, may occur with a pleomorphic histology and distortion of lymph node architecture. Frank malignant lymphoma may develop whether or not pseudolymphoma is present. In one study, the risk of malignant lymphoma in patients with Sjögren's syndrome was 44 times the normal rate.[75] The neoplasms are usually non-Hodgkin's lymphomas of B cell lineage, and they often produce IgMκ.[76]

Lymphoproliferative disorders that are associated with Sjögren's syndrome may require aggressive therapy. Pseudolymphoma usually responds to low doses of glucocorticoids and cyclophosphamide, but frank malignant lymphoma requires more aggressive therapy.

References

1. Textbook of Rheumatology. WB Saunders Co, Philadelphia, 1985, p 1070
2. Arthritis Rheum 17:1, 1974
3. Arthritis Rheum 21:37, 1978
4. Arthritis Rheum 21:798, 1978
5. Arthritis and Allied Conditions: A Textbook of Rheumatology, 10th ed. Lea & Febiger, Philadelphia, 1985, p 911
6. Am J Med 67:935, 1979
7. Systemic Lupus Erythematosus. Harvard University Press, Cambridge, Massachusetts, 1976
8. Am J Med 67:83, 1979
9. Am J Med 79:596, 1985
10. Am J Med 62:12, 1977
11. Am J Med 77:612, 1984
12. Ann Intern Med 96:718, 1982
13. Am J Med 75:382, 1983
14. Medicine (Baltimore) 55:323, 1976
15. Semin Arthritis Rheum 8:212, 1979
16. N Engl J Med 317:265, 1987
17. Angiology 36:431, 1985
18. Am Heart J 110(6):1257, 1985
19. Semin Arthritis Rheum 14:202, 1985
20. Chest 88:129, 1985
21. J Rheumatol 13:1, 1986
22. Ann Intern Med 100:388, 1984
23. Clin Rheum Dis 11:591, 1985
24. Arthritis Rheum 30:471, 1987
25. Arthritis Rheum 30:382, 1987
26. Ann Intern Med 106:524, 1987
27. Clin Rheum Dis 11:611, 1985
28. J Rheumatol 14:259, 1987
29. N Engl J Med 316:1135, 1987
30. Ann Intern Med 106:518, 1987
31. Arthritis and Allied Conditions: A Textbook of Rheumatology, 10th ed. Lea & Febiger, Philadelphia, 1985, p 936
32. Textbook of Rheumatology. WB Saunders Co, Philadelphia, 1985, p 1042
33. Medicine (Baltimore) 60:87, 1981
34. Rheumatic Disease Clinics of North America 13:37, 1987
35. Clin Rheum Dis 11:485, 1985
36. Medicine (Baltimore) 60:208, 1981
37. J Clin Invest 58:853, 1976
38. N Engl J Med 306:264, 1982
39. Am J Med 72:783, 1982
40. J Clin Invest 79:762, 1987
41. Arthritis Rheum 30:225, 1987
42. Arthritis Rheum 30:241, 1987
43. Semin Arthritis Rheum 10:255, 1981
44. Ann Intern Med 100:714, 1984
45. Arthritis Rheum 30:961, 1987
46. J Exp Med 164:50, 1986
47. Textbook of Rheumatology. WB Saunders Co, Philadelphia, 1985, p 1098
48. Am J Med 82:447, 1987
49. N Engl J Med 316:191, 1987
50. Arthritis Rheum 19:693, 1976
51. Ann Intern Med 96:728, 1982
52. N Engl J Med 314:614, 1986
53. Ann Intern Med 106:79, 1987
54. Rheumatic Disease Clinics of North America 13:47, 1987
55. Ann Intern Med 107:689, 1987
56. Ann Intern Med 105:58, 1986
57. N Engl J Med 308:186, 1983
58. Am J Med 75:602, 1983
59. Arthritis Rheum 25:601, 1982
60. Am J Med 75:382, 1983
61. Arthritis Rheum 25:612, 1982
62. Semin Arthritis Rheum 5:83, 1975
63. N Engl J Med 298:1157, 1978
64. Dermatology in General Medicine, 2nd ed. McGraw-Hill Book Co, New York, 1979, p 1273
65. Textbook of Rheumatology, Vol 1, 2nd ed. WB Saunders Co, Philadelphia, 1985, p 1115
66. Arthritis and Allied Conditions: A Textbook of Rheumatology, 10th ed. Lea & Febiger, Philadelphia, 1985, p 907

67. Dermatology in General Medicine, 2nd ed. McGraw-Hill Book Co, New York, 1979, p 784
68. Textbook of Rheumatology. WB Saunders Co, Philadelphia, 1985, p 1178
69. Textbook of Rheumatology. WB Saunders Co, Philadelphia, 1985, p 956
70. Arthritis and Allied Conditions: A Textbook of Rheumatology, 10th ed. Lea & Febiger, Philadelphia, 1985, p 1037
71. Ann Intern Med 103:344, 1985
72. Ann Intern Med 104:323, 1986
73. J Immunol 136:477, 1986
74. Am J Med 80:23, 1986
75. Arthritis Rheum 20:123, 1977
76. N Engl J Med 229:1215, 1978

Index

Myeloproliferative disorders, 405–411
  agnogenic myeloid metaplasia, 406–408
  chronic eosinophilic leukemia, 411–412
  chronic myeloid leukemia, 408–411
  essential thrombocythemia, 406
Myocardial infarction, acute, 141–166
  clinical features and diagnosis during initial phase
    echocardiography, 143
    electrocardiography, 142–143
    physical examination, 142
    prognosis, 143, 145
    symptoms, 142
  diagnosis during acute phase, 151–152
  epidemiology, 141
  hypertension associated with, 128
  initial treatment for, 145–151
    antithrombotic therapy, 151
    beta-blocking drugs, 145–146
    relief of pain, 145
    thrombolytic therapy, 146–150
  management of uncomplicated cases during convalescence, 163–166
  medically treatable complications of, 153–162
    accelerated idioventricular rhythm, 158
    atrial arrhythmias, 160
    bradyarrhythmias and conduction disorders, 154–155
    cardiac arrest, 158–160
    CHF and cardiogenic shock, 160–162
    extension and expansion of infarction, 153–154
    left ventricular mural thrombus, 154
    lidocaine therapy, 157–158
    pericarditis and Dressler's syndrome, 154
    primary versus secondary arrhythmia, 156
    recurrent ischemic pain, 153
    right ventricular infarction, 161
    venous thromboembolism, 154
    ventricular tachyarrhythmias and, 155–156
  non-Q wave, 164
  pathogenesis, 141–142
  prevention of recurrent, 165
  routine management in the CCU, 152–153
  surgically treatable complications of, 162–163
Myocardial ischemia, 164
  arrhythmias and, 19
Myxoma, cardiac, 575

Nadolol, 113, 115, 117
  dose in renal disease, 749
Nafcillin, 515, 525
  dose in renal disease, 736
Nalidixic acid, 491, 522
Naloxone
  dose in renal disease, 740
  for shock, 15
Naproxen, dose in renal disease, 762
Narcotics, dose in renal disease, 739–740
Neisseria gonorrhea infections, 589–598
  in acute PID, 599–603
  causative agent in, 589–590
  clinical features of, 590–592
  diagnosis of, 592–593
  epidemiology of, 590
  in homosexual men, 598
  treatment of, 509, 593–598
Neisseria meningitidis, 509, 804
Neoplasms. *See also* Leukemias
  fever caused by, 616
  pericardial, primary, 180–181
  pericardial effusion caused by, 177
Neostigmine, dose in renal disease, 760
Netilmicin, 542
  dosage of, 518
  dose in renal disease, 730
Neuromuscular blocking agents, dose in renal disease, 760
Neurotoxin poisoning, 646
Neutropenia, antibiotics and, 501
Nicardipine, dose in renal disease, 750

Nifedipine, 117
  in hypertensive emergencies, 125, 126
  dose in renal disease, 750
Nimodipine, dose in renal disease, 750
Nitrates, dose in renal disease, 753
Nitrendipine, dose in renal disease, 750
Nitrofurantoin, 555
  dose in renal disease, 735
Nitroglycerin, 145, 194
  dose in renal disease, 753
Nocardia, antimicrobials for, 512
Norepinephrine, for shock, 13
Norfloxacin, 522, 553
Nortriptyline, dose in renal disease, 745
Nosocomial bacteremia and shock, 451–454
Nutrition, enteral and parenteral, 301–330. *See also* Malnutrition
  for cancer, 323–324
  for cardiac failure, 322–323
  central vein infusions, 314–318
  complications of, 316–318
  determining requirements, 303–304
  in Crohn's disease, 255
  enteral tube feedings, 307–308, 312
  for hepatic disease, 319, 321–322
  home nutritional support, 326–328
  innovations in nutritional support, 328–330
  perioperative, 324–326
  peripheral vein infusions, 312–314
  for renal failure, 318–319
  respiratory failure and, 885
  in respiratory insufficiency, 323

Octreotide, dose in renal disease, 763
Ofloxacin, 554–555
  dosage, 522
  dose in renal disease, 737
Olsalazine, for ulcerative colitis, 243–244
Ondansetron, dose in renal disease, 763
Opioids, overdose of, 632–633